SECOND EDITION

MR and CT Imaging of the Head, Neck, and Spine

EDITED BY

RICHARD E. LATCHAW, M.D.
Neuroradiologist
Radiology Imaging Associates, P.C., and Colorado
  Neurological Institute
Englewood, Colorado
Clinical Professor of Radiology
University of Colorado
Denver Colorado

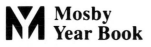
Mosby
Year Book

St. Louis Baltimore Boston Chicago London Philadelphia Sydney Toronto

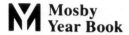
Mosby
Year Book

Dedicated to Publishing Excellence

Sponsoring Editors: James D. Ryan/Anne S. Patterson
Associate Managing Editor, Manuscript Services: Deborah
  Thorp
Production Project Coordinator: Carol A. Reynolds
Proofroom Manager: Barbara Kelly

1 2 3 4 5 6 7 8 9 0 CL PC 95 94 93 92 91

Library of Congress Cataloging-in-Publication Data
MR and CT imaging of the head, neck, and spine / [edited by Richard E.
  Latchaw.—2nd ed.
        p.   cm.
    Rev. ed. of: Computed tomography of the head, neck, and spine.
  c1985.
    Includes bibliographical references.
    Includes index.
    ISBN 0-8151-5330-9
    1. Central nervous system—Magnetic resonance imaging. 2. Central
nervous system—Tomography. 3. Head—Imaging. 4. Neck—Imaging.
5. Spine—Imaging.
    [DNLM: 1. Head—anatomy & histology. 2. Head—radiography.
3. Magnetic Resonance Imaging. 4. Neck—anatomy & histology.
5. Neck—radiography. 6. Spine—anatomy & histology. 7. Spine—
radiography. 8. Tomography. X-Ray Computed. WE 141 M9385]
RC386.6.M34M75 1991   90-6587
616.8′047572—dc20   CIP
DNLM/DLC
for Library of Congress

This book is dedicated to Dr. Lou Wener: unparalleled in MRI, a caring individual. . . he was my friend.

STEPHEN A. BERMAN, M.D., PH.D.
Fellow in EMG
Spinal Cord Injury Service
West Roxbury Veterans Administration Medical Center
Boston, Massachusetts

JAMES A. BRUNBERG, M.D.
Assistant Professor of Radiology, Neurology, and
  Neurosurgery
University of Michigan
Director, Division of MR Imaging
Co-director, Division of Neuroradiology
Department of Radiology
University of Michigan Hospitals
Ann Arbor, Michigan

R. NICK BRYAN, M.D., PH.D.
Profesor of Radiology and Neurosurgery
Johns Hopkins University
Director, Division of Neuroradiology
Department of Radiology
Johns Hopkins Hospital
Baltimore, Maryland

GLEN E. BURMEISTER, M.D.
Radiologist, Radiology Imaging Associates, P.C.,
  Musculoskeletal Radiologist and Swedish Medical
  Center
Englewood, Colorado

GEORGE F. CARR, D.M.D.
Prosthodontist
Allentown, Pennsylvania
Faculty Member
Michigan Implant Institute
Dearborn, Michigan

SYLVESTER H. S. CHUANG, M.D.C.M., D.A.B.R.,
C.S.P.Q., F.R.C.P.C.
Associate Professor of Radiology
University of Toronto
Neuroradiologist, Department of Radiology
Hospital for Sick Children
Toronto, Ontario, Canada

HUGH D. CURTIN, M.D.
Professor of Radiology and Otolaryngology
Chief, Department of Radiology
Eye and Ear Hospital
Medical and Health Care Division
University of Pittsburgh
Pittsburgh, Pennsylvania

RICHARD H. DAFFNER, M.D.
Professor of Radiologic Sciences
Medical College of Pennsylvania (Western Campus)
Clinical Professor of Radiology
University of Pittsburgh
Senior Staff Radiologist
Department of Radiology
Allegheny General Hospital
Pittsburgh, Pennsylvania

MONY J. DE LEON, B.A, M.A., M.ED., ED.D.
Associate Professor of Psychiatry
New York University
Director of the Neuroimaging Research Laboratory
New York University Medical Center
New York, New York

BURTON P. DRAYER, M.D.
Director, Magnetic Resonance Imaging and Research
Chairman, Division of Neuroimaging Research-
  Education
Barrow Neurological Institute
Phoenix, Arizona

ELIZABETH A. EELKEMA, M.D.
Radiologist, Department of Radiology
St. Clair Hospital
Pittsburgh, Pennsylvania

CHARLES R. FITZ, M.D.
Professor of Radiology and Pediatrics
George Washington University
Neuroradiologist, Department of Radiology
Children's National Medical Center
Washington, D.C.

AJAX E. GEORGE, M.D.
Professor of Radiology
New York University
Senior Attending Neuroradiologist
New York University Medical Center
New York, New York

ROBERT I. GROSSMAN, M.D.
Professor of Radiology and Neurosurgery
University of Pennsylvania
Chief of Neuroradiology
Department of Radiology
Hospital of the University of Pennsylvania
Philadelphia, Pennsylvania

DAVID GUR, SC.D.
Professor of Radiology and Radiation Health
Director, Division of Radiological Imaging
Department of Radiology
Medical and Health Care Division
University of Pittsburgh
Pittsburgh, Pennsylvania

L. ANNE HAYMAN, M.D.
Research Professor of Radiology
Baylor College of Medicine
Director of Neuroradiology
Department of Radiology
Ben Taub General Hospital
Houston, Texas

STEPHEN T. HECHT, M.D.
Assistant Professor of Radiology and Neurosurgery
University of California—Davis
Neuroradiologist, Department of Radiology
University of California Medical Center—Davis
Sacramento, California

ROBERT J. HERFKENS, M.D.
Associate Professor of Radiology
Stanford University School of Medicine
Chief of Body MRI
Stanford University Hospital
Stanford, California

VINCENT C. HINCK, M.D.
Emeritus, Professor of Radiology
Baylor College of Medicine
Houston, Texas

WILLIAM L. HIRSCH, JR., M.D.
Assistant Professor of Radiology
Neuroradiologist, Department of Radiology
Medical and Health Care Division
University of Pittsburgh
Pittsburgh, Pennsylvania

JEFFERY P. HOGG, M.D.
Assistant Professor of Radiology
Neuroradiologist, Department of Radiology
Medical and Health Care Division
University of Pittsburgh
Pittsburgh, Pennsylvania

BARRY HOROWITZ, M.D.
Director of Neuroradiology
The Methodist Hospital
Clinical Associate Professor of Radiology
Baylor College of Medicine
Houston, Texas

JOSEPH A. HORTON, M.D.
Professor of Radiology and Neurological Surgery
Chief, Division of Neuroradiology
Department of Radiology
Medical and Health Care Division
University of Pittsburgh
Pittsburgh, Pennsylvania

DAVID JENKINS, M.D.
Staff Radiologist
Department of Radiology
Lafayette General Hospital
Lafayette, Louisiana

DAVID W. JOHNSON, M.D.
Assistant Professor of Radiology
Neuroradiologist, Department of Radiology
Medical and Health Care Division
University of Pittsburgh
Pittsburgh, Pennsylvania

CHARLES A. JUNGREIS, M.D.
Assistant Professor of Radiology and Neurological
Surgery
Neuroradiologist, Department of Radiology
Medical and Health Care Division
University of Pittsburgh
Pittsburgh, Pennsylvania

EMANUEL KANAL, M.D.
Assistant Professor of Radiology
Chief, Division of Magnetic Resonance Imaging
Department of Radiology
Director, The Pittsburgh NMR Institute
Medical and Health Care Division
University of Pittsburgh
Pittsburgh, Pennsylvania

SUSAN S. KEMP, M.D.
Assistant Professor of Radiology
Neuroradiologist, Department of Radiology
Medical and Health Care Division
University of Pittsburgh
Pittsburgh, Pennsylvania

JOEL B. KIRKPATRICK, M.D.
Professor of Neuropathology
Department of Pathology
Baylor College of Medicine
Houston, Texas

RICHARD E. LATCHAW, M.D.
Neuroradiologist
Radiology Imaging Associates, P.C., and Colorado
Neurological Institute
Englewood, Colorado
Clinical Professor of Radiology
University of Colorado
Denver, Colorado
Formerly:
Professor of Radiology and
Neurological Surgery
Interim Chairman and Chief
of Neuroradiology
Department of Radiology
Medical and Health Care Division
University of Pittsburgh
Pittsburgh, Pennsylvania

L. DADE LUNSFORD, M.D.
Professor of Neurological Surgery, Radiology, and
Radiation Oncology
Neurosurgeon, Department of Neurological Surgery
Medical and Health Care Division
University of Pittsburgh
Pittsburgh, Pennsylvania

CHARLES W. McCLUGGAGE, M.D.
Neuroradiologist, Texas Children's and St. Luke's
  Episcopal Hospitals
Clinical Assistant Professor of Radiology
Baylor College of Medicine
Houston, Texas

THOMAS J. MASARYK, M.D.
Head, Section of Neuroradiology
Division of Radiology
Cleveland Clinic Foundation
Cleveland, Ohio

JOHN J. PAGANI, M.D.
Staff Radiologist
Department of Radiology
Park Plaza Hospital
Houston, Texas

MICHAEL J. PAINTER, M.D.
Associate Professor of Pediatrics and Neurology
Chief, Department of Neurology
Children's Hospital of Neurology
Medical and Health Care Division
University of Pittsburgh
Pittsburgh, Pennsylvania

STANLEY M. PERL, M.D.
Radiologist and Medical Director
Magnetic Resonance Imaging Associates
Clinton, Maryland

MARK J. PFLEGER, M.D.
Resident, Radiology
Department of Radiology
Baylor College of Medicine
Houston, Texas

ROBERT M. QUENCER, M.D.
Professor of Radiology, Neurological Surgery, and
  Ophthalmology
Medical Director
Division of Magnetic Resonance Imaging
Department of Radiology
University of Miami School of Medicine
Miami, Florida

JEFFREY M. ROGG, M.D.
Clinical Instructor
Radiation Medicine
Brown University
Director of Magnetic Resonance Imaging
Rhode Island Hospital
Providence, Rhode Island

HELEN M. N. ROPPOLO, M.D.
Clinical Associate Professor of Radiology
Neuroradiologist, Department of Radiology
Medical and Health Care Division
University of Pittsburgh
Pittsburgh, Pennsylvania

WILLIAM E. ROTHFUS, M.D.
Associate Professor of Radiologic Science
Medical College of Pennsylvania (Western Campus)
Senior Staff Radiologist
Department of Radiology
Allegheny General Hospital
Pittsburgh, Pennsylvania

JOACHIM F. SEEGER, M.D.
Professor of Radiology
University of Arizona
Head, Section of Neuroradiology
Department of Radiology
University of Arizona Health Sciences Center
Tucson, Arizona

CHARLES E. SEIBERT, M.D.
Neuroradiologist
Radiology Imaging Associates, P.C., Swedish Medical
  Center and Colorado Neurological Institute
Englewood, Colorado
Clinical Associate Professor of Radiology
University of Colorado
Denver, Colorado

KATHERINE SHAFFER, M.D.
Associate Professor of Radiology and Otolarygology
Medical College of Wisconsin
Radiologist, Department of Radiology
Milwaukee County Medical Complex
Milwaukee, Wisconsin

ELLEN K. TABOR, M.D.
Assistant Professor of Radiology
Head and Neck Radiologist, Department of Radiology
Medical and Health Care Division
University of Pittsburgh
Pittsburgh, Pennsylvania

ROBERT W. TARR, M.D.
Assistant Professor of Radiology
Case-Western Reserve University
Neuroradiologist, Department of Radiology
University Hospitals
Cleveland, Ohio

FELIX W. WEHRLI, PH.D.
Professor of Radiologic Science
University of Pennsylvania
Director of MR Education
Hospital of the University of Pennsylvania
Philadelphia, Pennsylvania

MEREDITH A. WEINSTEIN, M.D.
Staff Radiologist
Hill and Thomas
Cleveland, Ohio

LOUIS WENER, M.D. (DECEASED)
Formerly:
Radiologist and Medical Director
Magnetic Resonance Imaging Associates
Clinton, Maryland

GERALD L. WOLF, PH.D., M.D.
Professor of Radiology
Harvard Medical School
Director, Center for Imaging and Pharmaceutical
  Research
Massachusetts General Hospital
Boston, Massachusetts

HOWARD YONAS, M.D.
Assistant Professor of Neurological Surgery and
  Radiology
Neurosurgeon, Department of Neurological Surgery
Medical and Health Care Division
University of Pittsburgh
Pittsburgh, Pennsylvania

FOREWORD

Dr. Latchaw's previous effort in this area, *Computed Tomography of the Head, Neck, and Spine* (as the first edition was titled) was the definitive work to date on that subject. Knowing him well, I was captivated by his ongoing comments about producing the next edition. Magnetic resonance imaging has made such a massive impact on imaging practice in this area that it has become dominant, whereas computed tomography has faded somewhat, burgeoning, however, in its contribution to the evaluation of the abdomen and pelvis, and thus not losing much luster. However, its use is on the decline in neuroradiology.

Other authors and editors have had the same problem, that is, having to redo a book that was largely CT oriented, after MRI. Most of them have not fared well, either in the text or in the illustrations. They generally have attempted to add to their previous material rather than take on the whole new subject, and thus produce a lesser product, in some ways, than the first attempt. This book, however, is basically all new. The contents are massively MR oriented, with appropriate references to CT as indicated.

The book is profusely illustrated and provides references that are up-to-date to the point of printing. The discussions are excellent. In this day of constantly changing, moving-target technology, one expects that a book of this genre will be largely clinical, because patients and diseases remain stable fixation points. It *is* clinical, but it also is profusely and informatively technologic. There are insights here on contrast material and image quality that have not surfaced elsewhere, and which make the book worth reading for that reason alone. Brilliant explanations of pathophysiologic changes as manifested by images accompany these images and the text describing them.

A major work such as this is a real tour de force. Dr. Latchaw, a brilliant bundle of energy, left the university (academic) setting for a large private group practice adjacent to the Rockies. One would predict that he would have had difficulty in putting everything together. But no. He has prevailed, and brilliantly so. This is a superb effort and stands as the definitive text as well as an encyclopedia on the subject of brain, head, neck, and spine imaging, that is, neuroimaging. These efforts must be viewed to be appreciated. I commend Dr. Latchaw and his co-authors for a major, major contribution. While it may not overshadow Dick's beloved mountains, it is a great start.

DAVID O. DAVIS, M.D.
Professor and Acting Chairman
Department of Radiology
George Washington University Medical Center
Washington, D.C.

PREFACE

In the first edition of this book, entitled *Computed Tomography of the Head, Neck, and Spine,* we stressed the correlation of pathophysiology and CT imaging. We wanted our readers to understand why we see what we see on a CT scan. That approach was highly successful.

As we brought the first book to press, MRI was rapidly emerging. We wished to write as definitive a book on MRI as we had on CT, so we waited until MR contrast agents became available.

Throughout the late 1980s, it became apparent that MRI would become the imaging procedure of choice for many neurological diseases. However, in writing a book on MRI, we also wished to incorporate what we knew from CT. We had learned so much from CT that it was logical to carry it over to MR. For many of the diseases, CT and MR show similar types of findings, albeit with a slightly different appearance. In practice, the two are frequently intertwined: hence this book, which combines the two modalities.

The divisions of this book are similar to those of the first book, except for the addition of a chapter on certain physical principles of MRI. There has been no attempt to introduce a great deal of physics in this book; other books are far more proficient in that undertaking. Rather, the chapter stresses the optimization of the MR scan, demonstrating ways to obtain better contrast-to-noise and signal-to-noise ratios. We again ended the book with such exciting procedures as stereotactic neurosurgery on the MR scanner (just as we have performed on CT scanners). In between, there is a discussion of numerous clinical entities, comparing and contrasting their MR and CT appearances.

We sincerely hope that our readers will conclude that with the publication of the second edition of *MR and CT Imaging of the Head, Neck, and Spine,* we have accomplished our goals.

RICHARD E. LATCHAW, M.D.

ACKNOWLEDGMENTS

It is unnecessary that I say thank you in print to the co-authors of this monumental project. They need only read their colleagues' material to feel the same kind of pride that I do in a project well done. Rather, my thanks go to all of the unsung heros whose names do not appear in the list of contributors: all of those secretaries who labored so hard to get the final product into production. Without their help, a project like this could never have occurred.

There is one individual who deserves the highest level of praise: my wife Joan. Formerly, as my secretary at the University of Pittsburgh, Joan Roberge was of immense help in preparing *Computed Tomography of the Head, Neck, and Spine.*

We then began to tackle the second edition: *MR and CT Imaging of the Head, Neck, and Spine.* She has been my strength throughout its production, and has helped me gather figures, obtain references, and write and edit numerous chapters, and has put up with my continual modifications. During my tenure as Interim Chairman of the Department of Radiology at the University of Pittsburg, she, as Departmental Administrator, protected me, so that I could spend time with my favorite project. I was so enamored of her abilities that I decided to marry her. Now, it's our book.

RICHARD E. LATCHAW, M.D.

CONTENTS

CONTENTS

PART I

Physical Principles

Image Quality in Clinical Magnetic Resonance Imaging

Emanuel Kanal, M.D.

Felix W. Wehrli, Ph.D.

Magnetic resonance (MR) imaging has progressed remarkably throughout the past several years and is in the process of taking on the dominant role among the clinical imaging modalities. MR applications are especially prominent in neuroradiologic, musculoskeletal and pelvic imaging, providing diagnostic information never previously enjoyed by the medical community. Although frequently compared with computed tomography (CT) scanning in its applications and diagnostic capabilities, the similarities between these two modalities are limited, their principal commonality being their tomographic nature. Far more so than with many other imaging modalities, however, an in-depth comprehension of the physical principles underlying MR is a necessary prerequisite for understanding and interpreting the images.

The focus of the diagnostic workup should be directed toward the clinical goal, that is, the *accurate identification and diagnosis of pathologic versus normal structures*. This goal can only be realized if we achieve adequate *image quality*. Image quality is a complex composite of a multitude of parameters. Detailed knowledge of the effects of and interrelationships among the scanning parameters and their impact on image quality is critical for accurate image interpretation. This chapter discusses the practical clinical ramifications of the scan parameters chosen, notably as far as signal-to-noise, contrast, and spatial resolution are concerned, all essential to *lesion detectability*.

INTRINSIC AND EXTRINSIC PARAMETERS

Many parameters can affect tissue signal intensity and contrast in an MR image. While some of these parameters are operator-definable and thus *extrinsic*, others are not as readily manipulated. The *intrinsic* parameters represent those that are either essentially fixed or are tissue-specific, while the extrinsic parameters can generally be freely manipulated. This type of subdivision allows the user to determine rapidly which of the various factors are under his or her control and which are tissue-specific and thus given by nature. The principal intrinsic parameters are the *spin-lattice relaxation time (T1)*, the *spin-spin relaxation time (T2)*, and the *proton density [N(H)]*. The major extrinsic parameters are the *pulse timing intervals*—the determinants of image contrast—and, in addition, parameters that are also found in other imaging modalities and that include field of view (FOV), section thickness, matrix size, number of sections imaged, intersection spacing, etc.

Variations in section thickness, matrix size, FOV, and number of excitations may induce profound alterations in signal-to-noise ratio and resolving power and, thus, lesion detectability. Finally, as is the case with any digital imaging modality, the display parameters have a marked effect on the perceived image intensity and contrast and therefore lesion detectability.

It is the combination of intrinsic and operator-selected extrinsic imaging parameters that will determine the *outcome* of the entire *examination*, from diagnostic utility to scan time.

SIGNAL-TO-NOISE, CONTRAST-TO-NOISE, RESOLVING POWER

Study Objectives

The primary objective of any MR examination is to obtain the required diagnostic information in the least amount of scan time. What is considered necessary and sufficient can vary from patient to patient and among observers. There are several universal concepts, however, that tend to recur in all MR examinations. These include *signal intensity*, *contrast*, *noise*, *imaging volume*, *voxel volume*, and *scan time*, terms that will subsequently be defined in detail.[1]

As a simplification, the target tissue signal is to be perceived as that signal received from the tissue of interest. Noise is a complex variable, and can be random or structured. For the purposes of the rest of this chapter, *noise* will refer to a random fluctuation riding on signal and background. The ratio of signal intensity to the noise of the system is referred to as the *signal-to-noise ratio*, or *SNR*. Similarly, *contrast* is the difference in intensities between the signals from two tissues, while the *contrast-to-noise ratio (CNR)* is simply the ratio of this quantity to noise.[2]

The degree and order of importance of the CNR, voxel volumes, scan time, and imaging volume for each image set guide the scan parameter options appropriate for each image acquisition. For example, a study that seeks to identify very small structures (e.g., evaluation for pituitary microadenoma) may demand smaller voxel volumes (achieved by any combination of decreased FOVs, thinner slices, and larger matrix values). This selection will generally be at the expense of some other imaging objectives, for example, SNR, CNR or imaging time. Conversely, an examination whose goal is to evaluate gross changes in morphology and size of a known, several centimeter–sized intracranial neoplasm post-chemotherapy may be successfully accomplished with an entirely different set of imaging parameters, satisfying a different set of goal ordering. Here, for example, imaging time may be kept at a minimum with markedly shorter imaging times resulting from such choices as larger FOVs, smaller acquisition matrix size, and thicker sections. These

provide higher signal intensities, necessitating fewer excitations, thus permitting considerably shortened imaging times. It is the magnitude and ordering of the goals noted above that permits such vast differences in approaches to scan parameter selection.

SNR and Image Appearance

As noted above, the noise can be viewed as a random component added to or subtracted from the pixel intensity. Increased noise is equivalent to an increase in the amplitude of these random fluctuations. Noise results from essentially two sources: electronic noise from the receiver circuit and, especially at higher fields, from the excited tissue itself.

While there are multiple methods for measuring SNR[3] we will see that regardless of the methodology used in its measurement, SNR will be affected by variations of any of the major scanning parameters such as FOV, slice thickness, matrix size, number of excitations, pulse repetition time, echo time, and others. An illustration of the effect of SNR on the image is given in Figure 1–1 where two images are displayed, differing only in SNR. Note the grainier appearance of the noisier, lower SNR image rendering visualization of small structures such as the infundibulum or the aqueduct difficult.

CNR and Image Appearance

Contrast between structures on an MR image can be defined as the difference in signal intensities (I) for two structures A and B as follows:

$$C = \frac{I(A) - I(B)}{I(B)} \qquad (1a)$$

The denominator in equation (1a) is a normalization factor typically assigned to the background environment. It should be noted that contrast is a property that is intrinsic to the tissues and structures of interest, whereas SNR is instrumentation-dependent (preamplifier noise, coil characteristics, etc.).

While SNR is an important criterion for lesion detection, it is not sufficient. Even tissues with high SNR may not be detected, depending on the adjacent tissue intensities and geometry. To illustrate this point, imagine a bright white light emanating from an equally intense bright white back-

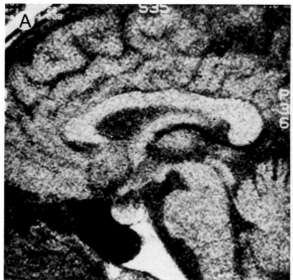 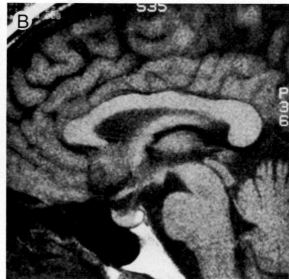

FIG 1–1.
Effect of noise on visual perception. Contrast in both images is the same but the CNR differs. It is lower in the image of Fig 1–2,A by a factor of 2. Note that the lower CNR primarily impairs visualization of small structures such as the aqueduct of Sylvius but has little effect on visual perception of large structures such as the corpus callosum.

ground. The fact that the SNR of both the light and the background is very high does not ensure that two adjacent structures can be differentiated. An additional criterion for detectability, therefore, is that of sufficient contrast between the target tissue and its adjacent structure(s). For example, even if the light in the previous example were of moderate intensity, if placed on a black background (such as in a completely darkened room), it would be highly detectable. This example is an illustration of a moderate SNR from the target "tissue" but a markedly lower SNR from the adjacent structures, resulting in a very pronounced contrast and CNR between the two and therefore successful detectability.

The detectability of any structure is determined, therefore, by a combination of contrast and SNR which is denoted CNR[2] and which is defined as:

$$CNR = SNR(A) - SNR(B) \qquad (1b)$$

where SNR(A) and SNR(B) refer to the SNR measured for tissues A and B. It therefore follows that only the difference in SNR determines CNR. A clinical example to illustrate this point (albeit in a musculoskeletal application) is that of a subcutaneous lymphangioma, adjacent to both subcutaneous fat and several muscular bundles of the forearm. Fat, with its associated short T1, can provide excel-

lent contrast with the long T1 of the tumor, provided that a pulse sequence is chosen which emphasizes the T1 differences between the two tissues. For the borders of this mass that abut the muscle, however, a study emphasizing T1 differences results in relatively poor contrast due to the similarly long T1 values of muscle and tumor. For such tissue contrast a study stressing T2 differences is superior for highlighting the long T2 tumor versus the short T2 muscle and even fat with its moderately short T2 value (Fig 1–2).

It is important to emphasize that excellent contrast between pathology and adjacent anatomy may be of no clinical utility if the CNR is too low. Despite the differences in their mean signal intensities, they may not be discernible as distinct entities due to the considerable overlap of their signal provided by the low SNR from each tissue.

It should be evident, therefore, that achieving optimal CNR between targeted structures is indeed a *primary objective* of every MR examination. This can be accomplished by designing a protocol to yield high contrast while maintaining sufficient SNR from at least one of the two tissues being contrasted.

Even CNR is itself necessary but not sufficient for lesion detection. To continue with the previous analogy of a light source on a dark background, assuming a fixed signal intensity, the discernibility will also be dependent upon the size of the light source to be detected. As with all digital imaging

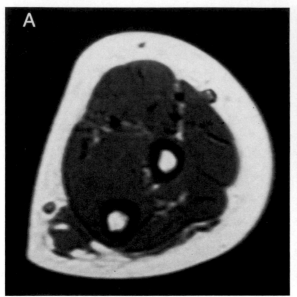
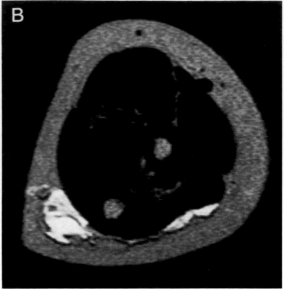

FIG 1–2.
Lymphangioma (surgically verified) within the subcutaneous tissues of the forearm, not extending into the adjacent muscle bundles. Whereas **A** has clearly superior overall SNR, it is diagnostically less useful as it demonstrates the tumor to be isointense with the adjacent muscle. **B** emphasizes signal T2 contrast between the tumor and the adjacent fat and muscle, allowing excellent delineation of the tumor margins. Furthermore, note the tongue-like projection of the tumor around the distal forearm that was not noticeable on **A.**

modalities, the MR image will be displayed in the form of a fixed grid of picture elements, or *pixels.* The number of pixels that represent the region of interest will be dependent upon the size of the lesion relative to the pixel size. In MR imaging pixel size is determined by such operator-definable parameters as slice thickness, FOV, and the number of matrix elements, N_p, and N_f.

The three-dimensional counterpart of the pixel is the *voxel* (volume element) which is the product of pixel area and slice thickness. Assuming that the total number of pixels is given (as is the lesion size relative to its background), the detectability of the lesion will also be determined by the specified voxel dimensions and volume since it is the latter that determines the signal per pixel. For digital imaging modalities, then, the number of pixels represented by the region of interest plays a role in lesion detection, akin to how object size determines the resolving ability in nondigital processes.

In what way do CNR and object size (or, in the case of digital imaging modalities, the number of pixels represented by the region of interest) interrelate to determine object discernibility? Each is a prime determinant in what has been referred to as the *resolving power* of the examination. As first pointed out and treated theoretically by Rose,[4] smaller objects demand higher CNRs than larger objects. As CNR decreases, smaller objects may therefore fall below the threshold of detectability, with only the largest objects remaining visible. This point has been illustrated with Figure 1–1 where smaller anatomic structures like the aqueduct are only poorly visualized in the lower SNR image (Fig 1–1,A).

Resolving Power

In a digital image the pixel dimensions determine the smallest theoretically discernible structure. Other factors contribute to the resolving power as well. These include the CNR and the point spread function of the system. These factors can only serve to decrease the maximum obtainable resolving power (i.e., increase the size of the smallest identifiable structure) which, however, can never exceed that characterized by the voxel volume (i.e., the smallest quantum of digitization).

It follows from the above that at any fixed voxel volume, increasing the CNR increases the resolving power of the image. It may therefore be possible to increase effective resolving power by increasing contrast. This may be more time-efficient than decreasing noise or increasing SNR by repeated signal averaging.

The specific parameter choices and sequence selections are of course determined by the specific pathologic entity being imaged, its surrounding structures with which it is to be contrasted, and the clinical constraints under which imaging must be performed in each particular case. Discussions of the individual scan parameters involved in modifying resolving power follow below.

Scan Time

Another study objective we always strive for is that of minimizing scan acquisition times. Shorter examinations satisfy several goals, including that of decreased patient discomfort and, secondarily, motion and increased through-put considerations. *Scan time* can be defined as the time required to successfully acquire a sufficient amount of data from which the desired image set can be reconstructed. The most widely used imaging technique today is 2-dimensional Fourier transform (2-D FT), where scan time (T_s) can be expressed as follows:

$$T_s = TR \times N_p \times NEX \qquad (2)$$

In equation (2) TR is the time interval between successive sequence repetitions, N_p refers to the number of phase-encoding increments (i.e., the number of pixels in phase-encoding direction), and NEX is the number of excitations (i.e., the number of times the acquisition of each line is repeated). It follows from equation (2) that modifications of any of these parameters—N_p, NEX, and TR—will linearly affect scan time. However, modifications of any one of these parameters will inevitably also affect the SNR, CNR, and resolving power of the study. It therefore follows that the scan time can be maintained by appropriate juggling of these three variables, but not without altering the CNR, SNR, or resolving power of the obtained images.

Consider the following example. Halving N_p from 256 to 128 (assuming that the FOV is held constant) and simultaneously doubling NEX from 2 to 4 will result in no change in total scan time, as per equation (2). Nevertheless, for reasons that will be discussed further below, this modification will result in a sequence that will yield a twofold increase in the overall SNR of the study as a whole.

PULSE SEQUENCE DEPENDENCE OF IMAGE CONTRAST

Relaxation Times

MR is a multiparametric modality and image contrast and therefore depends in a complex but quantifiable manner on a multitude of parameters.

The first group of parameters is called *intrinsic* because they are given by the chemical properties of tissue (essentially water in its different binding states). The three principal parameters are the spin relaxation times (T1 and T2) and the proton density (proton concentration) (N). T1 is the time constant for the return of the longitudinal magnetization to equilibrium (longitudinal or spin-lattice relaxation time). T2 is the time constant for the return of the transverse relaxation time to equilibrium (transverse or spin-spin relaxation time). T1 and T2 depend in a complex manner on the motional characteristics of molecules. In the free state (unimpeded translational and rotational motion), relaxation is relatively inefficient and, consequently T1 and T2 are long (examples: cerebrospinal fluid (CSF), synovial fluid, cystic liquids). Typically, however, water molecules are bound to the polar head groups of tissue proteins.[5] Since these water molecules are in rapid exchange with free water molecules, the observed T1s and T2s are weighted averages:

$$1/T1,2 = p_{free}/T1,2_{free} + p_{bound}/T1,2_{bound} \qquad (3)$$

where p_{bound} and p_{free} are the fractions of bound and free molecules, respectively (Fig 1–3).

Disease processes like edema, tumor, demyelination, abcess, etc., typically cause an increase in the free water concentration and hence an increase in T1 and T2. This is the basis of the detection of abnormalities by MR.

Extrinsic parameters, by contrast, relate to the pulse sequence timing parameters in conjunction with the specific pulse sequence used. Unlike the intrinsic parameters, they are under user control. It is therefore imperative that the user gain a thor-

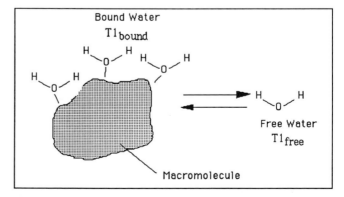

FIG 1–3.
Water molecules exist in at least two different states: free and bound. Any shift in the equilibrium increasing the free water concentration causes an increase in the observed T1 or T2 relaxation time.

ough understanding of the impact of the choice of these parameters on image signal and contrast. The most common among the extrinsic contrast parameters are the radiofrequency pulse timing parameters TR and TE which are defined in the next section.

Dependence of Signal and Contrast in Spin-Echo Imaging

This subject was dealt with early on during the evolution of clinical MR by a variety of authors[6–11] and has since been reviewed extensively.[1, 12, 13]

The simplest pulse sequence consists of a train of 90-degree radiofrequency (RQ) pulses which are applied every TR milliseconds (Fig 1–4). The RF pulse rotates the longitudinal magnetization into the transverse plane where it is detected. The resultant signal is proportional to the longitudinal magnetization immediately before the RF pulse. Immediately after the pulse the longitudinal magnetization is zero, but it grows back exponentially during the pulse repetition time as follows:

$$M_z(TR) = M_z(0)[1 - \exp(-TR/T1)] \qquad (4)$$

where $M_z(0)$ is the equilibrium magnetization.

According to equation (4), the signal received is a function of both the T1 of the tissue protons as well as the TR chosen. Hence, if we know T1 we can predict the relative signal intensities for any TR. For this purpose, let us consider three common tissues: white matter (WM), gray matter (GM), and CSF, for which the following is known: T1(WM)<T1(GM)<<T1(CSF). In addition, it turns out that the proton densities for the three tissues differ as follows: N(WM)<N(GM)<N(CSF). The effect of proton densities is more apparent at long TR, that is, once the spins are fully relaxed. From the plot in Figure 1–5,A we see that at TR = 0.5

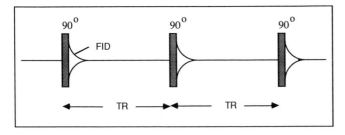

FIG 1–4.
RF pulse sequence consisting of train of 90-degree RF pulses spaced TR milliseconds apart. Each *RF* pulse produces a free induction decay *(FID)*.

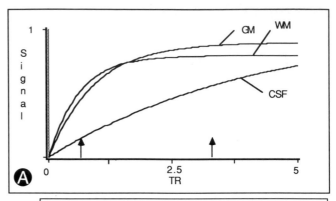

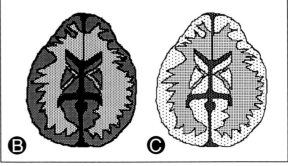

FIG 1–5.
A, MR signal calculated as a function of the pulse repetition time (TR) for gray matter (GM) (T1 = 0.9 seconds, N = 0.9), white matter (T1 = 0.6 seconds, N = 0.8) and CSF (T1 = 4 second, N = 1.0) assuming 90-degree pulses are applied every TR second and the signal is collected immediately thereafter. At short TR *(left arrow),* the relative signal intensities are: WM>GM>>CSF and the image **(B)** is said to be T1-weighted. At longer TR *(right arrow,* **A)** the relative signal intensities are: GM>WM>CSF. The image **(C)** is proton density–weighted with respect to GM and WM but still T1-weighted with respect to CSF.

second the relative signal intensities are as follows: WM>GM>>CSF; hence the relative signal intensities follow the inverse of the tissue T1 relaxation times. Such an image is often referred to as T1-weighted (Fig 1–5,B).

In order to overcome the adverse effects of magnetic field inhomogeneity a spin echo is generated. A 180-degree RF pulse follows TE/2 ms after the 90-degree excitation pulse. The 180-degree pulse causes refocusing of the spin isochromats to form an echo at time t = TE, as shown in the pulse sequence diagram of Figure 1–6.

The amplitude of the spin-echo signal is given approximately by the expression:

$$M_{xy} = M_{xy}°[1-\exp(-TR/T1)] \exp(-TE/T2) \qquad (5)$$

where M_{xy} and $M_{xy}°$ are the transverse magnetization at echo time and immediately following the 90-degree pulse, respectively and TE is the echo

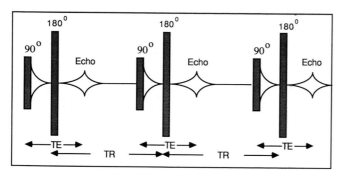

FIG 1–6.

Spin-echo pulse sequence: TE/2 ms after the 90-degree excitation pulse, a 180-degree phase reversal RF pulse is applied which causes the spins to refocus at time TE, creating what is denoted a *spin echo.*

delay. The longer TE the more the resultant images are T2-weighted. However, at very long TE the signal loss from transverse magnetization decay adversely affects CNR. Figure 1–7,A shows a plot of signal intensity as a function of the echo time *TE,* calculated for TR = 2 seconds.

A crucial feature of the signal intensity plot in

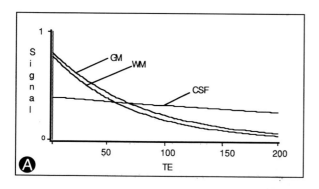

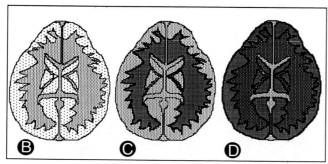

FIG 1–7.

A, brain signal versus echo time (TE), calculated at a pulse repetition time TR = 2 seconds. Note that *CSF* initially has much lower signal intensity because of its long TR. However, as TE increases it eventually surpasses that of *GM* and *WM* due to its very long T2 (approximately 1500 ms vs. 80 and 70 ms for GM and WM, respectively. The images in **B–D** correspond to TEs of approximately 20 ms (GM>WM>>CSF), 60 ms (GM=CSF>WM) and 100 ms (CSF>GM>WM). This last image is said to be T2-weighted.

Figure 1–7,A is the reversal of contrast between CSF on the one hand and GM and WM on the other hand. Further, at the TE where the two signal curves cross, contrast between the two anatomic entities vanishes. The TE at which contrast reversal occurs is dictated by the TR, since the initial hypointensity of CSF is caused by its long T1. Hence, increasing TR will, according to equation (5), cause an increase in the CSF signal and, consequently, the contrast reversal point will be shifted toward shorter TEs, as shown by the signal intensity curves in Figure 1–8, calculated for TR = 4 seconds.

Hence we see that the relative contrast is a sensitive function of the choice of the extrinsic parameters TR and TE. T1-weighted images are obtained at short TR (TR~ 0.5 second) and short TE (~10–20 ms). Proton density–weighted images, on the other hand, are typified by much longer TR (~2–4 second) and short TE (~10–20 ms). T2-weighted images typically require TRs of the order of 2 to 4 seconds and TEs of 60 to 100 ms. Finally, the contrast reversal point occurs at lower TE when a long TR is chosen.

The relationships between relative signal intensity and pulse sequence parameters are borne out by Figure 1–9 showing a matrix of images acquired on the same normal volunteer illustrating the TR and TE dependence of signal intensity and contrast with TE increasing from right to left and TR increasing from top to bottom.

There are several noteworthy features in these images. First, the SNR increases with increasing TR and decreases with increasing TE. Second, the increase in relative signal intensity with TR occurs

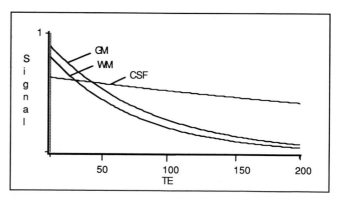

FIG 1–8.

Brain signal vs. echo time *TE,* calculated at a pulse repetition time TR = 4 seconds. Note that the longer TR causes an increase in the *CSF* signal intensity and hence a shift in the contrast reversal point between CSF on the one hand and gray *(GM)* and white matter *(WM),* on the other hand.

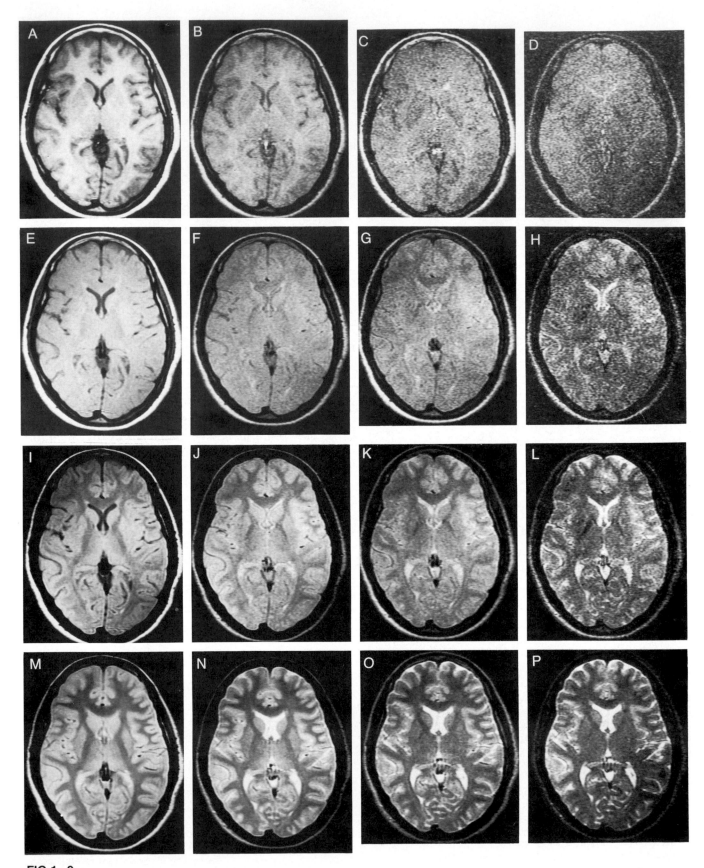

FIG 1–9.
Matrix of images with TR constant across rows and TE constant down columns: *Row 1:* TR = 500 ms. *Row 2:* TR = 1,000 ms. *Row 3:* TR = 2000 ms. *Row 4:* TR = 4,000 ms. *Row 5:* TR = 8000 ms. *Row 6:* TR = 12000 ms. From left to right. *Column 1:* TE = 25 ms. *Column 2:* TE = 50 ms. *Column 3:* TE = 75 ms. *Column 4:* TE = 100 ms.
(Continued.)

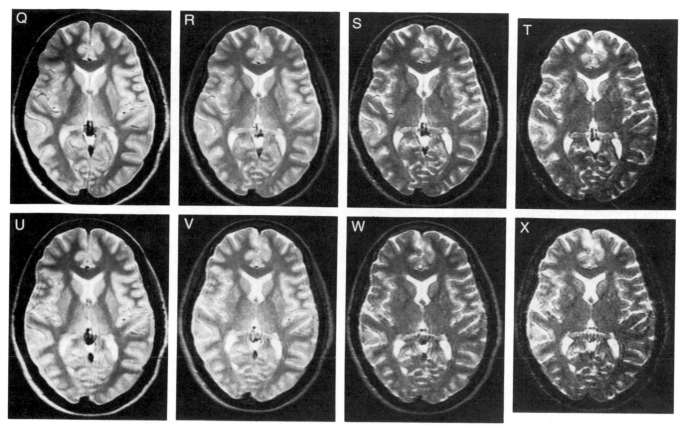

FIG 1–9   (cont.).

at different rates, being slowest for the structure with longest T1 (CSF). Third, contrast reversal between GM and WM on the one hand and CSF on the other hand, occurs at shorter TE as TR is increased. Figure 1–10 summarizes the relationships between relative signal intensity and extrinsic and intrinsic parameters.

The above rules are generally valid in clinical

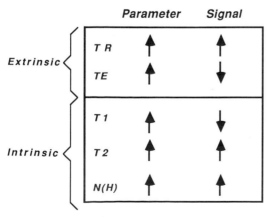

FIG 1–10.
Summary of relative signal dependence on intrinsic and extrinsic parameters.

situations as well since most pathologic tissues have relaxation properties similar to CSF. Therefore, CSF contrast is a good indicator for clinical contrast.

SPATIAL RESOLUTION AND ITS TRADE-OFF PARAMETERS

Effect of Scan Parameters on Resolving Power

The resolving power, or the ability to identify and discern adjacent objects, is equally dependent upon CNR between the object and its background as it is on the size of the target tissue on the image being examined. As with all digital modalities, the size of the target tissue (relative to its background, or adjacent tissue to which it is being contrasted) is dependent upon the dimensions of the imaging pixels. Therefore, the maximum theoretically attainable resolution is constrained by the dimensions of the imaging voxel itself. In other words, it is not possible to differentiate between two adjacent structures whose dimensions are the same as or less than those of the voxel itself. It therefore

SNR and voxel volume for typical settings as they are used in neuroimaging, demonstrating the large range of SNR and spatial resolution that are possible. In this comparison we have arbitrarily assigned a value of 100 for an FOV of 24 cm, 256 × 256 matrix, NEX = 1, a slice thickness of 5 mm, and a BW of 16 kHz as our standard parameter set. The scan time for this set of scan parameters is unity. Further, we assume the FOV to be rectangular ($D_x = D_y = D$).

It therefore becomes obvious from Table 1–1 that the dynamic range of SNR and spatial resolution achievable with the available choices of imaging parameters is very large, and a judicious choice of these parameters is required for attaining a particular clinical goal. Images corresponding to the parameter combinations listed in Table 1–1 are illustrated in Figure 1–11. Note, for example, that highest spatial resolution with retention of reasonable SNR exacts a substantial scan time penalty (Fig 1–11, E).

In a recent study it was shown that the perceived image quality is a composite of SNR and spatial resolution and that an image quality index can be defined as the product of SNR and the reciprocal voxel size. This image quality index was shown to correlate with reader preference.[15] Preference is therefore expected to be given to those images that combine high SNR with small voxel size. The reader may test this relationship by rating the images of Figure 1–11.

Choice of RF Coil

There are many different designs and implementations of body, head, and "surface" coils for the various clinical imaging systems today. While each has its benefits and limitations, it may be generalized that all surface or "local" coils provide inherently greater SNRs than circumferential body or head coils, albeit at the expense of a more limited reception profile. An excellent review of the subject has been provided by Schenck et al.[16] and Hyde et al.[17] At this point we will therefore only briefly review the most important characteristics:

1. Surface coils provide highest SNR near the surface to which they are applied, with a nonlinear falloff occurring with increasing distance from the coil as illustrated in Figure 1–12. At coil surface, the gain in SNR can be up to a factor of 4 to 6 relative to head and body coil at the same distance from the coil.

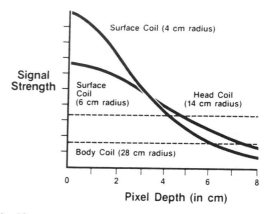

FIG 1–12.
Detection sensitivity plotted as a function of pixel depth for two circular surface coils, the head and body coil. (From Schenck JF, et al: *AJNR* 1985; 6:193–196. Used with permission.)

2. The penetration depth of a circular surface coil is about 1 radius. Hence, the more superficial a structure the smaller the coil radius that can be tolerated and therefore the better the SNR. This therefore permits the physician to trade some of the excess SNR for improved spatial resolution or shorter scan times.

3. Surface coils are typically of the receive-only design, with the body coil acting as a transmitter coil. However, in spite of excitation of tissue outside the physical boundaries, they do not typically cause wrap-around in small FOV imaging (due to their limited reception profile), as long as the two coils are decoupled from one another during the receive phase. Surface coils are therefore uniquely suited for smaller FOV ultrahigh-resolution applications such as imaging the orbit, temporomandibular joint, extremities, etc.

4. The limitation of volume of reception makes surface coils generally less susceptible to motion from distant parts of the body. This is particularly relevant when imaging such areas as the kidneys, adrenal glands, pancreas, or spine, where less image degradation from respiratory motion is detected since signals from (higher-amplitude) abdominal motion are not received.

Some of the distinguishing features of surface coils are illustrated in Figure 1–13,A and B with two cervical spine images obtained under identical conditions with a body coil and a surface coil, respectively. Note that while the cervical spinal cord itself is more clearly delineated (i.e., >SNR) on the surface coil image due to its proximity to the coil, the anterior anatomic regions more distant from the posteriorly placed surface coil (such as the

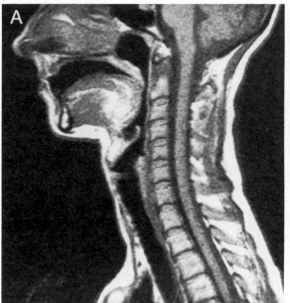 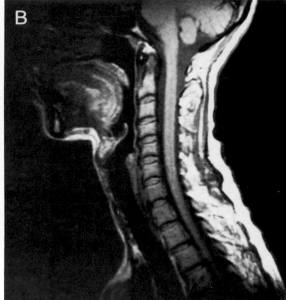

FIG 1–13.
Surface coil vs. body coil. Whereas the SNR in the region of the cervical spinal cord is superior in **B,** acquired with a 5½-in. round surface coil placed posterior to the patient's neck, the SNR is poor anteriorly where distance from the coil is great relative to its dimen- sions. The image in **A,** obtained with a body coil (of much larger dimensions), is much more homogeneous in SNR throughout the imaged volume but has less overall SNR than the image in **B** for areas adjacent to the surface coil.

mandible and tongue) are actually better appreciated on the body coil image.

Image Display Settings

Once the data have been acquired, they are stored as numerical values that represent (relative) signal intensities. The actual pixel intensity on the system monitor, however, depends on the display window and level settings. These permit operator control in scaling the data in such a way as to optimize desired image contrast and intensity. The window setting determines the intensity ranges that the pixel values fall into, while the level determines the mean brightness over which these values will be displayed. As each system has its own hardware-dependent constraints as far as brightness levels are concerned, a decrease in the display window will result in increased contrast of the structures of interest at the expense of a decrease in the display range. All pixels above the upper limit of the display window will have maximum intensity, while pixels below the lower limit of the window will appear at lowest or background intensity. The optimal display window setting is determined by the range of pixel values of the tissue(s) to be displayed. These relationships are illustrated in Figure 1–14 depicting a proton density-weighted image displaying a low-contrast parietal lobe lesion, filmed at four settings of the display window width. Note that as the display window is decreased, lesion conspicuity increases, albeit at the expense of an increase in image noise.

SUMMARY

The most powerful feature of MR imaging at present is its ability to demonstrate substantially greater tissue contrast than has been achievable by any other imaging modality. This property results from the intrinsic tissue parameters that determine MR signal intensity spanning a much wider range than, for example, x-ray attenuation coefficients in CT. The intricate, yet user-controllable, interdependence of these parameters has profound effects upon such image characteristics as SNR, image contrast, spatial resolution, and total study time. Before designing or selecting a protocol for a particular examination, decisions must be made relating to the structures to be imaged with respect to their adjacent tissues. Furthermore, it is critical to prospectively assess the relative importance of signal-to-noise, image contrast-to-noise, spatial resolution, and imaging time with respect to the suspected diagnoses under evaluation. Once these objectives have been placed in a relative order of importance, pulsing sequences can be established

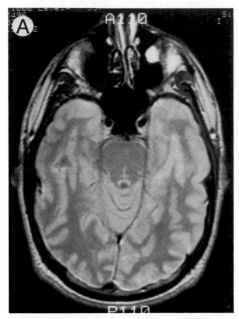

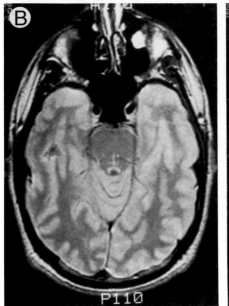

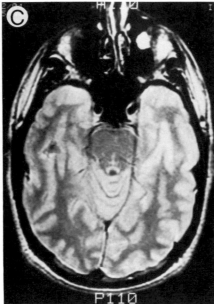

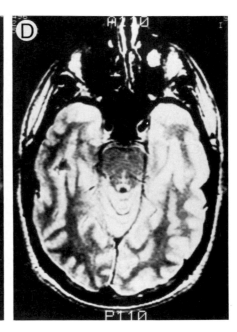

FIG 1–14.
Effect of display window on contrast. The same image, showing a low-contrast occult vascular malformation in the right parietal lobe, has been displayed at four different settings of the window width (WW): **A,** WW = 1000; **B,** WW = 750; **C,** WW = 500; **D,** WW = 250. Note that the lesion conspicuity (contrast) increases with decreasing display window setting while the image noise increases in the same order.

that will best accomplish these predefined goals. However, the heuristic nature of the problem should be recognized, which means that there is typically no single optimal set of scan parameters. Finally, with the continued development of new pulse sequence techniques such as fast low-flip-angle imaging and other techniques yet to be devised, there is even greater promise and utility in the role of MR imaging for clinical diagnosis and medical research.

REFERENCES

1. Kanal E, Wehrli FW: Signal-to-noise ratio, resolution and contrast, in Wehrli FW, Shaw D, Kneeland HB (eds): *Biomedical Magnetic Resonance Imaging: Principles, Methodology and Applications.* New York, VCH Publishers, 1988, pp 47–112.
2. Edelstein WA, Bottomley PA, Hart HR, et al: Signal, noise, and contrast in nuclear magnetic resonance (NMR) imaging. *J Comput Assist Tomogr* 1983; 7:391–401.
3. Kaufman L, Kramer DM, Crooks LE, et al: Measuring signal-to-noise ratios in MR imaging. *Radiology* 1989; 173:265–267.

4. Rose AA: *Vision: Human and Electronic.* New York, Plenum Press, 1973.

5. Fullerton GD, Cameron IL: Relaxation of biological tissues, in Wehrli FW, Shaw D, Kneeland HB (eds): *Biomedical Magnetic Resonance Imaging: Principles, Methodology and Applications.* New York, VCH Publishers, 1988, pp 115–151.

6. Bydder GM, Steiner RE, Young IR, et al: Clinical NMR imaging of the brain: 140 cases. *AJR* 1982; 139:215–236.

7. Crooks LE, Mills CM, Davis PL, et al: Visualization of cerebral and vascular abnormalities by NMR imaging: The effects of imaging parameters on contrast. *Radiology* 1982; 144:843–852.

8. Wehrli FW, MacFall JR, Shutts D, et al: Mechanisms of contrast in NMR imaging. *J Comput Assist Tomogr* 1984; 8:369–380.

9. Wehrli FW, MacFall JR, Glover GH, et al: The dependence of nuclear magnetic resonance (NMR) image contrast on intrinsic and pulse sequence timing parameters. *Magn Res Imaging* 1984; 2:3–16.

10. Mitchell MR, Conturo TE, Gruber TJ, et al: Two computer models for selection of optimal magnetic resonance imaging (MR) pulse sequence timing. *Invest Radiol* 1984; 19:350–360.

11. Hendrick RE, Nelson TR, Hendee WR: Optimizing tissue differentiation in magnetic resonance imaging. *Magn Res Imaging* 1984; 2:193–204.

12. Wehrli FW, MacFall JR, Newton TH, et al: Parameters determining the appearance of NMR images, in Newton TH, Potts DG (eds): *Modern Neuroradiology: Advanced Imaging Techniques.* San Anselmo, Calif, Clavadel Press, 1983.

13. Mitchell MR, Eisenberg A, Conturo TE, et al: MRI optimization strategies, in Partain LE, Price RR, Patton JA, et al (eds): *Magnetic Resonance Imaging.* Philadelphia, WB Saunders Co, 1988, pp 101–116.

14. Wehrli FW, MacFall JR, Prost JH: Impact of the choice of the operating parameters on MR images, in Partain LE, Price RR, Patton JA, et al (eds): *Magnetic Resonance Imaging.* Philadelphia, WB Saunders Co, 1988.

15. Owen R, Wehrli FW: Predictability and reader preference in clinical MR imaging. *Magn Res Imaging,* in press.

16. Schenck JF, Hart HR, Foster TH, et al: High-resolution magnetic resonance imaging using surface coils. in Kressel HY (ed): *Magnetic Resonance Annual,* vol 2. New York, Raven, 1986.

17. Hyde JS, Kneeland HB: High-resolution methods using local coils, in Wehrli FW, Shaw D, Kneeland HB (eds): *Biomedical Magnetic Resonance Imaging: Principles, Methodology and Applications.* New York, VCH Publishers, 1988, pp 189–222.

PART II

Anatomy

Atlas of the Adult Cerebrum

L. Anne Hayman, M.D.

Mark J. Pfleger, M.D.

Joel B. Kirkpatrick, M.D.

John J. Pagani, M.D.

This chapter provides consecutive brain images that can be matched to clinical axial images, thereby giving the reader quick access to the nomenclature of clinically important regions (Figs 2–1 through 2–38). It is indexed so that unfamiliar structures mentioned in other chapters can be quickly found. Magnetic resonance (MR) scans are correlated with myelin-stained, normal, whole-brain, histologic sections. These images were obtained on a 1.5T GE Signa unit with a long TR/TE (2,000/80) pulse sequence. A 24-cm field of view was used to obtain 5-mm contiguous scans with two averages on a single, normal volunteer.

The brain sections were obtained from the collection of Dr. Paul Yakolev at the Armed Forces Institute of Pathology. They were taken at selected intervals from serial axial sections of a formalin-fixed brain specimen. It should be noted that fixation has artificially enlarged the ventricles, sulci, and fissures. The distance of each brain slice from the base slice is indicated in millimeters. These measurements reflect the in vivo distance between the brain slices.

The level and angle of the anatomic and MR illustrations is indicated on adjacent, small schematic diagrams. Because it is not possible to exactly match anatomic sections and MR scans, the reader should compare the anatomic sections immediately before and after the section that is paired with each MR scan.

Anatomic structures of clinical significance in imaging are labeled on both the MR and brain sections. This information was garnered from diverse sources.[1–14]

REFERENCES

1. Curnes JT, Burger PC, Djang WT, et al: MR imaging of compact white matter pathways. *AJNR* 1988; 9:1061–1068.
2. Naidich TP, Daniels DL, Peck P, et al: Anterior commissure; Anatomic-MR correlation and use as a landmark in three orthogonal planes. *Radiology* 1986; 158:421–429.
3. Daniels DL, Haughton VM, Naidich TP: *Cranial and Spinal Magnetic Resonance Imaging: An Atlas and Guide.* New York, Raven Press, 1987.
4. Pernkopt E: *Atlas of Topographical and Applied Human Anatomy*, ed 2. Baltimore, Urban & Schwarzenberg, 1980.
5. Matsui T, Hirano A: *An Atlas of the Human Brain for Computed Tomography.* Tokyo, Igaku-Shoin, 1978.
6. Lockhart RD, Hamilton GF, Fyfe FW: *Anatomy of the Human Body.* Philadelphia, JB Lippincott Co, 1959.
7. Carpenter MB: *Human Neuroanatomy*, ed 7. Baltimore, Williams & Wilkins Co, 1979.
8. Roberts MP, Hanaway J, Morest DK: *Atlas of the Human Brain in Section*, ed 2. Philadelphia, Lea & Febiger, 1987.

9. Krieg WJS: *Functional Neuroanatomy,* ed 3. Evanston, Ill, Brain Books, 1966.

10. DeArmond SJ, Fusco MM, Dewey MM: *Structure of the Human Brain,* ed 3. New York, Oxford University Press, 1989.

11. Haines DE: *Neuroanatomy. An Atlas of Structures, Sections and Systems,* ed 2. Baltimore, Urban & Schwarzenberg, 1987.

12. Singer M, Yakovlev PI: *The Human Brain in Sagittal Section.* Springfield, Ill, Charles C Thomas, Publisher, 1954.

13. Schlesinger B: *The Upper Brainstem in the Human.* New York, Springer-Verlag, 1976.

14. Schnitzlein HN, Murtagh FR: *Imaging Anatomy of the Head and Spine.* Baltimore, Urban & Schwarzenberg, 1985.

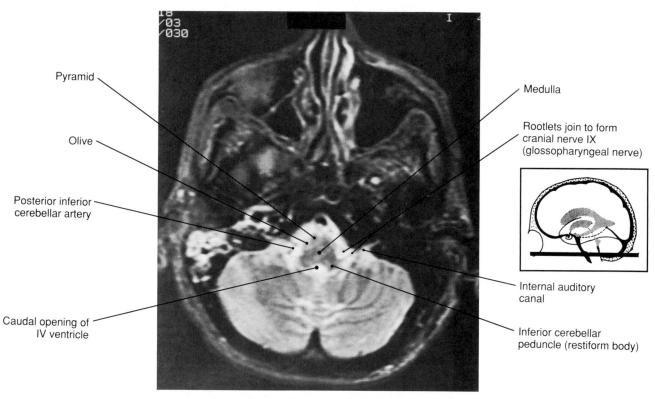

FIG 2–1.

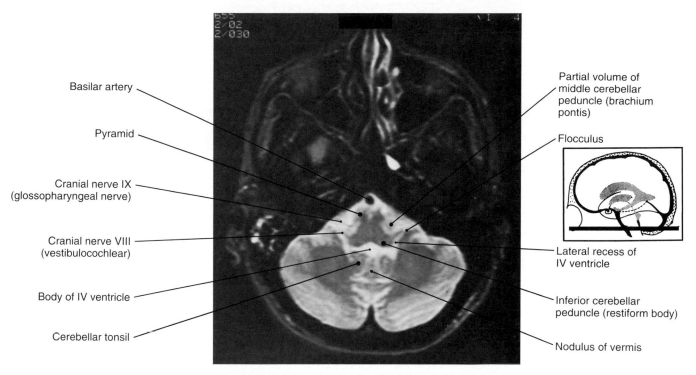

Basilar artery

Pyramid

Cranial nerve IX
(glossopharyngeal nerve)

Cranial nerve VIII
(vestibulocochlear)

Body of IV ventricle

Cerebellar tonsil

Partial volume of
middle cerebellar
peduncle (brachium
pontis)

Flocculus

Lateral recess of
IV ventricle

Inferior cerebellar
peduncle (restiform body)

Nodulus of vermis

FIG 2–2.

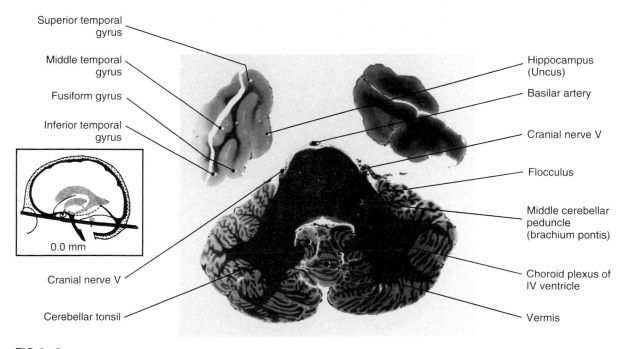

Superior temporal
gyrus

Middle temporal
gyrus

Fusiform gyrus

Inferior temporal
gyrus

0.0 mm

Cranial nerve V

Cerebellar tonsil

Hippocampus
(Uncus)

Basilar artery

Cranial nerve V

Flocculus

Middle cerebellar
peduncle
(brachium pontis)

Choroid plexus of
IV ventricle

Vermis

FIG 2–3.

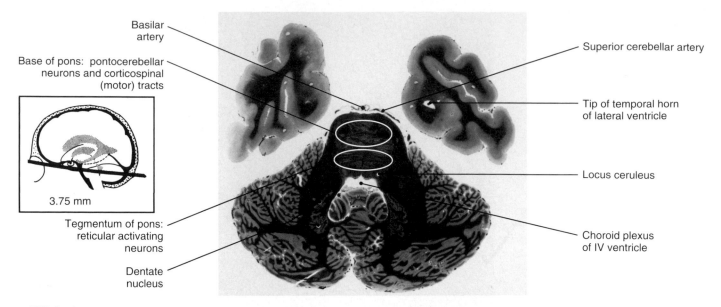

Basilar
artery

Base of pons: pontocerebellar
neurons and corticospinal
(motor) tracts

3.75 mm

Tegmentum of pons:
reticular activating
neurons

Dentate
nucleus

Superior cerebellar artery

Tip of temporal horn
of lateral ventricle

Locus ceruleus

Choroid plexus
of IV ventricle

FIG 2–4.

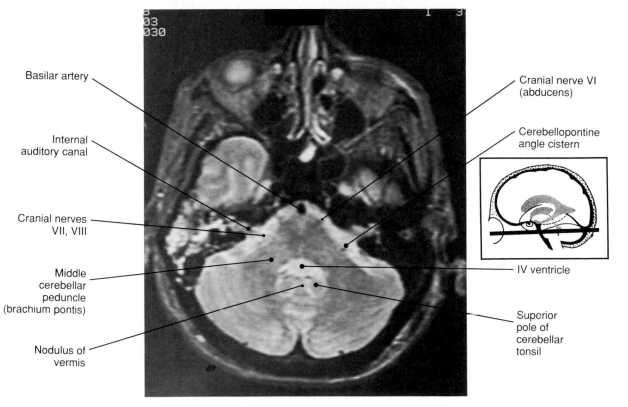

Basilar artery

Internal
auditory canal

Cranial nerves
VII, VIII

Middle
cerebellar
peduncle
(brachium pontis)

Nodulus of
vermis

Cranial nerve VI
(abducens)

Cerebellopontine
angle cistern

IV ventricle

Superior
pole of
cerebellar
tonsil

FIG 2–5.

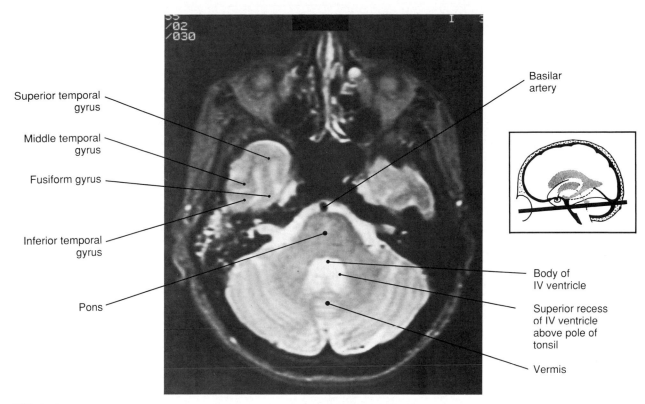

Superior temporal gyrus

Middle temporal gyrus

Fusiform gyrus

Inferior temporal gyrus

Pons

Basilar artery

Body of IV ventricle

Superior recess of IV ventricle above pole of tonsil

Vermis

FIG 2–6.

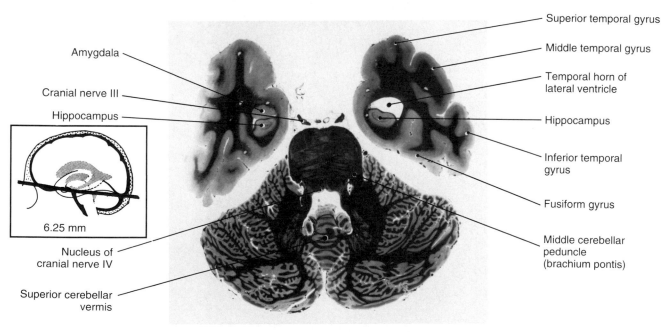

Amygdala

Cranial nerve III

Hippocampus

6.25 mm

Nucleus of cranial nerve IV

Superior cerebellar vermis

Superior temporal gyrus

Middle temporal gyrus

Temporal horn of lateral ventricle

Hippocampus

Inferior temporal gyrus

Fusiform gyrus

Middle cerebellar peduncle (brachium pontis)

FIG 2–7.

Gyrus rectus

Cranial nerve I
(olfactory)

Pituitary
infundibulum

Cranial nerve VI
(abducens)

7.5 mm

IV ventricle

Superior recess of
IV ventricle
above tonsil

Stem of internal
carotid artery

Posterior
communicating artery

Posterior cerebral
artery

Superior cerebellar
peduncle (brachium
conjunctivum)

Dentate nucleus

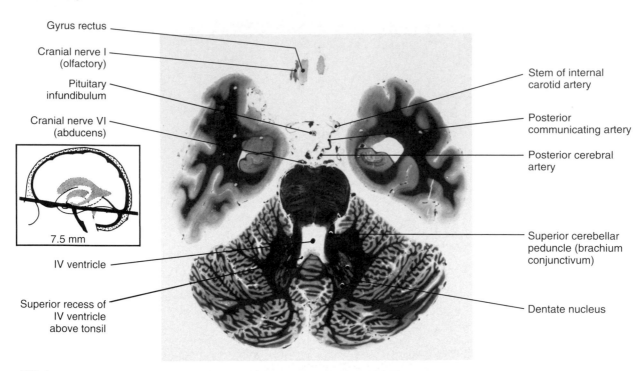

FIG 2−8.

Superior
temporal gyrus

Hippocampus

Middle
temporal gyrus

Inferior
temporal gyrus

Fusiform gyrus

IV ventricle

Dural wall of
cavernous sinus

Carotid artery entering
the cavernous
sinus

Basilar artery

Cranial nerve V
(trigeminal)

Stem of
petrosal vein

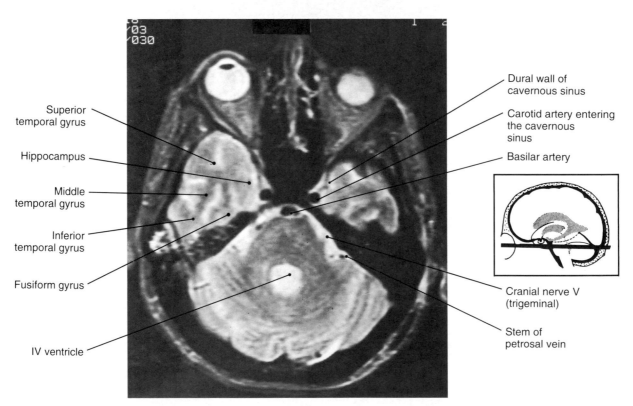

FIG 2−9.

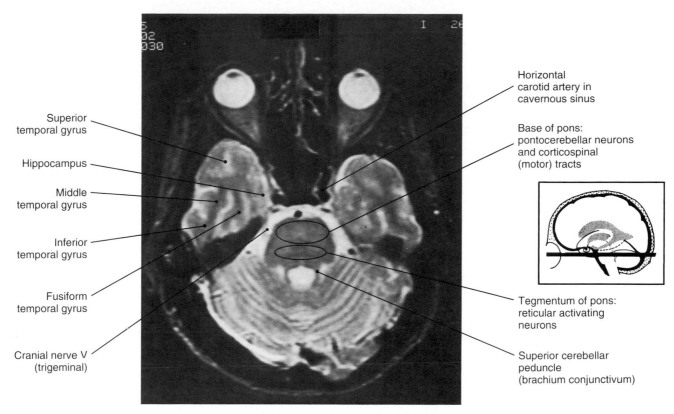

Superior temporal gyrus

Hippocampus

Middle temporal gyrus

Inferior temporal gyrus

Fusiform temporal gyrus

Cranial nerve V (trigeminal)

Horizontal carotid artery in cavernous sinus

Base of pons: pontocerebellar neurons and corticospinal (motor) tracts

Tegmentum of pons: reticular activating neurons

Superior cerebellar peduncle (brachium conjunctivum)

FIG 2–10.

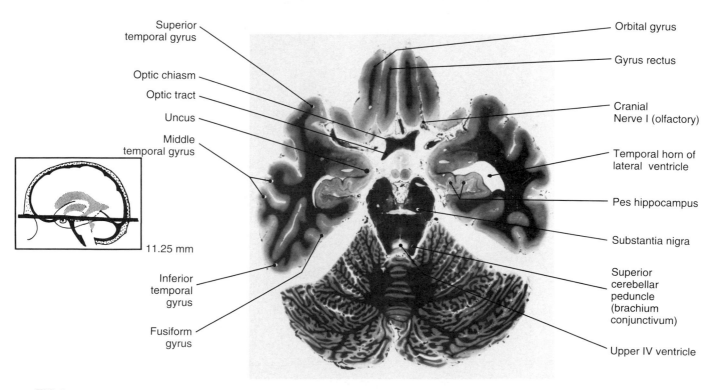

Superior temporal gyrus

Optic chiasm

Optic tract

Uncus

Middle temporal gyrus

11.25 mm

Inferior temporal gyrus

Fusiform gyrus

Orbital gyrus

Gyrus rectus

Cranial Nerve I (olfactory)

Temporal horn of lateral ventricle

Pes hippocampus

Substantia nigra

Superior cerebellar peduncle (brachium conjunctivum)

Upper IV ventricle

FIG 2–11.

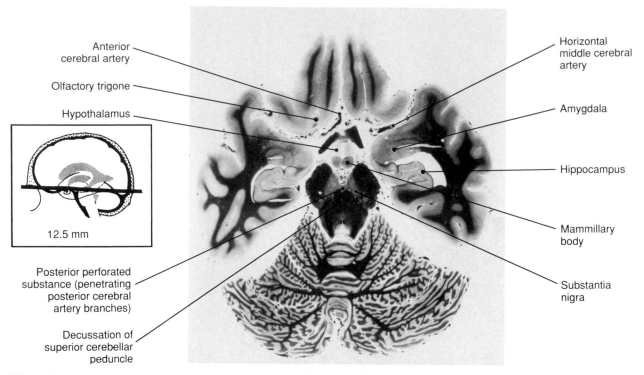

Anterior cerebral artery

Olfactory trigone

Hypothalamus

12.5 mm

Posterior perforated substance (penetrating posterior cerebral artery branches)

Decussation of superior cerebellar peduncle

Horizontal middle cerebral artery

Amygdala

Hippocampus

Mammillary body

Substantia nigra

FIG 2–12.

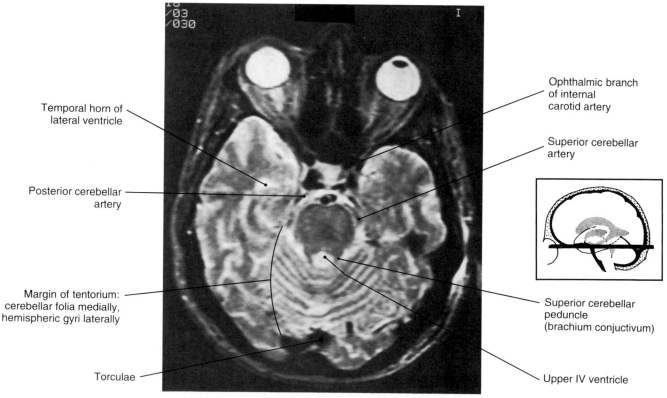

Temporal horn of lateral ventricle

Posterior cerebellar artery

Margin of tentorium: cerebellar folia medially, hemispheric gyri laterally

Torculae

Ophthalmic branch of internal carotid artery

Superior cerebellar artery

Superior cerebellar peduncle (brachium conjuctivum)

Upper IV ventricle

FIG 2–13.

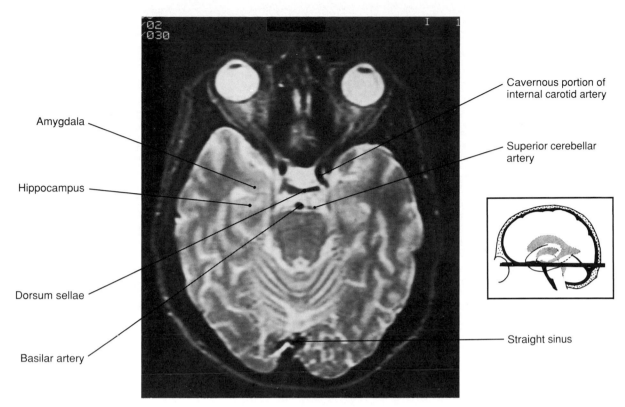

Amygdala

Hippocampus

Dorsum sellae

Basilar artery

Cavernous portion of internal carotid artery

Superior cerebellar artery

Straight sinus

FIG 2–14.

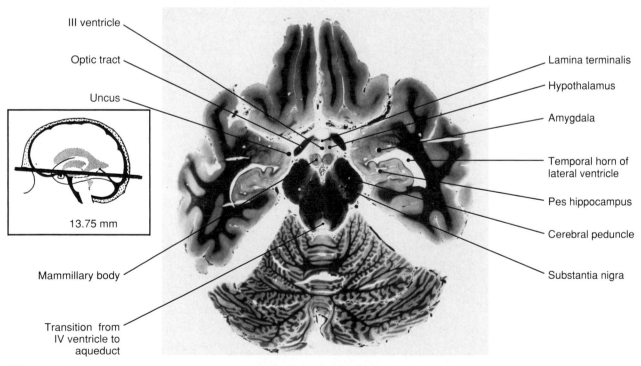

III ventricle

Optic tract

Uncus

13.75 mm

Mammillary body

Transition from IV ventricle to aqueduct

Lamina terminalis

Hypothalamus

Amygdala

Temporal horn of lateral ventricle

Pes hippocampus

Cerebral peduncle

Substantia nigra

FIG 2–15.

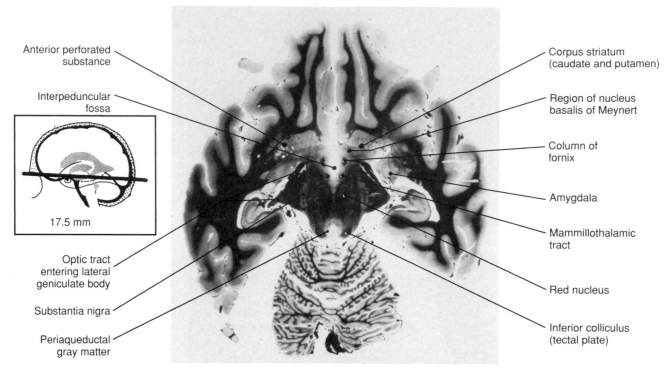

Anterior perforated substance

Interpeduncular fossa

17.5 mm

Optic tract entering lateral geniculate body

Substantia nigra

Periaqueductal gray matter

Corpus striatum (caudate and putamen)

Region of nucleus basalis of Meynert

Column of fornix

Amygdala

Mammillothalamic tract

Red nucleus

Inferior colliculus (tectal plate)

FIG 2–16.

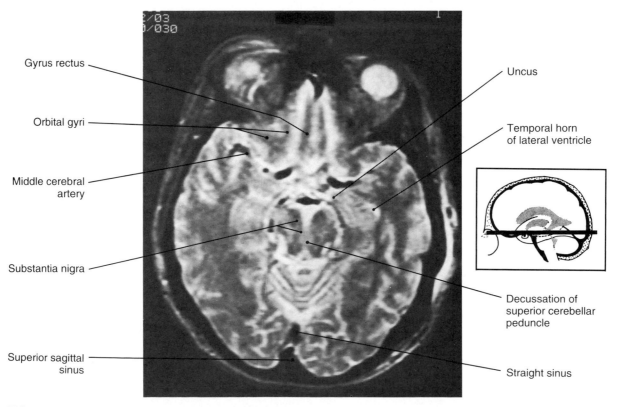

Gyrus rectus

Orbital gyri

Middle cerebral artery

Substantia nigra

Superior sagittal sinus

Uncus

Temporal horn of lateral ventricle

Decussation of superior cerebellar peduncle

Straight sinus

FIG 2–17.

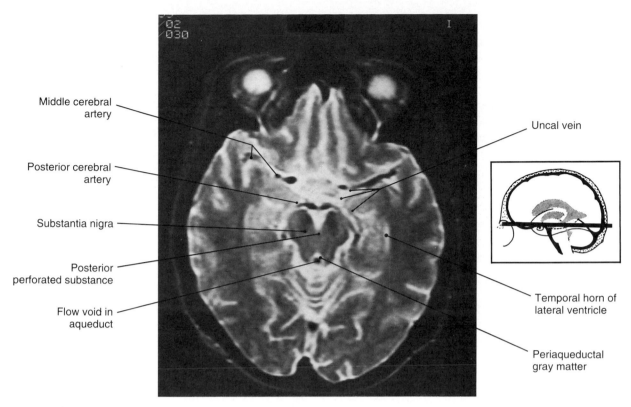

Middle cerebral artery

Posterior cerebral artery

Substantia nigra

Posterior perforated substance

Flow void in aqueduct

Uncal vein

Temporal horn of lateral ventricle

Periaqueductal gray matter

FIG 2–18.

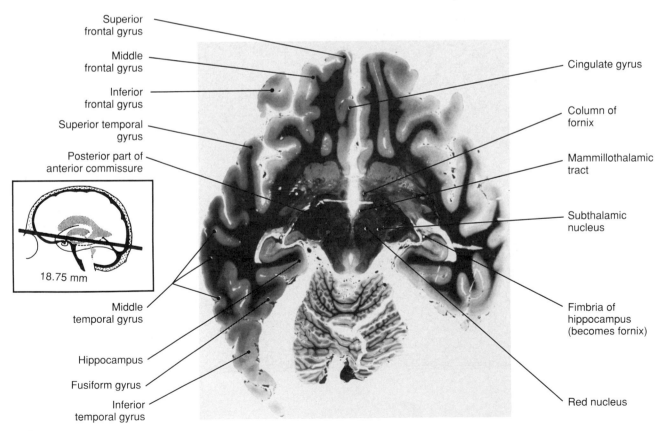

Superior frontal gyrus

Middle frontal gyrus

Inferior frontal gyrus

Superior temporal gyrus

Posterior part of anterior commissure

18.75 mm

Middle temporal gyrus

Hippocampus

Fusiform gyrus

Inferior temporal gyrus

Cingulate gyrus

Column of fornix

Mammillothalamic tract

Subthalamic nucleus

Fimbria of hippocampus (becomes fornix)

Red nucleus

FIG 2–19.

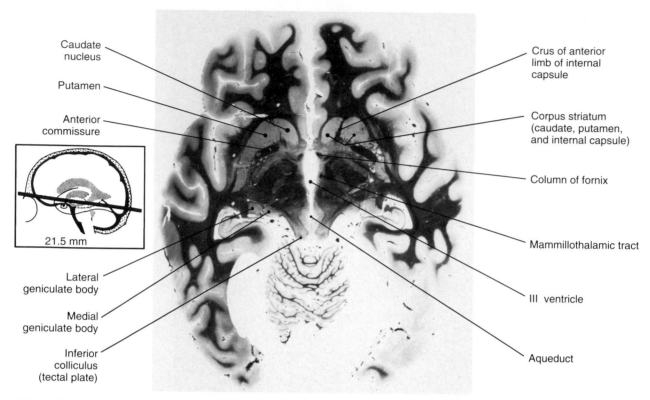

Caudate nucleus

Putamen

Anterior commissure

21.5 mm

Lateral geniculate body

Medial geniculate body

Inferior colliculus (tectal plate)

Crus of anterior limb of internal capsule

Corpus striatum (caudate, putamen, and internal capsule)

Column of fornix

Mammillothalamic tract

III ventricle

Aqueduct

FIG 2–20.

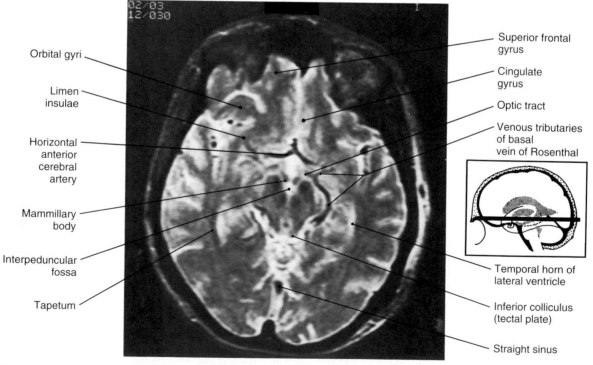

02/03
12/030

Orbital gyri

Limen insulae

Horizontal anterior cerebral artery

Mammillary body

Interpeduncular fossa

Tapetum

Superior frontal gyrus

Cingulate gyrus

Optic tract

Venous tributaries of basal vein of Rosenthal

Temporal horn of lateral ventricle

Inferior colliculus (tectal plate)

Straight sinus

FIG 2–21.

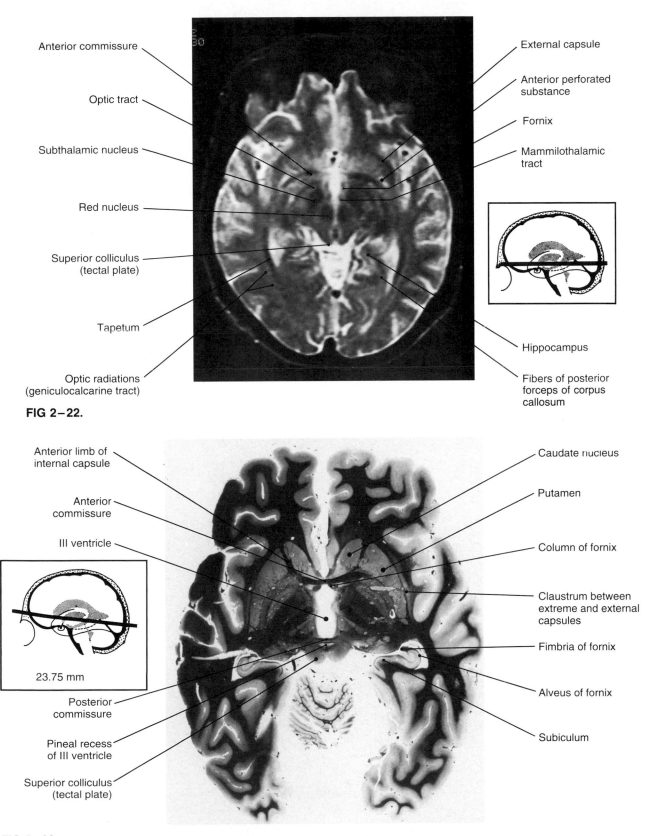

Anterior commissure

Optic tract

Subthalamic nucleus

Red nucleus

Superior colliculus
(tectal plate)

Tapetum

Optic radiations
(geniculocalcarine tract)

External capsule

Anterior perforated
substance

Fornix

Mammilothalamic
tract

Hippocampus

Fibers of posterior
forceps of corpus
callosum

FIG 2–22.

Anterior limb of
internal capsule

Anterior
commissure

III ventricle

23.75 mm

Posterior
commissure

Pineal recess
of III ventricle

Superior colliculus
(tectal plate)

Caudate nucleus

Putamen

Column of fornix

Claustrum between
extreme and external
capsules

Fimbria of fornix

Alveus of fornix

Subiculum

FIG 2–23.

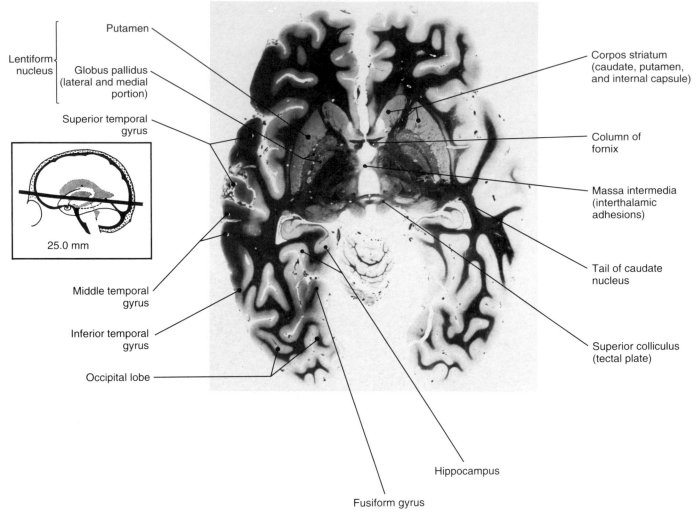

Lentiform nucleus {
- Putamen
- Globus pallidus (lateral and medial portion)

Superior temporal gyrus

25.0 mm

Middle temporal gyrus

Inferior temporal gyrus

Occipital lobe

Corpos striatum (caudate, putamen, and internal capsule)

Column of fornix

Massa intermedia (interthalamic adhesions)

Tail of caudate nucleus

Superior colliculus (tectal plate)

Hippocampus

Fusiform gyrus

FIG 2–24.

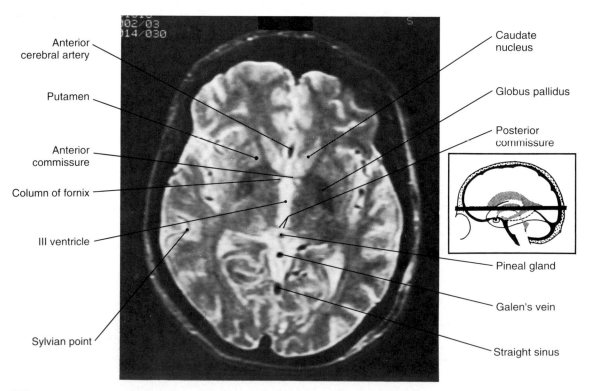

Anterior cerebral artery

Putamen

Anterior commissure

Column of fornix

III ventricle

Sylvian point

Caudate nucleus

Globus pallidus

Posterior commissure

Pineal gland

Galen's vein

Straight sinus

FIG 2–25.

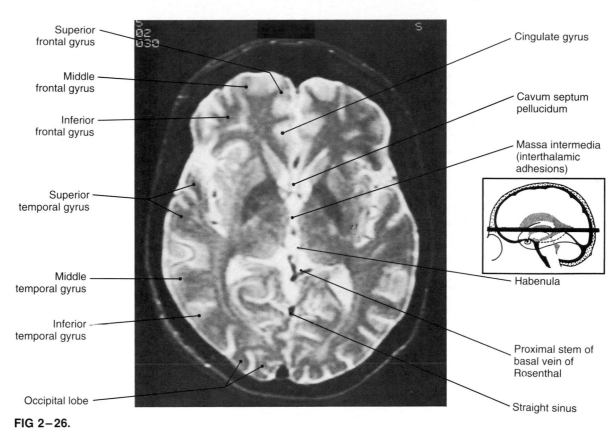

Superior frontal gyrus

Middle frontal gyrus

Inferior frontal gyrus

Superior temporal gyrus

Middle temporal gyrus

Inferior temporal gyrus

Occipital lobe

Cingulate gyrus

Cavum septum pellucidum

Massa intermedia (interthalamic adhesions)

Habenula

Proximal stem of basal vein of Rosenthal

Straight sinus

FIG 2–26.

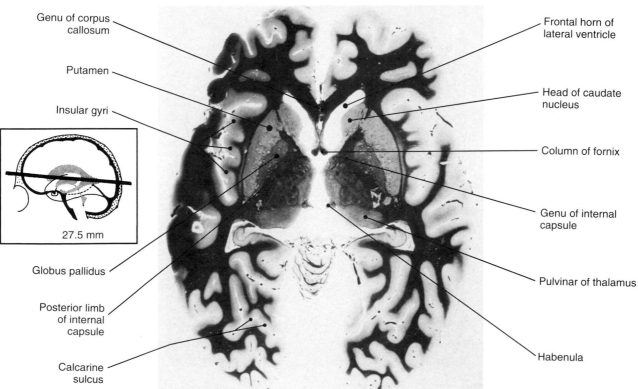

Genu of corpus callosum

Putamen

Insular gyri

27.5 mm

Globus pallidus

Posterior limb of internal capsule

Calcarine sulcus

Frontal horn of lateral ventricle

Head of caudate nucleus

Column of fornix

Genu of internal capsule

Pulvinar of thalamus

Habenula

FIG 2–27.

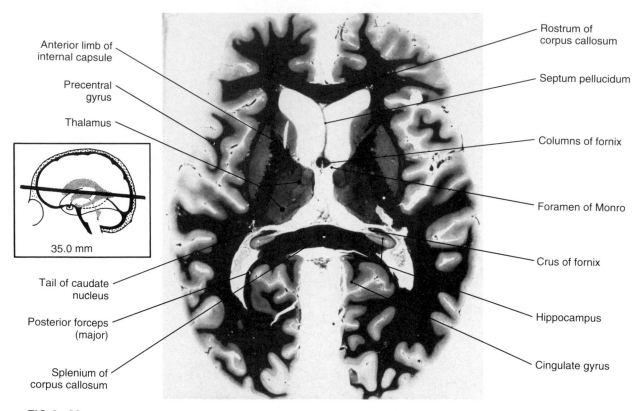

Anterior limb of
internal capsule

Precentral
gyrus

Thalamus

35.0 mm

Tail of caudate
nucleus

Posterior forceps
(major)

Splenium of
corpus callosum

Rostrum of
corpus callosum

Septum pellucidum

Columns of fornix

Foramen of Monro

Crus of fornix

Hippocampus

Cingulate gyrus

FIG 2–28.

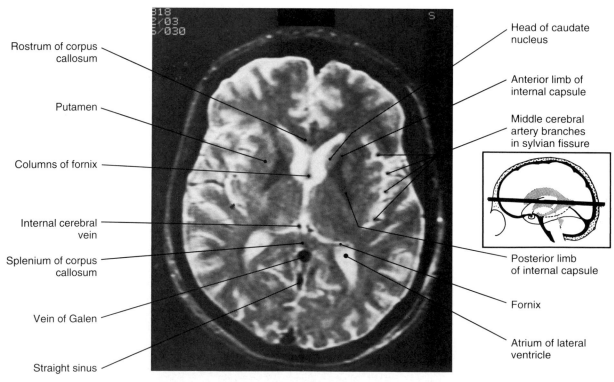

Rostrum of corpus
callosum

Putamen

Columns of fornix

Internal cerebral
vein

Splenium of corpus
callosum

Vein of Galen

Straight sinus

Head of caudate
nucleus

Anterior limb of
internal capsule

Middle cerebral
artery branches
in sylvian fissure

Posterior limb
of internal capsule

Fornix

Atrium of lateral
ventricle

FIG 2–29.

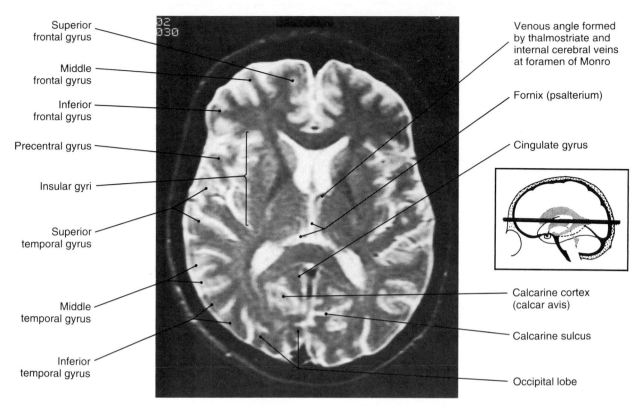

Superior frontal gyrus

Middle frontal gyrus

Inferior frontal gyrus

Precentral gyrus

Insular gyri

Superior temporal gyrus

Middle temporal gyrus

Inferior temporal gyrus

Venous angle formed by thalmostriate and internal cerebral veins at foramen of Monro

Fornix (psalterium)

Cingulate gyrus

Calcarine cortex (calcar avis)

Calcarine sulcus

Occipital lobe

FIG 2–30.

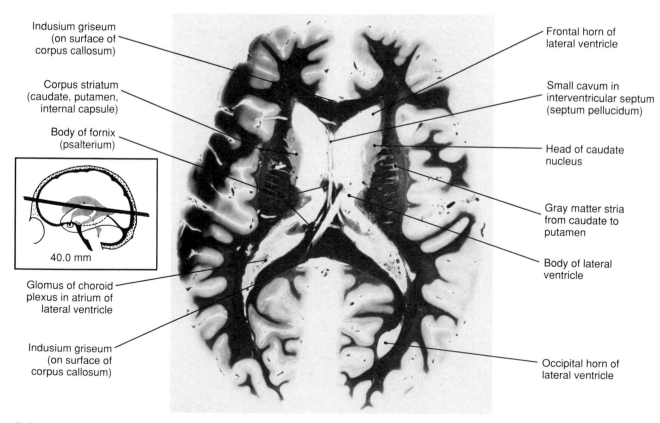

Indusium griseum (on surface of corpus callosum)

Corpus striatum (caudate, putamen, internal capsule)

Body of fornix (psalterium)

Glomus of choroid plexus in atrium of lateral ventricle

Indusium griseum (on surface of corpus callosum)

40.0 mm

Frontal horn of lateral ventricle

Small cavum in interventricular septum (septum pellucidum)

Head of caudate nucleus

Gray matter stria from caudate to putamen

Body of lateral ventricle

Occipital horn of lateral ventricle

FIG 2–31.

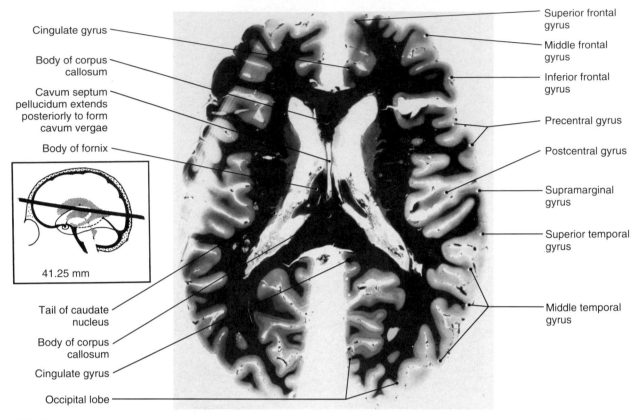

Cingulate gyrus

Body of corpus callosum

Cavum septum pellucidum extends posteriorly to form cavum vergae

Body of fornix

41.25 mm

Tail of caudate nucleus

Body of corpus callosum

Cingulate gyrus

Occipital lobe

Superior frontal gyrus

Middle frontal gyrus

Inferior frontal gyrus

Precentral gyrus

Postcentral gyrus

Supramarginal gyrus

Superior temporal gyrus

Middle temporal gyrus

FIG 2–32.

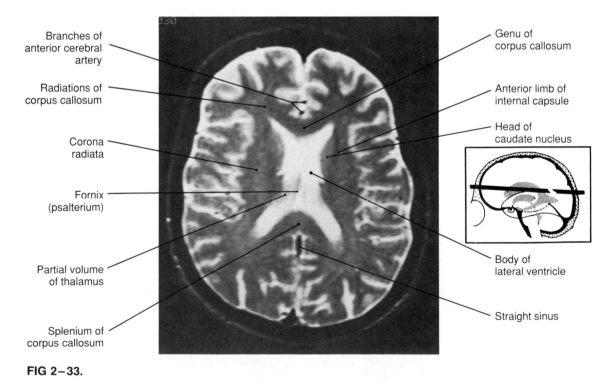

Branches of anterior cerebral artery

Radiations of corpus callosum

Corona radiata

Fornix (psalterium)

Partial volume of thalamus

Splenium of corpus callosum

Genu of corpus callosum

Anterior limb of internal capsule

Head of caudate nucleus

Body of lateral ventricle

Straight sinus

FIG 2–33.

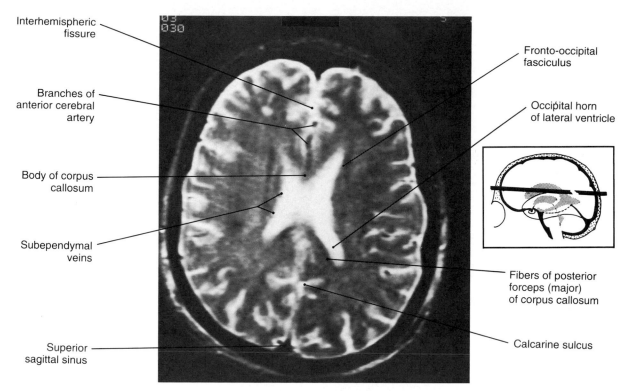

Interhemispheric fissure

Branches of anterior cerebral artery

Body of corpus callosum

Subependymal veins

Superior sagittal sinus

Fronto-occipital fasciculus

Occipital horn of lateral ventricle

Fibers of posterior forceps (major) of corpus callosum

Calcarine sulcus

FIG 2–34.

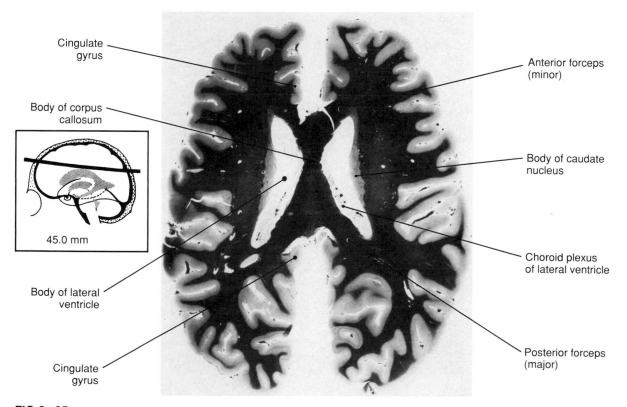

Cingulate gyrus

Body of corpus callosum

Body of lateral ventricle

Cingulate gyrus

Anterior forceps (minor)

Body of caudate nucleus

Choroid plexus of lateral ventricle

Posterior forceps (major)

45.0 mm

FIG 2–35.

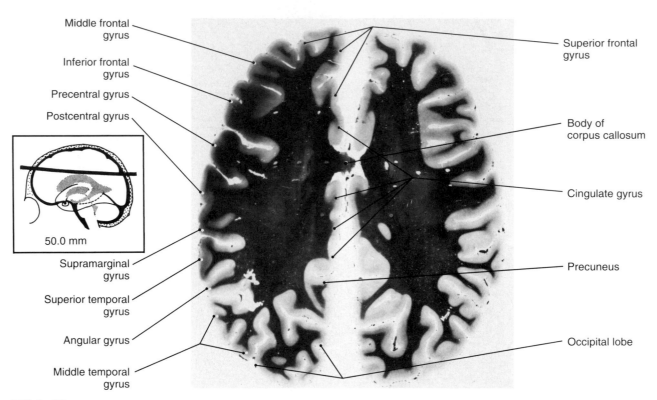

Middle frontal gyrus

Inferior frontal gyrus

Precentral gyrus

Postcentral gyrus

50.0 mm

Supramarginal gyrus

Superior temporal gyrus

Angular gyrus

Middle temporal gyrus

Superior frontal gyrus

Body of corpus callosum

Cingulate gyrus

Precuneus

Occipital lobe

FIG 2–36.

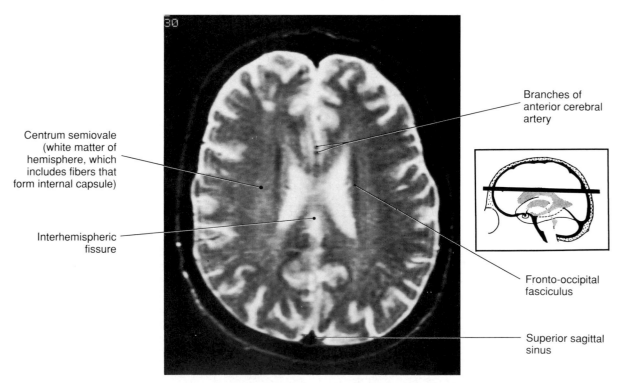

Centrum semiovale (white matter of hemisphere, which includes fibers that form internal capsule)

Interhemispheric fissure

Branches of anterior cerebral artery

Fronto-occipital fasciculus

Superior sagittal sinus

FIG 2–37.

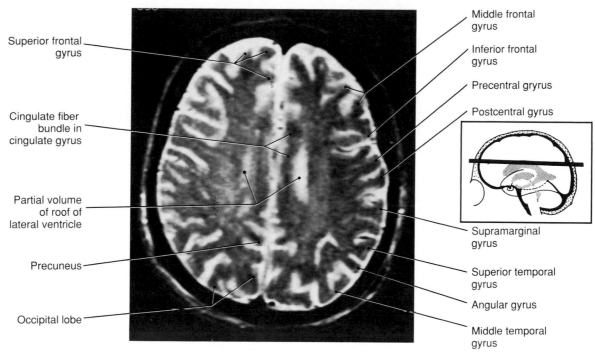

Superior frontal gyrus

Cingulate fiber bundle in cingulate gyrus

Partial volume of roof of lateral ventricle

Precuneus

Occipital lobe

Middle frontal gyrus

Inferior frontal gyrus

Precentral gryrus

Postcentral gyrus

Supramarginal gyrus

Superior temporal gyrus

Angular gyrus

Middle temporal gyrus

FIG 2–38.

INDEX TO THE ILLUSTRATIONS

Entries refer to figures in which the specific structures are labeled.

Structure	Figure No.
Geniculocalcarine tract	2–22
Globus pallidus	2–24, 2–25, 2–27
Gyrus, angular	2–36, 2–38
Gyrus, cingulate	2–19, 2–21, 2–26, 2–28, 2–30, 2–32, 2–35, 2–36, 2–38
Gyrus, frontal, inferior	2–19, 2–26, 2–30, 2–32, 2–36, 2–38
Gyrus, frontal, middle	2–19, 2–26, 2–30, 2–32, 2–36, 2–38
Gyrus, frontal, superior	2–19, 2–21, 2–26, 2–30, 2–32, 2–36, 2–38
Gyrus, fusiform	2–3, 2–6, 2–7, 2–9 to 2–11, 2–19, 2–24
Gyrus, insular	2–27, 2–30
Gyrus, orbital	2–11, 2–17, 2–21
Gyrus, postcentral	2–32, 2–36, 2–38
Gyrus, precentral	2–28, 2–30, 2–32, 2–36, 2–38
Gyrus, rectus	2–8, 2–11, 2–17
Gyrus, supramarginal	2–32, 2–36, 2–38
Gyrus, temporal, inferior	2–3, 2–6, 2–7, 2–9 to 2–11, 2–19, 2–24, 2–26, 2–30
Gyrus, temporal, middle	2–3, 2–6, 2–7, 2–9 to 2–11, 2–19, 2–24, 2–26, 2–30, 2–32, 2–36, 2–38
Gyrus, temporal, superior	2–3, 2–6, 2–7, 2–9 to 2–11, 2–19, 2–24, 2–26, 2–30, 2–32, 2–36, 2–38
Habenula	2–26, 2–27
Hippocampus	2–3, 2–7, 2–9, 2–10, 2–12, 2–14, 2–19, 2–22, 2–24, 2–28
Hippocampus, pes	2–11, 2–15
Hypothalamus	2–12, 2–15
Indusium griseum	2–31
Interhemispheric fissure	2–34, 2–37
Internal capsule	2–20, 2–24, 2–31, 2–37
Internal capsule, anterior limb	2–20, 2–23, 2–28, 2–29, 2–33
Internal capsule, genu	2–27
Internal capsule, posterior limb	2–27, 2–29
Interpeduncular fossa	2–16, 2–21
Interthalamic adhesions	2–24, 2–26
Lamina terminalis	2–15
Lentiform nucleus	2–24
Limen insulae	2–21

Structure	Figure No.
Locus ceruleus	2–4
Mammillary body	2–12, 2–15, 2–21
Mammillothalamic tract	2–16, 2–19, 2–20, 2–22
Massa intermedia	2–24, 2–26
Medulla	2–1
Nodulus of vermis	2–2, 2–5
Nucleus basalis of Meynert	2–16
Occipital lobe	2–24, 2–26, 2–30, 2–32, 2–36, 2–38
Olfactory trigone	2–12
Olive	2–1
Optic chiasm	2–11
Optic radiations	2–22
Optic tract	2–11, 2–15, 2–16, 2–21, 2–22
Periaqueductal gray matter	2–16, 2–18
Pineal gland	2–25
Pituitary infundibulum	2–8
Pons	2–6
Pons, base	2–4, 2–10
Pons, tegmentum	2–4, 2–10
Pontocerebellar neurons	2–10
Posterior commissure	2–23, 2–25
Posterior forceps major	2–28, 2–34, 2–35
Posterior perforated substance	2–12, 2–18
Precuneus	2–36, 2–38
Pulvinar of thalamus	2–27
Putamen	2–16, 2–20, 2–23 to 2–25, 2–27, 2–29, 2–31
Pyramid	2–1, 2–2
Red nucleus	2–16, 2–19, 2–22
Restiform body	2–1, 2–2
Reticular activating neurons	2–10
Septum pellucidum	2–28
Sinus, straight	2–14, 2–17, 2–21, 2–25, 2–26, 2–29, 2–33
Sinus, superior sagittal	2–17, 2–34, 2–37
Subiculum	2–23
Substance, anterior perforated	2–16, 2–22
Substance, posterior perforated	2–12, 2–18
Substantia nigra	2–11, 2–12, 2–15 to 2–18
Subthalamic nucleus	2–19, 2–22
Sylvian fissure	2–29

mised. Thus, when the rescuing vessel is compromised, territory outside the usual vascular limit is also compromised. MRI of completed infarctions may demonstrate the wallerian degeneration in fiber tracts that originated in the now absent or damaged neurons. Hence, the reader should pay particular attention to the section of the text that describes these tracts.

ANTERIOR CEREBRAL ARTERY TERRITORY

In Figures 3–1 and 3–2, the branches of the anterior cerebral artery have been divided into three groups: (1) the medial lenticulostriate arteries, (2) the pericallosal branches to the corpus callosum, and (3) the branches to the cerebral hemisphere. These illustrations were adapted from the atlas of Matsui and Hirano, and a detailed labeling of the anatomy can be found there.[1] Figure 3–3 is a companion diagram of the medial aspect of the right cerebral hemisphere. It is provided to localize the axial and coronal images of Figures 3–1 and 3–2. The regions supplied by the hemispheric branches and the cortical function of each region are shown.

Medial Lenticulostriate Arteries

The medial lenticulostriate arteries include the artery of Heubner and basal branches of the anterior cerebral artery. The artery of Heubner supplies the anterior aspects of the putamen and caudate nucleus as well as the anteroinferior part of the internal capsule. Infarction causes weakness of the contralateral face and arm without sensory loss. A transient aphasia is often seen in which spontaneous speech is lost while repetition and comprehension are preserved.[2] Occasionally there is dysarthria. Although the lower extremity is unaffected, there is a halting gait because of difficulty in initiating movements.[2, 3]

The basal branches supply the dorsal aspect of the chiasm and the hypothalamus. The anterior portion of the hypothalamus is supplied by small perforating branches from the anterior cerebral artery; infarctions in this area can cause abnormality in temperature regulation, fluid electrolyte balance, synchronization of sleep and wakefulness, and perhaps some aspects of cardiac rhythm. Infarction of the hypothalamus may cause transient memory disorders or more protean psychological manifestations of anxiety, agitation, or a feeling of weakness.[3]

If there is a bilateral occlusion of the lenticulostriate arteries, a profound alteration of mental activity develops, at times resulting in a state of akinetic mutism (a comalike condition in which the patient's eyes remain open and cause him to appear awake to superficial inspection). More commonly, a classic picture of coma evolves.[4, 5]

Infarction of the medial lenticulostriate arteries is much less common than hypertensive hemorrhage from these vessels. Unlike infarction, hemorrhage that arises medial to the putamen ignores vascular boundaries, destroys the hypothalamus, and ruptures into the ventricle. Therefore the radiologist can differentiate a hemorrhagic infarct, in which hemorrhage occurs secondarily, from a primary hemorrhage (intracerebral hematoma).

Callosal Branches

The callosal arteries arise from the pericallosal branch of the anterior cerebral artery, penetrate the upper surface of the corpus callosum, and extend thence inferiorly into the septum pellucidum. Usually there are 7 to 20 short callosal branches, although these are sometimes replaced by a single artery. Infarction can result in isolation of the language-dominant left hemisphere from the right hemisphere, which mediates function of the left side of the body. As a result, the patient experiences difficulty in moving the left side of his body in response to verbal commands (ideomotor apraxia), even though there may be no paralysis. Furthermore, the patient cannot recognize words written on the left side of his body, although his sensation may be unimpaired (tactile agnosia), and he has difficulty in writing with his left hand (left-sided agraphia).[6, 7]

Hemispheric Branches

There are usually nine hemispheric branches (Fig 3–3,A), each supplying a segment of the medial surface of the hemisphere. The medial surface of the hemisphere can be supplied in whole or in part by either anterior cerebral artery. (Sometimes both hemispheres are supplied by a single pericallosal artery, the so-called azygous artery, occlusion of which results in infarction of the medial surfaces of both hemispheres.)

In view of the large number of branches and numerous variations of cross-perfusion that can occur, one might expect that the compromise of hemispheric branches could lead to a wide variety of possible clinical sequelae. However, the patterns of infarction can be simplified by comparing the whole-brain schematics of the vascular territories of Figure 3–3,A with the functional areas in Figure 3–3,B.

For example, Figure 3–3,A and B reveals that the frontal association areas that mediate judgment, insight and mood receive arterial supply from the orbitofrontal, frontopolar, and anterior internal frontal arteries and, to a lesser extent, the middle internal frontal arteries.[8] (The posterior internal frontal and paracentral territories may sometimes include a small part of the frontal association area that mediates judgment, insight, and mood [Fig 3–3,B]). These functions would be impaired by occlusion of those branches. Some degree of aphasia (disturbance of language function) may develop because the arterial supply of subjacent white matter, related to the frontal speech area of Broca, is also disturbed (see the later discussion of aphasia, especially under the hemispheric branches of the middle cerebral artery territory). A release of grasping, groping, and sucking reflex patterns may be seen in addition to impairment of those functions indicated in Figure 3–3,B.[2]

Figure 3–3,A and B also shows that the motor synchronization area is supplied by the middle and posterior internal frontal branches and, to a small extent, by the anterior internal frontal and paracentral branches. Infarction of the anterior part of the motor synchronization areas affects contralateral conjugate eye deviation, while involvement of the posterior part affects coordination of contralateral eye, head, and trunk movement.[9]

Note that the motor function area is supplied by the paracentral branch. Unilateral damage thereof causes weakness of the contralateral lower extremity (marked "leg" on Fig 3–3). Bilateral damage causes incontinence as well.[8] Note further that the sensory area is supplied by the paracentral and superior and inferior parietal branches. Rarely a parieto-occipital branch (not shown in Fig 3–3,A) may supply the posterior part of this area. Damage to the anterior part of the sensory region impairs but does not abolish appreciation of primary sensory modalities such as touch and pain. Damage to the posterior part impairs more complex sensory appreciation such as recognition of objects by touch (stereognosis), recognition of shapes written on skin (graphesthesia), and two-point discrimination.[10]

The supply of the cingulate gyrus, which "controls" memory and emotion, comes from the pericallosal, orbitofrontal, frontopolar, posterior internal frontal, paracentral, and superior and inferior parietal arteries. The cingulum fiber tract within this area is part of the limbic system that is supplied by the posterior cerebral and anterior cerebral arteries. Therefore, memory and emotional disturbance may occur as a result of damage to either vascular territory.[2, 8]

Finally, infarction in the region of the parieto-occipital fissure (which is sometimes supplied by the parieto-occipital branch of the anterior cerebral artery) has been reported in one case of anterior cerebral artery compromise. In this instance, the patient experienced disturbance of recognition in the contralateral visual field (visual agnosia). The rarity of such cases can be ascribed to the fact that the same area is usually well supplied by the posterior circulation.[2]

MIDDLE CEREBRAL ARTERY TERRITORY

In Figures 3–4 and 3–5, branches of the middle cerebral artery have been divided into two groups: (1) the lateral lenticulostriate branches to the basal ganglia and adjacent fiber tracts and (2) the hemispheric branches to the cerebral convexity.[11] Figure 3–6 is a companion diagram of the lateral aspect of the *left* cerebral hemisphere. It is provided to localize the axial and coronal images of Figures 3–4 and 3–5. The regions supplied by the hemispheric branches and the cortical function of each region are shown.

Lateral Lenticulostriate Arteries

In 20% of cases the lateral lenticulostriate branches arise from one of the hemispheric branches of the middle cerebral artery. In the other cases they arise from the trunk of the middle cerebral artery. They supply the substantia innominata, the lateral part of the anterior commissure, most of the putamen and the lateral segment of the globus pallidus, the superior half of the internal capsule and adjacent corona radiata, and the body and head (except the anterior-inferior portion) of the caudate nucleus. Portions of the optic radiation (which originate from the lateral geniculate body) and the arcuate fasciculus are supplied by the striate branches.[12]

The largest area of the brain normally supplied

Anterior Cerebral Territory in Axial

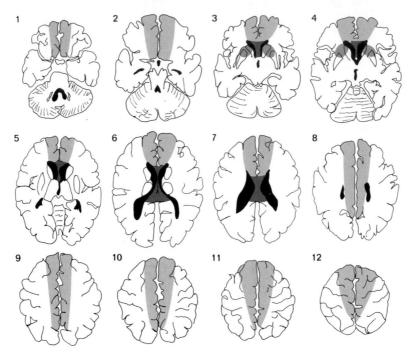

FIG 3–1.
Axial diagrams arranged in sequence from base to vertex. Angle and levels of scan planes are shown in Fig 3–3. Territory of anterior cerebral artery is divided into three regions: medial lenticulo-striate *(medium shading)*, callosal *(dark shading)*, and hemispheric *(light areas)*.

Cortical Branches

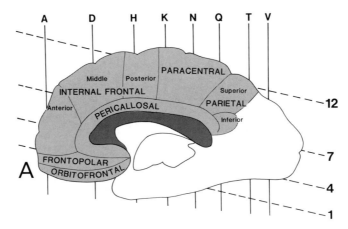

FIG 3–3.
A, regions supplied by nine hemispheric branches of anterior cerebral artery localized on medial view of cerebral hemisphere.

Anterior Cerebral Territory in Coronal

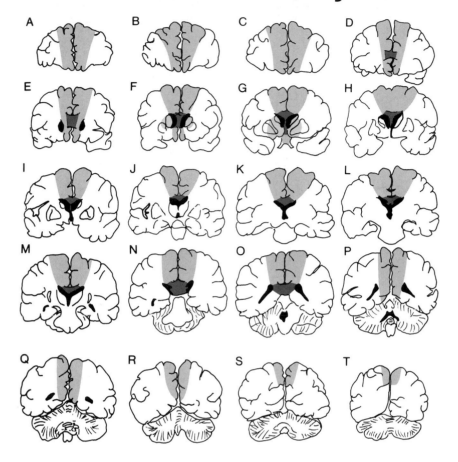

FIG 3–2.
Coronal diagrams arranged in sequence from front to back. Angle and levels of scan planes are shown in Fig 3–3. Territory of anterior cerebral artery is divided into three regions: medial lenticulo-striate *(medium shading),* callosal *(dark shading),* and hemispheric *(light areas).*

Cortical Functions

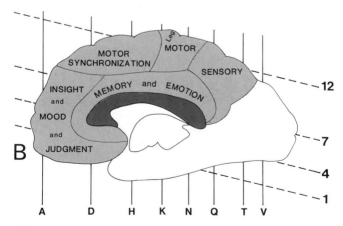

FIG 3–3 (cont.).
B, functional regions supplied by anterior cerebral artery localized on medial view of cerebral hemisphere. See axial and coronal diagrams in Figs 3–1 and 3–2 for correlation.

Middle Cerebral Territory in Axial

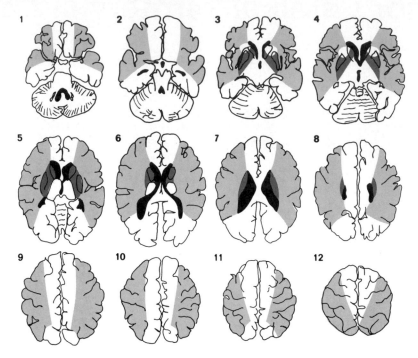

FIG 3–4.
Axial diagrams arranged in sequence from base to vertex. Angle and levels of scan planes are shown in Fig 3–6. Territory of middle cerebral artery is divided into two regions: lateral lenticulostriate *(medium shading)* and hemispheric *(light areas)*.

Cortical Branches

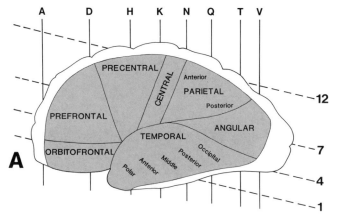

FIG 3–6.
Arterial territories and function correlated. **A,** regions supplied by hemispheric branches of middle cerebral artery on lateral view of left cerebral hemisphere. Axial and coronal scan levels marked in Figs 3–4 and 3–5 are indicated for cross-referencing.

Middle Cerebral Territory in Coronal

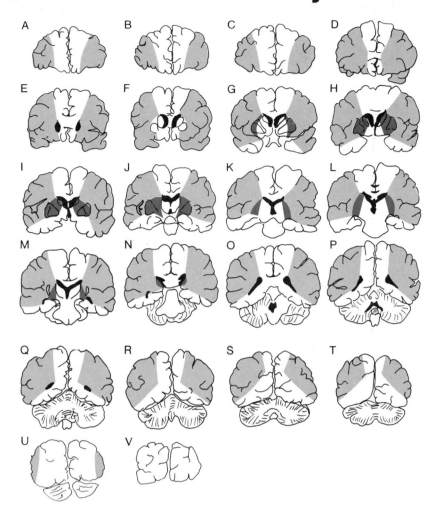

FIG 3–5.
Coronal diagrams arranged in sequence from front to back. Angle and levels of scan planes are illustrated in Fig 3–6. Territories of middle cerebral artery are identified as in Fig 3–4.

Cortical Functions

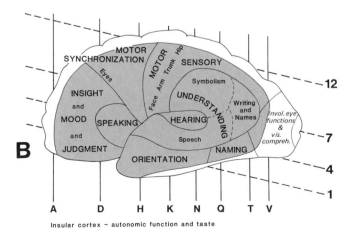

Insular cortex – autonomic function and taste

FIG 3–6 (cont.).
B, functional cortical regions supplied by middle cerebral artery localized on lateral view of left cerebral hemisphere. Areas labeled "speaking" and "understanding" are found only in dominant hemisphere (usually the left). These zones have poorly understood functions in nondominant hemisphere. Axial and coronal scan levels marked in Figs 3–4 and 3–5 are indicated for correlation.

Posterior Cerebral Territory in Axial

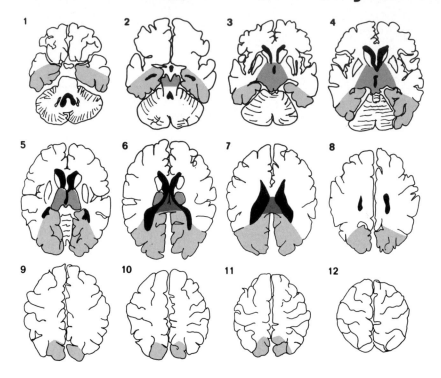

FIG 3–7.

Axial diagrams arranged in sequence from base to vertex. Angle and levels of scan planes are shown in Fig 3–9. Territory of posterior cerebral artery is divided into three regions: thalamic and mid- brain perforators *(medium shading)*, callosal *(dark shading)* and hemispheric *(light areas)*.

Cortical Branches

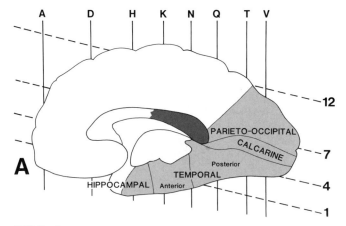

FIG 3–9.

A, regions supplied by the five hemispheric branches of posterior cerebral artery localized on medial view of right cerebral hemi- sphere.

Posterior Cerebral Territory in Coronal

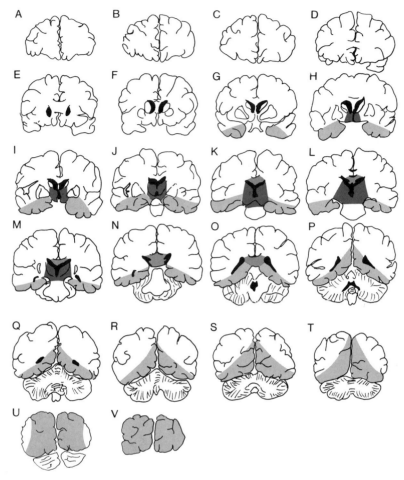

FIG 3–8.
Coronal CT scan diagrams arranged in sequence from front to back. Angle and levels of scan planes are shown in Fig 3–9. Territories of posterior cerebral artery are identified as in Fig 3–7.

Cortical Functions

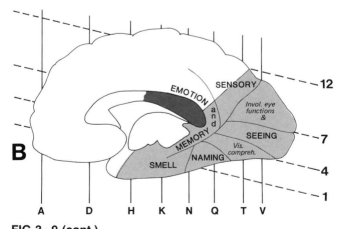

FIG 3–9 (cont.).
B, functional cortical regions supplied by posterior cerebral artery localized on medial view of right cerebral hemisphere. See axial and coronal scan levels in Figs 3–7 and 3–8 for correlation.

by the striate vessels is shown in Figures 3–4 and 3–5. It will be smaller if a large recurrent artery of Heubner, anterior choroidal artery, or both are present since these vessels may nourish the anterior inferomedial part of the striate territory (shown in Fig 3–4 and 3–5).

The striate branches of the middle cerebral artery are "end branches" in that they have few if any major anastomotic connections other than those of the capillary bed. They do not supply the claustrum and extreme capsule, which are nourished by the hemispheric branches that supply the insular cortex.[13]

Vascular lesions in the striate distribution can disturb four functions: (1) movement, (2) tactile sensation, (3) speech, and (4) vision. The deficiency of movement is that of contralateral hemiparesis of the face, arm,* and leg,* which is caused by damage to the motor fibers in the internal capsule. Weakness, slowness and changes in passive tone accompany the hemiparesis because the basal ganglia and extra pyramidal pathways are affected. A true parkinsonian syndrome is not a recognized feature of basal ganglia infarction. However, the slowness, increased tone and spasticity associated with capsular infarction may sometimes be mistaken for early parkinsonism. Indeed, the basal ganglia component of the hemiplegia seen in striate lesions may partly account for the greater degree of spasticity sometimes seen when these lesions are contrasted with hemispheric lesions that produce hemiplegia.[14]

The sensory tracts lie close to the motor tracts in the region of the internal capsule. Hence, both functions are commonly affected in lesions of the striate territory. *Pure* motor strokes (involving face, arm, and leg) sometimes occur with striate lesions.[15, 16] However, this is not diagnostic of a lesion in the striate area. *Pure* motor stroke may be seen with infarctions at (1) the base of the pons (due to occlusion of the paramedian branches of the basilar artery), (2) the medullary pyramids (vertebral branches), or (3) rarely at the cerebral peduncle (basilar or posterior cerebral artery).[15–19] Since the striate branches of the middle cerebral artery may not supply the entire posterior limb of the internal capsule, occlusion of the anterior choroidal artery may be the cause of identical deficits.[15, 17, 20] Occlusion of any of these vessels can cause a very small infarction that may be difficult to detect.

*In this chapter, the terms *arm* and *leg* are used to represent the upper and lower extremity, respectively.

Striate lesions that damage the sensory fibers in the posterior limb of the internal capsule can cause elevation of the threshold for primary modalities of touch, pain, temperature, and vibration in the contralateral face, arm and leg. Lesions in the posterior cerebral territory in subcortical or thalamic nuclei may mimic these findings. Finally, of course infarctions of the other vessesl that supply the posterior internal capsule can mimic striate artery lesions as previously discussed.

Lesions in the lateral striate territory may produce speech and language impairment. Damage to the nearby area of Broca (roughly the posterior portion of the third frontal gyrus) causes Broca's syndrome, which consists of reduced language output, impaired repetition and naming, along with (largely) preserved comprehension.[21, 22] Although Broca's area is supplied by the hemispheric branches (which we will discuss next), lateral striate infarction sometimes causes similar impairments, at least transiently.

Striate lesions may also involve the arcuate fasciculus. This subcortical fiber tract connects the area of the brain labeled "understanding" in Figure 3–6,B (the area of Wernicke) with the area labeled "speaking" (the area of Broca). Damage to this tract causes *conduction aphasia* (an impaired ability to repeat words or phrases).[22, 23]

The visual deficit produced by lesions in the striate territory is that of a contralateral homonymous hemianopsia that may be complete or subtle and difficult to detect clinically.[24, 25] This deficit is caused when there is damage to the optic radiations that traverse the striate territory as they originate from the geniculate body.

Hemispheric Branches

Twelve major cortical branches are illustrated in Figure 3–6,A. In view of the large number of branches, one might expect a great variety of clinical sequelae. The overall picture can be simplified by comparing the vascular territories of Figure 3–6,A with the functional areas of Figure 3–6,B. The areas marked "speaking" and "understanding" are present only in the dominant hemisphere, which is the left hemisphere in almost all right-handed patients and in about half of the left-handed patients. In the nondominant hemisphere these areas have no well-accepted clinically demonstrable function.

When we use the word "speaking" in this context we actually mean the complex language function associated with verbal output including speaking, writing and even sign language. This definition excludes the purely motor aspects of these functions such as movement of facial muscles or hands (which relate to the motor region for face or arm, respectively). Similarly, "understanding" means understanding of language whether written, spoken, sign, or Braille language and is conceptually separate from a loss of the sensory modalities of sight, hearing or touch, which can mediate language. More detail on this complex and fascinating subject can be gleaned from relevant papers and references.[21, 22, 26, 27]

The cortical area marked "hearing" receives impulses from both ears. Therefore, deficits in this area must be bilateral to cause clinical symptoms. The insular cortex is not shown in Figure 3–6,A or B since it lies buried within the sylvian fissure. This infolded cortex is supplied by the major hemispheric branches that course over its surface. Small branches arise from these surface vessels and penetrate the insular cortex, extreme capsule, and claustrum.

Damage to the insular cortex can produce the opercular syndrome of Foix-Chavany-Marie, which is characterized by impairments of speech, articulation (dysarthria) and clarity (dysphonia), swallowing (dysphagia), and chewing (dysmasesia).[28, 29] These problems are due to the interruption of signals to the 5th, 7th, and 9th through 12th cranial nerves. This syndrome is a type of pseudobulbar palsy.[28, 29]

The lateral surface of the frontal lobe mediates judgement, insight, and mood. It receives arterial supply from the orbitofrontal and prefrontal branches of the middle cerebral artery. (The medial surface of the frontal lobe contains the remainder of the judgment, insight and mood areas, which are supplied by the anterior cerebral artery.[12, 20, 24, 25]

The prefrontal and precentral arteries supply that area of the dominant hemisphere that is essential for "speaking" (Fig 3–6,B). Damage here causes Broca's (motor) aphasia, which, as previously noted, causes markedly reduced verbal output (agrammatic and telegraphic) and impaired ability to repeat sentences and phrases or name objects.[22, 23] The patient's ability to understand speech remains largely intact.[22, 23]

A much less common type of aphasia, transcortical motor aphasia, results from lesions rostral or superior to Broca's area.[22, 30] Infarctions of the territories of the orbitofrontal, prefrontal and precen-

tral middle cerebral arterial branches (Fig 3–6,A) or a watershed infarction of the zone between the anterior and middle cerebral arteries may produce this syndrome. The patient suffers an aphasia identical to Broca's except that repetition of sentences and phrases is not impaired.[23, 30]

As shown in Figure 3–6,A, the precentral artery also supplies those parts of the frontal lobe that facilitate "motor synchronization." One area in this region controls coordination of eye and head movement. Damage here deprives the patient of the ability to look in the direction opposite the side of the lesion.[31]

The cortex marked "motor" in Figure 3–6,B is supplied by the central branch of the middle cerebral artery. Damage in this territory causes contralateral weakness of the face, arm, trunk, and hip. The motor cortex of the medial surface of the frontal lobe that controls the leg is supplied by the anterior cerebral artery.[20] The leg, however, may be weakened after occlusion of the central branch of the middle cerebral artery. This occurs if the lesion also damages the motor fiber tracts to the leg as they travel downward beneath the cortical areas (marked "face" and "arm" in Fig 3–6,B). It may also occur when the cortical, middle cerebral lesion causes edema in the medial frontal lobe and this edema compresses the motor fiber tracts of the leg. The leg weakness associated with middle cerebral cortical lesions is usually less severe and more transient than that seen with cortical infarcts of the anterior cerebral artery, which controls motor function of the leg.[14, 24, 25, 31]

The cortex marked "sensory" in Figure 3–6,B is supplied by central and anterior parietal branches.[25] Damage to this region causes loss of high-order sensory functions in the face, arm, trunk, and hip. Occasionally the leg is involved, presumably by the mechanisms described previously. These lesions cause loss of (1) position sense; (2) tactile localization; (3) stereognosis (recognizing the object one is feeling); (4) ascertainment of shape, size, and texture; (5) two-point discrimination; and (6) recognition of letters or numbers written on the skin (graphesthesia).[14, 31, 32] This cortical sensory loss contrasts with the loss of primary sensory perception (pain, temperature, vibration, and touch) that is found with lesions in the lateral striate territory of the middle cerebral artery.

The posterior parietal, angular, occipital, and posterior temporal arteries (shown in Fig 3–6,A) vascularize a part of the cortex that, in the dominant hemisphere, mediates "understanding".[12, 25]

Damage to this region, which is known as Wernicke's area, causes striking neuropsychological symptoms.[14, 22, 25, 31] Involvement of the lower part of the area impairs perception and understanding of speech. Damage to the rest of it impairs written, visual, and auditory language integration.[22, 23] Lesions tend to involve the entire Wernicke area and produce an aphasia in which language comprehension, repetition, and naming are all severely affected, although the spontaneity and fluency of speech remain intact. As a result, the patient with Wernicke's aphasia speaks meaningless gibberish that has normal intonation and fluency, and he cannot understand written or spoken language.[22, 23]

Lesions in part of the dominant hemisphere supplied by the angular artery may produce a neuropsychological deficit known as Gerstsmann's syndrome in which the patient exhibits a variety of problems in understanding. Acalculia (loss of arithmetic ability), alexia (inability to read), finger agnosia (inability to identify one's fingers), and right-left confusion may be present.[33] Aphasia is sometimes also encountered.

Infarction of the parietal lobe occurs when there is occlusion of the central, anterior and/or posterior parietal arteries. In the *nondominant* hemisphere, it produces disturbances in the ability to utilize or synthesize geometric and spatial information (amorphosynthesis).[34] These disturbances can take many forms. Some of them are syndromes of unilateral neglect. For example, the patient may ignore the existence of the half of the world contralateral to the lesion. Only part of such neglect that produces a contralateral hemianopsia may be due to concomitant lesions of the sensory cortex or involvement of the optic radiations.[35] Other neglect syndromes are the denial of illness, hemiplegia, or pain in the contralateral body (anosagnosia). The patient may also have difficulty with clothing himself, which is often worse contralateral to the lesion (dressing apraxia). These syndromes cannot be explained by concomitant paralysis, sensory loss, or dementia. Another difficulty that may be encountered with nondominant parietal lesions is loss of orientation or spatial memory. In these instances, the subject has difficulty finding his way around town, house or room. All of the syndromes described for the nondominant parietal lobe may also be seen with lesions of the dominant parietal lobe, but they are difficult to detect because of concomitant aphasia.[35]

The anterior temporal and temporal polar arteries supply the inferior temporal areas and a portion of the insular cortex. Occlusion of these branches does not produce readily discernible clinical signs and symptoms although autonomic disturbances such as contralateral mydriasis (enlargement of the pupil) and hyperhydrosis (increased perspiration) may be associated with damage in this area.[35]

POSTERIOR CEREBRAL VASCULAR TERRITORY

In Figures 3–7 and 3–8, the branches of the posterior cerebral artery have been divided into three groups: (1) the penetrating arteries to the brain stem, thalamus, and other deep structures; (2) the splenial branch to the corpus callosum; and (3) the branches to the cerebral hemisphere.[36, 37] Figure 3–9 is a companion diagram of the medial aspect of the right cerebral hemisphere. It is provided to localize the axial and coronal images in Figures 3–7 and 3–8. The regions supplied by the hemispheric branches and the cortical function of each region are shown.

Penetrating Branches

Numerous very small branches arise from the proximal part of the posterior cerebral artery as it encircles the midbrain. These have arbitrarily been divided into one group that supplies the thalamus and hypothalamus and another that supplies the midbrain.[38]

Thalamus and Hypothalamus

The approximate origin and termination of the vessels that supply the thalamus are indicated in Figure 3–10,A. Each vessel in the drawing represents numerous very small branches. The pattern of arterial supply to the thalamus is variable. That shown in Figure 3–10,A is the most common and represents 30% of the brains studied.[38] In general, four groups of perforating vessels supply the thalamus: (1) premamillary, (2) thalamoperforating, (3) thalamogeniculate, and (4) posterior choroidal and cingulate.

As illustrated in Figure 3–10,A the *premamillary arterial group* supplies the anterior thalamus (the anterior, medial, ventral anterior, and ventral lateral nuclei). The anterior nucleus connects with the mamillary bodies and the hippocampus and is part of the memory and emotion circuit of Papez.[39, 40] The dorsal medial nucleus connects with the frontal lobe, the amygdala, and possibly

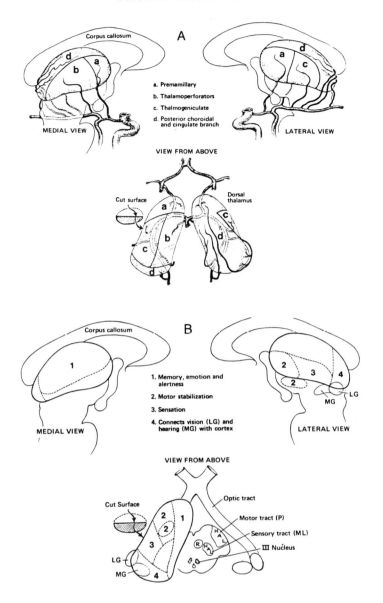

FIG 3–10.
A, schematic view of four vascular territories on thalamus. Each is represented by single arterial branch at approximate origin and termination of numerous small perforating branches: *(a)* premammillary, *(b)* thalamoperforator, *(c)* thalamogeniculate, and *(d)* posterior choroidal and cingulate branches. This pattern represents 30% of brains. Midbrain perforators (the largest of which is the quadrigeminal plate artery) are not illustrated. **B,** four functional relay areas of thalamus: (1) memory and emotion (anterior and dorsal medial nuclei), (2) motor stabilization (ventral anterior, ventral lateral, and subthalamic nuclei), (3) sensation (ventroposteromedial and ventroposterolateral nuclei), and (4) connections of visual (LG = lateral geniculate) and hearing (MG = medial geniculate) areas with the parietal cortex via the pulvinar. Unmarked areas are nonspecific association areas that are poorly understood. Lesions in area *1* result in neuropsychologic symptoms; in area *2* they result in hemiballismus (or curb Parkinson disease contralaterally); in area *3* they result in Dejerine-Roussy syndrome; and in area *4* they cause aphasia, if the left thalamus is affected. Midbrain sectioned at level below inferior colliculi shows major midbrain motor tract (P = pyramidal) and sensory tract (ML = medial lemniscus) divided into areas for head (H), arm (A), and leg (L) fibers. These tracts control side of body opposite lesion. Red nucleus (R) is pathway for fibers from cerebellum to thalamus. Lesions here affect coordination contralaterally.

the hypothalamus. Damage to either of these nuclei can cause profound memory loss and personality change (Fig 3–10,B). Usually the recent memory is most severely affected (Wernicke-Korsakoff syndrome).[41] The specific anatomic pathophysiology underlying these effects is a subject of controversy.[42, 43] The ventral anterior and lateral nuclei influence the motor system, particularly the extrapyramidal and cerebellar systems; their ablation may relieve some symptoms of Parkinson's disease.[44] The lateral nucleus helps coordinate motor and sensory impulses but has no clinically defined function (Fig 3–10,B).

In addition to the thalamus, the premamillary arteries supply the intermediate part of the hypothalamus, an area that forms the central one third of the walls of the third ventricle and the mamillary bodies. There is collateral supply to this area from internal carotid branches.[45] This part of the hypothalamus is the source of somatostatin[46] (which blocks the release of growth hormone and thyroid-stimulating hormone) and thyroid-releasing hormone.[47] Neuropathways carrying vasopressin and oxytocin to the posterior pituitary gland as well as pathways for luteinizing hormone–releasing factor, corticotropic-releasing factor, and prolactin-inhibitory factor travel through this region.[47] Therefore, lesions in this area can cause a complete loss of endocrine function that simulates total section of the pituitary stalk as well as hyperphasia, anorexia, and rage attacks.[46]

The premamillary artery, together with branches from the thalamoperforating arteries, supplies the posterior part of the hypothalamus.[45] Tumors in this area produce precocious puberty,[46] disturbances of temperature regulation,[48] and disturbances of consciousness with somnolence.[46] The anterior hypothalamus is supplied by the anterior cerebral artery. (Consult "Medial Lenticulostriate Arteries," earlier in this section.)

As illustrated in Figure 3–10,A, the *thalamoperforating arterial group* supplies the medial ventral part of the thalamus (centromedian and parafascicular nuclei). This territory mediates many aspects of arousal, attention, and alertness.[39] Thalamoperforating branches derived from one posterior cerebral artery commonly supply all or part of the contralateral territory as well as the ipsilateral territory.[49]

As illustrated in Figure 3–10,A, the *thalamogeniculate group* supplies the lateral ventral part of the thalamus (pulvinar, ventroposterior lateral, and ventroposterior medial nuclei). The pulvinar may coordinate visual and auditory information by receiving input from the lateral and medial geniculate bodies and projecting to the occipital and temporal lobes.[39] Lesions of the left pulvinar area can produce language dysfunction (aphasia or dysphasia).[50] The ventral posterior lateral and ventral posterior medial nuclei relay sensory information from body and face, respectively.[39] Lesions produce an initial insensitivity to pain that evolves over a period of months into spontaneous or inappropriately elicited pain in the affected body part. This has been named anesthesia dolorosa and is found in the Dejerine-Roussy (thalamic) syndrome[51] (see Fig 3–10).

The thalamogeniculate branches also supply the lateral geniculate body, the medial geniculate body, and structures below the anterior and medial part of the thalamus (e.g., the Forel fields in the subthalamic area). Lesions of the lateral geniculate body cause loss of sight in the half of the visual field opposite the lesion.[39] The medial geniculate body is part of the hearing pathway, but unilateral lesions of the medial geniculate body do not cause clinical hearing problems since there is bilateral representation of hearing at this level due to previous decussation. Lesions in the vicinity of the subthalamic area and Forel fields can cause violent flinging movements of the opposite extremities (hemiballismus) as well as uncontrollable jerking and writhing movements (choreoathetosis).[52, 53] However, only hemiballismus has good localizing value and suggests a lesion in the nucleus subthalamicus. Since the subthalamic region receives collateral supply from the anterior choroidal artery, these manifestations are rare in infarction but common in hemorrhage.[53]

As shown in Figure 3–10,A, the *choroidal and cingulate branches* supply the posterior and superior thalamus (anterior, medial, pulvinar, and habenular nuclei). There are extensive anastomoses in these areas, and infarction is rare.[49, 54] Symptoms resulting from lesions in the first three of these thalamic nuclei have been described in the previous discussion. There is no known specific clinical deficit produced by habenular lesions per se. In addition to the thalamus, the posterior choroidal branches supply the pineal gland, choroid plexus, crus, commissure and body of the fornix, part of the anterior columns of the fornix, and part of the lateral geniculate body.[49]

Midbrain

The second group of small penetrating branches supplies the midbrain.[54] They enter the midbrain substance perpendicularly, either directly at their point of origin from the posterior cerebral artery or after accompanying the parent artery around the midbrain for some distance.[54, 55] Others term these "thalamoperforators" and the syndromes produced by their occlusion "thalamoperforate syndromes."[56] Since this group of vessels does not supply the thalamus, it would be better to call them "midbrain perforators" and the associated syndromes "midbrain perforate syndromes."*

Damage to parts of the midbrain can lead to (1) third nerve paralysis, which causes symptoms in both eyes but most marked in the eye on the same side as the lesion; (2) disturbed sensation, strength, and/or coordination on the side opposite the lesion; (3) depression of consciousness; and (4) decerebrate rigidity. A detailed description of these deficits follows. The reader will find it helpful to refer to Figure 3–10,B to localize the third nerve nucleus, red nucleus, and motor and sensory tracts in the midbrain as these structures are discussed.

A total third nerve paralysis results in ptosis, a dilated unreactive pupil, and downward and outward deviation of the eye ipsilaterally. Injury to peripheral third nerve fibers (after they leave the brain stem or as they travel through the cisterns to reach the eye) causes some or all of these symptoms ipsilaterally. Brain stem lesions may cause third nerve symptoms bilaterally since the nuclei are close together. In fact, isolated brain stem lesions involving a single third nerve nucleus are therefore very rare (see Fig 3–10,B). Brain stem lesions may simulate peripheral third nerve lesions by compromising nerve fibers in the brain stem before they exit. Some authors state that third nerve paralysis without pupillary abnormality indicates infarction rather than compression by a mass, but this distinction is unreliable.[58–61]

There are fibers of the third nerve at the collicular level of the midbrain that can be damaged by tumor compression (e.g., pinealoma) so as to produce Parinaud's syndrome.[61, 62] This consists of a loss of upward gaze, impaired pupillary reactivity, and convergence nystagmus, which is not true nystagmus but rather a simultaneous contraction of all the extraocular muscles. Convergence results

because the medial recti muscles are the strongest in the group.[61]

Disturbances of sensation or movement are caused by damage to the major sensory tract (medial lemniscus) or motor tract (pyramidal) (see Figure 3–10,B). Lesions here cause contralateral hemianesthesia and/or hemiparesis and may affect the head, arm, or leg in varying degrees.[63]

Damage to the red nucleus, which coordinates cerebellar-thalamic fiber tracts (see Fig 3–10,B), results in impaired coordination and control of movement contralaterally.[64] There is tremor during movement (perpendicular to the direction of motion) that worsens as the target is approached. One also finds dysmetria, difficulty with rapidly alternating movements, and inability to check or stop a previously initiated movement.[62, 65, 66] Another related type of tremor, rubral tremor, may also be seen. This tremor is present at rest (although it increases during movement) and involves the limb more proximately than does the usual cerebellar tremor. A third type of tremor, seen only at rest, that is similar to that of Parkinson's disease may also be encountered.[62, 65, 66] In addition to the tremor, there may be contralateral hemiballismus and choreoathetosis (as described previously) if there is associated damage of the adjacent substantia nigra and/or subthalamic region.[56, 64, 65, 67]

Depression of consciousness is presumably caused by damage to the central or paramedian reticular midbrain activating system. It can also be caused by destruction or depression of the reticular system in the pons or medulla or by bilateral hemispheric dysfunction. Thus impairment of consciousness by itself is of little localizing value.[62]

Decerebrate rigidity can be produced in animals by lesions in the regulating structures between the quadrigeminal plate and the lateral vestibular nucleus in the pons.[62, 68] The subject assumes a position in which the legs are rigidly extended and the arms are extended, abducted, and hyperpronated.[60] This posture is not as reliable a localizing indicator in humans as it is in other animals.[58]

Callosal Branches

The callosal arteries are a plexus of small vessels that arise from the parieto-occipital or lateral choroidal branches and penetrate the upper surface of the posterior half of the corpus callosum. The plexus may be replaced by a single branch.[49]

---

*The midbrain contains many vital pathways and nuclei. Lesions here have a variety of clinical manifestations. Many midbrain syndromes have eponyms (e.g., Claude's, Nothnagel's, Weber's, and Benedikt's syndromes among others), but we feel that it is simpler and more fruitful to emphasize the functional anatomy. Familiarity with *combinations* of the deficits described in this chapter is the key to localizing lesions to the midbrain. Any isolated deficit can always be caused by a lesion outside of the midbrain, but if you look for the combinations of deficits we describe, you can frequently make an accurate localization of a lesion to the midbrain and/or find satisfying correlations between the CT anatomy and the clinical presentation. This is usually better than trying to fit the signs and symptoms to the eponymic syndromes (which are specific examples of combinations of deficits and which are worthy of attention after you are familiar with the basic functional anatomy).[54, 56, 57]

Infarction can result in separation of the language-dominant left hemisphere from the right hemisphere which mediates function of the left side of the body. If the patient's left occipital lobe and splenium are infarcted, he can speak, write, and understand speech, but he becomes unable to read with his remaining left visual field despite the fact that he can see the letters. (He cannot transfer the visual images received by the right occipital lobe for interpretation in the left hemisphere.) This is called alexia without agraphia. It is rare and may be partial.[69]

Hemispheric Branches

The posterior cerebral artery has five cortical branches. The patterns of infarction can be simplified by comparing the vascular territories (Fig 3–9,A) with corresponding functional areas (Fig 3–9,B). Infarction of cortical branches of the posterior cerebral artery is responsible for several interesting clinical syndromes. The calcarine artery (sometimes together with the parieto-occipital artery) supplies the calcarine cortex ipsilaterally. Infarction thereof causes homonymous hemianopsia of the contralateral visual fields. It is commonly stated that with lesions of the calcarine cortex, the central macular part of the visual field is spared due to collateral circulation.[70] A recent study reported macular sparing in 5 out of 25 cases of cortical blindness.[71]

Infarction of the calcarine cortex bilaterally may result in complete blindness. However, there is sometimes also an unusual constellation of symptoms known as Anton's syndrome in which the patient, although blind, is unaware of the blindness and denies it.[72] Sometimes he will construct elaborate descriptions of his surroundings. If allowed, he may walk into walls or trip over objects.

Apraxia of ocular movements (inability to shift the direction of gaze on command) may also be encountered. This may be accompanied by optic ataxia (poor control of movements, e.g., hand movements, performed under visual guidance) and decreased attention to the visual periphery. This combination of optic apraxia, optic ataxia, and peripheral visual inattention is called Balint's syndrome.[73] Many cases are actually due to bilateral tumors rather than vascular lesions.[73] It is in bilateral occipital infarction that macular sparing is most commonly reported. Macular sparing in these instances may actually represent partial recovery

from total blindness.[69] Damage to the calcarine cortex can also produce unformed visual hallucinations, metamorphopsia (distortion of shape), teleopsia (an illusion in which near objects appear to be at a great distance), distortion of visual outlines, and other aberrations of visual perception.[72]

Damage to the nondominant calcarine cortex as well as damage to the nondominant lingual gyrus, which are supplied by the calcarine and temporal branches (Fig 3–9,A), may produce topographic disorientation and prosopagnosia. Prosopagnosia is the inability to recognize familiar faces even though they can be clearly seen.[72]

Damage to the cortex above and below the calcarine fissure, particularly in the dominant hemisphere, destroys the visual association areas that control involuntary eye function and visual comprehension. These areas are supplied by the parieto-occipital and posterior temporal branches of the posterior cerebral artery. Patients with lesions in these areas may continue for several seconds to see the image of an object that is quickly removed from view. They may also not perceive an object in the damaged visual field if another identical object is simultaneously presented in the normal visual field. This phenomenon is called extinction.[72]

The anterior temporal branch supplies only the inferior aspect of the anterior temporal lobe; the tip of the temporal lobe is supplied by the middle cerebral artery. The cortex in this area is involved in naming objects.

The hippocampal branches of the posterior cerebral artery supply the hippocampal formation including its projections, the fornices, and the psalterium (see Fig 3–9,B). The most commonly observed clinical finding in patients with bilateral hippocampal infarcts is memory deficit. This may also be seen in unilateral deficits on the dominant side. Lesions in this area may also impair the sense of smell.[72] CT studies have suggested that damage to the anterior temporal lobe may cause both taste and smell dysfunctions.[74]

REFERENCES

1. Matsui T, Hirano A: *An Atlas of the Human Brain for Computerized Tomography.* Tokyo, Igaku-Shoin Medical Publishers, Inc, 1978, pp 314–547.
2. Critchley M: Anterior cerebral artery and its syndromes. *Brain* 1930; 53:120–165.
3. Denny-Brown D: The nature of apraxia. *J Nerv Ment Dis* 1958; 126:9–32.
4. Plum F, Posner JB, *The Diagnosis of Stupor and*

Coma, ed 2. Philadelphia, FA Davis Co, Publishers, 1972, pp 5–23.

5. Fisher CM: Clinical syndromes in cerebral arterial occlusion, in Fields WS (ed): *Pathogenesis and Treatment of Cerebrovascular Disease.* Springfield, Ill, Charles C Thomas, Publishers, 1961, pp 151–181.

6. Geschwind N, Kaplan E: A human cerebral disconnection syndrome: A preliminary report. *Neurology* 1962; 12:675–685.

7. Strub RL, Black FW: *The Mental Status Examination in Neurology.* Philadelphia, FA Davis Co, Publishers, 1977, pp 119–125.

8. Chusid JG: *Correlative Neuroanatomy and Functional Neurology,* ed 16. Los Altos, Calif, Lange Medical Publications, 1976, pp 1–13.

9. Cogan DG: *Neurology of the Ocular Muscles,* ed 2. Springfield, Ill, Charles C Thomas, Publishers, 1956, pp 92–96.

10. Critchley M: *The Parietal Lobes.* London, Edward Arnold Publishers, Ltd, 1953, pp 86–155.

11. Berman SA, Hayman LA, Hinck VC: Correlation of CT cerebral vascular territories with function: III. Middle cerebral artery. *AJR* 1984; 142:1035–1040.

12. Stephens RB, Stillwell DL: *Arteries and Veins of the Human Brain.* Springfield, Ill, Charles C Thomas, Publishers, 1969, pp 33–70.

13. Gibo H, Carver CC, Rhoton AL, et al: Microsurgical anatomy of the middle cerebral artery. *J Neurosurg* 1981; 54:151–169.

14. Vick N: *Grinker's Neurology,* ed 7. Springfield, Ill, Charles C Thomas, Publishers, 1976, pp 482–486.

15. Fisher CM: Capsular infarcts, the underlying vascular lesions. *Arch Neurol* 1979; 36:65–73.

16. Fisher CM, Curry HB: Pure motor hemiplegia of vascular origin. *Arch Neurol* 1965; 13:130–140.

17. Mohr JP: Lacunes. *Stroke* 1982; 13:3–11.

18. Ho K: Pure motor hemiplegia due to infarction of the cerebral peduncle. *Arch Neurol* 1982; 39:524–526.

19. Fisher CM: Lacunar strokes and infarcts: A review. *Neurology* 1982; 32:871–876.

20. Berman SA, Hayman LA, Hinck VC: Correlation of cerebral vascular territories with cerebral function by computed tomography. I. Anterior cerebral artery. *AJNR* 1980; 1:259–263; *AJR* 1980; 135:352–357.

21. Naeser MA, Hayward RW: Lesion localization in aphasia with cranial computed tomography and the Boston diagnostic aphasia exam. *Neurology* 1978; 28:545–555.

22. Benson DF, Geschwind N: The aphasias and related disturbances, in Baker AB, Baker LH (eds): *Clinical Neurology,* vol 1. Hagerstown, Md, Harper & Row, Publishers, Inc, 1971.

23. Goldstein K: *Language and Language Disturbances.* New York, Grune & Stratton, 1948.

24. Foix C, Levy M: Les ramollissement Sylviens, syn-

dromes des lesions en foyer du territories de l'artere Sylviens en de ses branches. *Rev Neurol (Paris)* 1927; 48:1–51.

25. Waddington MM, Ring BA: Syndromes of occlusion of middle cerebral artery branches. Angiographic and clinical correlation. *Brain* 1968; 91:685–696.

26. Geschwind N: Current concepts in aphasia. *N Engl J Med* 1971; 284:654.

27. Benson SF: *Aphasia, Alexia, and Agraphia.* New York, Churchill Livingstone, Inc, 1979.

28. Foix C, Chavany A, Marie P: Deplegie facio-linguo-masticatrice cortico-sous-corticale sans paralysie des membres. *Rev Neurol (Paris)* 1926; 33:214–219.

29. bruyn GW, Gathier JC: The operculum syndrome, in Vinken PJ, Bruyn GW (eds): *Handbook for Clinical Neurology,* vol 2. Amsterdam, Elsevier Science Publishers, 1969, pp 776–783.

30. Rubens AB: Transcortical motor aphasia, in Whitaker H, Whitaker HA (eds): *Studies in Neurolinguistics,* vol 1. New York, Academic Press, Inc, 1976, pp 293–306.

31. Adams RD, Victor M: *Principles of Neurology,* ed 2. New York, McGraw-Hill International Book Co, 1981, pp 534–538.

32. Dejerine J, Mouzon J: Un nouveau type de syndrome sensit corticale observe dans un cas de monoplegie corticale dissocies. *Rev Neurol (Paris)* 1914; 28:1265–1273.

33. Gerstmann J: Zur Symptomatologie der Himlaswness im Ubergangpgebiet der unteren Parietal und mittleren Occipitalunlung. *Nervenarzt* 1930; 3:691–695.

34. Denny-Brown D, Banker B: Amorphosynthesis from left parietal lesions. *Arch Neurol Psychiatry* 1954; 1:302–312.

35. Critchley M: *The Parietal Lobes.* London, Edward Arnold Publishers, Ltd, 1953.

36. Hayman LA, Berman SA, Hinck VC: Correlation of CT cerebral vascular territories with function: II. Posterior cerebral artery. *AJR* 1981; 137:13–19.

37. Matsui T, Hirano A: *An Atlas of the Human Brain for Computerized Tomography.* Tokyo, Igaku-Shoin, Medical Publishers, Inc, 1978; pp 400–451.

38. Schlesinger B: *The Upper Brainstem in the Human.* Berlin, Springer Publishing Co, 1976; pp 240–261.

39. Ingram WR: *A Review of Anatomical Neurology.* Baltimore, University Park Press, 1976; pp 309–344, 366.

40. Papez JW: A proposed mechanism of emotion. *Arch Neurol* 1937; 38:725–743.

41. Victor M: The amnestic syndrome and its anatomical basis. *Can Med Assoc J* 1969; 100:1115–1125.

42. Horel JA: The neuroanatomy of amnesia: A critique of the hippocampal memory hypothesis. *Brain* 1978; 101:403–445.

43. Scoville WB, Milner B: Loss of recent memory after bilateral hippocampal lesions. *J Neurol Neurosurg Psychiatry* 1957; 20:11–21.

44. Cooper IS: An investigation of neurosurgical allevi- ation of Parkinsonism, chorea, athetosis and dysto- nia. *Ann Intern Med* 1956; 45:381–392.

45. Haymaker W: Blood supplies of the human hypo- thalamus, in Haymaker W, Anderson E, Nauta WJH (eds): *The Hypothalamus.* Springfield, Ill, Charles C Thomas, Publishers, 1969, pp 210–212.

46. Zimmerman EA: Neuroendocrine disorder, in Rosenberg RN (ed): *Neurology.* New York, Grune & Stratton, 1980, pp 246–250.

47. Rudelli R, Deck JHN: Selective traumatic infarction of the human anterior hypothalamus. *J Neurosurg* 1979; 50:645–654.

48. Pelletier G, Leclerc R, Dube D: Morphologic basis of neuroendocrine function in the hypothalamus, in Tolis G, Labrie F, Martin J, et al (eds): *Clinical Neuroendocrinology: A Pathophysiological Ap- proach.* New York, Raven Press, 1979, pp 15–27.

49. Percheron G: The anatomy of the arterial supply of the human thalamus and its use for the interpreta- tion of the thalamic vascular pathology. *J Neurol* 1973; 205:1–13.

50. Brown JW: Language, cognition and the thalamus. *Appl Neurophysiol* 1974; 36:33–60.

51. Scherbel ME, Scherbel A: The basis of thalamic pain: A structurofunctional hypothesis. *Trans Am Neurol Assoc* 1969; 94:149–152.

52. Carpenter MB: *Human Neuroanatomy.* Baltimore, Williams & Wilkins, 1976, pp 515–517.

53. Whittier JR: Ballism and the subthalamic nucleus (nucleus hypothalamicus; corpus Luysi). *Arch Neu- rol* 1947; 58:672–692.

54. Zeal AA, Rhoton AL: Microsurgical anatomy of the posterior cerebral artery. *J Neurosurg* 1978; 48:534– 559.

55. Stephens RB, Stillwell DL: *Arteries and Veins of the Human Brain.* Springfield, Ill, Charles C Tho- mas, Publishers, 1969, pp 48–49, 60–65.

56. Merritt HH: *A Textbook of Neurology.* Philadel- phia, Lea & Febiger, 1967, pp 196–197, 200.

57. Walton JN: *Brain's Diseases of the Nervous System.* New York, Oxford University Press, 1977, p 335.

58. Plum F, Posner JB: *The Diagnosis of Stupor and Coma.* Philadelphia, FA Davis Co, Publishers, 1980, pp 67–69.

59. Sears ES, Franklin G: Diseases of the cranial nerves, in Rosenberg RN (ed): *Neurology.* New York, Grune & Stratton, 1980, pp 471–494.

60. Warwick R: Representation of the extra-ocular mus- cles in the oculomotor nuclei of the monkey. *J Comp Neurol* 1953; 98:449–495.

61. Gay AJ, Newman NM, Keltner JL, et al: *Eye Move- ment Disorders.* St Louis, CV Mosby Co, 1974, pp 139–140.

62. Fog M, Hein-Sorensen O: Mesencephalic syn- dromes, in Vinken PJ, Bruyn GW (eds): *Handbook of Clinical Neurology, vol 2, Localization in Clini- cal Neurology.* Amsterdam, Elsevier Science Pub- lishers, 1969, pp 272–285.

63. Walton C: *Basic Human Neuroanatomy.* Boston, Little Brown & Co, Inc, 1977, pp 25–26.

64. Aronson AE, Bastron JA, Brown JR, et al: *Mayo Clinic, Clinical Examinations in Neurology.* Phila- delphia, WB Saunders Co, 1971, pp 84–91.

65. Foix C, Masson A: Le syndrome de l'artere cere- brale posteriere. *Presse Med* 1923; 32:361–365.

66. Holmes G: The cerebellum of man. *Brain* 1939; 62:1–30.

67. De Jong R: *The Neurologic Examination.* Hager- stown, Md, Harper & Row, Publishers, Inc, 1979, pp 160.

68. Daube JR, Sandok BA: *Medical Neurosciences.* Bos- ton, Little Brown & Co, Inc, 1978, p 176.

69. Benson DF, Geschwind N: The alexias, in Vinken PJ, Bruyn GW (eds): *Handbook of Clinical Neurol- ogy,* vol 4. Amsterdam, Elsevier Science Publishers, 1969, pp 112–140.

70. Ross Russell RW: The posterior cerebral circula- tion. *J R Coll Physicians Lond* 1973; 7:331–346.

71. Aldrich MS, Alessi AG, Beck RW, et al: Cortical blindness: Etiology, diagnosis, and prognosis. *Ann Neurol* 1987; 21:149–158.

72. Walsh KW: Neuropsychology: A clinical approach. Edinburgh, Churchill Livingston, Inc, 1978, pp 229–245.

73. Hecaen H, DeAjuriaguerra J: Balint's syndrome (psychic paralysis of visual fixation and its minor forms). *Brain* 1984; 77:373–400.

74. Schellinger D, Henkin RT, Smirniotopoulos JG: CT of the brain in taste and smell dysfunctions. *AJNR* 1983; 4:752–754.

PART III

Physiology

4

Water-Soluble Iodinated Contrast Media for Imaging the Brain and Spinal Cord

L. Anne Hayman, M.D.

Vincent C. Hinck, M.D.

TYPES OF WATER-SOLUBLE CONTRAST MEDIA

Water-soluble iodinated contrast medium was first used in humans in 1927 by Egas Moniz. In his initial experiments, he injected a 70% solution of strontium bromide percutaneously into the carotid arteries of six patients, but obtained no suitable radiographs. However, the second patient in the series experienced severe pain during the injection; the fourth patient suffered a severe reaction and fever; and the sixth patient died 8 hours after the injection from a cerebral thrombosis.

Given these results, if Moniz were a modern-day radiologist, it is highly unlikely that he would have been permitted to continue his research and ultimately test the 25% solution of sodium iodide that enabled demonstration of the internal carotid artery and its branches. Because sodium iodide caused pain on injection, a colloidal preparation of thorium dioxide was introduced for carotid angiography. This radioactive agent, retained by the liver and at sites of extravasation that occurred during injection, induced fibrosis and neoplasia over time and was abandoned.[1]

Ionic Monomers

Thorium dioxide was supplanted by iodinated water-soluble compounds, which were originally introduced in 1928 for *intravenous* administration to visualize the urinary collecting system. None of these compounds (iodopyracet, sodium methiodal, and sodium iodomethamate) are in use today because of their toxic side effects. They were replaced in the early 1950s by ionic triiodo compounds, which are better tolerated and are commonly used today. Figure 4–1 shows the three variations of the triiodo structure of these ionic monomeric contrast agents. All of these agents are sodium or meglumine salts of a substituted monomeric triiodobenzoic acid and completely dissociate into ions in solution. There is evidence to suggest that varying the side chains that are attached to each molecule may significantly affect the behavior of these compounds in the clinical setting.[1] The compounds added to stabilize the solution also influence the reactions that will be manifested in clinical use. These media are referred to as *ionic* contrast media. They are toxic as a consequence of their electrical charge and this is certainly important where myelographic neurotoxicity is concerned. On the other hand, its importance in terms of general systemic toxicity is probably exaggerated.[2] They have a relatively high osmolarity, because each molecule of the salt has one cation (sodium or meglumine) and one anion (the iodinated benzoate radical) in solution. Only the anion has clinical relevance. The osmotic effect of the cation is undesirable.[3]

Nonionic Monomers

In 1969, Almen[4] proposed several chemical formulations that would produce fewer or no ions

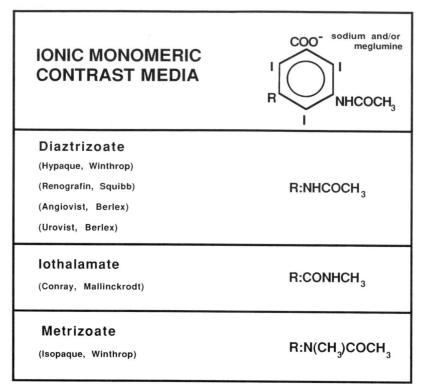

FIG 4-1.
Three ionic monomeric contrast media. All share the structure pictured in the category heading. They differ in the composition of the R chain that is pictured with each contrast medium. Diatrizoate, iothalamate, and metrizoate are available on the US market.

when in solution. Some of these compounds form the group of *nonionic* water-soluble contrast media. Note that the iodinated benzoic acid seen in Figure 4-2 has been converted into a molecule that will not dissociate in solution. The first of these agents, metrizamide, was introduced into the United States in 1978. They are traditionally described as "low-osmolality" media but, at high iodine concentrations, they have osmolalities two to three times that of plasma. Nonetheless, they are an improvement over their antecedent ionic monomers which are toxic because their osmolality may reach 7.5 times that of plasma.[2] Metrizamide may be removed from the US market since many of the agents listed in Figure 4-2 have now become available for myelography and angiography.

Ionic Dimers

Another way in which the osmolality of the contrast agent has been reduced is by connecting the two triiodobenzoic acid molecules (Fig 4-3). These agents were also referred to as low-osmolality media but, like the nonionic monomers, their osmolal-

ity at high iodine concentrations is two to three times greater than that of plasma. For this reason, they also are somewhat toxic.[2]

The meglumine salt of iothalamic acid (Dimeray) was introduced for use in myelography before metrizamide became available. It was withdrawn from the market after a short time because a number of serious neurotoxic reactions occurred. Dimeray was the first *ionic dimer* used in the United States. It had a lower osmolarity than conventional ionic agents, because it dissociated into three particles (one large iodinated dimeric anion and two cations) rather than the four particles (two anions and two cations) which would have resulted if a solution containing six iodine atoms were prepared using the ionic formula demonstrated in Figure 4-1.

Another contrast medium that is an ionic dimer is ioxaglate. It has been introduced to the US market by Mallinckrodt for use as an angiographic agent. The reduced osmolality of this medium appears to moderate the burning sensation that accompanies intracarotid injection of ionic contrast media. It does not reduce the retinal irritation produced by contrast injection.

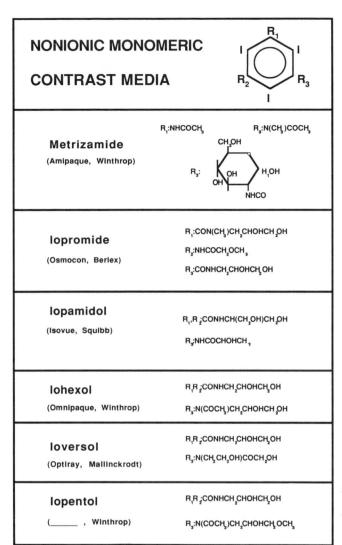

NONIONIC MONOMERIC CONTRAST MEDIA

Metrizamide (Amipaque, Winthrop)	R_1:NHCOCH$_3$ R_3:N(CH$_3$)COCH$_3$
Iopromide (Osmocon, Berlex)	R_1:CON(CH$_3$)CH$_2$CHOHCH$_2$OH R_2:NHCOCH$_2$OCH$_3$ R_3:CONHCH$_2$CHOHCH$_2$OH
Iopamidol (Isovue, Squibb)	R_1,R_2:CONHCH(CH$_2$OH)CH$_2$OH R_2:NHCOCHOHCH$_3$
Iohexol (Omnipaque, Winthrop)	R_1R$_2$:CONHCH$_2$CHOHCH$_2$OH R_3:N(COCH$_3$)CH$_2$CHOHCH$_2$OH
Ioversol (Optiray, Mallinckrodt)	R_1R$_2$:CONHCH$_2$CHOHCH$_2$OH R_3:N(CH$_2$CH$_2$OH)COCH$_2$OH
Iopentol (_____ , Winthrop)	R_1R$_2$:CONHCH$_2$CHOHCH$_2$OH R_3:N(COCH$_3$)CH$_2$CHOHCH$_2$OCH$_3$

FIG 4–2.
Six nonionic monomeric contrast media. All share the structure pictured in the category heading. They differ in composition of the three R chains that are pictured with each of the contrast media. Metrizamide, iopamidol, and iohexol are currently available on the US market.

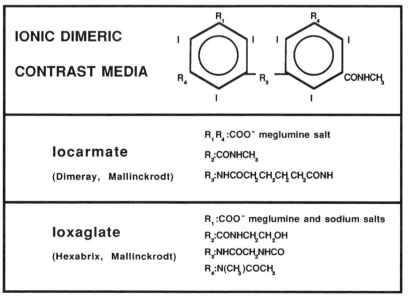

IONIC DIMERIC CONTRAST MEDIA

Iocarmate (Dimeray, Mallinckrodt)	R_1R$_4$:COO$^-$ meglumine salt R_2:CONHCH$_3$ R_3:NHCOCH$_2$CH$_2$CH$_2$CH$_2$CONH
Ioxaglate (Hexabrix, Mallinckrodt)	R_1:COO$^-$ meglumine and sodium salts R_2:CONHCH$_2$CH$_2$OH R_3:NHCOCH$_2$NHCO R_4:N(CH$_3$)COCH$_3$

FIG 4–3.
Two ionic dimeric contrast media. Both share the structure pictured in the category heading. They differ in composition of the three R chains that are pictured with each of them. Iocarmate was removed from the US market, and ioxaglate has been introduced to the US market.

Nonionic Dimers

Here we encounter a group of chemicals devoid of electrical charge and, accordingly, devoid of charge-related toxicity. If necessary, these chemicals can also be made iso-osmolar with plasma at all iodine concentrations by addition of saline, thereby eliminating osmolality-induced toxicity as well.[2]

Figure 4–4 displays structures of three nonionic dimers: iotrol, iodixanol, and iotrolan. These compounds may find important application in myelography where their large molecular size and higher viscosity offer advantages. Their lower osmolality may also enable improvement of image quality in intravenous (IV) digital subtraction angiography by permitting delivery of a more concentrated contrast bolus.[2] These agents have the basic structure of ionic dimers but they eliminate the cations by substituting two radicals.

Summary

All of these new dimers and the nonionic agents have succeeded in reducing the number of particles in solution from that originally encountered in solutions of the traditional monoacid ionic agents (see Fig 4–1) that contain the same amount of iodine. In reality, some of the new agents have an osmolality that is reduced to one third of that found in the ionic agents, although theoretically their structure should have reduced the osmolality less dramatically (Fig 4–5). This "exaggerated" effect can be ascribed to the fact that these molecules not only have fewer particles in solution but also aggregate in solution, thereby further diminishing the particle count and further reducing osmolality.[3]

With the development of these new compounds, the radiologist will be confronted with the need to select the safest and least costly contrast

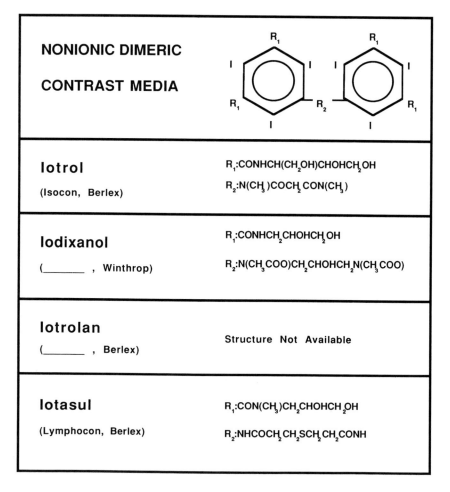

NONIONIC DIMERIC CONTRAST MEDIA	
Iotrol (Isocon, Berlex)	R_1:CONHCH(CH$_2$OH)CHOHCH$_2$OH R_2:N(CH$_3$)COCH$_2$CON(CH$_3$)
Iodixanol (_____ , Winthrop)	R_1:CONHCH$_2$CHOHCH$_2$OH R_2:N(CH$_3$COO)CH$_2$CHOHCH$_2$N(CH$_3$COO)
Iotrolan (_____ , Berlex)	**Structure Not Available**
Iotasul (Lymphocon, Berlex)	R_1:CON(CH$_3$)CH$_2$CHOHCH$_2$OH R_2:NHCOCH$_2$CH$_2$SCH$_2$CH$_2$CONH

FIG 4–4.

Four nonionic dimeric contrast media which share the structure pictured in the category heading. They differ in composition of the two R chains that are pictured with each of them. Iotrol, iodixanol, and iotrolan are under development as myelographic contrast media, whereas iotasul may be suitable for lymphography.

Physical Characteristics of
Iodinated Contrast Media

Generic Name	Trade Name	Mol. Wt.	mg/ml	mOsmol/kg	Refs.
Metrizamide	Amipaque	789	170	300	6,13,14,
Iopromide	Osmocon	791	300	600	*
Iopamidol	Isovue	777	200	413	7,15
Iohexol	Omnipaque	821	300	700	12
Ioversol	Optiray				*
Iopentol		836	226		*
Diatrizoate	Hypaque	614	292	1520	11,13
	Renografin		400	1909	
	Angiovist				
	Urovist				
Iothalamate	Conray	614	280	1500	5,13
Metrizoate	Isopaque	628	280	1460	13
Iotrolan	Isocon	1626	300	300	17
Iodixanol		1500	82		*
Iotasul	Lymphocon	1606	300		16
Iocarmate	Dimeray	1254	280	1040	5
Ioxaglate	Hexabrix	1269	280 320	490 600	8,9,10

FIG 4–5.
The physical characteristics of water-soluble iodinated contrast media. Each reference pertains to the specific contrast medium for which it is listed. * = information obtained from confidential company sources.

medium for a given procedure, to evaluate image quality with each agent, and possibly to encounter a new spectrum of complications. Preliminary uses for the new contrast media discussed can be found in Figure 4–6.

Experience teaches that the side effects caused by a given water-soluble contrast agent will vary according to route of administration (i.e., intrathecal, intralymphatic, or intravascular) and, of course, that the information gleaned from each approach is quite different from that developed by the others. Accordingly, discussion of the physiology and the practical clinical implications of the contrast agents will be divided into three sections discussing the available media for intrathecal, intravascular, and intralymphatic applications respectively.

PHYSIOLOGY OF WATER-SOLUBLE CONTRAST MEDIA INTRODUCED TO THE SUBARACHNOID SPACE

Normal Nervous System

Water-soluble contrast media are now introduced routinely to the subarachnoid space to define contours of the spinal cord, nerve root sheaths, and the cisterns surrounding the brain. Ionic contrast media were the first water-soluble agents to be used clinically for this purpose. They were introduced in Europe but were limited to studies of the lumbar canal because, above this level, they caused many side effects.[18] For this reason, they were never used in the United States. The incidence of side effects was reduced with the intro-

	Myelography	Angiography	Intravenous	Lymphography
Metrizamide (Amipaque)	*			
Iopromide (Osmocon)		√	√	
Iopamidol (Isovue)	√	√	√	
Iohexol (Omnipaque)	√	√	√	
Ioversol (Optiray)		√	√	
Iopentol	√	√	√	
Diatrizoate (Hypaque)		√	√	
Iothalamate (Conray)		√	√	
Metrizoate (Isopaque)			√	
Iotrol (Isocon)	√		√	
Iodixanol	√	√	√	
Iotrolan		√	√	
Iotasul (Lymphocon)				√
Iocarmate (Dimeray)	**			
Ioxaglate (Hexabrix)		√	√	

FIG 4–6.
Neuroradiologic uses for water-soluble iodinated contrast media in the United States. * = limited use may cause this compound to be removed from the US market; ** = has been removed from US market.

duction of an ionic dimer (Dimeray), which, though it contained the same amount of iodine, had a lower osmolality than the ionic media (see Fig 4–5). As we have already noted, Dimeray was withdrawn from the US market and metrizamide (Amipaque), a nonionic monomer, became the water-soluble agent of choice for examination of the subarachnoid space and the cerebral intraventricular compartments.

Neurotoxicity of Metrizamide

Metrizamide produces neurotoxic side effects (seizures, changes in mood or perception, nausea, and vomiting) that are dose-related[19] and that occur 4 to 10 hours after injection into the lumbar subarachnoid space. They appear to be related to entry of contrast agent into the brain substance (documented as computed tomographic [CT] contrast enhancement of the cortical surfaces after intrathecal administration). However, because patients who are clinically asymptomatic after intrathecal contrast injection have been noted on CT to display brain and spinal cord "blush" (i.e.,

central nervous system [CNS] contrast entry), other factors than just tissue penetration must be involved in the production of these toxic side effects, which appear to be more frequent in elderly patients and rarely occur in children.[20, 21] Caille and co-workers[22] have suggested that the amount of medium in the cisterns which is available to diffuse into the tissue is an important factor influencing toxicity seen after intrathecal injection.

Canine experiments have shown that the concentration of radiolabeled metrizamide in the brain correlates with the neurotoxic symptoms that can be observed clinically. Research has shown that puppies receiving the same dose of metrizamide as adult dogs will have a brain metrizamide concentration that is 2,500 times lower than that of the adult. This may explain why fewer neurotoxic side effects from metrizamide are noted in infants and children when compared with those in adult patients.[23] This reduced brain concentration of metrizamide appears to be due to two factors. First, the current clinical guideline for the maximum dose in infants and children is approximately twice that of the adult dose on the basis of body weight (kg). However, this increase does not fully correct for the greatly increased proportion of body weight contributed by the brain in children. When the recommended maximum dosages are recorrected on a *brain* weight basis, the maximum clinical dose recommended for children is less than 50% of the maximum adult dose. This failure to correct for brain weight differences is partially responsible for the reduced brain concentrations, but it does not fully account for the 2,500-fold decrease in brain metrizamide concentration. Physiologic differences are undoubtedly at work.

There may be a greater cerebrospinal fluid (CSF) clearance of metrizamide in the puppy as compared with the adult dog. This would prevent prolonged contact of the metrizamide with the puppy brain. One might also postulate differences in the brain itself that enable greater metrizamide penetration in the adult dog brain. Further studies are needed to determine precisely why these age-related differences exist.

While metrizamide penetration of the brain is well documented, the precise tissue compartment which it enters is unknown. In rabbits, IV perfusion studies (using ^{125}I-labeled metrizamide) were undertaken to determine its distribution but it was not possible to distinguish between the interstitial and intracellular components.[24] The presence of metrizamide in the extracellular fluid is *assumed*, because other compounds of similar molecular weight and size have been shown to enter the brain from the CSF by diffusing from the region of high CSF concentration at the brain surface to the lower concentration in the interstitial spaces. That the diffusion of metrizamide from the cisterns into the brain is altered by the composition of the brain surface has been demonstrated by CT scans. In surface areas composed of white matter (i.e., spinal cord, brain stem, corpus callosum, and nerve roots), the penetration of the medium is diffuse. These areas never achieve the high concentrations found in gray matter zones that are in direct contact with the CSF (i.e., cerebellar cortex, cerebral cortex, the putamen of the thalamus, the hypothalamus, and the inferior surfaces of the basal ganglia). These latter regions equilibrate with the cisternal metrizamide so readily that the brain CSF boundaries are obliterated at CT (Fig 4–7).[25]

The theory that metrizamide freely diffuses into brain extracellular space has been proposed by Winkler and Sackett[26] on the basis of experiments performed with other labeled tracers. The problem of where the metrizamide is located is complicated by the fact that there may be *two* extracellular compartments within the brain. Levin and associates[27] observed that tracers in the CSF equilibrated in an extracellular space that contains 14% to 14.7% of brain fluid. The same tracer given by the venous route equilibrated in a smaller, presumably perivascular space, which contained 1.9% to 5% of the brain fluid. There were no demonstra-

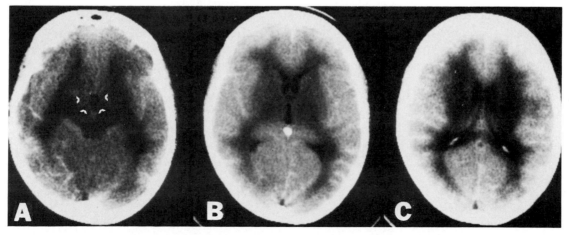

FIG 4–7.
CT scans of a 59-year-old woman 6 hours after metrizamide (290 mg/mL, 11 mL) administered by lumbar puncture for a cervical myelogram inadvertently entered the cranial cisterns. Within 8 hours, the patient was mute and semicomatose. Her condition returned to normal over 48 hours. Premedication with diphenylhydantoin (Dilantin) presumably averted overt seizure activity. **A,** note the general shape of the suprasellar cistern still preserved *(arrows)* as contrast agent penetrates the basal (surface) aspect of the basal ganglia, hypothalamic area, and the adjacent frontal and temporal cortex surrounding the third ventricle. Note that the cerebral peduncles are surrounded by contrast medium, yet they measure 10 to 30 Hounsfield units below those of the enhanced cortex. **B,** and **C,** note that the gyral type of pattern at the leading edge of the diffusion margin has almost disappeared.

ble connections between these extracellular compartments.

A recent study has demonstrated that the mean metrizamide distribution volume in the rabbit thoracic spinal cord is 12%. This smaller distribution volume may be related to (a) the larger effective size of the "associated" metrizamide molecules or (b) an interference with diffusion related to binding of the glucose carriers.[28]

There is indirect evidence that the extracellular compartments of the brain may communicate when the animal is dehydrated. In this situation, extracellular fluid is drawn into the cerebral vessels to counteract the increased blood osmolarity produced by the dehydration.[29] If the CSF contains metrizamide, the augmented brain penetration caused by this "bulk flow" may increase the brain concentration of the media and hence the incidence of toxic symptoms. This mechanism has been verified by a prospective study in which metrizamide myelogram patients who were hydrated had fewer side effects than those who fasted overnight.[30]

We do not know how injected metrizamide is cleared from the CSF in normal subjects. There are three theories:

1. The first postulates that the rate of metrizamide clearance from the CSF is closely related to the rate of CSF absorption by the arachnoid granulations.[31] Hence, changes in degree of hydration or level of CSF pressure (which would affect CSF absorption) would alter metrizamide clearance.

2. The second theory proposes reabsorption by cerebral vessels as another important factor in removal of the metrizamide. Autoradiographic findings (after giving huge doses of marker) indicate that clearance is different in gray and white matter. This may be due to the difference in density of vessels in the two tissues (Fig 4–8).

3. The third theory postulates that the bulk flow of fluid *from* the center of the brain *to* its surface prevents contraflow penetration of the contrast medium into the brain's depths and "washes it out" of the gray matter. This "flow" is postulated to be decreased in older subjects, thus perhaps accounting for the increased incidence of symptoms they experience after intrathecal metrizamide administration.

The following evidence, however, suggests that there is *no* bulk of CSF in *normal* brain: (1) Hydrostatic pressure in the perineuronal fluid space is lower than systemic blood pressure and

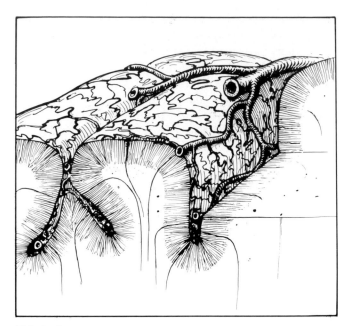

FIG 4–8.
The cortical surface vessels. Line drawing shows the angiographically invisible small arterial branches that form the pial vascular network. From the network, innumerable small vessels arise and penetrate the cortical gray matter. Each of them is surrounded by the CSF-filled perivascular space of Virchow-Robin. Note that only an occasional penetrating vessel continues into the white matter.

spinal CSF pressure; (2) the entry of tracers from CSF into brain is not affected by changes in CSF pressure.[32, 33] Under *normal* conditions, brain entry of most CSF tracers appears to occur by diffusion (sink action) at a rate determined by the tracer's diffusion constant. If, however, the tracer is injected through a cannula *into* the brain, it is transported away from the injection site by bulk flow, probably along perivascular channels. *Bulk flow* cannot, however, be demonstrated if the tracer is injected after the edema caused by cannula insertion has resolved.[34] Indeed, the bulk flow theory may explain why the brain blush has not been observed in patients and animals with acutely damaged brain. Evidence for bulk flow in the normal brain is at present controversial.

Neurotoxicity of New Nonionic Myelographic Media

Clinical studies using iohexol have established that it is less toxic than metrizamide. Except for early onset of headache, side effects of patients after lumbar puncture only were identical to those of patients after puncture plus intrathecal infusion of iohexol.[35] In another study which compared metrizamide to iotrol, the iotrol patients reported fewer adverse reactions.

None of the 19 iotrol patients in the sample displayed electroencephalographic (EEG) changes. In 7 of the 19 patients, the baseline EEG tracing did alter after injection of metrizamide.[36] This has also been noted in EEG studies of rabbits after the injection of metrizamide.[37] In yet another series it was noted that iotrol did not cause significant lengthening of visual response latency (measured 20 hours after injection). Changes in this parameter as well as more frequent and more severe headaches occurred in patients receiving metrizamide and iopamidol.[38]

A study comparing iopamidol and iohexol revealed no differences between the two agents.[39] Neither has been shown to cause the decreased production of carbon dioxide in neural tissue slices, which occurs when metrizamide is used.[40]

These studies have prompted some clinicians to increase the myelographic doses of the newer nonionic media. In one survey, high doses of iohexol (15–24 mL at a concentration of 180 mg/mL) produced contrast-related reactions which were only equal to those which occur after administration of routine doses of metrizamide.[41]

The lower toxicity of iotrol and iopamidol appears to depend upon their molecular structure rather than osmolality. Both iohexol and metrizamide penetrate canine brain substance in a statistically identical manner after intrathecal injection.[42] Iohexol has a slightly larger mean distribution volume (13%) in rabbit spinal cord compared with metrizamide (12%).[28] Neither iotrol nor iopamidol causes cerebral edema or blood-brain barrier (BBB) disruption after intrathecal injection in dogs.[42]

Abnormal Nervous System

Infarction

There is little experimental or clinical information available concerning the penetration of intrathecally administered contrast medium into the abnormal CNS. Drayer and co-workers have shown that metrizamide will not enter an area of acutely devitalized dog brain.[43] Perhaps (1) cytotoxic edema reduces the volume of extracellular space into which the contrast agent can diffuse, or (2) the vasogenic edema that follows infarction creates a "bulk flow" away from the lesion.[26]

Hydromyelia/Syringomyelia

Cavitation of the spinal cord, including hydromyelia and syringomyelia, has been studied using metrizamide CT. Observations of the lesion immediately after instillation of the contrast medium and again 6 to 11 hours later showed delayed enhancement of the cavity. This supports the theory that the fluid in some syrinx cavities arises in the subarachnoid space and passes through the spinal cord into the cavity.[44] Slow filling of the cyst through a very small central canal is a less likely explanation when one considers that metrizamide penetrates normal spinal cord tissue (Fig 4–9).[45]

Hydrocephalus

The CT findings of communicating hydrocephalus have been studied on delayed scans after ventricular injection of metrizamide. Opacification of low-attenuation areas adjacent to the dilated ventricles documents pathologic entry of the agent

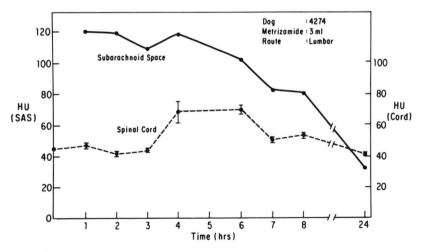

FIG 4–9.
Graph of CT units in the subarachnoid space (SAS) and spinal cord after injection of intrathecal metrizamide. Note the rise in Hounsfield units (HU) within the spinal cord. (Courtesy of Philip Dubois, M.D., Duke University, Durham, NC).

through the abnormally fenestrated ependymal lining of the ventricle. From here it passes into the enlarged periventricular extracellular spaces of the brain.[46] Following ventricular instillation of metrizamide in 17 children with known or suspected obstructive hydrocephalus, CT showed transependymal diffusion equally throughout the white and gray matter. This persisted for up to 6 days after instillation in cases in which adequate shunting was not performed (Fig 4–10).[47] The uniform distribution of the metrizamide seems to indicate that absorption by the numerous vessels of the gray matter did not occur in these children. Delayed scans after instillation of intrathecal metrizamide in elderly patients with a triad of acute-onset dementia, broad-based gait, and incontinence (i.e., normal-pressure hydrocephalus or NPH) showed patterns of media transit identical to those reported in radionuclide cisternography.[48] Because the latter test does not reliably predict which patients will show clinical improvement following a shunt procedure,[49] water-soluble contrast media are rarely used to investigate NPH.

Miscellaneous

We discovered no information in the literature concerning the CT enhancement patterns found after injection of metrizamide into the CSF of patients or animals with brain or spinal tumors. The dearth of such clinical reports is surprising because spinal punctures are frequently performed on patients whose small intracerebral tumors have been defined by CT prior to tap. Theoretically, the zones of vasogenic edema surrounding the tumor would prevent contrast medium from entering the edematous region. There is virtually no information in the literature concerning the interactions of metrizamide with other types of brain abnormality. This is particularly surprising in regard to pseudotumor cerebri because spinal tap is part of the treatment and the brain in this disease has an unusual form of edema that may be primarily cytotoxic. The degree of metrizamide brain penetration in these patients could be measured by CT scans. This information might reveal how the reduction in extracellular space affected the CT brain blush (i.e., the brain penetration of the contrast medium).

PHYSIOLOGY OF WATER-SOLUBLE CONTRAST MEDIA INTRODUCED TO THE VASCULAR SYSTEM

Normal Nervous System

In the United States nonionic media have joined the ionic contrast media for intravascular use in angiography, CT, and digital angiography. The high cost of the nonionic agents (which is mainly due to expensive but necessary purification procedures)[50] has limited their use as intravascular contrast agents even though the nonionic agents are better tolerated by experimental animals (Fig 4–11).

Intraarterial Route

Ionic monomeric contrast media cause severe, life-threatening complications in only 0.009% of patients.[51] The mechanism underlying these reactions is not understood but it is probably not mediated by a primary neurotoxic event. The ability of newer, costly nonionic media to reduce the incidence and severity of these reactions has not been demonstrated in a controlled environment. Actually such an extremely low reaction rate as indicated above makes it unlikely that a randomized, controlled study involving a statistically significant number of subjects could ever be conducted.

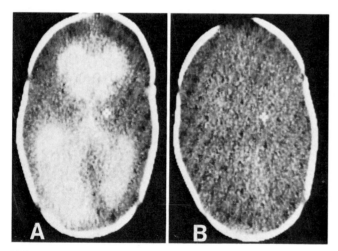

FIG 4–10.
CT scans in a 1-month-old child with aqueductal stenosis. **A,** scan shows transependymal absorption of the contrast medium into the periventricular white matter. (The brain density was 8 HU greater than on the precontrast scan.) **B,** repeat CT scan 48 hours later shows metrizamide throughout the brain with slightly less in the ventricles and the cortical rims. (The brain density was 11 HU greater than the precontrast scan.) The brain and ventricles showed no residual metrizamide 7 days after injection. It is worthwhile noting that this pattern may not be representative of the adult brain, which is composed of myelinated central white matter and has a lower water content than does that of a 1-month-old infant. (From Fitz CR, Harwood-Nash DC, Chuang S, et al: *Neuroradiology* 1978; 16:6–9. Used by permission.)

Contrast Agent	LD$_{50}$(g of Iodine/kg body weight)
Sodium meglumine ioglicate	8.72 (8.04-9.27)
Sodium meglumine ioxaglate	8.41 (7.70-9.13)
Metrizamide	12.97 (11.99-14.03)
Iohexol	~13
Iopromide	12.92 (11.70-14.22)
Nonionic dimer	16.05 (14.24-18.37)

FIG 4–11.

The lethal dose (LD$_{50}$: that dose producing death in 50% of test rats) for various *intravenous* water-soluble contrast agents. The 95% confidence limits are given in parentheses. (From Mutzel W: Properties of conventional contrast media, in Felix R, Kozner E, Wegener OH (eds): *Contrast Media Computed Tomography*. Amsterdam, Excerpta Medica, 1981, pp 19–30. Used by permission.)

Clinical studies have been unable to demonstrate any neurotoxic differences between iohexol, metrizamide, iopamidol, iothalamate meglumine, and diatrizoate meglumine. The lower-osmolality agents *did* produce less patient discomfort.[52–63] The nonionic contrast media produce an even smaller anticoagulant effect than the ionic agents.[64, 65] This, in turn, may account for the red blood cell aggregates which are found in the cerebral angiography syringe at the interface between blood and contrast agent. No clinical embolic complications have as yet been reported but precautions have been advised.

The neurotoxicity of intraarterial contrast media is currently ranked according to the amount of BBB damage induced in normal brain tissue by very prolonged or repeated intracarotid injections. This is at best an arbitrary test, because none of the ionic media in Figure 4–1 cause BBB damage in the normal brain at the formulations, injection rates, and doses used clinically. A nonionic agent, iopamidol, with the same iodine content as an ionic agent, iothalamate, can be given as a prolonged (1.5 mL/sec for *30 seconds*) intracarotid injection in dogs without inducing the BBB disruption that would be seen if iothalamate were used.[66] This presumably can be ascribed to the marked difference in the osmolalities of these agents (see Fig 4–5).[67] Whether or not this reduction in osmolality is of sufficient clinical advantage remains to be seen. The high cost of nonionic agents and the fact that they are clearly superior to ionic media only when given as *30-second* carotid injections may limit the application of nonionic media in carotid angiography.

Rarely, a situation arises in which an ionic contrast agent with an extremely high osmolality is unintentionally injected at cerebral angiography. The highly concentrated contrast medium induces changes on CT that are primarily the result of osmotic insult to the BBB. Sage and co-workers[68] reported a case in which 10 mL of Renografin 76 (osmolality of 1,940 mOsm/kg H$_2$O) was inadvertently used for a selective right carotid injection. Figure 4–12 shows the contrast enhancement and edema on a 45- to 60-minute delayed scan. The patient experienced a focal left body seizure that subsided without treatment but the EEG was abnormal 2 hours later. The mild left central facial weakness, initially noted 15 minutes after the seizure, resolved 3 hours later.[68] There were no permanent neurologic deficits.

Permanent damage can, however, be induced by intraarterial injection of concentrated ionic media. A very high dose of Renografin 76 given to a neurologically normal 20-month-old child during cardiac angiography preceded the onset of seizure, coma, and death. The CT scans at 1, 3, and 7 days after angiography showed persistent enhancement of both gray and white matter (Fig 4–13). The anuria that developed caused extremely high blood iodine levels for a prolonged period. Dialysis reduced the blood levels, but the abnormal brain enhancement could still be seen on CT 7 days later. The microscopic location of the contrast medium within the brain could not be determined. However, its persistence 7 days after the arteriography seems to indicate that "binding" of unknown nature and significance had occurred.

Use of the newer nonionic water-soluble

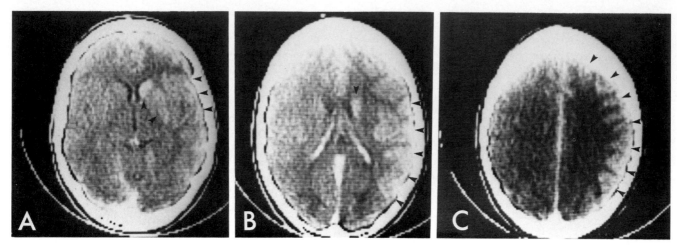

FIG 4–12.
Blood-brain barrier disruption of the right hemisphere of an adult after inadvertent intracarotid injection of Renografin 76 is seen on 45- to 60-minute delayed CT scans at three different levels **(A, B, C)**. Note enhancement of the cortex **(A, B, C,** *lateral arrowheads)* and basal ganglia **(A, B,** *medial arrowheads)* and edema of the white matter. Transient seizures and neurologic deficits were noted. (From Sage MR, Drayer BP, Dubois PJ, et al: *AJNR* 1981; 2:272–274. Used by permission.)

agents instead of the standard ionic agents (e.g., Renografin 76) for cardiac and arch angiography would eliminate the possibility that extremely hyperosmolar contrast media might inadvertently reach the brain and harm the patient. It is possible that the nonionic agents may be intrinsically less harmful than the ionic media for reasons other than the reduction in osmolality. Hydrophilic agents have been shown to be better tolerated in vivo than lipophilic agents. This generalization can only be made about compounds with a similar structure. Therefore, the evaluation of structurally dissimilar contrast media by their butanol coefficients (Fig 4–14) may not be predictive of toxicity.[67] (The butanol coefficient may be defined as a property of the contrast medium that measures the degree to which it is soluble in lipid and water at a given pH.)

Intravenous Route

Ionic monomeric contrast media have been reported to produce fatal reactions in the range of 1 in 40,000 to 1 in 66,502 patients receiving the contrast agent IV. The underlying mechanism which accounts for these reactions is not understood but it probably is not mediated by a primary neurotoxic event. The ability of new costly nonionic media to reduce these reactions has not been demonstrated. The extremely low reaction rate makes it unlikely that a controlled study of a statistically significant number of patients can ever be conducted.

Uncontrolled studies of the newer nonionic

media have claimed that their use reduces the incidence of the mild and moderate systemic reactions that are reported with ionic monomeric media infusions. However, these same reactions have been shown to be significantly reduced by steroid premedication (32 mg methylprednisone) given 12 and 2 hours before administration of the IV ionic medium.[69] Premedication is considerably less expensive than use of the newer lower-osmolality contrast agents.

The rate of entry and distribution of contrast medium in normal brain after maintaining a constant, prolonged (4-hour) contrast blood level by IV infusion has been calculated in the rabbit using labeled diatrizoate (an ionic contrast medium) and labeled metrizamide (a nonionic contrast medium). Regardless of the blood levels, there was no difference between these two agents as to *distribution* in normal brain tissue, both being generally more concentrated in gray than in white matter. Also, there was no difference in the slow rate and limited extent of entry of the contrast media. Both agents entered the brain and appeared to move through the gray matter by diffusion. They occupied a volume equal to 0.5% to 2.0% of the brain water.[24] This is the same size as the compartment that equilibrates with IV administered radioactive sodium, iodide, mannitol, chromium ethylenediamine tetraacetic acid (EDTA), or sucrose. While the ultrastructural site of this space is unknown, the Virchow-Robin space (that region around intracerebral vessels and inside the glial sheaths) has been proposed (Fig 4–15).[70]

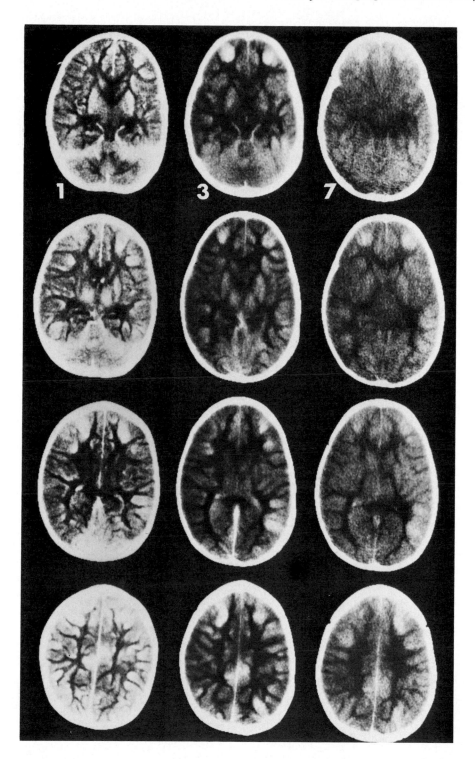

FIG 4–13.

Serial CT scans of a 20-month-old child after receiving an extremely high dose of Renografin 76 during cardiac angiography, which induced generalized blood-brain barrier (BBB) disruption, seizure, coma, renal failure, and death. The left column of scans, 1 day after angiography, shows intense enhancement of all gray matter structures. Some focal areas of particularly striking enhancement may have been caused by the additional BBB damage resulting from the seizures. The center column of CT scans, 3 days after angiography, continues to show enhancement of the brain in spite of dialysis to reduce the blood iodine level. The right column of scans, 7 days after angiography, shows persistent diffuse enhancement from contrast medium extravasation. No hemorrhage was present in the enhanced areas at autopsy. (Courtesy of Robert Peister, M.D., Philadelphia.)

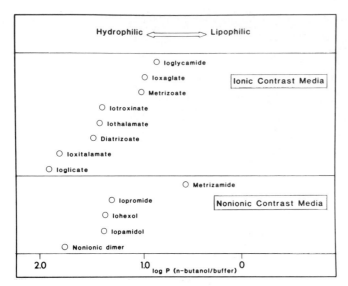

FIG 4–14.
Butanol/buffer partition coefficients of water-soluble ionic and nonionic contrast media (n=butanol/buffer, pH 7.6). Among similar compounds, those that are lipophilic produce more neurotoxic symptoms. The comparison of dissimilar contrast media on the basis of this measurement appears unproductive. (From Mutzel W: Properties of conventional contrast media, in Felix R, Kozner E, Wegener OH (eds): *Contrast Media Computed Tomography.* Amsterdam, Excerpta Medica, 1981, pp 19–30. Used by permission.)

If this site is correct, the contrast medium appears to have crossed normal, tight endothelial junctions that are the primary barrier against large particles (i.e., those with a diameter larger than 1.5 ng). Horseradish peroxidase with a molecular weight of 44,000 and albumin-bound Evans blue with a molecular weight of 69,000 are examples of commonly employed large molecules that are excluded from the perivascular space. Thus, it is possible that the smaller molecules of the contrast agents enter the perivascular space from the vessels (see Fig 4–15). If one assumes that there is only one extracellular compartment, the IV medium diffuses into the same space in the brain as the intrathecally administered agents. *If* this is true, we are left to wonder why one does not routinely encounter observable neurotoxic side effects in patients given IV ionic contrast media because ionic agents have devastating effects when they enter the brain (even in very low concentration) after intrathecal injection. Remember that it took only small amounts of an ionic contrast medium used in the lumbar subarachnoid region to induce such severe side effects that it was banned as a myelographic agent in the United States.

The extravasation of IV administered ionic

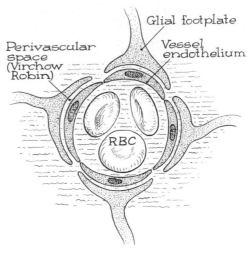

FIG 4–15.
Schematic cross section of a penetrating cerebral vessel such as that seen in Figure 4–7. The endothelial cells are connected at "tight junction points," which prevent the entry of large molecules into the perivascular space. Because contrast media are relatively small molecules that equilibrate with a small percentage of the brain water after IV infusion, it has been postulated that they may be free to enter the Virchow-Robin spaces. *RBC* = red blood cell.

contrast material documented in the previously cited animal study has been shown by CT to occur in normal human brain. The brain enhancement observed after IV contrast infusion cannot be explained by the volume of the vascular bed per se.[71] It appears to represent contrast medium that has escaped from the normal cerebral circulation.*

There is no rational way to rate the neurotoxicity of IV administered contrast media because minimal amounts of both nonionic and ionic agents enter the normal brain. Even in very high doses (1.1 g iodine/kg body weight), the contrast agent rapidly equilibrates with the plasma osmolality of approximately 280 to 300 mOsm/kg H_2O.[72] Hence, the neurologic symptoms seen in normal animals after prolonged or repeated intracarotid injections of contrast media are not seen after IV contrast. A previous study of dogs, which claimed to show generalized and focal BBB damage caused by high doses of IV contrast media,[73] could not be substantiated when repeated with dogs that were not under general anesthesia.[74]

*This precludes the use of iodinated contrast agents for measuring cerebral blood flow because the enhancement on CT represents not only the intravascular pool but also an unknown amount of extravascular agent. This is a particularly relevant problem in evaluating areas of abnormal brain (which are, after all, the regions of clinical interest).

Another (as yet untried) more precise way to rank vascular contrast media would be to measure the *rate constant* of brain entry for each agent and calculate the *Km*, which is a working measurement of each agent's BBB permeability.[70] Furthermore, the site at which the agents equilibrate could be determined by careful film and microscopic autoradiography using tritium-labeled contrast media.

All of the parameters listed could then be remeasured in normal brain of various ages and in abnormal brain to determine how the changes of extracellular fluid composition and alterations in glia and neurons caused by pathologic conditions contribute to the overall toxicity of each contrast agent. Until standardized techniques are developed and applied to various contrast media, our understanding of these compounds will remain, as presently, severely circumscribed.

Before moving on to discuss lesions that can be detected on CT scan through enhancement, it should be noted that the BBB is easily penetrated by contrast media in the region of the pineal gland, the posterior half of the pituitary gland, the choroid of the eye, the choroid plexus of the ventricles, and the dura. Therefore, these areas normally display intense contrast enhancement on CT.

Abnormal Nervous System

There is a profusion of experimental and clinical data in the literature concerning alteration of the BBB in the abnormal brain.[75] Detection of this alteration by IV infusion of water-soluble contrast media before CT scanning has provided the basis for many publications over the past 6 or 7 years. The enormous interest evident in this area can be ascribed to the fact that most neurologic disorders are associated with an increased permeability of CNS vessels, which is important to the pathophysiology, diagnosis, treatment, and perhaps even to the etiology of the disorders discussed. The advances made in the last several years will be discussed by category.

Infarction

Many clinical and experimental CT studies have examined the behavior of ionic vascular contrast media given after cerebral infarction. There are three contrast CT patterns that can be seen alone or in combination after an infarction. Each of

these will be discussed separately. The *first* is absence of normal gray matter enhancement, which can be seen throughout the evolution of the infarction. In the early stages, it indicates that the iodine transporting cerebral circulation does not adequately perfuse that portion of the brain. Later, it indicates a cystic or gliotic area traversed by capillaries that have developed a mature BBB. Absence of normal gray matter enhancement is a reliable sign of permanent cerebral destruction.[76]

The *second* pattern is only seen on scans done within 24 hours after onset of or sudden worsening of ischemic symptoms. The immediate contrast scan shows a variety of patterns that are not predictive of the ultimate viability of the tissue. The 3-hour delayed contrast CT scan has a characteristic pattern of slowly increasing, diffuse, heterogeneous enhancement that involves both white and gray matter without regard for differences in their vascular anatomy. In one study, three of the seven patients reported with this CT pattern were on heparin therapy or had a clotting disorder. These three and one other in the series subsequently developed massive confluent hemorrhagic infarction in areas that showed delayed CT enhancement. This pattern of enhancement may predict which patients run the risk of developing hemorrhagic infarctions. The contrast extravasation may represent accumulation in the zones of vasogenic edema that precede the hemorrhage (Fig 4–16).[77]

The *third* pattern is characterized by *immediate* contrast enhancement, which persists or intensifies on delayed CT scans. When this pattern is seen *4 or more days after the onset* of cerebral ischemia, most of it can be attributed to extravasation of contrast medium into damaged areas containing proliferating immature capillaries.[76, 78] It resolves when the new capillaries are surrounded by glial foot processes and develop an effective BBB.[79] Capillary maturation throughout the lesion can be a lengthy process, particularly in larger infarcts. Hence, enhancement may be seen as late as 150 days following cerebral infarction. Enhancement caused by this mechanism is not necessarily related to vasogenic edema because it can be observed long after the mass effect caused by edema has resolved.

While capillary proliferation adequately explains CT enhancement seen 4 or more days after infarction, it does not explain the persistent enhancement that has been reported by one study in patients after a very recent transient ischemic at-

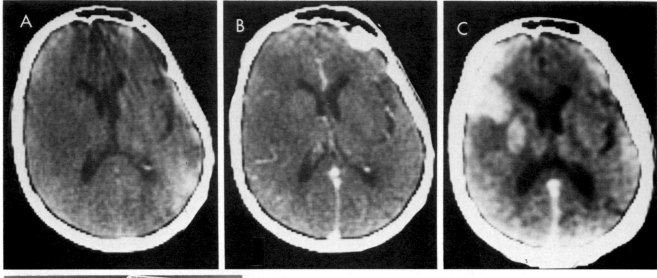

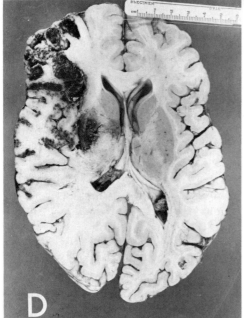

FIG 4–16.
Series of CT scans done 20 hours after cerebral embolization during a bout of atrial fibrillation: **A,** precontrast CT: obliteration of right sylvian fissure; compression of right lateral ventricle. **B,** immediate high-dose contrast CT: absence of gray matter enhancement in right operculum and posterior lateral right thalamus. **C,** filtered delayed high-dose contrast scan 3 hours later showing wedge enhancement that includes lentiform area and adjacent cortex. In addition, an adjacent zone of cortical nonenhancement is seen. The mass effect did not increase as enhancement developed. **D,** autopsy specimen obtained 8 days later. Hemorrhagic infarction is seen in the area of delayed enhancement, and anemic infarction (with a very small punctate zone of hemorrhage) in areas showing no gray matter enhancement. (From Hayman LA, Evans RA, Bastion FO, et al: *AJNR* 1981; 2:139–147. Used by permission.)

tack.[80]* Animal studies indicate that enhancement in such cases may be due to extravasation of the contrast medium into compromised but viable brain substance that is found *adjacent* to zones of cerebral infarction. Cats with acute middle cerebral artery infarction that were given IV ^{125}I-labeled meglumine iothalamate (Conray), technetium pertechnetate, or chlormerodrin Hg 203 showed tracer was surrounding *or possibly within*

*It is difficult to determine if areas of brain that were functionally silent or possessed abilities that are difficult to quantitate clinically may have been infarcted, thus producing the enhancement seen in the "transient ischemia" patients reported in this study.

viable neurons at the periphery of the infarct 2 hours after the infusion.[81, 82] The iothalamate and technetium studies were not supplemented by autoradiography. However, these tracers accumulated in areas of brain adjacent to the infarct at a time when dysautoregulation (which theoretically might increase tissue radioactivity by increasing the relative volume of tracer-containing blood) had subsided.[83] Therefore, evaluation of infarct size by measuring volume of enhancing tissue is unreliable because enhancement may indicate areas of transiently compromised viable brain.

In view of the above animal evidence of contrast extravasation into viable brain that surrounds infarcted brain, one would expect neurotoxic side effects from the contrast media to occur. Multiple studies have been done to detect contrast medium–induced side effects. Clinical observations indicate that patients with persistent gray matter enhancement on contrast CT after what appear to be transient ischemic attacks experience *no* clinically apparent reaction after a 42-g iodine infusion.[84] The authors have prospectively observed a series of 40 consecutive patients with cerebral infarction who received a high dose of contrast containing 80 g of iodine without experiencing any detectable clinical deterioration. This is particularly interesting because the number of enhancing infarctions in a given series can be increased by using higher doses of iodine.[85]

A large retrospective study has been done to examine the effect of contrast administration upon recovery from cerebral infarction. It suffered from the usual severe methodologic handicaps of a retrospective study. Nevertheless, *it failed to demonstrate any statistically significant deleterious effect from the contrast agent.* The lack of correlation was surprising because, according to the protocol, contrast medium (sodium iothalamate) was administered to patients with large infarctions and considerable mass effect (i.e., those with a poor prognosis) and withheld from those with normal preinfusion scans (i.e., those with an excellent prognosis).[86, 87] The authors of that study concluded that, although statistical proof was lacking, the *possibility* that contrast material *may* adversely affect potentially viable neuronal tissue should be kept in mind. The absence of documented contrast-induced side effects in these patients should prompt us to consider a theory that relates the toxicity of *vascular* contrast media to factors other than accumulation in the brain.

In summary, when the third pattern is found 0 to 4 days after infarction, it can be explained by extravasation of contrast medium from compromised vessels into areas that may not become necrotic. This occurs principally in gray matter, because, as we have already noted, the majority of cerebral vessels are in gray matter. Gradually, *no sooner than 4 days* after ischemia, the third pattern of contrast CT enhancement can be ascribed to extravasation of contrast media from immature capillaries. In the early stages, it also tends to predominate in gray matter because reanastomosis of iodine-containing circulation with the developing immature capillaries occurs more readily in the gray matter than in the sparsely vascularized white matter.

In theory, a *fourth* pattern of CT enhancement may occur. A very large increase in the blood volume caused by vasodilation in areas adjacent to an acute infarct might produce enhancement on the immediate contrast scan that would diminish or disappear on the delayed scan (as the blood iodine concentration diminished).[76] This pattern has not been reported in clinical material, perhaps because it is obscured by simultaneous extravasation, which creates the third pattern of CT enhancement.

The administration of contrast material to patients with cerebral infarction has advanced our understanding of the events that occur in human infarction, but it appears to have no value in the therapeutic context because enhancement does not appear to correlate with prognosis. To determine whether such a correlation exists would require a large series of patients in which all important parameters (i.e., age, sex, etiology, location and extent of infarction, presence or absence of collaterals, and a standardized mode of therapy) were precisely controlled.

Neoplasm

One of the most important uses for IV ionic contrast media in neuroradiology has been to enhance the CT visibility of CNS neoplasms. In 1975, Gado and associates[88] demonstrated that CT enhancement in two patients with intracranial neoplasms could not be explained by increased blood volume in the lesion. He did this by measuring the tissue-blood enhancement ratio and surmised that extravasation of contrast agent into the tumor was the cause of the tumor enhancement recorded by CT. Impairment of the BBB (which normally prevents the escape of all but a very small proportion of the intravascular contrast medium) is a well-known feature of neoplastic vessels. With the exception of low-grade gliomas, necrotic neoplasms, and patients on corticosteroid therapy, contrast administration commonly causes enhancement of neoplasms on CT. However, those neoplasms that have minimal BBB deficiency require higher doses of contrast agent to produce prolonged high blood iodine levels before they become visible (i.e., on *delayed* CT scans) (Fig 4–17).[89–93]

Multiple clinical papers have shown that traditional doses of IV contrast medium given immediately before CT sometimes fail to demonstrate BBB leakage (i.e., contrast enhancement).[89–93] One study of patients being followed by contrast CT after chemotherapy and radiotherapy for cra-

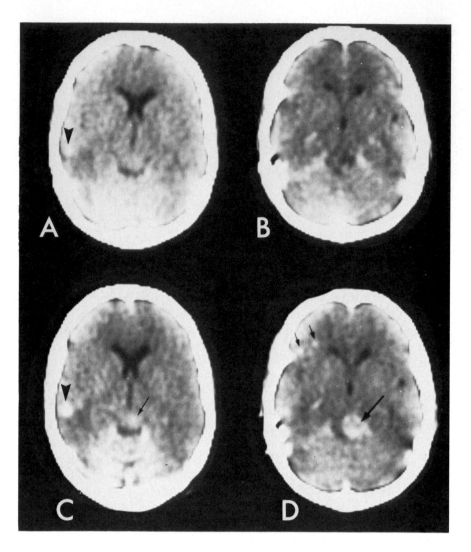

FIG 4–17.
A and **B**, immediate conventional dose postinfusion scans showing a subtle left temporal metastasis *(arrowhead)* from adenocarcinoma of the lung and surrounding focal cerebral edema. A scan 1 hour later failed to show the lesion. **C** and **D**, 1-hour delay high-contrast dose (80 g/L) scan of the same patient 1 day later showing additional lesions in brain stem and left frontal lobe *(arrows).*

Visualization of the left temporal lesion *(arrowhead)* is improved considerably. The large brain stem lesion was not visible on the immediate high-dose scan done that same day. (From Hayman LA, Evans RA, Hinck VC, et al: *Radiology* 1980; 136:677–684. Used by permission.)

nial tumors found that BBB damage was not detected in 11.5% of *treated* cases unless a 90-minute delayed scan was done.[91] Takeda and co-workers[94] have analyzed the dynamics of CT enhancement of 31 neoplasms by performing immediate CT scans followed by scans 1 and 2 hours after IV administration of contrast medium. They calculated tissue-blood contrast ratios and noted differences among meningiomas, pituitary adenomas, and neurinomas. They postulated that the mechanism of BBB disruption (i.e., increased pinocytosis or vascular endothelial fenestration) was different in each type of tumor. This resulted in different tissue-blood contrast ratios.

The precise location of the contrast medium that extravasates from the tumor vessels is not known. An autoradiographic study using IV tritium-labeled methotrexate (a chemotherapeutic agent) in mice with intracerebral implants of ependymoblastoma has shown vascular and interstitial tracer within the neoplasm 2 and 10 minutes after injection. Sixty minutes after injection, however, intracellular methotrexate was identified in the center of the neoplasm. Peripheral and infiltrating neoplastic cells showed comparatively little intracellular methotrexate. Uptake was higher in the edematous brain surrounding the neoplasm than in normal brain but not as high as that found in the neoplasm per se.[95] These results are intriguing because the molecular weight of the methotrexate is similar to that of the currently used ionic contrast agents. In fact, Neuwelt and co-workers[96] have shown that the concentrations of methotrexate and ionic contrast media can be correlated in brain after osmotic BBB disruption. If the autoradiography of methotrexate were comparable to that of contrast media, the initial CT enhancement of neoplasms might be explained by the vascular and interstitial component alluded to above, and the findings on delayed CT scan might be related to the intracellular entry of the contrast agent. Until contrast medium extravasation in neoplasms is autoradiographed, these issues will remain the subject of speculation.

The incidence of IV contrast medium–induced seizures is increased by six- to 19-*hundred*fold in patients with brain metastases compared with (presumably neurologically normal) patients receiving IV contrast infusion for pyelograms.[97–100] The risk of seizures after contrast administration in the neoplasia group is increased 30-*hundred*fold over the standard pyelogram group if the patient with a brain tumor also has a neoplasia-related seizure history or is undergoing (or has undergone) CNS antineoplastic therapy. Clearly, these patients have a seizure focus that predates contrast administration, and the administration of contrast medium triggers a seizure. Unlike the seizures induced in patients receiving intrathecal contrast material, the entry of the agent into the brain after the IV infusion does not appear to be the precipitating factor. Witness the fact that in Scott's series,[99] three of the seven patients with contrast-induced seizures had no detectable enhancement on CT. Conversely, there was no correlation between seizure induction and the presence of massive CT enhancement of metastases in the series of 188 cases of Pagani and co-workers.[97]

Fischer[101] has postulated that the vasogenic edema associated with brain neoplasms produces local slowing of the circulation around these lesions and this phenomenon has been well documented on contrast CT scans.[102] Fischer believes that the prolonged exposure of the vascular endothelium to contrast medium gives the chemical an opportunity to exert a *direct* "permeability changing effect," thus causing seizures in patients with metastatic disease.[101] The pattern was indeed detected by Pagani and associates[97] in several patients (Fig 4–18), but they did not suffer seizures. It would appear, therefore, that extravasation of

contrast medium, manifested as cortical enhancement, was not the cause of contrast-induced seizures in this group.[97]

The intraarterial injection of contrast material in patients with brain neoplasm is primarily directed at defining the vascularity of the lesion and its immediately surrounding area in order to gauge the location and extent of tumor and thereby to assist in planning the neurosurgical approach. In recent studies, patients with intracerebral neoplasms have been given an intracarotid infusion of 25% mannitol (to disrupt the BBB) and then an infusion of chemotherapeutic agent. Interposed 2 minutes after the infusion of mannitol, a high dose of ionic contrast medium (containing approximately 80 g of iodine) has been given IV. Amazingly intense enhancement has been seen in both normal brain and neoplasm in areas perfused by the carotid that received the mannitol injection. Enhancement with CT after osmotic insult to the BBB persisted longer than that seen using the same dose of contrast agent in the absence of the osmotic insult (Fig 4–19). Despite the exceptionally high, prolonged levels of intracerebral contrast agent to which normal brain tissue was subjected, the incidence of seizure induction in the high-risk patients reported by Neuwelt and colleagues[96] does not appear to have been greater than that reported by others who have examined similar high-risk subjects.

As we have seen, the intraarterial injection of contrast media with an osmolality similar to 25% mannitol (e.g., Renografin 76) induces seizures (see Fig 4–12) and death if given in sufficiently large doses (see Fig 4–13). It is surprising that osmotic disruption of the cerebral BBB with the intracarotid injection of mannitol induced no EEG changes or visible seizures.[96] This must mean that the osmotic disruption caused by the contrast medium is insufficient alone to cause the toxic manifestations noted.

It is equally interesting that the IV infusion of a high dose of ionic contrast agent (containing approximately 80 g of iodine) 2 minutes after intracarotid mannitol did not produce a higher incidence of neurotoxic side effects, because it did produce amazingly high contrast levels in the brain. These observations support the suggestion of Pagani and co-workers,[97] that the amount of extravasation of intravascular media per se is not the key to neurotoxicity as it appears to be with intrathecally administered contrast media.

One theory to explain the data would be to suggest that damaging the BBB sets in motion a

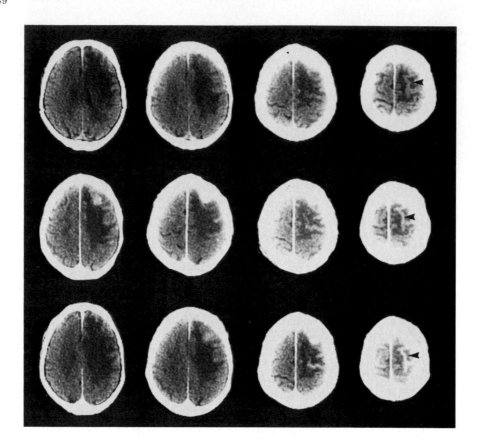

FIG 4–18.
Noncontrast CT scans of an 83-year-old man with edema secondary to a metastasis in the left cerebral hemisphere *(top row)*. A high-dose contrast CT scan done 1 hour after infusion reveals the metastatic focus. An *arrow* indicates enhancement of the motor cortex *(center row)*, which intensified on the 2-hour delayed scans *(bottom row)*. Despite the persistent accumulation of contrast medium in the motor cortex, the patient did not seize. (Window settings are adjusted to maximize enhancement. The intensity of the contrast enhancement should be compared with the normal cortex of the right hemisphere.) (From Pagani JJ, Hayman LA, Bigelow RH, et al: *AJNR* 1983; 4:67–72. Used by permission.)

chain of events that alters the extracellular fluid, glia, and neurons and that these changes in turn protect the brain from the effects of the contrast medium. The changes must, of course, occur (or be substantially underway) within 2 minutes after disruption of the BBB because, as indicated above, massive CT contrast enhancement has been recorded when the IV contrast infusion was started 2 minutes after BBB disruption.

These changes would not have had time to develop if it was the contrast agent per se that disrupted the BBB because intracarotid injections of hyperosmolar contrast media *simultaneously* produce BBB disruption and contrast extravasation. Protective mechanisms would not, in such circumstances, have had a chance to become activated. This theory (of protective changes rapidly induced by BBB disruption prior to contrast extravasation) could also explain why intrathecally administered contrast material that enters the brain at much lower concentrations (as documented on CT) causes seizures. In the case of intrathecal administration, the protective BBB mechanisms are not invoked before the contrast agent contacts the normal brain tissue.

Another, but less likely, possibility is that contrast medium that enters the brain from the vascular system enters a space different from the one occupied by contrast medium that enters from the subarachnoid space.[27]

While it is not clear how contrast agents trigger seizures, it has been shown that giving adequate levels of diphenylhydantoin does not prevent seizures induced by IV administered contrast media in high-risk tumor patients. However, it does appear to protect "normal" brain patients who receive subarachnoid nonionic contrast for myelographic studies. Prophylactic doses of diazepam, on the other hand, have been found to significantly reduce the incidence of seizures caused by IV con-

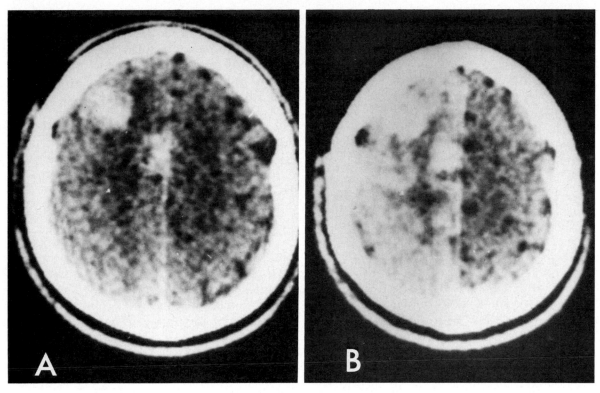

FIG 4–19.
A, 30-minute delayed contrast scan showing extravasation of contrast medium into two areas of a malignant neoplasm in the right hemisphere. **B,** repeat 30-minute delayed contrast scan several days later. Scan was obtained after intracarotid mannitol was infused to disrupt the blood-brain barrier. The contrast medium was given 2 minutes after the mannitol infusion. Note the extensive extravasation of contrast medium in tumor and adjacent motor cortex. The patient did not seize. (From Neuwelt EA, Diehl JT, Vu LH, et al: *Ann Intern Med* 1981; 94:449–453. Used by permission.)

trast administration.[97] Considerable work has yet to be done to determine precisely how toxic side effects are induced by different agents given by the intravascular and intrathecal routes.

Infection

The pattern of CT enhancement following IV infusion of ionic contrast agents in subjects with *bacterial* cerebritis and abscess has been studied in both patients and laboratory animals. The early detection of these lesions has enabled timely therapy, thereby reducing the mortality rate in this condition.[103] Enzmann and co-workers[104] studied the CT contrast patterns in dogs after injection of α-streptococcus into the brain (traumatic abscess formation). They identified four stages of CT enhancement: (1) *Early cerebritis* appeared as an illdefined area of enhancement (contrast extravasation) which intensified and enlarged on delayed CT scans 1 hour after bolus infusion of contrast agent. (2) *Late cerebritis* appeared as an area of ring enhancement that filled in centrally on delayed CT scans. The enhancement achieved great-

est intensity 10 to 20 minutes after the contrast infusion and plateaued during the remainder of the 60-minute scan session. (3) *Early capsule formation* appeared as a smaller width of ring enhancement than that described above. The intensity of enhancement peaked 5 to 10 minutes after infusion and began to fade after 30 minutes. (4) *Late capsule formation* appeared as a still smaller ring or nodule which no longer filled centrally on delayed scans. The enhancement intensity was greatest early and faded rapidly. The fact that the pattern of CT enhancement changes over time (i.e., amount and timing of entry and resorption of contrast agent) indicates an orderly progression of pathophysiologic processes that could be mapped. This is important because patients with cerebritis may respond well to medical management with antibiotics and corticosteroids and not require surgical intervention. Britt and colleagues[105] suggest that these patients can be recognized as having a ring-shaped enhancing pattern that fills in on 30-minute postcontrast scans. Conversely, the patients with abscesses requiring surgical therapy will have enhancing rings that do not fill in on delayed contrast CT scans.

The CT pattern in immunosuppressed patients with brain abscesses is atypical. The ring enhancement is absent, presumably because of an alteration in host response to infection. It is a poor prognostic sign.[106] Immunologically compromised patients may also be infected with papovavirus, which is thought to produce progressive multifocal leukoencephalopathy. Enhancement with CT has been reported in some of these patients.[107]

It has been noted that medical therapy with corticosteroids reduces lesion enhancement on CT and that lesion enhancement will intensify after corticosteroids are withdrawn. These findings have no apparent clinical significance. In fact, lesion enhancement appears to persist after antibiotic therapy has obliterated a focus of infection.[103]

The CT enhancement seen after cerebral infection is caused by contrast extravasation from the new vessels found at the boundary zone surrounding cerebritis and abscess. These vessels develop more slowly if an experimental lesion is induced with septic emboli (i.e., the usual route of nontraumatic clinical infections) rather than by direct traumatic injection because the embolic lesions are associated with infarction.[105]

Pathologic correlation of other types of brain infection with contrast CT patterns has not yet been reported in laboratory animals. Tuberculous, cysticercotic, and fungal lesions seen on CT scans of patients resemble pyogenic abscess, presumably because they also induce neovascularity with a deficient BBB.[108]

An unusual contrast CT scan appearance in a case of herpes simplex viral encephalitis has been reported in an infant. It was associated with persistent, apparently irreversible contrast enhancement (i.e., extravasation) in the gray matter of the brain. The infant's poor condition precluded determining if this contrast retention ("binding") contributed to clinical deterioration.[109]

Congenital

Angiography and CT with and without contrast infusion are the primary diagnostic methods of evaluating patients for congenital vascular malformation and aneurysm. Noncontrast CT is superior to angiography in detecting small hemorrhages, small areas of adjacent infarction, subarachnoid blood, and calcification. Contrast CT can provide information not revealed by the arteriogram concerning thrombosed or partially thrombosed le-

sions. Thrombosed areas can be visible on contrast CT for three reasons: (1) The scanner is sensitive to smaller amounts of contrast entering the lesion than are detectable at angiography. (2) Small vessels in the walls of giant aneurysms have a defective BBB, which allows contrast extravasation.[110] (3) Areas of resolving hemorrhage have new vessels with an immature BBB, which allows contrast extravasation. Contrast CT scan can also detect zones of ischemic infarction in uninvolved adjacent brain that can appear "normal" on the noncontrast scan.[111]

Trauma

In general, contrast CT and arteriography are not necessary in the evaluation of patients examined after acute trauma unless an underlying brain disorder is suspected clinically. The noncontrast scan adequately detects cerebral contusions as well as intra- and extracerebral blood. The authors have noted one case in which a high dose of contrast material was given to a patient within 48 hours after acute head trauma, and extremely intense gray matter enhancement was seen on immediate scan (Fig 4–20). A scan 3 hours later demonstrated contrast extravasation within a zone of edema. This was not associated with alteration of clinical status of the patient, who was alert and oriented throughout. Intraventricular pressure, which was recorded throughout the period, was not altered. This case suggests that preexistence of a BBB defect created by acute brain concussion may protect the patient from the effects of massive contrast extravasation. (See Neoplasm above for a discussion of this theory.)

Contrast administration is necessary for the occasional patient in whom the unenhanced scan shows an isodense mass that could represent resolving subacute subdural hematoma. This situation is encountered less frequently with newer-generation scanners. When it does occur, bolus infusion of contrast medium can be used to enhance the brain surfaces and thereby differentiate subdural collection from brain swelling.[112]

Amendola and Ostrum[113] reported that some subdural collections enhance on delayed contrast CT (Fig 4–21). The cause of delayed subdural enhancement is unknown. It may indicate that a membrane has formed and the subdural collection must be removed surgically. However, electron microscopy of the inner surface of the normal dura has revealed that it has no tight junctions[114] to prevent contrast medium from entering the CSF or,

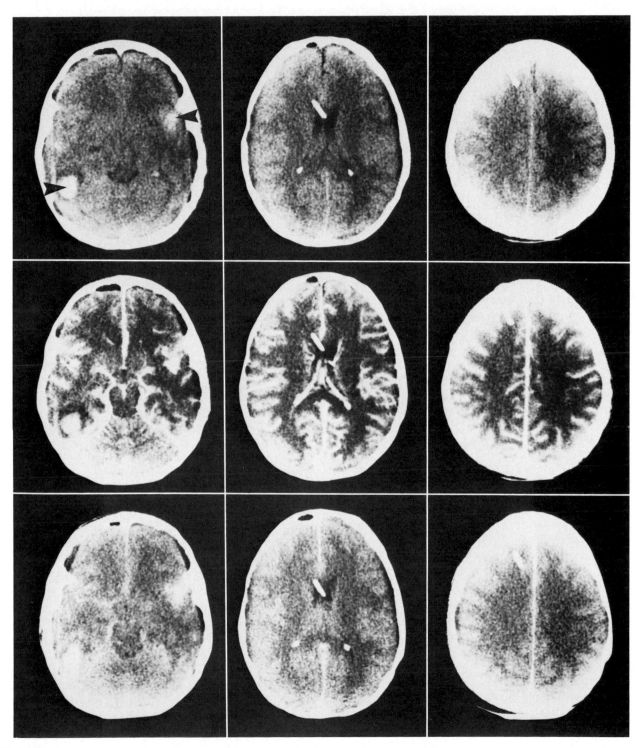

FIG 4–20.

Top row, CT scan 48 hours after head trauma showing two intracerebral hematomas *(arrowheads)* and an intraventricular pressure cannula. *Center row,* CT scans immediately after IV ionic contrast medium (diatrizoate) infusion show extremely intense enhancement of gray matter structures presumably caused by the cerebral concussion. *Bottom row,* CT scan 3 hours later shows residual enhancement of a broad area surrounding the gray matter and enhancement of the crescent of edema formerly seen anterior to the right temporal hematoma. No neurologic sequelae or change in intracranial pressure was noted during or 24 hours after these scans.

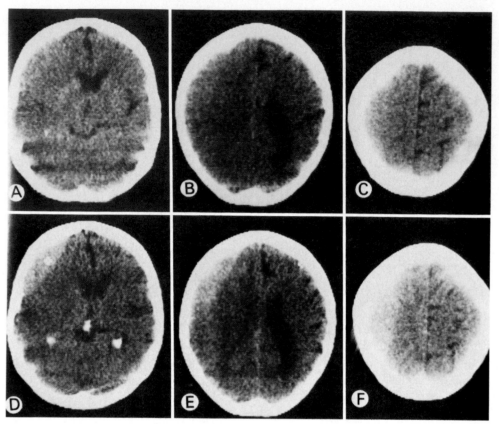

FIG 4–21.
A–C, CT scans 5 minutes after administration of contrast media in a 65-year-old man. Effacement of sulci in the right hemisphere is evident. **D–F,** delayed scans 6 hours later showing contrast ex- travasation into the right frontal subdural hematoma. (From Amendola MA, Ostrum BJ: *AJR* 1977; 129:693–697. Used by permission.)

theoretically, the subdural collection. Surgical pathologic correlation would be necessary to determine the mechanism by which delayed subdural enhancement occurs.

Miscellaneous

Osmotic Brain Injury.—The degree of osmotically induced BBB disruption can be quantitated by serially measuring intensity of enhancement on serial CT scans after IV infusion of Renografin 60.[115] Animal experiments have suggested that nonionic agents such as metrizamide may not be as effective as the traditional high-osmolality ionic agents in producing contrast enhancement on CT. Neuwelt and associates[116] examined phenobarbital-sedated dogs after 25% mannitol was injected into the carotid artery to disrupt the BBB. They showed that the CT enhancement produced by iothalamate meglumine (Conray 60) was greater and persisted longer after intravascular administration than the enhancement caused by metrizamide. However, CT scans of dogs that received radiation therapy

for brain tumors have shown that the absolute uptake of contrast medium was identical for iohexol (nonionic monomeric) and iothalamate (ionic monomeric) at 5, 10, 15, and 30 minutes.[117] Additional studies comparing CT enhancement after intravascular administration of ionic and nonionic media must be done in patients with commonly encountered clinical types of brain lesions before one can determine if ionic agents produce equivalent CT brain enhancement.

Radiation and Drug-Induced Brain Injury.— Normal brain exposed to prophylactic intrathecal methotrexate or radiotherapy can develop necrosis of deep hemispheric white matter that can be fatal. These areas can be detected on contrast CT scans as enhancing foci.[118] These areas may be mistaken as neoplastic foci and biopsied. The CT appearance in the early stages of this condition is poorly documented.

Marked CT contrast enhancement of the spinal cord and roots have been reported in children who

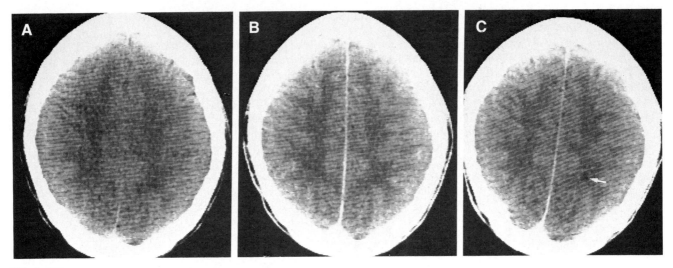

FIG 4–22.
Low-density multiple sclerosis plaque seen only on high-dose delayed scan, **A,** unenhanced scan appears normal. **B,** immediate standard contrast CT scan appears normal. **C,** 1-hour delayed scan after a high dose of contrast medium in the patient shows low-density plaque in the left centrum semiovale *(arrow).* (From Vinuela FV, Fox AJ, Debrun GM, et al: *AJR* 1982; 139:123–127. Used by permission.)

received 1,200 to 2,400 rad to the spine 1 month to 4½ years prior to the scan. Subclinical damage to the BBB has been postulated as the cause of this phenomenon.[119]

Multiple Sclerosis.—Disruption of the BBB occurs in vessels of the white matter and, less commonly, in the cortical and subcortical regions of the brain in patients with acute and relapsing multiple sclerosis. The number of lesions detected by CT can be dramatically increased if high IV doses of contrast medium are used and the scan is delayed for 1 hour. This allows time for the maximum amount of ionic contrast medium to accumulate in lesions having minimal BBB damage.[120, 121] Chronic multiple sclerosis lesions can usually be identified as nonenhancing low-density zones in the white matter. Occasionally, a chronic lesion will be isodense on noncontrast scans but identified as a zone of nonenhancement surrounded by normal diffuse white matter enhancement in delayed contrast scans (Fig 4–22).[120]

PHYSIOLOGY OF WATER-SOLUBLE CONTRAST MEDIA INTRODUCED TO THE LYMPHATIC SYSTEM

A new water-soluble contrast agent, iotasul (see Fig 4–4), has been tested in dogs. Injection of this agent into the tissues of the neck resulted in opacification of the regional lymphatic system.[16]

This agent, used with CT, could have a substantial impact on the staging of tumor spread. The difficulty in producing the substance lies mainly in purifying the product. Once this problem has been solved, this agent will be tested clinically in humans.

SUMMARY

We have tried to recapitulate the development of water-soluble contrast agents, review present knowledge concerning the physiology of existing contrast media, and define four important areas that merit further investigation. In summary, these are to (1) define the BBB for contrast media directly instead of relying on extrapolated data obtained by using markers of different molecular size and characteristics, (2) determine why intrathecal administration is more toxic than intravascular administration, (3) isolate those factors other than osmolarity that cause the neurotoxic side effects of contrast media, and (4) determine the macro- and microscopic location of those contrast molecules that enter both normal brain (at all ages) and abnormal brain.

REFERENCES

1. Fischer HW: Contrast media, in Newton TH, Potts DG (eds): *Radiology of the Skull and Brain: An-*

giography, vol 2, book 1. St Louis, CV Mosby Co, 1974, pp 893–907.

2. Dawson P, Howell M: The non-ionic dimers: A new class of contrast agents. *Br J Radiol* 1986; 59:987–991.

3. Grainger RG: Osmolality of intravascular radiological contrast media. *Br J Radiol* 1980; 53:739–746.

4. Almen T: Contrast agent design: Some aspects on the synthesis of water-soluble contrast agents of low osmolality. *J Theor Biol* 1969; 24:216–226.

5. Amundsen P: Water-soluble myelographic agents, in Miller R, Skucas J (eds): *Radiographic Contrast Agents.* Baltimore, University Park Press, 1977, pp 437–448.

6. Bertoni JM, Schwartzman RJ, vanHorn G, et al: Asterixis and encephalopathy following metrizamide myelography: Investigations into possible mechanisms and review of the literature. *Ann Neurol* 1981; 9:366–370.

7. Bonati F, Felder EE, Tirone P: Iopamidol: New preclinical and clinical data. *Invest Radiol* 1980; 15:s310–s316.

8. Grainger RG: Intravascular contrast media—The past, the present, and the future. *Br J Radiol* 1982; 55:1–18.

9. Gonsette RE: Animal experiments and clinical experiences in cerebral angiography with a new contrast agent (ioxaglic acid) with a low hyperosmolality. *Ann Radiol* 1978; 21:271–273.

10. Gonsette RE, Liesenborgh L: New contrast media in cerebral angiography: Animal experiments and preliminary clinical studies. *Invest Radiol* 1980; 15 (suppl 6):270–274.

11. Hoppe JO, Archer S: X-ray contrast media for cardiovascular angiography. *Angiology* 1960; 11:244–254.

12. Lindgren E: Iohexol. *Acta Radiol [Suppl] (Stockh)* 1980; 362:9–11.

13. Olin TB, Redman HC: Experimental evaluation of contrast media in the vertebral circulation. *Acta Radiol [Suppl] (Stockh)* 1967; 270:216–227.

14. *Physician's Desk Reference,* ed 34. Oradell, NJ, Medical Economics Co, 1980, pp 2039–2041.

15. Pitre D, Felder E: Development, chemistry and physical properties of iopamidol and its analogues. *Invest Radiol* 1980; 15:s301–s309.

16. Siefert HM, Mutzel W, Schobel C, et al: Iotosul: A water-soluble contrast agent for direct and indirect lymphography. *Lymphology* 1980; 13:150–157.

17. Sovak M, Ranganathan R, Speck U, et al: Nonionic dimer: Development and initial testing of an intrathecal contrast agent. *Radiology* 1982; 142:115–118.

18. Skalpe IO: Adverse effects of water-soluble contrast media in myelography, cisternography, and ventriculography. *Acta Radiol [Suppl] (Stockh)* 1977; 355:359–370.

19. Peeters FLM: Myelography with metrizamide. *Radiol Clin* 1977; 46:203–213.

20. Drayer BP, Rosenbaum AE, Reigel DB, et al: Metrizamide computed tomography cisternography: Pediatric applications. *Radiology* 1977; 124:349–357.

21. Sleven D: Personal communication, 1983.

22. Caille JM, Guibert-Trainer F, Howa JM, et al: Cerebral penetration following metrizamide myelography. *J Neuroradiol* 1980; 7:3–12.

23. Hayman LA, Pagani JJ, Anderson GM, et al: Concentration of intrathecal[3]H labeled metrizamide in normal dog brain: I. Age related differences. *AJNR* 1983; 4:1091–1096.

24. Fenstermacher JD, Bradbury MW, duBoulay G, et al: The distribution of[125]I-metrizamide and ^{125}I-diatrizoate between blood, brain, and cerebrospinal fluid in the rabbit. *Neuroradiology* 1980; 19:171–180.

25. Hayman LA, Hinck VC, Pagani JJ, et al: Regional differences in permeability of the cisternal spaces of the normal brain. In preparation.

26. Winkler SS, Sackett JF: Explanation of metrizamide brain penetration: A review. *J Comput Assist Tomogr* 1980; 4:191–193.

27. Levin E, Arieff A, Kleeman CR: Evidence of different compartments in the brain for extracellular markers. *Am J Physiol* 1971; 221:1319–1326.

28. Holtas S, Morris TW, Ekholm SE, et al: Penetration of subarachnoid contrast medium into rabbit spinal cord: Comparison between metrizamide and iohexol. *Invest Radiol* 1986; 21:151–155.

29. Weed LH, McKibben PS: Pressure changes in the cerebro-spinal fluid following intravenous injection of solutions of various concentrations. *Am J Physiol* 1919; 48:512–530.

30. Eldevick OP, Nakken KO, Haughton VM: The effect of dehydration on the side effects of metrizamide myelography. *Radiology* 1978; 129:715–716.

31. Potts DG, Gomez DG, Abbott GF: Possible causes of complications of myelography with water-soluble contrast medium. *Acta Radiol [Suppl] (Stockh)* 1977; 355:390–402.

32. Cuypers J, Matakas F, Potolicchio SJ Jr: Effect of central venous pressure on brain tissue pressure and brain volume. *J Neurosurg* 1976; 45:89–94.

33. Matakas F, Stechele S, Keller F: Microcirculations within the cerebral extracellular space, in Cervol-Navarro J, Betz E, Ebhardt G, et al (eds): *Advances in Neurology.* New York, Raven Press, 1978, pp 125–131.

34. Cserr HF, Ostrach LH: Bulk flow of interstitial fluid after intracranial injection of blue dextran 2000. *Exp Neurol* 1974; 45:50–60.

35. Sand T, Stovner LJ, Dale L, et al: Side effects after diagnostic lumbar puncture and lumbar iohexol myelography. *Neuroradiology* 1987; 29:385–388.

36. Malnor MD, Houston LW, Strother CM, et al: Iotrol versus metrizamide in lumbar myelography: A double-blind study. *Radiology* 1986; 158:845–847.

37. Maly P, Almen T, Golman L, Olivecrona H: Excitative effects in anaesthetized rabbits from subarachnoidally injected iso- and hyperosmolar solutions of iohexol and metrizamide. *Neuroradiology* 1984; 26:131–136.

38. Broadbridge AT, Bayliss SG, Brayshaw CI: The effect of intrathecal iohexol on visual evoked response latency: A comparison including incidence of headache with iopamidol and metrizamide in myeloradiculography. *Clin Radiol* 1987; 38:71–74.

39. Hoe JWM, Ng AMN, Tan LKA: A comparison of iohexol and iopamidol for lumbar myelography. *Clin Radiol* 1986; 37:505–507.

40. Ekholm SE, Morris TW, Fonte D, et al: Iopamidol and neural tissue metabolism: A comparative in vitro study. *Invest Radiol* 1986; 21:798–801.

41. Simon JH, Elholm SE, Kido DK, et al: High dose iohexol myelography. *Radiology* 1987; 163:455–458.

42. Wood AK, Kundel HL, McGrath JT, et al: Computed tomography, magnetic resonance imaging, and pathologic observations of the effects of intrathecal metrizamide and iohexol on the canine central nervous system. *Invest Radiol* 1987; 22:672–677.

43. Drayer BD, Dujovny M, Boehnke M, et al: The capacity for computed tomography diagnosis of cerebral infarction. *Radiology* 1977; 125:393–402.

44. Barnett HJM, Fox A, Vinuela F, et al: Delayed metrizamide CT observations in syringomyelia (abstract). *Ann Neurol* 1980; 8:116.

45. Dubois PJ, Drayer BP, Sage M, et al: Intramedullary penetrance of metrizamide in the dog spinal cord. *AJNR* 1981; 2:313–317.

46. Hiratsuka H, Fujiwara K, Okada K, et al: Modification of periventricular hypodensity in hydrocephalus with ventricular reflux in metrizamide CT cisternography. *J Comput Assist Tomogr* 1979; 3:204–208.

47. Fitz CR, Harwood-Nash DC, Chuang S, et al: Metrizamide ventriculography and computed tomography in infants and children. *Neuroradiology* 1978; 16:6–9.

48. Hindmarsh T: Computed cisternography for evaluation of CSF flow dynamics. *Acta Radiol [Suppl] (Stockh)* 1977; 355:269–279.

49. Symonn L, Hinzpeter T: The enigma of normal pressure hydrocephalus: Tests to select patients for surgery and to predict shunt function. *Clin Neurosurg* 1976; 24:285–315.

50. Bettman MA: Angiographic contrast agents. Conventional and new media compared. *AJR* 1982; 139:787–794.

51. McClennan BL: Low-osmolality contrast media: Premises and promises. *Radiology* 1987; 162:1–8.

52. Kido DK, Potts DG, Bryan RN, et al: Iohexol cerebral angiography: Multicenter clinical trial. *Invest Radiol* 1985; 20 (suppl):S55–S57.

53. Amundsen P, Dugstad G, Presthus J, et al: Randomized double-blind cross-over study of iohexol and amipaque in cerebral angiography. *AJNR* 1983; 4:342–343.

54. Pelz D, Fox AJ, Vinuela F, et al: Clinical trial of iohexol vs. Conray 60 for cerebral angiography. *AJNR* 1984; 5:565–568.

55. Bird CR, Drayer BP, Velaj R, et al: Safety of contrast media in cerebral angiography: Iopamidol vs. methylglucamine iothalamate. *AJNR* 1984; 5:801–803.

56. Hindmarsh T, Bergstrand G, Ericson Kl, et al: Comparative double-blind investigation of meglumine metrizoate, metrizamide, and iohexol in carotid angiography. *AJNR* 1983; 4:347–349.

57. Grainger RG: A clinical trial of new low osmolality contrast medium: Sodium and meglumine ioxaglate (Hexabrix) compared with meglumine iothalamate (Conray) for carotid arteriography. *Br J Radiol* 1979; 52:781–786.

58. Norman D, Brant-Zawadzki M, Sobel D: Neuroangiography: Tolerability and efficacy of Hexabrix in cerebral angiography. *Invest Radiol* 1984; 19:S306–S307.

59. Robertson WD, Nugent RA, Russell DB, et al: Clinical experience with Hexabrix in cerebral angiography. *Invest Radiol* 1984; 19:S308–S311.

60. Matozzi F, Turski PA, Gentry LR, et al: Cerebral angiography: Clinical comparison of iopamidol and Conray-60. *Invest Radiol* 1984; 19:S219–S221.

61. Pinto RS, Berenstein A: The use of iopamidol in cerebral angiography. *Invest Radiol* 1984; 19:S222–S224.

62. Bryan RN, Miller SL, Roehm JOF, et al: Neuroangiography with iohexol. *AJNR* 1983; 4:344–346.

63. Drayer BP, Velaj RV, Bird R, et al: Comparative safety of intracarotid iopamidol, iothalamate, meglumine, and diatrizoate meglumine for cerebral angiography. *Invest Radiol* 1984; 19:S212–S218.

64. Stormorken H, Skalpe IO, Testart MC: Effect of various contrast media on coagulation, fibrinolysis and platelet function: An in vitro and in vivo study. *Invest Radiol* 1986; 21:348–354.

65. Dawson P, Hewitt P, Mackie IJ, et al: Contrast, coagulation, and fibrinolysis. *Invest Radiol* 1986; 21:248–252.

66. Sage MR, Wilcox J, Evill CA, et al: Comparison of blood brain barrier disruption following intracarotid metrizamide and methylglucamine iothalamate (Conray 280). *Australas Radiol,* 1982; 26:225–228.

67. Mutzel W: Properties of conventional contrast media, in Felix R, Kazner E, Wegener OH (eds): *Contrast Media in Computed Tomography.* Amsterdam, Excerpta Medica, 1981, pp 19–30.

68. Sage MR, Drayer BP, Dubois PJ, et al: Increased permeability of the blood-brain-barrier after carotid Renografin-76. *AJNR* 1981; 2:272–274.

69. Lasser EC, Berry CC, Talner LB, et al: Pretreatment with corticosteroids to alleviate reactions to intravenous contrast material. *N Engl J Med* 1987; 317:845–849.

70. Bradbury M: *The Concept of a Blood-Brain Barrier.* New York, John Wiley & Sons, Inc, 1979, pp 38–58.

71. Caille JM, Billerey J, Renou AM, et al: Cerebral blood volume and water extraction from cerebral parenchyma by hyperosmolar contrast media. *Neuroradiology* 1978; 16:579–582.

72. Feldman S, Hayman LA, Hulse M: Pharmacokinetics of low and high dose intravenous diatrizoate contrast media administration. *Invest Radiol* 1984; 19:54–57.

73. Zamani AA, Kido DK, Morris JH, et al: Permeability of the blood brain barrier to different doses of diatrizoate meglumine-60. *AJNR* 1982; 3:631–634.

74. Hayman LA, Pagani JJ, Serur JR, et al: Impermeability of the blood barrier to intravenous high-iodine-dose meglumine diatrizoate in the normal dog. *AJNR* 1984; 5:409–411.

75. Sage MR: Blood-brain barrier: Phenomenon of increasing importance to the imaging clinician. *AJNR* 1982; 3:127–138.

76. Hayman LA, Sakai F, Meyer JS, et al: Iodine enhanced CT patterns after cerebral arterial embolization in baboons. *AJNR* 1980; 1:233–238.

77. Hayman LA, Evans RA, Bastion FO, et al: Delayed high dose contrast CT: Identifying patients at risk of massive hemorrhagic infarction. *AJNR* 1981; 2:139–147.

78. DiChiro G, Timins EL, Jones AE, et al: Radionuclide scanning and microangiography of evolving and completed brain infarction. A correlative study in monkeys. *Neurology* 1974; 24:418–423.

79. Cancilla PA, Frommes SP, Kahn LE, et al: Regeneration of cerebral microvessels: A morphologic and histochemical study after local freeze-injury. *Lab Invest* 1979; 40:74–82.

80. Kinkel WR, Jacobs L, Kinkel PR: Grey matter enhancement: A computerized tomographic sign of cerebral hypoxia. *Neurology* 1980; 30:810–819.

81. Dudley AW, Lunzer S, Heyman A: Localization of radioisotope (chloromerodrin Hg-203) in experimental cerebral infarction. *Stroke* 1970; 1:143–148.

82. Anderson DC, Coss DT, Jacobson RL, et al: Tissue pertechnetate and iodinated contrast material in ischemic stroke. *Stroke* 1980; 11:617–622.

83. O'Brien MD, Jordan MM, Waltz AG: Ischemic cerebral edema and the blood brain barrier. *Arch Neurol* 1974; 30:461–465.

84. Kinkel W: Personal communication, 1980.

85. Valk J: High dose contrast injections and cerebral infarctions, in *Computed Tomography and Cerebral Infarctions with an Introduction to Practice and Principles of CT Scan Reading*, New York, Raven Press, 1980, pp 45–46.

86. Kendall BE, Pullicino P: Intravascular contrast injection in ischemia lesions: II. Effect on prognosis. *Neuroradiology* 1980; 19:241–243.

87. Pullicino P, Kendall BE: Contrast enhancement in ischemia lesions. I. Relationship to prognosis. *Neuroradiology* 1980; 19:235–239.

88. Gado MH, Phelps ME, Coleman RE: An extravascular component of contrast enhancement in cranial computed tomography: Part II. Contrast enhancement and the blood-tissue barrier. *Radiology* 1975; 117:595–597.

89. Crocker EF, Zimmerman RA, Phelps ME, et al: The effect of steroids on the extravascular distribution of radiographic contrast material and technetium pertechnetate in brain tumors as determined by computed tomography. *Radiology* 1976; 119:471–474.

90. Davis JM, Davis KR, Newhouse J, et al: Expanded high iodine dose in computed cranial tomography: A preliminary report. *Radiology* 1979; 131:373–380.

91. Shalen PR, Hayman LA, Wallace S, et al: Protocol for delayed contrast enhancement in computed tomography for cerebral neoplasia. *Radiology* 1981; 139:397–402.

92. Hayman LA, Evans RA, Hinck VC: Delayed high iodine dose contrast computed tomography: Cranial neoplasms. *Radiology* 1980; 136:677–684.

93. Raininko R, Majurin ML, Virtama P, et al: Value of high contrast medium dose in brain CT. *J Comput Assist Tomogr* 1982; 6:54–57.

94. Takeda N, Tanaka R, Nakai O, et al: Dynamics of contrast enhancement in delayed computed tomography of brain tumors: Tissue-blood ratio and differential diagnosis. *Radiology* 1982; 142:663–668.

95. Tator CH: Chemotherapy of brain tumors: Uptake of tritiated methotrexate by a transplantable intracerebral ependymoblastoma in mice. *J Neurosurg* 1972; 37:1–8.

96. Neuwelt EA, Maravilla KR, Frenkel EP, et al: Osmotic blood-brain barrier disruption: Computerized tomographic monitoring of chemotherapeutic agent delivery. *J Clin Invest* 1979; 64:684–688.

97. Pagani JJ, Hayman LA, Bigelow RH, et al: Diazepam prophylaxis of contrast media-induced seizures during computed tomography of patients with brain metastases. *AJNR* 1983; 4:67–72.

98. LoZito JC: Convulsions: A complication of contrast enhancement in computerized tomography. *Arch Neurol* 1977; 34:649–650.

99. Scott WR: Seizures: A reaction to contrast media for computed tomography of the brain. *Radiology* 1980; 137:359–361.

100. Pagani JJ, Hayman LA, Bigelow RH, et al: Prophylactic diazepam in prevention of contrast media associated seizures in glioma patients undergoing cerebral computed tomography. *AJNR* 1983; 4:67–72.

101. Fischer HW: Occurrence of seizure during cranial computed tomography. Opinion. *Radiology* 1980; 137:563–564.

102. Penn RD, Walser R, Kurtz D, et al: Tumor volume, luxury perfusion, and regional blood volume changes in man visualized by subtraction computerized tomography. *J Neurosurg* 1976; 44:449–457.

103. Whelan MA, Hilal SK: Computed tomography as a guide in the diagnosis and followup of brain abscesses. *Radiology* 1980; 135:663–671.

104. Enzmann DR, Britt RH, Yeager AS: Experimental brain abscess evolution: Computed tomographic and neuropathologic correlation. *Radiology* 1979; 133:113–122.

105. Britt RH, Enzmann DR, Yeager AS: Neuropathological and computerized tomographic findings in experimental brain abscess. *J Neurosurg* 1981; 55:590–603.

106. Enzmann DR, Brant-Zawadzki M, Britt RH: CT of central nervous system infections in immunocompromised patients. *AJR* 1980; 135:263–267.

107. Heinz ER, Drayer BP, Haenggeli CA, et al: Computed tomography in white matter disease. *Radiology* 1979; 130:371–378.

108. Whelan MA, Stern J: Intracranial tuberculoma. *Radiology* 1981; 138:75–81.

109. Junck L, Enzmann DR, DeArmond SJ, et al: Prolonged brain retention of contrast agent in neonatal herpes simplex encephalitis. *Radiology* 1981; 140:123–126.

110. Pinto RS, Kricheff II, Butler AR, et al: Correlation of computed tomographic, angiographic and neuropathological changes in giant cerebral aneurysms. *Radiology* 1979; 132:85–92.

111. Hayman LA, Fox AJ, Evans RA: Effectiveness of contrast regimens in CT detection of vascular malformations of the brain. *AJNR* 1981; 2:421–425.

112. Hayman LA, Evans RA, Hinck VC: Rapid high-dose contrast computed tomography of isodense subdural hematoma and cerebral swelling. *Radiology* 1979; 131:381–383.

113. Amendola MA, Ostrum BJ: Diagnosis of isodense subdural hematomas by computed tomography. *AJR* 1977; 129:693–697.

114. Nabeshima S, Reese TS, Landis DMD, et al: Junctions in the meninges and marginal glia. *J Comp Neurol* 1975; 164:127–169.

115. Drayer BP, Schmeckel DE, Hedlund LW, et al: Radiographic quantitation of reversible blood-brain barrier disruption in vivo. *Radiology* 1982; 143:85–89.

116. Neuwelt EA, Maravilla KR, Frenkel EP, et al: Use of enhanced computerized tomography to evaluate osmotic blood-brain barrier disruption. *Neurosurgery* 1980; 6:49–56.

117. Fike JR, Cann CE, Turowski K, et al: Contrast enhancement of brain tumors and irradiated normal brain: A comparison of iohexol and iothalamate. *Neuroradiology* 1986; 28:61–64.

118. Shalen PR, Ostrow PT, Glass PJ: Enhancement of the white matter following prophylactic therapy of the central nervous system for leukemia. *Radiology* 1981; 140:409–412.

119. Pettersson H, Harwood-Nash DCF, Fitz CR, et al: Contrast enhancement of the irradiated spinal cord in children. *AJNR* 1981; 2:581–584.

120. Vinuela FV, Fox AJ, Debrun GM, et al: New perspectives in computed tomography of multiple sclerosis. *AJR* 1982; 139:123–127.

121. Sears ES, McCammon A, Bigelow R, et al: Maximizing the harvest of contrast enhancing lesions in multiple sclerosis. *Neurology* 1982; 32:815–820.

5

Paramagnetic Contrast Agents for MR Imaging of the Brain

Gerald L. Wolf, Ph.D., M.D.

Upon discovering new territory, the explorers who have visited the region often describe more than they have actually seen. The Fountain of Youth and regions of untold wealth beyond the next barrier alternate with tales of fierce savages and extraordinary dangers. Although this makes for entertaining stories, subsequent reality debunks many of these myths. In prior times, the spreader of such inaccurate information might have produced a few decades of ignorance before the truth was revealed. Of late, the lifetimes of myths in medicine have been much shorter.

The early myths of nuclear magnetic resonance (NMR) seem quite human in this context (Table 5–1). None of these dogmatic statements by excellent investigators have held up because they were predictions rather than documented measurements. It is clear that the injection of contrast agents would be avoided if they were unnecessary. Tomorrow's science may realize this dream, but today's reality indicates that magnetic resonance (MR) contrast agents can be extremely helpful in MR imaging (MRI) of the central nervous system (CNS) and adjacent structures.

The use of paramagnetic agents to increase proton relaxation and shorten experiment time began almost at the same time as the NMR phenomenon was described. Felix Bloch and colleagues described the use of ferric nitrate to increase the relaxation rate of protons in water.[1] The chelates of paramagnetic metals were seriously reviewed by Dwek et al in 1971,[2] but the first report of biological efficacy was based upon $MnCl_2$ perfusion of tissues by Lauterbur et al.[3] Independently, Schering and Mallinckrodt began to explore paramagnetic chelates as potential MR contrast agents in 1980. My laboratory worked closely with Mallinckrodt, and we were first to report the effects of gadolinium–diethylenetriamine pentaacetic acid (Gd-DTPA) upon tissue proton relaxation in an abstract submitted in December 1982.[4]

The Schering group made the first MR images with Gd-DTPA on May 5, 1982,[5] and sent their compounds to Dr. Robert Brasch of the University of California, San Francisco in June 1982, where the first images in this country were made on rats.[6,7] In December 1983, the first human trials were begun in Germany,[8] and 1 year later Dr. Kenneth Maravella began clinical trials in the United States. European experience with Gd-DTPA reached several thousand cases by the time that Berlex submitted its completed clinical trial of 458 cases to the Food and Drug Administration (FDA) in August 1986. The FDA approval process took 22 months for a single clinical indication—neoplasms of the brain.

There are numerous other paramagnetic chelates that could be useful in the CNS, including Gd-DOTA (tetraazacyclododecane-tetraacetic acid) and relatives, iron desferroximine (S-FDF, SALUTAR), and nonionic compounds. In the historical context, it is appropriate to recognize the development of organic paramagnetics by Brasch et al.[9] and the first use of ferrite agents by Wolf et al.,[10] even though these compounds do not have current utility in the CNS.

TABLE 5–1.

NMR Myths of Our Youth

Signals too weak for imaging
Long wavelengths preclude anatomic resolution
Radiofrequency penetration inadequate above 15 MHz
MRI will always be slow
MRI will never need contrast agents
No tissue contrast above 100 MHz

TABLE 5–2.

Stimulated Nuclear Relaxation Requirements

Close encounter with another magnetic field
  (<10 Å for another proton)
Right magnetic field
  (same frequency or a multiple)
Adequate time for effective interaction
  (microseconds at body temperature)

BASIC PRINCIPLES OF NUCLEAR RELAXATION ENHANCEMENT BY PARAMAGNETICS

Nuclear relaxation is basically a stimulated process somewhat similar to the laser phenomenon. Relaxation mechanisms are somewhat different for nuclei with spin $>\frac{1}{2}$, so we will focus chiefly on proton relaxation. A single excited proton located well away from other nuclei would require many years to relax. Relaxation is facilitated if there is another magnetic field nearby that can influence the stable orientation of a single proton in a strong magnetic field (Fig 5–1).

Table 5–2 shows the necessary characteristics for the two magnetic fields to mutually interact. The tiny magnetic moment of a proton generates a

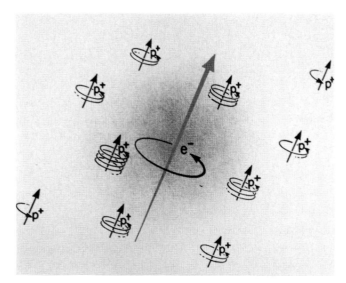

FIG 5–1.
Although there are many protons in an aqueous sample, they have a small field *(p)* and brief close encounters. In pure water, proton T1 and T2 times are about 4,000 ms. An unpaired electron *(e–)* creates a very large field, and this enhances the proton relaxation rate. (From Brasch RC: Contrast enhancement in NMR imaging, in Newton TH, Potts DG (eds): *Modern Neuroradiology*, vol 2: *Advanced Imaging Techniques.* San Anselme, Calif, Clavet Press, 1983, p 66. Used by permission.)

very small sphere of influence because magnetic field strength falls off by the third power of the distance from the nucleus, or by $1/r^6$ in the case of three dimensions.[11] For two protons, the magnetic fields must approach within a few angstroms to be effective. For the fields to effectively interact, the frequencies must be the same or in multiples thereof. Finally, the magnetic interaction must continue for a relatively long time (microseconds).

Pure water has numerous protons that precess at the same frequency, and this makes close approaches common. In water, there is another proton only a few angstroms away. Close encounters between protons, however, are usually quite brief, with a statistical average duration of only picoseconds. Thus, water usually has a very long T1 and an equally long T2. Adding large molecules that tumble slowly seemingly slows the proton movement in close proximity to the macromolecule, and this increases the proton contact time and efficiency of proton interaction. In biological tissue, water protons have T1 relaxation 3 to 12 times faster and T2 relaxation 10 to 80 times faster.

Paramagnetic substances have electrons with unpaired spin and thus generate a magnetic field around them, but this field is 657 times as large as the magnetic field around a proton. This huge field makes it more likely that the proton will remain within distance for the necessary microseconds to stimulate proton relaxation (see Fig 5–1). The mathematics of this is compelling: 0.1 nmol/mL of Gd will double the proton relaxation rate of water!

There are many metals that have one or more unpaired electrons (Fig 5–2), and all will increase proton relaxation in water. It only remains for a chemist to ensure safety and appropriate targeting. Many of the potential paramagnetics are too weak, too insoluble, too toxic, unstable in their chelates, or not available in practical form for clinical use. Chelates of Fe^{3+}, Mn^{2+}, and Gd^{3+} are currently favored.

The relaxation of protons associated with proteins or other molecules is field and temperature

Atomic No.	Ion	Electronic Configuration		Magnetic Moment (Bohr Magnetons)
		3d	4f	
24	Cr^{3+}	↑ ↑ ↑		3.8
25	Mn^{2+}	↑ ↑ ↑ ↑ ↑		5.9 (weak field)
26	Fe^{3+}	↑ ↑ ↑ ↑ ↑		5.9 (weak field)
29	Cu^{2+}	↑↓ ↑↓ ↑↓ ↑↓ ↑		1.7–2.2
63	Eu^{3+}		↑↓ ↑ ↑ ↑ ↑ ↑ ↑	(6.9)
64	Gd^{3+}		↑ ↑ ↑ ↑ ↑ ↑ ↑	7.9
66	Dy^{3+}		↑↓ ↑↓ ↑ ↑ ↑ ↑ ↑	(5.9)

Note.—Upright arrow denotes an electron with a spin of $+\frac{1}{2}$; downward arrow denotes an electron with a spin of $-\frac{1}{2}$.

FIG 5–2.
Parmagnetic metals with unpaired electrons. Relaxation effects will be increased if there are more unpaired electrons and if the magnetic moment is large. (From Runge VM, Clanton JA, Lukehart CM, et al: *AJR* 1983; 141:1209–1215. Used by permission.)

dependent. For clinical circumstances, we usually ignore temperature as a variable. The influence of the paramagnetic is also field dependent (Fig 5–3).

The Gd ion is potentially very toxic. It may penetrate the cell through calcium channels, bind avidly to protein, and cause enough distortion in tertiary structure to impair the function of that protein. The damaged protein-Gd complex is often carried to the liver for degradation. This subjects the liver to excess Gd and can create the risk of hepatotoxicity. There are body homeostatic systems for Fe and Mn. Normally, the body has huge stores of organic iron in hemoglobin, myoglobin, and transferrin but absorbs dietary iron poorly and usually in direct proportion to its need. Internal iron is recirculated, but inorganic iron ions are toxic, and the body is poorly prepared to deal with a large amount of soluble inorganic iron. Fortunately, iron is not very soluble at body pH. Because excretory mechanisms have low capacity, a few hundred milligrams of soluble ferric iron injected parenterally could be dangerous. On the other hand, manganese homeostasis usually allows much more manganese absorption and manganese excretion, principally via the hepatobiliary route, and this is much more efficient. Because Mn^{2+} is more soluble, more potent, and less toxic than Fe^{3+} simple Mn salts could be useful. Mn does accumulate in the brain and heart to cause toxicity, but conclusions about the unsuitability of $MnCl_2$ for safe and effective use in humans may be premature. (Mea culpa—I said it too!)[12]

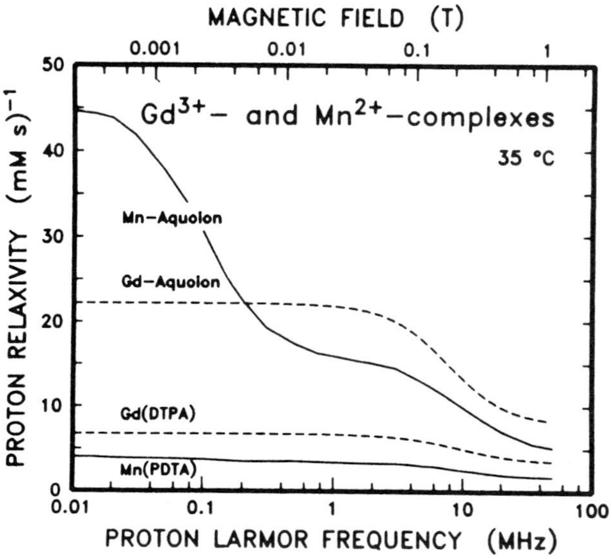

Nuclear medicine had developed a large number of chelates for metals to enable effective organ imaging with ^{59}Fe, [54]Mn, ^{51}Cr, ^{99m}Tc, ^{111}In, or [153]Gd. It was only natural to use these chelates for stable paramagnetic isotopes. Chelation is expected to decrease toxicity—often by restricting penetration of the metal into cells and/or by increasing clearance. Chelation could further alter tissue biodistribution in useful ways. Both of these properties would require the paramagnetic metal-chelate complex to be quite stable.[13] In vivo, the relative abundance of other metal cations in the body creates the opportunity for competitive displacement of the more toxic paramagnetic metal. Time, pH, solubility, metabolism, and concentration of the competitors are important variables. It has been possible to create very stable Gd chelates (DTPA, DOTA, NOTA [triazacyclononanetriacetic acid]), Fe chelates (EHPG [ethylene bis-(2-hydroxyphenylglycine)], desferroxamine), and Mn chelates (porphyrins), but current CNS interest is focused on Gd-DTPA.

When gadolinium is effectively captured in-

FIG 5–3.
Field dependence of hydrated metal ions (aquoions) and metal chelates. Relaxivity is expressed as 1/T1 per millimole of agent to show patency. Aquoions are much more powerful at very low field. Chelation reduces relaxivity of the paramagnetic metal and also reduces field dependency. (From Koenig SH, Spiller M, Brown RD III, et al: *Nucl Med Biol* 1988; 15:23–29. Used by permission.)

side the chelate, the Gd toxicity is reduced a hundredfold, and biodistribution is dominated by the DTPA. Unfortunately, the chelate binds many of the paramagnetic electrons and reduces the opportunity for water protons to closely approach the remaining unpaired electrons. Thus, potency (effect per milligram) is reduced. Chelates of paramagnetic metals are less potent than aquoions are, and the chelate also has a field-dependent effect (Fig 5–4). We model the structure of Gd-DTPA as shown in Figure 5–5.[14]

With all these caveats, why is Gd-DTPA so useful in brain imaging? First, the median lethal dose (LD_{50}) is reduced to approximately 10 to 20 mmol/kg (species and method dependent).[15] Not only is Gd tightly bound ($K_{sp} \sim 10^{27}$; there is 10^{27} bound ions for every one that is free), but DTPA is large enough to keep the Gd out of cells and small enough to ensure rapid renal excretion.[13, 14] In general, hepatobiliary excretion requires penetration of the hepatocyte, and Gd-DTPA is a poor biliary agent.[14] Although Gd-DTPA detection is device dependent (field, signal-noise ratio, pulse parameters) and local accumulation varies with the extracellular fluid (ECF) volume and vascular permeability, the effective imaging dose of Gd-DTPA is approximately 0.1 mmol/Kg. Thus, the relative

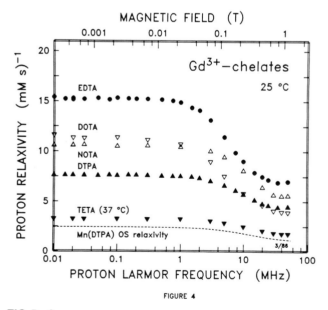

FIG 5–4.
Field dependence of some chelates of gadolinium. Ethylenediaminetetraacetic acid (EDTA) does not bind as many electrons, thus leaving more opportunity for a water proton to closely approach an unpaired electron, but Gd-EDTA is much more toxic. DOTA, NOTA, and TETA (5-nitrogen analog of NOTA) are other chelates for gadolinium. (From Koenig SH, Baglin C, Brown RD III, et al: *Magn Reson Med* 1984; 1:496–501. Used by permission.)

Na$_2$[Gd DTPA]

OCTADENTATE CHELATE

FIG 5–5.
The general structure of Gd-DTPA is schematically shown. Five of the seven unpaired 4f orbitals are bound by the chelate. Two electrons are free and must be balanced by cations—two sodiums here, but two meglumines in Magnevist. (From Goldstein EJ, Burnett KR, Hansell JR, et al: *Physiol Chem Phys Med NMR* 1984; 16:97–104. Used by permission.)

safety index for Gd-DTPA is much greater for imaging the damaged blood-brain barrier (BBB) with MRI than when using water-soluble x-ray contrast agents and computed tomography (CT).

Gd-DTPA has a net −2 charge that is balanced by two meglumine ions in the Magnevist formulation. The resulting clinical product has the characteristics shown in Table 5–3. In comparison with Renografin-76, the formulation is equally hypertonic, less viscous, less concentrated, and of lower density. At high concentration the Gd-DTPA will form layers vs. less dense solutions, but this is chiefly seen in the urinary bladder.[16] As an extra-

TABLE 5–3.

Magnevist Injection (Brand of Gadopentatate Dimeglumine)

Composition	469 mg Gd-DTPA
	0.4 mg meglumine
	0.2 mg DTPA (0.5 mol/L)
Molecular weight	938
pH	6.5–8.0
Osmolality	1.94 mOsm/kg
Viscosity	2.9 centipoise
Density	1.199 g/mL

TABLE 5–4.

Enhancement Agents for Brain Imaging: Mechanism

Modality	Agent	Mechanism
CT	Iodine	Absorption
MRI	Gadolinium	Enhanced relaxation
SPECT*	Technetium	Radiation

*SPECT = single-photon emission computed tomography.

cellular agent, Gd-DTPA will be rapidly distributed following bolus injection (plasma half-life [$T\frac{1}{2}$] about 12 minutes) and rapidly excreted by normal kidneys (excretion $T\frac{1}{2}$ about 60 minutes).[8, 14]

Because Gd-DTPA remains extracellular, it has little opportunity to influence the protons on lipids that are predominantly intracellular. The ECF space is large but normally much smaller than a cell diameter. Visualize the normal ECF as a huge film of fluid. In most current brain applications, Gd-DTPA is excluded from the ECF in circulations where there are tight capillary junctions, i.e., brain, spinal cord, retina, anterior chamber of the eye. The mechanism of Gd-DTPA enhancement of MR images is indirect. Most other imaging devices directly detect the contrast agent (Table 5–4).

MRI DETECTOR AND MR PARAMAGNETIC CONTRAST INTERACTION

Current imaging instruments are sensitive to proton concentration, proton T1 and T2 relaxation times, and motion. Paramagnetic agents increase both T1 and T2 proton relaxation within their small sphere of influence.[16–18] Actually T2 is shortened about 15% more than T1. In most imaging sequences, more rapid proton T1 relaxation *increases* signal when pulse repetition is <4 T1, and rapid proton T2 relaxation *decreases* signal when image intensity varies with echo time (TE). Most available MRI devices have minimal TE above 20

ms and use T2-weighted scans to detect abnormality. Due to this complex and competitive effect upon MRI signal, Gd-DTPA enhancement is both dose and detector (MRI instrument) sensitive.

Without Gd-DTPA, T2-weighted sequences are designed to reduce the influence of T1 and emphasize proton density and T2. In this circumstance, Gd-DTPA would have little benefit because T1 relaxation is nearly complete between pulses, and this could lead to a loss of T2-dependent signal. Note that proton density is not affected by Gd-DTPA, although signal obtained from protons is affected. A plot of Gd-DTPA concentration vs. dose with any sequence where T1 and T2 influence signal oppositely will show an inflection point where Gd-DTPA reduces the MRI signal (Fig 5–6). T1-weighted sequences still have some but less T2 weighting, and the inflection point for Gd-DTPA will be shifted to a higher dose. Some have loosely stated that T2 is not affected at a low dose of Gd-DTPA. This is incorrect.

Thus, the local tissue concentration of Gd-DTPA and the imaging parameters necessarily influence the detection of Gd-DTPA. When the detector is appropriately programmed, the detection of Gd-DTPA is exquisitely sensitive as shown in Figures 5–7 and 5–8. Further, the ratio of lethal dose to effective imaging dose is much better with Gd-DTPA than with x-ray agents (Table 5–5).

Using motion-sensitive pulse sequences such as spin-echo techniques can cause a flow void where proton motion is rapid relative to interpulse time. MRI signal is absent because there is no detectable transverse magnetization and thus Gd-DTPA cannot create more signal. In imaging circumstances where strong signal is present due to the continuous entrance of fully magnetized protons between pulses ("paradoxical enhancement"), Gd-DTPA will also be ineffective because these "fresh" protons are fully relaxed. Thus, rapidly moving blood usually shows no Gd-DTPA effect at reasonable doses. Where blood is stagnant or mov-

TABLE 5–5.

Contrast Agents for Brain Imaging: Safety

Modality	Agent	Imaging Dose	Lethal Dose	Safety Index
CT	Iodine (as iothalamute)	600 mg I/kg	9,000 mg I/kg	15
MRI	Gadolinium (as gadopentatate)	0.1 mmol/kg	15 mmol/kg	150
Gamma camera	Technetium (as technopentatate)	10 mg/kg	—	—

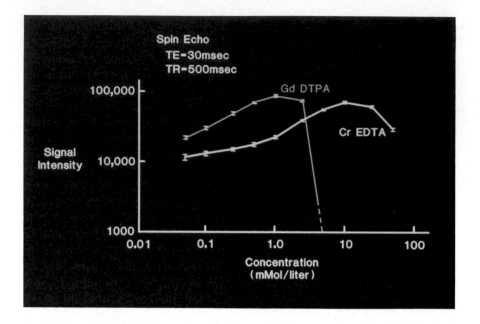

FIG 5-6.
With the MRI device set to have a short repetition time (TR) and relatively short TE, MR signal intensity increases with the concentration of Gd-DTPA in this log-log graph. When the T2 of the solution begins to approach 30 ms, the signal loss is so great that Gd-DTPA solutions have *less* intensity than do solutions with very low concentration. (From Runge VM, Clanton JA, Lukehart CM, et al: *AJR* 1983; 141:1209–1215. Used by permission.)

ing slowly enough that actual blood T1 and T2 times are reflected in the images, then the presence of Gd-DTPA will also be visible in the resulting images.

The purpose of an administered contrast agent is to differentially change one of two or more tissues. The major use of Gd-DTPA in the CNS is to demonstrate a region where the BBB is leaky. With respect to the BBB, Gd-DTPA and water-soluble xray contrast agents behave identically, and most radiologists will have an instinct for appropriate use. From the foregoing, a few caveats emerge. First, properly performed MRI will detect the recommended dose of Gd-DTPA with much greater sensitivity than will CT with its contrast agents. Due to detector-indicator interaction, the breach in

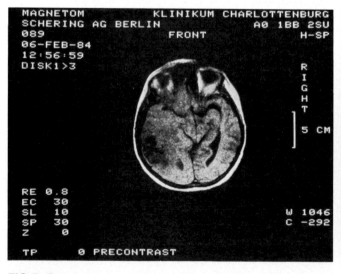
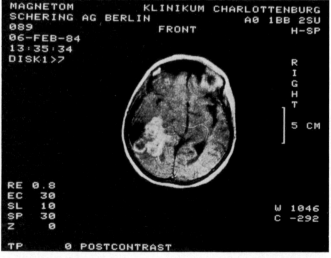

FIG 5-7.
An early patient study from the Schering trials in Germany. **A,** an axial slice (TR 800, TE 30, 10-mm slice) of a patient with a left glioma done Feb 6, 1984. **B,** the same patient after Gd-DTPA/dimeglumine. (Courtesy of F. Niendorf.)

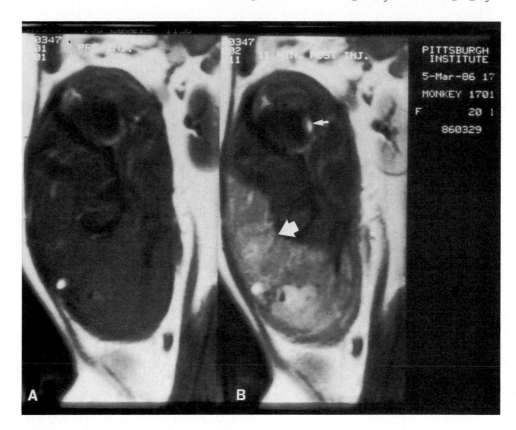

FIG 5–8.

Sagittal image of a pregnant monkey before **(A)** and 11 minutes after 0.05 mmol/kg Gd-DTPA **(B).** The placenta has a large ECF space **(B,** *large arrow)* and shows early opacification (within 45 seconds) and slow washout. However, some Gd-DTPA crosses the placenta and is excreted by the fetal genitourinary system. The Gd-DTPA is seen in the fetal bladder **(B,** *small arrow).* The monkey is actually supine, and the Gd-DTPA layers dependently.

the BBB could be missed due to inappropriate pulse parameters, too little *or* too much Gd-DTPA, or inappropriate timing.

Fortunately, the concern over too much Gd-DTPA causing signal loss due to excess T2 shortening is compensated for by the pathophysiology we are trying to detect. A disease that damages the barrier causes excess accumulation of ECF (Gd-DTPA does not enter intact cells), and this causes the local voxel T1 and T2 to be prolonged. We model the result in Table 5–6. (Note that the accumulated ECF has a much longer T2 than does gray or white matter). In our example, white matter and the region with excess ECF-like fluid will be indistinguishable on T1-weighted scans but fairly well distinguished on T2-weighted scans (however, gray and white matter are poorly distinguished).

TABLE 5–6.

Gd-DTPA and CNS Proton Relaxation

	Before Gd-DTPA				After Gd-DTPA			
			MR Intensity*				MR Intensity	
Tissue	T1	T2	T1W†	T2W†	T1	T2	T1W	T2W
Gray matter	850	75	0.29	0.31	800	73	0.30	0.31
White matter	680	65	0.14	0.28	675	64	0.14	0.27
Extracellular fluid 250	400	0.15	0.55	500	80	0.42	0.36	—

* MR intensity is calculated from the relation $(1 - e^{-\frac{TR}{T1}})\, e^{-\frac{TE}{T2}}$: T1W = TR 400 ms, TE 20ms; T2W = TR 2000ms, TE 80ms.

† T1W = T1 weighted; T2W = T2 weighted.

When we add Gd-DTPA, the abnormal zone will accumulate Gd-DTPA and lower both T1 and T2, the latter slightly more. However, since the T2 of the abnormal fluid was prolonged initially, the MR intensity change is well maintained, and there is superb characterization of all three tissues on T1-weighted and still excellent distinction on T2-weighted images. Note that gray and white matter change minimally due to an intact BBB. Edema without BBB leak will also be uninfluenced. Thus, the long T2 of the abnormal zone protects us from the shortening of T2 due to Gd-DTPA while still obtaining the benefits of the shortened T1.

Areas without a BBB will enhance in proportion to the permeability of the capillary to Gd-DTPA, the plasma level, the size of the ECF space, and the temporal relation between concentration gradients favoring outward diffusion (early) and inward diffusion (late). Thus, many normal tissues will enhance (Table 5–7). It is important to emphasize that Gd-DTPA moves through the ECF space by diffusion but the images reflect accumulation within a potentially small fraction of the tissue voxel. If the tissue with Gd-DTPA permeability has little ECF, it will be difficult to detect. A thickened, edematous structure that is permeable will have a stronger Gd-DTPA effect. With Gd-DTPA leaking into the lesion from the periphery and moving slowly centrally in proportion to diffusion—usually measured in centimeters per hour—time is important. Figure 5–9 is a striking example of this phenomenon.

Rapidly moving blood may not enhance, but slower-moving blood will. The effects of motion

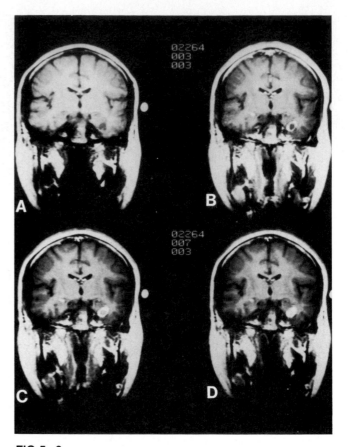

FIG 5–9.
Coronal T1-weighted scans (TR 500, TE 20) of a patient with a small left temporal glioma. **A,** before Magnevist. **B,** 3 minutes after; **C,** 30 minutes after; and **D,** 55 minutes after 0.1 mmol/kg Magnevist. The first Gd-DTPA accumulates at the rim of the tumor, but the center of the tumor is slowly opacified by diffusion of the contrast agent.

TABLE 5–7.
Enhancement of Normal Tissues With Gd-DTPA

Tissue	Enhancement (%)
Sinus mucosa	
Nasopharynx	100–200
Cavernous sinus	
Retinal choroid	
Infundibulum	
Pituitary gland	50–100
Choroid plexus	
Petrous carotid artery	
Falx	
Paraspinal muscle	
Parotid gland	10–50
Fat	
Gray matter	
White matter	0–5
CSF	
Large blood vessels	

vary with speed, direction relative to the gradients, and the exact imaging technique used. In general, any blood region with a moderate signal (not a "paradoxically" enhanced region) will give a stronger signal on T1-weighted scans for about two plasma half-lives, or about 15 to 30 minutes. Enhancement in the venous and cavernous sinus is expected.[19]

We can also negatively contrast a structure with slower accumulation of Gd-DTPA with a faster-enhancing structure (usually normal). As Table 5–7 shows, normal pituitary enhances, and pituitary adenoma or infarct usually enhances less and/or more slowly (Fig 5–10).

The available speed of dynamic MRI makes it possible to change the usual presentation of before and after images (still frames) into a "moving" picture of several frames that captures the local pharmacokinetics of Gd-DTPA (as shown in Fig 5–11).

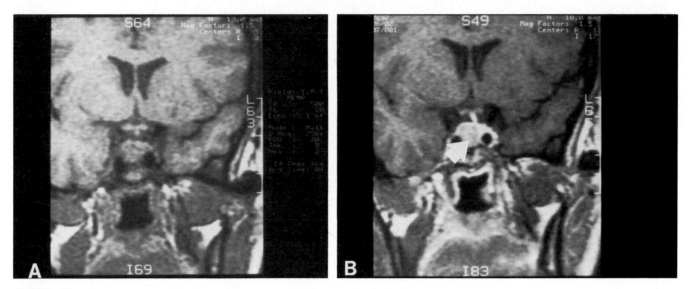

FIG 5–10.
Patient with pituitary microadenoma before **(A)** and several minutes after Gd-DTPA **(B).** The normal pituitary enhances more than the adenoma (**B,** *arrow*). (Courtesy of V. Haughton.)

The strong circulatory component of Gd-DTPA accumulation provides a physiologic sequence that may allow the radiologist to follow tumor response to antineoplastic intervention with much better sensitivity than by measuring tumor shrinkage.

THE MAGNEVIST CLINICAL TRIAL

In order to expedite FDA approval, Berlex made several choices for conducting its investigational new drug trials, and these have an impact on the data available to guide clinical use. A new drug application (NDA) must document safety and efficacy for a particular clinical indication. Because the FDA had not reviewed an agent from this drug class, a decision was made to seek approval for a single indication (brain neoplasm) at a single dose (0.1 mmol/kg) in trials in the United States. A very small placebo group was included for safety comparison. All patients were thought to have neoplasms—based upon clinical information and

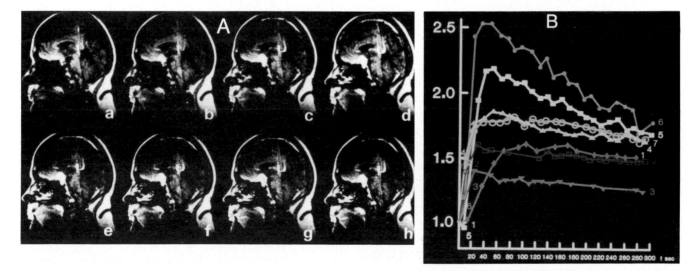

FIG 5–11.
Serial 10-second scans **(A)** before *(a)* and after *(b–h)* Gd-DTPA in a patient with sphenoid wing meningioma. These rapid pictures were obtained with the FLASH technique. The dynamic change in signal intensity for several meningomas **(B)** shows a common pattern of rapid opacification due to rapid circulation and a large ECF with no BBB. (Courtesy of R. Felix.)

TABLE 5–8.

Adverse Effects of Magnevist in U.S. Clinical Trials

Reaction	Drug	Number of Patients			
		Total	Percentage	Drug Related	Percentage
Headache	Gd-DTPA	40	9.8	20	4.9
	Placebo	5	17.9	0	
Nausea	Gd-DTPA	17	4.1	14	3.4
	Placebo	1	3.6	0	
Vomiting	Gd-DTPA	17	1.7	6	1.5
	Placebo	1	3.6	0	
Hypertension	Gd-DTPA	4	1.0	1	0.2
	Placebo	1	3.6	0	
Dizziness	Gd-DTPA	4	1.0	3	0.7
	Placebo	0		0	
Rash	Gd-DTPA	4	1.0	2	0.5
	Placebo	0		0	
Local Pain	Gd-DTPA	7	1.7	1	0.2
	Placebo	0		0	
Total Patients	Gd-DTPA	410			
Placebo		28			

other imaging studies including CT—and were studied with a rigid protocol: both T1- and T2-weighted unenhanced scans, slow injection of Magnevist over a period of 2 minutes, followed by T1 weighting at 3, 30, and 55 minutes and T2 weighting at 8 and 35 minutes. Voluminous safety indices were collected. Any adverse effect was recorded and judged to be drug related or not by the investigator.

Table 5–8 summarizes the adverse effects that were recorded with a 1% or greater incidence. Headache was the most common side effect. It was rarely severe and occurred more often with placebo. Clearly the noise and confinement of MRI and the likely presence of neoplasms of the brain in the study patients were confounding factors. Nausea, vomiting, change in vital signs, and dizziness were little different from placebo, albeit the small number of placebo patients makes comparison hazardous. Regrettably, MRI patients who often had contrast enhanced CTs were not asked to compare the two experiences. The investigating team was impressed with the apparently innocuous nature of the drug at this dose in these patients. Rash and local pain were encouragingly infrequent.

About 15% of female patients and 30% of male patients had a transient increase in serum iron above normal and 1% to 3% of patients had a transient increase in serum bilirubin levels. These responses are consistent with a small amount of he-

molysis. One may speculate this is due to the hypertonicity of the formulation. To my knowledge, serum iron has not been serially followed after intravenous administration of x-ray contrast agents.

Since Gd-DTPA enhancement is easily detected and radiologists have an exceptional memory for their own cases, a subset of complete cases was blindly read by an independent team of MRI experts. For some sessions, only the T1- or T2-weighted unenhanced or enhanced scans were presented and independently interpreted. Later, the entire series was presented. The benefits of Gd-DTPA from this exercise are summarized in Table 5–9.

The series had few patients without a BBB abnormality, and thus sensitivity was very high. In many cases histologic proof was absent, so specificity is uncertain. A relative comparison of the interpretation of unenhanced vs. enhanced scans is

TABLE 5–9.

Summary of Diagnostic Efficacy of Magnevist

Diagnosis was facilitated in 66% of cases
Additional diagnostic information was found in 74% of cases
Diagnosis was possible in 73% of uncertain cases on unenhanced scans
More lesions were found in 24% of studies
Diagnosis was changed in 28% of studies
Diagnostic confidence was increased in 76% of cases

more powerful and shows striking benefits in facilitating diagnosis, providing additional diagnostic information, establishing a diagnosis in cases uncertain without enhancement, and detecting more lesions. Of special note in this restricted study is the considerable change in final diagnosis and the marked increase in diagnostic confidence. This was found despite the expertise of the overreaders.

CLINICAL USES OF Gd-DTPA

From the foregoing, it is apparent that Gd-DTPA can be used to anatomically delineate a leaky BBB, to enhance slowly moving blood, and to identify differential enhancement in regions where two tissues have no BBB but have different perfusion rates or ECF volumes. In all these areas, Gd-DTPA is behaving the same as water-soluble x-ray contrast agents, and its clinical use is tempered only by its greater safety, greater detectability (given appropriate pulse sequences), and failure to enhance rapidly moving fluids.

Gd-DTPA improves CNS diagnosis with MRI in about the same proportion as x-ray contrast agents improve CT[20] and for identical reasons (Table 5–10). Enhancement occurs early, is easily detectable, and lasts for a long time (Table 5–11). Since unenhanced MRI is usually better than un-enhanced CT because of the soft-tissue contrast, enhanced MRI will be correspondingly better than enhanced CT. Unenhanced MRI and enhanced CT are about equal but clearly inferior to enhanced MRI.

The availability of Gd-DTPA adds another dimension to planning an MRI examination—and there were already plenty of alternatives. Although the clinical trials of Gd-DTPA show major benefit, it is unclear how the new agent should be incorporated into routine clinical practice.

HOW SHOULD Gd-DTPA BE USED?

There is no certain answer to this question, chiefly because the clinical trial was small and inclusions and exclusions restricted entry to a very select population. The imaging was done in a rigidly proscribed manner, and neither time nor cost was a consideration. An accurate recommendation for routine clinical use awaits reports of utility in such a setting.

If Gd-DTPA is to be cost-effective, it should provide appropriate value when added to a complete unenhanced MRI series, replace other studies, and/or reduce imaging time. The ultimate

TABLE 5–10.

Sensitivity of MRI in Extra-axial Tumors

Without Gd-DTPA	With Gd-DTPA
74%	89%

TABLE 5–11.

Time of the Maximum Enhancement in Cerebral Neoplasms*

	Minutes		
	<15	15–45	>45
All study patients	60%	32%	8%

Time of Diagnostic Enhancement in Cerebral Neoplasms*

Neoplasm	Time (min)
Meningiomas	<5
Neuromas	<5
Gliomas	
Grades II–IV	<5
Grade I†	<10
Metastases	5–10

* Assumes short TR/short TE and 0.1 mmol/kg dose.
† Some low-grade gliomas do not enhance.

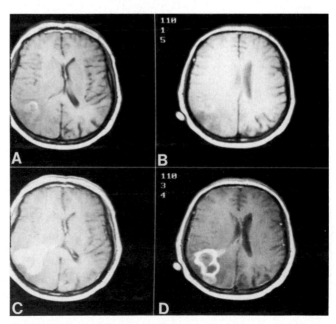

FIG 5–12.
Paramagnetic materials from a subacute hemorrhage look like Gd-DTPA. **A,** a T1-weighted scan before Gd-DTPA shows internal hemorrhage in this tumor. Images **B** (3 minutes), **C** (30 minutes), and **D** (55 minutes) show the accumulation of more paramagnetic material representing the arrival and diffusion of Gd-DTPA.

throughput utility would be to perform a single T1-weighted enhanced scan 5 to 45 minutes after administering Gd-DTPA in the waiting room. First caveat: some intense lesions on T1-weighted enhanced scans are *not* due to Gd-DTPA—fat in an unexpected location, hemorrhage in its paramagnetic stage, some artifacts (Figs 5–12 to 5–14). Second caveat: T2-weighted scans and other planes have incremental value. Some experts would accept enhanced T1-weighted scans as sufficient in following a known abnormality and for a few lesions that have been fairly well characterized by CT or angiography.

Nearly every other clinical circumstance is uncharacterized. There are some uses of Gd-DTPA in the brain that are not often considered. It could be used as the best available screen for pathology in serious diagnostic dilemmas or in the following nonideal circumstances: patient cooperation restricts total imaging time, historical and clinical information provided is unclear or of uncertain accuracy, the MRI device is performing at less than optimum, or the interpreter needs extra assistance to improve his accuracy. Many other scenarios are expected to evolve as creative practioners gain access to the agent.

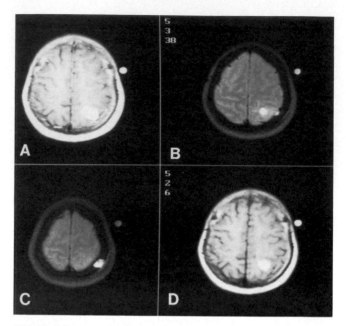

FIG 5–14.
A spectacular case showing the need for pre-Gd images to evaluate the Gd-DTPA effect. **A,** a T1-weighted image 3 minutes after Gd-DTPA. However, **D** shows the preimage. On the T2-weighted multislice preimages at two other levels, a strong signal is seen in the subdural space and on the surface of the brain (**C** and **B,** respectively). This patient had a tissue biopsy 5 days before the MRI.

THE FUTURE OF MR CONTRAST AGENTS FOR BRAIN IMAGING

Magnevist is FDA approved for MRI use in patients with suspected BBB abnormality or abnormal vascularity. There are many additional uses that are known but for which an NDA application for approval has not been made. These include pediatric use, numerous applications in the spine,[21] relative tissue perfusion (including serial studies of response to interventions),[22–26] and subarachnoid or intrathecal use.[27] New agents in the same category are also anticipated.

There are efforts to develop agents that are lipid soluble and could measure useful properties of brain disease other than BBB damage or slow perfusion. Likewise, some large-exit pathways exist that would allow very complicated MR contrast agents such as monoclonal antibodies or cell receptor markers to be used. Because superparamagnetic or ferromagnetic particles are more potent and detectable at still lower doses than paramagnetic chelates, this class of MR contrast agents could become useful. Figure 5–15 summarizes a

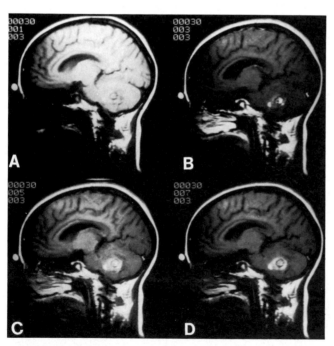

FIG 5–13.
A hemangioblastoma on a T1-weighted image before **(A)** and 3 minutes **(B)**, 30 minutes **(C)**, and 55 minutes **(D)** after Gd-DTPA. It is the change from pre- to postimages that reveals the leak of Gd-DTPA.

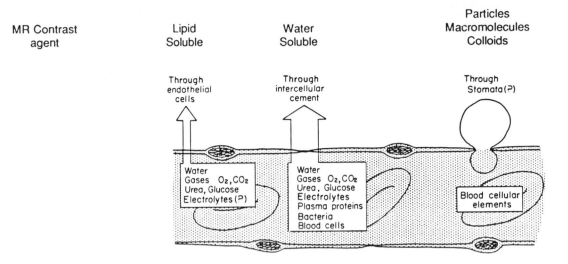

FIG 5–15.

Other opportunities for MR contrast agent development. Water-soluble paramagnetic chelates leave the vascular space through capillary junctions. Lipid-soluble agents could penetrate through cells. Many normal vascular beds and nearly all tumor circulations have capillary pores large enough to allow molecules of several thousand molecular weight to enter. Monoclonal antibodies tagged to ferrite particles could be useful as highly targeted MR contrast agents.

very active period of further research that will make an extraordinary detector still more valuable for human studies.

REFERENCES

1. Block F, Hansen WW, Packard M: The nuclear induction experiment. *Physiol Rev* 1946; 70:474–485.
2. Dwek RA, Richards RE, Morallee KG, et al: Lanthanide cations as probes in biological systems. Proton relaxation enhancement studies for model systems and lysozyme. *Eur J Biochem* 1971; 211:204–209.
3. Lauterbur PC, Mendonca-Dias MH, Rubin AM: Augmentation of tissue water proton spin-lattice relaxation rates by the in vivo addition of paramagnetic ions, in Dulton PO, Leigh JS, Scarpa A (eds): *Frontiers of Biological Energetics.* New York, Academic Press, Inc, 1978, p 752.
4. Fobben E, Wolf GL: Gadolinium DTPA—a potential NMR contrast agent. Effects upon tissue proton relaxation and cardiovascular function in the rabbit. Presented at the Association of University Radiologists, March 1983. *Invest Radiol* 1984; 19:324–328.
5. Laniado M, Weinmann HJ, Schorner W, et al: First use of GdDTPA/dimeglumine in man. *Physiol Chem Phys Med NMR* 1984; 16:157–165.
6. Brasch RC, Weinmann HJ, Wesbey GE: Contrast enchanced NMR imaging: Animal studies using gadolinium DTPA complex. *AJR* 1984; 142:625–630.
7. Harrocks WD, Sipe JP: Lanthanide shift reagents: A survey. *J Am Chem Soc* 1971; 93:6800–6804.
8. Weinmann HJ, Laniado M, Mutzel W: Pharmacokinetics of GdDTPA/dimeglumine after intravenous injection into healthy volunteers. *Physiol Chem Phys Med NMR* 1984; 16:167–172.
9. Brasch RC, London DA, Wesbey GE, et al: Nuclear magnetic resonance study of a paramagnetic nitroxide contrast agent for enhancement of renal structures in experimental animals. *Radiology* 1983; 147:773–779.
10. Wolf GL, Burnett KR, Goldstein EJ, et al: Contrast agents for magnetic resonance imaging, in Kressel HY (ed): *Magnetic Annual 1985.* New York, Raven Press, 1985, pp 231–266.
11. Bloembergen N: Proton relaxation times in paramagnetic solutions. *J Chem Phys* 1957; 27:572–588.
12. Wolf GL, Baum L: Cardiovascular toxicity and tissue proton T1 response to manganese injection in the dog and rabbit. *AJR* 1983; 141:193–197.
13. Fornasiero D, Bellen JC, Baker RJ, et al: Paramagnetic complexes of manganese (II), iron (III), and gadolinium (III) as contrast agents for magnetic resonance imaging. The influence of stability constants on the biodistribution of radioactive aminopolycarboxylate complexes. *Invest Radiol* 1987; 22:322–327.
14. Goldstein EJ, Burnett KR, Hansell JR, et al: Gadolinium DTPA (an NMR proton imaging contrast agent): Chemical structure, paramagnetic properties, and pharmocokinetics. *Physiol Chem Phys Med NMR* 1984; 16:97–104.
15. Weinmann HJ, Brasch RC, Press WR, et al: Characteristics of gadolinium-DTPA complex: A potential NMR contrast agent. *AJR* 1984; 142:619–624.

16. Gadian DG, Payne JA, Bryant DJ, et al: Gadolinium DTPA as a contrast agent in MR imaging—theoretical projections and practical observations. *J Comput Assist Tomogr* 1985; 9:245–251.

17. Wolf GL, Joseph PM, Goldstein EJ: Optimal pulsing sequences for MR contrast agents. *AJR* 1986; 147:367–371.

18. Koenig SH, Baglin C, Brown RD III, et al: Magnetic field dependence of solvent proton relaxation by Gd^{+3} and Mn^{+2} complexes. *Magn Reson Med* 1984; 1:496–501.

19. Kilgore DP, Breger RK, Daniels DL, et al: Cranial tissues: Normal MR appearance after intravenous injection of gadolinium-DTPA. *Radiology* 1986; 160:757–761.

20. Breger RK, Papke RA, Pojunas KW, et al: Benign extraaxial tumors: Contrast enchancement with Gd-DTPA. *Radiology* 1987; 163:427–429.

21. Sze G, Abramson A, Krol G, et al: Gadolinium-DTPA in the evaluation of intradural extramedullary spinal disease. *AJNR* 1988; 9:153–163.

22. Virapongse C, Mancuso A, Quisling R: Human brain infarcts: GdDTPA-enhanced MR imaging. *Radiology* 1986; 161:785–794.

23. Grossman RJ, Joseph PM, Wolf G, et al: Experimental intracranial septic infarction: Magnetic resonance enhancement. *Radiology* 1985; 155:649–653.

24. Schorner W, Laniado M, Niendorf HP, et al: Time-dependent changes in image contrast in brain tumors after gadolinium-DTPA. *AJNR* 1986; 7:1013–1020.

25. Dwyer AJ, Frank JA, Doppman JL, et al: Pituitary adenomas in patients with Cushing disease: Initial experience with GdDTPA-enhanced MR imaging. *Radiology* 1987; 164:421–426.

26. Davis PC, Hoffman JC Jr, Malko JA: Gadolinium-DTPA and MR imaging of pituitary adenoma: A preliminary report. *AJNR* 1987; 8:817–823.

27. DiChiro G, Knop RH, Girton ME, et al: MR cisternography and myelography with GdDTPA in monkeys. *Radiology* 1985; 157:373–377.

6

Xenon/CT Cerebral Blood Flow Analysis

Howard Yonas, M.D.

David Gur, Sc.D.

David W. Johnson, M.D.

Richard E. Latchaw, M.D.

The imaging of blood flow within the brain became possible in the early 1970s due to the application of modern computers to radiology. While a number of approaches for acquiring tomographic cerebral blood flow (CBF) have been developed in the past decade, each has specific advantages and disadvantages. Currently none fulfills the ideal criteria of being (1) easily interpretable, with direct anatomic reference and high resolution; (2) readily accessible; (3) relatively simple and safe to obtain; (4) quantitative, providing blood flow values that correlate with physiologic thresholds for function and survival; and (5) able to survey the whole brain.

Stable xenon computed tomographic (Xe/CT) CBF imaging has been under development at the University of Pittsburgh since 1978 and has undergone extensive clinical use since 1984. Despite its limitations, Xe/CT is a CBF technique that we believe comes closest to fulfilling the above criteria for clinical usefulness. Following a brief review of the history of CBF measurements and a review of cerebrovascular physiology as it specifically relates to tomographic CBF measurements, this chapter will focus on the Xe/CT CBF method and its clinical application.

HISTORY OF CBF MEASUREMENT IN CLINICAL MEDICINE

Kety and Schmidt mathematically characterized the Fick principle for the measurement of CBF in 1948.[1] Nitrous oxide, a metabolically inert and highly lipid soluble gas, was initially used as the tracer of flow. The Fick principle had stated that the quantity of a gas taken up by a tissue per unit of time is equal to the quantity entering the tissue via the arterial blood minus the quantity leaving in the venous blood. Knowing the time course of the change in the inert gas concentration in the arterial blood entering the brain and in the venous blood leaving it as well as the blood partition coefficient (λ), Kety and Schmidt calculated the average CBF. This measurement of global CBF with nitrous oxide as well as all later methods using other tracers were based on the assumptions that blood flow is in a steady state during the period of study and is not affected by the tracer and that the value of the partition coefficient of the inert gas is representative of the tissue being studied.

A major advance toward the clinical application of CBF measurement came with the substitution of radiolabeled ^{133}Xe for nitrous oxide and the use of external scintillation counting as a means of directly measuring the regional movement of the tracer within the brain.[2] Clinical application of the methodology was later broadened after Obrist developed a method to introduce xenon by inhalation[3] instead of by direct arterial injection. Regional CBF (rCBF) determined by the ^{133}Xe method, however, has a number of limitations.[4] Counts arising from extracranial tissue provide a signal contamination, as do emissions arising from deeper structures (i.e., the neck and pharynx). The ^{133}Xe technique is dependent on the use of a "normal" partition coefficient, which, in diseased states, can significantly alter the CBF. This technique also can falsely detect flow in brain regions with no flow when counts from adjacent hyperemic tissues numerically overshadow the area of no flow. This phenomenon was a major disadvantage of the technique and prompted the development of a tomographic imaging system for ^{133}Xe. While devices utilizing ^{133}Xe as the radioactive source for single-photon–emission computed tomography (SPECT) are now commercially available, they still have relatively poor resolution, lack anatomic correlation, and continue to depend on "normalized" partition coefficient values.

Additional quantitative and regionally specific tomographic techniques for blood flow determination have also been developed in the past decade. CBF measurement techniques using water-soluble tracers (N-isopropyl-^{123}I-p-iodoamphetamine [IMP],[5] Hm-PAO) that have a high tissue affinity to neuronal binding sites during their initial arterial passage through the cerebral circulation are now available and adaptable to both dedicated tomographic and rotating Anger camera technologies. While this method has the advantage of providing CBF data at all brain levels, it provides no direct anatomic reference, and quantitative data are provided only if arterial blood sampling is performed to correct for tracer recirculation. While the binding of iodoamphetamine is predictable within normal tissues, it is less predictable in diseased states.[6] Another approach to blood flow determination uses the tomographic reconstruction of positron-emitting markers. Positron-emission tomography (PET) supplies regionally specific flow information, which, coupled with studies of metabolism, offers a unique way to study normal and altered physiologic states. Although PET adds a valuable approach to brain imaging, the technology demands the on-site efforts of a team of scientists, and the equipment is expensive to acquire and support, thereby limiting its availability to relatively few research institutions. PET also provides no anatomic reference, it has poor resolution in most existing units, and serious questions as to its quantitative capability have been raised.[6] Magnetic resonance imaging (MRI) currently has no capacity to quantitate tissue perfusion, although it can accurately calculate unidirectional flow within large blood vessels.

In the early 1980s the use of rapid CT scanning before, during, and after iodine injection was proposed for the study of CBF. The major advantages of using iodine are that it provides a high degree of image enhancement and, in delayed scanning, qualitative diagnostic information on defects in blood-brain barrier permeability.[7] Its major disadvantages are the difficulties in obtaining meaningful quantitative absolute flow values and in correlating such data with tissue perfusion. In addition, usually only one brain level at a time can be studied.[8] Xe/CT CBF measurements became possible in the late 1970s with the observation by Winkler and colleagues that xenon was radio dense.[9] The method will be more fully presented later in the chapter.

CEREBRAL BLOOD FLOW PHYSIOLOGY

Although different methods have been used to arrive at *normal CBF* values, the resulting values have been surprisingly similar. The single-compartment measurement of 54 ± 12 cc/100 g/min derived by Kety and Schmidt,[1] which is the average of all flow compartments, is not significantly different from values derived by ^{133}Xe,[10] Xe/CT,[11, 12] or PET[13] techniques. Average flow values of about 80 cc/100 g/min for gray matter and 20 cc/100 g/min for white matter also have been recorded consistently.[10–13]

CBF, however, is not constant; both global and local CBF constantly vary due to changes in levels of neuronal activity and acid-base balance. Normally, CBF is coupled directly with *metabolism,* so increased metabolic activity is associated with an increase in CBF.[14] Everyday activities such as hand movement, reading, or speaking are accompanied by a very rapid local increase in CBF in the specific cortical area in which these activities are controlled.[15, 16] Severe anxiety or pain can cause a global increase in CBF. At the extremes of metabolic activity, seizures are accompanied by a 50%

elevation of flow values,[17] while coma is accompanied by a reduction of similar magnitude.[18, 19] Alterations in the partial pressure of *carbon dioxide* (pCO_2) have the most potent, direct effect on CBF.[20] In normal individuals, CBF varies by 3%/mm Hg CO_2; therefore if pCO_2 suddenly increases from the normal of 40 to 60 mm Hg, CBF rises dramatically, and in the head-injured patient, intracranial pressure (ICP) also may be elevated.[21] A pCO_2 greater than 60 mm Hg is associated with maximal vasodilatation, whereas values at or below 20 mm Hg can cause ischemia due to severe vasoconstriction.[22] Not only does the manipulation of pCO_2 have direct therapeutic implications, but the recording of pCO_2 during CBF measurement is essential for the interpretation of CBF information. Among normal spontaneously breathing subjects initial pCO_2 levels have varied from 32 to 48 mm Hg; thus the results of flow analysis are less meaningful unless this physiologic parameter is considered. Also, CBF information obtained from a person at different times cannot be compared unless corresponding differences in pCO_2 also are considered. To deal with this problem, some clinicians have attempted to standardize all CBF values at a "normal" pCO_2 level of 40 mm Hg; however, this is a questionable clinical practice because, in diseased states, the degree of CBF activation can be significantly different from 3%/mm Hg CO_2.

Variations of *blood viscosity* can also have a significant influence on CBF. An elevated viscosity resulting from a hematocrit of 50% will lower CBF 20% to 30% below normal *rheology*.[23] Conversely, the therapeutic reduction of the hematocrit from 50% to 30% can be used to raise CBF. Thus, the awareness of this parameter is important for the study of CBF.

Autoregulation refers to the proportional change in vascular resistance that maintains a stable CBF as the cerebral perfusion pressure changes.[24] Normally, CBF is consistent at mean arterial pressures (MAPs) ranging from 60 to 150 mm Hg. Below a MAP of 60 mm Hg, however, CBF falls because the vessels are maximally dilated and unable to compensate for a further drop in MAP. At a MAP greater than 150 mm Hg, despite maximal vasoconstriction, CBF rises and potentially can cause cerebral edema and hemorrhage. The recording of blood pressure during CBF studies is important because in injured tissues that may have lost autoregulation, blood flow can vary directly with even subtle changes in blood pressure.

Studies of blood flow, blood volume, oxygen extraction, and metabolism during a progressive reduction in perfusion pressure have clarified the manner in which the brain responds to hemodynamic compromise. The initial response to a gradual lowering of blood pressure is vasodilation with an accompanying increase in blood volume.[25] Upon maximal vasodilation, oxygen extraction steadily increases as CBF begins to fall; metabolism is altered only at the extreme of hemodynamic decompensation when values approach 20 cc/100 g/min. Because of these findings, CBF studies obtained before and after a vasodilatory challenge are believed to provide information about not only the vasodilatory status of cerebral vasculature but also the hemodynamic and metabolic status of the brain. The administration of 3% to 5% CO_2[26, 27] or the intravenous injection of 1 g acetazolamide (Diamox)[28, 29] have been used to produce a vasodilatory challenge. Although the response to inhaling CO_2 can vary, CBF normally rises 30% to 40% in all brain regions 20 minutes after acetazolamide is administered. A significant rise in CBF suggests that the vasculature was not maximally dilated and that adequate reserves were available to increase supply as metabolic activity increased. Conversely, the inability of one or more vascular territories to elevate flow suggests that vessels already were maximally dilated in these regions and that flow reserves were severely compromised.

Blood flow and metabolism can become uncoupled in some clinical situations. An acute infarction resulting from embolic occlusion of the cerebral vessels accompanied by a lack of collateral flow will cause an absence of both CBF and metabolism; however, weeks later, flow values within the infarction often increase more than required by the metabolic activity. This return of flow apparently is related to the neovascularization of the infarct during the resolution phase. This "relative" luxury perfusion, with low flow values greater than metabolic demand, is part of the normal process of stroke resolution. If reperfusion occurs within minutes or hours after an ischemic injury due to embolus migration, hyperemia occurs, with flow values greater than normal and far in excess of metabolic demand. This condition has been called "absolute" luxury perfusion.[30]

In two common situations, the supply of blood flow can be inadequate to meet the metabolic demands. During seizure activity, a greatly elevated metabolic demand may surpass the ability of the blood supply to provide adequate nutrition.[17] Conversely, if blood flow falls below 20 cc/100 g/min, neuronal conductance ceases.[31] However, irreversible cellular damage does not occur unless CBF values fall below 6 to 8 cc/100 g/min.[32] An important relationship also exists between the depth and the duration of the ischemic challenge, so flow values of 2 to 3 cc/100 g/min can be tolerated for only a few minutes while values of 15 cc/100 g/min may be tolerable for an hour prior to irreversible infarctions.[33] In either case, permanent neuronal damage can be avoided if CBF is restored. Another complicating variable is the greater vulnerability to ischemia in certain brain regions. This *selective vulnerability* explains why, despite "successful" resuscitation, cardiac arrest can cause the neocortex to be severely injured while the brain stem and basal ganglia are relatively spared.

Xe/CT CBF THEORY AND APPLICATIONS

We and others have pursued the development of Xe/CT-derived CBF because it (1) can be performed in any hospital with a late-generation CT scanner at relatively low cost; (2) provides high-resolution CBF information coupled with CT-derived anatomic images; and (3) is rapidly accessible, obtained in conjunction with routine CT imaging in as little as 20 minutes.

Theoretical Basis for Xe/CT CBF

The Xe/CT CBF technique requires a number of departures from other CBF methods to derive the information essential to solve the Kety-Schmidt equation. Although various approaches to this equation have been reported, this chapter will focus on the methodologic choices made by our group at the University of Pittsburgh and subsequently incorporated within the GE 9800 CT system (General Electric Medical Systems Division, Milwaukee).

1. –*Arterial buildup.* The arterial curve is characterized indirectly by using the end-tidal xenon concentration to measure the arterial buildup. Although a mass spectrometer can be used to record xenon concentrations,[34] a thermoconductivity analyzer is similarly accurate at normal breathing rates and is less expensive and more stable.[35]

2. –*Tissue buildup.* Because only a limited number of images separated by relatively long intervals can be obtained by using the CT technology, initially we were forced to assume that re-

gions of interest (ROIs) as small as $0.1 \times 0.1 \times 0.5$ mm^3 are each a *single-flow compartment*.[36, 37] The higher resolution and greater image stability provided by new scanners have validated our assumptions.[38, 39] By using buildup information, we were also able to limit the time required for exposure to xenon and thus minimize the physiologic side effects of the gas.

3. –*Partition coefficient.* The partition coefficient (λ) can be measured directly with stable xenon and CT imaging either until all brain structures are saturated with xenon or until enough data are acquired to be able to mathematically extrapolate λ.[37, 39, 40] The latter approach has provided good flow information during a 4½-minute examination, a length of time comfortable for most patients.

4. –*CBF calculation.* Although some investigators have calculated CBF by using a single enhancement point and others have assumed a "normative λ", a two-variable approach using the best fit for data has greatly reduced errors associated with the Xe/CT CBF calculation.[39, 41–43] With the latter approach, computer programs have made possible the determination of CBF for every CT voxel,[11, 40] and high-resolution maps of flow can be generated.

5. –*Signal-to-noise ratio (SNR) vs. clinical tolerance.* A major clinical limitation of Xe/CT CBF measurement has been the marginal SNR that results when the lower, more clinically acceptable concentrations of xenon are used. Although 100% xenon provides about 30 Hounsfield units of tissue enhancement, the inhalation of this concentration for even a single breath can be dangerous.[44] Concentrations of 50% to 60% consistently cause sedation and have been associated with bronchospasm. Our initial observations suggested that concentrations ranging from 24% to 50% could be tolerated,[45] but our experience in more than 2,500 patients has convinced us that concentrations of xenon at or below 33% are preferable and cause few transient ill effects in most people.[46] The relatively low noise level and high image stability of the GE 9800 scanner has made these lower concentrations acceptable for calculating CBF.

Xe/CT Clinical Methodology

The current Xe/CT method has been used at the University of Pittsburgh since 1984. CT scanners equipped to measure CBF continue to function in their normal imaging capacity, and with only 5 minutes of preparation they can be prepared also to acquire CBF information. A CBF study can usually be accomplished within 30 to 40 minutes, allowing the time necessary for xenon washout. Routine CBF studies can be obtained 20 minutes later in order to test responses to proposed therapies or physiologic stress tests.

In our institution studies proceed as follows: the patient is fully informed of the possible transient sensory disturbances that can occur during xenon inhalation. The importance of remaining completely still during the study is stressed because the examination can require up to 7 minutes from the time the baseline images are obtained to the end of xenon inhalation.

The patient is then positioned within the scanner, and an initial set of images is taken to select the apparent levels for CBF analysis. It is essential to select levels that have minimal artifact. Because our studies are currently limited to three brain levels, it is essential that levels are chosen from the most appropriate brain region to address the clinical question. The patient's blood pressure and end-tidal CO_2 are monitored throughout the study. We also have found an oximeter useful, especially when studying critically ill patients. Next, the patient is fitted with either a face mask or a mouthpiece (accompanied by firm nasal compression). The patient continues to breathe room air delivered through a ventilation system as two baseline scans are obtained at each level of study. Once this is completed, the patient automatically is switched to a xenon/oxygen mixture delivered from a 60-L plastic bag through a nonrebreathing system.

The end-tidal xenon concentration mixture is monitored by a thermoconductivity detector that displays a single value with each breath. The value for each breath is stored in a computer to derive the exponent that characterizes the end-tidal curve and, indirectly, the arterial curve. Patients indicate their tolerance of xenon gas inhalation throughout the examination by predetermined toe movements. Comatose patients who require ventilatory support can be studied by connecting the delivery system outflow to the intake of a volume ventilator. An "external-pressure" sensor inserted on the delivery side of the ventilator is used to maintain correct timing of end-tidal sampling.

Multiple brain levels are studied during one inhalation period by using programmed incremental table movements between CT images obtained at 20-second intervals.[47] Up to three levels now can be examined during a single study; the number of levels currently is limited by the heat-loading constraints of the CT x-ray tube. Xenon end-tidal values obtained from the thermoconductivity detector and the recorded xenon percentage are converted into an estimated time-dependent CT enhancement of arterial blood by using the following relationship:

$$Ca(u) = C \, Xe \, CT \, (1 + 1.1 \, Hct)$$

where $Ca(u)$ = the instantaneous arterial Xe concentration; $C = kVp$, the dependent conversion constant; $Xe \, CT$ = end-tidal Xe concentrations; and Hct = hematocrit.

Sequential CT images are used to characterize the local buildup of xenon in tissue for the calculation of local CBF. The two baseline scans obtained before xenon inhalation are averaged to reduce the noise level, and this averaged baseline image is subtracted from each image obtained during xenon inhalation. Each voxel measuring $1 \times 1 \times 5$ or $1 \times 1 \times 10$ mm^3 subsequently is defined by a series of ΔCT values as a function of time. These data are combined with the measured arterial concentrations over time to solve the Kety-Schmidt equation:

$$\Delta CT(t) = f\int_0^t \Delta Ca(u)e^{-k(t-u)}du, \text{ where } f = k \cdot \lambda$$

A weighted least-squares fit routine is used to derive estimates of two parameters, flow (f) and lambda (λ), by using an iterative approach. A centrally weighted, three-pixel, bell-shaped smoothing routine is used before the computation to reduce pixel-to-pixel noise, and a centrally weighted, 9×9 or 7×7 bell-shaped smoothing routine is used after the computation. When a data set cannot be fit to the xenon buildup curve within the limits of allowable error, the system automatically averages values from the adjacent eight voxels and substitutes that value. More than 20,000 values are derived from each CT level and displayed on a quantitative gray scale.

Flow values can be analyzed in a number of ways. Given the large number of calculations acquired, the mean and standard deviation of flow values for any desired region can be displayed. For example, in Figure 6–1, a continuous quantitative gray scale is used to display the flow data. In this map, the average flow value of the 16 ROIs (2 cm

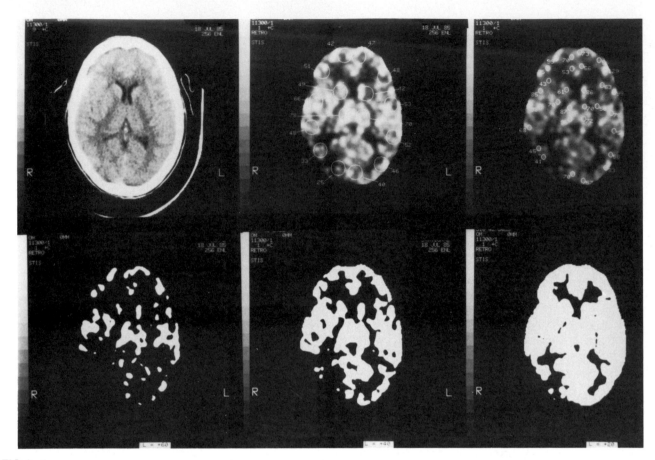

FIG 6–1.

The CT image in the *upper left* is the baseline anatomy from which the same CBF data on the *right* and *below* are displayed in different formats. The gray scale for the *center top* image is our standard of 0 to 100 cc/100 g/min, and 2-cm ROIs are placed within the cortical mantle and basal ganglia. The gray scale on the *top* *right* was altered to 1 to 150 cc/100 g/min so that the flow values from the high–flow peak 5-mm ROIs could be more easily seen. The three images across the *bottom* from *left to right* are flow thresholds at 60, 40, and 20 cc/100 g/min. All values above the indicated flow threshold are displayed in white and below in black.

in diameter each) was 49 cc/100 g/min; values for each ROI depended both on its arbitrary placement and on the mix of tissue within it. The selective placement of 5-mm ROIs within CT-defined gray matter areas provided values ranging from 41 to 129 cc/100 g/min, with a mean of 74.8 cc/100 g/min; the associated white matter mean for similarly generated ROIs was 19.2 cc/100 g/min. The gray-white ratio in this study of normal subjects was 3.9 : 1.

The CBF database for each CT level can be analyzed in many ways: histograms can be created, flow information can be demonstrated as thresholds above and below a certain level, and all blood flow values within any specified region can be analyzed directly.

While the analysis of CBF within a single CT voxel measuring $1 \times 1 \times 5$ mm or $1 \times 1 \times 10$ mm^3 is theoretically possible, the error inherent in such a measure, especially in white matter, can be very high. Within ROIs of 8 to 12 mm in diameter the variability of measurements approaches 10% to 12%, while with ROIs greater than 2 cm in diameter the variability is less than 10%. Rather than focusing on smaller regions with higher inherent errors we have turned to the averaging of flow values within large vascular or anatomic regions or the averaging of multiple circular ROIs within the cortical mantle and basal ganglia that can later be grouped by the reader as to physiologically defined regions. The fact that the standard duration of the flow values within any larger region of the brain is relatively large, i.e., 50 ± 25 to 30 cc/100 g/min, should not, however, be surprising because this is the mean flow value and standard deviation of the many voxels within an ROI. While the mean of such an ROI would be highly stable, the standard deviation depicts only the presence of both normally high and low flow regions within the ROI.

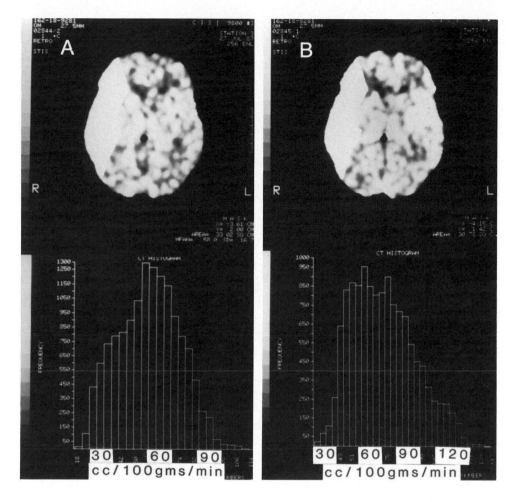

FIG 6–2.
A, a normal CBF study is displayed above with a *cursor* overlying the right cortical distribution of the middle cerebral artery. The mean flow value within this ROI was 58 cc/100 g/min. *Below* is a histogram of all flow values within the ROI *above*. Note that very few voxels are normally below 10 or above 100 cc/100 g/min. **B,** 20 minutes after the intravenous injection of 1 g of Diamox a repeat flow study shows a mean of 73 cc/100 g/min with shift of the flow values toward higher values.

Laboratory Validation

The validity of the Xe/CT CBF technique has been shown through studies that have demonstrated consistency and reproducibility[48] as well as an appropriate physiologic response to challenges designed to alter CBF (e.g., CO_2, Diamox) (Fig 6–2).[49] The method has also shown significant correlations in simultaneous comparisons to techniques using microspheres[50, 51] (Fig 6–3) and[14]C-iodoantipyrine[52] and in a series of phantom studies.[53] All of these assessments indicate that the technique provides adequate information for many investigational[48, 54] and clinical applications.[49, 55, 56] Its unique ability to demonstrate low flow or no flow in small tissue volumes has also been confirmed in a series of in vivo measurements in baboons that had permanent[48] or reperfused[57] (Fig 6–4) small and well-defined strokes as well as in hemorrhagic shock states.[52]

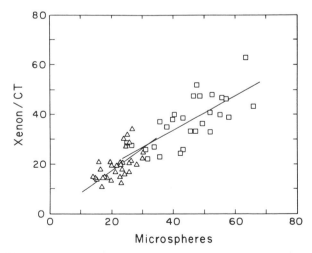

FIG 6–3.
Strong correlations between flow values obtained by the Xe/CT CBF and microsphere methods were found in this study conducted in a series of baboons.

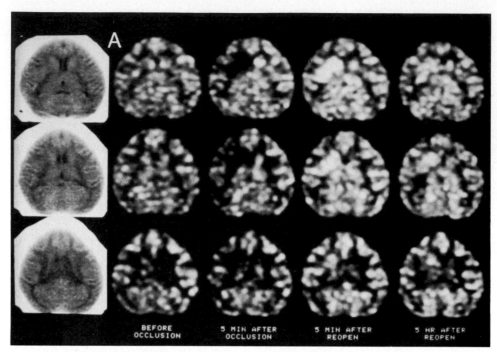

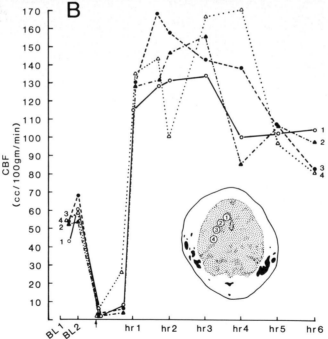

FIG 6-4.
A, sequential sets of three blood flow studies at the CT-defined anatomic levels were obtained in this baboon prior to, during, and following selective temporary occlusion of the right lateral striate arteries of a baboon. **B,** vessel occlusion consistently produced a near no-flow state within the basal ganglia that on reopening became severely hyperemic for 3 to 6 hours. Flow values near zero for 1 hour were consistently accompanied by pathologically defined infarctions.

Clinical Experience

We have found the Xe/CT system we have utilized to be a useful diagnostic tool that adds an important dimension to the information provided by CT imaging. The major uses for this technique that we have pursued have involved the study of patients with acute and chronic occlusive vascular disorders, arteriovenous malformations (AVMs), vasospasm from subarachnoid hemorrhage, and head trauma. Other clinical applications for Xe/CT CBF, including the study of patients with dementia,[56] malignancy,[58] normal-pressure hydrocephalus,[59] and aging,[60] have also been reported.

This discussion will focus on the role of the technique in acute decision making. The keys to this application are (1) the rapid accessibility of flow information, (2) the clinical impact of being able to record zero flow, and (3) the ability after only a brief pause (20 minutes) to repeat studies in order to evaluate CBF response to changes in therapy or physiologic challenges.

Cerebrovascular Disorders

Early Stroke Diagnosis.—The role of the CT scan in the early evaluation of stroke victims is to rule out a mass lesion or hemorrhage. Infarctions generally are not apparent on CT within a day after injury. Adding a Xe/CT CBF study to the first examination, ideally within a few hours after the deficit is manifested, provides additional valuable in-

formation, potentially within a time frame in which therapeutic efforts can be beneficial. Information about the location and size of the injury or whether flow in the injured area is abnormally high or absent, as distinguished from low or normal, has had direct clinical impact (Fig 6–5).[61] Although this type of information has been the goal of many technologies, Xe/CT CBF provides quantitative local CBF information throughout a spectrum of flow possibilities ranging from near zero to significantly greater than 100 cc/100 g/min. When values near zero or high flow focally[48, 61] or globally[55] (Fig 6–6) have been recorded with stable Xe/CT, they have been highly predictive of later CT alteration consistent with infarction and/or brain death. Clearly, measures to augment flow by rheologic manipulation, induced hypertension, or clot lysis would be useless and potentially harmful if a significant portion of the hemisphere initially had flow values near zero. Efforts would be better directed toward the need to treat the massive swell-

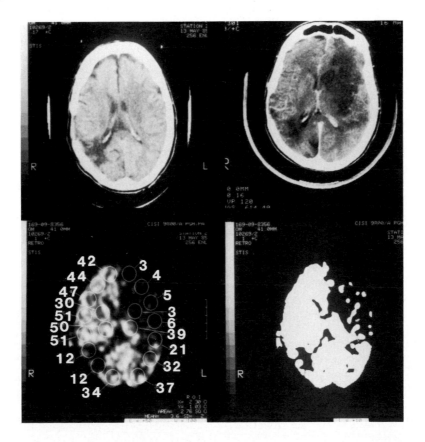

FIG 6–5.

One hour after an uneventful left carotid endarterectomy, this woman awoke with a dense right hemiplegia. Although the emergent CT scan was not abnormal *(top left)*, the accompanying CBF study *(lower left)* revealed a near absence of flow within the left anterior and middle cerebral artery distributions. In the *lower right* im-

age, values from the image on the *left* above 10 cc/100 g/min are displayed as *white* and below as *black*. Note the agreement between cortical regions with initial flow values below 10 cc/100 g/min and the CT-defined region of infarction observed 3 days later *(upper right)*.

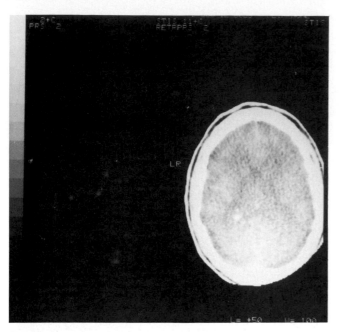

FIG 6–6.
This individual with hepatic failure was being maintained on full medical supports as a candidate for liver transplant despite a comatose state. The ability to resolve "no" blood flow within all cranial compartments was useful in discontinuing hopeless medical efforts. The CBF map on the *left* is essentially black. The average of all flow values was 1 ± 1 cc/100 g/min.

ing that often accompanies large infarctions, especially in young patients.

In a sizable number of stroke patients, CBF studies obtained within a few hours of deficit onset have shown injured brain regions to be hyperemic, presumably because the embolus had migrated and allowed reperfusion[61] (Fig 6–7). The finding of regions with flow values well above normal (absolute luxury perfusion) suggests that, in this situation also, steps to augment blood flow are inappropriate and could be harmful. The acute finding of low flow within the injured area, however, would indicate a suitable candidate for aggressive medical or surgical intervention to augment blood.[62]

Chronic Occlusive Vascular Disease.—Unfortunately, a single blood flow study provides relatively limited insight about the hemodynamic status of the cerebral circulation, except in the extreme instances of very high or absent flow. The problem is that low flow values may be due to either reduced metabolism or a compromised blood supply (low supply). An infarction within the thalamus can cause reduced metabolism due to disconnection in deafferentation of more peripheral areas,[63] with reduced blood flow values within the

entire hemisphere by 20%, while a lesion in the centrum semiovale commonly is accompanied by lower flow values only within the overlying cortex.

To gain an understanding of the intracranial hemodynamics from a CBF measurement, a second blood flow study is required after a "stress test" of blood flow reserves. Because of its simplicity, safety, and consistency in producing a CBF challenge, we have used acetazolamide, 1 g intravenously, and have found that normal blood flow values routinely are increased by 20% to 50% in most individuals 20 minutes after its administration. Most of our studies have in fact revealed normal flow values that were augmented dramatically, despite angiographic evidence of severe unilateral or bilateral vascular disease (Fig 6–8). Such studies have been useful in steering us away from efforts to augment blood flow and have led us to reexamine the vascular anatomy in patients who are recurrently symptomatic. The reassessment consistently has pointed to previously unrecognized embolic sources. Five percent to 10% of patients with recurrent symptoms of ipsilateral carotid vascular disease, however, have exhibited reduced flow values and a minimal or even paradoxical response to acetazolamide (Fig 6–9). These were usually patients whose symptoms were produced by standing or sitting. Efforts to increase CBF reserves seem most appropriate for this group of patients.

Intracranial Vasospasm.—Angiographically diagnosed vasospasm, seen as vascular narrowing, occurs in 60% to 80% of patients who have subarachnoid hemorrhage due to aneurysm rupture. In contrast, symptomatic vasospasm occurs in only 20% of patients with aneurysm rupture and happens only when flow values fall below the level required to maintain neuronal function.

Blood flow measurements have provided valuable information for the management of patients with aneurysms. Studies have shown that CBF information can aid in deciding when to operate and whether physiologically significant clinical vasospasm is present. Single or double studies following CBF challenges via blood pressure manipulation also have guided treatment once it has been started. In patients who are neurologically intact following subarachnoid hemorrhage, the finding of low blood flow values (<30 cc/100 g/min) has been useful in predicting that clinical vasospasm will follow and that patients will not tolerate surgical intervention.[64, 65] The high resolution of Xe/CT CBF images has been reported to be capable of

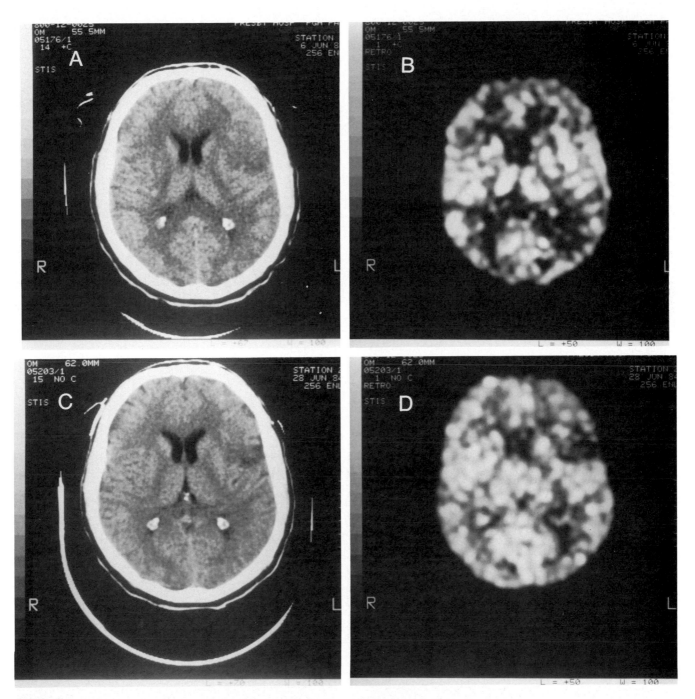

FIG 6–7.
This individual fell while jogging and developed a right hemiplegia and aphasia. While the initial CT scan 4 hours later showed mild increased density in the left frontoparietal region **(A)**, the accompanying CBF study **(B)** showed marked hyperemia in the same re-gion despite a very tight ICA stenosis due to dissection. The follow-up studies (**C** and **D**) 3 weeks later on the right show only loss of tissue volume and only a small region with low flow despite persistent severe ICA stenosis.

identifying not only an overall reduction of flow but also a pattern of irregularly high and low flow values, which may indicate a small-vessel spasm possibly preceding a severe spasm[66] (Fig 6–10).

The use of daily transcranial Doppler (TCD) studies and less frequent CBF studies offers a better means to detect the development of vasospasm than was previously possible by clinical evaluation alone.[67] With the early recognition of worsening vasospasm has come the ability to begin earlier,

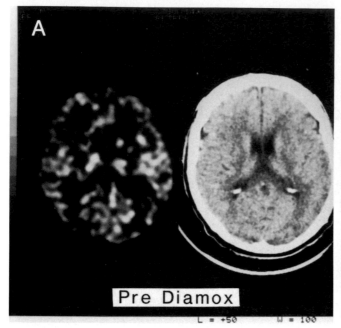

FIG 6–8.
A, relatively low flow values were encountered on the baseline blood flow study in this 70-year-old man who has sustained multiple strokes in the past. His arteriogram showed bilateral internal carotid artery occlusions. **B,** 20 minutes after Diamox injection the repeat flow study demonstrated markedly elevated values in all ter-ritories. This capacity to dramatically elevate flow with chemical stress reveals that this individual did not have a compromise of blood supply at this time but instead reduced metabolism due to prior injuries.

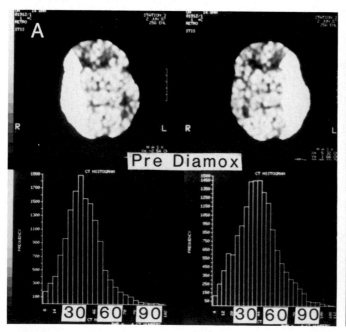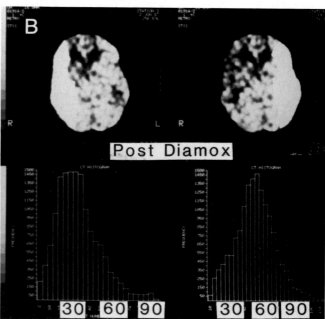

FIG 6–9.
A, this individual sustained a left-sided transient ischemic attack and was found to have a 99% right cervical carotid stenosis. The same blood flow study is displayed *above* with ROIs on the patient's right and left cortical middle cerebral artery territories. Note that the distribution of flow values peaks near 30 cc/100 g/min in the right and near 50 in the left hemisphere. **B,** 20 minutes after 1 g of intravenous Diamox a slightly higher peak of flows is seen in the left hemisphere, but markedly lower flows are seen in the right hemisphere. This individual sustained a large right middle carotid artery infarction 2 days later while awaiting surgery.

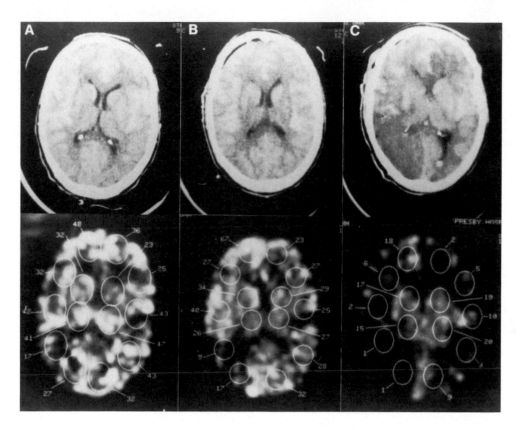

FIG 6–10.
This 60-year-old woman sustained a subarachnoid hemorrhage from an anterior communicating aneurysm and presented to our hospital as Hunt and Hess grade 1 on the fourth day postbleed. Her initial CT and CBF study on the fifth day postbleed **(A)** showed an irregular pattern of high and low blood flow in all territories. **B,** obtained the next day 3 hours after the aneurysm was successfully clipped but when the patient was slow to awaken. Lower flow values were then evident in the left hemisphere with severely reduced flow in the right parietal region. She remained comatose for the next 2 days when the study in **C** was obtained. Areas that had flow values less than 10 cc/100 g/min in **B** had then progressed to CT-defined infarction. At this time flow values were severely reduced in all cortical distributions. The CBF study in **C** predicted the last study on day 10 postbleed, which showed *no* flow in any territory and confirmed the diagnosis of brain death.

aggressive medical measurements for its treatment. Serial Xe/CT studies have also been able to predict regions with irreversible ischemia[68] (Fig 6–11). In addition, the inappropriate use of such measures can be avoided by distinguishing between vasospasm and other causes of clinical deterioration (Fig 6–12). TCD studies alone, however, have not proved to be consistently predictive of symptomatic vasospasm because TCD is insensitive to narrowing in second- and third-order vessels.

After hypertensive therapy has been started for a significant flow compromise, a second blood flow study can be performed to test its effectiveness and to monitor the effects of altering (raising or lowering) the blood pressure support. Such studies have helped to determine when aggressive medical therapy can be discontinued.

Testing of the Competence of the Circle of Willis.—Xe/CT CBF studies have been incorporated within our evaluation of an individual to tolerate occlusion of a carotid artery during, for example, aneurysm or skull base surgery. Following the clinical examinations of patients during balloon trial occlusion (BTO) of the intracranial artery (ICA), patients who do not develop a deficit undergo a flow study with the balloon inflated and deflated.[69] In this way we have identified an additional 10% to 20% of individuals who, while maintaining flow above the 20-cc/100 g/min level needed to maintain neuronal function, may have severely compromised reserves with flow values only slightly above this threshold, thus allowing no additional tolerance for blood pressure reduction (Fig 6–13). Medical efforts to maintain CBF or surgical efforts to reconstruct vessels have been utilized in these patients.

Head Trauma
Rapidly accessible tomographic CBF information also has become an integral part of managing head trauma victims.[70] The ability to record CBF

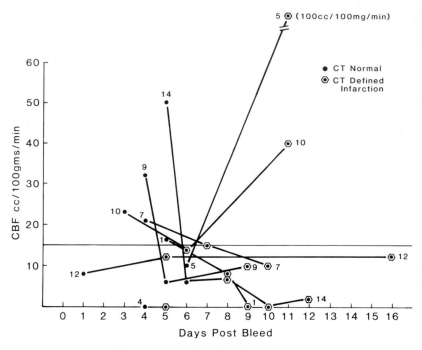

FIG 6–11.

These eight individuals with symptomatic vasospasm developed CT-defined infarctions concurrent or subsequent to the identification of flow values below 15 cc/100 g/min. In *case 5*, CT conver-

sion to infarction occurred along with high flow values, which indicated that reperfusion had most likely occurred within this previously ischemic region due to the resolution of vasospasm.

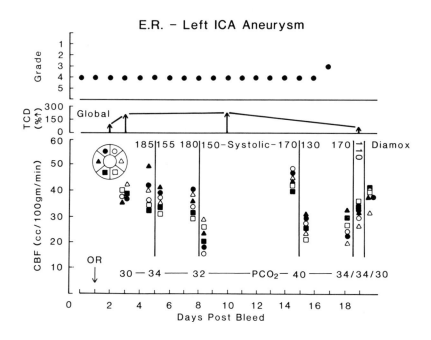

FIG 6–12.

This 72-year-old woman presented in grade 4 after a severe subarachnoid hemorrhage from a large internal carotid artery *(ICA)* aneurysm. Transcranial Doppler readings *(above)* indicated a progressive rise of velocities beginning on the third day postbleed. Average flow values for each vascular territory are plotted *below* at one or two blood pressure levels. Blood pressure was altered by decreasing the rate of dopamine infusion between CBF studies

performed at 20-minute intervals. A loss of autoregulation was found on days 8 and 15, with intact autoregulation on days 5 and 19 postbleed. The last study indicated that raising the blood pressure with dopamine reduced blood flow when given to an individual with regained autoregulation. The presence of flow reserves was validated by a CBF rise following intravenous Diamox.

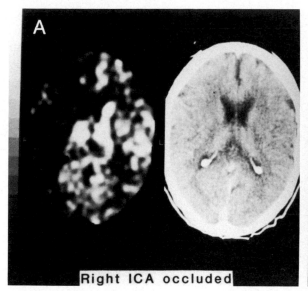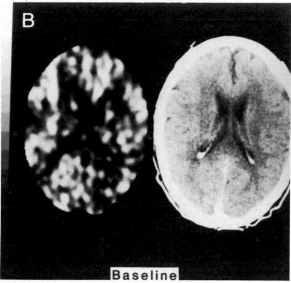

FIG 6–13.
This man with a right skull base tumor underwent a CBF study with balloon occlusion of the right internal carotid artery *(ICA)* **(A)** and a repeat study 20 minutes after its deflation **(B).** While this individual displayed no neurologic deficit with ICA occlusion, flow values in the ipsilateral anterior and middle cerebral territories fell below 20 cc/100 g/min. This information was useful in guiding the surgical team to surgically augment right hemispheric flow prior to sacrifice of the right ICA.

with the first CT scan has had an immediate influence on treatment decisions, for example, when an absence of cerebral perfusion with values near zero are identified in one or more vascular territories[71] (Fig 6–14). The finding of hyperemia within areas of low CT density also has been important for guiding ventilatory management (Fig 6–15). Increased flow values in a patient with elevated ICP frequently has guided management toward more aggressive ventilation therapy. In severe closed head injuries, however, the "blind" lowering of ICP by hyperventilation, without local CBF information, can lead to ischemia in normal tissues and a "steal" to abnormal tissues.[72] Repeated Xe/CT CBF studies after pCO_2 manipulation have proved to be very useful to determine the most appropriate level of hyperventilation treatment.

Limitations and Problems

Several features of xenon warrant discussion: its anesthetic properties, the associated effect on blood flow, and radiation exposure.

Although the incidence of intolerance to xenon inhalation appears to be low at a concentration of about 30% for 4 minutes and 20 seconds, there are individual exceptions. Some people are very sensitive to xenon and experience an early anesthetic effect of agitation that is often manifested by laughter or brief unresponsiveness. In 1,750 studies performed at nine institutions, significant side effects included respiratory slowing in 3%, seizures in 0.2%, delayed headache in 0.4%, and nausea or vomiting in 0.2%.[46]

The effect of xenon on blood flow has been evaluated by a number of investigators. Although one study in rats suggested a significant differential elevation of neocortical flows only,[73] no one else has found the same extent or pattern of flow augmentation. Radiolabeled microsphere studies in nonhuman primates demonstrated either no flow alteration or up to a 17% homogeneous increase in flow in all brain regions.[50] An examination of CBF alterations in normal subjects who received[133]Xe identified a wider range of flow enhancement that averaged 30% during a 4- to 5-minute period of xenon inhalation.[74] Because the flow values actually derived from the stable Xe/CT method do not appear to deviate as severely from established normal values, the true significance of these measurements is yet to be defined. The only trend noted in comparative studies is for Xe/CT-derived values to be higher than either iodoantypyrine- or microsphere-derived values. After examining 3,000 CBF examinations from clinical and animal studies, our impression is that an increase of flow, to whatever extent it may influence the calculation of CBF, is acceptable. Further, we believe

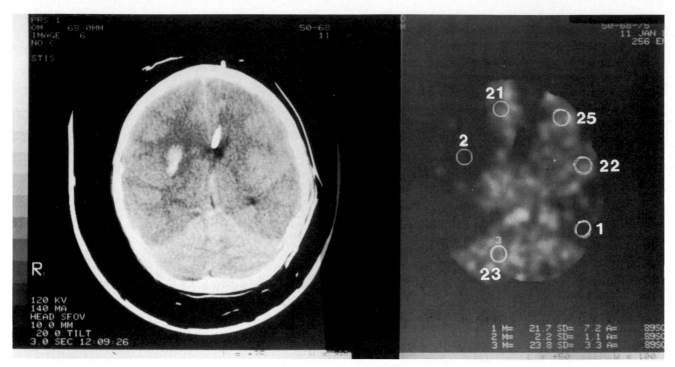

FIG 6–14.
This 3-year-old sustained a severe closed head injury and had a Glasgow coma score of 6 when a CT scan and CBF study was obtained. While the CT scan only demonstrated a moderate-size deep hematoma, the CBF study provided valuable insight that an injury of the ICA had probably occurred and caused an infarction of the right middle cerebral artery territory. Herniation with bilateral posterior cerebral artery compromise probably accounted for no flow within both posterior temporal regions. This study guided the treating team of physicians away from the emergent surgical intervention that had been planned.

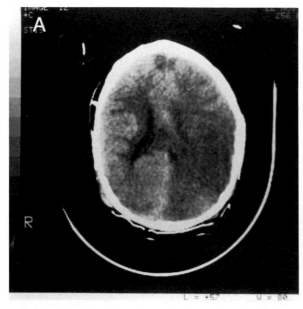

FIG 6–15.
This 8-year-old lad suffered a closed head injury and was comatose 2 days later when the CT scan **(A)** showed mass effect and low density within the left hemisphere. Despite an elevated ICP of 28 mm Hg, intravenous mannitol, and hyperventilation to a pCO_2 of 22 mm Hg, severe hyperemia was still encountered **(B)**. This study guided the treating physicians to reduce cerebral perfusion by initiating barbiturate coma.

that such an increase in CBF may be clinically useful and serve as a challenge of flow reserves similar to that obtained by inhaling added pCO_2. In addition, the only possible effect of elevated CBF during xenon inhalation is to elevate measured flow values, thus increasing the clinical relevance of the very low flow values that Xe/CT CBF can uniquely record.[55, 57, 61, 68]

The tendency of xenon to elevate CBF is of concern in patients with increased ICP and decreased compliance. Although we found no ICP increase during xenon inhalation in our initial observations of head-injured patients undergoing hyperventilation therapy,[71] the elevation of ICP due to an increase in CBF is theoretically possible.[75] Patients with elevated ICP will require careful monitoring until the extent of xenon-associated ICP elevation is fully defined under all clinical parameters.

A severely limiting aspect of high-resolution flow imaging is that no motion can be tolerated during the time required for acquiring baseline and all enhanced scans. When image resolution is relatively high, considerable misregistration can occur with as little as a few millimeters of movement in any plane.

Radiation exposure is another aspect of the method that must be considered when undertaking Xe/CT studies. Depending on the exposure factors, the dose of radiation per CT image can range from 2 to 3.5 rad. A flow study will deliver 8 to 28 rad to each level studied, depending on the number of baseline and enhanced scans obtained. Although these are considered to be clinically acceptable levels for other radiographic procedures such as cerebral angiography, this dose of radiation is of significance. However, the radiation field is highly collimated, and contiguous slices are avoided to minimize higher doses in overlapping bands. In addition, direct exposure of the lens of the eye is avoided. The brain is also considered less radiosensitive than many other body organ systems; therefore, the risk associated with even the highest possible exposure from a single or multiple Xe/CT CBF study is relatively low.

Direct measurements of the radiation dose to the lens of the eyes indicate that during a typical study the dose is not likely to exceed 0.2 cGy (200 mrad). The addition of a "scout view" will increase this exposure by approximately 0.05 cGy (50 mrad). If an organ dose is calculated for brain tissue, the average dose to the brain from a typical (eight-image) study of an adult is 4.32 cGy (rad) when utilizing the recommended protocol. Because of the radiation levels associated with this method, repeated studies in normal adults and investigational studies in children are not recommended without careful considerations of potential risks and benefits.

RECENT ADVANCES, POTENTIAL IMPROVEMENTS, AND FUTURE DIRECTIONS

With the improvement in computer power in recent years, several advances have been implemented in the Xe/CT CBF technology, and others are being investigated. These include but are not limited to the following: (1) the use of washin and washout (clearance) of xenon gas to allow for more data points to be acquired; (2) estimation of arterial concentration by double exponentials to improve the input function for the solution of the Kety-Schmidt equation (some attempts have been made to completely eliminate curve fitting of the arterial buildup; (3) the use of "lookup" tables rather than iterative least-square computation allowing extremely rapid derivation of flow values in each voxel of interest, thereby significantly reducing the time required to obtain and display flow maps; and (4) the reduction of the amount of xenon used in each study by adding rebreathing systems.

Some of these advances have made the technology easier to use in the clinical environment, while others have resulted in computational improvements. However, the two most important factors in increasing the likelihood for reliable, high-quality studies are lack of patient motion and an increase in SNR per unit of radiation dose. As noted, the first of these problems is being addressed, in part through the development of better head holders specifically designed for this application. The SNR of current CT scanners is consistently being upgraded through new detection systems, more stable x-ray tubes, and better signal-collecting electronics. There is no doubt that improvements in SNR per unit dose will have a direct impact on the quality of blood flow images and the ability to choose to reduce either the radiation dose or the inhaled xenon concentration.

In the future, high-heat-loading x-ray tubes will enable the study of more levels of the brain during a single Xe/CT examination. In addition, simple modifications of currently used protocols are likely to reduce bone artifacts, thus permitting better measurements of CBF in the low posterior and anterior regions of the brain (e.g., posterior fossa and temporal lobes).

There is no doubt that other improvements are possible and forthcoming. The clinical and experimental uses of this technique remain to be fully explored. However, as long as we believe that most acute and many chronic cerebral abnormalities are tissue perfusion driven, the most important chapter on this tissue-specific, clinically accessible, and anatomically correlatable CBF method is yet to be written.

REFERENCES

1. Kety SS, Schmidt CF: The nitrous oxide method for the quantitative determination of cerebral blood flow in man: Theory, procedure, and normal values. *J Clin Invest* 1948; 27:476–483.
2. Lassen NA, Ingvar DH: The blood flow of the cerebral cortex determined by radioactive krypton 85. *Experientia* 1961; 17:42–43.
3. Obrist WD, Thompson HK, King CH, et al: Determination of regional cerebral blood flow by inhalation of 133-xenon. *Circ Res* 1967; 20:124–135.
4. Ewing JR, Robertson WM, Brown GG, et al: ^{133}Xenon inhalation: Accuracy in detection of ischemic cerebral regions and angiographic lesions, in Wood JH (ed): *Cerebral Blood Flow: Physiologic and Clinical Aspects.* New York, McGraw-Hill International Book Co, 1987, pp 202–219.
5. Kuhl DE, Barrio JR, Huang SC, et al: Quantifying local cerebral blood flow by N-isoproply-p-(^{123}I)-iodoamphetamine (IMP) tomography. *J Nucl Med* 1982; 23:196–203.
6. Welch KMA, Levine SR, Ewing JR: Viewing stroke pathophysiology: An analysis of contemporary methods. *Stroke* 1986; 17:1071–1077.
7. Heinz ER, Dubois P, Osborne D, et al: Dynamic computed tomography study of the brain. *J Comput Assist Tomogr* 1979; 3:641–649.
8. Norman D, Axel L, Berninger WH, et al: Dynamic computed tomography of the brain: Techniques, data analysis, and applications. *AJR* 1981; 136:759–770.
9. Winkler S, Holden J, Sackett J, et al: Xenon inhalation as an adjunct to computerized tomography of the brain. Preliminary study. *Invest Radiol* 1977; 12:15–18.
10. Ingvar DH, Cronqvist S, Ekberg R, et al: Normal values of regional cerebral blood flow in man, including flow and weight estimates of gray and white matter. *Acta Neurol Scand* 1965; 41(suppl 14):72–78.
11. Segawa H: Tomographic cerebral blood flow measurement using xenon inhalation and serial CT scanning: Normal values and its validity. *Neurosurg Rev* 1985; 8:27–33.
12. Yonas H: Normative blood flow values by Xe/CT CBF obtained from normal population. In preparation, 1989.
13. Alpert NM, Ackerman RH, Correia JA, et al: Measurement of cerebral blood flow and oxygen metabolism in transverse section—preliminary results. *Acta Neurol Scand* 1979; 60(suppl 72):196–197.
14. Raichle ME, Grubb RL, Gado MH, et al: Correlation between regional cerebral blood flow and oxidative metabolism: In vivo studies in man. *Arch Neurol* 1976; 33:523–526.
15. Ingvar DH, Philipson L: Distribution of cerebral blood flow in the dominant hemisphere during motor ideation and motor performance. *Ann Neurol* 1977; 2:230–237.
16. Leniger-Follert E, Hossman K-A: Microflow and evoked potentials in the somatomotor cortex of the cat brain during specific sensory activation. *Acta Neurol Scand* 1979; 60(suppl 72)10–11.
17. Plum F, Posner JB, Troy B: Cerebral metabolic and circulatory response to induced convulsions in animals. *Arch Neurol* 1968; 18:1–13.
18. Ingvar DH, Haggendal E, Nilsson NJ, et al: Cerebral circulation and metabolism in a comatose patient. *Arch Neurol* 1964; 11:13–21.
19. Malmlund HO: Cerebral blood flow and oxygen consumption in barbiturate poisoning. *Acta Med Scand* 1968; 184:373–377.
20. Raichle ME, Plum F: Hyperventilation and cerebral blood flow. *Stroke* 1972; 3:566–575.
21. Gelmers HJ: *Regional Cerebral Blood Flow: Regulation, Measurement and Changes in Diseases.* The Netherlands Van Grocum Assoc 1978.
22. Sorensen SG: Theoretical considerations on the potential hazards of hyperventilation during anaesthesia. *Acta Anaesthesiol Scand Suppl* 1978; 67:106–110.
23. Wood JH, Polyzoidis KS, Epstein CM, et al: Quantitative EEG alterations after isovolemic-hemodilutional augmentation of cerebral perfusion in stroke patients. *Neurology* 1984; 34:764–768.
24. Olesen J: Quantitative evaluation of normal and pathologic cerebral blood flow regulation to perfusion pressure. *Arch Neurol* 1973; 28:143–149.
25. Gibbs JM, Wise RJS, Leenders SKL, et al: Evaluation of cerebral perfusion reserve in patients with carotid artery occlusion. *Lancet* 1984; 28:182–186.
26. David SM, Ackerman RH, Correia JA, et al: Cerebral blood flow and cerebrovascular CO_2 reactivity in stroke-age normal controls. *Neurology* 1983; 33:391–399.
27. Yamamoto M, Meyer JS, Sakai F, et al: Aging and cerebral vasodilator responses to hypercarbia. Responses in normal aging and in persons with risk factors for stroke. *Arch Neurol* 1980; 37:489–496.
28. Ehrenreich DL, Burns RA, Alman RW, et al: Influ-

ence of acetazolamide on cerebral blood flow. *Arch Neurol* 1961; 5:227–232.

29. Vorstrup S, Henriksen L, Paulson OB: Effect of acetazolamide on cerebral blood flow and cerebral metabolic rate for oxygen. *J Clin Invest* 1984; 74:1634–1639.

30. Lassen NA: The luxury perfusion syndrome and its possible relation to acute metabolic acidosis localized within the brain. *Lancet* 1966; 2:1113–1114.

31. Sundt TM Jr, Sharbrough FW, Anderson RE, et al: Cerebral blood flow measurements and electroencephalograms during carotid endarterectomy. *J Neurosurg* 1974; 41:310–320.

32. Astrup J, Symon L, Branston NM, et al: Cortical evoke potential and extracellular K^+ and H^+ at critical levels of brain ischemia. *Stroke* 1977; 8:51–57.

33. Morawetz RB, DeGirolami U, Ojeamann RG, et al: Cerebral blood flow determination by hydrogen clearance during middle cerebral artery occlusion in unanesthetized monkeys. *Stroke* 1978; 9:143–149.

34. Dhawan V, Goldiner P, Ray C, et al: Mass spectrometric measurement of end-tidal xenon concentration for clinical stable xenon/computerized tomography cerebral blood flow studies. *Biomed Mass Spectrom* 1982; 9:241–245.

35. Gur D, Herron HM, Molter BS, et al: Simultaneous mass spectrometry and thermoconductivity measurements of end-tidal xenon concentrations. *Med Phys* 1984; 11:208–212.

36. Drayer BP, Gur D, Yonas H, et al: Abnormality of the xenon brain-blood partition coefficient and blood flow cerebral infarction: An in vivo assessment using transmission computed tomography. *Radiology* 1980; 135:349–354.

37. Meyer JS, Hayman LH, Yamamoto M, et al: Local cerebral blood flow measured by CT after stable xenon inhalation. *AJR* 1980; 135:239–251.

38. Kishore PR, Rao GU, Fernandez RE, et al: Regional cerebral blood flow measurements using stable xenon enhanced computed tomography: A theoretical and experimental evaluation. *J Comput Assist Tomogr* 1984; 8:619–630.

39. Gur D, Good WF, Wolfson SK Jr, et al: In vivo mapping of local cerebral blood flow by xenon-enhanced computed tomography. *Science* 1982; 5:1267–1268.

40. Dhawan V, Haughton VM, Thaler HT, et al: Accuracy of stable xenon/CT measurements of regional cerebral blood flow: Effect of extrapolated estimates of brain-blood partition coefficients. *J Comput Assist Tomogr* 1984; 8:208–212.

41. Good WF, Gur D, Shabason L, et al: Errors associated with single-scan determinations of regional cerebral blood flow by xenon-enhanced CT. *Phys Med Biol* 1982; 27:531–537.

42. Gur D, Yonas H, Jackson DL, et al: Simultaneous measurements of cerebral blood flow by the xenon/

CT method and the microsphere method: A comparison. *Invest Radiol* 1985; 20:672–677.

43. Thaler HT, Baglivo JA, Lu HC, et al: Repeated least squares analysis of simulated xenon computed tomographic measurements of regional cerebral blood flow. *J Cereb Blood Flow Metab* 1982; 2:408–414.

44. Winkler S, Turski P: Potential hazards of xenon inhalation. *Am J Neuroradiol* 1985; 6:974–975.

45. Yonas H, Grundy B, Gur D, et al: Side effects of xenon inhalation. *J Comput Assist Tomogr* 1981; 5:591–592.

46. Latchaw RE, Yonas H, Pentheny SL, et al: Adverse reactions to xenon-enhanced CT cerebral blood flow determination. *Radiology* 1987; 163:251–254.

47. Gur D, Yonas H, Herbert DL, et al: Xenon enhanced dynamic computed tomography: Multilevel cerebral blood flow studies. *J Comput Assist Tomogr* 1981; 5:334–340.

48. Yonas H, Gur D, Claassen D, et al: Stable xenon enhanced computed tomography in the study of clinical and pathologic correlates of focal ischemia in baboons. *Stroke* 1988; 19:228–238.

49. Yonas H, Latchaw RE, Johnson DW, et al: Xenon-enhanced CT: Evaluating cerebral blood flow. *Diagn Imag* 1988; 10:88–94.

50. Gur D, Yonas H, Jackson DL, et al: Measurements of cerebral blood flow during xenon inhalation as measured by the microsphere method. *Stroke* 1985; 16:871–874.

51. Panos PP, Fatouros R, Kishore PRS, et al: Comparison of improved stable xenon/CT method for cerebral blood flow measurements with radiolabelled microspheres technique. *Radiology* 1985; 158:334.

52. Wolfson SK Jr, Clark J, Greenberg JH, et al: Xenon-enhanced computed tomography compared with [^{14}C] iodoantipyrine for normal and low cerebral blood flow states in baboons. *Stroke* 1990; 21:751–757.

53. Good WF, Gur D, Herron JM, et al: The development of a xenon/computed tomography cerebral blood flow quality assurance phantom. *Med Phys* 1987; 14:867–869.

54. Wolfson S, Safar P, Reich H, et al: Multifocal dynamic cerebral hypoperfusion after prolonged cardiac arrest in dogs, measured by the stable xenon-CT technique. *Crit Care Med* 1988; 16:390.

55. Darby JM, Yonas H, Gur D, et al: Xenon-enhanced computed tomography in brain death. *Arch Neurol* 1987; 44:551–554.

56. Tachibana H, Meyer JS, Okayasu H, et al: Xenon contrast CT-CBF scanning of the brain differentiates normal age-related changes from multi-infarct dementia and senile dementia of Alzheimer type. *J Gerontol* 1984; 39:415–423.

57. Yonas H, Gur D, Claassen D, et al: Stable xenon-enhanced CT measurement of cerebral blood flow

in reversible focal ischemia in baboons. *J Neurosurg* 1990; 73:266–273.

58. Tachibana H, Meyer JS, Rose JE, et al: Local cerebral blood flow and partition coefficients measured in cerebral astrocytomas of different grades of malignancy. *Surg Neurol* 1984; 21:125–131.

59. Meyer JS, Kitasawa Y, Tanahashi N, et al: Pathogenesis of normal-pressure hydrocephalus— preliminary observations. *Surg Neurol* 1985; 23:121–133.

60. Tachibana H, Meyer J, Kitagawa Y, et al: Xenon contrast CT-CBF measurements in parkinsonism and normal aging. *J Am Geriatr Soc* 1985; 33:413–421.

61. Hughes R, Yonas H, Gur D, et al: Stable xenon-enhanced CT in the first eight hours of cerebral infarction; 12th international joint conference on stroke and cerebral circulation. *Stroke* 1987; 18:283.

62. Hakim AM, Pokrupa RP, Villanueva J, et al: The effect of spontaneous reperfusion on metabolic function in early human cerebral infarcts. *Ann Neurol* 1987; 21:279–289.

63. Rappata S, Cambon HA, Samson Y, et al: Remote metabolic effects of thalamic and capsular stroke: Clinical-topographical correlations. *J Cereb Blood Flow Metab* 1987; 7:542.

64. Ferguson GG, Farrar JK, Meguro K, et al: Serial measurements of CBF as a guide to surgery in patients with ruptured intracranial aneurysms. *J Cereb Blood Flow Metab* 1981; 1(suppl 1):518.

65. Knuckey NW, Fox RA, Surveyor I, et al: Early cerebral blood flow and computerized tomography in predicting ischemia after cerebral aneurysm rupture. *J Neurosurg* 1985; 62:850–855.

66. Grahm TW, Hodak JA, Spetzler RF, et al: Patchy hyperemia as a predictor of symptomatic vasospasm. *J Cereb Blood Flow Metab* 1987; 7(suppl):663.

67. Sekhar LN, Wechsler LR, Yonas H: The value of

transcranial Doppler examination in the diagnosis of vasospasm following subarachnoid hemorrhage. *Neurosurgery*, in press.

68. Yonas H, Sekhar L, Johnson DW, et al: Xe/CT CBF determination of irreversible ischemia in patients with symptomatic vasospasm. *Neurosurgery* 1989; 24:368–372.

69. Erba SM, Horton JA, Latchaw RE, et al: Balloon test occlusion of the internal carotid artery with stable xenon/CT cerebral blood flow imaging. *Am J Neuroradiol* 1988; 9:533–538.

70. Latchaw RE, Yonas H, Darby JM, et al: Xenon/CT cerebral blood flow determination following cranial trauma. *Acta Radiol Suppl* 1986; 369:370–373.

71. Darby JM, Yonas H, Peitzman A, et al: Xenon-enhanced computed tomography in head injury. Presented at a conference on Intracranial Pressure and Brain Injury, June 19–23, Ann Arbor, Mich, 1988, in press.

72. Darby JM, Yonas H, Marion DW, et al: Local "inverse steal" induced by hyperventilation in head injury. *Neurosurgery* 1988; 23:84–88.

73. Rottenberg DA, Lu HC, Kearfott KJ: The in vivo autoradiographic measurement of regional cerebral blood flow using stable xenon and computerized tomography: The effect of tissue heterogeneity and computerized tomography noise. *J Cereb Blood Flow Metab* 1982; 2:173–178.

74. Obrist WD, Jaggi JL, Harel D, et al: Effect of stable xenon inhalation on human CBF. *J Cereb Blood Flow Metab* 1985; 5(suppl):557–558.

75. Harrington TR, Manwaring K, Hodak J: Local basal ganglia and brainstem blood flow in the head injured patient using stable xenon-enhanced CT scanning, in Miller JD, Teasdale GM, Rowan JV, et al (eds): *Intracranial Pressure*. New York, Springer Publishing Co, Inc, 1986.

7

Magnetic Resonance Flow Effects: Adaptations to Vascular Imaging

Thomas J. Masaryk, M.D.

Robert J. Herfkens, M.D.

Radiologists have come to appreciate magnetic resonance imaging (MRI) for its high contrast, multiplaner imaging capability, sensitivity to edema, ischemia and blood breakdown products, and responsiveness to patient motion, which is primarily manifested as artifacts.[1-10] While the sensitivity of magnetic resonance (MR) to motion was recognized more than 30 years before the use of MR as an imaging technique, radiologists and physicists have only recently struggled to master the sequelae of physiologic motion (cardiac, respiratory, cerebrospinal fluid [CSF] and blood flow).[10-12] This report will attempt to briefly outline MR flow phenomena and the means by which they are adapted to noninvasive, angiographic imaging of the central nervous system.

BASIC PRINCIPLES OF FLOW

Positively charged protons (hydrogen nuclei) exhibit spin and thus induce a magnetic field. A superimposed magnetic field (in this instance the imager) will cause the spinning atoms to become aligned and precess at a frequency dependent on the magnitude of the superimposed field. This simple, linear relationship underlies the entire imaging process and is described by the Larmor equation:

$$\lambda = \gamma \, G_0$$

where λ = the Larmor frequency; γ is a (known) constant, the gyromagnetic ratio (42 mHz/tesla); and G_0 is the (known) field strength. A radio frequency (RF) pulse applied at exactly this frequency will cause the spinning protons to change their alignment (typically 90 or 180 degrees) with the main magnetic field (G_0). Such RF pulses are often referred to as "excitation pulses." Following excitation to a higher energy state (i.e., unaligned with the magnetic field), the realignment of these spinning protons with the original superimposed magnetic field (B) will produce (emit) an RF current in a receiver coil that samples the RF signal at the same field-dependent frequency.

From the simplistic description above, one can appreciate that the basic imaging process consists of two essential components: (1) excitation in the form of an RF pulse and (2) spatial encoding and sampling of signal to form the MR image. The presence of motion (blood flow) during either excitation or spatial encoding and sampling results in two types of corresponding effects: (1) time-of-flight effects and (2) spin-phase phenomena. Detailed descriptions of MR flow effects can be found in the articles by Axel and by Bradley and Waluch but a brief description follows.[13, 14]

Time-of-flight effects depend upon the type of RF pulse sequence used for imaging. In selective spin-echo imaging (used in conventional brain imaging), protons *must* experience both the 90-degree excitation and 180-degree refocusing RF pulse in order to contribute to the measured signal. If there is motion through the selected slice during excitation such as blood in the internal carotid arteries of an axial image at the midbrain, spins initially present in the slice at the time of the first pulse may no longer be present at the time of the second, being replaced by inflowing unexcited spins (Fig 7–1). The obvious net result is a progressive loss of signal from the vessel that is most marked when flow is fast enough to completely replace all the blood protons in the time between the 90-and 180-degree pulses. This phenomenon is commonly referred to as "flow void" or "high-velocity signal loss."

The effect of flow is decidedly different for other pulse sequences such as the gradient-echo or "fast-scan" techniques. With these techniques only a single RF pulse is used (typically ≤90 degrees; however, ≥90 degrees can also be used) to generate the sampled signal. Once again (assuming that the RF pulses are slice selective and the transverse magnetization is dephased prior to the application

of each RF pulse), stationary tissue within the image receives repetitive excitations that will generate signal to the extent that stationary protons realign with the main magnetic field between pulses and are then available to generate signal following the application of the next pulse. This realignment is dependent upon the T1 relaxation constant of the tissue, which if not complete before the next pulse results in submaximal signal. Under these circumstances the stationary tissue is said to be partially or completely "saturated." Alternatively, with protons flowing through the image plane (e.g., carotid arteries in an axial fast scan of the cervical spine), saturated spins are continually replaced by freshly inflowing, fully magnetized (aligned) protons so that each spin experiences only one or at most several RF pulses. Under these circumstances, the vessel gains signal intensity and reaches a maximum when the blood velocity is such that all spins within the vessel are replaced between pulse repetitions (Fig 7–2). This time-of-flight effect is known as "flow-related enhancement" and is primarily seen in gradient-echo imaging. (It should be noted that flow-related enhancement can be observed on spin-echo scans

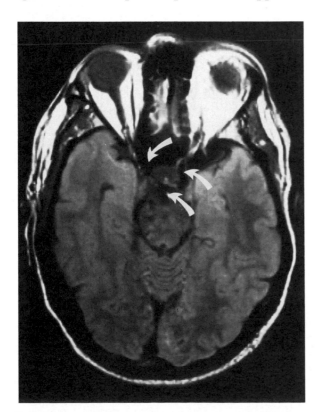

FIG 7–1.
An axial spin-echo image (600/30) at the level of the midbrain demonstrates "flow void" (or "high-velocity signal loss") within the juxtasellar carotid arteries and the basilar tip *(arrows)*.

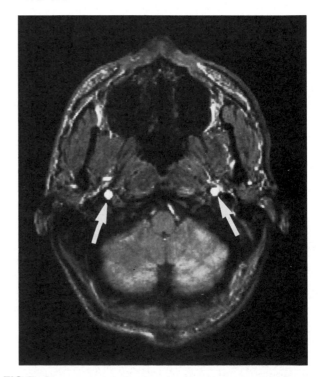

FIG 7–2.
An axial gradient echo scan (FISP 60/8/40) at the level of the medulla demonstrates marked flow-related enhancement *(arrows)* within the distal cervical carotid arteries.

with very short echo times. Under these conditions, the 90- and 180-degree pulses are temporally paired such that, relative to the repetition time (i.e., echo time [TE]/2 $<<$ repetition time [TR]), they act almost as a single pulse with negligible high-velocity signal loss occurring between.) Most commonly this is recognized on multislice two-dimensional scans at the proximal vessel as the so-called entry-slice phenomenon. By appropriately aligning the scan plane to be perpendicular (relative) to the direction of flow and adjusting the pulse sequence TR and flip angle, it is possible to manipulate the degree of flow-related enhancement relative to stationary signal saturation, thereby maximizing the contrast-to-noise (C/N) ratio between the vessels and the stationary background.

An appreciation of the flow effects related to signal sampling (i.e., spin-dephasing phenomena) requires an understanding of the means by which the MR signal is spatially encoded and sufficient data to generate an anatomic image. In effect, the scanner operates much like a combination metronome/multichannel radio capable of determining timing (phase) and frequency of the signal produced by resonating tissue protons. Sampling and spatial localization of the MR signal within the imager exploits the relationship described by the Larmor equation and the use of known gradient magnetic fields, i.e., a magnetic field stronger on one side of the magnet and weaker at the other. In order to localize signal in three-dimensional space, scanners use three orthosonal sets of gradients (Fig 7–3,A and B).

In conventional spin-echo imaging a slice-selecting gradient is applied at the time of the excitation pulse. If the excitation pulse is of a finite-frequency bandwidth, then according to the Larmor equation only those protons in the plane that are spinning at the same frequency (as determined by the slice-selection gradient) will be affected (Fig 7–3,C). Protons at other frequencies will not be affected. The result of this procedure is that only the protons residing in a single plane of tissue, the image slice, will be excited by the RF pulse and subsequently contribute to the measured signal.

Subsequently, a gradient in a second direction (phase-encoding gradient) is briefly applied and momentarily shifts the precessional frequency such that, once discontinued, protons returning to the same frequency will be out of phase, i.e., at different points in their arc of precession. The amount these spins are out of phase is predefined and determined by the duration and amplitude of the gradient pulse and the location of the spins with respect to the direction of the applied gradient. By successively incrementing the phase of the spins along the second direction, frequency (hence location) information with respect to this direction is obtained following a Fourier transform of this data. For a fixed gradient duration, the amplitude and number of increments acquired are determined by the required field of view (FOV) and resolution of the phase-encoded direction. Much like a metronome, the imager can appreciate these discrepancies in timed precession and adjust the gradient such that it is only synchronized to the phase of a narrow line of signal within the plane of the image, hence the term phase-encoding gradient (Fig 7–3,D).

Finally, a gradient field is applied along the third direction (the second axis of the digital image matrix) during the period when the signal emitted by the body is read (sampled) by the imager. As predicted by the Larmor equation, protons along each point of the gradient will generate a different frequency signal. Because the gradient field magnitude is known, it is possible (by using the Fourier transform) to localize the signal along the direction of the gradient on the basis of the Larmor relationship between field strength and frequency. The imager thus behaves as a multichannel radio receiver; as might be expected, the third gradient is referred to as the frequency encode or read gradient (Fig 7–3,E). Remember also that as a metronome it receives only one synchronized line of signal during each pulse sequence repetition. Thus, to create a 256 × 256 digital image matrix, the pulse sequence must be repeated 256 times to generate 256 lines (phase-encoding steps), which are read out with a frequency gradient of a bandwidth capable of providing 256 frequency points for a given FOV and sampling time. Note that the spins lying at different locations with respect to the readout direction will begin to dephase upon application of the read gradient and this will lead to rapid signal loss. Consequently, an additional "dephasing" compensation gradient is applied in this direction prior to sampling such that during sampling (i.e., readout) the spins will rephase to form a gradient echo, i.e., time of maximum signal (with the exception of T2 decay), typically at the center of the sampling interval and will thus be "in phase."

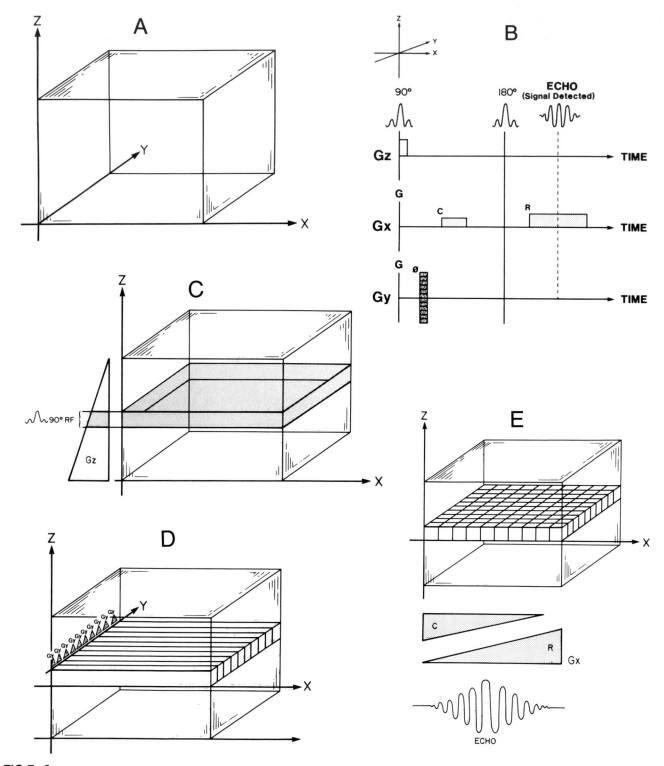

FIG 7–3.
A and **B,** three-dimensional space **(A)** within the MR imager is defined and localized by a series of three parameters **(B),** one for each direction: G_z = slice-select gradient, G_x = frequency-encode or readout gradient, and G_y = phase-encode gradient. **C,** the slice-select gradient is applied during the 90-degree excitation pulse. According to the Larmor equation, only protons spinning at the same frequency along the gradient as the bandwidth of the RF excitation pulse would be excited *(shaded area).* Thus, as the name suggests, the combination of excitation pulse and slice-select gradients selects out the image slice. **D,** the phase-encode gradient is applied for a brief period during each pulse sequence repetition; protons along the gradient change frequency momen-

With the basic mechanisms of signal sampling defined, what then is the effect of motion in the presence and direction of these gradient fields? The sequela of motion along an imaging gradient is that the linear relationship predicted by the Larmor equation for stationary tissue no longer exists for moving protons—frequency, hence phase, now changes geometrically, with field strength depending upon the character of the flow, i.e., constant velocity, accelerating, turbulent, etc. For a proton moving at constant velocity, the associated change in phase at the time of the echo is

$$\Delta I_V = \gamma \, G \, \Delta V \, (TE/2)^2,$$

where ΔI_V is the velocity-induced phase difference within the pixel that results from the velocity distribution ΔV across the voxel with respect to the direction of the applied gradient (G), γ is the gyromagnetic ratio, and TE is the echo time (i.e., time between the center of RF excitation and the center of the readout interval). Returning to the example of blood flowing in vessels within an MR image (e.g., the proximal middle cerebral artery in an axial brain scan), the distribution of velocities (and higher-order motion terms) within the digital image volume element (voxel) that corresponds to the vascular lumen will result in a distribution of spin phases that produces spatial misregistration in the phase-encode direction (i.e., ghosting) in addition to the uniform spatial shift due to the finite time required between phase encoding and readout that occurs when flow along a paraxial in the plane direction is present. Spin dephasing within the voxel also leads to partial or complete cancellation of the associated signal (Fig 7–4,A–C). One should note that these adverse effects will be most prominent in the presence of fast flow, large voxels, and gradients that are applied over a relatively long time period (i.e., read.) In summary, the net effects of motion in the presence of conventional signal sampling gradients, which occurs simultaneously with but independent of time-of-flight effects and is known as spin-phase phenomena, are ghosting and signal loss.

FLOW IMAGING

Angiography Based on Phase Manipulation

Macovski postulated the use of motion-induced phase contrast and subtraction as a method of producing projective MR angiograms (MRAs) in 1982.[15] Close scrutiny of the equation (above) that describes spin-phase phenomena reveals the means by which phase changes induced by motion may be manipulated or minimized in everyday imaging of patients. The single most effective method would be the reduction of TE, which would produce a geometric reduction in the amount of signal loss. The velocity distribution term ΔV may be modified by cardiac gating so that signal is sampled only in diastole or systole. A combination of short TE scanning with gating provides images of high vascular signal (diastolic) or low vascular signal (systolic) but identical signal for soft tissues. The technique of acquiring and subtracting two such gated images was originally reported by Wedeen et al. and was the first method used to produce angiographic images with MR.[16]

Another variable that can be changed is the gradient fields (G). Moran first described the use of precisely timed and configured compensation gradients that negate the phase change and hence signal loss induced by motion at the time of signal sampling (Fig 7–5,A and B).[17] Assuming otherwise constant scanning parameters (TE/TR), scans with and without the special compensation gradients can be obtained where, again, stationary tissue has the same signal and subtraction images (magnitude subtraction) appear as angiograms.[17] Analogous gradient modifications have been employed by Dumoulin and others to produce MRAs with both spin-echo and gradient-echo sequences.[18–25] Advantages of this method include the ability to visualize slowly moving protons (i.e., venous anatomy) as well as its high vascular contrast. Implementation of such gradients can be accomplished in either the slice-select, read, or phase-encode directions but requires additional gradients and hence more time prior to signal readout, which will prolong the TE. The latter is particularly disadvanta-

---

tarily such that once the gradient is discontinued protons in this direction will be spinning at different points along their arc of rotation, i.e., they will be at different phases. The imager is capable of recognizing this and is synchronized only to a single "line" of protons within the image plane. The remaining protons within the image plane will be out of phase. In this way, the imager is able to monitor the timing of spinning protons in a fashion analogous to a metronome. **E,** during the time that the signal, or "echo," is recorded by the receiver coil, the readout gradient is applied in order to spatially localize signal in the second direction of the image plane according to frequency. A compensation gradient is applied earlier in the pulse sequence in the same direction and corrects or compensates for phase shifts induced in stationary spins during the application of the read gradient.

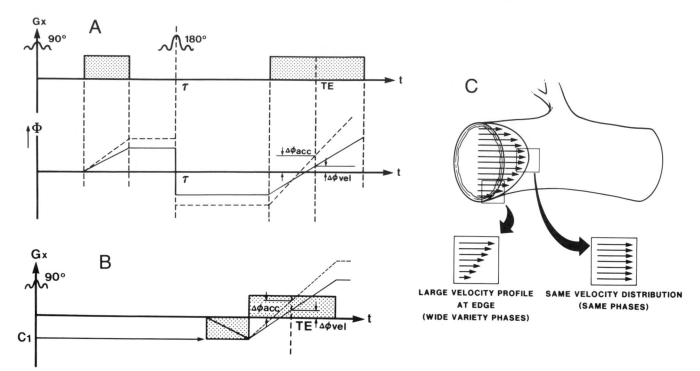

FIG 7–4.

A, spin-phase phenomenon shown by a schematic representation of a readout gradient of a standard spin-echo sequence *(above)* and a phase plot *(below)* of spins moving in the direction of the gradient at constant velocity *(solid line)* and constant acceleration *(dashed line)*. The horizontal axis represents time, while the vertical axis represents the magnitude of the gradients and phase shift, respectively. Note that during the application of the read gradient the phase shift produced by moving spins is no longer linear as described by the Larmor equation but is now a geometric change in phase such that the initial compensation gradient is no longer effective in synchronizing the signal at the time of the echo readout. In effect, the phase changes induced by motion cause the signal of moving spins to be out of synchronization with the imager, the net result of which is artifact and signal loss. **B,** a similar readout gradient diagram and phase plot for constant acceleration and constant velocity spins in a gradient-echo pulse sequence. In gra-dient-echo imaging, there is no 180-degree refocusing RF pulse. Instead, the compensation/readout gradient combination is bipolar. Occasionally this form of imaging is also referred to as "gradient-reversal" imaging. Notice that like spin-echo imaging the phase and frequency change for spins moving in the direction of the readout gradients is no longer linear as described by the Larmor equation. When the echo is sampled at the center of the readout, the signal of moving spins is no longer synchronous with the imager. **C,** a diagramatic representation of the velocity profile in a blood vessel demonstrates that even for laminar flow, particularly at the peripheral portions of the lumen, a large variety of velocities are present. If flow in this vessel were directed along the gradients shown in Figure 7–2,A or 7–2,B, the result is a larger variety of phase changes secondary to motion that result in cancellation or negation of signal and thus signal loss.

geous in regions of fast nonuniform motion and in all gradient-echo imaging. In addition, three such data sets (i.e., rephase/dephase pairs) must be acquired independently in the direction in which the motion compensation gradients are applied (e.g., read, slice, or phase differing for each) in order to detect flow in any direction. Corresponding rephase/dephase images are subtracted. The three subtraction images can be analyzed on their own and/or added to generate the final angiographic image.

Angiography Based on Radio Frequency Sequence Manipulation

Time-of-flight MR flow-imaging methods are designed to exploit longitudinal magnetization by utilizing tagging techniques (typically relaxation, inversion, or subtraction) to distinguish previously unexcited, hence unsaturated protons flowing into the imaging volume from surrounding stationary tissue.[26–33]

Dixon et al. are now recognized as the first to utilize time-of-flight effects as a means of providing vascular contrast to create angiographic images.[26] Using a method of adiabatic fast passage (known primarily to spectroscopists), they were

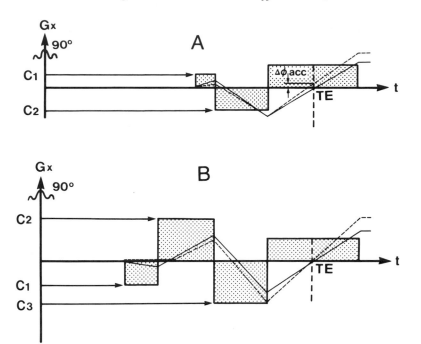

FIG 7–5.
A, read gradient configuration and a phase plot of constant acceleration and constant velocity spins for a gradient-echo scan compensated for velocity in the frequency-encode (read) direction. Notice that the insertion of an additional gradient lobe prior to the bipolar readout gradient can negate the change in phase induced by constant velocity. **B,** read gradient configuration and phase plot for gradient-echo pulse sequence compensated for both constant acceleration and constant velocity spins. With the use of three compensation gradients, it is now possible to negate the phase shifts of motion and synchronize the signal of spins with constant acceleration, constant velocity, and stationary tissue. Nevertheless, the gradient rise/fall times, switching delay times, etc., used to implement these flow compensations will by neccessity lengthen the TE. To some extent then, the use of gradient refocusing is counterproductive to minimizing gradient-induced phase shifts. The optimal compromise appears to be the use of velocity compensation gradients in the read and slice-select directions while attempting to use the shortest TE possible.

able to selectively tag incoming carotid flow with a special RF coil placed low in the neck and subsequently imaging at the level of the bifurcation by using a head coil. Originally, stationary tissue signal was suppressed through the use of special gradient ("twister") pulses, while more recent iterations of this technique have adopted stationary tissue RF saturation/inversion schemes.[34]

Nishimura and colleagues have had considerable success with another time-of-flight technique that utilizes thick-slab (so-called projection) images generated with a locally placed coil at the carotid bifurcation.[27] However, unlike Dixon's RF coil, which was used for spin labeling low in the neck, this method utilizes the local surface coil for RF receiving (sampling) signal only. Contrast is provided with gating and by controlling the signal of spins washing into the region of interest, with inverting (180-degree) pulses locally placed at and then also below the bifurcation and a separate transmitter coil on alternate image acquisitions. Angiograms are subsequently created by subtracting the two data acquisitions. Time-of-flight effects can be optimized by gating and by varying the timing between inverting pulses (TI), while phase effects secondary to high flow are minimized with extremely short TEs and gating. In this manner, high-quality images can be obtained.[27]

In 1986 and 1987 Wehrli et al. and Gullberg and colleagues reported on the possibility of examining blood vessels with sequential two-dimensional Fourier transform (2DFT) gradient-echo scans oriented perpendicular to the direction of flow on the basis of the considerable flow-related enhancement produced.[28, 29] Signal loss secondary to motion-induced spin-phase phenomena was minimized with motion compensation gradients and relatively short TEs. Additionally, short TRs made it possible to cover an area as large as the cervical carotid arteries while maintaining acceptable vascular contrast. Perhaps because at the time the data could not be easily viewed in a conventional angiographic format, this work received little immediate interest.

Subsequently Laub, Ruggieri, and colleagues reported their experience with a different selective saturation recovery time-of-flight angiography technique that used three-dimensional Fourier transform (3DFT) sequences.[30, 31] They attempted to maximize flow-related enhancement by utilizing a transmit/receive head coil (to localize the region of excitation/saturation) and optimizing the scan orientation relative to flow, the TR, and the flip angle. Also, in addition to flow compensation gradients and short TEs, unique to Laub's work were the extremely thin slices (and thus small voxels) available with 3DFT imaging, which theoretically may affect motion-induced phase change leading to signal loss. Note that it is the variability of phase within an image voxel that leads to the effective cancellation of proton signal. If a smaller voxel is used and, effectively, a narrower range of velocity (and ΔG)-induced phase change per voxel, then signal loss may be minimized. Typically, a thick slab of tissue (volume) is excited. The 3D pulse sequence is similar to 2D with the exception of the application of an additional phase-encoding gradient along the slice-select direction to spatially encode the signal in this direction. A 3DFT is used to reconstruct the final imaging. When using this technique, it is possible to produce 3D scans with voxel dimensions of 1 mm^3.[30, 31] Note that overall scan time is increased with 3D (relative to 2D); however, as compared with its 2D counterpart, each 3D slice benefits from a square root of NS increase in the signal-to-noise ratio, where NS is the number of slice-select phase-encoding steps or 3D slices acquired. T2* effects are also reduced in 3D vs. 2D.

Also novel to this approach was the implementation of automated postprocessing (maximum-intensity projection) software capable of selectively displaying vessels in any degree of obliquity based on their high signal relative to that of the stationary surround (because of flow-related enhancement into the imaging volume) and without the need for subtraction schemes (Fig 7–6). This not only provided 3D angiographic display but also limited acquisition time so that such sequences can be implemented as part of routine brain imaging. One potential drawback of this approach is the appearance of blood at high fields. The paramagnetic effect of methemoglobin within a stationary hematoma may appear as an area of active flow with these postprocessing techniques (Fig 7–7).

Preliminary clinical experience utilizing volume (3DFT), gradient-echo pulse sequences to produce MRAs of the intracranial and extracranial vasculature indicates that they can provide accurate, reproducible images of the cerebral circulation. These techniques are rapid and can be likened to an additional pulse sequence to be acquired in conjunction with conventional parenchymal MRI examinations (Fig 7–8). Such information should be useful not only in the routine diagnosis and management of stroke and transient ischemic attack (TIA) but also in clarifying the natural history of cerebrovascular complications of sickle cell anemia, neurologic deficit associated with extracorporeal membrane oxygenation (ECMO) therapy, and the epidemiology of cerebral aneurysms (Fig 7–9). Thus, valuable ancillary information can be obtained in both symptomatic patients requiring a brain study as well as in patient populations where the risk of intra-arterial angiography is deemed too great.

Nevertheless, initial clinical trials also indicate that further work may be required to completely eliminate artifacts such as signal loss resulting from complex motion (i.e., turbulence) in the presence of imaging gradients with this technique. One other drawback to the 3DFT time-of-flight method is the eventual saturation of moving spins as they reside longer (farther) in the region of excitation. Thus, present 3DFT methods are limited to relatively small regions of high flow (i.e., arteries of the head and neck).

Recognizing the drawback of "moving-spin saturation" with large-volume 3DFT techniques as well as the virtues of computer postprocessing to limit scan time and improve display, several groups have resurrected the work of Wehrli and Gullberg. Edelman et al. have used sequential, contiguous 2DFT scans with selectively applied saturation pulses to produce both arteriograms and venograms in the abdomen, while Keller et al. have generated impressive angiographic images of the carotid bifurcation.[32, 33] While spatial resolution in the slice-select direction (and thus voxel size) is not comparable to 3DFT imaging, this approach is not limited by slow flow or region of interest.

Future approaches to MR flow imaging that may solve some or all of these difficulties include the use of pulse sequences with even shorter TEs in order to avoid overestimation of stenoses. New, faster forms of data acquisition may make possible more rapid 2D scanning with subsequent 3D reformatting. For vessels oriented perpendicular to such scans, flow-related enhancement (and thus visualization) should still be possible even for slow-flow regions. Additionally, the use of intravascular contrast agents with such scans may also provide information regarding tissue perfusion analogous to that of xenon computed tomography (CT).[35] The implementation of saturation pulses with angiography pulse sequences should allow for the selection of vascular territories, or arteriograms and venograms.[36]

QUANTIFICATION OF FLOW

The signal variations produced by time-of-flight phenomena and motion-induced phase shifts can not only be used to modify (enhance) vascular signal intensity and anatomy in conventional magnitude imaging but can also be exploited to provide quantitative measurements of flow. Specifically, for a given gradient structure (amplitude and timing) the mathematical relationship between constant velocity (for example) and the associated phase term at the echo is known. Consequently, it is possible to obtain quantitative velocity measurements from phase data.

With the advent of numerous gradient schemes for modification of the phase of flowing spins, several investigators have implemented and assessed the accuracy of these techniques. Early on, Bryant et al. modified standard MRI gradients and compared flow measurements of carotid arteries based on measured phase shifts with those obtained by Doppler ultrasound.[37] Pettigrew and colleagues also attempted similar experiments with conventional spin-echo imaging verified by in vivo electromagnetic flowmeters in experimental animals with good results.[38, 39] Nevertheless, there are

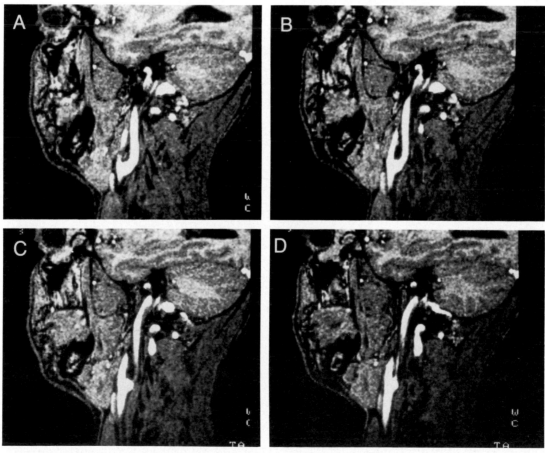

FIG 7–6.
A–D, 3DFT, or volume imaging, with parameters set to maximize flow-related enhancement and minimize phase dispersion yields a "stack" or "slab" of thin-section (1-mm-thick) images in which vascular structures have the highest signal intensity of any tissue. This particular example demonstrates such a sequence with serial sagittal images through the region of the carotid bifurcation.

Continued.

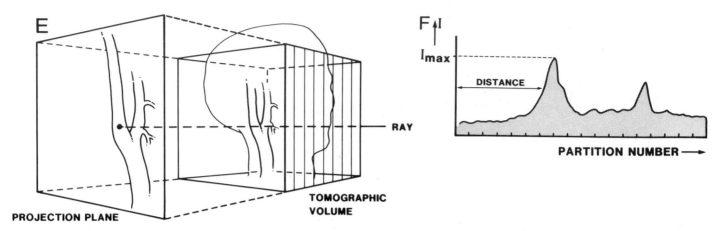

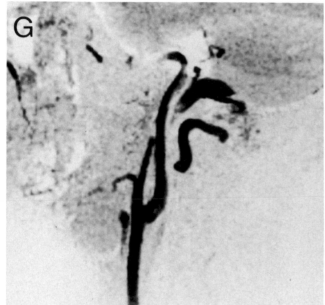

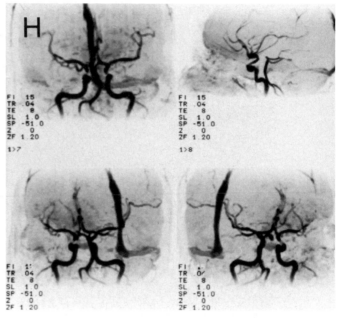

FIG 7–6   (cont.).

E, subsequently, the data are processed by using computerized ray-tracing algorithms in which the signal intensity of each voxel through the slab is traced along a ray through each individual image partition at an arbitarily selected angle of projection. **F,** the signal intensity (I) plot of such a ray is depicted by this graph, which plots intensity vs. image partition number. Vascular structures are represented by the peaks. The projected image eventually selected by the computer projects only the maximum-intensity structures such that the end result of the ray-tracing projection is

an angiogram **(G). H,** multiple postprocessed views of a single data acquisition of the intracranial circulation, again attempting to maximize flow-related enhancement while minimizing motion-induced spin-phase phenomenon and signal loss. From the *upper left* to the *lower right* one can appreciate the anteroposterior, lateral, and both oblique views of the intracranial circulation. **(A–G,** from Masaryk TJ, Modic MT, Ruggieri PM, et al: *Radiology* 1989; 171:801–806. Used by permission.)

drawbacks to these measurements, including (1) the need to recalibrate the sequence for different gradient strengths (i.e., slice thickness and FOV), (2) sensitivity to phase distortion from other sources of magnetic field inhomogeneity, and (3) the potential for rapid flow to produce large phase shifts (i.e., ≥360 degrees) that result in signal loss and aliasing of measured phase shifts to erroneously low values. Consequently, each sequence must be calibrated and each gradient structure optimized to provide maximum sensitivity over the

velocity range of interest. Flow compensation with gradient motion refocusing provides a partial solution to this last problem by suppressing large flow-related phase shifts (e.g., apply flow compensation in a direction other than that of interest and/or reduce or eliminate higher-order, i.e., acceleration, motion terms).[40]

Further refinements through the use of rapid-acquisition, short-TR, gradient-echo techniques have produced several methods that optimize signal contrast between moving spins and stationary

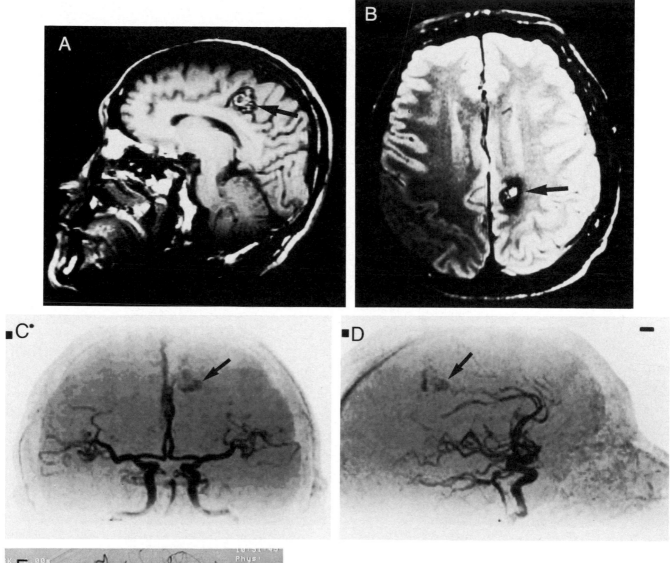

FIG 7–7.
A and **B,** sagittal T1-weighted and axial spin-density spin-echo images demonstrate chronic hemorrhage with both methemoglobin and hemosiderin *(arrows)* in the left parietal lobe in a young male with new onset of a seizure disorder. **C** and **D,** frontal and lateral 3DFT MRA performed by utilizing time-of-flight techniques and maximum pixel intensity postprocessing suggests the presence of an active parietal lobe arteriovenous malformation *(arrows).* **E,** a lateral left carotid angiogram fails to demonstrate the fistulas; thus it is a false-positive MRA based on the maximum-intensity projection program mistaking paramagnetic T1 shortening for flow-related enhancement.

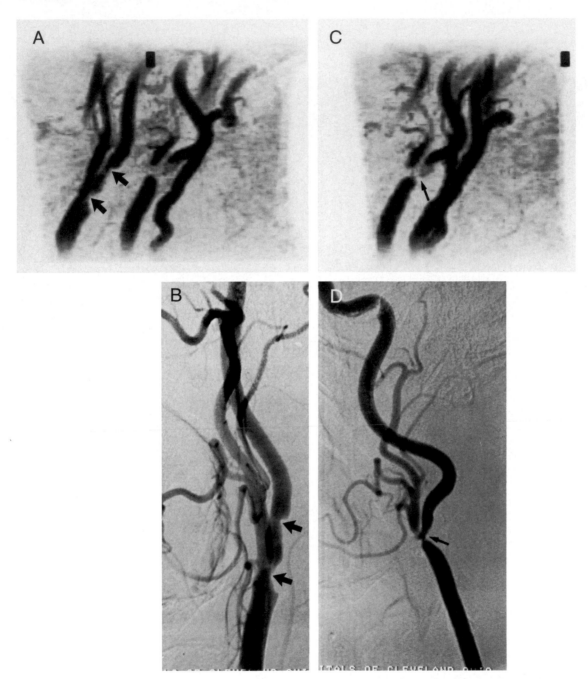

FIG 7–8.
A, 3DFT time-of-flight MRA of the right carotid bifurcation demonstrates a severe shelflike stenosis *(arrows)*. **B,** corresponding conventional intra-arterial angiogram. **C,** 3DFT time-of-flight MRA in the same patient as **A** and **B** demonstrates a severe stenosis of the contralateral bifurcation *(arrow)* with corresponding intra-arterial digital subtraction angiogram (**D**). Note the slight signal loss at the lesion (likely secondary to phase cancellation from higher-order motion) that exaggerates the severity of disease.

tissue, permit quantitative measurement of rapid flow, and may allow time-resolved measurements over the cardiac cycle.[41, 42]

Several time-of-flight schemes have been used to measure flow. One such technique involves the use of spin-echo imaging with a 90-degree excitation RF pulse applied at one point and a 180-degree refocusing pulse placed farther downstream (the experiment is repeated with different placement of the refocusing pulse to approximate a range of flows). Gradient-echo variations of this method have also been developed where a 90-degree excitation pulse is placed perpendicular to the flow and then the signal is read out in the slice-

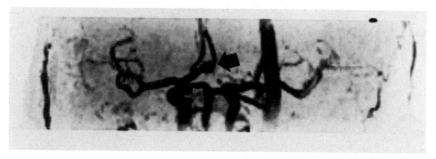

FIG 7–9.
Frontal projection of 3DFT time-of-flight MRA of a patient with an azygous anterior cerebral artery and an aneurysm *(arrow)*.

select direction; the relative displacement of the tagged bolus during the TR time reflects the flow rate.[43, 44] Phase encoding can be employed in one or two additional directions and the data reconstructed by using 2DFT or 3DFT. However, due to poor RF slice profile and T2* decay, the poor edge definition of the tagged region limits the accuracy of quantitative measurements. Another drawback to these methods is the potential for significant signal loss secondary to T2 or T2* effects at longer TEs. This inability to use longer TEs in turn restricts the ability of these techniques to detect and measure slow flow. A possible solution to such problems has been the implementation of a three-pulse-stimulated echo technique.[45]

Another time-of-flight alternative for physiologic flow measurement has been the use of presaturation bolus tracking. Borrowing from the technique of low flip angle gradient-echo cineangiography used in the heart, a series of images covering the length of the vessel of interest is rapidly acquired over the cardiac cycle immediately following a series of preparatory RF saturation pulses confined to a small region within the vessel.[46] When the images are played back in cine fashion, the bolus can visually be followed as it flows down the vessel, and quantitative measurements can be calculated on the basis of the known scan timing parameters. Once again, edge definition limits of a saturated region due to poor RF undermines the accuracy of quantitative measurements.

In summary, preliminary research and recent clinical experience indicates that MRA and flow measurements can play a role in routine scanning by providing useful information regarding the anatomy of the cerebral circulation. Used in conjunction with conventional spin-echo studies it may improve the overall sensitivity and specificity of MRI. Its role deserves further investigation into possible technical refinements, accuracy relative to other diagnostic studies, and impact upon patient management.

REFERENCES

1. Bryan RN, Willcott MR, Schneiders NJ, et al: NM evaluation of stroke in the rat. *AJNR* 1983; 4:242–244.
2. Brant-Zawadzki M, Percira B, Weinstein P, et al: MR imaging of acute experimental ischemia in cats. *AJNR* 1986; 7:7–11.
3. Unger E, Gado M, Fulling K, et al: Acute cerebral infarction in monkeys: An experimental study using MR imaging. *Radiology* 1987; 162:789–795.
4. Gomori JM, Grossman RI, Goldberg HI, et al: Intracranial hematoma: Imaging by high-field MR. *Radiology* 1985; 157:87–93.
5. Atlas SW, Grossman RI, Goldberg HI, et al: Partially thrombosed giant intracranial aneurysms: Correlation of MR and pathologic findings. *Radiology* 1987; 162:111–114.
6. Olsen WL, Brant-Zawadzki M, Hodes J, et al: Giant intracranial aneurysms: MR imaging. *Radiology* 1987; 163:431–435.
7. Lemme-Plaghos L, Kucharczyk W, Brant-Zawadzki M, et al: MRI of angiographically occult vascular malformations. *AJR* 1986; 146:1223–1228.
8. New PFJ, Ojemann RG, Davis KR, et al: MR and CT of occult vascular malformations of the brain. *AJR* 1986; 147:985–993.
9. Kucharczyk W, Lemme-Plaghos L, Uske A, et al: Intracranial vascular malformations: MR and CT imaging. *Radiology* 1985; 156:383–389.
10. Haacke EM, Patrick JL: Reducing motion artifacts in two-dimensional Fourier transform imaging. *Magn Reson Imaging* 1986; 4:359–376.
11. Surjan G: Nuclear resonance in flowing liquids. *Proc Indian Acad Sci* 1951; 33:107–113.
12. Alfidi RJ, Masaryk TJ, Haacke EM, et al: MR angiography of peripheral, carotid, and coronary arteries. *AJR* 1987; 149:1097–1109.

13. Axel L: Blood flow effects in magnetic resonance imaging. *AJR* 1984; 143:1157–1166.

14. Bradley WG, Waluch V: Blood flow magnetic resonance imaging. *Radiology* 1985; 154:443–450.

15. Macovski A: Selection projection imaging: Applications to radiology and NMR. *IEEE Trans Med Imaging* 1982; 1:42–47.

16. Wedeen VJ, Meuli RA, Edelman RR, et al: Projective imaging of pulsatile flow with magnetic resonance imaging. *Science* 1985; 230:946–948.

17. Moran PR: A flow velocity zeugmatographic interlace for NMR imaging in humans. *Magn Reson Imaging* 1982; 1:197–203.

18. Axel L, Morton D: A method for imaging blood vessels by phase compensated/uncompensated difference images. *Magn Reson Imaging* 1986; 4:153.

19. Pattany PM, Marino R, McNally JM: Velocity and acceleration desensitization in 2DFT MR imaging. *Magn Reson Imaging* 1986; 4:154–155.

20. Naylor W, Firmin DN: Multislice MR angiography. *Magn Reson Imaging* 1986; 4:156.

21. Dumoulin CL, Hart HR: Magnetic resonance angiography. *Radiology* 1986; 161:717–720.

22. Masaryk TJ, Ross JS, Modic MT, et al: Carotid bifurcation: MR imaging. *Radiology* 1988; 166:461–466.

23. Lenz GW, Haacke EM, Masaryk TJ, et al: In-plane vascular imaging: Pulse sequence design and strategy. *Radiology* 1988; 166:875–882.

24. Laub G, Kaiser W: MR angiography with gradient motion refocussing. *J Comput Assist Tomogr* 1988; 12:377–382.

25. Dumoulin CL, Souza SP, Walker MF, et al: Three-dimensional phase contrast angiography. *Magn Reson Med* 1989; 9:139–149.

26. Dixon WT, Du LN, Gado M, et al: Projection angiograms of blood labeled by adiabatic fast passage. *Magn Reson Med* 1986; 3:454–462.

27. Nishimura DG, Macovski A, Pauly JM, et al: MR angiography by selective inversion recovery. *Magn Reson Med* 1987; 4:193–202.

28. Wehrli FW, Shimakawa A, Gullberg GT, et al: Time-of-flight MR flow imaging: Selective saturation recovery with gradient refocussing. *Radiology* 1986; 160:781–785.

29. Gullberg GT, Wehrli FW, Shimakawa A, et al: MR vascular imaging with fast gradient refocussing pulse sequence and reformatted images from transaxial sections. *Radiology* 1987; 165:241–246.

30. Ruggieri PM, Laub GA, Masaryk TJ, et al: Intracranial circulation: Pulse sequence considerations in three-dimensional (volume) MR angiography. *Radiology* 1989; 171:785–791.

31. Masaryk TJ, Modic MT, Ruggieri PM, et al: Three-dimensional (volume) gradient-echo imaging of the carotid bifurcation: Preliminary clinical experience. *Radiology* 1989; 171:801–806.

32. Edelman RR, Wentz KU, Mattle H, et al: Projection arteriography and venography: Initial clinical results with MR. *Radiology* 1989; 172:351–357.

33. Keller PJ, Drayer BP, Fram EK, et al: MR angiography with two-dimensional acquisition and three-dimensional display. *Radiology* 1989; 173:527–532.

34. Sardashti M, Schwartzberg DG, Stomp GP, et al: Spin labeling angiography of the carotids by presaturation and adiabatic inversion. Presented at the Eighth Annual Meeting of the Society of Magnetic Resonance in Medicine. Amsterdam, The Netherlands, Aug 12–18, 1989.

35. Schmiedl U, Ogan M, Paajanen H, et al: Albumin labeled with Gd-DTPA as an intravascular, blood-pool enhancing agent for MR imaging: Biodistribution and imaging studies. *Radiology* 1987; 162:205–210.

36. Edelman RR, Wentz KU, Mattle HP, et al: Intracerebral arteriovenous malformations: Evaluation with selective MR angiography and venography. *Radiology* 1989; 173:831–837.

37. Bryant DJ, Payne JA, Firmin DN, et al: Measurement of flow with NMR imaging using a gradient pulse and phase difference technique. *J Comput Assist Tomogr* 1984; 8:588–593.

38. Pettigrew RI, Dannels W: Use of standard gradients with compund oblique angulation for optimal MR flow imaging in oblique vessels. *AJR* 1987; 148:405–409.

39. Pettigrew RI, Dannels W, Galloway JR, et al: Quantitative phase-flow MR imaging by using standard sequences: Comparison with in vivo flow-meter measurements. *AJR* 1987; 148:411–414.

40. Moran PR, Moran RA, Karstaedt N: Verification and evaluation of internal flow and motion. *Radiology* 1985; 154:433–441.

41. Hennig J, Muri M, Brunner P, et al: Quantitative flow measurement with the fast Fourier flow technique. *Radiology* 1988; 166:237–240.

42. Meir D, Maier S, Bosiger P: Quantitative flow measurements on phantoms and blood vessels with MR. *Magn Reson Med* 1988; 8:25–34.

43. Shimizu K, Matsuda T, Sakurai T, et al: Visualization of moving fluid: Quatitative analysis of blood flow velocity using MR imaging. *Radiology* 1986; 159:195–199.

44. Matsuda T, Shimizu K, Sakurai T, et al: Measurement of aortic blood flow with MR imaging: Comparative study with Doppler ultrasound. *Radiology* 1987; 162:857–861.

45. Foo T, Perman WH, Poon CS, et al: Projection flow imaging by bolus tracking using stimulated echoes. *Magn Reson Med* 1989; 9:203–218.

46. Edelman RR, Mattle HP, Kleefield J, et al: Quantification of blood flow with dynamic MR imaging and presaturation bolus tracking. *Radiology* 1989; 171:551–556.

PART IV

Infarction, Trauma, and Hemorrhage

8

Cerebral Ischemia and Infarction

Stephen T. Hecht, M.D.

Elizabeth A. Eelkema, M.D.

Richard E. Latchaw, M.D.

Cerebral ischemia and infarction represent states of nutritional deprivation of the brain. Ischemia is a temporary deprivation state resulting in reversible neurologic dysfunction. Infarction is the result of nutritional deprivation so prolonged that the affected neurons die and a region of brain necrosis ensues. Both processes may be focal, multifocal, or generalized. The resources of brain cells struggling in an ischemic state can be exhausted over time, resulting in cell death. If ischemic cells experience re-establishment of normal nutrient levels, however, they can recover completely to resume normal function. The most common cause of ischemia and infarction is oxygen deprivation, usually due to hypoperfusion, although glucose deprivation can also be a cause. Brain infarction is a result of the relation between the degree and the duration of hypoperfusion as well as selective vulnerability to hypoperfusion of the brain's various structures and cell types.[1, 2] Severe hypoperfusion of short duration can cause infarction, as can less severe hypoperfusion sustained for longer duration. Absolute cerebral blood flow (CBF) arrest cannot be tolerated under usual circumstances for longer than 10 minutes.

Focal cerebral ischemia can be due to vascular disorders (arterial or venous), connective tissue disorders, embolism, or hematologic disorders (Table 8–1). Global cerebral ischemia can be a result of decreased cardiac output, decreased peripheral vascular resistance, increased intracranial pressure, metabolic disorders, anemia, or respiratory failure (Table 8–2). In the case of cerebral venous thrombosis (Fig 8–1), obstruction of venous outflow causes increased venous pressure, which results in decreased perfusion pressure, thus causing ischemia.

Protective mechanisms to help ensure adequate cerebral perfusion include (1) autoregulation; (2) arterial anastomotic networks (circle of Willis, external of the internal carotid collaterals, muscular to the vertebral artery collaterals, leptomeningeal collaterals); (3) augmented oxygen and glucose extraction from circulating blood; and (4) systemic redistribution of blood flow to the brain at the expense of other organs. When hypoperfusion overwhelms the protective mechanisms, ischemia and/or infarction occurs.

The clinical analogues of ischemia and infarction are transient ischemic attack (TIA) and stroke. TIAs are brief episodes of focal neurologic dysfunction (monocular blindness [amaurosis fugax]; speech disturbances; numbness and/or weakness of the hand, arm, leg, and/or face) that resolve within a few minutes (rarely longer than 30 minutes). Ischemic episodes that last many hours are generally associated with emboli, with return of normal neurologic function as the emboli fragment under the pressure of blood pulsation. Strokes are long-lasting or permanent sudden-onset neurologic deficits and are associated with brain infarction. Atherosclerosis is the most common cause of TIAs and strokes.[3] The underlying cause of neurologic dysfunction in atherosclerosis is vascular narrowing with severe blood flow reduction, emboli generated by injured vessels, or a combination of both.

TABLE 8–1.

Causes of Focal Ischemia

Arterial disease
  Atherosclerosis
  Fibromuscular dysplasia
  Trauma
  Vasospasm
  Hypertensive arterial change (hyalinosis)
  Arteritis
    Giant-cell arteritis
    Periarteritis nodosa
    Granulomatous angiitis
    Systemic lupus erythematosus
    Moyamoya disease
    Takayasu arteritis
  Arterial dissection
  Aneurysm
  Migraine
  Meningitis
    Tuberculous
    Fungal
    Luetic
    Bacterial
Embolism
  Extracranial arterial disease
  Valvular heart disease
    Congenital
    Rheumatic
    Mitral valve prolapse
    Prosthetic valves
  Infective endocarditis
  Cardiac thrombus
  Tumor embolism
  Fat embolism
  Air embolism
Venous disease
  Cerebral Venous Thrombosis
    Otitis media
    Mastoiditis
    Orbital cellulitis
    Meningitis
    Oral contraceptives
    Pregnancy
    Puerperium
    Dehydration
    Trauma
    Tumor invasion or compression
    Sickle cell disease
    Polycythemia
    Paroxysmal nocturnal hemoglobinuria
Connective tissue disorders
  Ehlers-Danlos
  Pseudoxanthoma elasticum
Hematologic disorders
  Thrombocytosis
  Hyperviscosity
  Sickle cell disease
  Leukemia
  Idiopathic thrombocytopenic purpura
  Thrombotic thrombocytopenic purpura
  Paroxysmal nocturnal hemoglobinuria
  Hypercoagulable states (oral contraceptives)

TABLE 8–2.

Hemodynamic Causes of Global Cerebral Ischemia

Decreased cardiac output
  Cardiac arrest
  Arrhythmias
  Valvular heart disease
  Cardiac failure
  Pulmonary embolism
  Syncope
  Hypovolemia
  Cardiac tamponade
Decreased peripheral vascular resistance
  Autonomic insufficiency
  Vasovagal episode
  Septic shock
Metabolic disorders
  Fabry disease
  Homocystinuria

The continuum of clinical states associated with cerebral ischemia/infarction also includes reversible ischemic neurologic deficit (RIND) and partially reversible ischemic neurologic deficit (PRIND),[4] both of which represent clinical conditions intermediate between TIA and stroke. The most common clinical states associated with cerebral hypoperfusion are TIA and stroke. There is no clear correlation between the spectrum of clinical ischemia/infarction states and the spectrum of brain tissue changes associated with ischemia/infarction as depicted by cross-sectional imaging methods.

There are definite distribution patterns of atherosclerotic changes in the cervicocerebral arteries. The most common site is the proximal internal carotid artery, followed in prevalence by the carotid siphon. Atherosclerotic changes in the ipsilateral proximal internal carotid and carotid siphon represent the so-called tandem lesion, which reduces cerebral perfusion much more than either lesion would alone. Proximal external carotid stenoses are commonly seen and may have hemodynamic significance insofar as they reduce the potential for external to internal carotid anastomoses in the presence of severe ipsilateral internal carotid artery disease. Vertebrobasilar atherosclerosis is less common than carotid atherosclerosis. In the posterior circulation the proximal intracranial vertebral artery is the most common site for atherosclerotic changes, and narrowings are also often seen along the basilar artery.

Ischemia/infarction can be an epiphenomenon of other major disease processes. Aneurysmal subarachnoid hemorrhage can incite severe vaso-

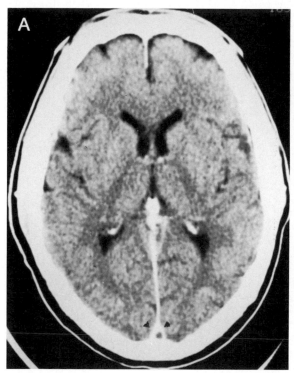 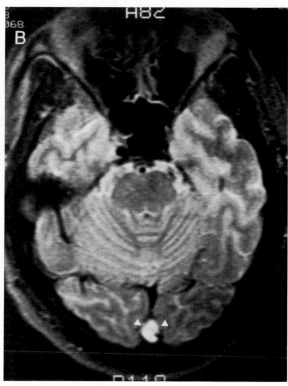

FIG 8–1.
Dural venous sinus thrombosis. **A,** a contrast-enhanced CT scan demonstrates the delta sign. The contrast-enhancing leaves of the dura that form the superior sagittal sinus *(black arrowheads)* sur- round the thrombus within. **B,** MRI (transverse, spin-echo [SE], 2,500/75) demonstrates the clot within the dural sinus *(white arrow-heads).*

spasm, which then restricts CBF and secondarily causes infarctions (Fig 8–2).

Cerebral infarctions can be bland or, when vessel walls rupture due to necrosis, hemorrhagic. Sudden onset of a focal neurologic deficit can also accompany cerebral hemorrhage of other etiology (hypertension, aneurysm [berry, mycotic], arteriovenous malformation, vasculitis, tumor, coagulopathy).

In acute cerebral ischemia and/or infarction the goals of cross-sectional brain imaging are to (1) demonstrate the location and extent of injury and, if possible, determine whether the injury is reversible or permanent; (2) demonstrate the absence or presence of hemorrhage and, if present, attempt to determine the etiology; and (3) exclude entities that mimic ischemia (e.g., intracerebral or extracerebral mass lesions). In the subacute to chronic state the goals are to (1) define the location and extent of infarction and (2) determine whether low flow to the affected area is a result of inflow restriction (in which case flow-augmenting intervention may be useful) or decreased demand (in which case flow-augmenting intervention would be of doubtful benefit and may be harmful).

In addition to the assessment of the brain, several cross-sectional imaging modalities can be useful in the assessment of extracranial vascular disease. Duplex ultrasound scanning is the easiest, least expensive, and most accurate noninvasive technique for evaluating the extracranial carotid arteries.[5, 6] Thin-section dynamic computed tomography (CT) of the carotid bifurcations has the potential to noninvasively image the carotid bifurcations in an accurate fashion.[7–9] Magnetic resonance imaging (MRI) also is capable of depicting the vascular system,[10–14] although MR angiography is not yet in routine clinical use.

Since a TIA does not cause any permanent neuronal damage, CT and MRI usually show no brain changes referable to that TIA. Reversible changes are rarely seen on CT and MRI of the brain that are referable to a single TIA. The more typical case, however, is that since people who have TIAs are more likely than the general population to have vascular disease, they are more likely to have evidence of previous infarction. Infarctions in TIA patients may represent previous ischemic events in clinically silent regions of the brain.

The initial pathologic change associated with

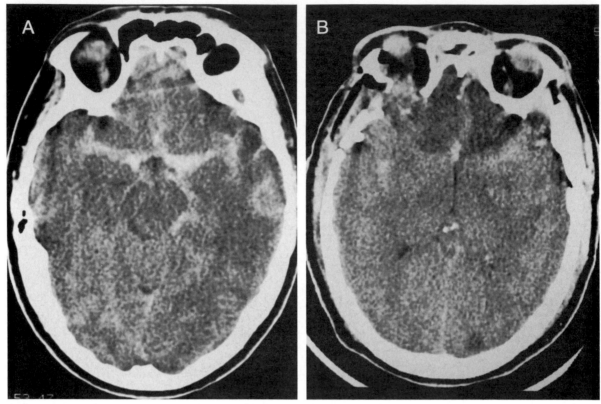

FIG 8–2.
Infarctions secondary to vasospasm. **A,** a CT scan without intravenous contrast at the time of ictus demonstrates subarachnoid hemorrhage. **B,** 4 days later, following clipping of the aneurysm and development of extensive vasospasm, bilateral anterior cerebral artery distribution infarctions have occurred.

cerebral ischemia/infarction is edema, first intracellular but ultimately intracellular and extracellular. The ischemic changes detectable by nonenhanced CT and proton MRI relate to the increased water content of affected tissues. Intravenous contrast-enhanced CT and MRI detect abnormalities of the blood-brain barrier.

COMPUTED TOMOGRAPHY

The earliest noncontrast CT changes associated with cerebral infarction are detectable within 24 hours and include subtle mass effect, loss of the distinction between the densities of gray matter and white matter, and slight hypodensity (Fig 8–3).[15] With high-quality CT scanners, the changes can be detected within 6 to 8 hours of ictus, with the more profound and larger lesions seen the earliest. Smaller infarctions and those in artifact-prone areas (e.g., the posterior fossa) may require a longer time to be detectable by CT. Cytotoxic edema, with its attendant hypodensity (Fig 8–4), reaches a maximum at 3 to 5 days and resolves by 2 to 3 weeks following infarction. At its peak, when large areas are infarcted, brain swelling can be severe enough to cause marked midline shift, ventriculomegaly due to compression of the aqueduct of Sylvius, and even herniation (Fig 8–5).[16] Herniation can cause compression and secondary ischemia in the compressed regions of brain (Fig 8–6). Infarctions and their associated parenchymal edema are generally restricted to vascular distributions (see Chapter 3) (Fig 8–7).

Infarcts can become isodense with normal brain at 2 to 3 weeks and then revert to hypodensity, the so-called fogging effect (Fig 8–8).[17] Fogging can occur in all or part of an infarct and represents the phase of phagocytization of necrotic brain after resolution of edema. Areas involved by fogging enhance intensely.

In time, as the dead neurons degenerate and undergo phagocytosis, the low density of the infarction becomes more sharply marginated. Ultimately there is parenchymal volume loss (encephalomalacia) and gliosis, with attendant dilatation of

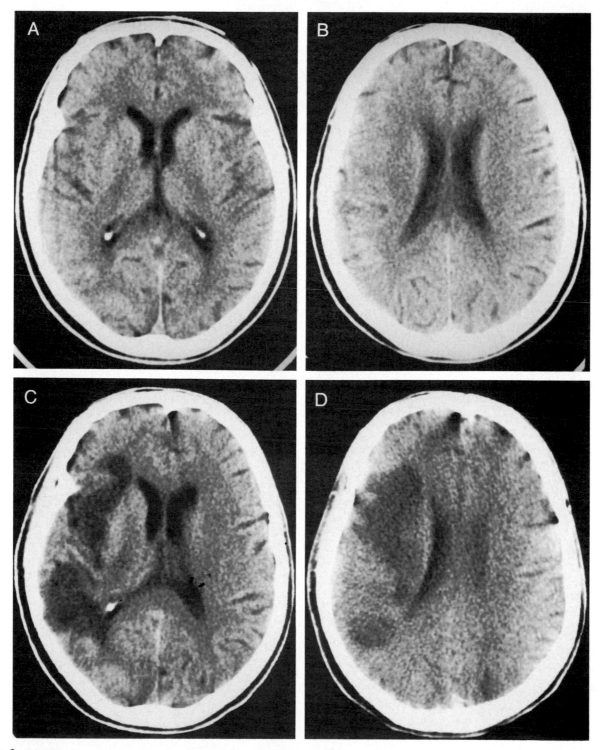

FIG 8–3.
Acute infarction. **A** and **B,** CT scans without intravenous contrast obtained at the time of ictus show minimal effacement of the right-sided cortical sulci, which reflects a slight mass effect. There is no definite hypodensity, nor is there loss of the gray-white distinction. **C** and **D,** CT scans without intravenous contrast obtained 4 days following ictus show extensive hypodensity and mass effect due to edema in the right middle cerebral artery distribution. The preservation of normal density in the right basal ganglia implies that the right lenticulostriate arteries remain patent.

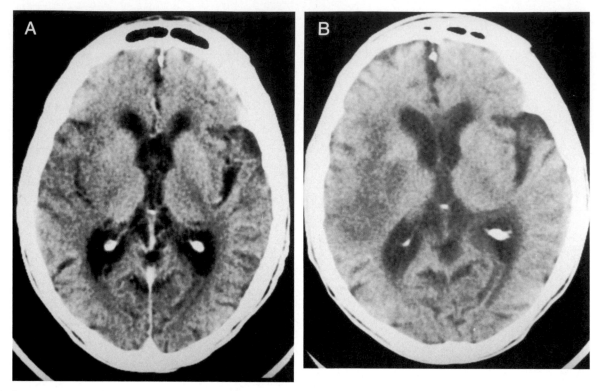

FIG 8–4.
Acute infarction. **A,** a contrast-enhanced CT scan at time of ictus shows effacement of the right sylvian cistern with slight hypodensity in the right globus pallidus and putamen. **B,** a CT scan without intravenous contrast 4 days later shows hypodensity in the right middle cerebral artery distribution, with hypodensity in the right globus pallidus and putamen more pronounced than on the previous examination. There has also been increased mass effect in the interval since the prior examination, as evidenced by complete obliteration of the right sylvian cistern.

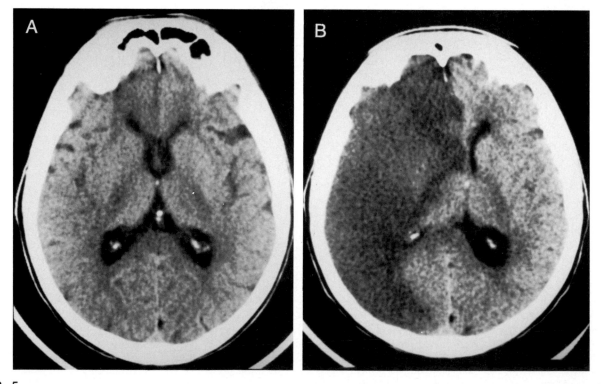

FIG 8–5.
Herniation secondary to mass effect from infarction. **A,** a CT scan without intravenous contrast at the time of ictus shows normal anatomy. **B,** a CT scan without intravenous contrast 1 day following ictus shows hypodensity involving the right anterior and middle cerebral artery territory, with severe mass effect and shift effacing the right lateral ventricle and causing a subfalcine herniation.

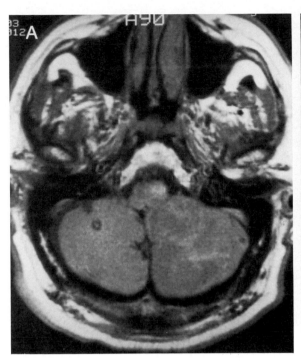
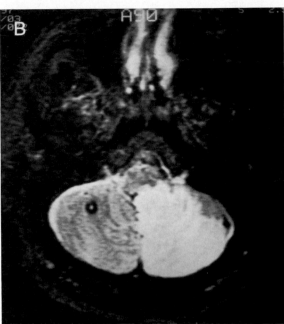

FIG 8–6.
Cerebellar infarction with mass effect compressing the medulla. **A,** MRI (transverse, SE 800/20) shows hypointensity and swelling in the right cerebellar hemisphere with compression of the medulla. **B,** MRI (transverse, SE, 2,500/100) shows the extensive left cerebellar edema with medullary compression. The small, low-intensity foci of hemosiderin deposition in both cerebellar hemispheres suggest previous multiple hemorrhagic infarctions, most likely secondary to tiny emboli.

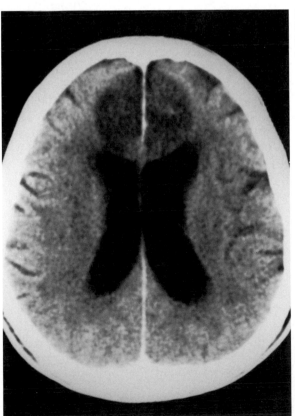

FIG 8–7.
Bilateral anterior cerebral artery infarctions. Contrast-enhanced CT shows mass effect effacing the frontal horns bilaterally. The vascular distribution is very clearly delineated.

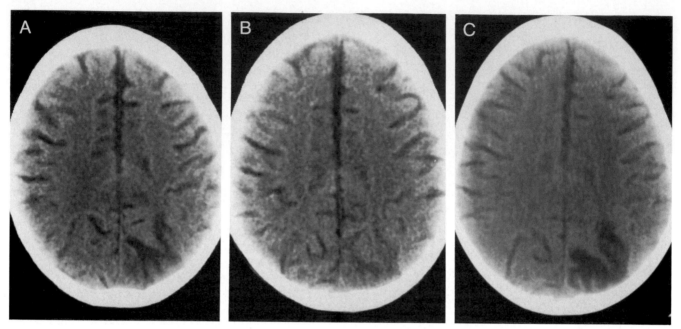

FIG 8–8.
Fogging effect. **A,** CT without intravenous contrast 1 week following ictus shows an area of low attenuation in the left parieto-occipital region. **B,** 2 weeks following ictus the left parieto-occipital lesion is less apparent on noncontrast CT. **C,** 3 weeks following ictus the left parieto-occpital lesion is again more apparent on noncontrast CT. The serial examinations demonstrate the isodense phase of infarctions between the low density from edema and the low density from developing encephalomalacia.

overlying sulci and cisterns and subjacent ventricles (Fig 8–9). Cavitation can also occur, particularly with deep infarctions. Calcification is relatively rarely associated with infarction (Fig 8–10).

Temporary generalized cerebral hypoperfusion can result in infarctions in the border zones between the anterior, middle, and posterior cerebral artery territories (so-called watershed infarctions) (Fig 8–11). Watershed infarctions are more accurately called arterial border zone or distal perfusion zone infarctions, are often associated with preexistent cerebral vascular disease (usually atherosclerotic and/or hypertensive),[18] and are often bilateral. Gray matter is metabolically more active than white matter and therefore has higher oxygen demands. On the basis of metabolic demand, gray matter should be more susceptible to ischemia than white matter. However, white matter is more distal in the arterial tree than grey matter. Therefore, in spite of its relatively decreased oxygen demand, white matter is often more susceptible to watershed infarction than gray matter since hypoperfusion affects the most distal perfusion zones most severely.

During the period when cytotoxic edema is severe there is little contrast enhancement. Contrast enhancement with intravenous iodinated contrast media starts to appear after a minimum of 24 to 36 hours following infarction, peaks at 1 to 2 weeks, and resolves by 6 to 8 weeks, although persistence for 3 months and longer is occasionally seen.[19] More prolonged enhancement raises the differential diagnostic possibility of tumor. Contrast enhancement reflects a damaged blood-brain barrier and therefore tends to be most prominent peripherally, at the interface between viable and infarcted brain in regions where neovascular capillaries are growing into the devitalized tissue. Enhancement often assumes a ring or gyriform pattern (Fig 8–12).[20]

Blood-brain barrier damage sufficient to allow the leakage of contrast material and thus enhancement requires at least 24 hours.[21] In the initial 24 hours following ictus, CT without contrast is adequate to exclude the presence of hemorrhage (which would preclude anticoagulation) (Fig 8–13) and to detect the changes of early infarction. Unenhanced CT is the most sensitive imaging modality for the detection of acute cerebral hemorrhage, and intravenous contrast can obscure or confuse the diagnosis of subtle hemorrhage. Paradoxically, contrast enhancement of hypodense infarctions can make them isodense with normal brain, thereby masking their presence. If CT without contrast suggests the presence of a focal mass, either intra- or extra-axial, then CT with contrast is useful for

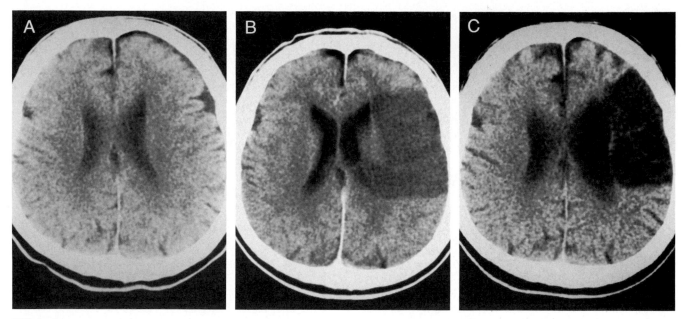

FIG 8-9.
Natural history of infarction on CT. **A,** CT without intravenous contrast at the time of ictus has negative findings. **B,** contrast enhanced CT 1 day following ictus shows low density due to edema in the left middle cerebral artery territory with associated mass effect. **C,** CT without intravenous contrast 6 months following ictus shows well-demarcated encephalomalacia in the left middle cerebral artery territory, with dilatation of the subjacent lateral ventricle on an ex vacuo basis.

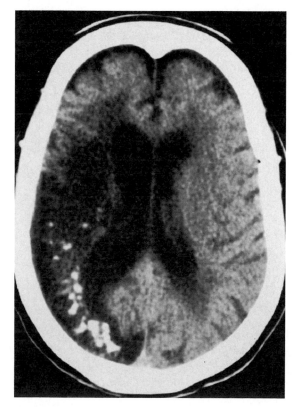

FIG 8-10.
Calcification in a chronic infarction. A noncontrast CT scan demonstrates a large right cerebral infarction with dilatation of the subjacent right lateral ventricle. Calcification in the dorsal portion of the infarcted parenchyma is rarely associated with old infarctions.

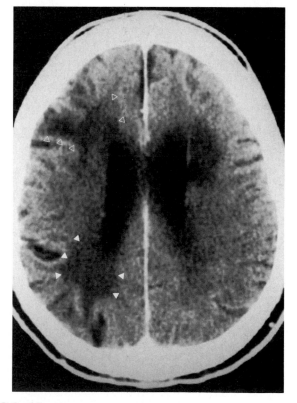

FIG 8-11.
Arterial border zone infarctions. A CT scan with contrast shows old infarctions in the right anterior arterial border zone, between the anterior and middle cerebral artery perfusion zones *(open arrowheads),* and the right posterior arterial border zone, between the right middle and posterior cerebral artery perfusion zones *(filled arrowheads).* The left periventricular infarction is not in a distal perfusion zone distribution.

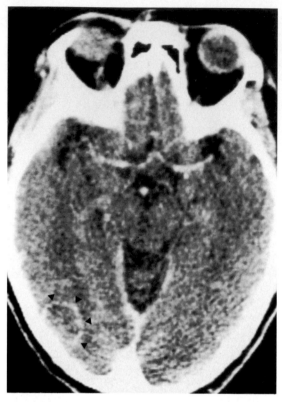

FIG 8–12.
Ring enhancement of an infarction. A CT scan with intravenous contrast shows an area of ring enhancement in the posterior right temporal lobe *(arrowheads)*. Histology by stereotactic biopsy was infarction.

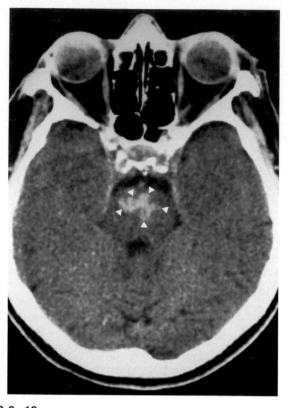

FIG 8–13.
Hemorrhagic infarction in a hypertensive patient. A CT scan without intravenous contrast demonstrates increased attenuation *(arrows)* within the pons that represents hemorrhage.

further characterization. In a study of stroke patients who had CT, recovery was better among those who had no intravenous contrast than among those who received intravenous sodium iothalamate,[22] which suggests that contrast that crosses the blood-brain barrier may damage potentially viable brain tissue. Newer, nonionic contrast media are less neurotoxic and may represent less of a threat to impaired but viable brain tissue.

Emboli can sometimes be imaged directly with CT, in addition to making their presence known indirectly by causing infarctions. An acute embolus is represented as hyperdense intra-arterial contents on noncontrast CT[23] (Fig 8–14) and is most commonly appreciated in the horizontal (M1) segment of the middle cerebral artery and in the basilar artery. Larger emboli generally break up in 1 to 5 days following ictus. With loss of autoregulation in the infarcted brain tissue, the hyperemia associated with reperfusion of devitalized brain can result in parenchymal hemorrhage (Fig 8–15). Hemorrhage detectable by CT may occur in more than 40% of ischemic infarctions,[24] usually as asympto-

matic petechial hemorrhages in the second week, but with symptomatic hemorrhages presenting in the first week after ictus.

Numerous unilateral infarctions in the middle and anterior cerebral artery territories suggest atherosclerotic disease in the ipsilateral carotid bifurcation with repeated embolization. Because most of the internal carotid blood flow goes to the middle cerebral artery, most carotid emboli go to the middle cerebral territory.

Lacunar infarcts are small (15 mm or less) infarcts, most often located in the basal ganglia, periventricular regions, and brain stem. They result from occlusive disease of small, deep arterioles, most commonly lenticulostriates and transmedullary arteries to the periventricular regions. Vascular occlusive disease is commonly associated with hypertension and diabetes. Since they are the result of systemic disease, lacunar infarcts tend to be multiple and bilateral. Many lacunar infarcts (or lacunae) are in silent areas of the brain and are therefore asymptomatic. When located in portions of the internal capsule or the brain stem, however, lacunae can cause dramatic symptoms. Acutely,

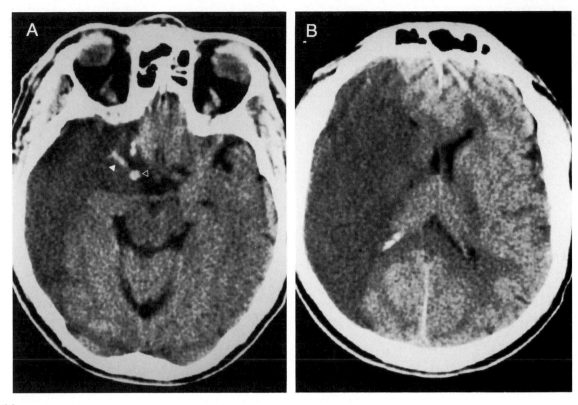

FIG 8–14.
Arterial embolus. A patient awoke with left hemiparesis following cardiac surgery. **A** and **B,** a CT scan without intravenous contrast shows a high-density embolus within the distal right internal carotid *(open arrowhead)* and in the right middle cerebral artery *(filled ar-* *rowhead)*. There is extensive hypodensity in the right middle cerebral artery distribution, with associated mass effect, shift, and subfalcine herniation.

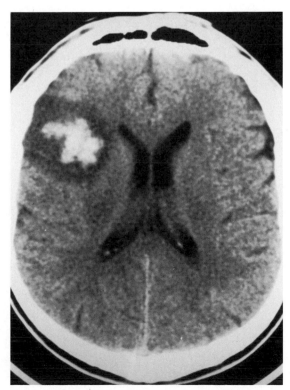

FIG 8–15.
Hemorrhagic infarction. A CT scan without intravenous contrast performed 1 day following ictus shows a high-density hemorrhage within the low density of the edematous, infarcted region of brain.

small lacunae are generally not imaged on CT, usually becoming apparent after weeks, when low-density cavitary changes become obvious (Fig 8–16). The accuracy of CT imaging is improved by the use of thin slice thickness, which reduces image degradation by partial volume averaging. Even with thin sections, however, CT is much less sensitive for visualization of lacunae than is MRI (Fig 8–17).[25] Larger lacunes follow the typical CT patterns of infarcts. Prominent perivascular (Virchow-Robin) spaces can mimic lacunes on CT and MRI (Fig 8–18).[26] MRI helps to distinguish them insofar as it demonstrates that the prominent perivascular spaces have signal characteristics precisely like those of cerebrospinal fluid (CSF) on multiple acquisitions and in multiple planes. Anatomically, prominent perivascular spaces tend to be restricted to the inferior third of the corpus striatum (especially the putamen), the thalami, and the mesial temporal lobes and superficially in gyri over the convexities.

Infants and children suffering from hypoxemia often have a CT appearance of diffusely decreased attenuation throughout the cerebral hemispheres, with preservation of normal-appearing parenchymal density in the basal ganglia, brain stem, and cerebellar hemispheres (Fig 8–19). The normal-appearing density on CT does not reflect normal cellular metabolism since the cells of the basal ganglia, brain stem, and cerebellar hemispheres may ultimately undergo necrosis; the normal density may instead reflect hyperemia secondary to ischemia.[27]

MAGNETIC RESONANCE IMAGING

In this chapter, the term short repetition time (TR), short echotime (TE) images will denote images acquired by using a two-dimensional Fourier transform (2DFT) spin-echo (SE) technique employing TRs of 1,000 ms or less and TEs of 30 ms or less. The term long TR, long TE images will denote images acquired by using a 1.5-tesla 2DFT SE technique employing TRs of 2,000 ms or longer and TEs of 80 to 120 ms.

Proton MRI detects mobile proton density. In the human body mobile protons are most abundant in the form of water. MRI is exquisitely sensitive to alterations in tissue water content, more so than any other currently available imaging modality. As previously mentioned, the initial pathologic tissue changes associated with cerebral infarction involve changes in tissue water content. It follows, then, that MRI is the most sensitive method for imaging the early pathologic changes of cerebral infarction.[28–30]

FIG 8–16.
Lacunar infarctions. Contrast-enhanced CT shows sharply marginated, bilateral foci of low attenuation in the periventricular regions that represent cavitated lacunar infarctions.

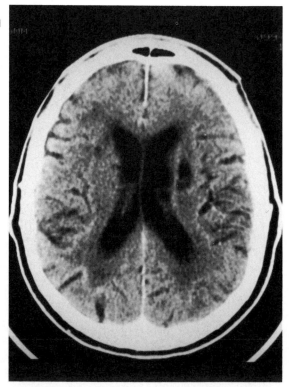

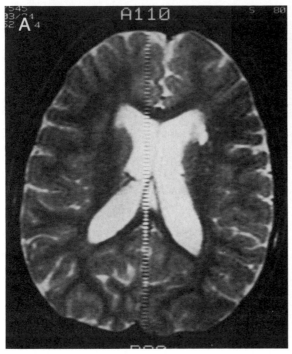 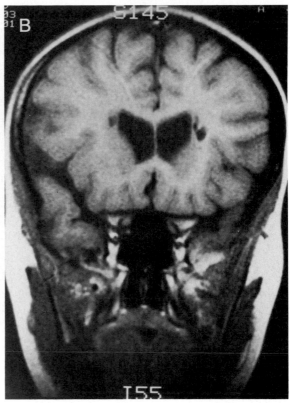

FIG 8–17.
MRI of lacunar infarctions. **A,** transverse (SE, 3,000/100). Regions of increased signal intensity adjacent to both frontal horns represent lacunar infarctions. The zipperlike artifact traversing the image is due to an RF leak. **B,** coronal (SE, 600/20). The bilateral la-cunar infarctions adjacent to the ventricles are cavitated since their signal characteristics follow the signal characteristics of ventricular CSF on both short TR, short TE and long TR, long TE images.

An increase in the bulk water content of tissue causes prolongation of both T1 and T2 relaxation times.[31] Tissue water molecular structure may also have an effect on relaxation times.[32] The subtle low density seen on CT in the first few hours after infarction is represented on MRI as low intensity on short TR, short TE images and dramatic, obvious hyperintensity on long TR, long TE images (Figs 8–20 and 8–21). Long TR, long TE images are more sensitive than are short TR, short TE images for the detection of changes associated with tissue edema.[33] Experimental work on animals suggests that MRI can detect brain tissue changes within 1 hour following vascular occlusion if there is a large area of infarction.[34] MRI can also depict changes in ischemic tissues before infarction occurs,[35] although the distinction between ischemia and infarction is not made.

Without intravenous contrast media MRI does not adequately distinguish between the intact and the damaged blood-brain barrier, although the presence of extensive edema implies an injured blood-brain barrier. With intravenous gadolinium–diethylenetriamine pentaacetic acid (DTPA), however, the status of the blood-brain barrier can be more accurately assessed (Fig 8–22). Experimental work with cats indicates that the time sequence of MRI enhancement patterns with gadolinium-DTPA does not follow precisely the time sequence with enhanced CT. Gadolinium-DTPA enhancement is first imaged at 16 to 18 hours and is maximal in the first 3 days.[36, 37] Following the development of edema and mass effect, contrast enhancement is reduced. Poor perfusion of an infarcted area can reduce delivery of intravenous contrast and thereby confound contrast enhancement of a damaged blood-brain barrier.

At high field strengths MRI, acute hemorrhage has relatively low intensity on long TR, long TE images due to shortening of the T2 relaxation time by magnetic susceptibility of the deoxyhemoglobin within the intact red blood cells of a fresh clot[38, 39] (see Chapter 9). At lower field strengths the distinction between brain tissue edema and acute

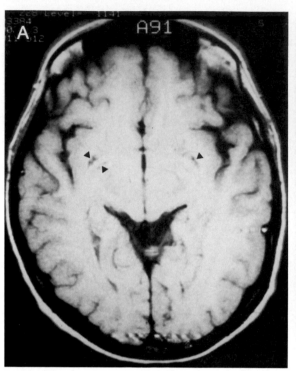
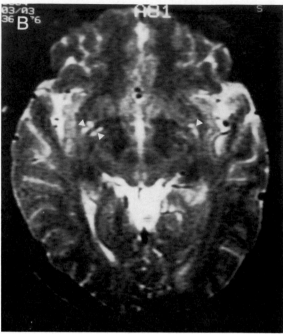

FIG 8–18.
Prominent perivascular (Virchow-Robin) spaces. **A,** MRI, transverse, 600/20. **B,** MRI, transverse, 3,000/100. The small lesions bilaterally (*black arrowheads* on the short TR, short TE MRI; *white arrow points* on the long TR, long TE MRI) have signal characteristics precisely like the signal characteristics of CSF. Their location in the inferior aspect of the basal ganglia bilaterally suggests that they represent prominent perivascular spaces rather than lacunar infarctions.

FIG 8–19.
Diffuse infarction due to hypoxemia in an infant. CT with intravenous contrast shows decreased attenuation in the cerebral parenchyma, particularly in the parietal and occipital regions. There is preservation of normal-appearing density within the basal ganglia. The normal CT attenuation of the basal ganglia does not mean that the basal ganglia function normally at a cellular level.

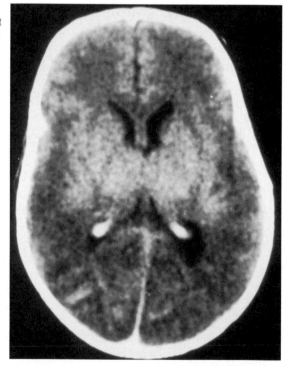

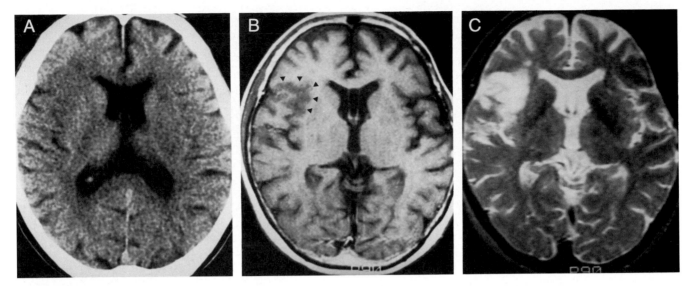

FIG 8–20.
Acute infarction. **A,** noncontrast CT at the time of ictus is normal. **B,** MRI, transverse (SE, 600/20). Short TR, short TE acquisition shows low intensity in the anterior right middle cerebral artery distribution *(arrowheads)*. The right sylvian cistern is effaced. **C,** MRI, transverse (SE, 3,000/80). Long TR, long TE acquisition demonstrates dramatic increased signal intensity in the anterior right middle cerebral artery distribution due to edema.

hemorrhage is less reliably made on the basis of signal intensities alone. Subacute hemorrhage is sensitively imaged by MRI at all field strengths and is characterized by methemoglobin-induced T1 relaxation time shortening and T2 relaxation time lengthening, which causes marked hyperintensity on both short TR, short TE images and long TR, long TE images. The peripheral hemosiderin

in chronic extracellular blood collections causes hypointensity on both short TR, short TE images and long TR, long TE images (Fig 8–23). Although CT detects acute hemorrhage more accurately than MRI does, the sequelae of subacute and chronic hemorrhages are more apparent on MRI.

Small foci of T2 prolongation in the deep white matter of elderly patients are commonly imaged

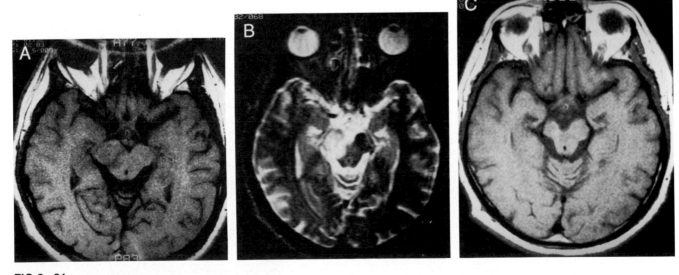

FIG 8–21.
Acute and chronic infarction, right midbrain. **A,** MRI, transverse (SE, 600/25). Short TR, short TE images 2 days following ictus show low density and swelling in the right cerebral peduncle. **B,** MRI, transverse (SE, 3,500/120). Long TR, long TE images show the increased signal intensity of acute infarction. **C,** MRI, transverse (SE, 600/20). Short TR, short TE acquisition 2½ years following ictus shows atrophy of the right cerebral peduncle.

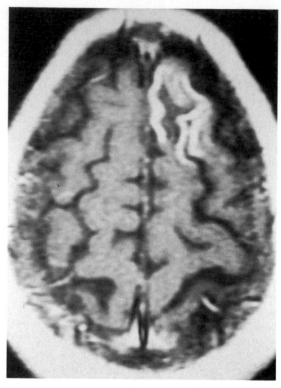

FIG 8–22.
Gyriform enhancement of subacute infarction following gadolinium administration: MRI, transverse (SE, 500/20). Noncontrast short TR, short TE images of the same patient at the same time showed no increased intensity.

(Fig 8–24), more commonly than are so called lacunes as imaged by CT. The discrepancy is due to the superior sensitivity of MRI to alterations in tissue water content, but it also points out the lack of specificity of MRI since edema, gliosis, and demyelination all cause T2 prolongation and result in hyperintensity on long TR, long TE, images.[40] The

small foci of increased intensity on long TR, long TE images in the brains of elderly people (who may be neurologically asymptomatic) do not necessarily indicate brain edema associated with acute lacunar infarction and may reflect gliosis or demyelination associated with chronic ischemia.[41] The presence of foci of increased signal intensity on

FIG 8–23.
Chronic hemorrhagic infarction on MRI. MRI (transverse, SE, 2,500/100) shows low-intensity hemosiderin *(arrowheads)* within the increased intensity of the old right middle cerebral artery infarction. There are also numerous other periventricular foci of T2 prolongation that are compatible with old ischemic changes.

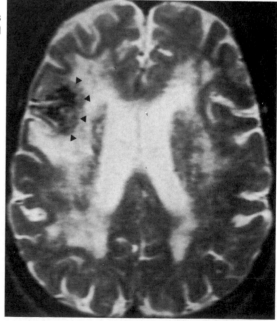

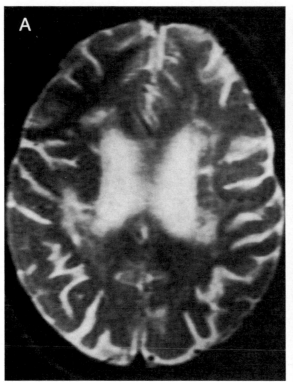
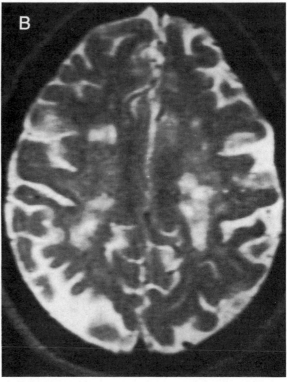

FIG 8–24.
Periventricular changes in an elderly patient. **A** and **B,** MRI, transverse (SE, 3,000/100). Numerous bilateral periventricular foci of T2 prolongation are common, nonspecific changes in the elderly. The foci of T2 prolongation do not necessarily correlate with neurologic or intellectual deficit.

long TR, long TE images does not correlate with cognitive function or cerebrovascular risk factors but does correlate strongly with age.[42] Subcortical arteriosclerotic encephalopathy (SAE) causes numerous, often confluent bilateral foci of T2 prolongation in the basal ganglia and the subcortical and deep cerebral white matter.[43] Binswanger's disease is a triad of dementia, hypertension, and multiple deep microinfarctions. Both SAE and Binswanger's disease are clinical and pathologic diagnoses and require more than just an MRI appearance.

MRI changes related to wallerian degeneration following infarction become apparent at approximately 4 weeks,[44] with hypointense signal in the corticospinal tracts on long TR, long TE images representing myelin protein breakdown. After 10 to 14 weeks the corticospinal tract changes and becomes hyperintense as a result of myelin lipid breakdown, gliosis, and increased water content. After several years unilateral brainstem atrophy reflects volume loss due to selective neuronal death (Fig 8–25).

MRI is useful for characterizing the contents of cavitary lesions. The CSF in cavitated infarctions of any size has signal characteristics like those of CSF in expected locations (e.g., the ventricles and cisterns) (Fig 8–26). If a fluid collection is isodense with CSF on CT but has relative hyperintensity when compared with CSF on long TR, long TE images, then increased protein content in the fluid is suggested, which is more typical of tumors.[45] The relative hyperintensity of proteinaceous fluids as compared with the intensity of CSF on long TR, long TE images is an example of the influence of T1 effects on long TR, long TE images. Proteinaceous fluids do not have T2 relaxation times longer than that of CSF. They are hyperintense on long TR, long TE images because they have T1 relaxation times shorter than that of CSF and therefore recover more longitudinal magnetization between radio frequency (RF) pulses. Due to their short T1 relaxation times, proteinaceous fluids start their decay processes with much more signal than does CSF. Even though their signals decay at a more rapid rate than that of CSF, when sampled at TEs for standard long TR, long TE images, proteinaceous fluids still have more signal than CSF has.

MRI also depicts vascular morphology and

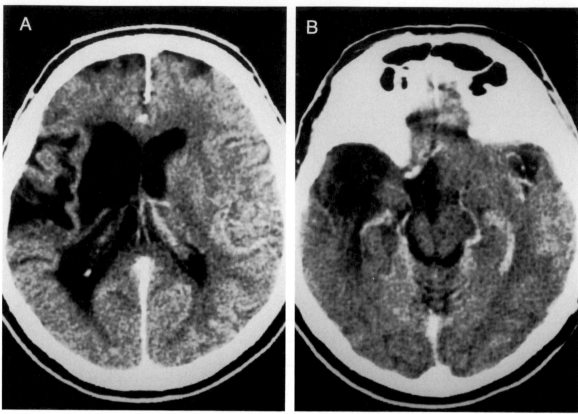

FIG 8–25.
Wallerian degeneration. **A,** CT with intravenous contrast of a remote right middle cerebral artery infarction shows encephalomalacia with dilatation of the subjacent right lateral ventricle. **B,** the right cerebral peduncle is atrophic, representing wallerian degeneration related to the old right middle cerebral artery infarction. Note also the encephalomalacia in the anterior right temporal lobe.

flow patterns to greater advantage than does contrast-enhanced CT. MRI distinguishes between rapid flow, slow flow, and vascular occlusion (although care must be taken to avoid diagnostic errors due to entry slice phenomenon, even echo rephasing, and other flow-related phenomena) (Figs 8–27 and 8–28).[46–51] Subintimal hemorrhage in arterial dissection can also be accurately imaged with MRI (Figs 8–29 and 8–30).[52]

Proton MRI requires a longer time period for imaging than does CT, so motion artifact causes more problems with MRI than with CT. With the development of pulse sequences allowing shorter acquisition times, degradation of MR images by patient motion will become a minor problem. MR images are not degraded by bone artifact, so posterior fossa ischemia/infarction is more accurately assessed with MRI than with CT (Fig 8–31).

In vivo MR spectroscopy and spectroscopic imaging of phosphorus-containing compounds (including adenosine triphosphate [ATP] and adenosine diphosphate [ADP]) allow quantitation of local brain metabolism in ischemic states.[53] Preliminary work is encouraging,[54] but the method is not yet readily available for clinical human imaging.

MRI of sodium (rather than of protons) is also possible.[55] Since the changes in intracellular and extracellular sodium concentrations parallel the initial changes in intracellular and extracellular water following infarction[56] and because MRI of sodium is confounded by its rarity in the body (sodium is 1/4,000 as common as hydrogen), sodium MRI has relatively little clinical advantage at present.

PHYSIOLOGIC ASSESSMENT OF CEREBRAL ISCHEMIA

Static CT and MRI scans, without and with intravenous contrast, provide no information regarding CBF dynamics. Dynamic bolus CT involves rapid acquisition of a series of CT images during the first pass through the cerebral vasculature of

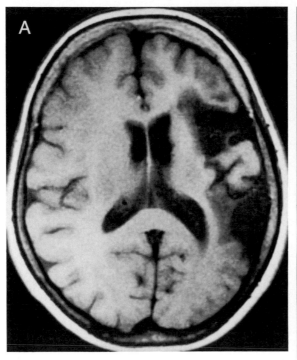
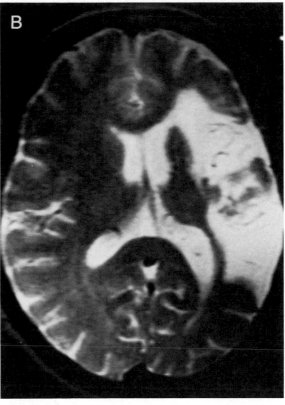

FIG 8–26.
Remote cerebral infarction: MRI, transverse. **A,** SE, 600/25; **B,** SE, 300/90. There is severe encephalomalacia associated with the left middle cerebral artery infarction. The destroyed brain has been re- placed by CSF. Note the similarity of the signal characteristics of the ventricular CSF and the fluid in the old infarct.

intravenous contrast, and this allows the detection of decreased circulation times.[57–59] Most CT scanners require at least 1 to 2 seconds per slice, with additional time required for table translation, so the process is too slow to generate enough data to accurately depict cerebral hemodynamics at multiple levels. Accurate measurements can be made if numerous cuts are obtained at a single level. Selecting the proper level to image with dynamic bolus CT is problematic in acute stroke patients who have normal or equivocal CT scan findings. Dynamic bolus CT scanning has been most useful for the study of subacute infarction, when the plain and/or intravenous contrast-enhanced CT scan findings are abnormal, and for guiding selection of the proper level for the dynamic series.

Xenon-enhanced CT CBF mapping uses inhaled stable xenon as an intravascular radiographic contrast agent (see Chapter 6). Xenon is soluble in blood and readily crosses the intact blood-brain barrier. The xenon atom is small, lipophilic, and nonionic and therefore is an excellent perfusion agent since it passes quickly into the cerebral pa-

renchyma in normal and diseased states. Its high Z number makes it a good radiographic contrast agent, similar to iodine. Iodinated contrast agents are not as good for cerebral perfusion studies; because of their molecular size, their passage through the vasculature measures circulation time rather than perfusion.

Xenon-enhanced CT CBF mapping defines the extent and degree of ischemia better than CT or MRI.[60] Xenon CT has better spatial resolution than do other perfusion mapping modalities (single photon emission computed tomography [SPECT], positron emission tomography [PET]),[61–63] and the data are rapidly acquired and processed, so they provide CBF maps in a period of time short enough to be clinically germane.[64] The quantitation of CBF by xenon-enhanced CT CBF mapping allows the prediction of whether a region of ischemic brain has the potential to recover or whether it is so severely damaged that it will surely die. The distinction between reversible ischemia and injury so severe as to cause certain infarction is critically important in the clinical

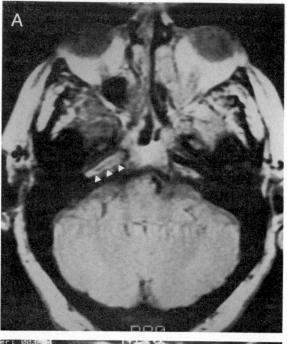

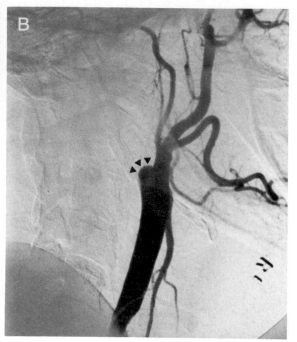

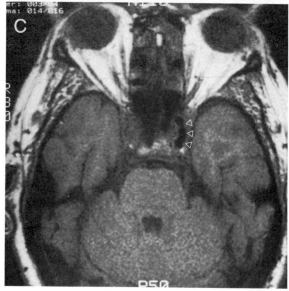

FIG 8–27.
Right carotid artery occlusion. **A,** a right common carotid arteriogram demonstrates occlusion of the right carotid artery at its origin *(arrowheads).* **B,** MRI, transverse (SE, 2500/25). Increased signal intensity in the right carotid canal *(arrowheads)* indicates the thrombosed right internal carotid artery. Note the signal void caused by flowing blood in the left carotid canal. **C,** MRI, transverse (SE, 600/20). The signal void caused by flowing blood in the left cavernous carotid artery is indicated by *arrowheads.* The absence of signal void in the right cavernous carotid artery is secondary to the right internal carotid artery thrombosis.

management of acute cerebral ischemia patients. CBF augmentation, both medical (including hemodilution and hypertension) and surgical, may be beneficial for patients with reversible ischemia, but for those whose ischemia is so severe that they will surely develop infarction, blood flow augmentation will not help and can cause severe complications (e.g., hemorrhage into necrotic brain). Xenon-enhanced CT CBF mapping can accurately depict cerebral hypoperfusion very early while CT images are still normal (Fig 8–32).[65] The threshold for cerebral infarction is approximately 15 to 18 mL/100 g/min, with lower values progressing to in-

farction and higher values maintaining the potential to recover. The duration of hypoperfusion plays an important role in the development of infarction in addition to the degree of hypoperfusion.[66]

One obvious limitation of all CBF methods is that they only provide CBF data for a single point in time. A region may have a flow of 20 mL/100 g/min at the time of examination but 30 minutes later may be down to 10 mL/100 g/min. A further and related problem is that cerebral metabolism is not directly coupled to CBF in the acute ischemic state. Regional hyperperfusion (CBF in excess of

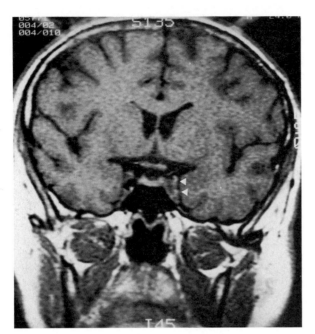

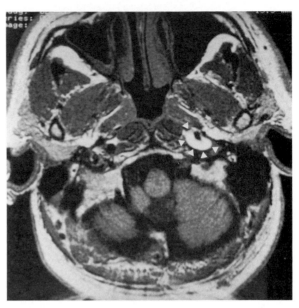

FIG 8–28.
Thrombosed left internal carotid artery: MRI, coronal (SE, 400/20). The absence of signal void in the left cavernous sinus *(arrow points)* is due to thrombosis of the left cavernous carotid artery. Note the normal signal void caused by the right cavernous carotid artery.

FIG 8–29.
Carotid artery dissection: MRI, transverse (SE, 600/20). The increased signal intensity surrounding the left internal carotid artery *(arrow points)* is a perivascular clot associated with left internal carotid artery dissection. The low-intensity region within the clot represents signal void caused by flowing blood in the irregular residual lumen of the left internal carotid artery.

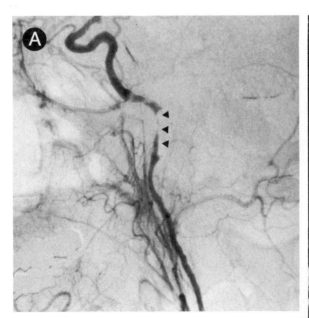

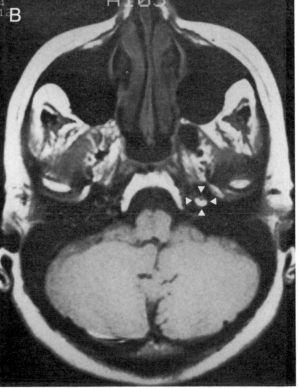

FIG 8–30.
Carotid artery dissection. **A,** an arteriogram shows irregularity due to dissection along the entire length of the left internal carotid artery. Particularly high grade stenosis at the skull base is indicated by *arrowheads*. **B,** MRI (transverse, SE, 600/20) shows increased signal intensity in the region of the left internal carotid artery at the skull base *(arrowheads)* that represents clot associated with the left internal carotid artery dissection. The small area of decreased signal intensity in the anterior portion of the clot represents the small residual lumen of the left internal carotid artery.

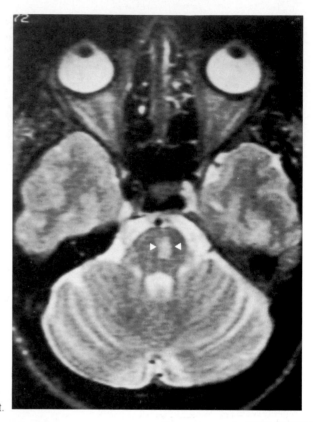

FIG 8–31.
Brain stem infarction: MRI, transverse (SE, 2,500/100). A small pontine infarction is represented as an area of T2 prolongation (between the *arrowheads*) in this 31-year-old woman with a history of vasculitis. CT of the same lesion was severely degraded by posterior fossa streak artifact.

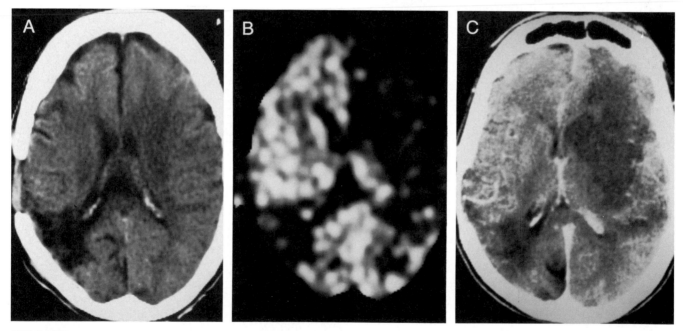

FIG 8–32.
Xenon-enhanced CT CBF mapping of acute ischemia. **A,** CT immediately following ictus shows an old right posterior arterial border zone infarction. The left anterior and middle and cerebral artery territories appear normal. **B,** Xenon-enhanced CT CBF map performed at the same time as **A.** The decreased blood flow in the old right posterior border zone infarction was expected. The large area of hypoperfusion in the left anterior and middle cerebral artery territories was not expected based upon the CT. **C,** CT with intravenous contrast 3 days following ictus. Vasogenic edema in the left anterior and middle cerebral artery territory infarction is causing marked hypodensity and shift.

100 mL/100 g/min) is pathologic, representing reactive hyperemia, and indicates that the involved brain tissue may progress to infarction.

In the subacute and chronic ischemic states xenon-enhanced CT CBF mapping accurately defines the distribution of blood flow. CBF is coupled with metabolism in chronic ischemia, but a single flow measurement does not distinguish whether hypoperfusion is due to decreased blood supply with normal cellular demand or due to decreased cellular demand. In order to acquire information regarding oxygen demand of tissues receiving decreased perfusion, a double study is performed, both before and after intravenous administration of 1 g acetazolamide (Diamox).[67] Diamox is a cerebral vasodilator that increases blood flow in patients who have adequate functional reserves. In areas with low CBF due to the lack of cellular demand, local CBF will increase with intravenous Diamox. In low-CBF areas with more demand than supply, local CBF will not increase with intravenous Diamox since the vascular reserves are being used maximally. The Diamox test, therefore, quickly and accurately defines areas that may benefit from flow augmentation.

REFERENCES

1. Jones TH, Morawetz RB, Crowell RM, et al: Thresholds of focal cerebral ischemia in awake monkeys. *J Neurosurg* 1981; 54:773–782.
2. Welsh FA: Regional evaluation of ischemic metabolic alterations. *J Cereb Blood Flow Metab* 1984; 4:309–316.
3. Kricheff II: Atherosclerotic ischemic cerebrovascular disease. *Radiology* 1987; 162:101–109.
4. Latchaw RE, Wechsler LR: Strokes and transient ischemia attacks, in Straub WH (ed): *Manual of Diagnostic Imaging: A Clinician's Guide to Clinical Problem Solving*, ed 2. Boston, Little Brown & Co, Inc, 1989.
5. Taylor KJW, Burins PN, Wells PNT (eds): *Clinical Applications of Doppler Ultrasound*. New York, Raven Press, 1988.
6. DeWitt LD, Wechsler LR: Transcranial Doppler. *Stroke* 1988; 19:915–921.
7. Heinz ER, Pizer SM, Fuchs H, et al: Examination of the extracranial carotid bifurcation by thin-section dynamic CT: Direct visualization of intimal atheroma in man (part 1). *AJNR* 1984; 5:355–359.
8. Heinz ER, Fuchs J, Osborne D, et al: Examination of the extracranial carotid bifurcation by thin-section dynamic CT: Direct visualization of intimal atheroma in man (part 2). *AJNR* 1984; 5:361–366.
9. Tress BM, Davis S, Lavain J, et al: Incremental dynamic computed tomography: Practical method of imaging the carotid bifurcation. *AJR* 1986; 146:465–470.
10. Masaryk TJ, Ross JS, Modic MT, et al: Carotid bifurcation: MR imaging: Work in progress. *Radiology* 1988; 166:461–466.
11. Dumoulin CL, Hart HH: Magnetic resonance angiography. *Radiology* 1986; 161:717–720.
12. Valk PE, Hale JD, Kaufman L, et al: MR imaging of the aorta with three-dimensional vessel reconstruction: Validation by angiography. *Radiology* 1985; 157:721–725.
13. Wedeen VJ, Rosen BR, Buxton R, et al: Projective MRI angiography and quantitative flow-volume dosimetry. *Magn Reson Med* 1986; 3:226–241.
14. Miller DL, Reinig JW, Volkman DJ: Vascular imaging with MRI: Inadequacy in Takayasu's arteritis compared with angiography. *AJR* 1986; 146:949–954.
15. Wall SD, Brant-Zawadzki M, Jeffrey RB, et al: High frequency CT findings within 24 hours after cerebral infarction. *AJNR* 1981; 2:553–557.
16. Kirshner HS, Staller J, Webb W, et al: Transtentorial herniation with posterior cerebral artery territory infarction. *Stroke* 1982; 13:243–246.
17. Becker H, Desch H, Hacker H, et al: CT fogging effect with ischemic cerebral infarcts. *Neuroradiology* 1979; 18:185–192.
18. Wodarz R: Watershed infarctions and computed tomography: A topographical study in cases with stenosis or occlusion of the carotid artery. *Neuroradiology* 1980; 19:245–248.
19. Inoue Y, Takemoto K, Miyamoto T, et al: Sequential computed tomography scans in acute cerebral infarction. *Radiology* 1980; 135:655–662.
20. Houser WO, Campbell JK, Baker HL Jr, et al: Radiologic evaluation of ischemic cerebrovascular syndromes with emphasis on computed tomography. *Radiol Clin North Am* 1982; 20:123–142.
21. Kuroiwa T, Seida M, Tomida S, et al: Discrepancies among CT, histological, and blood-brain barrier findings in early cerebral ischemia. *J Neurosurg* 1986; 65:517–524.
22. Kendall BE, Pullicino P: Intravascular contrast injection in ischemic lesions: II. Effect on prognosis. *Neuroradiology* 1980; 19:241–243.
23. Pressman BD, Tourje EJ, Thompson JR: An early CT sign of ischemic infarction: Increased density in a cerebral artery. *AJNR* 1987; 8:645–648.
24. Horning CR, Dorndorf W, Agnoli AL: Hemorrhagic cerebral infarction: A progressive study. *Stroke* 1986; 17:176–184.
25. Brown JJ, Hesselink JR, Rothrock JF: MR and CT of lacunar infarcts. *AJNR* 1988; 9:477–482.
26. Jungreis CA, Kanal E, Hirsch WL, et al: Normal perivascular spaces mimicking lacunar infarction: MR imaging. *Radiology* 1988; 169:101–104.
27. Latchaw RE, Johnson DW, Hecht ST, et al: Multi-

focal cerebral hypoperfusion after cardiac arrest studied with Xe/CT blood flow analysis: Methodology and results. Presented at the annual meeting of the American Society of Neuroradiology, Orlando, Fla, March 1989.

28. Brant-Zawadzki M: MR imaging of the brain. *Radiology* 1988; 166:1–10.

29. Bryan RN, Willcott MR, Schneiders NJ: Nuclear magnetic resonance evaluation of stroke: A preliminary report. *Radiology* 1983; 149:189–192.

30. Kertesz A, Black SE, Nicholson L, et al: The sensitivity and specificity of MRI in stroke. *Neurology* 1987; 37:1580–1585.

31. Naruse S, Horikawa Y, Tanaka C, et al: Proton nuclear magnetic resonance studies on brain edema. *J Neurosurg* 1982; 56:747–752.

32. Unger E, Littlefield J, Gado M: Water content and water structure in CT and MR signal changes: Possible influence in detection of early stroke. *AJNR* 1988; 9:687–691.

33. Brant-Zawadzki M, Norman D, Newton TH, et al: Magnetic resonance imaging of the brain: The optimal screening technique. *Radiology* 1984; 152:71–77.

34. Brant-Zawadzki M, Pereira B, Weinstein P, et al: MR imaging of acute experimental ischemia in cats. *AJNR* 1986; 7:7–11.

35. Bell BA, Symon L, Branston NM: CBF and time thresholds for the formation of ischemic cerebral edema, and effects of reperfusion in baboons. *J Neurosurg* 1985; 62:31–41.

36. McNamara MT, Brant-Zawadzki M, Berry I, et al: Acute experimental cerebral ischemia: MRI enhancement using Gd-DTPA. *Radiology* 1986; 158:701–705.

37. Imakita S, Nishimura T, Naito H, et al: Magnetic resonance imaging of human cerebral infarction: Enhancement with Gd-DTPA. *Neuroradiology* 1987; 29:422–429.

38. Gomori JM, Grossman RI, Goldberg HI, et al: Intracranial hematomas: Imaging by high field MR. *Radiology* 1985; 157:87–93.

39. Hecht-Leavitt C, Gomori J, Grossman RI: High-field MRI of hemorrhagic cortical infarction. *AJNR* 1986; 7:581–585.

40. Virapongse C, Mancuso A, Quisling R: Human brain infarcts: Gd-DTPA–enhanced MR imaging. *Radiology* 1986; 161:785–794.

41. Marshall VG, Bradley WG Jr, Marshall CE, et al: Deep white matter infarction: Correlation of MR imaging and histopathologic findings. *Radiology* 1988; 167:517–522.

42. Hendrie HC, Farlow MR, Austrom MG, et al: Foci of increased T2 signal intensity on brain MR scans of healthy elderly subjects. *AJNR* 1989; 10:703–707.

43. Kertesz A, Black SE, Tokar G, et al: Periventricular and subcortical hyperintensities on magnetic resonance imaging: Rims, caps, and unidentified bright objects. *Arch Neurol* 1988; 45:404–408.

44. Kuhn MJ, Mikulis DJ, Ayoub DM, et al: Wallerian degeneration after cerebral infarction: Evaluation with sequential MR imaging. *Radiology* 1989; 172:179–182.

45. Kjos BO, Brant-Zawadzki M, Kucharczyk W, et al: Cystic intracranial lesions: Magnetic resonance imaging. *Radiology* 1985; 155:363–369.

46. Wedeen VJ, Rosen BR, Chester D, et al: MR velocity imaging by phase display. *J Comput Assist Tomogr* 1985; 9:530–536.

47. Waluch V, Bradley WG: NMR even echo rephasing in slow laminar flow. *J Comput Assist Tomogr* 1984; 8:594–598.

48. Bradley WG, Waluch V: Blood flow: Magnetic resonance imaging. *Radiology* 1985; 154:443–450.

49. Shimizu K, Matsuda T, Sakura T, et al: Visualization of moving fluid: Quantitative analysis of blood flow dynamics using MR imaging. *Radiology* 1986; 159:195–199.

50. Von Schulthess GK, Higgins CB: Blood flow imaging with MR: Spin-phase phenomena. *Radiology* 1985; 157:687–695.

51. Fox AJ, Bogousslavsky J, Carey LS, et al: Magnetic resonance imaging of small medullary infarctions. *AJNR* 1986; 7:229–233.

52. Goldberg HI, Grossman RI, Gomori JM, et al: Cervical internal carotid artery dissecting hemorrhage: Diagnosis using MR. *Radiology* 1986; 158:157–161.

53. Levine SR, Welch KMA, Helpern JA, et al: Prolonged deterioration of ischemic brain energy metabolism and acidosis associated with hyperglycemia: Human cerebral infarction studied by serial ^{31}PNMR spectroscopy. *Ann Neurol* 1988; 23:416–418.

54. Maudsley AA, Hilal SK, Simon HE, et al: In vivo MR spectroscopic imaging with P-31: Work in progress. *Radiology* 1984; 153:745–750.

55. Hilal SK, Maudsley AA, Simon HE, et al: In vivo NMR imaging of tissue sodium in the intact cat before and after acute cerebral stroke. *AJNR* 1983; 4:245–249.

56. Gotoh O, Asano T, Koide T, et al: Ischemic brain edema following occlusion of the middle cerebral artery in the rat, I: The time courses of the brain water, sodium and potassium contents and blood-brain permeability to ^{125}I-albumin. *Stroke* 1985; 16:101–106.

57. Jinkins JR: Dynamic CT of micro- and macroangiopathic states of the cerebrum. *Neuroradiology* 1988; 30:22–30.

58. Norman D, Axel L, Berninger WH, et al: Dynamic computed tomography of the brain: Techniques, data analysis and applications. *AJNR* 1981; 136:759–770.

59. Traupe H, Heiss WD, Hoeffken W, et al: Hyperperfusion and enhancement in dynamic computed to-

mography of ischemic stroke in patients. *J Comput Assist Tomogr* 1979; 3:627–632.

60. Hughes RL, Yonas H, Gur D, et al: Stable xenon-enhanced CT in the first eight hours of cerebral infarction. *Stroke* 1987; 18:283.

61. Holman BL, Hill TC: Perfusion imaging with single-photon emission computed tomography, in Wood JH (ed): *Cerebral Blood Flow.* New York, McGraw-Hill International Book Co, 1987, pp 243–256.

62. Lee RGL, Hill TC, Holman L, et al: Predictive value of perfusion defect since using *N*-isopropyl-^{125}I-*p*-iodoamphetamine emission tomography in acute stroke. *J Neurosurg* 1984; 61:449–452.

63. Heiss W-D, Herholz K, Bocher-Schwarz HG, et al: PET, CT, and MR imaging in cerebrovascular disease. *J Comput Assist Tomogr* 1986; 10:903–911.

64. Yonas H, Good WF, Gur D, et al: Mapping cerebral blood flow by xenon-enhanced computed tomography: Clinical experience. *Radiology* 1984; 152:435–442.

65. Yonas H, Gur D, Claassen D, et al: Stable xenon enhanced CT measurement of cerebral blood flow in reversible focal ischemia in baboons. *J Neurosurg* 1990; 73:266–273.

66. Yonas H, Gur D, Good BC, et al: Stable xenon CT blood flow mapping for evaluation of patients with intracranial-extracranial bypass surgery. *J Neurosurg* 1985; 62:324–333.

67. Rogg J, Rutigliano M, Yonas H, et al: The acetazolamide challenge: A method using imaging techniques to evaluate cerebral blood flow reserve. *AJNR* 1989; 10:803–810.

9

Intracranial Hemorrhage

Robert I. Grossman, M.D.

IMAGING TECHNIQUES AND GENERAL FINDINGS

Computed Tomography

One of the most striking and important developments in radiology occurred with the first images of intracranial hemorrhage viewed on an 80 × 80 matrix (Fig 9–1). These images appear very crude by today's standards; however, in 1974 they represented a dramatic and important breakthrough in medicine. Prior to the advent of computed tomography (CT), hemorrhagic events in the central nervous system were almost entirely imaged indirectly by displacements of cerebral structures. It was an extremely rare observation to demonstrate extravasation of contrast material on an arteriogram (Fig 9–2). It is difficult to imagine what practice was like before CT. With the first CT images of hemorrhage radiologists embarked on fertile ground for clinical investigation and attempted to understand the appearance of many hemorrhagic conditions on this new modality. In the next approximately 8 years a plethora of literature appeared that was devoted to hemorrhagic topics. Just as we began to understand and could diagnose most hemorrhagic conditions on CT, a new technology became available that both significantly complicated and enriched our lives. Magnetic resonance imaging (MRI), like CT, represented a quantum leap in capability and difficulty. Initially it appeared that we could only visualize subacute hemorrhage. Subsequently, with the development of higher-field strength units and more sophisticated pulse sequences the various shades of hemorrhage became visible. MRI is an exciting and rewarding modality for investigating the biochemical and physical chemical properties and events associated with various hemorrhagic states. It has and will continue to provide significant insights into hemorrhagic conditions. This chapter will discuss the mechanisms responsible for the images of hemorrhagic conditions on both CT and MRI.

Blood is composed of cells and proteins that, in a variety of different circumstances, may extravasate from the circulatory system. When this occurs in the central nervous system, the event is usually recognized by the abrupt onset of a neurologic deficit or a significant symptom ("the worst headache of my life!"). This situation demands prompt attention including appropriate imaging diagnosis. CT has played a remarkable role in the diagnosis of acute hemorrhage. Why CT is so useful in acute hemorrhage is based on an appreciation of its principles. The x-ray attenuation values of a substance or a structure determines its visibility on CT. There is a linear relationship between CT attenuation values and hematocrit (Hct).[1] New and Aronow measured the attenuation of whole blood with an Hct of 45% and found it to have an attenuation of approximately 56 Hounsfield units (HU) (their original measurement was 28 EMI units).[2] Normal gray matter ranges from 37 to 41 HU, and normal white matter is from 30 to 34 HU. Thus freshly extravasated blood in a patient with a normal Hct could be immediately demonstrated on CT. The increased attenuation of whole blood is based primarily upon the protein concentration (globin portion) of the blood. If one is imaging hemorrhage in an anemic patient, whatever the eti-

171

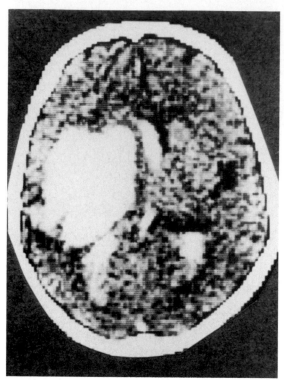

FIG 9–1.
Original EMI CT (80 × 80 matrix) of an acute hypertensive hemorrhage with dissection of the blood into the ventricles. (Courtesy of Kenneth R. Davis, M.D.)

ology, there is a possibility that the acute hemorrhage will be isodense to brain.[3] Values of hemoglobin below 10 g/dL may be undetectable on the basis of density alone.

Following the extravasation of blood a clot forms with a progressive increase in the attenuation of the hemorrhage over approximately 72 hours. This is a result of clot formation and retraction, with the extrusion of low-density serum and a subsequent increase in hemoglobin concentration. After approximately the third day the attenuation values of the clot begin to decrease, and over the next few weeks the hemorrhage fades to isodensity. After 1 month (rarely 2 months) there should be no high intensity demonstrated from a single intraparenchymal hemorrhage. The hemorrhage loses density from the periphery to the central region. This is the result of the biochemical changes that are occurring in the clot. The red blood cells (RBCs) containing desaturated hemoglobin are undergoing lysis, dilution, and subsequent digestion of the blood products by peripheral macrophages. It is obvious from our understanding of MRI (see below) that a hemorrhage does not disappear in

the brain just because it has become isointense on CT.

In a simple intraparenchymal hemorrhage the initial low attenuation surrounding the high-density hemorrhage is secondary to the serum from the retracted clot. This hypodense rim is not large. The circumferential hypodensity increases and reaches a maximum at approximately 5 days. Vasogenic edema is responsible at this time for the surrounding low absorption. After approximately 2 months there is usually just a little hypodense slit representing the residua of the hemorrhagic event. With an uncomplicated hemorrhage less atrophy is seen than with infarction. The CT picture of gradual fading of the high-absorption hemorrhage is very different from the MRI picture in which certain hallmarks persist indefinitely. Interestingly, late (approximately 1 to 2 months postictus) precontrast CT scans have occasionally noted high-absorption rims in some cases. This actually represents hemosiderin deposition and can be detected by CT.[4] Thus, CT offers the ability to see acute and subacute hemorrhage in the nonanemic patient. It is fast, relatively easy to perform, not cumbersome, and accurate in most regions of the brain. Less favorable situations occur when the hemorrhage is small, thin, or in the lower brain stem and posterior fossa. Lesions in the brain stem may be obscured by artifact. Thin flat collections of blood (particularly subarachnoid and extracerebral hemorrhages) may not be visualized because of partial volume averaging. Thin sectioning perpendicular to the clot provides the best method for detection.[5] The collection must be twice the width of the slice thickness to not be affected by partial volume averaging. This is usually not a significant problem since axial imaging is perpendicular to the falx and major cisterns.

The use of intravenous iodinated contrast material in hemorrhage is unnecessary in most situations. However, it is useful acutely when one is dealing with a small hemorrhage associated with mass effect out of proportion to that hemorrhage. Here the differential diagnosis involves hemorrhage into a tumor, either primary or metastatic, venous infarction, or arterial hemorrhagic infarction. Venous or arterial hemorrhagic infarction characteristically follows a vascular distribution. In these cases one need not give contrast. The diagnosis of tumor with hemorrhage often requires contrast both to verify the presence of tumor and perhaps to identify additional lesions.

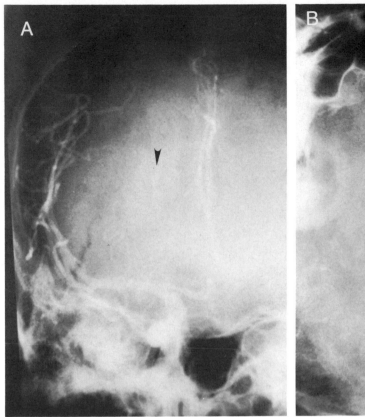
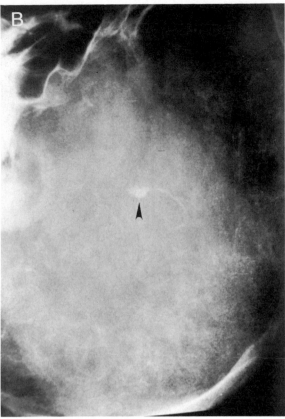

FIG 9–2.
A, a right carotid anteroposterior (AP) arteriogram demonstrates hemorrhage from a lenticulostriate artery *(arrowhead).* **B,** a lateral arteriogram shows a late capillary phase revealing the extrava- sated blood. Note that the patient is supine and the hemorrhage has layered out *(arrowhead).* (Courtesy of Herbert I. Goldberg, M.D.)

An enhancing ring in an uncomplicated intraparenchymal hemorrhage may appear from approximately 6 days to 6 weeks following the initial event (Fig 9–3).[6] This has been unassociated with mass effect and disappears from 2 to 6 months after the first scan. Diagnostically a problem arises if the patient, for whatever reason, was not scanned within the first week or so after the ictal event. One is then presented with a ring-enhancing lesion, the differential diagnosis of which includes tumor (primary or metastatic), abscess and other inflammatory conditions, infarction, and multiple sclerosis. This situation may be clarified somewhat by appropriate history and clinical findings as well as repeat CT. Serial imaging is then useful in differentiating hemorrhage from tumor and abscess since hemorrhage will decrease in mass effect and enhancement over time without treatment. MRI, however, will definitively separate hemorrhage from the nonhemorrhagic ring-enhancing lesion.

Magnetic Resonance Imaging

MRI has dramatically changed the way we look at hemorrhage. Not only can we detect acute hemorrhage, but we have the ability to detect subacute, chronic, and ancient hemorrhagic events. MRI will indicate the abnormality well after the CT findings of acute hemorrhage have faded away. The biochemical changes occurring in hemorrhage have their unique signature for the various biochemical stages. Therefore MRI has expanded our classification of the timing of hemorrhagic events. This is clearly important in cases where the longitudinal history of hemorrhagic events may help diagnose conditions such as hereditary occult cerebrovascular malformations (OCVM), child abuse, and amyloid angiopathy.

Protons and electrons are charged particles and are magnetic dipoles behaving as a bar magnet with the North and South poles separated by a finite distance. They also have angular momentum,

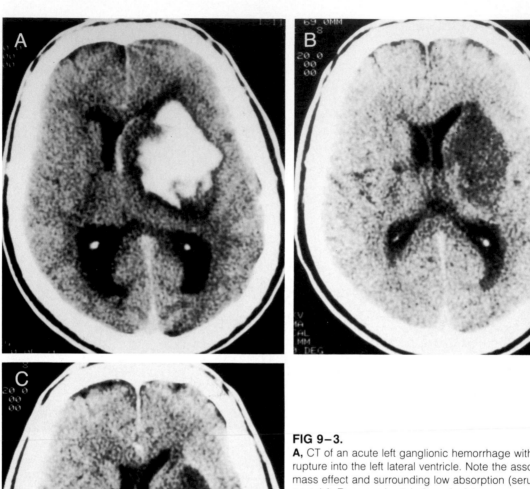

FIG 9–3.
A, CT of an acute left ganglionic hemorrhage with rupture into the left lateral ventricle. Note the associated mass effect and surrounding low absorption (serum acutely). **B,** approximately 3 weeks later an unenhanced scan demonstrates a low-absorption abnormality in the left basal ganglionic region, now without much mass effect. One of the pitfalls of CT as compared with MRI is the lack of specificity of this stage of the hemorrhage. Taken by itself one is hard-pressed to call this low-absorption lesion a hemorrhage. **C,** following intravenous contrast the intraparenchymal hemorrhage demonstrates ring enhancement.

with the electron possessing 1,000 times more momentum than the proton secondary to the relative differences in mass. The proton and the electron are constrained by quantum mechanics to align with or against an applied magnetic field. Protons realign with the magnetic field (relax), in the absence of unpaired electrons, via fluctuations in their local magnetic field that are caused by the motion of adjacent protons. However, when unpaired electrons are present, their large magnetic moment (lighter mass) produces significant fluctuations in the local magnetic field. These fluctuations enhance the ability of water proton relaxation. This effect, proton-electron dipolar-dipolar (PEDD) proton relaxation enhancement (PRE) interaction, occurs at short distances (~3 Å). Thus, a water proton must approach the electron distribution in the molecular orbital to efficiently relax (Fig 9–4).

Paramagnetic substances (those with unpaired electrons) have no intrinsic magnetic fields. How-

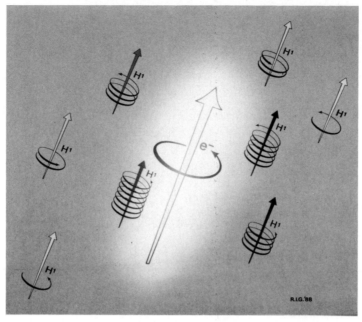

FIG 9–4.
The PEDD PRE interaction occurs when water protons approach within ~3 A of the unpaired electron. In this situation relaxation is facilitated with shortening of the relaxation times T1 and T2.

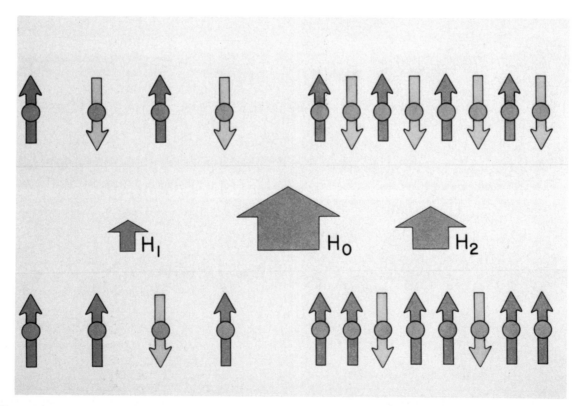

FIG 9–5.
Electron moments pointing randomly *(top line)*. Moments on the right have twice the number of electrons as those on the left. When an H_0 magnetic field is applied, more moments align with the magnetic field *(lower line)*. The main magnetic field (H_0) is augmented by H_1 on the left and by H_2 on the right. Notice that the augmentation of H_0 is proportional to the number of unpaired electrons ($H_2 > H_1$).

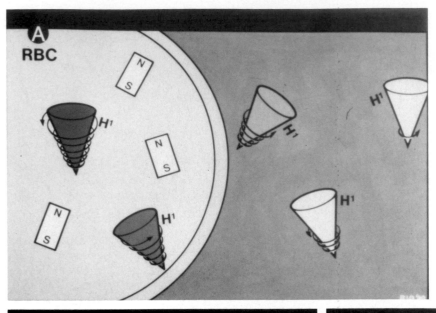

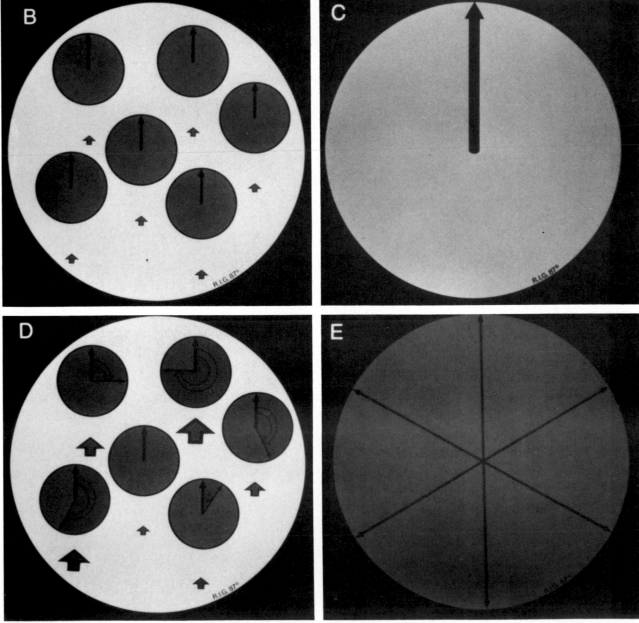

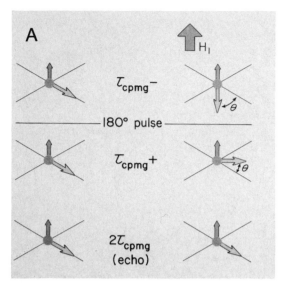

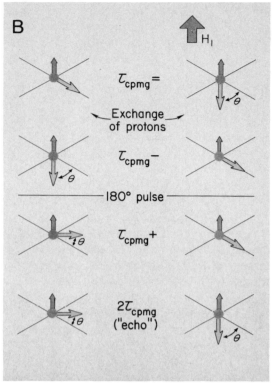

FIG 9–7.

Situations without diffusion **(A)** and with diffusion **(B)** in which water protons encounter a heterogeneous field (H_1). **A,** in this case no diffusion of water protons takes place. The *left side* represents the proton precessing in the rotating frame of reference H_0 while the right side demonstrates the additional phase (θ) produced by the higher field H_1. Notice at the time of the echo (2 τ_{cpmg}) the protons are back in phase. This coherence was produced by the 180-degree pulse and the absence of diffusion (the water protons stayed in the same field). **B,** in this case we have added diffusion indicated by the exchange of protons to different fields. Note that the protons do not regain phase coherence at the time of their echo in spite of being subjected to the same 180-degree pulse. CPMG=Carr-Purcell-Meiboom-Gill.

ever, when placed in an extrinsic magnetic field they locally augment the external field. This is indicated in Figure 9–5 where in the absence of a magnetic field the unpaired electrons are pointing randomly (top line). Placed in the magnetic field H_0 these unpaired electrons will augment the main field by H_1 or H_2 ($H_2 > H_1$) depending on the concentration of unpaired electrons. The magnetic susceptibility of a substance is a measure of how easily a substance can be magnetized or the ratio of the additional field strength to the strength of the applied field. If a paramagnetic substance has N unpaired electrons, then its magnetic susceptibility is proportional to $(N)(N + 2)$. In the case of

paramagnetic substances one deals with the augmented magnetic field produced by the paramagnetic. Where a heterogeneous distribution of paramagnetic substance (i.e., intracellular deoxyhemoglobin, intracellular methemoglobin, intralysosomal hemosiderin) exists, the magnetic fields demonstrate local variability. Water protons diffusing across a red cell membrane would experience slightly different fields (Fig 9–6). The water protons would precess at slightly different rates secondary to the different local field strengths (produced by local susceptibility differences). The diffusing water protons are precessing at slightly different rates (Larmor frequencies) because they

FIG 9–6.

A, water protons diffusing across the cell membrane experience different local magnetic fields between the inside and outside of the RBC. These local field differences cause the protons to precess at different rates that are proportional to the local field strengths. The inside of the RBC, in this case, contains a paramagnetic such as deoxyhemoglobin and thus has a greater local magnetic field than the outside of the cell. The water protons diffusing across the red cell membrane experience this higher field and precess faster. **B,** a voxel of tissue with no differences in susceptibili-

ties. *Short arrows* (magnetic field) indicate that each water proton *(gray circle)* is "experiencing" the same field. Notice that all protons are in phase. **C,** the sum of the phases in the voxel is a coherent signal (long T2). **D,** a voxel containing regions of heterogeneous magnetic susceptibility. Notice that the water protons "experience" locally varying fields and have precessed at different rates depending upon the strength of the local field. **E,** sum of the phases in this heterogeneous field. Notice that the spins are out of phase with each other and cancel each other (short T2).

are experiencing different magnetic fields. This phase spread, related to diffusion, cannot be corrected by the 180-degree pulse in the spin-echo pulse sequence (Fig 9–7). The loss of such phase coherence is responsible for the "short T2" observed in regions that contain a heterogeneous distribution of a paramagnetic substance.

The diffusion effects increase as the proton is allowed to sample differing fields, i.e., as the time between 180-degree pulses increases (interecho time) (Fig 9–8). When this occurs, water protons lose phase coherence with each other. Another way of thinking about this is to appreciate that as the number of echoes in a particular pulse sequence is decreased, the T2 shortening increases, i.e., the fourth echo when using an echo time (TE) of 25-ms pulse sequence is less effective at producing T2 shortening than is a single echo of a TE at 100 ms. This is secondary to the protons having greater time to sample heterogenous magnetic fields with associated loss of phase coherence. The diffusion effects vary as the square of the main magnetic field strength, the square in the variation of magnetic susceptibility (the concentration of paramagnetic), and the interecho time.

In contrast, PEDD PRE relaxation shortens both T1 and T2 and varies little with magnetic field. However, the water proton must be able to approach to within 3 $\overset{\circ}{A}$ of the electron to facilitate the PEDD PRE (see Fig 9–4). If the unpaired electrons are shielded from this approach and the

paramagnetic substance is heterogeneously distributed, it will only produce selective T2 relaxation.

Thus, paramagnetic substances have two separate relaxation mechanisms: (1) PEDD PRE and (2) T2 PRE. The difference between them is related to the ability of water protons to approach within 3 $\overset{\circ}{A}$ of the unpaired electrons.

The maximum heterogeneity of hemorrhage will occur with an Hct of 50%. The heterogeneity factor can be expressed mathematically by the expression $(1 - Hct/100) \times (Hct/100)$. If one assumes a 5% Hct (as in subarachnoid hemorrhage), then its heterogeneity factor will be $(1 - 0.05) \times (0.05) = .0475$. The heterogeneity factor for an Hct of 50% is $(1 - 0.5) \times (0.5) = .25$. Thus, a hemorrhage of Hct 5% will only have 19% of the T2 shortening when compared with a hemorrhage of 50% (.0475/.25).[7]

In a fresh hemorrhage, RBCs containing saturated hemoglobin extravasate into the brain parenchyma. Oxyhemoglobin, with iron in the ferrous (Fe^{2+}) state, does not contain any unpaired electron spins and is not paramagnetic. Thus, if such a hyperacute hemorrhage is evaluated by MRI, its appearance on short repetition time (TR) images is of isointensity to slight hypointensity secondary to the water/protein content of the extravasated whole blood. On long TR images the hemorrhage becomes higher in intensity. This is also related to the increased water/protein content of the blood. In this situation one cannot distinguish hemorrhage from any other lesion with a long T1 and a long T2. Fortunately the noncirculating RBCs become desaturated over a few hours (and clearly by 24 hours), and the subsequent deoxyhemoglobin (Fe^{+2}) has four unpaired electrons; however, these electrons are shielded from direct interaction with water protons. Intracellular deoxyhemoglobin will consequently produce susceptibility change only and shorten T2 alone. Therefore, acute hemorrhage containing deoxyhemoglobin will be isointense or slightly hypointense on short TR images and very hypointense on long TR images (Fig 9–9).[8–10]

The pO_2 of the hemorrhagic milieu is of critical importance in the detection of acute hemorrhage. In subarachnoid hemorrhage the pO_2 of cerebrospinal fluid (CSF) is approximately 43 mm Hg, which produces an approximate percent saturation of 72% (Fig 9–10). This results in only 28% deoxyhemoglobin. The amount of T2 shortening varies as the square of the concentration of the

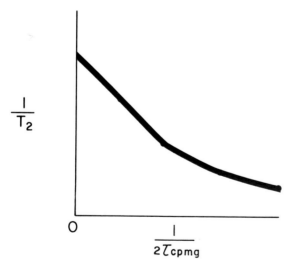

FIG 9–8.
Relationship of interecho time 2 τ_{cpmg} and relaxation time T2. As the interecho time increases, the relaxation time decreases. This graph is a plot of 1/T2 (relaxation rate) and 1/2 τ_{cpmg} (reciprocal of the interecho time).

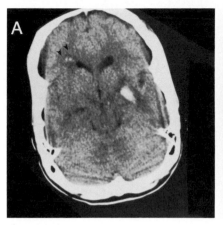
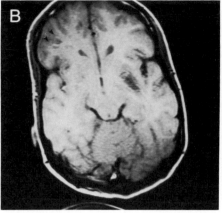
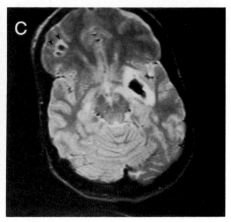

FIG 9–9.
Acute hemorrhage in the left basal ganglionic region. Note the high absorption on CT **(A)**, the slight hypointensity on the short TR image **(B)**, and the marked hypointensity on a long TR/long TE im- age with surrounding high intensity (edema and/or serum)**(C)**. There is also a small region of hemorrhage lateral to the right fron- tal horn that is seen on all the images *(arrowheads).*

paramagnetic so that $(.28)^2 \times 100\% = 7.8\%$ of the T2 shortening that one would expect with 100% deoxyhemoglobin (Fig 9–11). Lysis of RBCs may also play a role in the inability to demonstrate T2 shortening. This may occur within the first 12 hours following hemorrhage, and some susceptibil- ity changes may therefore be lost.

The pO_2 may also be important in other clini- cal situations as well. The low oxygen tension in tu- mors will give rise to increased quantities of deoxy-

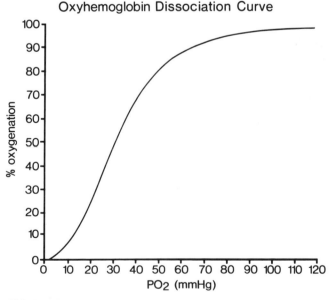

FIG 9–10.
Oxyhemoglobin dissociation curve. At approximately 43 mm Hg (approximate pO_2 of CSF) 72% of the hemoglobin is saturated, and therefore only 28% is in an unsaturated state.

hemoglobin and greater hypointensity.[11] With the lower oxygen tension there is some persistence in the deoxyhemoglobin state. In hemorrhagic corti- cal infarction there is luxury perfusion that may in- crease the tissue pO_2. If this situation did occur, the acute hemorrhage in the infarction might not be as hypointense as expected because of the in- creased saturation of the hemoglobin.[12] Acute neo- natal hemorrhage might be difficult to detect if there were a large amount of fetal hemoglobin. The fetal hemoglobin has a higher affinity for oxy- gen and shifts the oxyhemoglobin dissociation curve to the left, which would decrease the amount of deoxyhemoglobin present. Thus, the pO_2 of the tissue into which the hemorrhage has oc- curred affects the appearance of acute hemorrhage. Low pH and high pO_2 also shift the oxyhemoglo- bin dissociation curve to the right (Bohr effect). Therefore hemorrhage into areas containing a low pH will have more unsaturated hemoglobin (deoxy- hemoglobin) and will presumably be more hypoin- tense.

The intracellular deoxyhemoglobin is oxidized to methemoglobin. The process begins in the pe- riphery of the hemorrhage and occurs from about 3 days to a week. The periphery of the hemorrhage appears to have the optimal pO_2 and pH for this oxidation process. The iron in methemoglobin is in the ferric state (Fe^{3+}) with five unpaired electrons. Unlike deoxyhemoglobin, these electrons are ac- cessible to water protons. The result is a PEDD PRE interaction, and its appearance on short TR images is that of high intensity.[13, 14] The high in-

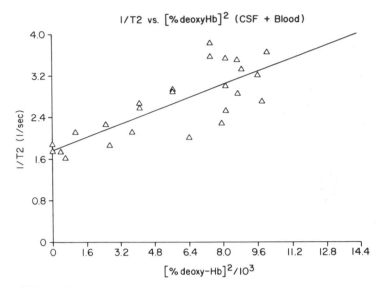

FIG 9–11.

This graph demonstrates the linear relationship between the T2 relaxation rate and the square of the concentration of deoxyhemoglobin; correlation coefficient 0.79.

tensity is initially noted in a ring (Fig 9–12). The center of the ring still contains deoxyhemoglobin and will be isointense or slightly hypointense on short TR images. The slight central hypointensity is really the effect of T2 shortening on the short TR images (the intensity will be decreased by the factor $e^{-TE/T2}$). The deoxyhemoglobin-to-methemoglobin conversion proceeds throughout the he-

matoma. The PEDD PRE mechanism shortens both the T1 and T2 in parallel. In addition, when methemoglobin is intracellular, there are susceptibility effects present (heterogeneous distribution of a paramagnetic) that also shorten T2. Thus intracellular methemoglobin will produce high intensity on short TR images and low intensity on long TR, long TE images.

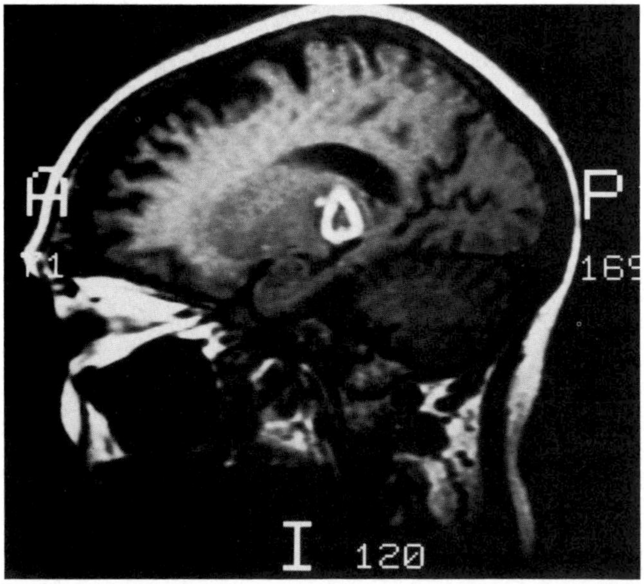

Cells containing the methemoglobin then lyse, and the hematoma contains free methemoglobin. The lysis of the RBC eliminates the heterogeneity in the distribution of paramagnetic and thus significantly increases the T2 of the hematoma. The free methemoglobin still possesses a PEDD PRE (producing a short T1 and T2), but there is now lack of the significant T2 shortening from the loss of heterogeneity. The net effect of the loss of heterogeneous susceptibility but the continued presence of T2 shortening (PEDD PRE) of methemoglobin is to have a somewhat higher intensity as compared with normal brain. This is due, in part, to the effect of the proton density of the clot, which will produce increased intensity and the important loss of heterogeneity.[15]

The appearance of subacute hemorrhage is variable. One must evaluate the hemorrhage by its appearance on both T1-weighted, proton density-weighted, and T2-weighted pulse sequences.[16] On the short TR/short TE pulse sequences the subacute hemorrhage will have high intensity secondary to the T1 shortening of the paramagnetic meth-

FIG 9–12.

Six-day-old hemorrhage demonstrating a methemoglobin ring (high intensity) with an isointense center on a short TR sagittal image.

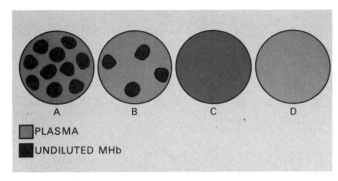

PLASMA

UNDILUTED MHb

FIG 9–13.
Diagrammatic representation of the four basic conditions that may arise in subacute hemorrhage. From *left to right:* **A,** undilute intracellular methemoglobin; **B,** dilute intracellular methemoglobin; **C,** free concentrated methemoglobin; and **D,** dilute free methemoglobin.

emoglobin. The proton density (long TR/short TE) image will be variable due to differences in dilution. Variable intensities on the T2 (long TR/long TE)-weighted images are related to differences in dilution and variations in the selective T2 relax-

ation, the latter being a result of different degrees of cell lysis. The free (extracellular) methemoglobin decreases the susceptibility differences between the inside and outside of the remaining cells. This decreases the heterogeneous suscepti-

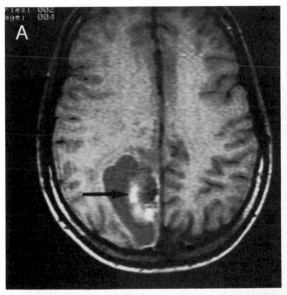

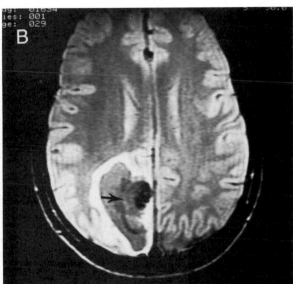

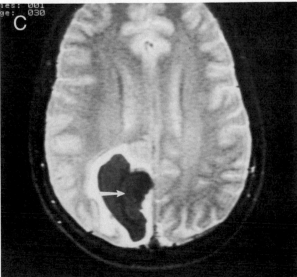

FIG 9–14.
A, an *arrow* points to undilute intracellular methemoglobin, which has high intensity on short TR images. **B,** methemoglobin is isointense on long TR/short TE *(arrow)* and **(C)** hypointense on long TR/long TE images *(arrow).*

bility and produces a marked decrease in the T2 shortening because such shortening varies as the square of the variation in susceptibility. Cell lysis thus is more effective in decreasing the selective T2 relaxation than is simple dilution because of this significant decrease in susceptibility differences. The effect of dilution produces minimal changes in the heterogeneous distribution of intracellular methemoglobin until the Hct is greater than 90% or less than 10%. The proton density of undiluted (after plasma resorption) intracellular methemoglobin or deoxyhemoglobin (Hct of 90% or more) is similar to that of gray matter.

Let us now attempt to evaluate some of the different situations that may arise in subacute hemorrhage and determine their MRI appearance. These changes are summarized in Figure 9–13. Undiluted intracellular methemoglobin will be hyperintense on short TR/short TE images, isointense on long TR/short TE images, and very hypointense on long TR/long TE images (Fig 9–14). Dilute intracellular methemoglobin will display increased intensity on short TR/short TE images, increased intensity on the long TR/short TE images, and decreased intensity on the long TR/long TE images (Fig 9–15). The decrease in the PEDD PRE

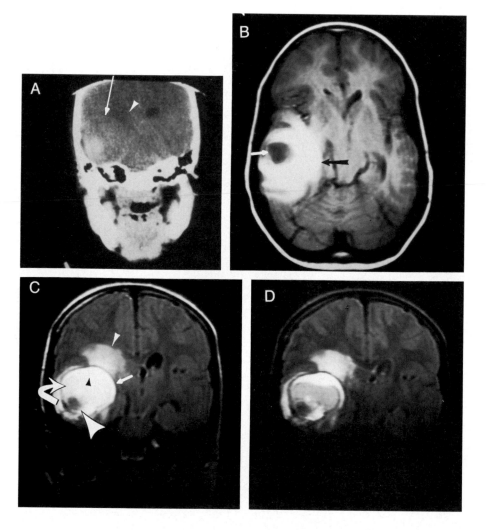

FIG 9–15.
Example of dilute intracellular methemoglobin in a complex hemorrhage 2 and 12 days old. **A,** coronal CT showing the extent of subacute hemorrhage (isodense on CT) *(arrow)* and surrounding edema *(arrowhead)*. Note that the 2-day-old hemorrhage is hyperdense. **B,** short TR axial image showing acute hemorrhage slightly hypointense to gray matter *(white arrow)* and the high intensity of a subacute hemorrhage *(black arrow)*. **C,** long TR/short TE image showing acute hemorrhage *(large white arrowhead)*. The *curved arrow* represents dilute intracellular methemoglobin, which is mildly hyperintense. The *black arrowhead* is dilute, free methemoglobin. One can also discern hemosiderin *(arrow)* and edema *(white arrowhead)*. **D,** long TR/long TE image showing that the dilute intracellular methemoglobin has decreased intensity. Deoxyhemoglobin is also decreased in intensity. Dilute, free methemoglobin has high intensity. The hemosiderin rim is more hyperintense.

by dilution is compensated for by the increase in proton density until there is a great degree of dilution. The decrease in the selective T2 will only be apparent at an Hct less than 10%. Dilute, free methemoglobin reveals hyperintensity on all spin-echo pulse sequences (Fig 9–15,C and D). This is secondary to the shortening of T1 and T2 by the PEDD PRE of free methemoglobin and the absence of susceptibility effects due to the loss of the cellular (heterogeneous) distribution of the paramagnetic. The diluteness of the solution accounts for the increased proton density. The T1 shortening and high proton density of dilute, free methemoglobin dominate the signal intensity because TR is much longer than TE and not much longer than T1 while TE is usually shorter than T2. Undiluted, free methemoglobin will be hyperintense on short TR/short TE images, isointense on long TR/short TE images, and isointense on long TR/long TE images.

There are many other combinations that may occur. Free and intracellular methemoglobin will reveal high intensity on the short TR/short TE images, variable intensity (depending on dilution) on proton-density images, and variable hypointensity (depending on the heterogeneity of magnetic susceptibility). A hemorrhage containing intracellular deoxyhemoglobin and intracellular methemoglobin will be variably hyperintense on short TR/short TE images. The proton-density–weighted

images will depend upon the diluteness of the hemorrhage, and the long TR/long TE images will be hypointense. These are not all of the possible combinations but serve as examples of the variety of intensity patterns one might encounter in subacute hemorrhage.

The most common situation visualized occurs when the hemorrhage becomes high intensity on short and long TR images. At that time we note the appearance of a peripheral rim of hypointensity, most noticeable on the long TR images (Fig 9–16). This is secondary to the formation of intralysosomal hemosiderin. Hemosiderin is formed by lysosomal degradation of the protein shell of ferritin. Ferritin consists of a soluble protein shell surrounding a core of ferric (Fe^{+3}) oxyhydroxide. Hemosiderin is water insoluble and sits in lysosomes of macrophages. In the brain it appears that hemosiderin-laden macrophages cannot be mobilized. This is secondary to re-establishment of the blood-brain barrier following simple hemorrhage. An absence or persistent dysfunction of the blood-brain barrier permits mobilization of the iron. In the body such mobilization requires entry of chelators or reducing agents into the lysosome to effect solubilization. Most importantly, the hemosiderin core contains approximately 2,000 Fe^{+3} atoms each with five unpaired electrons, thus a total of up to 10,000 electrons per hemosiderin molecule, shielded from PEDD PRE interaction, but clearly

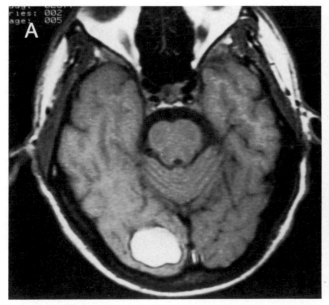
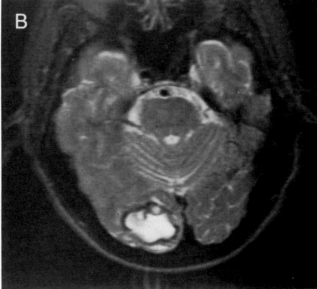

FIG 9–16.
The central high intensity on short TR/short TE **(A)** and long TR/long TE images represents free dilute methemoglobin **(B).** Note the rim of hypointensity in **A** but better seen in **B** (more T2 weighted).

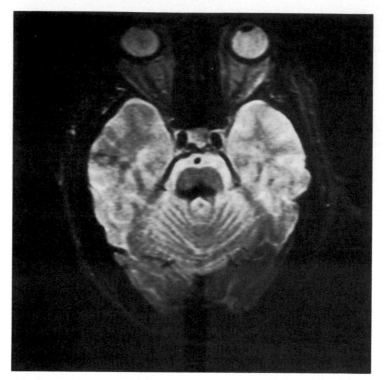

FIG 9–17.
Long TR/long TE image revealing residual hemosiderin from a very old pontine hemorrhage.

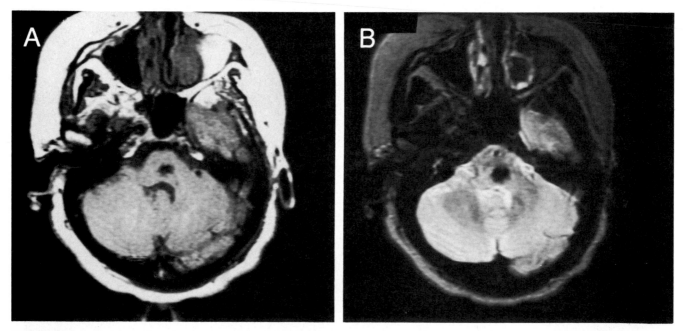

FIG 9–18.
A, old pontine hemorrhage containing hemosiderin. It is hypointense on short TR/short TE pulse sequences and becomes markedly hypointense on long TR/long TE sequences **(B).**

able to produce significant susceptibility changes on long TR/long TE images. In fact the T2 shortening effect is so powerful that we see hypointensity on short TR and long TR/short TE images (Fig 9–16,A).

Over a period of months the methemoglobin is gradually resorbed, and one is left with a rim containing hemosiderin-laden macrophages (Fig 9–17). These deposits will remain indefinitely in the brain parenchyma as an indelible marker of the hemorrhagic event and will be detected on spin-echo pulse sequences as hypointensity on long TR/long TE pulse sequences. One can determine the presence of susceptibility effects by observing increasing hypointensity as the images become more T2 weighted (i.e., as the TE is increased) (Fig 9–18).

The role of the gradient-echo image in hemorrhage is one of a useful adjunct in certain situations. These partial–flip angle scans are considerably more sensitive than spin-echo images to susceptibility differences. This sensitivity is partic-

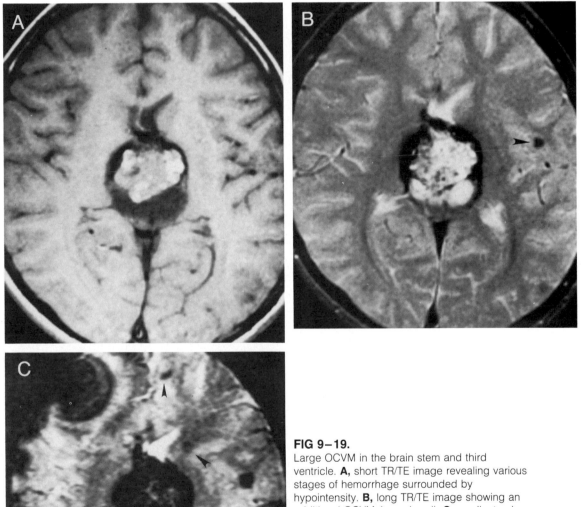

FIG 9–19.
Large OCVM in the brain stem and third ventricle. **A,** short TR/TE image revealing various stages of hemorrhage surrounded by hypointensity. **B,** long TR/TE image showing an additional OCVM *(arrowhead)*. **C,** gradient-echo image with *arrowheads* identifying additional OCVM not seen on long TR/TE images.

ularly important with lower-field strength magnets where the diffusion effects (selective T2 shortening) are proportional to the square of the applied magnetic field. At any field strength the gradient echo has increased sensitivity to susceptibility differences that are on the order of an imaging voxel (1 mm) rather than the diffusion distance of water during the spin-echo interecho interval (approximately 0.01 mm). This sensitivity is a double-edged sword. It permits detection of areas of susceptibility differences, yet one loses the sensitivity to the distance over which the heterogeneity is manifested if it is below the size of a voxel. Boundaries between different susceptibilities will demonstrate T2 shortening regardless of whether or not hemosiderin is present. This may cause some problems because the presence of incomplete rims of hemosiderin is suggestive of hemorrhagic tumor. The gradient-echo image would appear as a complete rim of hemosiderin secondary to the boundary effect and might mislead the observer.

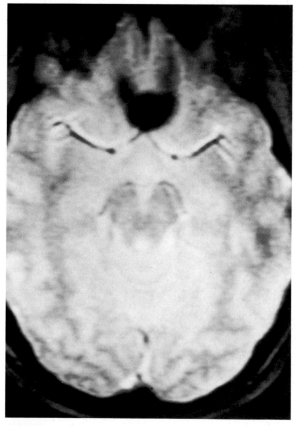

FIG 9–20.
Gradient-echo image demonstrating susceptibility changes in the inferior frontal region secondary to air in the sphenoid and ethmoid sinuses (diamagnetic susceptibility). Such changes may obscure regions of possible abnormalities.

In addition, the extensive hypointensity might also hide surrounding high intensity, another finding in intratumoral hemorrhage. The fast scan is useful in patients with OCVMs to reveal additional lesions and suggests that this is a familial condition (Fig 9–19). It may also play a role in patients with seizures and a normal spin-echo study to increase the sensitivity of detecting a small OCVM. At the present time diamagnetic susceptibility differences between air and tissue in the frontal region and in the petrous region produce significant artifact to discourage its use as a screening modality (Fig 9–20).

DIFFERENTIAL DIAGNOSIS OF MRI FINDINGS AND POTENTIAL PROBLEMS IN INTERPRETATION

In acute hemorrhage we note isointensity on short TR images and hypointensity on long TR images. Calcification may appear as hypointensity. However, the hypointensity if secondary to calcium alone does not change as one increases the T2 weighting. Iron, on the other hand, will reveal greater hypointensity and will appear more extensive the more T2 weighted the images are. One can clearly show this by observing hypointensity changes from long TR/short TE to long TR/long TE images. Unfortunately, iron and calcium may be deposited together, and one will then be unable to separate the two.

Flow voids may be confused with the hypointensity of hemosiderin and perhaps deoxyhemoglobin. This situation may occur when there is enough hemosiderin present to significantly shorten T2 on a short TR/short TE image. The flow void will be hypointense on all pulse sequences, but the hypointensity will not vary (assuming no flow-related intensity changes) by increasing the TE. There are a number of other methods to separate hemosiderin or deoxyhemoglobin from flow. The easiest method for detecting blood flow is to perform a gradient-echo image that emphasizes flow. The parameters of such a scan vary from machine to machine, yet the effect of single slices sequentially acquired produces fully relaxed spins (secondary to flow) entering each slice. These fully relaxed spins will cause the higher intensity noted on the gradient-echo image and can unambiguously separate flow from other causes of hypointensity. Other findings to appreciate with flow are even-echo rephasing and flow-related enhancement. The former is due to dephasing of isochromats on the odd echoes and rephasing of them on even echoes of a multiecho sequence. It is best demonstrated in situations with slow laminar flow.[17] Demonstration of even-echo rephasing rules out vascular thrombosis. Flow-related enhancement produces high intensity in a vessel or CSF perpendicular to the imaging plane as unsaturated (fully magnetized) protons enter the first slices of a multislice volume. This phenomenon is noted in regions with slowly flowing blood and is greatest in stationary tissues with relatively long T1 and pulse sequences using short TR intervals. This combination maximizes the degree of tissue unsaturation and the relative high signal from the unsaturated

flowing protons. If the velocity of the flowing blood is such that the protons leave the imaging slice prior to the 180-degree pulse (time-of-flight effects), then the intensity of the blood flow is significantly decreased with associated signal loss (high-velocity signal loss).[18]

Melanotic melanoma can be confused, on short TR images, with the high intensity of methemoglobin in subacute hemorrhage. The source of the high intensity may either be the free radicals in melanin or chelated metal ions (Fig 9–21).[19] On long TR images melanotic melanomas are hypointense but not as hypointense as intracellular methemoglobin because of its lack of susceptibility effects. Fat also has high intensity on short TR pulse

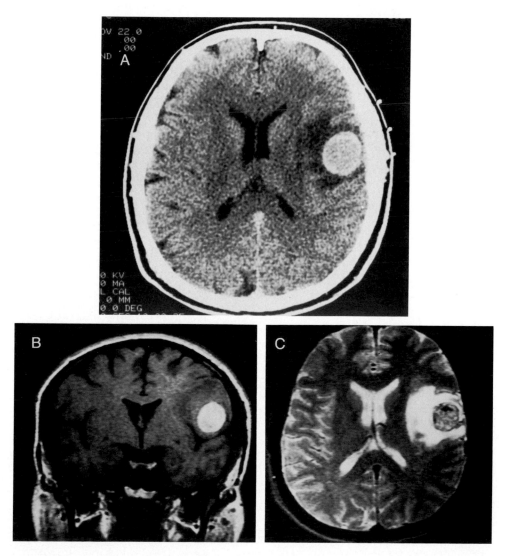

FIG 9–21.
A, nonenhanced CT of pathologically proved melanoma metastasis. Note the high absorption in the left frontal region. **B,** short TR/short TE image revealing high intensity similar to that of methemo-

globin. **C,** long TR/long TE image demonstrating isointensity and the slight hypointensity of melanotic melanoma. This is not as hypointense as intracellular methemoglobin.

sequences and is hypointense on long TR images. It too may be confused with subacute hemorrhage. Chemical shift imaging can be useful in differentiating fat from hemorrhage.

Although there may be occasional ambiguity in the diagnosis of intraparenchymal hemorrhage on MRI, in the vast majority of cases the diagnosis is rather straightforward. In the next section we will discuss specific hemorrhagic pathologic entities and apply the imaging principles we have already considered.

HEMORRHAGIC CONDITIONS

Intraparenchymal Hemorrhage

Spontaneous intraparenchymal hemorrhage is responsible for approximately 10% of strokes. The most common etiology of intraparenchymal hemorrhage is hypertension, which accounts for approximately 50% of spontaneous intraparenchymal hemorrhages. Another 40%, in descending order of occurrence, are secondary to aneurysm, arteriovenous malformation, blood dyscrasias, and bleeding diathesis including anticoagulation, hemorrhagic

tumors (melanoma, choriocarcinoma, hypernephroma, bronchogenic carcinoma), hemorrhagic infarction, and cerebral arteritis (collagen vascular disease, amyloid, drug abuse including cocaine and methamphetamine abuse). Approximately 10% have no known etiology. With the early diagnosis of hypertension and its treatment the incidence of intraparenchymal hemorrhage has been noted to decline since 1945. The most common site for hypertensive hemorrhage to occur is the putamen, followed by the thalamus, lobar white matter, pons, and cerebellum. The incidence of intraventricular hemorrhage is variable.

The sources of bleeding in hypertensive hemorrhage are from penetrating arteries at the base of the brain (lenticulostriate and thalmoperforating arteries, the paramedian branches of the basilar artery), and from microaneurysms. The so-called Charcot-Bouchard aneurysms (0.05 to 2 mm in diameter) are found in up to 50% of hypertensive patients as compared with 10% of normotensive patients (Fig 9–22). The location of microaneurysms corresponds to the relative sites of hemorrhage. Eighty-five percent of patients with hypertension and intracerebral hemorrhage have microaneurysms.

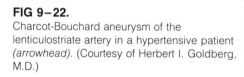

FIG 9–22.
Charcot-Bouchard aneurysm of the lenticulostriate artery in a hypertensive patient *(arrowhead).* (Courtesy of Herbert I. Goldberg, M.D.)

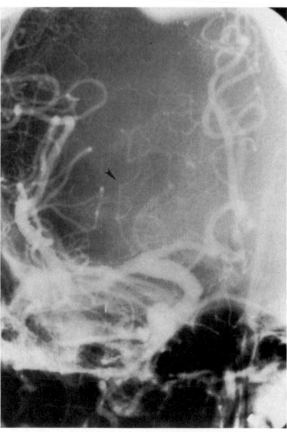

Lobar intracerebral hemorrhage occurs in the subcortical white matter and has a propensity for the parietotemporal and posterior half of the brain.[20] As opposed to putaminal hemorrhage, the lobar hemorrhages have a lower incidence of hypertension (approximately 33%).[21] Other etiologies include arteriovenous malformation, tumor, and coagulopathy. These patients tend to have a better prognosis than those with ganglionic hemorrhages.

Cerebral amyloid angiopathy is a cause of intraparenchymal hemorrhage in the normotensive elderly population. It is associated with dementia.[22] The most common vessels affected are small and medium-sized arteries of the cerebral cortex and meninges in the occipital and temporal lobes.[23] The bleeding is thought to be a result of the rupture of microaneurysms and the loss of elasticity of the vessels secondary to amyloid deposition.[24] One may suggest the diagnosis in superficial cortical hemorrhages in the appropriate location. Cerebral amyloid hemorrhage has a propensity for recurrence.

From the radiologic point of view acute intraparenchymal hemorrhage may be equally well diagnosed by CT or MRI. The limiting factors are the accessibility of the particular scanner and the condition of the patient. The poorer the condition, the more likely the patient is to undergo CT. MRI has the ability to detect small hemorrhages and those in the posterior fossa that might be missed by CT. In hemorrhages that are over a week old MRI is the more sensitive modality. The MRI intensity changes of intraparenchymal hemorrhage are summarized in Figure 9–23.

Subarachnoid and Intraventricular Hemorrhage

At the present time CT is clearly the imaging procedure of choice for detecting subarachnoid and intraventricular hemorrhage. This is secondary to the inability of MRI to detect oxyhemoglobin (nonparamagnetic). As stated earlier, the appearance of acute hemorrhage is dependent upon the concentration of deoxyhemoglobin present. The CSF has a higher pO_2 than the interstices of a parenchymal hemorrhage, and therefore the RBCs in CSF would be bathed in fluid with a relatively higher pO_2 and, consequently, less deoxyhemoglobin and more oxyhemoglobin. Other factors that may also limit the appearance of subarachnoid and intraventricular hemorrhage on MRI are CSF pulsations, a relatively low Hct lysis of RBCs, and reabsorption of RBCs by the pacchionian granulations. The etiologies of this type of hemorrhage include ruptured aneurysm, trauma, arteriovenous malformation, hypertension, and hemorrhagic diathesis. Intraventricular hemorrhages were most often produced by ruptured aneurysms of the anterior cerebral artery or its branches.[25] Both patients with subarachnoid and intraventricular hemorrhage have a better prognosis if no obvious source of the hemorrhage is identified. The outcome of intraventricular hemorrhage is not as bleak as was once considered. In one study 21% of patients returned to normal or had only mild disability. Associated with subarachnoid and intraventricular hemorrhage is enlargement of the ventricles. This is a result of the RBCs producing a communicating hydrocephalus by impairing resorption of CSF in the pacchionian granulations.[26] Ventricular dilatation may be seen within the first 2 weeks of the hemorrhage.[27, 28] There is a direct correlation between the clinical status of the patient and the size of the ventricles.

MRI is also useful in subarachnoid hemorrhage in cases in which multiple aneurysms are found angiographically and CT and angiography are inconclusive in determining the aneurysm that has bled.[29] MRI will reveal a localized collection of blood contiguous with the aneurysm that has hemorrhaged (Fig 9–24).

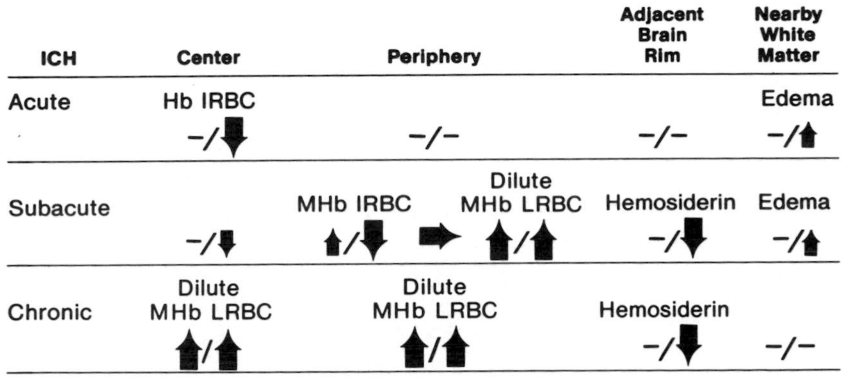

ICH	Center	Periphery			Adjacent Brain Rim	Nearby White Matter
Acute	Hb IRBC −/↓	−/−			−/−	Edema −/↑
Subacute	−/↓	MHb IRBC ↑/↓	→	Dilute MHb LRBC ↑/↑	Hemosiderin −/↓	Edema −/↑
Chronic	Dilute MHb LRBC ↑/↑	Dilute MHb LRBC ↑/↑			Hemosiderin −/↓	−/−

FIG 9–23.
MRI intensity findings in an intraparenchymal hemorrhage. Short TR, short TE intensities separated (/) from long TR, long TE intensities. *Arrows pointing up* indicate increased intensity. *Arrows pointing down* indicate decreased intensity. *Thicker arrows* indicate more pronounced effects.

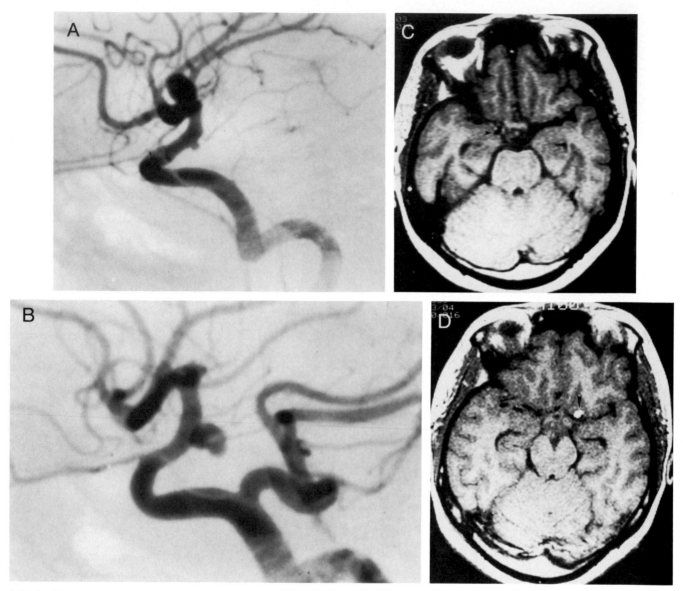

FIG 9–24.
Patient with multiple aneurysms. **A,** lateral arteriogram with a large left distal internal carotid aneurysm and a small posterior communicating aneurysm. **B,** right lateral view demonstrating a large posterior communicating artery aneurysm and a persistent trigeminal artery. **C,** axial short TR MRI showing a right posterior communicating artery aneurysm *(arrowhead).* **D,** slightly higher section with high intensity (methemoglobin) on the right posterior communicating artery aneurysm which bled *(arrowhead).*

Hemorrhagic Cortical Infarction

Hemorrhagic infarction occurs in approximately 20% of all infarctions and is confined to the cortex.[30] The hemorrhage is most often noted in the deeply infolded cortical gyri. Hemosiderin deposition may be detected pathologically from 2 to 10 days.[31] The hemorrhage occurs following a loss of perfusion to the cerebral parenchyma and subsequent reperfusion. There are several postulated reperfusion mechanisms: (1) lysis of an embolus, (2) collateral flow around an embolus, (3) re-establishment of blood flow following a period of

hypotension, and (4) intermittent obstruction of the posterior cerebral artery following transtentorial herniation.[32, 33] The MR images of hemorrhagic cortical infarction vary little from that of intraparenchymal hemorrhage. As stated previously, the acute hemorrhage may not be as hypointense on long TR images as an acute intraparenchymal hemorrhage secondary to early vascular recanalization and luxury perfusion. The evolution of the hemorrhage is similar to intraparenchymal hemorrhage (Fig 9–25). Chronic intraparenchymal hemorrhage demonstrates evidence of atrophy and he-

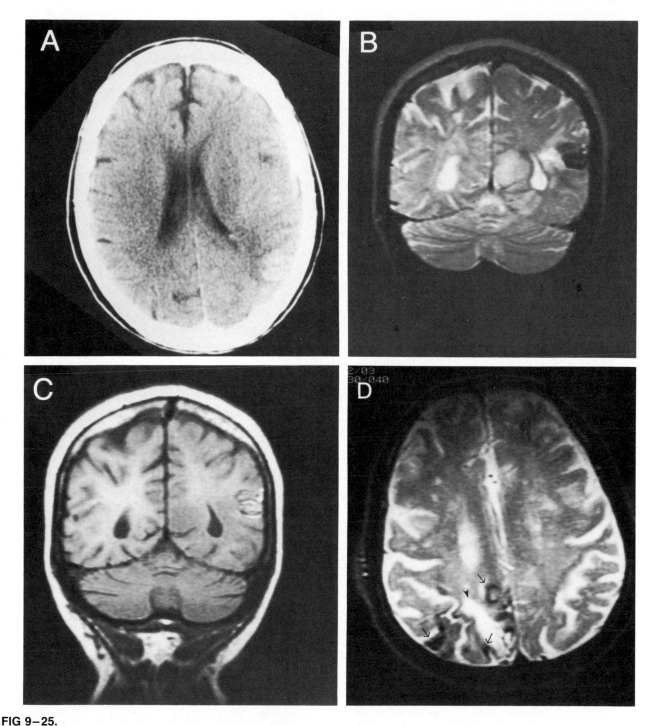

FIG 9–25.

Acute hemorrhagic cortical infarction. **A,** CT shows a high-absorption left parietal cortical hemorrhage associated with mass effect and edema out of proportion to the hemorrhage. This is in the distribution of the middle cerebral artery. **B,** coronal long TR/long TE image with marked hypointensity of the acute hemorrhage (deoxy-hemoglobin). **C,** subacute stage with evolution of acute hemorrhage to methemoglobin, which has high intensity on this short TR image. **D,** long TR/long TE image of another patient with hemosiderin deposition *(arrows),* evidence of an old infarct *(arrowhead),* and secondary atrophy.

mosiderin deposition. The hemosiderin remains in the brain parenchyma as a marker of the hemorrhage. The hemosiderin is also more hypointense than deoxyhemoglobin is.

CT findings in hemorrhagic infarction demon-strate low absorption and mass effect in a vascular distribution manifested by effacement of the corti-cal sulci (Fig 9–25,A). The mass effect is usually out of proportion to the amount of hemorrhage seen. The differential diagnosis in this case is of a hemorrhagic tumor or perhaps hemorrhagic venous infarction.

The question of which imaging modality to use in acute cases is problematic. Either MRI or CT will be able to detect a significant hemorrhage, which is the important clinical question to answer. With a large hemorrhage the patient will not undergo anticoagulation. MRI is more sensitive than CT for detecting small, probably clinically insignificant hemorrhages. In the subacute or chronic stage (~4 days or more) MRI is clearly superior to CT.

Venous Thrombosis

Cerebral venous thrombosis has been a difficult diagnosis to substantiate prior to the advent of MRI. It can be seen in a variety of disorders and at different ages. In the pediatric population it is associated with dehydration following gastroenteritis or viral syndromes. In adults it may be seen in patients who are hypercoaguable, septic, or dehydrated. The presentation usually occurs with the abrupt onset of seizures and neurologic deficit. Venous infarcts tend to be very epileptogenic and may be associated with parenchymal hemorrhage. In patients with the appropriate history one must

be sensitized to this diagnosis and carefully evaluate the images.

On CT one may discern the appearance of a thrombosed cortical vein by demonstrating a punctate high-absorption abnormality on an unenhanced scan ("cord sign") (Fig 9–26). Associated with this cord sign, at times, is an area of low absorption that represents associated edema and/or infarction. The appearance of acute thrombosis of a major sinus may be seen as an area of high absorption on a plain scan (Fig 9–27). It is important to scan in the plane perpendicular to the sinus to fully appreciate the thrombus. Thus, anterior sagittal sinus thrombosis is best imaged by using coronal scanning, whereas the posterior sagittal sinus and torcular regions are best demonstrated on axial images. Another popular but somewhat inaccurate sign described for posterior sagittal sinus thrombosis is the "delta sign" or "empty triangle sign."[34] In approximately 1 week the blood in an acute posterior sagittal sinus thrombus becomes isodense. Following intravenous contrast the region around the thrombus will enhance (Fig 9–28). The enhancement represents the normal enhancement of the dura plus additional venous collateral around the thrombus outlining the isodense clot. Additional findings associated with thrombosis is the appearance of collateral venous pathways around the tentorium or throughout the white matter (di-

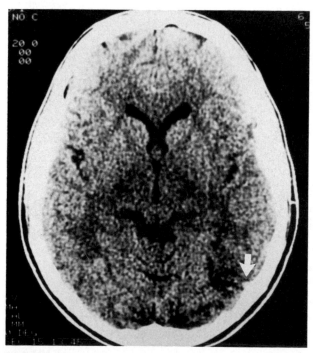

FIG 9–26.
Thrombosed cortical vein *(arrow)* demonstrating high absorption on unenhanced CT ("cord sign").

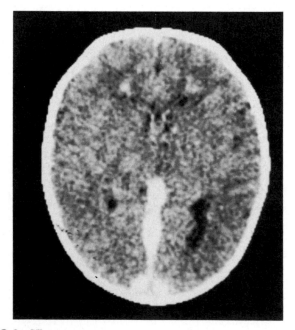

FIG 9–27.
Unenhanced CT with high absorption in the vein of Galen, straight sinus, and torcula representing thrombosis.

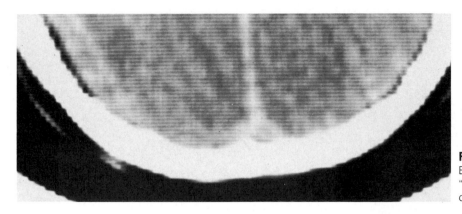

FIG 9–28.
Enhanced CT of the "empty triangle" or "delta" sign with a sagittal sinus clot (isodense) surrounded by enhancement.

lated medullary veins).[35] These present as enhancing serpentine structures around the tentorium.

In acute thrombosis we note the absence of the flow void on the short TR image (Fig 9–29,A). On the long TR image the appearance of the acute thrombus is of low intensity (deoxyhemoglobin), which may be similar to flowing blood (Fig 9–29,B). Thus, acutely it is most important to appreciate the isointensity (as opposed to the flow void) on short TR images. As with intraparenchymal hemorrhage, the isointensity converts to high intensity on both short and long TR images as deoxyhemoglobin is converted to methemoglobin (Fig 9–30). This usually occurs over a few days. The difference between chronic intraparenchymal

hemorrhage and and chronic venous thrombosis is that in the latter hemosiderin is *not* deposited. Instead, the thrombus lyses, and the flow void is reestablished.[36] One does not see hemosiderin deposition in venous thrombosis or, for that matter, in vascular dissection.

Vascular Dissection

Vascular dissection is an often overlooked etiology of stroke. Prior to MRI the diagnosis was made by angiography with demonstration of a narrowed irregular vessel. As opposed to aortic dissection, the false lumen is virtually never visualized. Today angiography is still the gold standard; how-

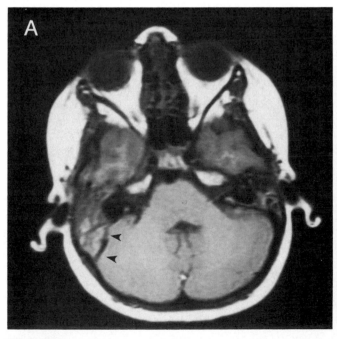
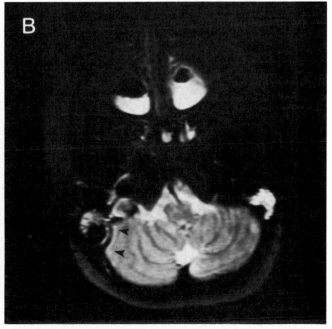

FIG 9–29.
A, acute thrombosis of the right sigmoid sinus. Note the absence of a flow void on short TR images. **B,** low intensity on long TR/long TE images of deoxyhemoglobin. The curvilinear structure around the sinus represents collateral flow *(arrowheads).*

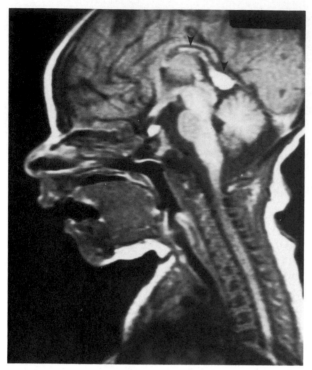

FIG 9–30.
High intensity on short TR images in a thrombosed internal cerebral vein and the vein of Galen represents the methemoglobin stage of a clot *(arrowheads).*

ever, MRI using a surface-coil technique appears to be the study of choice to rule in the diagnosis. Presently, if MRI findings are positive, we do not perform an angiogram. The MRI findings follow the same pattern as venous thrombosis. One may appreciate the intramural hemorrhage as well as the residual lumen (Fig 9–31). When using MRI the resorption of the hemorrhage and restoration of the full lumen can also be demonstrated noninvasively.[37] The most common etiology of vascular dissection is blunt trauma to the artery. This can occur following manipulation of the neck, rapid forceful turning of the neck, or a direct blow to the neck. Fibromuscular disease may predispose to dissection. The complications usually arise from cerebral emboli that are formed on the irregular intima. Most often the vessel is not completely occluded, and impairment to flow is usually not hemodynamically significant.

Extracerebral Collections

CT had a major impact in identifying extracerebral collections.[38] MRI has enhanced the diagnostic acumen because of its increased sensitivity in detecting isodense, posterior fossa, and peritento-

rial collections. The vast majority of these collections occur secondary to traumatic events. On CT the epidural hematoma has a biconvex shape. Most epidural hematomas are associated with skull fractures, although they may be seen without visible evidence of the fracture. They are a result of tears in the middle meningeal artery, vein, or the dural sinuses. The latter is seen in the pediatric population. The hemorrhage may be either arterial or venous. The most common location is over the cerebral convexities, and the hemorrhage is limited by the dural attachments at the suture lines. Acute epidural hemorrhage may be life-threatening and demand prompt drainage. The vast majority of acute epidural hemorrhages have high absorption; however, there are circumstances in which severe blood loss creates a situation of significant anemia with subsequent isodensity of the hemorrhage on CT.[39] The CT diagnosis is made by demonstrating a lenticular-shaped high-absorption peripheral convexity mass in the usual setting of head trauma (Fig 9–32). There is associated compression of the brain and, at times, low absorption (edema) in the subjacent brain areas. As with other extra-axial masses, the white matter is observed to be buckled, but the gray/white interface is well defined.[40]

Subdural hematomas are somewhat more enigmatic, particularly the subacute and chronic ones. They may be categorized as acute, subacute, or chronic based on the interval between trauma and imaging. Unfortunately, this is quite difficult since there may be a lack of historical data in many individuals, particularly alcoholic and demented patients. Subdural hemorrhage occurs in a potential space (subdural space) as a result of a tear or shear in the bridging veins that run from the brain into the fixed venous sinuses. These veins tether the mobile brain to the fixed sinuses and may be sheared in the process of acceleration/deceleration injuries. Acute subdural hematomas are high-absorption concave structures that usually occupy the entire hemisphere. In the acute situation they are usually associated with significant parenchymal injury, and the subdural lesion itself is usually not as significant as the parenchymal damage.[41] The subdural hemorrhage as opposed to the epidural is not confined by dural attachments and can thus spread out throughout the entire potential space. The age at which an acute subdural hemorrhage becomes isointense varies from days to 1 to 3 months.[42] Without rebleeding subdural hematomas become low density as compared with brain in approximately 4 weeks.[43]

The problems in CT diagnosis occur with the

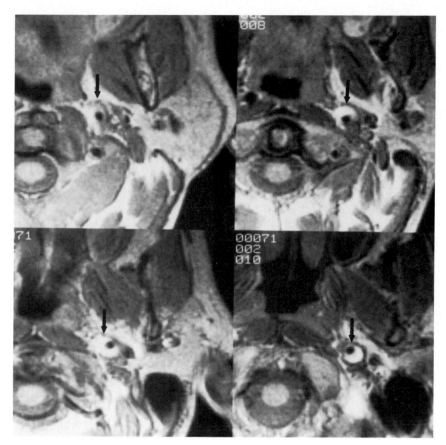

FIG 9–31.
Short TR/short TE images of a left carotid dissection *(arrows)*. Note the intramural hemorrhage (high intensity) and the residual lumen (low intensity) secondary to flowing blood.

isodense subdural hematoma. In one series 25% of subdural hematomas were isointense to normal brain.[44] Analysis of the CT scan should be performed compulsively to detect the absence of a normal sulcal pattern (particularly in the elderly population), extra-axial mass effect, and compression of the ventricles (abnormally small ventricles for age). Bilateral isodense collections are confusing because of the associated symmetry of the brain and lack of a contralateral shift of the midline structures. Following intravenous contrast administration, medial displacement of a cortical vein may be recognized.[45] In addition, the isodense subdural hematoma may demonstrate contrast enhancement if the scan is somewhat delayed (~30 minutes). A neocapillary bed in the external dura is formed after hemorrhage and is responsible for the increased vascular permeability (enhancement) and the propensity for rebleeding.[46] On unenhanced images levels of various densities may be observed, and there may be membranes with loculated collections. The dependent portion containing the cells and high protein content is usually isodense to high density, while the supernatant has low density and is free of cells.

Acute subdural hematomas usually have concave or straight margins with the adjacent brain, while subacute and particularly chronic collections, although most often concave, may at times become convex as fluid is absorbed into the hematoma.[47] Rarely large acute subdural hematomas may be convex.

Peritentorial subdural hematomas may be difficult to diagnose on CT because their appearance may simulate an intra-axial lesion.[48] These collections are seen following traumatic delivery and in adult trauma cases. They present acutely with a sheetlike high-absorption region with a well-defined medial margin that tapers laterally and conforms to the tentorial anatomy (Fig 9–33). They are the result of tearing of bridging veins that drain into the straight, transverse, or petrosal sinuses.[49] Coronal imaging is helpful in placing the lesion in the tentorium.

MRI has essentially made the diagnosis of isodense subdural hematoma a moot point. One may

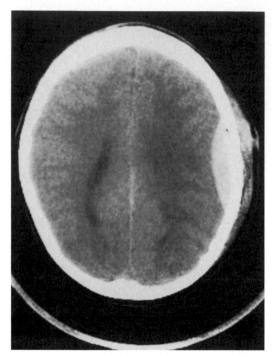

FIG 9–32.
CT of a left acute epidural hematoma consisting of a left high-absorption extracerebral lenticular mass. Note that the gray-white junction is preserved.

unambiguously demonstrate an extracerebral collection that has higher intensity on short TR images than the contiguous brain (Fig 9–34). Peritentorial hemorrhage is easy to visualize both in the axial and coronal images. The MRI sequence of intensity pattern changes is similar to intraparenchymal hemorrhage with the exception that hemosiderin deposition is unusual because of the absence of a blood-brain barrier. MRI is clearly the imaging modality of choice for diagnosing extracerebral collections.

Occult Cerebrovascular Malformations

OCVMs are vascular lesions, most likely cavernous hemangiomas. They are not usually shown on angiography, hence the term *occult*. These lesions are subject to small recurrent hemorrhages with significant deposition of hemosiderin.[50] Prior to MRI the diagnosis of OCVM was very difficult to make unambiguously. On CT the lesion may appear as a high-absorption (calcified) region without edema or mass effect that enhances following intravenous contrast administration (Fig 9–35). However, this is nonspecific, and such a lesion may be a calcified tumor, granuloma, hamartoma,

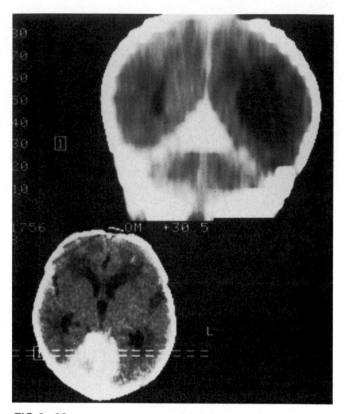

FIG 9–33.
Axial and reconstructed coronal CT of a peritentorial subdural hematoma. Note the tapering of the subdural hematoma laterally and its conformation to the tentorium.

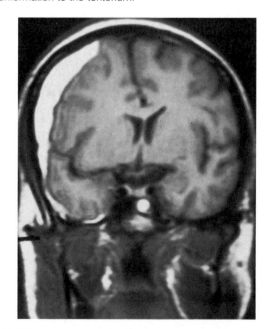

FIG 9–34.
Obvious subacute right subdural hemorrhage on short TR image with high intensity (methemoglobin) and displacement of underlying brain. Notice that the hemorrhage dissects under the temporal lobe. Subtemporal subdural hemorrhages are much easier to detect with MRI rather than CT.

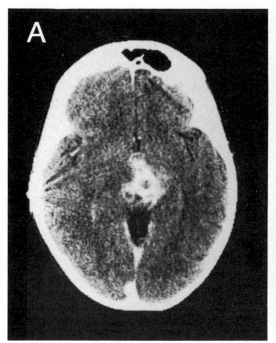
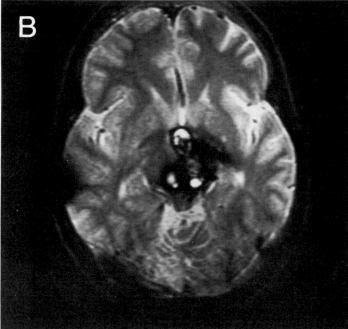

FIG 9–35.
A, CT of a large midbrain mass with high absorption and enhancement. **B,** long TR/long TE MRI showing hemosiderin surrounding various hemorrhagic regions. No edema surrounding the hemosiderin is present. These findings are rather specific for OCVMs.

or old hemorrhage. At times such lesions were irradiated as possible low-grade tumors. MRI has a rather specific appearance. The key to the diagnosis is the presence of peripheral hemosiderin accumulation (low intensity on long TR images) surrounding various stages of hemorrhage (high- and low-intensity regions) (Fig 9–35). To be certain that this is not a hemorrhage into a tumor there should be a complete rim of hemosiderin and no associated edema (Fig 9–36).[51] If there is associated edema, which may occur if the OCVM has recently hemorrhaged, then follow-up imaging is important to show resolution of the edema. OCVM may be multiple in 16% to 33% of patients and may have a familial tendency.[49] The gradient-echo technique may be useful in identifying small OCVMs, which could be an etiology of a seizure disorder and not identified on spin-echo technique. MRI is strongly recommended prior to surgical intervention or radiation therapy.

Intratumoral Hemorrhage

Significant hemorrhage into malignant neoplasms occurs in approximately 3% to 14% of brain metastases and 1% to 3% of primary gliomas.[52–55] Microscopic hemorrhages may be commonly seen pathologically. Metastatic lesions with a propensity for hemorrhage include melanoma, choriocarcinoma, bronchogenic carcinoma, renal cell carcinoma, and thyroid carcinoma. The etiology of intratumoral hemorrhage may be related to regions of rapid growth with subsequent necrosis, invasion

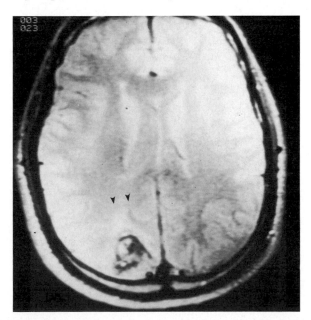

FIG 9–36.
Patient with an incomplete rim of hemosiderin and associated anterior edema *(arrowheads)* in a hemorrhagic astrocytoma. This appearance could be confused with an OCVM but for the edema and incomplete hemosiderin rim.

of cerebral vessels by tumor, and tumor neovascularity.

MRI findings of intratumoral hemorrhage differ from intraparenchymal hemorrhage in that there is more signal heterogeneity, often associated with nonhemorrhagic tumor.[54] Hemosiderin deposition is irregular and not consistent (Fig 9–37). The circumferential hemosiderin distribution is often lacking, and incomplete hemosiderin rings may be present. There is usually surrounding persistent edema (high intensity on long TR images). The above findings should increase the suspicion that one is not dealing with a simple intraparenchymal hemorrhage. The intensity pattern is also somewhat different. Acute hematomas may be more hypointense than a normal intraparenchymal hemorrhage (Fig 9–38). Since tumors are known to be more hypoxic, acute hemorrhage into this environment will contain more desaturated hemoglobin. Associated with the increased hypointensity is a delay in the hematoma evolution to the subacute pattern.

On CT contrast enhancement is useful in revealing nonhemorrhagic regions of enhancement that represent the tumor. At times the hemorrhage

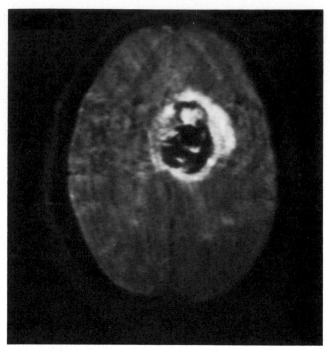

FIG 9–38.
Acute hemorrhage into a glioma. Long TR/long TE MRI reveals marked hypointensity presumed secondary to relative tumor hypoxia with increased amounts of deoxyhemoglobin.

may completely obliterate the evidence of tumoral enhancement. Other signs of tumor are mass effect out of proportion to the hemorrhage and significant low absorption in the white matter (edema). In uncertain diagnostic situations repeat scanning in about 4 weeks is strongly recommended.

Siderosis of the Central Nervous System

Superficial siderosis of the central nervous system consists of hemosiderin deposits in reactive macrophages in the leptomeninges, in subpial tissue, and on cranial nerves secondary to massive or recurrent subarachnoid hemorrhage.[56–61] Prior to the advent of MRI this condition was almost exclusively made at autopsy. MRI beautifully demonstrates the marked hypointensity on long TR, long TE images around the leptomeninges and on the cranial nerves (Fig 9–39).[62] This has also been noted on the ventricular ependyma following neonatal intraventricular hemorrhage (Fig 9–40).[63]

The clinical syndrome consists of hearing loss, cerebellar dysfunction, pyramidal tract signs and progressive mental deterioration. It is associated with repeated hemorrhages over 3 to more than 20 years' duration. Cranial nerves II, V, VII, and VIII

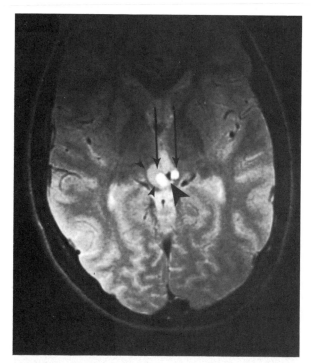

FIG 9–37.
Hemorrhage into a pineal region tumor. A long TR/long TE image demonstrates very high intensity of hemorrhage (methemoglobin) *(arrows)* in a tumor (high intensity region) *(arrowheads)*. Note the absence of hemosiderin surrounding the hemorrhage. Low intensity represents the calcified shifted pineal body *(large arrowhead)*.

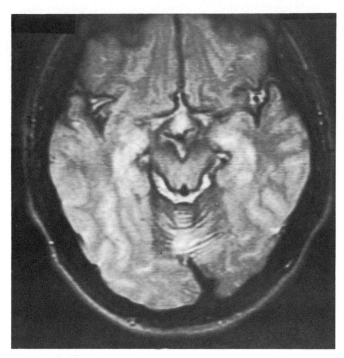

FIG 9–39.
Long TR/long TE MRI illustrates hemosiderin deposition manifested by marked hypointensity throughout the leptomeninges. This followed recurrent subarachnoid hemorrhages secondary to a spinal ependymoma and represents siderosis of the central nervous system.

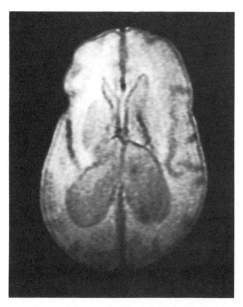

FIG 9–40.
Long TR/long TE MRI of ventricular siderosis following germinal matrix hemorrhage. One can appreciate the hypointensity of hemosiderin outlining the frontal horns of the ventricles.

are particularly involved, with VIII having an unusually long course through the subarachnoid space, which making it more sensitive to hemosiderin deposition.

Intracranial Hemorrhage in Premature Infants

The periventricular-intraventricular hemorrhage is the most common and potentially severe of all neonatal hemorrhages. Forty percent to 70% of infants with birth weights of less than 1,500 g or ages less than 35 weeks' gestation have been shown by CT to have such hemorrhages.[64–66] These hemorrhages originate in the germinal matrix, which is a structure located beneath the ventricular ependyma and is thickest in the region between the head of the caudate and thalamus. It is the origin of neuroblasts that migrate during development. It contains vascular structures, principally capillaries, and reaches its maximum size at approximately 32 to 34 weeks' gestation, after which it involutes. It is easy to appreciate that such subependymal hemorrhages may secondarily rupture into the ventricles or, when large, into the cerebral parenchyma. Sequelae of such hemorrhages include hydrocephalus and porencephalia.

The pathogenesis of these hemorrhages is related to the distribution and regulation of cerebral blood flow (asphyxia), vascular factors (fragility of

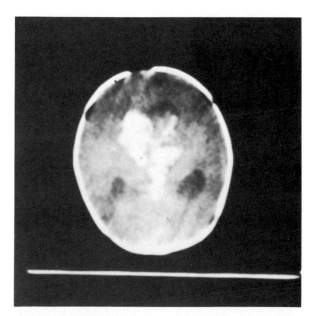

FIG 9–41.
CT of an acute germinal matrix hemorrhage with associate rupture into the lateral and third ventricles.

the vessels of the germinal matrix), and extrinsic factors (presence of excessive amount of fibrinolytic activity in the periventricular regions).[67] Prematurity is the cause of these hemorrhages. The clinical picture may vary from catastrophic deterioration to saltatory changes depending upon the extent of the hemorrhage.

At this time the major imaging techniques for detecting germinal matrix hemorrhage and its sequelae are CT and ultrasonography. Real-time sonography has been shown to be as accurate as CT and more accurate at 7 to 10 days posthemorrhage when the hemorrhage is isodense.[68] CT initially demonstrates the extent of the hemorrhage and its sequelae (Fig 9–41). MRI has been shown to be sensitive to the residual hemosiderin on the ependyma (see Fig 9–40). At the present time the logistics of MRI are suboptimal for imaging premature infants.

REFERENCES

1. Scott WR, New PFJ, Davis KR, et al: Computerized axial tomography of intracerebral and intraventricular hemorrhage. *Radiology* 1974; 112:73–80.
2. New PFJ, Aronow S: Attenuation measurements of whole blood and blood fractions in computed tomography. *Radiology* 1976; 121:635–640.
3. Smith WP, Batnitzky S, Rengachary SS: Acute isodense subdural hematomas: A problem in anemic patients. *AJNR* 1981; 2:37–40.
4. Som PM, Patel S, Nakagawa N, et al: The iron rim sign. *J Comput Assist Tomogr* 1979; 3:109–112.
5. Lim ST, Sage DJ: Detection of subarachnoid blood clot and other thin, flat structures by computed tomography. *Radiology* 1977; 123:79–84.
6. Zimmerman RD, Leeds NE, Naidich TP: Ring blush with intracerebral hematoma. *Radiology* 1977; 122:707–711.
7. Grossman RI, Kemp SS, Yu Ip C, et al: The importance of oxygenation in the appearance of acute subarachnoid hemorrhage on high field magnetic resonance imaging. *Acta Radiol Suppl* 1986; 369:56–58.
8. Thulborn KR, Waterton JC, Matthews PM, et al: Oxygenation dependence of the transverse relaxation time of water protons in whole blood at high field. *Biochim Biophys Acta* 1982; 714:265–270.
9. Singer JR, Crooks LE: Some magnetic sudies of normal and leukemic blood. *J Clin Eng* 1978; 3:237–243.
10. Fabry TL, Reich HA: The role of water in deoxygenated hemoglobin solutions. *Biochem Biophys Res Commun* 1966; 22:700–93.
11. Gatenby RA, Coia LR, Richter MP, et al: Oxygen tension in human tumors: In vivo mapping using CT-guided probes. *Radiology* 1985; 156:211–214.
12. Hecht-Leavitt C, Gomori JM, Grossman RI, et al: High-field MRI of hemorrhagic cortical infarction. *AJNR* 1986; 7:581–585.
13. Eisenstadt M: NMR relaxation of protein and water protons in methemoglobin solutions. *Biophys J* 1981; 33:469–474.
14. Koenig SH, Brown RE, Lindstrom TR: Solvent and the heme region of methemoglobin and fluoromethemoglobin. *Biophys J* 1981; 34:397–408.
15. Hackney DB, Atlas SW, Grossman RI, et al: Subacute intracranial hemorrhage: Contribution of spin density to appearance on spin-echo MR images. *Radiology* 1987; 165:199–202.
16. Gomori JM, Grossman RI, Hackney DB, et al: Variable appearances of subacute intracranial hematomas on high-field spin-echo MR. *AJNR* 1987; 8:1019–1026.
17. Waluch V, Bradley WG: NMR even-echo rephasing in slow laminar flow. *J Comput Assist Tomogr* 1984; 8:594–598.
18. Bradley WG, Waluch V: Blood flow: Magnetic resonance imaging. *Radiology* 1985; 154:443–450.
19. Gomori JM, Grossman RI, Shields JA, et al: Choroidal melanomas: Correlation of NMR spectroscopy and MR imaging. *Radiology* 1986; 158:443–445.
20. Kase CS, Williams JP, Wyatt DA, et al: Lobar intracerebral hematomas: Clinical and CT analysis of 22 cases. *Neurology* 1982; 32:1146–1150.
21. Ropper AH, Davis KR: Lobar cerebral hemorrhages: Acute clinical syndromes in 26 cases. *Ann Neurol* 1980; 8:141–147.
22. Glenner GG, Henry JH, Fujihara S: Congophilic angiopathy in the pathogenesis of Alzheimer's degeneration. *Ann Pathol* 1981; 1:120–129.
23. Patel DV, Hier DB, Thomas CM, et al: Intracerebral hemorrhage secondary to cerebral amyloid angiopathy. *Radiology* 1984; 151:397–400.
24. Lee SS, Stemmermann BN: Congophilic angiopathy and cerebral hemorrhage. *Arch Pathol Lab Med* 1978; 102:317–321.
25. Graeb DA, Robertson WD, Lapointe JS, et al: Computed tomographic diagnosis of intraventricular hemorrhage. *Radiology* 1982; 143:91–96.
26. Kibler RF, Couch RSC, Crompton MR: Hydrocephalus in the adult following spontaneous subarachnoid haemorrhage. *Brain* 1961; 84:45–61.
27. Vassilouthis J, Richardson AE: Ventricular dilatation and communicating hydrocephalus following spontaneous subarachnoid hemorrhage. *J Neurosurg* 1979; 51:341–351.
28. Menon D, Weir B, Overton T: Ventricular size and cerebral blood flow following subarachnoid hemorrhage. *J Comput Assist Tomogr* 1981; 5:328–333.
29. Hackney DB, Lesnick JE, Zimmerman RA, et al:

MR identification of bleeding site in subarachnoid hemorrhage with multiple intracranial aneurysms. *J Comput Assist Tomogr* 1986; 10:878–880.

30. Goldberg HI: In Lee SH, Rao KCVG (eds): *Cranial Computed Tomography.* New York, McGraw-Hill International Book Co, 1983, pp 583–657.

31. Stehbens WE: *Pathology of the Cerebral Blood Vessels.* St Louis, CV Mosby Co, 1972, pp 131–155.

32. Fisher CM, Adams RD: Observations on brain embolism with special reference to the mechanism of hemorrhagic infarction. *J Neuropathol Exp Neurol* 1951; 10:92–94.

33. Adams RD, Sidman RI: *Introduction to Neuropathology.* New York, McGraw-Hill International Book Co, 1968.

34. Buonanno FS, Moody DM, Ball MR, et al: Computed cranial tomographic findings in cerebral sinovenous occlusion. *J Comput Assist Tomogr* 1978; 2:281–290.

35. Banna M, Groves JT: Deep vascular congestion in dural venous thrombosis on computed tomography. *J Comput Assist Tomogr* 1979; 3:539–541.

36. Macchi PJ, Grossman RI, Goldberg HI, et al: High field MR imaging of cerebral venous thrombosis. *J Comput Assist Tomogr* 1986; 10:10–15.

37. Goldberg HI, Grossman RI, Gomori JM, et al: Cervical internal carotid artery dissecting hemorrhage. Diagnosis using MR. *Radiology* 1986; 158:157–161.

38. Ambrose J: Computerized transverse axial scanning (tomography): Part 2. Clinical application. *Br J Radiol* 1973; 46:1023–1047.

39. Rieth KG, Schwartz FT, Davis DO: Acute isodense epidural hematoma on computed tomography. *J Comput Assist Tomogr* 1979; 3:691–693.

40. George AE, Russell EJ, Kricheff II. White matter buckling: CT sign of extra-axial intracranial mass. *AJNR* 1980; 1:425–430.

41. Jameson KG, Yelland JDN: Surgically treated traumatic subdural hematomas. *J Neurosurg* 1972; 3:137–149.

42. Kwang KS, Hemmati M, Weinberg P: Computed tomography in isodense subdural hematoma. *Radiology* 1978; 128:71–74.

43. Evaluation of the age of subdural hematomas by computerized tomography. *J Neurosurg* 1977; 47:311–315.

44. Moller A, Ericson K: Computed tomography of isoattenuating subdural hematomas. *Radiology* 1979; 130:149–152.

45. Kim KS, Hemmati M, Weinberg PE: Computed tomography in isodense subdural hematoma. *Radiology* 1978; 128:71–74.

46. Weir B, Gordon P: Factors affecting coagulation: Fibrinolysis in chronic subdural fluid collections. *J Neurosurg* 1983; 58:242–245.

47. Forbes GS, Sheedy PF, Piepgras DG, et al: *Radiology* 1978; 126:143–148.

48. Lau LSW, Pike JW: The computed tomographic findings of peritentorial subdural hemorrhage. *Radiology* 1983; 146:699–701.

49. Stehbens WE: *Pathology of the Cerebral Blood Vessels.* St Louis, CV Mosby Co, 1972, pp 471–558.

50. Gomori JM, Grossman RI, Goldberg HI, et al: Occult cerebrovascular malformations: High-field MR imaging. *Radiology* 1986; 158:707–713.

51. Atlas SW, Grossman RI, Gomori JM, et al: Hemorrhagic intracranial malignant neoplasms: Spin-echo MR imaging. *Radiology* 1987; 164:71–77.

52. Zimmerman RA, Bilaniuk LT: Computed tomography of acute intratumoral hemorrhage. *Radiology* 1980; 135:355–359.

53. Mandybur TI: Intracranial hemorrhage caused by metastatic tumors. *Neurology* 1977; 27:650–655.

54. Leeds NE, Elkin CM, Zimmerman RD: Gliomas of the brain. *Semin Roentgenol* 1984; 19:27–43.

55. Russell DS, Rubenstein LJ: *Pathology of Tumors of the Nervous System.* Baltimore, Williams & Wilkins, 1977.

56. Neumann MA: Hemochromatosis of the central nervous system. *J Neuropathol Exp Neurol* 1948; 7:19–34.

57. Neumann MA: Hemochromatotic pigmentation of the central nervous system. *Arch Neurol* 1957; 76:355–369.

58. McGee DA, Van Patten HJ, Morotta HL, et al: Subpial cerebral siderosis. A report of two cases. *Neurology* 1962; 12:108–113.

59. Tomlinson BE, Walton JN: Superficial haemosiderosis of the central nervous system. *J Neurol Neurosurg Psychiatry* 1964; 27:332–339.

60. Oppenheimer DR, Griffith HB: Persistent intracranial bleeding as a complication of hemispherectomy. *J Neurol Neurosurg Psychiatry* 1966; 29:229–240.

61. Hughes JT, Oppenheimer DR: Superficial siderosis of the central nervous system. A report on nine cases with autopsy. *Acta Neuropathol (Berl)* 1969; 13:56–74.

62. Gomori JM, Grossman RI, Bilaniuk LT, et al: High-field MR imaging of superficial siderosis of the central nervous system. *J Comput Assist Tomogr* 1985; 9:972–975.

63. Gomori JM, Grossman RI, Goldberg HI, et al: High-field spin-echo MR imaging of superficial and subependymal siderosis secondary to neonatal intraventricular hemorrhage. *Neuroradiology* 1987; 29:339–342.

64. Burstein J, Papile L, Burstein R: Intraventricular hemorrhage and hydrocephalus in premature newborns: A prospective study with CT. *AJR* 1979; 132:631–635.

65. Papile LA, Burstein J, Burstein R, et al: Incidence and evolution of subependymal and intraventricular hemorrhage: A study of infants with birth

weights less than 1500 gm. *J Pediatr* 1978; 92:529–534.

66. Lee BCP, Grassi AE, Schectner S, et al: Neonatal intraventricular hemorrhage: A serial computed tomography study. *J Comput Assist Tomogr* 1979; 3:483–490.

67. Volpe JJ: Neonatal intraventricular hemorrhage. *N Engl J Med* 1981; 304:886–890.

68. Johnson ML, Rumack CM, Mannes EJ, et al: Detection of neonatal intracranial hemorrhage utilizing real-time and static ultrasound. *JCU* 1981; 9:427–433.

10

Head Trauma

Elizabeth A. Eelkema, M.D.

Stephen T. Hecht, M.D.

Joseph A. Horton, M.D.

Trauma is a major public health problem in the United States; it is the leading cause of death between the ages of 1 and 44 years.[1] Head injuries cause or contribute to death in most trauma fatalities.[2, 3] Head injuries requiring hospitalization occur at a rate of 200 per 100,000 population per year[4]; more than 73,000 of these result in long-term disability.[5] Motor vehicle accidents (MVAs) are the leading cause of head injury followed by falls, assaults, sports and recreation accidents, and firearm wounds.[5] Head injuries sustained in MVAs tend to be more severe than head injuries sustained in other types of trauma, require longer hospital stays, and have higher economic costs.[4]

Head trauma causes a spectrum of brain injuries ranging from transient physiologic dysfunction manifested by short periods of confusion and amnesia to severe, immediate, irreversible neuronal damage and death. The primary goal of imaging the trauma patient is to quickly and accurately identify treatable lesions before secondary injury to the brain occurs. Computed tomography (CT) is ideally suited to evaluate patients immediately after trauma and has, since its advent and widespread use, made significant contributions to the care and survival of trauma patients. Magnetic resonance imaging (MRI) is useful to assess patients who are stable but neurologically impaired in the days to months after trauma.[6-8]

CT is widely available and rapid, permits close monitoring of unstable patients, is compatible with respirators and other mechanical support devices, and can be used with patients whose medical and occupational histories are not available. It is very sensitive in detecting acute hematomas (Fig 10–1) and depressed fractures (Fig 10–2) that require emergency surgery. CT is less sensitive in the detection of nonhemorrhagic white matter injuries.[7, 8] The brain stem and posterior fossa are difficult to evaluate with CT due to beam hardening artifacts from surrounding dense bone.

MRI is not well suited to assess acutely injured patients. Routine MRI requires more time to perform than CT and is more susceptible to patient motion artifact. The necessity for specially adapted life support equipment and difficulty in closely monitoring patients impose additional technical problems. The lack of signal from cortical bone and the relative inability to differentiate fresh hemorrhage from normal brain impair MRI's ability to detect fractures and acute hematomas and therefore limit its usefulness in acute head trauma. MRI is far superior to CT in detecting nonhemorrhagic white matter injuries and in demonstrating hemorrhagic injuries more than a few days old.[7-9] MRI is also more sensitive than CT in detecting small or subacute extra-axial fluid collections[9, 10] and in evaluating the brain stem and posterior fossa (Fig 10–3).[8, 11]

All head injuries are the result of shearing, tensile, and compressive forces applied to the skull, dura, and brain. The type and extent of injury that

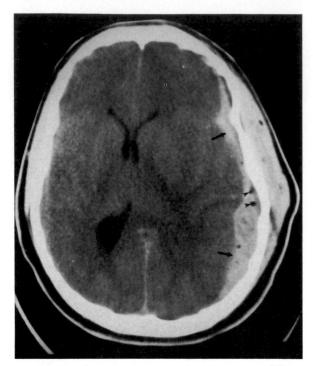

FIG 10–1.
Acute subdural hematoma. An unenhanced CT scan shows a crescentic, hyperdense blood collection *(arrows)* compressing the left cerebral hemisphere. The mass effect of the subdural hematoma causes complete effacement of the atrium of the left lateral ventricle and a shift of the midline structures to the right. The subdural hematoma contains several air bubbles *(arrowheads)* due to a mastoid fracture (not shown).

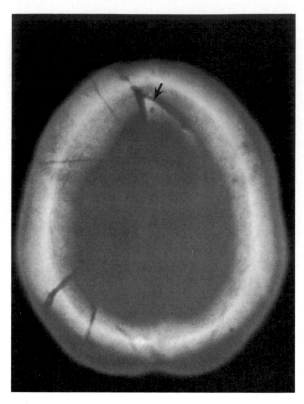

FIG 10–2.
Depressed skull fracture seen by unenhanced CT of an elderly alcoholic patient who rolled down concrete steps. There are multiple fractures of the calvarium, including a depressed frontal fracture *(arrow).*

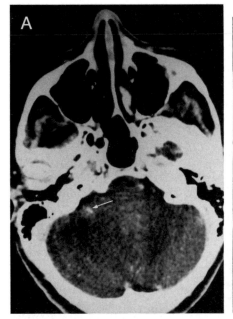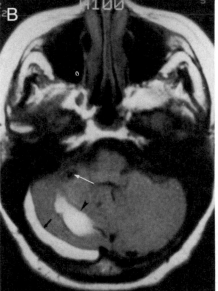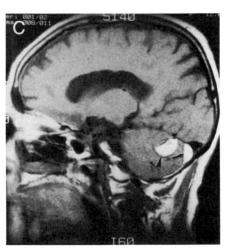

FIG 10–3.
Subacute posterior fossa subdural hematoma due to a ruptured arteriovenous malformation (AVM). **A,** contrast-enhanced axial CT shows a small area of enhancement in the right cerebellopontine angle. *(arrow);* this was shown later at angiography to be a small AVM. Artifact from the dense bone at the skull base obscures the details of the brain structure. **B** and **C,** 13 days after CT. **B,** axial MRI: TR=700, TE=20. Blood that is hyperintense relative to brain is demonstrated in the posterior fossa subdural space *(black arrow)* and in the horizontal fissure of the cerebellum *(arrowhead).* The AVM is shown as a signal void due to flowing blood *(white arrow).* **C,** sagittal MRI: TR = 600, TE = 20. The location of the hyperintense blood collections in the subdural space *(arrow)* and in the horizontal fissure *(arrowhead)* is more easily appreciated on the sagittal image.

results from the applied forces are dependent on many factors, including the mechanism of injury (e.g., a moving or resting head, blunt or penetrating trauma), the nature of the injuring force (static vs. dynamic, impact vs. impulse loading), the magnitude and rate of application of the injuring force, and the age and volume of the brain and skull.

Recent experimental work has emphasized the importance of angular acceleration forces and resultant shear strain in the etiology of many types of head injury, including subdural (SDH) and intraparenchymal (IPH) hematomas, contusions, lacerations, and diffuse axonal injury.[12–14] Direct contact or impact loading is required only for fractures and epidural hematoma (EDH).[15] All other types of head injury may be produced by impulse or inertial loading with resultant acceleration forces alone. Impulse or inertial loading occurs when the head is abruptly set into motion or abruptly stopped without direct contact.[15] Impact injury that imparts motion to a resting head or stops a moving head will also have inertial or acceleration components.

Neural tissue, vascular structures, and bone fail differently with different types of deforming forces and with different magnitudes and rates of stress application. For example, angular acceleration applied to the head at a fairly high rate will disrupt the bridging veins at the brain's surface and cause an SDH, while acceleration of the same magnitude that is applied at a lower rate will injure deeper neural tissue and result in diffuse axonal injury.[14] Tissue response to injury also varies with patient age.

IMAGING TECHNIQUES

For most head CT studies performed to evaluate patients immediately following trauma, unenhanced studies alone are adequate and appropriate. Acute hematomas and depressed fractures that may require immediate surgery are well demonstrated by unenhanced scans. The administration of intravenous contrast material requires a short but potentially critical amount of time, and rarely, enhancement of an unsuspected, pre-existing lesion may be confused with hemorrhage. The administration of intravenous contrast material usually adds little to the initial evaluation of acute head injury but may be of value in follow-up.[16]

Once emergent lesions are treated, either CT or MRI may be used to follow the evolution of primary lesions and to detect secondary complications and long-term sequelae of brain injury. To follow acute hemorrhagic lesions, demonstrate herniation, and assess fracture relationships and ventricle size, unenhanced CT studies are usually sufficient. Contrast enhancement is helpful in certain situations such as the demonstration of chronic hematoma membranes, displaced dura and cortical vessels, or secondary infections. The decision to administer intravenous contrast material should be made on an individual case basis.

Spinal and cranial injuries often coexist. Therefore, trauma patients should not be repositioned or manipulated until stability of the cervical spine is established. Head CT scans may be obtained with the patient on a backboard with a definite but acceptable decrease in the quality of the CT image. In patients with suspected basilar fractures, thin (<3.0 mm) sections through the skull base should be obtained (Fig 10–4). Coronal scans are useful to demonstrate basilar, orbital, and facial fractures (Fig 10–5).

One of the main advantages of MRI is its ability to image in multiple anatomic planes. Coronal

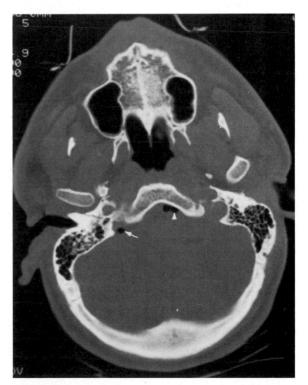

FIG 10–4.
Basal skull fracture with pneumocephalus seen by unenhanced, 3-mm-thick slice, axial CT with an edge enhancement algorithm. The right temporal bone fracture crosses a mastoid air cell and results in pneumocephalus. Air is present in the right cerebellopontine angle *(arrow)* and prepontine cistern *(arrowhead)*.

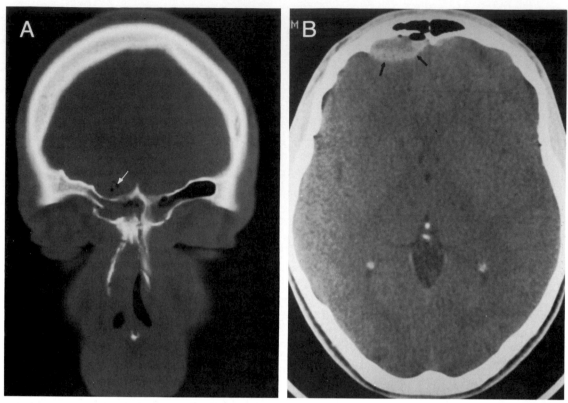

FIG 10–5.
Nasal and sinus fractures, acute EDH. **A** and **B,** unenhanced CT. **A,** coronal, edge enhancement algorithms. A bilateral frontal sinus, nasal fractures, and a left frontonasal fracture are shown. The fron- tal sinus fracture has resulted in pneumocephalus *(arrow).* **B,** Axial MRI. The intracranial air is within a small frontal EDH *(arrows).*

and sagittal scans are very useful to detect superficial cortical contusions, injuries to the body of the corpus callosum, and extra-axial fluid collections along the floor of the anterior or middle cranial fossae or adjacent to the tentorium (Fig 10–6). The location and nature of these lesions are often confusing on axial images. Because the sequential stages of evolving hemorrhage have markedly varied signal intensities with different pulse sequences and long TR images are more sensitive in detecting nonhemorrhagic lesions, both short and long TR conventional spin-echo techniques should be obtained.[8] Gradient-echo scans may be useful in detecting hemosiderin deposits in remote hemorrhagic injuries.[17] The role of gadolinium enhancement in the assessment of trauma patients is not yet established but will probably parallel the use of intravenous contrast material with CT.

FORMS AND APPEARANCES OF INJURIES

Head injuries can be broadly categorized as focal (extra-axial and intraparenchymal hematomas, contusion, laceration, and fracture) or diffuse (diffuse axonal injury [DAI], diffuse swelling and edema). While each type of injury will be discussed separately, two or more frequently coexist.

Epidural Hematoma

The cranial dura is a tough, fibrous capsule closely applied to the inner surface of the skull. Meningeal arteries and veins course between the dura and grooves in the inner table of the skull. A blow to the head may cause focal skull deformity that separates the dura from the calvarium, with or without associated fracture.[18, 19] Bleeding from the disrupted meningeal vessels collects in and enlarges the epidural space that is created as the dura and calvarium are separated. EDHs are not common in the elderly, whose dura is very adherent to the bone.[19]

The CT features of an acute EDH reflect the confined blood clot lying between the inner table of the skull and the underlying depressed dura and compressed brain. An acute EDH is typically well defined, biconvex, and of higher attenuation (ap-

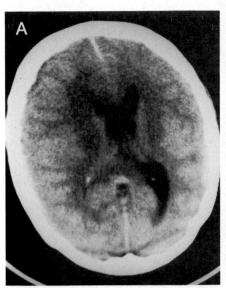

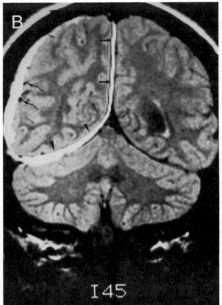

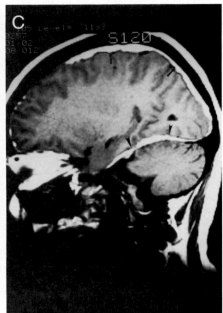

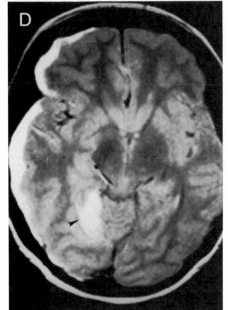

FIG 10–6.

Subacute SDH in a young woman with minor head trauma 14 days before CT and 24 days before MRI. **A,** unenhanced CT shows only mass effect, effacement of the right lateral ventricle, and a shift of the midline structures to the left. **B,** coronal MRI: TR = 2,000, TE = 30. A thin, hyperintense SDH encircles the right cerebral hemisphere. Blood in the interhemispheric fissure *(arrows)* and above the tentorium *(arrowheads)* is well shown. Cortical vessels that are inwardly displaced by the SDH appear as signal-free structures *(wavy arrows).* **C,** sagittal MRI: TR = 600, TE = 20. The extensive, but thin and uniform layer of hyperintense subdural blood extends over the convexity *(arrows)* and above the tentorium *(arrowheads).* **D,** Axial MRI: TR = 2,000, TE = 30. The subacute SDH is also hyperintense to brain on the spin density or "mixed image." The portion of the SDH adjacent to tentorium is shown *(arrowhead),* but its location relative to the tentorium (above or below) cannot be determined as easily on the axial image as on the coronal or sagittal images. (Courtesy of William S. Owen, M.D., Warren, Ohio.)

proximately 40 to 80 Houndsfield units [HU]) than normal gray matter (25 to 40 HU) (Fig 10–7). The high attenuation of a fresh intracranial blood clot is due to the protein component (globin) of the hemoglobin molecule and not the iron moiety.[20] An acute EDH is usually of homogeneous high density but may contain areas of lower attenuation due to unclotted blood or serum extruded during clot formation (Fig 10–8).[21, 22] EDH exerts a mass effect on the underlying brain that is characterized by sulcal effacement, ventricular compression, and a shift of the midline structures. Coexistent intra-

dural injuries are common and contribute to the mass effect.

Linear fractures are commonly associated with EDH (64% to 93% in adults[19, 23–25]) but need not be present. EDH without fracture is more common in children,[26] and depressed fractures are rarely associated with EDH.[27]

The most common acute EDH is temporal in location (70% to 75%)[23, 25] (Figs 10–7 and 10–8) and is usually caused by bleeding from a torn middle meningeal artery. Other common locations are frontal (see Fig 10–5), parietal, occipital, at the

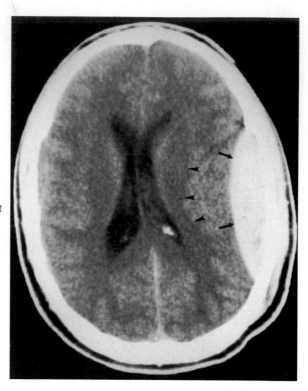

FIG 10–7.
Acute EDH. A well-defined, biconvex, high-attenuation blood collection *(arrows)* compresses the left cerebral hemisphere. There is inward displacement of the gray-white junction *(arrowheads)* and slight effacement and displacement of the left lateral ventricle.

vertex, and in the posterior fossa (Fig 10–9). Acute EDH occasionally occurs along the floor of the middle cranial fossa. On axial images a hematoma in this location may appear similar to a temporal pole contusion. Coronal CT images, the administration of intravenous contrast material, or MRI may help distinguish the two (Fig 10–10). Coronal and/or sagittal reformatted CT images help demonstrate a vertex EDH from a direct blow to the top of the head (Fig 10–11). EDH may be small or multiple or contain air if a paranasal sinus or mastoid fracture is present (see Fig 10–5). An extra-axial hematoma that crosses the attachment of the falx must be epidural in location (Fig 10–12).

Common clinical signs of supratentorial EDH include decreased consciousness, pupillary abnormalities, and limb weakness.[23] Most EDH will cause symptoms immediately or within hours. The classic history of deterioration following initial unconsciousness and a "lucid interval" occurs in a minority of patients with EDH (12% to 42%).[24, 25] An EDH that exerts enough mass effect to compromise cerebral function by direct compression or herniation is a neurosurgical emergency. A small EDH in a patient without focal neurologic symptoms may be managed conservatively (Figs 10–8 and 10–13).[28, 29] Delayed presentation (after several days) of an EDH may occur. In most of these cases, no bleeding site is identified at surgery, and

the delay in onset of symptoms is attributed to slower accumulation of blood from presumed venous bleeding.[30, 31]

As an EDH ages, its CT appearance changes. With clot retraction and liquefaction a peripheral decrease in attenuation develops. With further clot lysis and hemoglobin degradation the density of the entire collection decreases; it fades from hyperdensity (compared with the adjacent portions of the brain) through isodensity to hypodensity (Fig 10–13).

A resolving EDH, conservatively managed, will usually progressively decrease in size, although a temporary expansion of the collection between the 5th and 16th day has been observed.[29] The inner margin of the hematoma becomes vascularized over a few weeks.[21] The innermost margin of an EDH is dura; this normally enhances (see Fig 10–10), but the enhancing margin becomes more prominent as the vascular membrane develops (Fig 10–14).[21] The displaced dura commonly calcifies, and this can occur within days (see Figs 10–8 and 10–13). As an EDH shrinks, it assumes a more crescentic shape as the underlying brain "re-expands" and regains its normal contour (see Fig 10–8).

While arterial bleeding due to trauma is the leading cause of EDH, it may also result from torn meningeal veins, dural venous sinuses, emissary

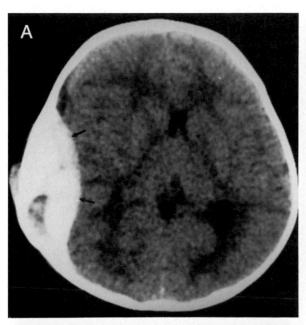

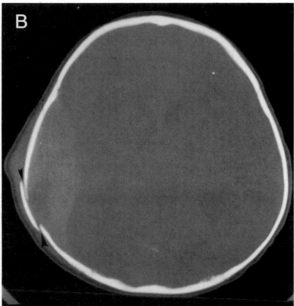

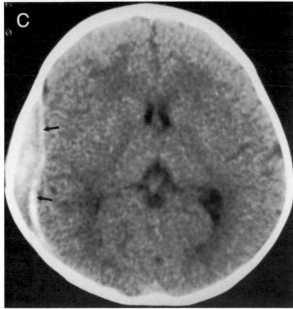

FIG 10–8.

Acute EDH in a 9-month-old boy who fell down stairs. He had swelling over the right parietal area but was neurologically normal. **A** and **B,** unenhanced CT immediately after injury. **A,** a hyperdense, acute EDH *(arrows)* compresses the right cerebral hemisphere. The atrium of the right lateral ventricle is effaced, and the midline is shifted to the left. The EDH is nonuniform, with a low-density region that may be serum or unclotted blood. **B,** the same slice as **A,** processed with an edge enhancement algorithm, shows the comminuted right parietal fracture that is slightly elevated by the EDH *(arrowheads).* Because the child was asymptomatic, he was managed conservatively. **C,** unenhanced CT 11 days after injury. The EDH has decreased in size and density and has assumed a more crescentic shape with tapering margins. The displaced dura is calcified *(arrows).* The residual mass effect of the hematoma is shown by effacement of the ipsilateral lateral ventricle, but the shift of midline structures is much less than on the previous scan.

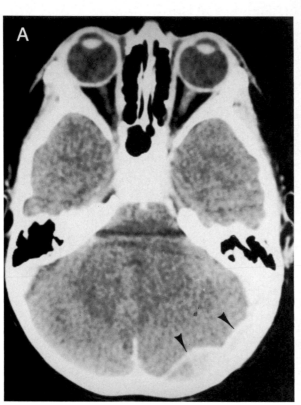

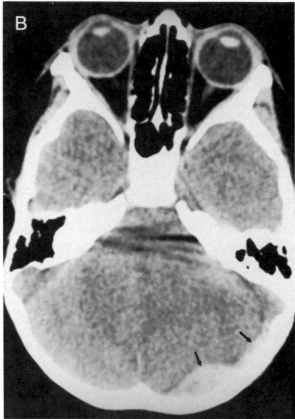

FIG 10–9.
Posterior fossa EDH in a 3-year-old child with a closed head injury. **A,** unenhanced axial CT shows two small, biconvex epidural blood collections in the left posterior fossa *(arrows).* **B,** axial CT with in- travenous contrast material shows enhancement of the elevated dura *(arrowheads).*

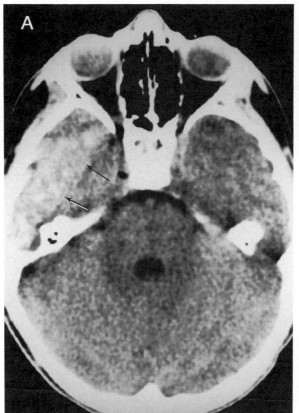

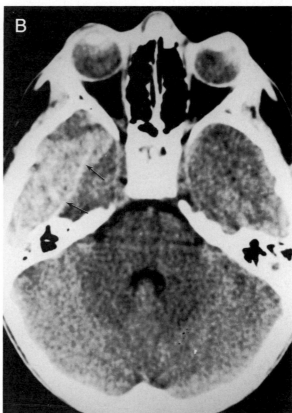

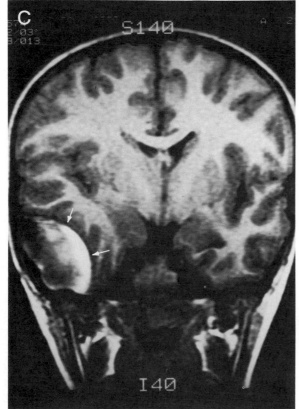

FIG 10–10.
Subtemporal EDH in a 5-year-old boy who struck his right temple on a coffee table. **A,** unenhanced axial CT shows a heterogeneous, but predominantly hyperdense abnormality in the right middle cranial fossa *(arrows)*. The density is that of fresh hemorrhage, but the location of the blood (intraparenchymal vs. extra-axial) is not clear. **B,** after intravenous contrast material is given, there is enhancement of the displaced dura *(arrows),* which indicates that the blood collection is in the epidural space. **C,** coronal MRI 6 days after CT (TR = 2,000, TI = 800, TE = 20). The coronal image clearly demonstrates the epidural location of the nonuniform subacute hematoma. The elevated dura is demonstrated as a linear, signal-free structure *(arrows).*

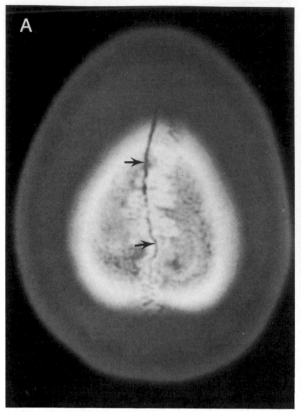

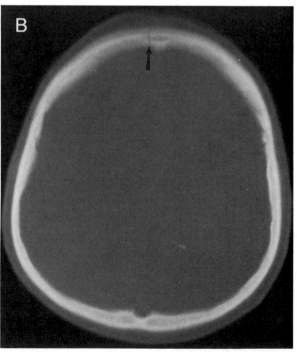

FIG 10–11.

EDH at the vertex in a 26-year-old man whose motorcycle collided with a deer. **A,** axial CT filmed with a wide window. A linear, sagittal fracture *(arrow)* crosses the sagittal suture. There is diffuse scalp swelling. **B,** coronal reformatted image. A hyperdense fluid collection at the vertex crosses the attachment of the falx *(arrow)*, and this indicates that the blood is epidural in location.

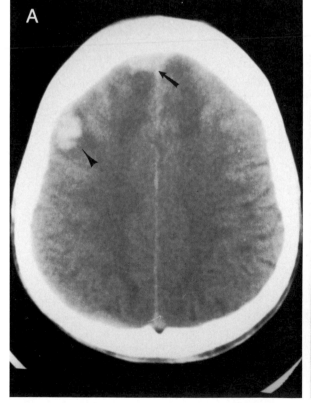

FIG 10–12.

Acute frontal EDH, cortical contusion. **A** and **B,** unenhanced axial CT. **A,** a small frontal EDH crosses the anterior attachment of the falx *(arrow)*. A right frontal cortical contusion is present *(arrow-head)*. **B,** filmed with wide window width, the CT scan shows a linear, nondisplaced frontal fracture *(arrow)*.

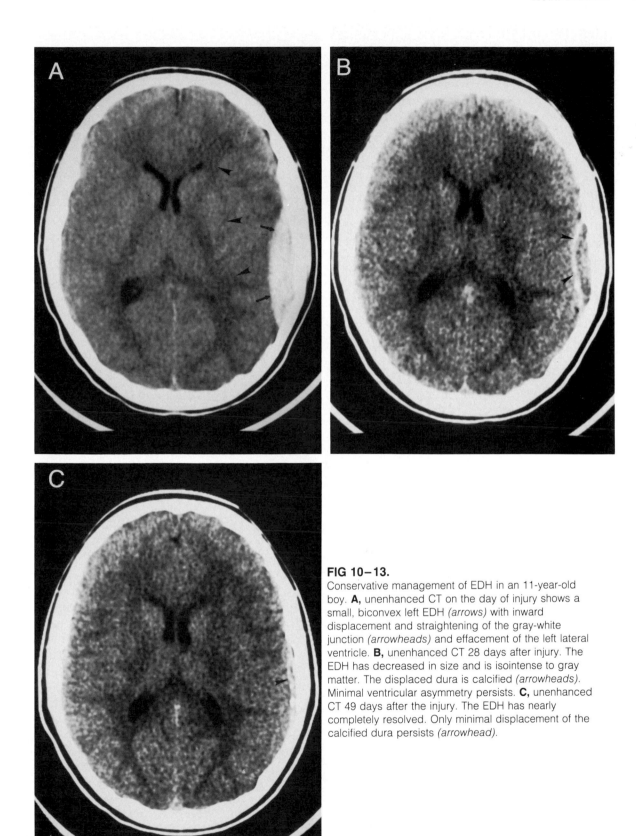

FIG 10–13.
Conservative management of EDH in an 11-year-old
boy. **A,** unenhanced CT on the day of injury shows a
small, biconvex left EDH *(arrows)* with inward
displacement and straightening of the gray-white
junction *(arrowheads)* and effacement of the left lateral
ventricle. **B,** unenhanced CT 28 days after injury. The
EDH has decreased in size and is isointense to gray
matter. The displaced dura is calcified *(arrowheads)*.
Minimal ventricular asymmetry persists. **C,** unenhanced
CT 49 days after the injury. The EDH has nearly
completely resolved. Only minimal displacement of the
calcified dura persists *(arrowhead)*.

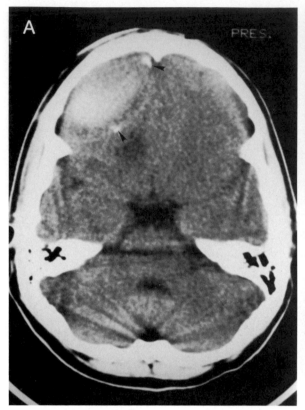
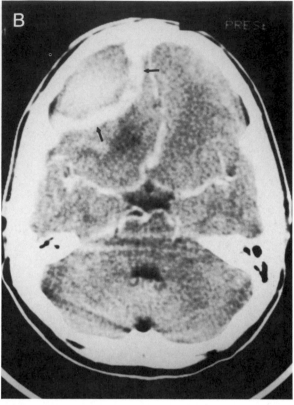

FIG 10–14.
Membrane enhancement in a 4-week-old EDH. **A,** unenhanced axial CT shows the right frontal epidural blood collection that is slightly hyperdense to brain. The displaced dura shows scattered calcification *(arrowheads).* **B,** CT with intravenous contrast material. There is dense enhancement at the rim of the EDH *(arrows)* due to enhancement of the membranes that surround chronic hematomas and normal enhancement of the dura.

veins, or calvarial fractures (see Fig 10–11). EDH also develops following cranial surgery for reasons other than trauma or after evacuation of other extra-axial or intraparenchymal hematomas.[32] EDH is commonly associated with SDH or IPH, and other parenchymal injuries (35% to 47%) (Figs 10–12 and 10–15).[19, 23–25]

Subdural Hematoma

The subdural space (normally a potential space) occurs at the rather loose inner dura-arachnoid interface that covers the outer surface of the brain, including the interhemispheric surfaces and the surfaces above and below the tentorium (see Fig 10–6). Unlike the epidural space, the subdural space is easily dissected.

The CT appearance of an SDH reflects the location, distribution, and age of the hemorrhage. Although the attenuation characteristics of an SDH correlate imperfectly with the age of the collection, a fairly accurate classification divides SDH into three groups: *acute* (higher attenuation than normal gray matter, 40 to 70 HU) (see Fig 10–1), *subacute* (isodense to normal gray matter, 25 to 40 HU) (Fig 10–16), and *chronic* (lower attenuation than normal gray matter, 16 to 25 HU) (Fig 10–17).[33, 34] Practically, however, patients with acute traumatic SDHs differ so significantly in the severity of brain compression and associated injuries from patients with chronic SDHs that division into these two groups is more appropriate and clinically useful.[35, 36]

Acute SDH commonly occurs in patients sustaining high-velocity deceleration injuries in MVAs or falls (Figs 10–1 and 10–18).[37] Thin-walled veins bridge the subdural space as they pass from their subarachnoid location on the brain's surface to the dural venous sinuses. Rupture of a superficial bridging vein is a common cause of acute SDH. It is less well known that branches of superficial cerebral arteries also penetrate the dura, and a disrupted penetrating artery is a common source of acute SDH.[38–40] Brain contu-

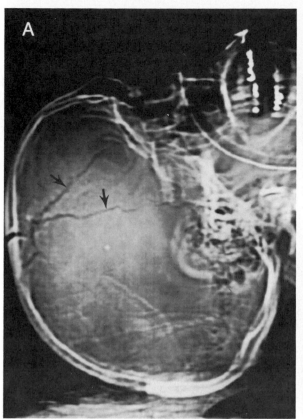
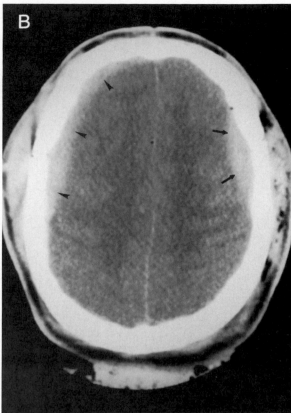

FIG 10–15.
Concurrent acute SDH and EDH. **A,** the lateral "scout" or localizer CT image of the head shows bilateral, frontal, and temporal fractures *(arrows).* **B,** unenhanced axial CT. A well-localized, biconvex acute EDH is present on the left *(arrows).* On the right, a more diffuse, crescent-shaped acute SDH is shown *(arrowheads).*

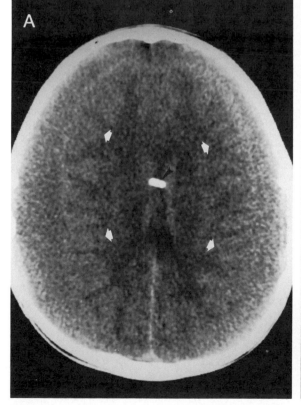
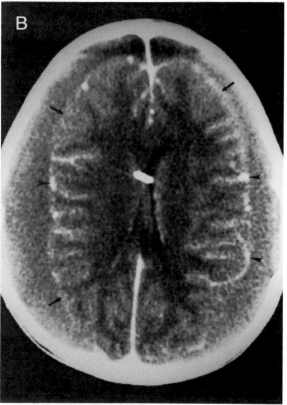

FIG 10–16.
Isodense SDH following shunting for obstructive hydrocephalus. **A,** unenhanced CT shows inward displacement of the gray-white junction *(arrows)* bilaterally by chronic SDHs that are isodense to the adjacent cortical gray matter. A shunt tube is present in the effaced ventricles *(arrowhead).* **B,** CT with intravenous contrast material. Faint enhancement of the membrane that surrounds the chronic subdural hematoma is shown *(arrows).* The displaced cortical veins enhance more brightly *(arrowheads).*

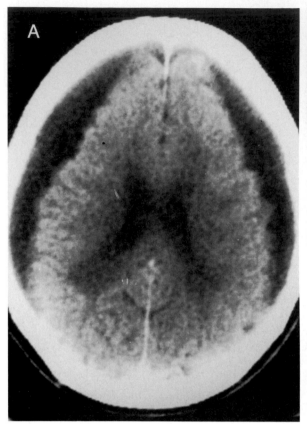

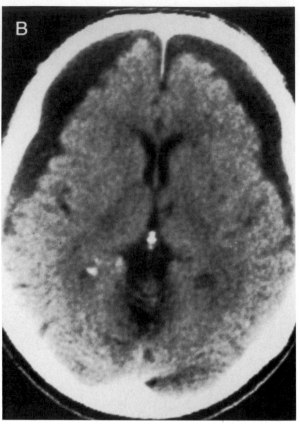

FIG 10–17.
Bilateral chronic SDH in an 81-year-old male with dementia. **A** and **B,** unenhanced axial CT. There are low-attenuation fluid collections that are isodense to CSF over both cerebral hemispheres. The frontal lobes have a peaked configuration. The lateral ventricles are narrow and compressed parallel to the midline.

sions, lacerations, and ruptured aneurysms (Fig 10–19) or AVMs (see Fig 10–3) are less frequent sources of SDH.[39, 41] Some authors designate an acute SDH in direct continuity with an IPH or laceration as a "burst" or "pulped" lobe (usually frontal or temporal) (Fig 10–20).[27, 42] Concomitant parenchymal injuries or edema is more common with acute SDH (45% to 56%) (Fig 10–21) than with EDH.[35, 36, 43] Approximately 36% of patients with SDH have associated skull fractures.[37] The mortality rate of acute SDH is approximately 50%.[39, 40, 43]

An acute SDH typically appears on CT as a hyperdense crescent-shaped collection conforming to the inner surface of the skull (Figs 10–19 and 10–21). Although the volume of blood demonstrated on each image may be small, the total volume of an SDH distributed over the hemisphere is often large enough to exert considerable mass effect. A characteristic deformity of the ipsilateral lateral ventricle results, with medial displacement and compression of the entire ventricle, posterior displacement of the frontal horn, and anterior dis-

placement of the occipital horn and choroid plexus of the atrium (see Fig 10–18). Inward displacement and straightening of the gray-white junction ("buckling") (see Fig 10–18), effacement of sulcal spaces underlying the hematoma, and a shift of the midline structures also reflect an extra-axial mass effect (Fig 10–21). Cerebral edema and contusion often contribute to the mass effect. Subfalcine or transtentorial herniation caused by a large hematoma may kink the foramen of Monro or aqueduct with dilatation only of the contralateral (noncompressed ventricle) (Fig 10–21).

A small SDH may not be visible with the narrow window widths usually used in cranial CT. Widening the window width is necessary to distinguish a small SDH from the dense bone of the skull. For this reason all "trauma head" CTs should be viewed or filmed at three different windows: narrow window width for brain, midrange window width for subdural blood, and maximum window width for bone (Fig 10–22).

Acute SDHs, typically are of homogeneous high

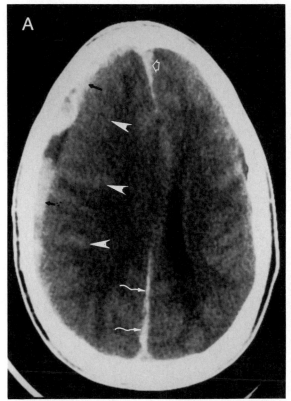

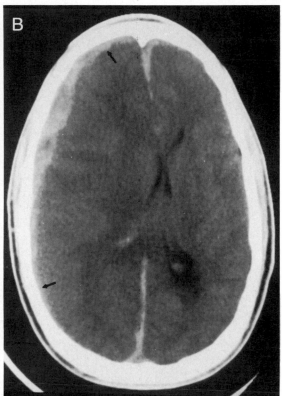

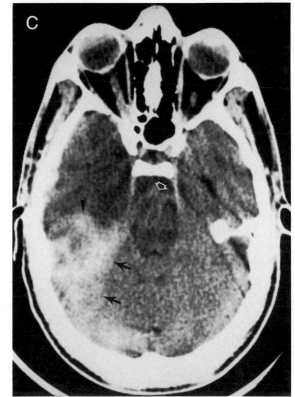

FIG 10–18.
Acute SDH in a 17-year-old male injured in an MVA.
A–C, unenhanced axial CT. **A,** an image filmed at a relatively narrow window width (usual "brain window") shows an acute SDH *(arrows)* compressing the right cerebral hemisphere. The gray-white junction is buckled inward *(arrowheads).* The collection is of fairly uniform thickness and contains an area of lower density due to unclotted blood or extruded serum. The right SDH extends into the posterior portion of the interhemispheric fissure *(wavy arrows).* The anterior interhemispheric fissure contains a small left SDH *(open arrow).* **B,** image inferior to **A,** filmed at a wider window width ("blood or subdural window"). At the wider window, the tapering margins of the SDH are more easily appreciated *(arrows).* The right lateral ventricle is compressed, with anterior and medial displacement of the atrium and posterior and medial displacement of the frontal horn. **C,** an image at the level of the midbrain shows a sheet of blood above the tentorium *(arrows)* that extends into the right middle cranial fossa *(arrowhead).* SAH is present in the prepontine cistern *(open arrow).*

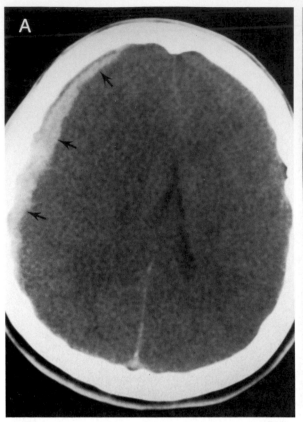

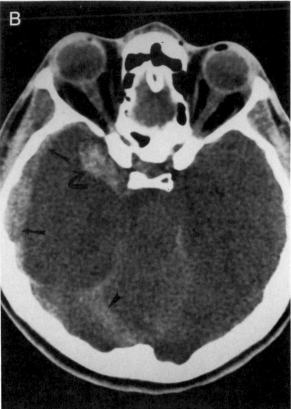

FIG 10–19.
Acute SDH due to a ruptured aneurysm in a 38-year-old female found unresponsive after calling paramedics for assistance. **A** and **B,** unenhanced axial CT. **A,** a typical thin, crescent-shaped hyperdense acute SDH *(arrows)* overlies the right cerebral hemisphere. The lateral ventricles are effaced and displaced to the left. **B,** a more inferior image shows subdural blood in the middle cranial fossa *(arrows),* with components above the tentorium *(arrowhead)* and in the parasellar area *(curved arrow).* At autopsy, a ruptured right posterior communicating artery aneurysm and extensive subdural but no intraparenchymal blood was found.

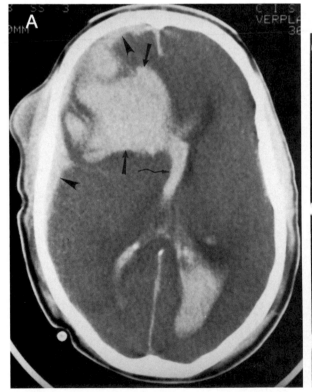

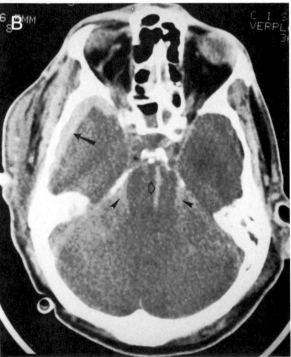

FIG 10–20.
"Pulped" frontal lobe in a 45-year-old male following severe head trauma. **A** and **B,** unenhanced axial CT. **A,** there is a large hematoma in the right frontal lobe *(arrows)* in continuity with subdural *(arrowheads)* and intraventricular *(wavy arrow)* hemorrhage. **B,** a more inferior image shows subdural blood in the right middle cranial fossa *(arrow),* SAH in the basal cisterns *(arrowheads),* and a slitlike "Duret" hemorrhage in the brain stem *(open arrow).* The sphenoid sinus contains blood from a fracture of the sinus wall (not shown).

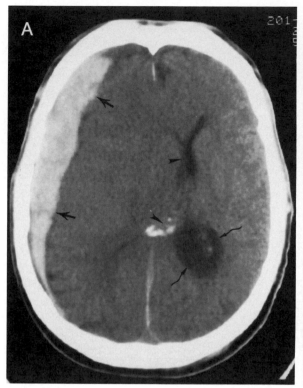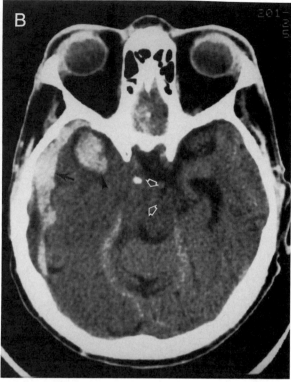

FIG 10–21.
Acute SDH with subfalcine and uncal herniation. **A** and **B**, unenhanced axial CT. **A,** an image at the level of the lateral ventricles shows the large acute SDH *(arrows)* over the right hemisphere. There is considerable mass effect with marked compression and displacement of the right lateral ventricle *(arrowheads).* Due to the brain distortion and obstruction of CSF outflow, the left lateral ventricle is dilated *(wavy arrows).* **B,** a more inferior image shows the subdural blood extending into the right middle cranial fossa *(arrow)* and an IPH in the right temporal pole *(arrowhead).* Note that the hematoma is nearly completely surrounded by brain, and compare with Figure 10–19. The right uncus *(open arrows)* is herniated into the suprasellar cistern, and there is compression of the midbrain.

attenuation, but other appearances are common. An acute SDH may be inhomogeneous with irregular areas of low density due to unclotted blood, serum extruded during clot formation, or pockets of cerebrospinal fluid (CSF) contained within the collection (see Figs 10–18 and 10–21).[44, 45] The most important "atypical" appearance of an acute SDH is isodensity (25 to 40 HU) to brain. Patients who are anemic may develop SDHs that are acutely isodense to brain.[46] In isodense SDH the secondary signs of the characteristic ventricular deformity, sulcal effacement, displacement of the gray-white junction, and midline shift should suggest the presence of an SDH.[47–49] Even with bilateral isodense SDH the characteristic parallel and narrowed configuration of the lateral ventricles should raise suspicion for SDH (Fig 10–23). Intravenous contrast material will enhance the cerebral cortex and displaced cortical vessels and will usually help demonstrate or exclude an isodense SDH (see Fig 10–16).[48] Occasionally a "hyperacute"

SDH (those imaged within a few hours of trauma) are more focal in distribution and may mimic an EDH (Fig 10–24). It is postulated that adhesions prevent the even distribution of blood in the subdural space.[50]

SDH is most frequently found over the cerebral convexities and is usually widely distributed over the hemisphere (see Figs 10–6 and 10–18). SDH also occurs in the interhemispheric fissure. An interhemispheric SDH has a straight medial margin abutting the falx and a convex margin laterally compressing the adjacent brain (Fig 10–25). Extension of a convexity SDH into the fissure curves smoothly over the brain (Fig 10–26). The well-defined margin of the hematoma, the typical hyperdense appearance of fresh blood (40 to 70 HU), and the presence of subdural blood along the tentorium help distinguish an acute interhemispheric SDH from other causes of an abnormally dense or prominent falx. Subarachnoid hemorrhage (SAH) appears as fine, linear densities in the

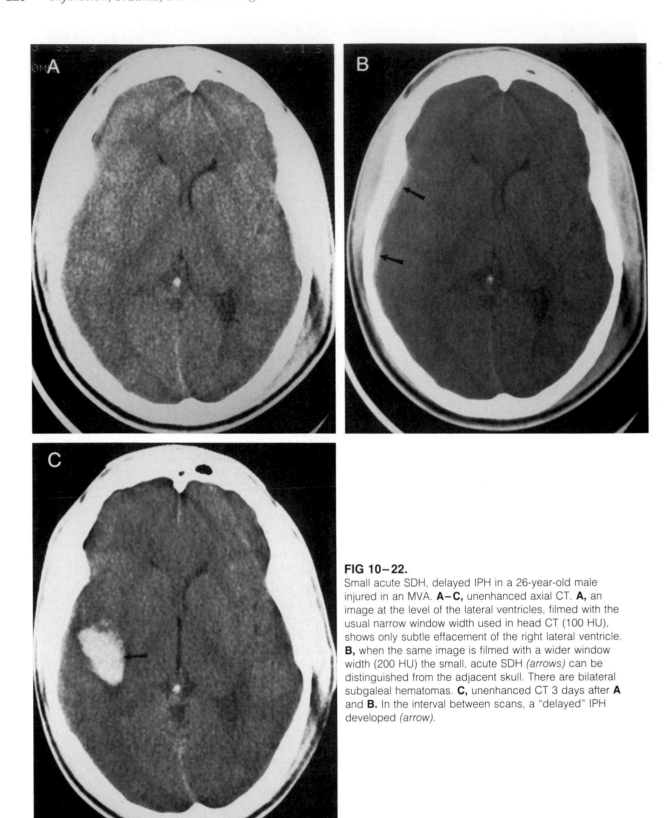

FIG 10–22.
Small acute SDH, delayed IPH in a 26-year-old male injured in an MVA. **A–C,** unenhanced axial CT. **A,** an image at the level of the lateral ventricles, filmed with the usual narrow window width used in head CT (100 HU), shows only subtle effacement of the right lateral ventricle. **B,** when the same image is filmed with a wider window width (200 HU) the small, acute SDH *(arrows)* can be distinguished from the adjacent skull. There are bilateral subgaleal hematomas. **C,** unenhanced CT 3 days after **A** and **B.** In the interval between scans, a "delayed" IPH developed *(arrow).*

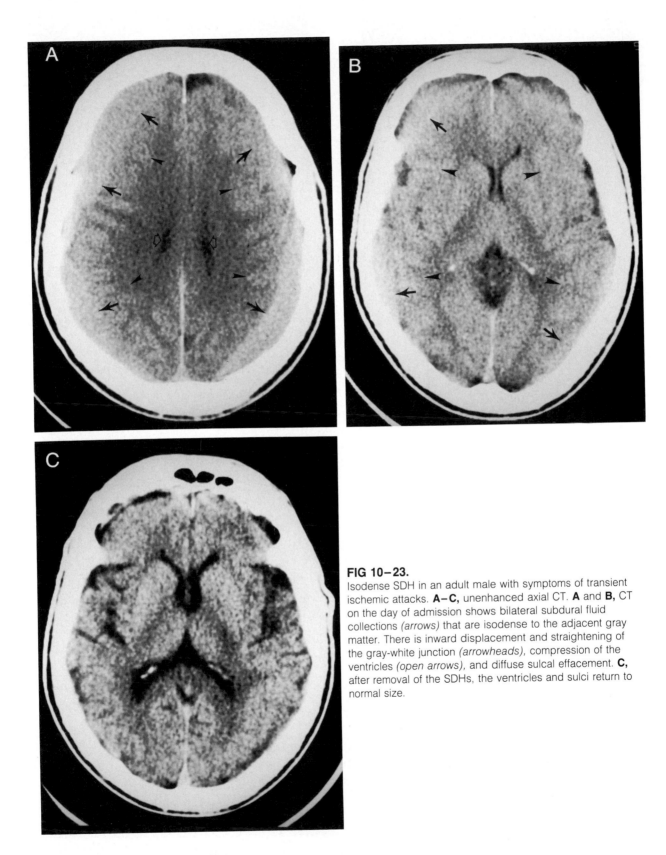

FIG 10–23.
Isodense SDH in an adult male with symptoms of transient ischemic attacks. **A–C,** unenhanced axial CT. **A** and **B,** CT on the day of admission shows bilateral subdural fluid collections *(arrows)* that are isodense to the adjacent gray matter. There is inward displacement and straightening of the gray-white junction *(arrowheads),* compression of the ventricles *(open arrows),* and diffuse sulcal effacement. **C,** after removal of the SDHs, the ventricles and sulci return to normal size.

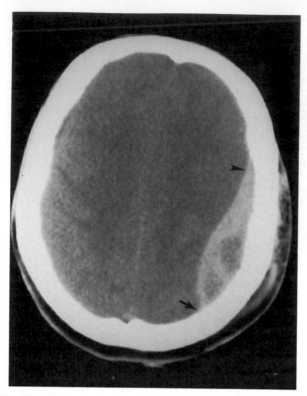

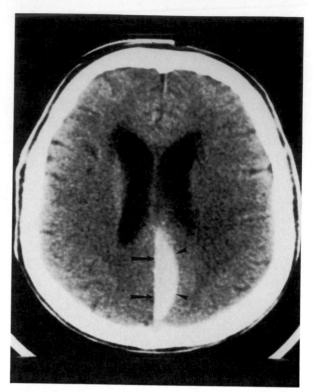

FIG 10–24.
Acute SDH mimicking EDH in unenhanced axial CT. A nonuniform hyperdense extra-axial blood collection overlies and compresses the left cerebral hemisphere. The collection has a wider "waist," and the posterior margin of the collection forms a more acute angle *(arrow)* with the skull than is typical of acute SDH. The anterior gradually tapering margin is more typical of acute SDH *(arrowhead)*. At operation an acute subdural hematoma was removed.

FIG 10–25.
Interhemispheric SDH seen by unenhanced CT. The hyperdense acute SDH in the left side of the interhemispheric fissure has a straight margin adjacent to the falx *(arrows)*. The lateral margin is outwardly convex *(arrowheads)* and compresses the occipital lobe.

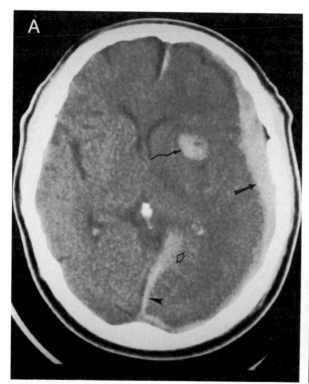

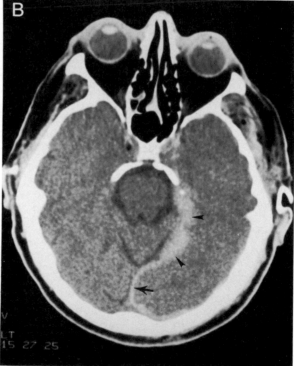

FIG 10–26.
Acute SDH and IPH. **A** and **B,** unenhanced CT. **A,** a typical crescent-shaped, hyperdense acute SDH overlies the left cerebral hemisphere *(arrow)*. The hematoma extends into the interhemispheric fissure *(arrowhead)* and above the tentorium *(open arrow)*.

There is an intraparenchymal hematoma in the left basal ganglia *(wavy arrow)*. **B,** a more inferior image shows the SDH in the posterior interhemispheric fissure *(arrow)* and along the superior surface of the tentorium *(arrowheads)*.

parasagittal sulci, while dural calcifications are more focal and generally very dense.[51] Interhemispheric fissure SDHs are more common in the posterior aspect of the fissure. Children subject to shaking trauma may develop interhemispheric SDH.[52] In children, edema of adjacent brain structures may cause the falx to appear very prominent, and follow-up scans may be required to prove or exclude an interhemispheric SDH.[51]

Acute SDHs above or below the tentorium produce a band of hyperdensity conforming to the contour of the tentorium (see Figs 10–18 and 10–26).[53] On axial images it is often difficult to determine whether a peritentorial SDH is present and whether the blood is above or below the tentorium. The presence of blood in the interhemispheric fissure or middle cranial fossa is a clue to a supratentorial location (see Fig 10–18). Contrast enhancement of the tentorium may aid in distinguishing infratentorial and supratentorial collections.[54] Coronal CT and MRI are very helpful in defining a peritentorial SDH (see Fig 10–6).

A posterior fossa SDH may result from disruption of bridging veins over the cerebellum, torn dural venous sinuses, or cerebellar contusions.[36] Like convexity SDHs, acute posterior fossa SDHs are demonstrated by CT as hyperdense collections conforming to the inner table of the skull (Fig 10–27).

As an SDH ages, the clot liquifies, and the hemoglobin protein is lysed and removed. The density of the SDH decreases. It gradually becomes isodense to gray matter over a period of 2 or 3 weeks (see Figs 10–16 and 10–23).[55] Occasionally the denser elements of a subacute SDH layer posteriorly and result in a "hematocrit effect." A vascular granulation tissue membrane that enhances with intravenous contrast material encircles the hematoma within a few weeks, and this can help prove the presence of an isodense SDH (see Fig 10–16). Displaced cortical vessels also enhance and are distinguished from an enhancing membrane by their presence on only one or two images.[48] Because of the vascular membrane, contrast material can enter the collection. On delayed scans obtained 3 to 6 hours after intravenous contrast material is given, subacute or chronic SDH may show increased attenuation when compared with precontrast scans.[47, 56]

A chronic SDH is defined as one that has been present for 3 weeks or more. Chronic SDH most commonly affects the elderly population and occurs with an incidence of 1 to 2 per 100,000 per year.[57] Rupture of a vein that bridges the parasagittal subdural space is the most common cause of chronic SDH. This is facilitated by cerebral volume loss that places the thin-walled bridging veins under increased tension. Chronic SDH is more common after minor trauma such as a fall or assault than after high-speed trauma such as an MVA. The trauma is often so minor as to be forgotten. Since a history of trauma is often not elicited and the symptoms caused by a chronic SDH may mimic those of a neoplasm, transient ischemic attack, stroke, or dementia, it is not unusual to detect an SDH on a study requested because a different condition is suspected (see Fig 10–23).[58] Sixteen percent to 20% of chronic SDHs are bilateral.[37] Fracture is associated with chronic SDH in fewer than 10% of cases.[58, 59]

Chronic SDH is typically of lower attenuation than is brain tissue (see Fig 10–17). In an older patient SDH initially displaces CSF from enlarged subarachnoid spaces around atrophic brain. Because of the cerebral volume loss, brain compression and midline shift are less than would occur due to a collection of equal volume occurring over a younger, fuller brain. Sulcal effacement, inward displacement, and straightening of the gray-white junction do, however, also occur in chronic SDH.

A chronic SDH is characteristically surrounded by a well-defined capsule.[60] This results in a more focal or "wider" collection with a straighter medial edge than the typically crescent-shaped acute SDH has (Fig 10–28). The capsule is very vascular, enhances with intravenous contrast material (Figs 10–28 and 10–29), often calcifies, and rarely ossifies (Fig 10–30). Bleeding and effusion of protein through the capsular vessels is the currently accepted mechanism of enlargement of chronic SDH.[58] This process results in a collection of increased density when compared with the typical hypodense chronic SDH (see Fig 10–29). The increased density may occur uniformly and result in a collection that is isodense to the brain, or the newer, denser blood may layer dependently and create a "hematocrit effect" (Fig 10–31). The characteristic medially displaced, narrow, parallel lateral ventricles or a brain that looks "too good" for the patient's age should suggest bilateral isodense SDH (see Fig 10–23).

Low-density chronic SDH should not be confused with prominent CSF spaces due to atrophy or cerebral volume loss. A chronic SDH compresses and effaces convexity sulci and the ventricular system. By contrast, patients with diffuse

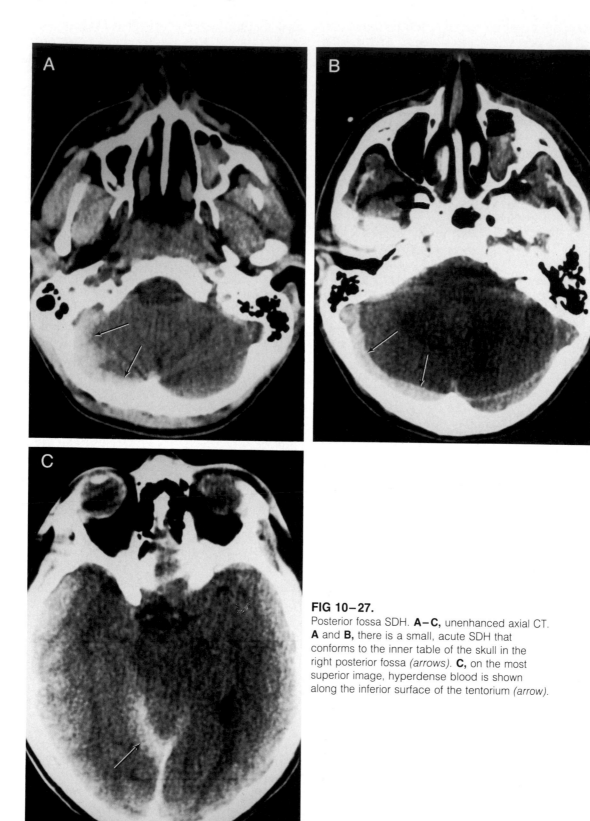

FIG 10–27.
Posterior fossa SDH. **A–C,** unenhanced axial CT. **A** and **B,** there is a small, acute SDH that conforms to the inner table of the skull in the right posterior fossa *(arrows).* **C,** on the most superior image, hyperdense blood is shown along the inferior surface of the tentorium *(arrow).*

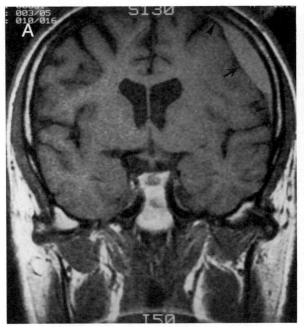
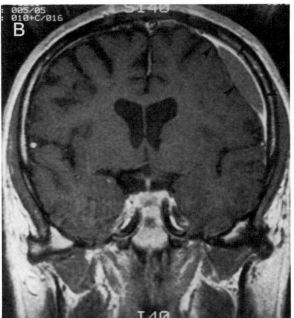

FIG 10–28.
Chronic SDH with membrane enhancement. **A,** unenhanced coronal MRI (TR = 600, TE = 20). The subdural hematoma *(arrow)* compressing the left cerebral hemisphere is hyperintense to CSF. The SDH has characteristically tapering margins *(arrowheads)* but a relatively wide "waist" as is typical of chronic SDHs. **B,** gadolinium-enhanced coronal MRI (TR = 600, TE = 20). The membrane encircling the chronic SDH enhances brightly *(arrowheads).*

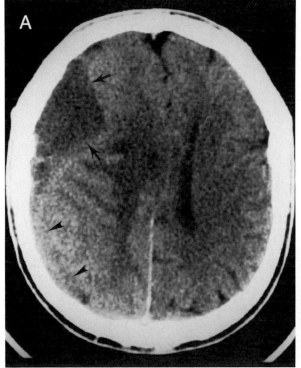
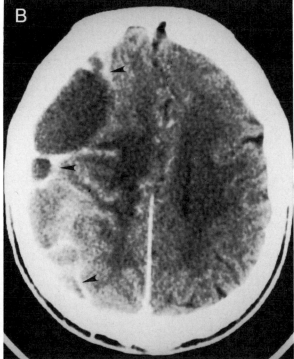

FIG 10–29.
Membrane enhancement in chronic SDH in a 64-year-old man with a previous stroke. **A,** unenhanced CT shows a nonuniform extra-axial fluid collection compressing the right hemisphere. The anterior portion of the collection *(arrows)* is hypodense relative to gray matter, while the posterior portion of the collection is hyperdense *(arrowhead)* due to recent hemorrhage. **B,** when intravenous contrast material is given, the membranes encircling the chronic SDH enhance *(arrowheads).*

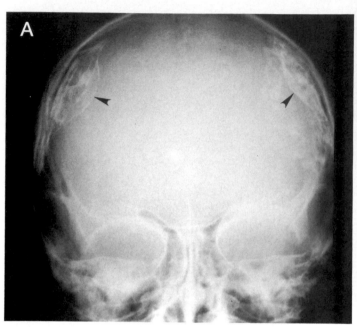

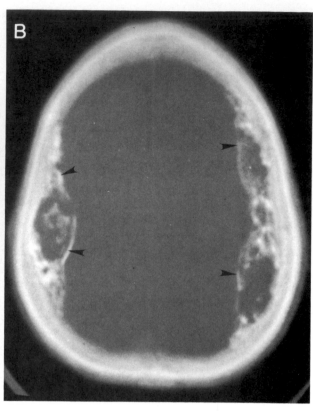

FIG 10–30.
Calcified SDH in a 17-year-old male with chronic, bilateral SDH. **A,** a frontal view of the skull shows bilateral, lens-shaped calcification adjacent to the inner table of each parietal bone *(arrowheads)*. **B,** unenhanced CT filmed with wide windows shows the bilateral cal- cified SDH *(arrowheads)*. The chronic SDH have a fairly straight medial margin and are of a more uniform width than is typical of acute SDH.

FIG 10–31.
Rebleed into a chronic SDH in an 82-year-old man with symptoms suggesting thrombotic stroke. Unenhanced CT shows bilateral subdural fluid collections, with a dependent hyperdense layer representing fresh blood elements within a chronic, low-density SDH.

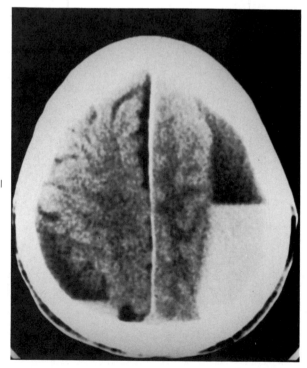

atrophy display prominent sulcal spaces, basal cisterns, and ventricles. Overly rapid decompression of obstructive hydrocephalus and craniotomy for nontraumatic reasons may precipitate SDH. Patients with cerebral volume loss, shunts, alcoholism, coagulopathies, anticoagulant use, or hemodialysis are all at increased risk for SDH developing.[37]

Subdural Hygroma

Low-attenuation subdural fluid collections can develop after head trauma without antecedent hematoma and are referred to as subdural hygromas. Rarely, such collections develop immediately after trauma and are under increased pressure, and clear, xanthochromic, or slightly blood-tinged fluid is found at surgery.[61] These collections are thought to be due to small arachnoid tears that act as one-way valves allowing CSF to collect in the subdural space.[37, 61] More commonly, subdural hygromas develop after a short delay (2 to 14 days) and probably result from effusion of fluid across injured leptomeningeal capillaries. These hypodense subdural fluid collections are most often frontal in location (Fig 10–32) and resolve spontaneously within several months.[62]

Subarachnoid Hemorrhage

Post-traumatic SAH is common and often associated with cortical contusion or laceration and extra-axial or intra-axial hematomas (see Fig 10–18). SAH is often an isolated finding following trauma and is then usually limited to a few sulci or fissures (Fig 10–33). CT is not very sensitive to a small SAH (unless blood replaces more than 70% of the CSF in any location, the subarachnoid fluid will be isodense to normal CSF or brain).[63] An SAH that is detectable by CT appears as linear zones of abnormally high density in the sulci, fissures, or basal cisterns. Extensive SAH may result in a "cisternogram effect," with vessels and cranial nerves appearing as low-density filling defects in the dense subarachnoid blood.

MRI of Extra-axial Hemorrhage

The morphologic features of epidural and subdural hematomas are similar on MRI and CT (see Figs 10–10 and 10–28). MRI does have several advantages that make it more sensitive than CT in detecting extra-axial hematomas. Direct coronal

and sagittal images are easily obtained with MRI. Hematomas in a predominately axial orientation, such as those adjacent to the tentorium, and subtemporal or subfrontal hematomas are much more clearly shown on coronal or sagittal than axial images (see Fig 10–10). The lack of signal from cortical bone increases the sensitivity of MRI for small subdural and epidural hematomas. Small fluid collections are easier to detect when adjacent to black cortical bone, as occurs in MRI as opposed to CT, where partial volume averaging of dense cortical bone may obscure small hematomas.[6, 11] Also, the demonstration of displaced dura or cortical vessels as signal-free structures on MRI helps to demonstrate small extra-axial collections and aids in distinguishing SDH from EDH or intra-axial from extra-axial lesions without injected contrast material (Fig 10–34).[6]

The MRI appearance of intracranial hemorrhage is very complex and is fully addressed in Chapter 9. Acute extra-axial hematomas can be demonstrated with MRI because of the subtle but detectable signal intensity differences between blood and adjacent bone and brain (Fig 10–35). Unless very small, such collections are usually easily demonstrated with CT. The clear superiority of MRI lies in the detection of subacute and chronic fluid collections that are isodense to brain on CT (see Fig 10–6). Subacute hematomas (those at least approximately 3 days old) have very high signal intensity, initially on short TR images, then later on both short and long TR images (Fig 10–35).[10, 64] The characteristic hyperintensity of subacute hemorrhage on conventional spin-echo techniques helps make MRI more sensitive than CT in detecting subacute hematomas. MRI is extremely sensitive to the signal-altering effects of even small amounts of blood or hemoglobin oxidation products. Chronic SDH will be hyperintense to CSF on short TR images for at least several months, long after chronic SDHs are isodense to CSF on CT (Fig 10–36).[65]

MRI is less sensitive than CT in detecting SAH. Unless a focal clot forms (Fig 10–37), SAH differs little in signal intensity from normal CSF or adjacent brain.

Focal Parenchymal Injuries, Contusions, and Hematomas

Cerebral contusions are very common following head trauma. These consist of heterogenous areas of hemorrhage, edema, and necrosis. If suffi-

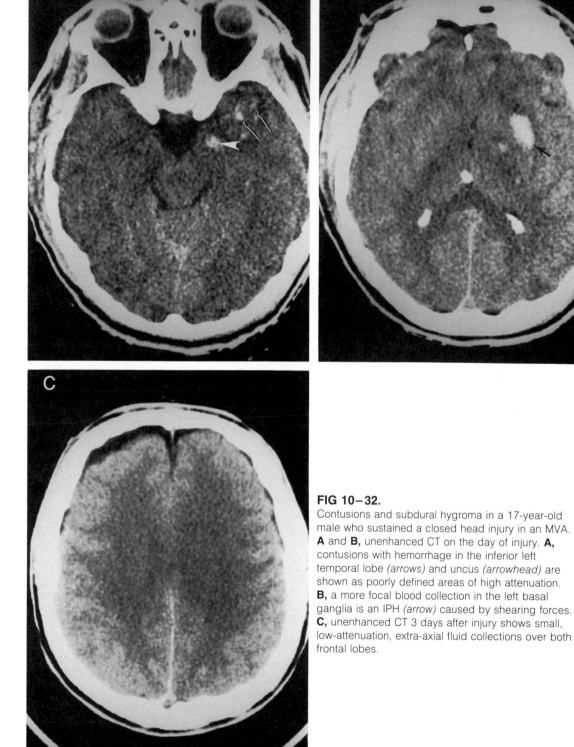

FIG 10–32.
Contusions and subdural hygroma in a 17-year-old
male who sustained a closed head injury in an MVA.
A and **B,** unenhanced CT on the day of injury. **A,**
contusions with hemorrhage in the inferior left
temporal lobe *(arrows)* and uncus *(arrowhead)* are
shown as poorly defined areas of high attenuation.
B, a more focal blood collection in the left basal
ganglia is an IPH *(arrow)* caused by shearing forces.
C, unenhanced CT 3 days after injury shows small,
low-attenuation, extra-axial fluid collections over both
frontal lobes.

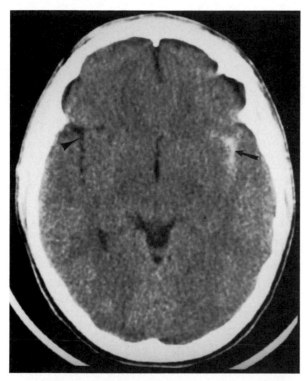

FIG 10–33.
SAH, unenhanced CT of a 30-year-old female who was injured when her car struck a tree shows a high-attenuation, fresh SAH in the left sylvian fissure *(arrow).* The normal right sylvian fissure contains CSF *(arrowhead).* Because there was a question of loss of consciousness prior to the accident and possible aneurysm rupture, an angiogram was performed and was negative.

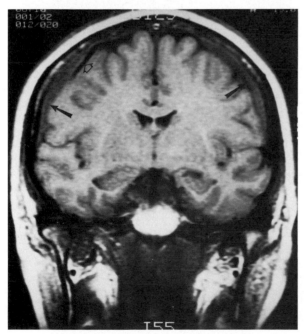

FIG 10–34.
Bilateral, chronic SDH: unenhanced coronal MRI (TR = 700, TE = 20). There are subdural fluid collections *(closed arrows)* that are mildly hyperintense to the CSF in the ventricles. A cortical vein that is inwardly displaced by the chronic SDH is shown as a signal-free structure *(open arrow).*

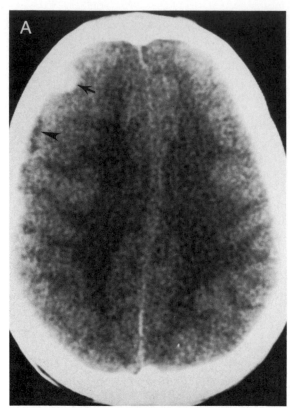

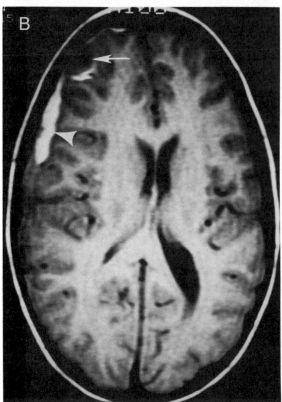

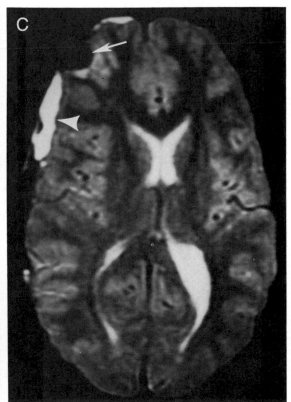

FIG 10–35.
Acute and subacute SDH in a 13-year-old girl with paroxysmal nocturnal hemoglobinuria and recent headaches. **A,** unenhanced CT shows a nonuniform SDH on the right, with a hyperdense, fresher component anteriorly *(arrow)* and a lower-attenuation older portion posteriorly *(arrowhead)*. **B** and **C,** unenhanced axial MRI. **B,** TR = 600; TE = 20. **C,** TR = 2,750; TE = 80. The nonuniform right SDH is shown. On both long and short TR sequences, the fresher blood anteriorly is hypointense relative to brain *(arrows)*, whereas the older, subacute posterior component is markedly hyperintense *(arrowheads)*.

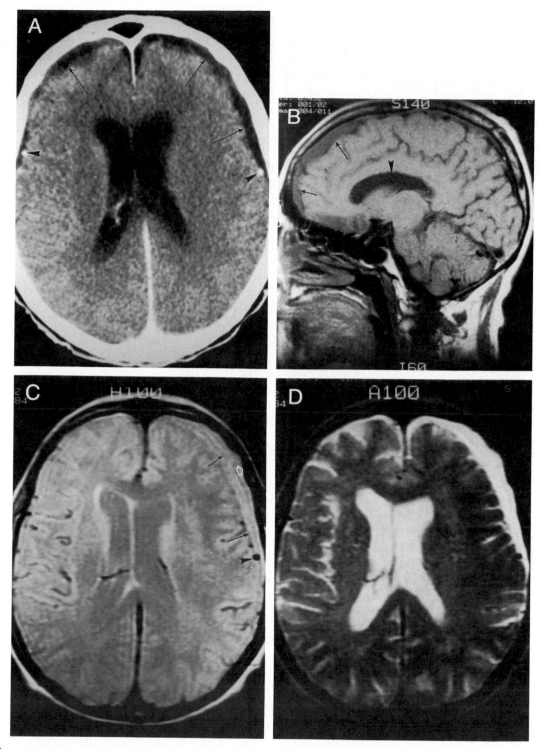

FIG 10–36.

Chronic SDH. **A,** CT with intravenous contrast material. There are bilateral subdural fluid collections *(arrows)* with a density equal to CSF. The enhanced cortical veins *(arrowheads)* are displaced from the inner table by the chronic SDH. **B,** unenhanced sagittal MRI (TR = 600, TE = 20). Sagittal MRI (to the *left* of the midline) shows the subdural fluid *(arrows)* over the left frontal lobe to be mildly hyperintense to CSF in the ventricles *(arrowhead)*. **C,** unenhanced axial MRI (TR = 2,500, TE = 25). On the spin-density or "mixed" image the subdural fluid *(arrows)* is isointense to the adjacent gray matter of the cerebral cortex but still clearly evident between the signal-free calvarium *(open arrow)* and displaced cortical vessels *(arrowhead)*. **D,** unenhanced axial MRI (TR = 2,500, TE = 100). On the long TR, long TE, or "T2-weighted" image the chronic SDH and CSF are of equal intensity, and both are markedly hyperintense relative to brain tissue.

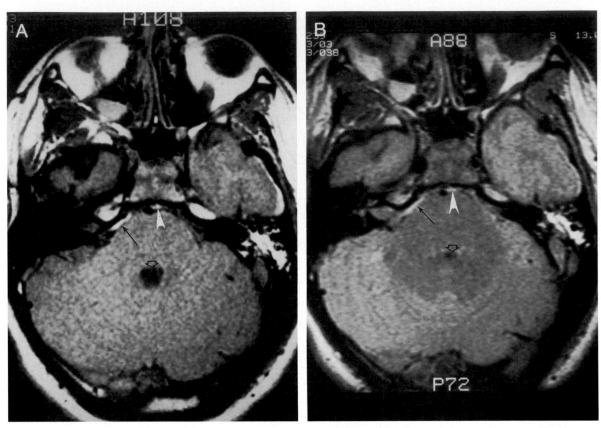

FIG 10-37.
SAH in a 17-year-old male with recent head trauma. **A** and **B**, unenhanced axial MRI. **A,** TR = 851, TE = 20. **B,** TR = 2,609, TE = 20. On both the long and short TR sequences, the subarachnoid blood in the prepontine *(arrowheads)* and right cerebellopontine angle *(arrows)* cisterns is hyperintense to brain and to CSF in the fourth ventricle *(open arrows)*.

cient blood is extravasated into the cerebral cortex or white matter, poorly defined areas of irregular high attenuation are demonstrated by CT (see Fig 10–32). Contusions in which edema and necrosis predominate may not be demonstrated initially by CT but commonly appear days later as areas of low attenuation due to edema. They may also have a "salt-and-pepper" appearance caused by edema mixed with delayed or coalescent hemorrhage (Fig 10–38).

Most contusions result from sudden contact of the dura-lined skull with the cortical surface. Contusions have often been designated as "coup" or "contrecoup" in type; "coup" refers to those lesions that occur in brain directly beneath the impact site (Fig 10–39), and "contrecoup" refers to those that occur in brain 180 degrees removed from the impact site. Direct impact is, however, not necessary for contusion to occur. Recent experimental work has emphasized the importance of angular acceleration forces in the development of contusions.[12] Angular acceleration causes differential movement of the brain within the skull and may result in sliding of the cortical surface along the inner table.[66] Because the floors of the anterior and middle cranial fossae are very irregular, frontal and temporal contusions predominate regardless of the site of impact or whether impact occurs (see Fig 10–32). Cortical contusions are less frequent in infants and young children because of the smooth inner surface of the skull.

Resolving contusions gradually fade in density as blood products are absorbed (Fig 10–40), and they may enhance with intravenous contrast material.[67] Old or healed contusions appear as areas of low attenuation representing encephalomalacia or porencephalia. Hemorrhage into an area of contusion is thought to account for most delayed IPHs.[68] Lacerations are injuries that disrupt the pia-glial membrane and are almost always associated with contusions.

IPHs are focal collections of blood within the substance of the brain. An acute IPH appears on CT as a focal, fairly well marginated area of blood density (60 to 80 HU) (see Figs 10–21 and 10–22). Within several hours low attenuation due to edema

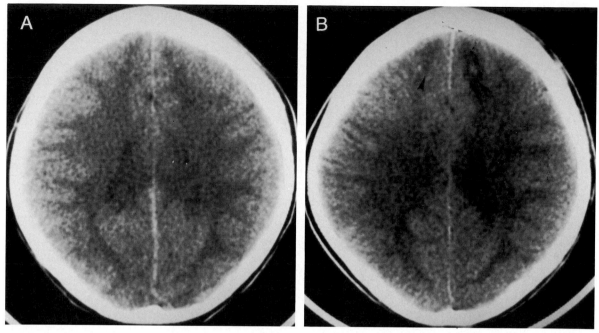

FIG 10–38.
Cerebral contusions in an 11-year-old girl injured in an MVA. **A,** unenhanced CT a few hours after injury is normal. **B,** unenhanced CT 6 days later shows low attenuation due to edema in both frontal lobes *(arrowheads)* that surrounds tiny, high-density hemorrhage.

develops in the brain structures surrounding the hematoma. Depending on its size and location, an IPH may exert considerable mass effect on the adjacent brain structures, with sulcal effacement of the cortex overlying the hematoma, shift of midline structures, and possible subfalcine or transtentorial herniation.

A hematoma that is not evacuated will gradually decrease in size and density (Fig 10–40).[69] A subacute or resolving hematoma may display a ring of enhancement after intravenous contrast material is given. It can be difficult to differentiate a resolving IPH from an abscess or neoplasm without prior scans or clinical history. After healing of an IPH, CT demonstrates a well-defined area of low density due to gliotic scarring or porencephaly (Fig 10–40), or the CT appearance may return to normal.

Traumatic hematomas have a similar distribution to cortical contusions and occur most frequently in the frontal and temporal lobes (Figs 10–40 and 10–41). While most IPHs are demonstrated on the first CT scan obtained after trauma, the development of "delayed" IPH is not uncommon and is thought to be due to hemorrhage into areas damaged previously by hypoxia or contusion (see Fig 10–22).[68] Delayed IPH may develop after decompression of EDH or SDH or reperfusion of a damaged area that lacks normal autoregulation of cerebral blood flow (CBF).

Post-traumatic cerebral contusions and hematomas are frequently found together (Fig 10–40) and often coexist with extra-axial hematomas (see Figs 10–12, 10–21, and 10–26). "Burst" temporal or frontal lobes are large IPHs in continuity with subdural hemorrhage (see Fig 10–20).

MRI of Contusion and Intraparenchymal Hematomas

The MRI appearance of cerebral contusion and hematoma is dependent on the age of the lesion.[64, 70] A full discussion of the MRI appearance of intracranial hemorrhage is given in Chapter 9. Hemorrhagic contusions and parenchymal hematomas undergo sequential changes in MRI signal characteristics on both short and long TR images. Simplistically, acute intracranial hemorrhage that contains deoxyhemoglobin will be isointense to slightly hypointense on short TR images and markedly hypointense on long TR images (Fig 10–42). Subacute hematomas are of much higher signal intensity than brain is; this is true initially on short TR images and then also on long TR images (Fig 10–43). These changes are ascribed to the paramagnetic effects of first intracellular and then ex-

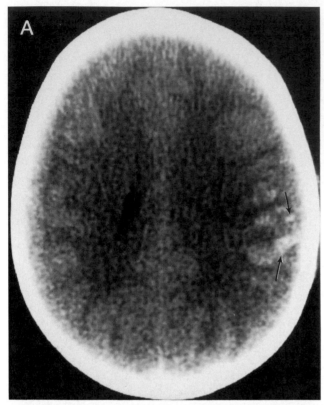

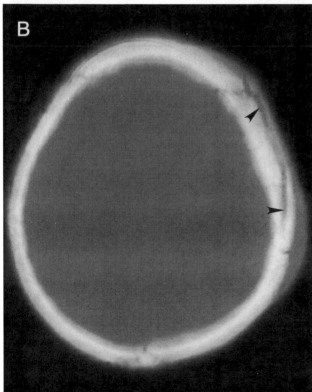

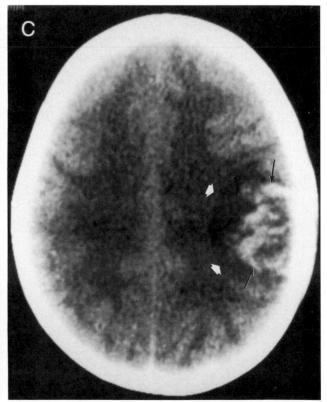

FIG 10–39.
Cortical contusion in a 7-year-old boy struck in the head with a baseball. **A–C,** unenhanced axial CT. **A,** the hemorrhagic component of the left parietal cortical contusion is shown as poorly defined scattered areas of high density in the cortical gyri *(arrows).* **B,** the same image as **A** but filmed with wide bone windows shows a left parietal fracture *(arrowheads),* and scalp swelling. **C,** 24 hours after the initial scan, unenhanced CT shows more extensive cortical hemorrhage *(black arrows)* and surrounding edema *(white arrows).*

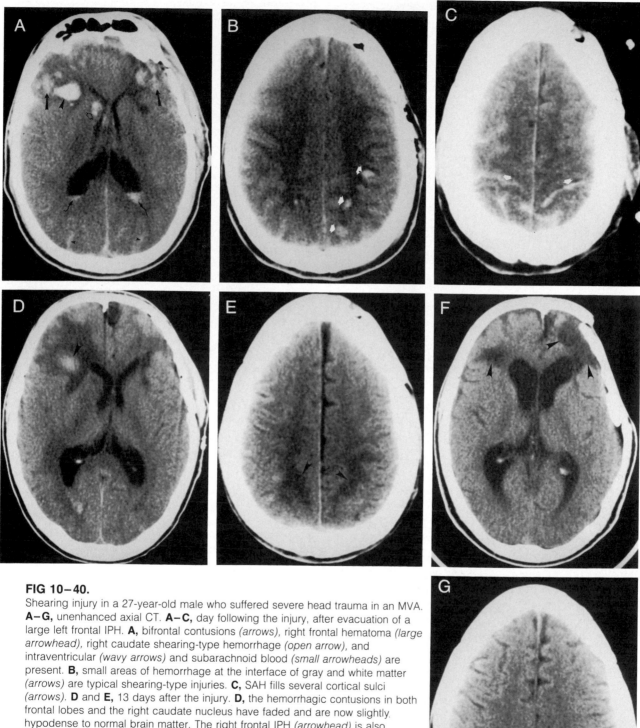

FIG 10−40.
Shearing injury in a 27-year-old male who suffered severe head trauma in an MVA.
A−G, unenhanced axial CT. **A−C,** day following the injury, after evacuation of a
large left frontal IPH. **A,** bifrontal contusions *(arrows),* right frontal hematoma *(large
arrowhead),* right caudate shearing-type hemorrhage *(open arrow),* and
intraventricular *(wavy arrows)* and subarachnoid blood *(small arrowheads)* are
present. **B,** small areas of hemorrhage at the interface of gray and white matter
(arrows) are typical shearing-type injuries. **C,** SAH fills several cortical sulci
(arrows). **D** and **E,** 13 days after the injury. **D,** the hemorrhagic contusions in both
frontal lobes and the right caudate nucleus have faded and are now slightly
hypodense to normal brain matter. The right frontal IPH *(arrowhead)* is also
smaller and less dense and surrounded by an area of low attenuation and mass
effect due to edema. **E,** the gray-white junction hemorrhages have also faded.
Edema, shown by low-density change and swelling *(arrowheads),* persists. **F** and
G, 14 weeks after the injury. The hemorrhage and edema have resolved.
Well-defined areas of low attenuation without mass effect in both frontal lobes
(large arrowheads) and the gray-white interface *(small arrowheads)* represent
permanent scars of gliosis and encephalomalacia. The ventricles and sulci have
enlarged.

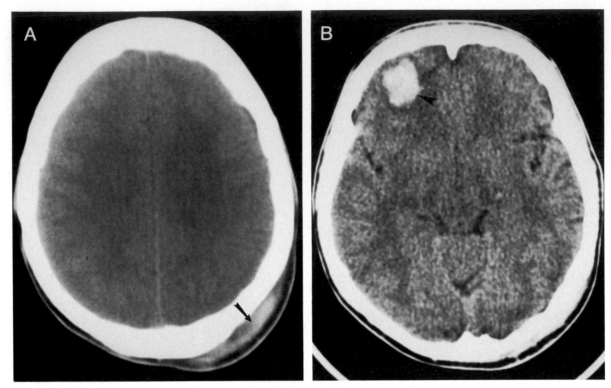

FIG 10–41.
Intraparenchymal, "contre-coup" hematoma in a 34-year-old female who struck the back of her head in a fall. **A** and **B,** unenhanced axial CT. **A,** there is a subgaleal hematoma *(arrow)* at the impact site. **B,** there is an IPH in the right frontal lobe *(arrowhead)* due to shearing forces generated in the fall and impact.

tracellular methemoglobin. Further degradation to hemosiderin results again in low signal intensity with long TR sequences that is most evident on later echo images.[64]

The MRI signal characteristics of brain surrounding an IPH also change over time.[64] Edematous brain surrounds an acute hematoma. Long TR, long TE images are most sensitive to this change and demonstrate edema as areas of high signal intensity (Fig 10–42), while on short TR images edema may appear as areas of mild hypointensity (Fig 10–43). In acute hematomas, there is vivid contrast between low-intensity deoxyhemoglobin and high-intensity edematous brain on long TR images. However, in the extracellular methemoglobin stage, the high-intensity hematoma merges with high-intensity edematous brain structures on long TR images. At this stage short TR images show more contrast between high-intensity hematoma and low-intensity edema (Fig 10–43).[7, 64]

Hemosiderin is deposited in the brain at the periphery of a hematoma; this results in markedly low signal intensity on long TR images.[64] This effect is more pronounced with long echo delay times (Fig 10–44) and higher field strengths. Sig-

nal loss due to hemosiderin may persist indefinitely as a marker of previous hemorrhage. Due to the magnetic susceptibility effects of hemosiderin, gradient-echo scans are more sensitive to the presence of hemosiderin than are conventional spin-echo techniques.[17]

The appearance of cerebral contusions on MRI is also quite variable and depends on the relative amounts of hemorrhage and edema present.[70] Hemorrhagic contusions evolve with signal characteristics similar to hematomas but have less uniform signal intensity due to the heterogeneous mixture of hemorrhage, edema, and necrosis. Acute nonhemorrhagic contusions, or those in which tissue edema and necrosis predominate, will be shown on long TR, long TE images as areas of increased signal intensity relative to normal brain.[7, 8, 70] Short TR images may be unremarkable or show areas of slight hypodensity (Figs 10–42 and 10–45).[70] The signal characteristics of these lesions are nonspecific and resemble many pathologic intracranial processes that prolong T1 and T2 values. MRI (particularly long TR sequences) is much more sensitive to the presence of nonhemorrhagic contusions than CT is. Coronal scans are

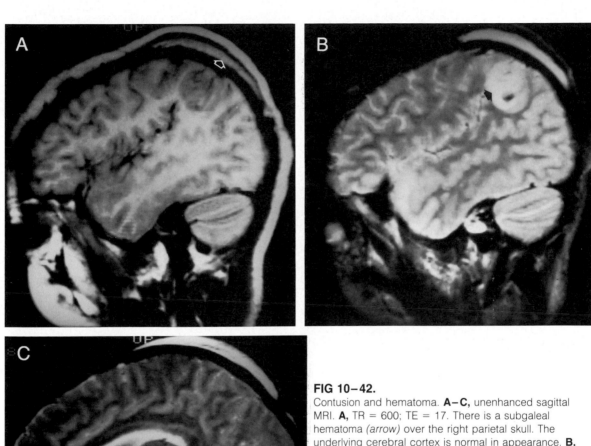

FIG 10–42.
Contusion and hematoma. **A–C,** unenhanced sagittal MRI. **A,** TR = 600; TE = 17. There is a subgaleal hematoma *(arrow)* over the right parietal skull. The underlying cerebral cortex is normal in appearance. **B,** same location as **A** (TR = 2,500, TE = 90). On the more "T2-weighted" image a cortical contusion *(arrow)* is hyperintense to normal brain. The high-signal subgaleal hematoma is again demonstrated. **C,** TR = 2,500; TE = 90. A slice to the left of the midline shows a small, acute hematoma in the left frontal lobe *(arrow)*. The marked hypointensity is thought to be due to the presence of deoxyhemoglobin. Edema surrounding the hematoma is of high signal intensity. (Courtesy of Patrick N. Connaughton, M.D., Lancaster, Penn.)

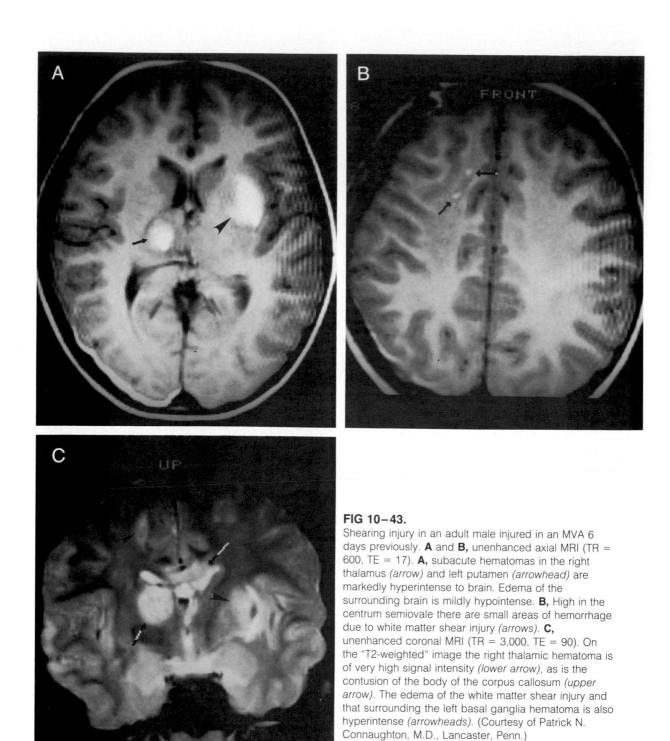

FIG 10–43.
Shearing injury in an adult male injured in an MVA 6 days previously. **A** and **B,** unenhanced axial MRI (TR = 600, TE = 17). **A,** subacute hematomas in the right thalamus *(arrow)* and left putamen *(arrowhead)* are markedly hyperintense to brain. Edema of the surrounding brain is mildly hypointense. **B,** High in the centrum semiovale there are small areas of hemorrhage due to white matter shear injury *(arrows).* **C,** unenhanced coronal MRI (TR = 3,000, TE = 90). On the "T2-weighted" image the right thalamic hematoma is of very high signal intensity *(lower arrow),* as is the contusion of the body of the corpus callosum *(upper arrow).* The edema of the white matter shear injury and that surrounding the left basal ganglia hematoma is also hyperintense *(arrowheads).* (Courtesy of Patrick N. Connaughton, M.D., Lancaster, Penn.)

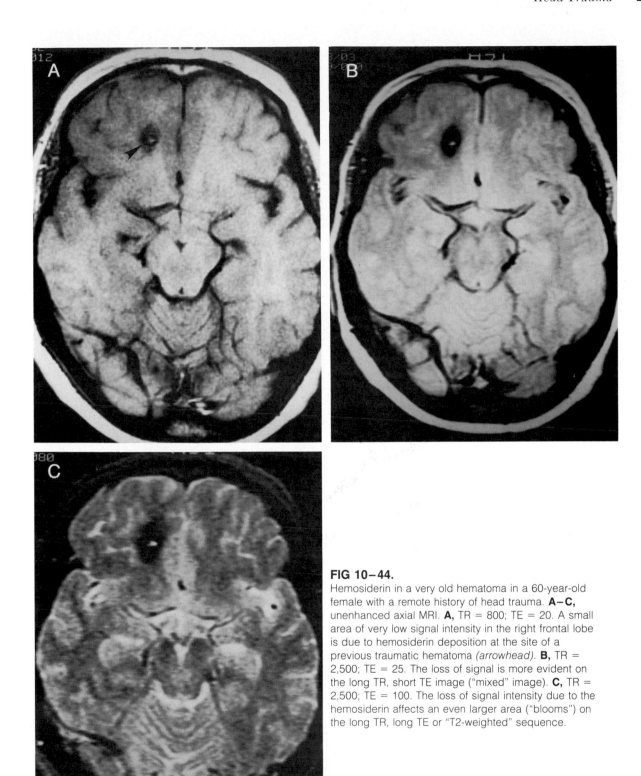

FIG 10–44.
Hemosiderin in a very old hematoma in a 60-year-old
female with a remote history of head trauma. **A–C,**
unenhanced axial MRI. **A,** TR = 800; TE = 20. A small
area of very low signal intensity in the right frontal lobe
is due to hemosiderin deposition at the site of a
previous traumatic hematoma *(arrowhead).* **B,** TR =
2,500; TE = 25. The loss of signal is more evident on
the long TR, short TE image ("mixed" image). **C,** TR =
2,500; TE = 100. The loss of signal intensity due to the
hemosiderin affects an even larger area ("blooms") on
the long TR, long TE or "T2-weighted" sequence.

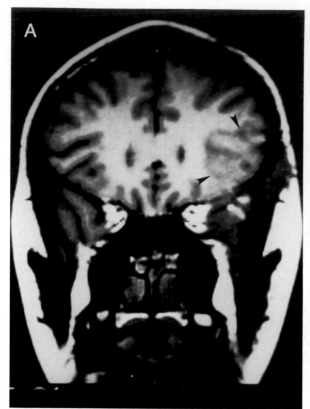

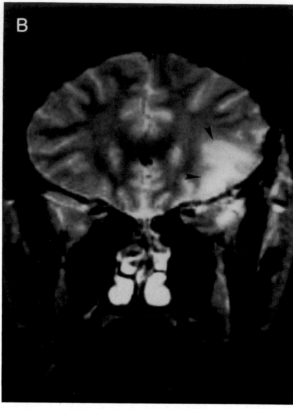

FIG 10–45.

Cortical contusion in a 28-year-old female injured in an MVA. **A** and **B,** unenhanced coronal MRI. **A,** TR = 600; TE = 17. The left frontal gyri are swollen *(arrowheads),* and the subcortical white matter is hypointense to normal white matter. **B,** TR = 2,104; TE = 90. The left frontal contusion is evident as an area of abnormally high signal intensity involving both the gray and white matter *(arrowheads).* (Courtesy of Patrick N. Connaughton, M.D., Lancaster, Penn.)

very helpful in demonstrating the superficial location of cortical contusions (Fig 10–46) and the variable involvement of subjacent white matter (Fig 10–45).

Diffuse Brain Injury

Head trauma that involves moderate to high rates of angular acceleration, typical of that caused by MVAs, may result in diffuse axonal injury (DAI).[13, 14] These "shearing injuries" result from differences in elastic and inertial properties between different but adjacent tissues. They are characterized by disruption of neuronal continuity and are particularly common at the gray-white interfaces, corpus callosum, anterior commissure, basal ganglia, and brain stem (Figs 10–40, 10–43, and 10–47).[71, 72] In the brain stem, shearing injuries commonly affect the dorsal lateral quadrant of the upper pons, the upper midbrain, and the cerebral peduncles. DAI has a poor prognosis, particularly if the brain stem is involved. The subtle CT

changes that follow DAI belie the severity of this type of injury. In more severe cases, vascular as well as neuronal structures are disrupted,[15] and CT then shows scattered hemorrhage (see Figs 10–40, 10–47, and 10–72). CT findings are often normal in the early post-trauma period, however, and may not demonstrate any changes until diffuse cerebral atrophy occurs due to extensive axonal loss.[73]

MRI is much more sensitive than CT is in detecting DAI.[7–9, 11, 70] The pathologic sequelae of shearing injury are axonal disruption, reactive axonal swelling, and infiltration with debris-laden macrophages.[60] Because vascular structures often remain intact, the MRI appearance of most axonal injuries reflects the prolonged T1 and T2 values of increased tissue fluid (edema). Nonhemorrhagic DAI therefore appears on MRI as scattered small areas that are mildly hypointense or isointense to brain on short TR images and hyperintense on long TR images.[8] Long TR sequences are more sensitive than are short TR sequences for detecting

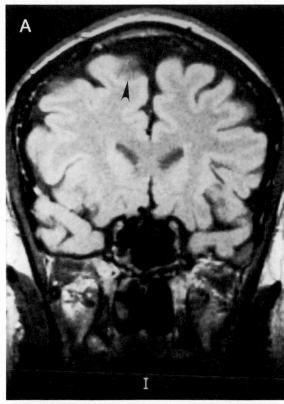

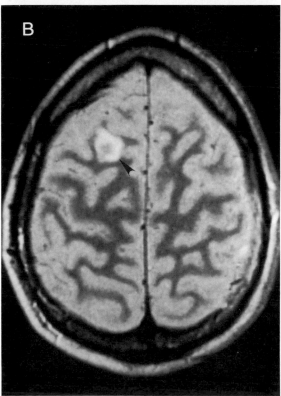

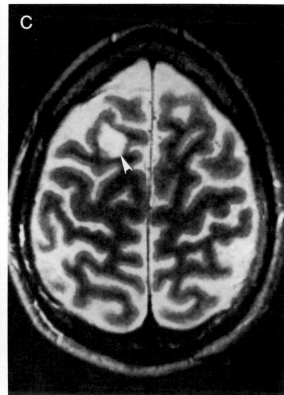

FIG 10–46.
Cortical contusion. **A–C,** unenhanced MRI. **A,** coronal;
TR = 1,000; TE = 40. The contused right posterior
frontal cortex is enlarged and of abnormally low signal
intensity *(arrowhead).* **B** and **C,** axial; TR = 3,000. **B,** TE
= 40. **C,** TE = 80. The cortical contusion is evident as
an area of increased signal intensity *(arrowheads)* on
the long TR sequences. (Courtesy of Peter J. Fedyshin,
M.D., Pittsburgh.)

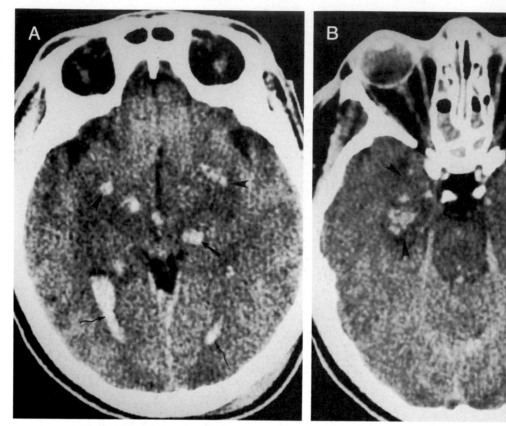

FIG 10–47.
Cerebral contusion and shearing injury in a 46-year-old woman 2 days after a head injury. **A** and **B,** unenhanced axial CT. **A,** there are multiple areas of hemorrhage in the thalamus *(arrow)* and basal ganglia *(arrowheads)* bilaterally due to shearing injury. Intraventricular hemorrhage *(wavy arrows)* is present in both occipital horns. **B,** a more inferior image shows the hemorrhagic contusions in the left inferior temporal gyrus *(arrows)* and right uncus *(arrowheads)*. Low attenuation due to edema in the 2-day-old injuries is well demonstrated.

nonhemorrhagic axonal injuries (Fig 10–48). Sagittal and coronal MRI is particularly helpful in demonstrating lesions of the body of the corpus callosum, while axial scans display abnormalities of the genu and splenium of the corpus callosum, the pons, the midbrain, and the cerebral peduncles to best advantage.

Diffuse Cerebral Swelling and Edema

Diffuse cerebral swelling (DCS) and edema are common although poorly understood sequelae of head trauma. DCS usually occurs in the early post-trauma period and appears on CT as widespread effacement of CSF spaces, including the convexity sulci, basal cisterns, and ventricles, by an enlarged brain that is of normal or slightly increased density (Fig 10–49).[74] While the mechanisms that trigger DCS are not well understood, increased CBF and intracranial blood volume have been demonstrated in both clinical and experimental settings and are presumed to result from a failure of normal autoregulation of cerebral perfusion and the resultant hyperemia.[75, 76] For unknown reasons, DCS is much more common in children than adults.

Brain enlargement in DCS is due to increased blood volume, while in cerebral edema it is due to increased tissue fluid. The increased fluid may be intracellular or extracellular. Cerebral edema may be vasogenic (due to damage of the blood-brain barrier), cytotoxic (due to neuronal damage), hydrostatic (due to a sudden increase in intravascular or perfusion pressure), obstructive (due to transependymal fluid flow in obstructive hydrocephalus), or hypo-osmotic (secondary to serum hypo-osmolality).[77] Cerebral edema after cranial trauma may result from any one or a combination of these mechanisms.

Cerebral edema can be global or focal. Widespread edema often follows regional swelling; this elevates the intracranial pressure (ICP) and com-

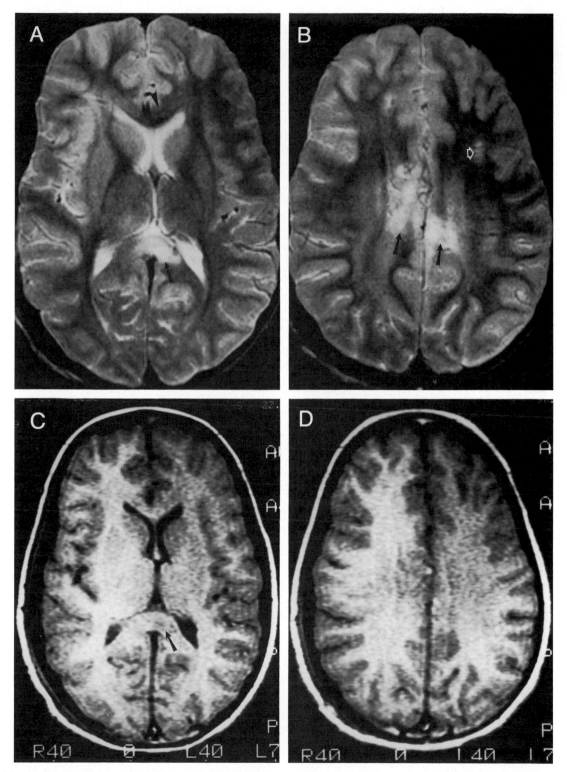

FIG 10–48.
Shearing injury of the corpus callosum. **A–D,** axial unenhanced MRI. **A** and **B,** TR = 2,800; TE = 80. **A,** the shearing injury of the splenium of the corpus callosum *(arrow)* is of markedly increased signal intensity when compared with the normal genu *(arrowhead).* **B,** increased signal marks the shearing injury of the body of the corpus callosum *(arrows)* and gray-white interface *(open arrow).* **C** and **D,** TR = 500; TE = 20. The short TR images (same locations as **A** and **B**) are nearly normal and demonstrate only a subtle region of low signal intensity in the splenium of the corpus callosum *(arrow).* (Courtesy of Orest Boyko, M.D., Durham, NC.)

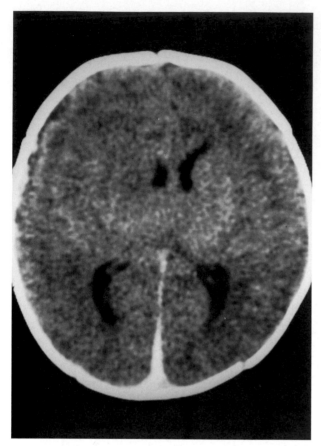

FIG 10–49.
Cerebral swelling in a 2-year-old child injured in an MVA. Unenhanced axial CT on the day of injury shows subtle high density in the white matter and a loss of distinction of the gray-white border in the right frontal lobe. The swollen right frontal lobe slightly effaces the right frontal horn.

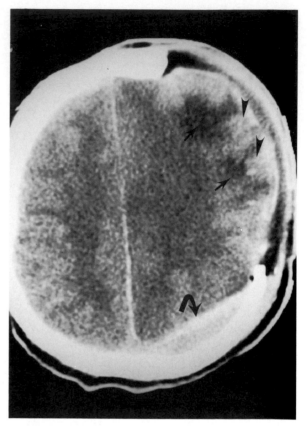

FIG 10–50.
Focal cerebral swelling and postoperative EDH in a 23-year-old male injured in an MVA 2 weeks prior to CT. On the day of injury, a left SDH was removed. Unenhanced axial CT shows the markedly swollen left frontoparietal cortex protruding through the craniectomy site. The swollen brain contains areas of low-density edema *(arrows)* and high-density hemorrhage *(arrowheads)*. The small posterior left EDH *(curved arrow)* developed after removal of the acute SDH.

promises CBF, which leads to diffuse tissue hypoxia. Focal edema occurs in areas of contusion, hematoma, or ischemia (Fig 10–50). In contrast to DCS in which the brain is of normal or slightly increased density, cerebral edema produces abnormal low attenuation in the brain parenchyma on CT, often affecting the central white matter more than the cortical gray matter. In severe edema, however, the gray matter is also abnormally low in density, and this blurs the distinction between gray and white matter (Fig 10–51). Like DCS, diffuse edema causes effacement of the sulci, fissures, and basal cisterns.

DCS usually develops very rapidly after trauma, while diffuse edema develops somewhat more slowly (over a period of hours to days).[78] The two may coexist. The degree of effacement of the basal cisterns on scans obtained within 48 hours of trauma has prognostic significance. Severe swelling or edema implies a poor prognosis. Compressed or absent basal cisterns herald an increased mortality rate.[79]

With resolution of cerebral swelling or edema, low-attenuation subdural effusions may develop over the cerebral hemispheres. These collections are usually self-limited and resolve within several months.[62]

Penetrating Trauma

Penetrating injuries are those in which the integrity of the skull has been disrupted and the brain penetrated by a foreign object (Fig 10–52). Gunshot wounds are a common cause of severe penetrating cranial trauma. Laceration of brain by the bullet and penetrating fragments of dura and bone, blunt force of the bullet's impact with the

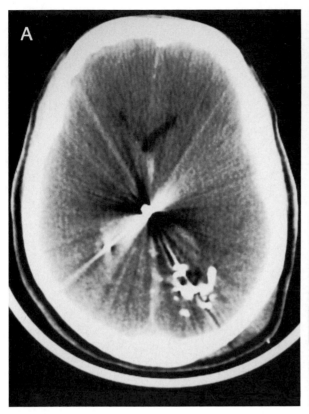

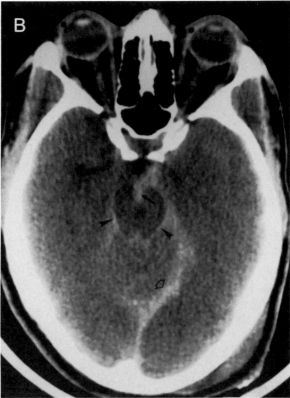

FIG 10–51.
Diffuse cerebral edema and extensive SAH due to a gunshot wound to the head. **A** and **B,** unenhanced axial CT. **A,** the multiple bullet fragments cause considerable streak artifact. **B,** there is a complete loss of distinction between the gray and white matter.

The entire brain is of abnormally low attenuation and diffusely swollen with marked sulcal effacement. Extensive SAH is present in the interpeduncular *(arrow)* and ambient cisterns *(arrowheads)* and along the tentorium *(open arrow).*

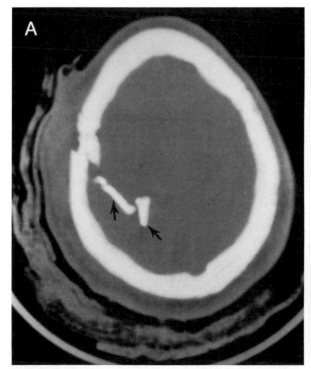

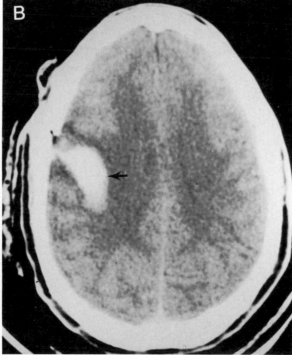

FIG 10–52.
Penetrating injury in a 26-year-old man struck by an airplane propellor. **A** and **B,** unenhanced axial CT on the day of injury. **A,** the propeller and bone fragments *(arrows)* are embedded in the brain.

B, a hematoma is present at the site of penetration *(arrow).* (Courtesy of Helen Roppolo, M.D., Pittsburgh.)

skull, blast effect of propellent gas received from wounds inflicted at close range, and transiently increased intracranial pressure all contribute to brain injury sustained in cranial gunshot wounds.[80] Bullets that fragment cause more extensive injury than do bullets that remain intact. Cranial CT demonstrates the bullet fragments, fractures, lacerations, hematomas, cerebral swelling, and edema (see Fig 10–51). Metal foreign bodies cause considerable streak artifact, and a scan plane angle should be selected that will minimize the number of images that include them. In patients who survive the initial gunshot wound, indriven fragments of devitalized bone, skin, and hair may lead to brain abscess formation.[35]

Penetrating injuries (other than gunshot wounds) in which a moving object strikes the stationary head differ from moving head injuries in

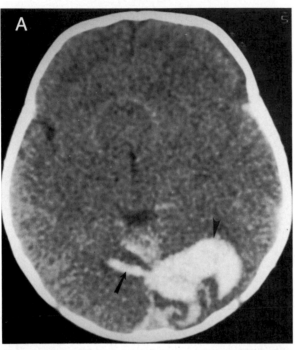

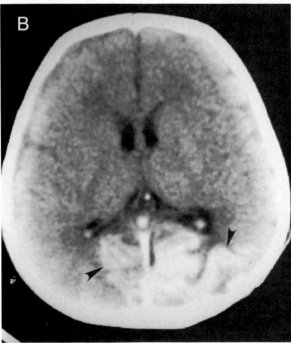

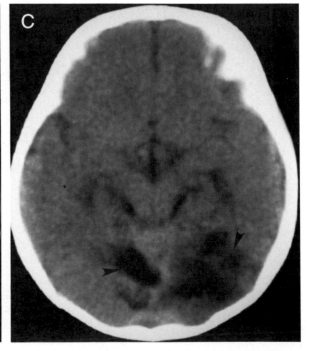

FIG 10–53.
Infarct due to a stab wound in a 3-month-old girl stabbed in the head. **A,** unenhanced CT on the day of injury shows a laceration of the right occipital lobe *(arrow)* and a left occipital hematoma *(arrowhead).* **B,** contrast-enhanced CT 9 days after the injury shows gyral enhancement in the bilateral occipital infarctions *(arrowheads).* **C,** unenhanced CT 2 months after the injury shows bioccipital encephalomalacia and porencephaly *(arrowheads).* The infarcted tissue is replaced with CSF-density fluid.

the extent of potential cerebral damage. In moving head injuries the entire brain is subject to damage by shearing and compressive forces, while in stationary head trauma the primary injury is limited to tissues damaged directly. Penetrating objects (knives, propellers, glass, etc.) cause laceration along the path of entry and may cause extensive bleeding or infarction due to direct vascular injury (Fig 10–53). Open wounds carry the added risk of infection. Nonleaded glass or other foreign material may not be well demonstrated by CT if their attenuation values are similar to brain tissue. On CT wood is usually hypodense to brain (Fig 10–54).[81]

Pneumocephalus

The presence of intracranial air on a CT scan or plain skull films obtained after trauma implies an open fracture or a fracture of an air-containing structure (mastoid air cells, paranasal sinus, or nose) (see Fig 10–4). Intracranial air may be in the subdural (see Fig 10–1), subarachnoid (see Fig 10–4), or epidural spaces (see Fig 10–5) or may be intraventricular (Fig 10–55) or intraparenchymal. To collect in the subarachnoid or subdural spaces, air introduced via a fracture must also cross a dural tear. Pneumocephalus usually resolves within a few weeks unless the dural rent is very large and

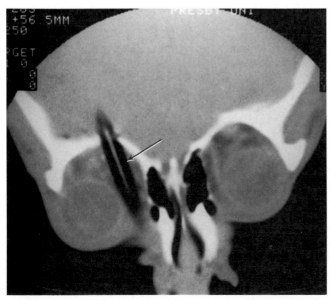

FIG 10–54.
Wooden foreign body in a 13-year-old male with a pencil stuck in his right orbit. Unenhanced coronal CT shows the pencil passing through the right orbit, penetrating the skull, and piercing the right frontal lobe. The wood of the pencil is isodense to air *(arrow).*

persistent. If the tear does not heal, a persistent CSF leak and recurrent meningitis may result (Fig 10–55).

Skull Fractures

CT provides very fine anatomic bone detail when viewed at a wide window width (1,000 to 4,000 HU), especially when bone reconstruction algorithms and thin sections (≤3 mm) are used. CT readily identifies fractures (see Figs 10–11 and 10–39), depressed fragments (see Fig 10–2), and diastatic sutures and can usually replace skull radiographs. A large cooperative study has questioned the efficacy of skull radiographs in trauma patients considered to be at low risk of significant intracranial injury.[82] While nondepressed linear skull fractures did occur in this group of patients, the fractures warranted no specific treatment, and no significant intracranial injuries were detected in the low-risk group. In patients with moderate or high risk of intracranial injury after trauma, CT detects intracranial injuries and usually any skull fractures that may be present. The only fractures likely to escape detection by CT are those parallel to the scan plane. The electronic localizer image provides a reasonable plain lateral view of the skull and should always be inspected for calvarial fractures (see Fig 10–15).

Most skull fractures are linear fractures of the calvarium.[37, 83] Depressed fractures are those in which a fragment is displaced inward an amount equal to or greater than the calvarium's thickness. This may occur as inward bending of both tables (Fig 10–56) or as an abrupt "step-off" (see Fig 10–2). The presence of intracranial air or fluid in the middle ear, mastoid, or sphenoid sinuses should prompt a careful search for basilar skull fractures (see Figs 10–4 and 10–55).

Fractures of the petrous portion of the temporal bone occur parallel to the long axis of the petrous ridge (longitudinal) or perpendicular to the petrous ridge (transverse). Longitudinal fractures are more common, often disrupt the ossicular chain, and in 20% of cases have associated facial paralysis. Transverse fractures are less common, but 50% have associated facial paralysis, and sensorineural hearing loss due to damage of the eighth cranial nerve or inner ear is frequent.[84]

Facial and orbital fractures are also well shown by CT. Coronal images are superior to axial images in demonstrating fractures of the orbital floor and roof. "Blowout" fractures in which a large blunt

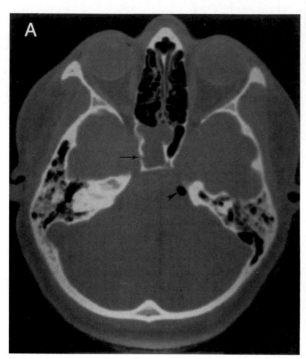

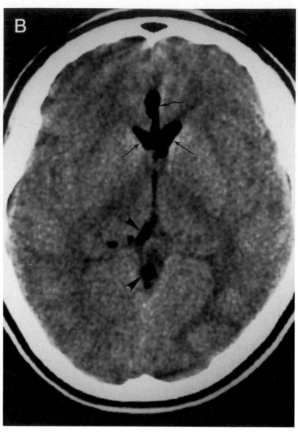

FIG 10–55.
Basal skull fracture, CSF leak, and pneumocephalus in a 15-year-old female with a head injury 1 month earlier and CSF rhinorrhea. **A** and **B,** unenhanced axial CT. **A,** the wide-window image shows a fracture of the wall of the fluid-filled right sphenoid sinus *(arrow)* and a small air bubble near the left petrous apex *(arrowhead)*. **B,** air is present in the ventricles *(arrows)*, retrothalamic cistern *(arrowheads)*, and interhemispheric fissure *(wavy arrow)*.

object strikes the eye usually involve the inferior and medial orbital walls. CT is ideal to assess the extent of the fracture and associated herniation of fat or muscle.

Extracalvarial Soft-Tissue Injury

CT and MRI display acute subgaleal hematomas as fairly well defined but often widespread fluid collections between the skull and skin (Figs 10–22 and 10–57). Elevated, bruised, or avulsed soft tissue is well displayed by CT, as are metal foreign bodies and small air collections in scalp lacerations.

SEQUELAE OF CRANIAL TRAUMA

Patients who survive the primary injuries sustained during head trauma may develop secondary or long-term complications. These include cerebral herniation, vascular compromise, infection, CSF leak, leptomeningeal cyst, hydrocephalus, and atrophy.

Cerebral Herniation

The brain tissue, blood, and CSF that comprise the normal intracranial contents are confined by the supratentorial and infratentorial cavities of the skull. An increase in the volume of one component such as in cerebral swelling, edema, or hematoma necessitates a decrease in the volume of the other components. Since the brain itself is essentially incompressible, the vascular and CSF spaces must compensate for intracranial mass lesions by decreasing in volume. When the "buffering capacity" of these spaces is exceeded, the brain will be displaced around the rigid falx and tentorium. Herniation may occur beneath the falx cerebri (subfalcine), through the tentorial notch (transtentorial), or through the foramen magnum. Symptoms of her-

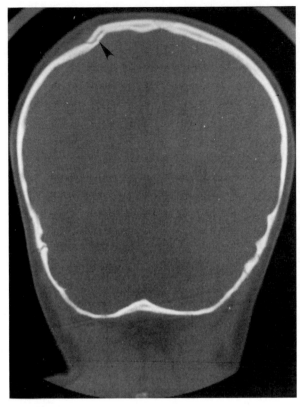

FIG 10–56.
Depressed skull fracture: unenhanced coronal CT. The "bone window" image shows the buckled, depressed right parietal fracture *(arrowhead).*

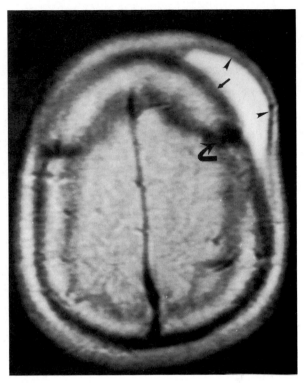

FIG 10–57.
Subgaleal hematoma: unenhanced axial MRI (TR = 2,500, TE = 25). A hyperintense left frontal subgaleal hematoma is interposed between the low-intensity galea *(arrowheads)* and outer table of the skull *(arrow).* The hematoma crosses the coronal suture *(curved arrow).*

niation are due to direct compression of herniated brain and adjacent brain, cranial nerves, and blood vessels.[15, 27, 37, 60]

In subfalcine herniation, the cingulate gyrus is forced beneath the falx. Subfalcine herniation is most easily recognized on coronal images, with tilting of the corpus callosum and compression of the cingulate gyrus against and beneath the falx (Fig 10–58). On axial images, subfalcine herniation is demonstrated by the distortion of the genu of the corpus callosum and lateral ventricle and by a shift of midline structures (Figs 10–21 and 10–58). Compression of the pericallosal artery between the falx and herniated cingulate gyrus may cause infarction in the distribution of the anterior cerebral artery.

The tentorium separates the cerebrum and supratentorial compartment from the infratentorial cerebellum and posterior fossa. The midbrain transverses the tentorial notch. The uncus and hippocampus of the medial temporal lobe rest along the superior surface of the tentorial edge. A supratentorial space-occupying process may cause her-

niation of the uncus or hippocampus over the free edge of the tentorial notch (Fig 10–59). Obliteration of the mesencephalic cistern, medial displacement of the herniated tissue, and distortion of the midbrain are demonstrated on CT[85] or MRI (see Fig 10–21). The ipsilateral oculomotor nerve and posterior cerebral artery are commonly compressed by unilateral uncal herniation, and this causes pupillary dilatation and infarction of the inferior temporal and medial occipital lobes. Compression of the midbrain on the side of the herniation may cause contralateral hemiparesis. Compression of the contralateral cerebral peduncle against the tentorial edge results in hemiparesis ipsilateral to the temporal herniation. This explains the apparent paradox of a dilated pupil ipsilateral to a hemiplegia. The impression the tentorium creates in the contralateral peduncle is known as Kernohan's notch.

Posterior or tectal herniation, in which the parahippocampal gyrus impinges on the midbrain tectum, may produce drowsiness, ptosis, and impaired upward gaze. More severe central transten-

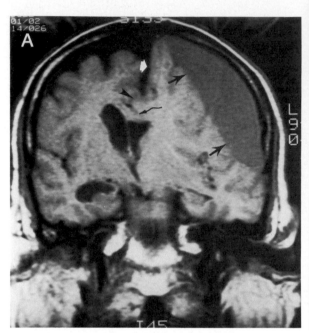

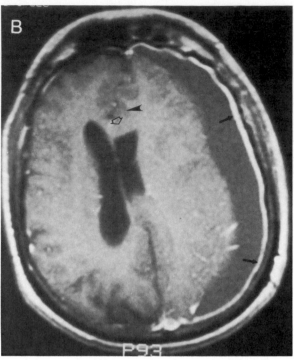

FIG 10–58.
Subfalcine herniation due to SDH. **A,** unenhanced coronal MRI. A large chronic SDH *(black arrows)* compresses the left cerebral hemisphere. The left cingulate gyrus *(arrowhead)* is herniated beneath the falx *(white arrow)*. The corpus callosum is distorted and displaced *(wavy arrow)*. **B,** axial MRI with intravenous gadolinium (TR = 517, TE = 30). The enhanced membrane surrounding the chronic SDH is thicker laterally *(arrows)*. Distortion and displacement of the cingulate gyrus *(arrowhead)* and the corpus callosum *(open arrow)* are shown but are less evident than on the coronal image. (Courtesy of David Shoemaker, M.D., Buffalo.)

torial herniation occurs if the third ventricle and midbrain are displaced downward through the tentorial incisura. As with uncal herniation, the oculomotor nerve and posterior cerebral artery may be compressed. Caudal displacement and compression of the mesencephalon impairs consciousness and respiratory and cardiac function. A downward axial shift of the brain stem can cause stretching and tearing of central perforating basilar artery branches with resultant brain stem ischemia or hemorrhage (Duret hemorrhages).

Severe central transtentorial herniation or a posterior fossa mass may force the cerebellar tonsils downward through the foramen magnum. Herniated tonsils compress the medulla and cause respiratory depression, bradycardia, and hypertension. Posterior fossa masses may also cause upward herniation of the cerebellar hemisphere or vermis through the tentorial notch (Fig 10–60).

Vascular Injuries

Blunt or penetrating injuries to the head, neck, or tonsillar fossa may damage cervical and cerebral vessels.[86] Hyperextension and rotation injuries stretch the internal carotid or vertebral arteries over the lateral masses of C1 and C2.[87] The vertebral artery may be damaged by stretching against the atlantoaxial or atlanto-occipital membranes or foramina transversaria.[88] Basilar fractures may damage the petrous internal carotid artery (ICA),[89] and vertebral fracture at any level above C6 may involve the vertebral artery. Dissection or intimal damage of the cerebral arteries due to stretching or compression may lead to thrombosis or thromboembolism and infarction. Symptoms are commonly delayed for several hours or days after trauma (Fig 10–61).[37, 87, 89]

Cerebral arteries may also be damaged by compression against the falx or tentorium in cerebral herniation. A pseudoaneurysm may develop at the sites of previous arterial lacerations or dissection. Intradural post-traumatic aneurysms are most common in superficial middle cerebral artery (MCA) branches.[60] Traumatic aneurysms may be distinguished from congenital aneurysms by their peripheral location between branch points and the absence of a neck. Post-traumatic cervical pseudo-

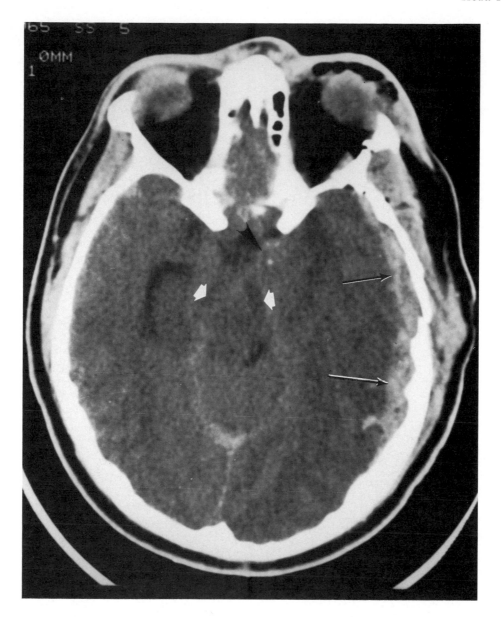

FIG 10–59.
Uncal herniation: unenhanced axial CT (same patient as shown in Fig 10–1). An acute left SDH *(black arrows)* compresses the left cerebral hemisphere, and this causes herniation of the uncus of the temporal lobe *(arrowhead)* over the tentorial edge. The midbrain *(white arrows)* is compressed.

aneurysms of the ICA or vertebral artery also occur.

Trauma is the cause of 75% of direct carotid cavernous fistulas (CCFs),[37] an abnormal communication between the cavernous internal carotid artery or its branches and the venous cavernous sinus. These are usually the result of a frontal impact with sphenoid fracture.[60] Less commonly, CCF results from rupture of an intracavernous carotid aneurysm or dural AVM. Changes of CCF on CT include a convex outer margin of the cavernous sinus, dilated superior ophthalmic vein, enlarged extraocular muscles, and proptosis (Fig 10–62).[90] Symptoms of CCF include orbital bruit, chemosis, and pulsatile exophthalmos.[37]

Cerebrospinal Fluid Leaks

Skull fractures accompanied by lacerations of the dura and arachnoid may be complicated by CSF otorrhea or rhinorrhea (see Fig 10–55). Petrous temporal bone fractures may lead to either otorrhea (via a ruptured tympanic membrane) or rhinorrhea (via the eustachian tube). Fractures of

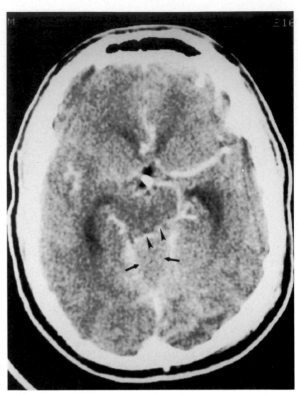

FIG 10–60.
Upward cerebellar herniation: contrast-enhanced axial CT. Due to swelling of the left cerebellar hemisphere following retromastoid craniectomy, the superior cerebellar vermis is herniated upward through the tentorial notch *(arrows)*. The herniated vermis compresses the midbrain tectum *(arrowheads)*.

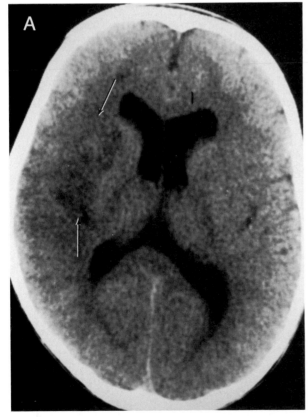

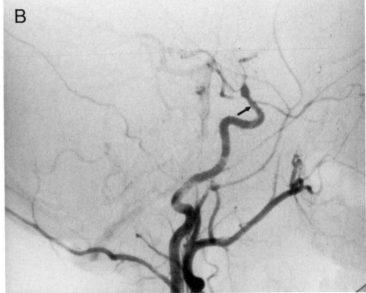

FIG 10–61.
Cerebral artery dissection in a 5-year-old boy with a head injury and intermittent left arm and leg weakness. A dense left hemiparesis developed 9 days after the injury. **A,** unenhanced CT 9 days after the injury shows subtle low attenuation in the right middle cerebral artery distribution *(arrows)*. **B,** an angiogram (right common carotid artery injection) on same day as CT shows irregularity of the distal right ICA *(arrow)* and severe stenosis of the middle and anterior cerebral arteries.

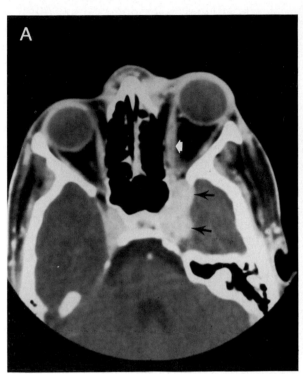

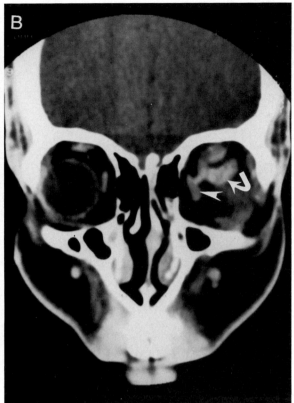

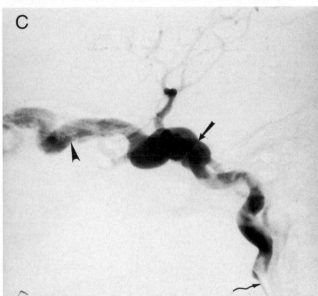

FIG 10–62.
Carotid cavernus sinus fistula in a 17-year-old girl with a head injury and multiple facial fractures 6 months prior to CT. **A,** axial CT with intravenous contrast material. The left cavernous sinus is markedly enlarged, with a lobulated, convex lateral border *(arrows)*. The left globe is proptotic, and the left medial rectus muscle is enlarged *(white arrow)*. **B,** coronal CT with intravenous contrast material shows a dilated and tortuous left superior opthalmic vein *(curved arrow)* and the enlarged medial rectus muscle *(arrowhead)*. **C,** a lateral view of the left internal carotid angiogram demonstrates abnormal opacification of the enlarged left cavernus sinus *(arrow)* and enlarged superior opthalmic vein *(arrowhead)* due to the carotid artery cavernous sinus fistula. The catheter tip is in the high cervical ICA *(wavy arrow)*.

the frontal sinus posterior wall, cribriform plate, or sphenoid sinus also cause CSF rhinorrhea. These patients complain of watery discharge or suffer recurrent bouts of meningitis as infecting organisms ascend from the paranasal sinuses, nose, or ear. Some CSF leaks, especially those occurring in the early post-trauma period, close spontane-

ously.[37] Others require surgery to repair the dural defect.[37, 91]

CT cisternography will often identify the site of leakage. Five milliliters of water-soluble contrast material is placed in the subarachnoid space via lumbar or cervical puncture, and the patient is placed head down for several minutes and imme-

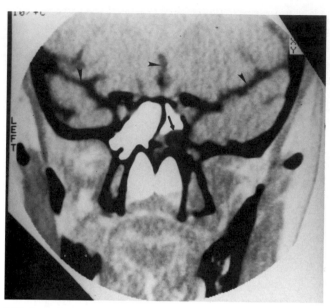

FIG 10–63.
CSF leakage on a cisternogram: coronal CT with contrast material in the subarachnoid space, filmed in reverse mode. Contrast material (which appears dark on the reverse mode) fills the cerebral fissures *(arrowheads)* and has collected in the left sphenoid sinus due to CSF leakage into the sinus *(arrow).*

diately scanned. Coronal scans with the patient prone are preferred. High-attenuation fluid in the sphenoid, frontal, or ethmoid sinuses, nose, or ear locates the leakage site (Fig 10–63). This procedure may be combined with radionuclide cisternography.

Infections

Meningitis and cerebral abscess are potential sequelae of head trauma (especially penetrating trauma) or sinus and skull base fractures associated with dural disruption (Fig 10–64).[37] Pieces of devitalized tissue that are retained in the brain may serve as sources of infection and lead to meningitis, empyema, abscess, or ependymitis.[35]

Leptomeningeal Cyst

Occasionally a calvarial fracture and associated dural tear fail to heal. Protrusion of the leptomeninges (or very rarely brain) through the dural and bone defect may follow.[37, 92] Constant, repeti-

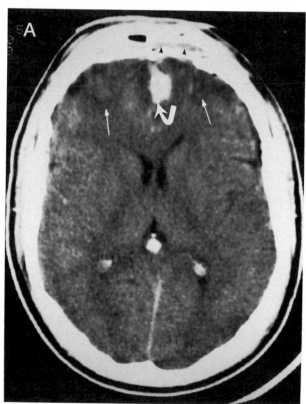

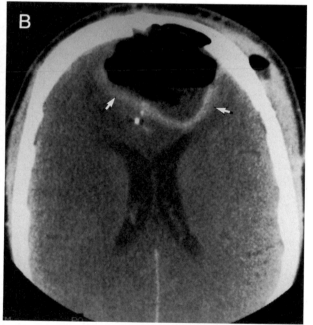

FIG 10–64.
Cerebral abscess. **A,** unenhanced axial CT 2 days after a head injury shows bifrontal edema *(arrows)* and a left frontal IPH *(curved arrow).* There is blood in the left frontal sinus *(arrowheads)* from a sinus fracture (not shown). **B,** CT with intravenous contrast material 1 month after the injury shows an air-containing rim-enhancing cerebral abscess *(arrows).*

tive CSF or vascular pulsations gradually enlarge the defect and cause a "growing" skull fracture or leptomeningeal cyst. The encysted mass of fluid does not communicate freely with the subarachnoid space.[92, 93] These rare lesions, which are probably always associated with significant head injury and contusion of the underlying brain, are found almost exclusively in children.[94] CT or MRI will demonstrate the calvarial defect and protruding soft-tissue mass (Fig 10–65).

Hydrocephalus

Ventricular dilation that develops at the time of or soon after trauma is due to obstructive hydrocephalus.[95] Obstruction may occur at several levels. A posterior fossa hematoma or cerebellar tonsillar herniation can obstruct the fourth ventricle or its outlets. Transtentorial herniation is often associated with compression of the cerebral aqueduct. SAH may block the absorption of CSF at the arachnoid villi, with resultant communicating hydrocephalus developing less acutely but usually within 2 weeks of trauma. DCS or edema compresses the ventricles, but if the process is symmetrical, the ventricles are not displaced. As the swelling or edema resolves, the ventricles "re-expand" and return to normal size, and this stage may be confused with communicating hydrocephalus. Acute communicating hydrocephalus is characterized by rounding of the frontal horns, a prominence of the third ventricle, effacement of cortical sulci, and periventricular lucency due to transependymal passage of CSF.

Atrophy

Loss of brain substance is a common sequela of head injury. Cerebral atrophy may be focal such as a parenchymal scar, porencephalia, or encephalomalacia due to a previous hematoma, contusion, or infarct. Neuronal death or axonal separation with wallerian degeneration of distal axons results in focal volume loss along the nerve's path. Cerebral volume loss after trauma may also be generalized following DAI, ischemia, or severe cerebral edema.[95] Generalized atrophy is manifested on CT and MRI by dilatation of the ventricles, fissures, sulci, and cisterns. Marked atrophy after DAI often reflects a severely debilitating injury (Fig 10–66).[96]

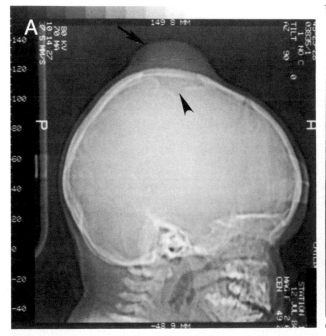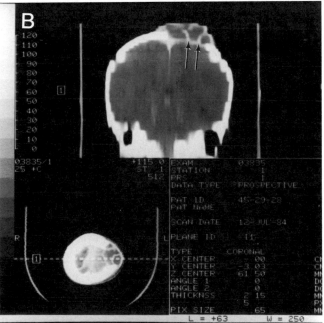

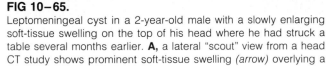

FIG 10–65.
Leptomeningeal cyst in a 2-year-old male with a slowly enlarging soft-tissue swelling on the top of his head where he had struck a table several months earlier. **A,** a lateral "scout" view from a head CT study shows prominent soft-tissue swelling *(arrow)* overlying a cranial defect *(arrowhead).* **B,** the coronal image reformatted from the axial CT, with intravenous contrast material, shows enhancing septations *(arrows)* in the loculated, fluid-filled mass.

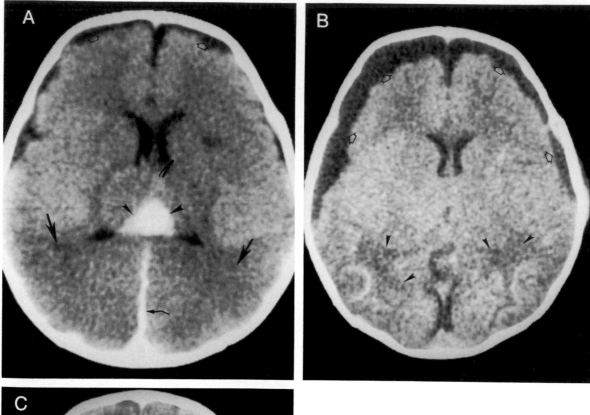

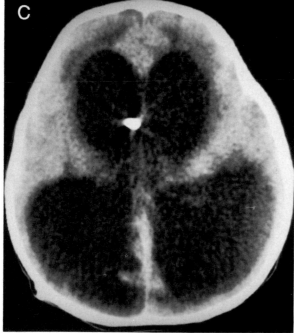

FIG 10–66.
Cerebral edema, subdural hygromas, and post-traumatic atrophy in a 5-month-old girl injured in an MVA. **A–C,** unenhanced axial CT. **A,** CT 1 day after the injury shows low attenuation and sulcal effacement in both occipital lobes due to cerebral swelling and edema *(arrows)*. SAH fills the cistern velum interpositum *(arrowheads)*, and subdural blood fills the posterior interhemispheric fissure *(wavy arrow)*. Acute, low-attenuation bifrontal fluid collections are present *(open arrows)*. **B,** CT 10 days after the injury shows larger bilateral subdural hygromas *(open arrows)*. The occipital gray matter is more well defined, and some of the swelling has resolved. Edema in the white matter persists *(arrowheads)*. **C,** 45 days after the injury severe cerebral atrophy is shown by marked ventricular dilation that persisted despite shunt tube placement. The volume loss is most severe in the occipital lobes.

PEDIATRIC HEAD TRAUMA AND CHILD ABUSE

Children are subject to the same types of head trauma as adults, especially MVAs, but are also uniquely subject to two other forms of trauma, namely, the trauma sustained during birth and that inflicted by caretakers. It is estimated that 1.5 million children are the victims of physical abuse in the United States each year and that 2,000 of these children die as a result of their injuries.[97] Cranial injuries occur in 13% to 25% of abused children and are the leading cause of death in child abuse.[98–100]

As the history of abuse is seldom volunteered and often denied, the clinician and radiologist must consider child abuse when the observed injuries are out of proportion to the history given or when a history of unusual or unlikely trauma is obtained (Fig 10–67). The clinical presentation of abused infants commonly includes lethargy, irritability, breathing difficulties, poor feeding, seizures, and hypotonia.[101, 102] Both impact and nonimpact (or shaking) trauma may cause severe intracranial damage with little external evidence of trauma (Fig 10–68). Shaking trauma with rapid acceleration and deceleration of the head can produce retinal hemorrhages.[103] While retinal hemorrhages are fairly frequently present in newborns due to the process of birth and delivery, these usually resolve within a few days.[104] Retinal hemorrhages occurring in infants more than a few days old should suggest abuse by shaking. The long-term sequelae of cranial trauma in physically abused children can be devastating and include blindness, porencephaly, encephalomalacia, and atrophy. Mental retardation may result from cumulative axonal injury in battered infants.[103]

While no single CT feature is diagnostic of physical abuse, some types of injury have been observed in abused children more often than those subject to accidental trauma and should raise suspicion of abuse. Interhemispheric SDHs have been associated with child abuse, but with a highly variable frequency (8% to 58%).[100, 101] Interhemispheric SDH generally occurs posteriorly. A very small acute interhemispheric SDH may be difficult to differentiate from a normal but prominent falx. SAH or cerebral edema of the parasagittal brain also may mimic interhemispheric SDH.[105] In some cases follow-up scans are required to make the diagnosis. Convexity SDHs are also fairly common in abused children with head injuries.[93]

Occasionally the head CT of an infant will demonstrate bilateral, low-attenuation, subdural fluid collections; widened cerebral sulci; and prominent ventricles, fissures, and basal cisterns.[106] This appearance mimics diffuse cerebral volume loss or atrophy, but clinical examination reveals a tense fontanelle and macrocrania,[106, 107] and the subdural fluid typically has a high protein content.[108] This condition is referred to as benign subdural effusion of infancy (Fig 10–69). Affected infants are typically 3 to 6 months of age.[106, 108] While trauma or meningitis may precede subdural effusion in some cases, in the majority no specific etiology for the effusions can be determined.[108]

Skull fractures are common findings in abused

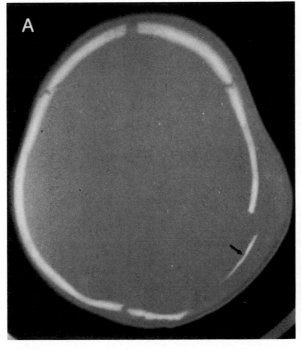 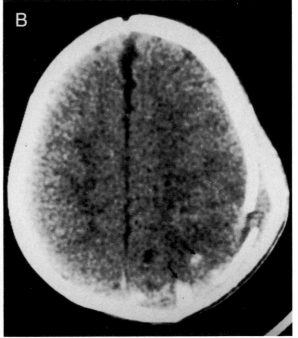

FIG 10–67.
Child abuse in a 5-month-old girl who "fell down stairs." **A** and **B,** unenhanced axial CT. **A,** the "bone window" image shows a comminuted, elevated left parietal fracture *(arrow)* and scalp swelling.

B, swollen brain with small areas of hemorrhage *(arrows)* elevates and protrudes through the fractured skull.

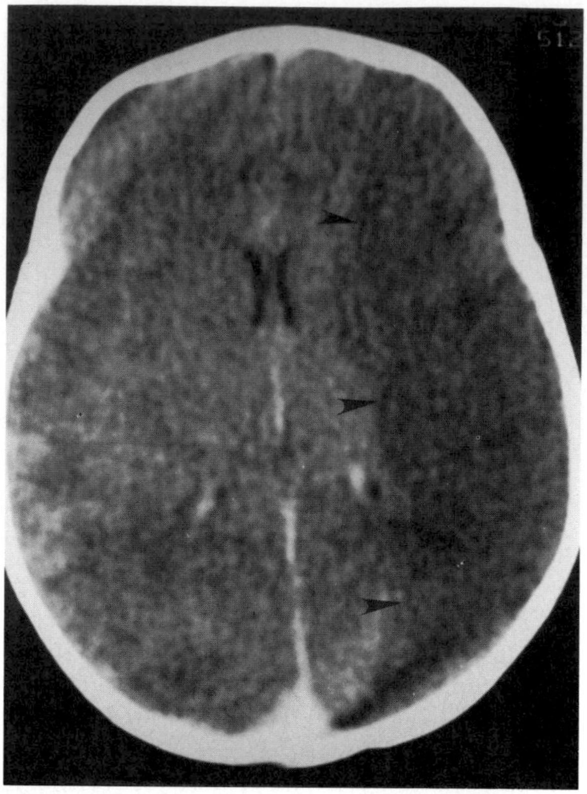

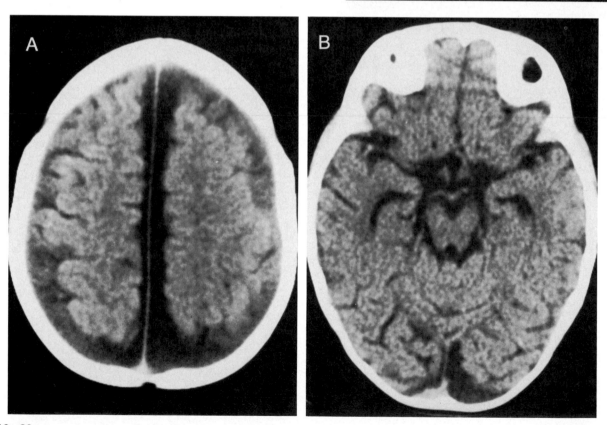

FIG 10–68.
Child abuse in a 5-year-old boy who was shaken. Unenhanced axial CT shows low density and mass effect of an acute left MCA infarct *(arrowheads)*.

FIG 10–69.
Benign subdural effusion of infancy in a 10-month-old male with a large head. **A** and **B,** unenhanced axial CT. **A,** hypodense subdural fluid collections overlie both cerebral hemispheres. **B,** the peri-mesencephalic and suprasellar cisterns, lateral ventricle temporal horns, and cortical sulci are all prominent.

children with head injuries. While the majority (88%) are simple linear fractures, fractures that are multiple or bilateral or cross sutures result more often from child abuse than accidental injuries (Fig 10–70).[109] SAH is very common in abused children with head injuries.[105]

Children who sustain accidental or intentional trauma may demonstrate any of the parenchymal, extra-axial, or extracranial injuries described in previous sections. There are, however, differences in the way the pediatric and more mature brain respond to trauma. The pediatric brain will more frequently develop severe swelling or edema. Either process may be focal, multifocal, or diffuse (Fig 10–70). Severe edema may be evident on CT as the "reversal sign"—a pattern in which the gray matter has lower attenuation than the white matter.[105] DCS associated with increased CBF and blood volume causes diffuse brain enlargement with normal to slightly increased attenuation. While the pathophysiology of cerebral swelling and edema is poorly understood, uncontrollable cerebral edema is a common cause of death in children with severe head injuries.[102]

An injury nearly unique to the young brain is nonhemorrhagic tear (also called contusional tear) of the white matter. These white matter rents usually spare the overlying cortex and occur in patients under 5 months of age.[60, 93] Cortical contusions and IPHs are less common in infants and young children than in older patients due to the relatively smooth inner surface of the skull.[93]

Infants may suffer cranial injury during delivery. During labor and birth, the infant's head is molded to allow its passage through the birth canal. Pressure and molding forces may be sufficient to cause fracture or subarachnoid, intraparenchymal, or subdural hemorrhages (Fig 10–71). "Ping-Pong ball fractures, named for their resemblance to dents in a Ping-Pong ball, result from pressure of the infant's head against the maternal pelvis.[94] These fractures usually do not resolve spontaneously.[37] The molding forces commonly produce tears of the falx and/or tentorium, and this produces focal collections of blood between the leaves of the dura that resolve spontaneously.

Diffuse SAH in infants may be caused by a traumatic delivery or hypoxic-ischemic insults.[110]

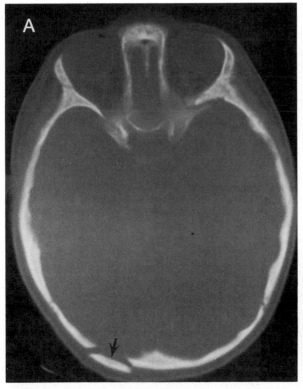 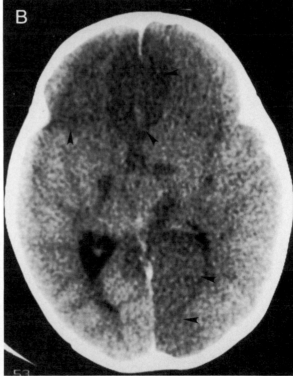

FIG 10–70.
Child abuse in a 1-year-old girl. **A** and **B,** unenhanced axial CT. **A,** a bone algorithm (edge enhancement) image shows a comminuted, elevated occipital fracture *(arrow).* **B,** there are widespread, multifocal areas of low attenuation and mass effect due to cerebral edema *(arrowheads).*

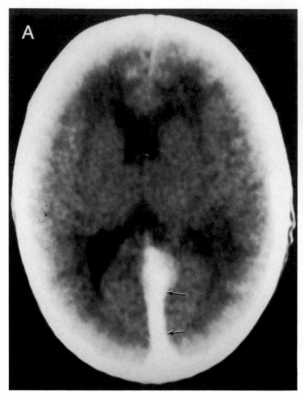

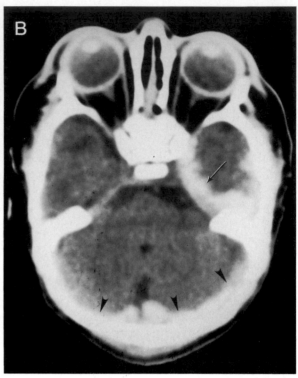

FIG 10–71.
Birth trauma in a full-term baby boy following a difficult vaginal delivery. **A** and **B,** unenhanced axial CT. **A,** an acute, hyperdense SDH occupies the posterior interhemispheric fissure *(arrows).* **B,** the subdural hematoma extends into the left middle cranial fossa *(arrow).* Bilateral posterior fossa subdura hematomas are present *(arrowheads).*

FIG 10–72.
Choroid plexus hemorrhage in a full-term infant with recurrent apnea and bloody CSF following a traumatic delivery. Unenhanced axial CT shows bilateral, hyperdense enlargement of the choroid plexus bilaterally *(arrows)* due to hemorrhage. There is intraventricular hemorrhage as well *(arrowhead).*

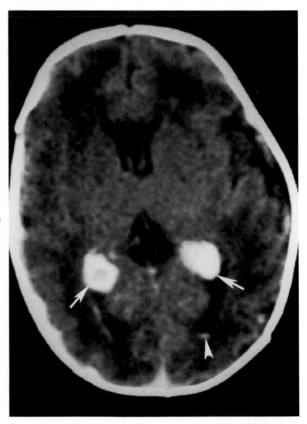

Cerebellar hemorrhages and posterior fossa SDHs in infants are usually associated with traumatic deliveries and occur with full-face presentations because the occiput and neck are hyperextended around the pelvic outlet. In full-term neonates hemorrhage into the cerebral hemispheres may occur without a history of trauma or hypoxia.[110, 111] Choroid plexus hemorrhages are more common in full-term than premature infants (Fig 10–72).[93]

Extracranial manifestations of the delivery pro-

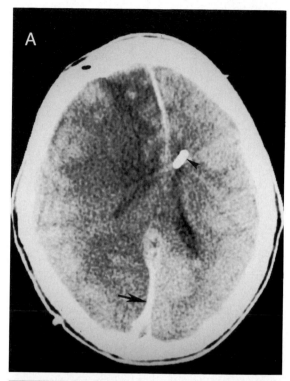

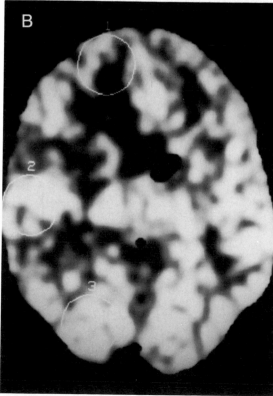

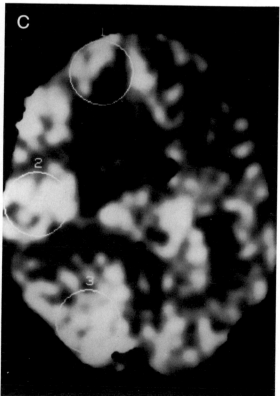

FIG 10–73.
Loss of cerebral autoregulation in a 21-year-old male who had a large right SDH evacuated 1 day previously. **A,** unenhanced axial CT shows marked swelling and edema of the right cerebral hemisphere, a small residual interhemispheric SDH *(arrow)*, and a shunt tube in the left lateral ventricle *(arrowhead)*. **B** and **C,** xenon-enhanced CBF CT study. **B,** $pCO_2 = 38$. With a normal level of pCO_2 there is diffuse hyperemia. CBF in the right MCA *(region of interest no. 2)* measures 81.8 cc/100 g tissue per minute. In the corresponding area *on the left,* the blood flow measures 79.2 cc/100 g/min. **C,** $pCO_2 = 29$. After hyperventilation, the left cerebral hemisphere responds in the expected way, with a reduction in blood flow to 45.8 cc/100 g/min. The perfusion of the injured right brain *(region of interest no. 2)* that lacks normal antoregulatory mechanisms does not change (75.4 cc/100 g/min).

cess include caput succedaneum and cephalohematoma. Caput succedaneum is rather diffuse scalp swelling over the presenting part of the head, while cephalohematoma is a localized accumulation of blood beneath the periosteum, usually of the parietal bone. Because of its subperiosteal location, cephalohematoma is well defined and limited to one cranial bone's outer surface by the periosteal attachment at the suture. Periosteum elevated by a cephalohematoma may quickly calcify.

XENON/CT IN CRANIAL TRAUMA

CT accurately demonstrates anatomic changes that result from cranial trauma but provides limited physiologic information. The xenon/CT method of CBF determination (XE/CT CBF) provides a prompt, quantitative perfusion measurement that may be used to guide therapy. A full discussion of the method is presented in Chapter 6. Extra-axial or intraparenchymal hematomas or diffuse enlargement of the cerebral hemispheres may compromise CBF locally by direct compression or herniation or diffusely by elevated ICP.

Increased ICP is a common problem in patients with head injuries. The management of elevated ICP often includes hyperventilation in an attempt to limit cerebral swelling and edema by controlling cerebral perfusion. Hyperventilation causes a decrease in pCO_2, which in turn normally decreases CBF. There is, however, wide individual variation in the response to hyperventilation, and even moderate reductions in pCO_2 can significantly compromise CBF.[112] Also, damaged tissue with abnormal CBF autoregulation may not respond to hyperventilation (Fig 10–73). XE/CT CBF studies may be easily obtained at different levels of pCO_2 and used to select the proper level of ventilation.

Severe hyperemia in the early post-trauma period despite hyperventilation reflects severe dysfunction with a loss of autoregulation of CBF[113] and often presages a poor clinical outcome.[114, 115] Xenon/CT CBF studies may aid in documenting brain death by demonstrating a lack of blood flow in all cerebral compartments.

REFERENCES

1. Baker SP, O'Neill B, Karpf RS: *The Injury Fact Book*. Boston, DC Health & Co., 1984.
2. Baker CC, Oppenheimer L, Stephens B, et al: Epidemiology of trauma deaths. *Am J Surg* 1980; 140:144–150.
3. Jagger J, Vernberg K, Jane JA: Air bags: Reducing the toll of brain trauma. *Neurosurgery* 1987; 20:815–817.
4. Kalsbeek WD, McLaurin RL, Harris BSH, et al: The national head and spinal cord injury survey: Major findings. *J Neurosurg* 1980; 53:519–531.
5. Kraus JF: Epidemiology of head injury, in Cooper PR (ed): *Head Trauma*, ed 2. Baltimore, Williams & Wilkins, 1987, pp 1–19.
6. Han JS, Kaufman B, Alfidi R, et al: Head trauma evaluated by magnetic resonance and computed tomography: A comparison. *Radiology* 1984; 150:71–77.
7. Zimmerman RA, Bilaniuk LT, Hackney DB, et al: Head injury: Early results of comparing CT and high-field MR. *AJNR* 1986; 7:757–764.
8. Gentry LR, Godersky JC, Thompson B, et al: Prospective comparative study of intermediate-field MR and CT in the evaluation of closed head trauma. *AJNR* 1988; 9:91–100.
9. Kelly AB, Zimmerman RD, Snow RB, et al: Head trauma. Comparison of MR and CT—Experience in 100 patients. *AJNR* 1988; 9:699–708.
10. Snow RB, Zimmerman RD, Gandy SE, et al: Comparison of magnetic resonance imaging and computed tomography in the evaluation of head trauma. *Neurosurgery* 1986; 18:45–52.
11. Wilberger JR Jr, Deeb ZL, Rothfus WE: Magnetic resonance imaging in cases of severe head injury. *Neurosurgery* 1987; 20:571–576.
12. Ommaya AK, Faas F, Yarnell P: Whiplash injury and brain damage. *JAMA* 1968; 204:285–289.
13. Gennarelli TA, Thibault LE, Adams JH, et al: Diffuse axonal injury and traumatic coma in the primate. *Ann Neurol* 1982; 12:564–574.
14. Gennarelli TA, Thibault LE: Biomechanics of acute subdural hematoma. *J Trauma* 1982; 22:680–686.
15. Gennarelli TA, Thibault LE: Biomechanics of head injury, in Wilkins RH, Rengachary SS (eds): *Neurosurgery*. New York, McGraw-Hill International Book Co, 1985, pp 1531–1535.
16. Mauser HW, Nieuwenhiuzen OV, Veiga-Pires JA: Is contrast-enhanced CT indicated in acute head injury? *Neuroradiology* 1984; 26:31–32.
17. Atlas SW, Mark AS, Grossman RI, et al: Intracranial hemorrhage: Gradient-echo MR imaging at 1.5T. *Radiology* 1988; 168:803–807.
18. Ford LE, McLaurin RL: Mechanisms of extradural hematomas. *J Neurosurg* 1963; 20:760–769.
19. Gallagher JP, Browder EJ: Extradural hematoma. Experience with 167 patients. *J Neurosurg* 1968; 29:1–12.
20. New PFJ, Aronow S: Attenuation measurements of whole blood and blood fractions in computed tomography. *Radiology* 1976; 121:635–640.

21. Zimmerman RA, Bilaniuk LT: Computed tomographic staging of traumatic epidural bleeding. *Radiology* 1982; 144:809–812.

22. Petersen OF, Espersen JO: How to distinguish between bleeding and coagulated extradural hematomas on the plain CT scanning. *Neuroradiology* 1984; 26:285–292.

23. McLaurin RL, Ford LE: Extradural hematoma. Statistical survey of forty-seven cases. *J Neurosurg* 1964; 21:364–371.

24. Jamieson KG, Yelland JDN: Extradural Hematoma. Report of 167 cases. *J Neurosurg* 1968; 29:13–23.

25. Cordobes F, Ramiro DL, Rivas JJ, et al: Observations on 82 patients with extradural hematoma. Comparison of results before and after the advent of computerized tomography. *J Neurosurg* 1981; 54:179–186.

26. Singounas EG, Volikas ZG: Epidural haematoma in a pediatric population. *Childs Brain* 1984; 11:250–254.

27. Miller JD, Becker DP: General principles and pathophysiology of head injury, in Youmans JR (ed): *Neurological Surgery*. Philadelphia, WB Saunders Co, 1982, pp 1896–1937.

28. Weaver D, Pobereskin L, Jane JA: Spontaneous resolution of epidural hematomas. Report of two cases. *J Neurosurg* 1981; 54:248–251.

29. Pang D, Horton JA, Herron JM, et al: Nonsurgical management of extradural hematomas in children. *J Neurosurg* 1983; 59:958–971.

30. Iwakuma T, Brunngraber CV: Chronic extradural hematomas. A study of 21 cases. *J Neurosurg* 1973; 38:488–493.

31. Sparacio RR, Khatib R, Chiu J, et al: Chronic epidural hematoma. *J Trauma* 1972; 12:435–439.

32. Fukamachi A, Koizumi H, Nageseki Y, et al: Postoperative extradural hematomas: Computed tomographic survey of 1105 intracranial operations. *Neurosurgery* 1986; 19:589–593.

33. Scotti G, Terbrugge K, Melancon D, et al: Evaluation of the age of subdural hematomas by computerized tomography. *J Neurosurg* 1977; 47:311–315.

34. Williams AL: Trauma, in Williams AL, Haughton VM (eds): *Cranial Computed Tomography. A Comprehensive Text*. St Louis, CV Mosby Co, 1985, pp 37–87.

35. Becker DP, Miller JD, Youry HF, et al: Diagnosis and treatment of head injury in adults, in Youmans JR (ed): *Neurological Surgery*. Philadelphia, WB Saunders Co, 1982, pp 1938–2083.

36. Cooper PR: Traumatic intracranial hematomas, in Wilkins RH, Rengachary SS (eds): *Neurosurgery*. New York, McGraw-Hill International Book Co, 1985, pp 1657–1666.

37. Dacey RG Jr, Jane JA: Craniocerebral trauma, in Joynt RJ (ed): *Clinical Neurology*. Philadelphia, JB Lippincott, 1988, pp 30–31.

38. O'Brien PK, Norris JW, Tator CH: Acute subdural hematomas of arterial origin. *J Neurosurg* 1974; 41:435–439.

39. Jones NR, Blumbergs PC, North JB: Acute subdural haematomas. Aetiology, pathology and outcome. *Aust NZ J Surg* 1986; 56:907–913.

40. Shenkin HA: Acute subdural hematoma. Review of 39 consecutive cases with high incidence of cortical artery rupture. *J Neurosurg* 1982; 57:254–257.

41. Rengachary SS, Szymanski DC: Subdural hematomas of arterial origin. *Neurosurgery* 1981; 8:166–172.

42. Adams JH: The neuropathology of head injuries, in Vinken PJ, Bruyn GW (eds): *Handbook of Clinical Neurology. Injuries of the Brain and Skull. Part I*. Amsterdam, North Holland Publishing Co, 1975, p 35.

43. Fell DA, Fitzgerald S, Moiel RH, et al: Acute subdural hematomas. Review of 144 cases. *J Neurosurg* 1975; 42:37–42.

44. Reed D, Robertson WD, Graeb DA, et al: Acute subdural hematomas; atypical CT findings. *AJNR* 1986; 7:417–421.

45. Greenberg J, Cohen WA, Cooper PR: The "hyperacute" extraaxial intracranial hematoma: Computed tomographic findings and clinical significance. *Neurosurgery* 1985; 17:48–56.

46. Smith WP, Batnitzky S, Rengachary SS: Acute isodense subdural hematomas: A problem in anemic patients. *AJNR* 1981; 2:37–40.

47. Amendola MA, Ostrum BJ: Diagnosis of isodense subdural hematomas by computed tomography. *AJR* 1977; 129:693–697.

48. Kim KS, Hemmati M, Weinberg PE: Computed tomography in isodense subdural hematoma. *Radiology* 1978; 128:71–74.

49. Moller A, Ericson K: Computed tomography of isoattenuating subdural hematomas. *Radiology* 1979; 130:149–152.

50. Braun J, Borovich B, Guilburd JN, et al: Acute subdural hematoma mimicking epidural hematoma on CT. *AJNR* 1987; 8:171–173.

51. Zimmerman RD, Russell EJ, Yurberg E, et al: Falx and interhemispheric fissure on axial CT: II. Recognition and differentiation of interhemispheric subarachnoid and subdural hemorrhage. *AJNR* 1982; 3:635–642.

52. Zimmerman RA, Bilaniuk LT, Bruce D, et al: Interhemispheric acute subdural hematoma: A computed tomographic manifestation of child abuse by shaking. *Neuroradiology* 1978; 16:39–40.

53. Lau LSW: The computed tomographic findings of peritentorial subdural hemorrhage. *Radiology* 1983; 146:699–701.

54. Naidich TP, Leeds NE, Kricheff II, et al: The tentorium of axial section. II. Lesion localization. *Radiology* 1977; 123:639–648.

55. Bergstrom M, Ericson K, Levander B, et al: Varia-

tions with time of the attenuation values of intracranial hematomas. *J Comput Assist Tomogr* 1977; 1:57–63.

56. Karasawa H, Tomita S, Suzuki S: Chronic subdural hematomas. Time-density curve and iodine concentration in enhanced CT. *Neuroradiology* 1987; 29:36–39.

57. Fogelholm R, Waltiro O: Epidemiology of CSFH. *Acta Neurochir (Wien)* 1975; 32:247–250.

58. Markwalder TM: Chronic subdural hematomas: A review. *J Neurosurg* 1981; 54:637–642.

59. Cameron M: Chronic subdural haematoma: A review of 114 cases. *J Neurol Neurosurg Psychiatry* 1978; 41:834–839.

60. McCormick WF: Pathology of closed head injury, in Wilkins RH, Rengachary SS (eds): *Neurosurgery*. New York, McGraw-Hill International Book Co, 1985, pp 1544–1569.

61. Hoff J, Bates E, Barnes B, et al: Traumatic subdural hygroma. *J Trauma* 1973; 13:870–876.

62. Kishore PRS, Lipper MH, Domingues de Silva AA, et al: Delayed sequelae of head injury. *CT: J Comput Tomogr* 1980; 4:287–295.

63. Chakeres DW, Bryan RN: Acute subarachnoid hemorrhage: In vitro comparison of magnetic resonance and computed tomography. *AJNR* 1986; 7:223–228.

64. Gomori JM, Grossman RI, Hackney DB, et al: Variable appearances of subacute intracranial hematomas on high-field spin-echo MR. *AJR* 1988; 150:171–178.

65. Sipponen JT, Sepponen RE, Sivula A: Chronic subdural hematoma: Demonstration by magnetic resonance. *Radiology* 1984; 150:79–85.

66. Dawson SL, Hirsch CS, Lucas FV, et al: *Hum Pathol* 1980; 11:155–166.

67. Tsai FY, Huprich JE: Further experience with contrast-enhanced CT in head trauma. *Neuroradiology* 1978; 16:314–317.

68. Gudeman SK, Kishore PRS, Miller JD, et al: The genesis and significance of delayed traumatic intracerebral hematoma. *Neurosurgery* 1979; 5:309–313.

69. Dolinskas CA, Bilaniuk LT, Zimmerman RA, et al: Computed tomography of intracerebral hematomas. I. Transmission CT observations on hematoma resolution. *AJR* 1977; 129:681–688.

70. Hesselink JR, Dowd CF, Healy ME, et al: MR imaging of brain contusions: A comparative study with CT. *AJNR* 1988; 9:269–278.

71. Strich SJ: Diffuse degeneration of the cerebral white matter in severe dementia following head injury. *J Neurol Neurosurg Psychiatry* 1956; 19:163–185.

72. Zimmerman RA, Bilaniuk LT, Genneralli T: Computed tomography of shearing injuries of the cerebral white matter. *Radiology* 1978; 127:393–396.

73. Lobato RD, Sarabia R, Rivas JJ, et al: Normal computerized tomography scans in severe head injury. Prognostic and clinical management implications. *J Neurosurg* 1986; 65:784–789.

74. Zimmerman RA, Bilaniuk LT, Bruce D, et al: Computed tomography of pediatric head trauma: Acute general cerebral swelling. *Radiology* 1978; 126:403–408.

75. Bruce DA, Alavi A, Bilaniuk L, et al: Diffuse cerebral swelling following head injuries in children: The syndrome of "malignant brain edema." *J Neurosurg* 1981; 54:170–178.

76. Langfitt TW, Tannanbaum HM, Kassell NF: The etiology of acute brain swelling following experimental head injury. *J Neurosurg* 1966; 24:47–56.

77. Adams JH, Corsellis JAN, Duchen LW: Hydrocephalus, in Adams JH, Corsellis JAN, Duchen LW (eds): *Greenfield's Neuropathy*, ed 4. New York, John Wiley & Sons, Inc, 1984, pp 67–84.

78. Ito U, Tomita H, Yamazaki S, et al: Brain swelling and brain edema in acute head injury. *Acta Neurochir* 1986; 79:120–124.

79. Toutant SM, Klauber MR, Marshall LF, et al: Absent or compressed basal cisterns on first CT scan: Ominous predictors of outcome in severe head injury. *J Neurosurg* 1984; 61:691–694.

80. Selden BS: Craniocerebral wound ballistics. *Indiana Med* 1987; 80:150–152.

81. Healy JF: Computed tomography of a cranial wooden foreign body. *J Comput Assist Tomogr* 1980; 4:555–556.

82. Masters SJ, McClean PM, Arcarese JS, et al: Skull x-ray examinations after head trauma. *N Engl J Med* 1987; 316:84–91.

83. Thomas LM: Skull fractures, in Wilkins RH, Rengachary SS (eds): *Neurosurgery*. New York, McGraw-Hill International Book Co, 1985.

84. Swartz JD: *Imaging of the Temporal Bone*. New York, Theme Medical Publishers, Inc, 1986.

85. Osborn AG: Diagnosis of descending transtentorial herniation by cranial computed tomography. *Radiology* 1977; 123:93–96.

86. Youmans JR, Mims TJ Jr: Trauma to the carotid arteries, in Youmans JR (ed): *Neurological Surgery*. Philadelphia, WB Saunders Co, 1982.

87. Giannotta SL, Ahmadi J: Vascular lesions with head injury, in Wilkins RH, Rengachary SS (eds): *Neurosurgery*. New York, McGraw-Hill International Book Co, 1985, pp 1678–1687.

88. Katirji MB, Reinmuth OM, Latchaw RE: Stroke due to vertebral artery injury. *Arch Neurol* 1985; 42:242–248.

89. Morgan MK, Besser M, Johnston I, et al: Intracranial carotid artery injury in closed head trauma. *J Neurosurg* 1987; 66:192–197.

90. Merrick R, Latchaw RE, Gold LH: Computerized tomography of the orbit in carotid-cavernous sinus fistulae. *CT: J Comput Tomogr* 1979; 4:127–131.

91. Spetzler RF, Wilson CB: Management of recurrent

CSF rhinorrhea of the middle and posterior fossa. *J Neurosurg* 1978; 49:393–397.

92. Scarff TB, Fine M: Growing skull fractures of childhood, in Wilkins RH, Rengachary SS (eds): *Neurosurgery.* New York, McGraw-Hill International Book Co, 1985, pp 1627–1628.

93. McLaurin RH, McLennon JE: Diagnosis and treatment of head injury in children, in Youmans JR (ed): *Neurological Surgery.* Philadelphia, WB Saunders Co, 1982, pp 2084–2136.

94. Bruce DA, Schut L, Sutton LN: Pediatric head injury, in Wilkins RH, Rengachary SS (eds): *Neurosurgery.* New York, McGraw-Hill International Book Co, 1985, pp 1600–1604.

95. Meyers CA, Levin HS, Eisenberg HM, et al: Early versus late lateral ventricular enlargement following closed head injury. *J Neurol Neurosurg Psychiatry* 1983; 46:1092–1097.

96. Kishore PRS, Lipper MH, Miller JD, et al: Posttraumatic hydrocephalus in patients with severe head injury. *Neuroradiology* 1978; 16:261–265.

97. Behrman RE, Vaughan VC: Abuse and neglect in children, in Nelson WE (ed): *Textbook of Pediatrics,* ed 12. Philadelphia, WB Saunders Co, 1983, p 100.

98. Tsai FY, Zee C, Apthorp JS, et al: Computed tomography in child abuse head trauma. *CT: J Comput Tomogr* 1980; 4:277–286.

99. Merten DF, Osborne DRS, Radkowski MA, et al: Craniocerebral trauma in the child abuse syndrome: Radiological observations. *Pediatr Radiol* 1984; 14:272–277.

100. Zimmerman RA, Bilaniuk LT, Bruce D, et al: Computed tomography of craniocerebral injury in the abused child. *Radiology* 1979; 130:687–690.

101. Ludwig S: Shaken baby syndrome: A review of 20 cases. *Ann Emerg Med* 1984; 13:104–107.

102. Duhaime AC, Gennarelli TA, Thibault LE, et al: The shaken baby syndrome: A clinical, pathological, and biomechanical study. *J Neurosurg* 1987; 66:409–415.

103. Caffey J: The whiplash shaken infant syndrome: Manual shaking by the extremities with whiplash-induced intracranial and intraocular bleeding, linked with residual permanent brain damage and mental retardation. *Pediatrics* 1974; 54:396–403.

104. Sezen F: Retinal haemorrhages in newborn infants. *Br J Ophthalmol* 1970; 55:248–253.

105. Cohen RA, Kaufman RA, Myers PA, et al: Cranial computed tomography in the abused child with head injury. *AJNR* 1985; 6:883–888.

106. Robertson WC Jr, Chun RWM, Orrison WW, et al: Benign subdural collections of infancy. *J Pediatr* 1979; 94:382–385.

107. Mori K, Handa H, Itoh M, et al: Benign subdural effusion in infants. *J Comput Assist Tomogr* 1980; 4:466–471.

108. Till K: Subdural haematoma and effusion in infancy. *Br Med J* 1968; 3:400–402.

109. Meservy CJ, Towbin R, McLaurin RL, et al: Radiographic characteristics of skull fractures resulting from child abuse. *AJR* 1987; 149:173–175.

110. Fenichel GM, Webster DL, Wong WKT: Intracranial hemorrhage in the term newborn. *Arch Neurol* 1984; 41:30–34.

111. Bergman I, Bauer RE, Barmada MA, et al: Intracerebral hemorrhage in the full-term neonatal infant. *Pediatrics* 1985; 75:488–496.

112. Overgaard J, Tweed WA: Cerebral circulation after head injury. Part 1: Cerebral blood flow and its regulation after closed head injury with emphasis on clinical correlations. *J Neurosurg* 1974; 41:531–541.

113. Latchaw RE, Yonas H, Darby JM, et al: Xenon/CT cerebral blood flow determination following cranial trauma. *Acta Radiol Suppl (Stockh)* 1986; 369:370–373.

114. Uzzell BP, Obrist WD, Dolinskas CA, et al: Relationship of acute CBF and ICP findings to neuropsychological outcome in severe head injury. *J Neurosurg* 1986; 65:630–635.

115. Darby JM, Yonas H, Gur D, et al: Xenon-enhanced computed tomography in brain death. *Arch Neurol* 1987; 44:551–554.

11

Nontraumatic Intracranial Hemorrhage

Robert W. Tarr, M.D.

Stephen T. Hecht, M.D.

Joseph A. Horton, M.D.

Every neuroimager will be faced with patients who have experienced an abrupt change in neurologic status. Computed tomography (CT) of the brain without intravenous contrast is the examination of choice for patients who experience a sudden ictus. Noncontrast CT facilitates the diagnosis of intracerebral hemorrhage, which is often associated with abrupt neurologic decompensation. Nontraumatic intracranial hemorrhage requires the neuroimager to make critically important diagnoses. The most common causes of nontraumatic intracerebral hemorrhage are aneurysm, arteriovenous malformation (AVM), hypertension, amyloid angiopathy, coagulopathy, tumor, infarction, drug abuse,[1-3] septic emboli, and germinal matrix hemorrhage (GMH). The distinction is based upon the history, the age of the patient, and the CT and magnetic resonance imaging (MRI) appearances.

The initial decision in the analysis of imaging studies in nontraumatic hemorrhage is the determination of the location (type) of hemorrhage. Spontaneous brain hemorrhages are generally in the subarachnoid space (SAH) or are intraparenchymal (IPH), intraventricular (IVH), or a combination. Subarachnoid blood may rarely enter the subdural space.

INTRACRANIAL HEMORRHAGE

Subarachnoid Hemorrhage

SAH often presents with a sudden onset of severe headache in an otherwise healthy person. On CT scans without intravenous contrast, blood in the subarachnoid space initially is seen as increased density in the cisterns, sulci, and fissures of the brain. The degree of increased density is related to the hematocrit and the amount of blood released into the subarachnoid space. If a patient is scanned within the first 24 hours, unenhanced CT detects more than 90% of SAHs. By the end of the first week it can still detect more than 50%.[4-7] The detection rate decreases with time because CT effectively depicts the increased attenuation of clotted blood, and as the clot resolves over time, its attenuation (and therefore its conspicuousness) decreases. After the first week, SAH is usually not imaged well by CT. If SAH is obvious on CT more than 1 week following the initial event, rebleeding has probably occurred. When examining the CT scans of patients with suspected SAH careful attention must be paid to the subarachnoid spaces at bone-brain interfaces since the high density of bone can mask the density of the hemorrhage. Examination of CT scans at wider windows and levels intermediate between brain and bone can enable detection of subtle SAHs.

Although some authors have reported the ability of MRI to detect acute SAHs,[8] this technique is generally unsuccessful in detecting SAH in the acute stage.[9] The reason for the limited success of MRI probably relates to the higher partial pressure of oxygen within the cerebrospinal fluid (CSF) as compared with brain parenchyma,[10] which delays the conversion of oxyhemoglobin to deoxyhemoglobin (and subsequently to methemoglobin) and prevents the acute hemorrhage from significantly altering the relaxation rates of surrounding protons within the CSF.[11] Thus, uncontrasted CT without intravenous contrast remains the imaging modality of choice for suspected acute SAH.

MRI is excellent at detecting subacute and chronic SAH. In the subacute stage SAH is characterized by hyperintensity (see Chapter 9). Subpial deposition of hemosiderin occurs in the chronic stage and results in superficial siderosis.[12, 13] This latter MRI appearance is one of marked hypointensity along the parenchymal surface and is best seen on long repetition time (TR)/long echo time (TE) sequences (Fig 11–1).

Negative CT or MRI findings do not exclude SAH. There is no relation between the amount of SAH in the intracranial subarachnoid space and the amount of blood in the spinal subarachnoid space.[14] If there is no contraindication to it, lumbar puncture should be performed on a patient suspected of having SAH, particularly if he has negative brain CT scan findings.

Intraparenchymal Hemorrhage

Pathologically, IPH can be divided into four stages: acute (1 to 3 days), subacute (4 to 8 days), capsule (9 to 13 days), and organization (greater than 13 days).[15, 16] In the acute stage the hematoma consists of intact red blood cells that undergo progressive crenation. There may be mild perivascular inflammation. In the subacute stage there is lysis of red blood cells, and hemosiderin-laden macrophages appear. Inflammation peaks at the subacute stage and reactive astrocytosis in the surrounding parenchyma begins. During the capsule stage, vascular proliferation is seen at the margin of the hematoma, inflammation regresses, and reactive astrocytosis becomes pronounced. In the organization stage a dense collagenous capsule forms around the hematoma, and hemosiderin-laden macrophages and less well organized collagen are found within the hematoma.

The CT appearance of IPH varies with time and correlates with the neuropathologic changes described above (Fig 11–2). Acutely, nonenhanced CT demonstrates a well-marginated hyperdense mass due to the high protein content of intact red blood cells. There may be some low density in the surrounding brain due to perivascular inflammation and edema. As erythrocytes lyse and progressively lose hemoglobin in the subacute stage, the hematoma becomes progressively isodense with brain parenchyma. In the early organi-

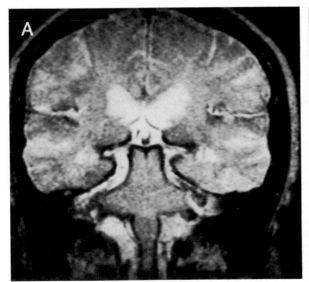
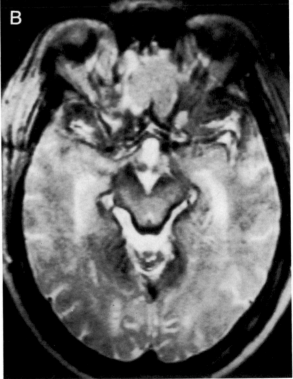

FIG 11–1.
Subpial hemosiderin deposition from a previous SAH. **A,** coronal MRI (spin-echo [SE], 2,500/80). **B,** axial MRI (SE, 2,500/80). MRI was performed in a patient with a history of SAH several years previously secondary to aneurysm rupture. There is signal hypointensity lining the sylvian fissures, inferomedial aspect of the temporal lobes, brain stem, cerebellum, and upper cervical spinal cord due to subpial deposition of hemosiderin. (Courtesy of Michael Kuharik, M.D., Indianapolis.)

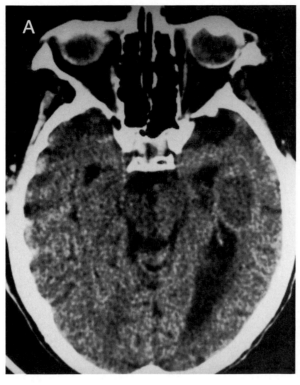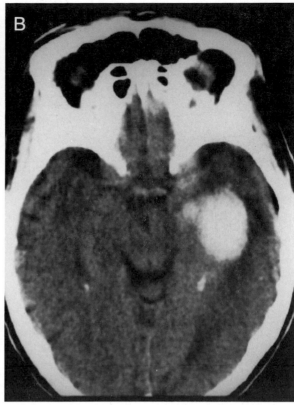

FIG 11–2.

Evaluation of hemorrhagic infarction. **A,** an uncontrasted CT scan demonstrates an acute hemorrhagic infarction involving the anterior portion of the left temporal lobe. **B,** an uncontrasted CT scan 3 months after the initial ictus (capsule stage) demonstrates decrease in size of the hematoma. The center of the hematoma has become hypodense when compared with brain parenchyma. A hyperdense rim surrounds the hematoma and represents the dense collagenous capsule.

zation stage the filling of the acellular hematoma with a vascularized matrix may cause the hematoma to again be slightly hyperdense when compared with brain structures. Eventually, an area of encephalomalacia is seen as a low-density area with negative mass effect.[15, 16]

Enhancement of the hematoma is first seen in the subacute stage and is related to perivascular inflammation. The enhancement pattern is initially a complete or almost complete ring around the periphery of the hematoma. In the capsule and early organizational stage the developing neovascularity contributes to the ring enhancement pattern. The ring of enhancement gradually decreases in diameter and becomes more irregular and more intense. Eventually, the ring pattern of enhancement is replaced by a nodular pattern due to filling in the center of the hematoma by developing neovascularity (Fig 11–3).[15, 16]

The enhancement pattern, especially the nodular enhancement of nonneoplastic hemorrhage, may be mistaken for the pattern seen with hemorrhagic neoplasms. Typically there is less mass ef-

fect with a nonneoplastic hemorrhage than with a tumoral hemorrhage in the subacute stage. Also, the volume of enhancement decreases over time with nonneoplastic IPHs, in contradiction to the volume of enhancement in neoplastic hemorrhages, which may increase over time.

The MRI appearance of IPH depends upon both the age of the hemorrhage and the field strength of the magnet.[17–19] During the first 24 hours, the findings are somewhat variable on short TR/short TE images, but long TR/long TE images demonstrate nonspecific hyperintensity due to reactive brain edema. Beyond 24 hours, MRI becomes increasingly specific for IPH, regardless of field strength. After 24 hours the hemorrhage becomes heterogeneous, and signal intensities vary with time. From 1 to 3 days areas of hypointensity develop on long TR/long TE images due to deoxyhemoglobin. After 3 days, areas of hyperintensity on short TR/short TE images and hypointensity on long TR/long TE images develop due to intracellular methemoglobin formation, a finding that is specific for hemorrhage. In the chronic state (beyond 2

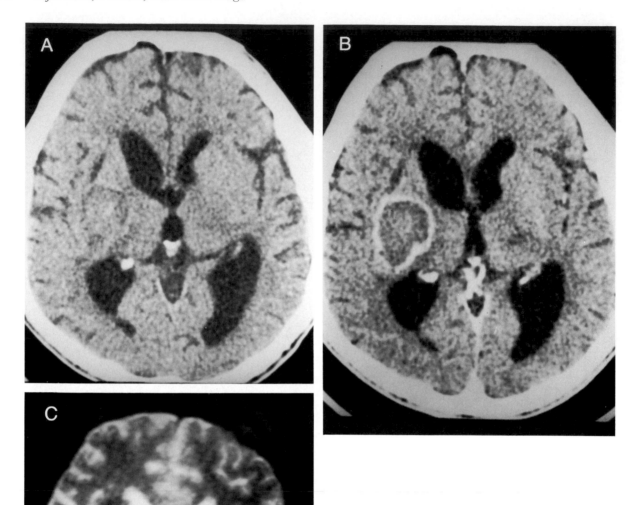

FIG 11–3.
Organization stage, hypertensive right basal ganglion hemorrhage. **A,** unenhanced CT demonstrates a slightly lucent central portion of the hematoma surrounded by a hyperdense rim consisting of collagenous capsule. **B,** following contrast administration, there is ring enhancement due to the neovascularity of the collagen capsule. A small nodule of enhancement in the central portion of the hematoma is also due to neovascularity. **C,** axial MRI scan (SE, 2,500/100) demonstrates a hyperintense central portion of the hematoma due to extracellular methemoglobin. The peripheral rim of hypointensity is due to hemosiderin deposition. Incidental note is made of high signal intensity in the left basal ganglion due to prior nonhemorrhagic ischemic change.

weeks), MRI is usually more sensitive than CT in detecting hemorrhage. In chronic hemorrhages, MRI may show residual areas of hyperintensity on both short TR/short TE and long TR/long TE images; these represent extracellular methemoglobin. In addition, hemosiderin may cause a markedly hypointense rim best seen on long TR/long TE images (Fig 11–3).

Intraventricular Hemorrhage

CT depicts IVH as dense blood within one or more ventricles. Acutely, blood in the lateral ventricles usually layers dependently. Thus, when patients are scanned in the supine position, a blood/CSF level may be seen in the occipital horns of the lateral ventricles. If the IVH is massive enough, the entire ventricular system may be filled with clotted blood. With time the clotted blood retracts and eventually disappears.

The limitations of MRI in the detection of acute IVH are similar to SAH. As with SAH, the T1 shortening effect of deoxyhemoglobin and methemoglobin may be delayed due to the high partial pressure of oxygen in the CSF. Subependymal siderosis may be detected as a subependymal rim of hypointensity on long TR/long TE sequences in cases of chronic IVH.[13]

ANEURYSMS

The most frequent nontraumatic cause of intracranial hemorrhage is rupture of an aneurysm, which accounts for 72% to 80% of all cases of nontraumatic intracranial hemorrhage.[20] It has been estimated from reviews of autopsy data that the incidence of aneurysm in the general population is approximately 2% (range, 0.2% to 9%).[21, 22] Approximately 40% of aneurysms found at autopsy have ruptured.[23, 24] Mortality figures for surgically untreated ruptured aneurysms vary between 41% and 61% at 6 months following the initial rupture.[25–27] Four percent of patients with untreated ruptured aneurysms rebleed within 24 hours of the initial aneurysm rupture. An additional 16% of patients rebleed within 2 weeks of the initial event.[28] Overall, in the first 6 months following aneurysm rupture the rate of rebleeding of an untreated aneurysm approaches 50%. Thereafter, the rebleeding rate is approximately 3% per year.[29]

Most aneurysms form at branch points of intracranial vessels. The most common aneurysm locations are the junction of the anterior cerebral artery and the anterior communicating artery (30%), the junction of the internal carotid artery and the posterior communicating artery (25%), the middle cerebral artery bi/trifurcation (13%), the supraclinoid carotid-ophthalmic junction and bifurcation of the supraclinoid segments (15%), and the vertebrobasilar system (5%).[24] Ninety-five percent of aneurysms are supratentorial. Multiple aneurysms occur with a frequency of 15% to 22%.[30]

The pathogenesis of aneurysm formation is somewhat controversial.[31] Proponents of the "congenital" theory have stated that intrinsic structural weaknesses in the walls of cerebral arteries predispose to aneurysm formation.[32–34] Morphologic studies have shown that there is an increase in the number of fenestrations in the internal elastic membrane and media at the apex of branching cerebral arteries.[33, 34] The increased number of fenestrations is felt to represent a congenital structural weakness from which aneurysms arise. Proponents of the degeneration theory assert that hemodynamic stresses by the axial impingement of the blood stream upon branch points of arteries reduce tensile strength, which predisposes to microaneurysm formation.[31, 35]

It is probable that a combination of factors plays a role in aneurysm formation. Hemodynamic stresses, whether applied to points of intrinsic structural weaknesses or even to normal artery wall, can induce degenerative arterial changes that can lead to aneurysm formation.[35] Once a tiny aneurysm is formed, the stress on the aneurysm wall is greater than on the adjacent arterial wall since the aneurysm wall is thinner and has less elasticity. This increased stress produces further structural fatigue and degenerative changes. This cycle predisposes to aneurysm growth and rupture.

Aneurysms that are peripheral or unusual in location can result from vasculitis, tumors such as atrial myxoma and choriocarcinoma, sepsis, and trauma. Aneurysms are also associated with systemic diseases like fibromuscular dysplasia,[36] polycystic kidney,[37] Marfan's syndrome,[38] and other collagen deficiencies. Aneurysm development is associated with high flow states (e.g., on arteries feeding AVMs).[39] Aneurysms associated with AVMs may regress following AVM treatment.

Most aneurysms are in the subarachnoid space. It follows that when they bleed, they usually cause SAH. Aneurysms arising from the cavernous segment of the internal carotid artery are an exception, usually being extra-arachnoid and within the leaves of the dura. Cavernous carotid aneurysms present with cranial nerve deficits due to the mass effect of the aneurysm or with a carotid cavernous fistula due to rupture.

Aneurysms can bleed into brain parenchyma, especially if they have become adherent to the pial surface, but a pure IPH without subarachnoid blood is rare. Aneurysms can also bleed into the ventricles, particularly when anterior communicating artery aneurysms rupture through the lamina terminalis. Blood can also enter the ventricular system via the choroidal fissures and the foramina of Luschka and Magendie. Entry through these foramina is most common with aneurysms of the posterior circulation, especially of the posterior inferior cerebellar artery.

The location of blood (particularly parenchymal hemorrhage) following aneurysm rupture often provides useful information regarding aneurysm location.[40] Septal hemorrhage is associated with anterior communicating artery aneurysm rupture (Fig 11–4). Temporal lobe hematomas are usually associated with middle cerebral artery aneurysm, although medial temporal lobe hematomas may also be due to posterior communicating or internal carotid artery aneurysms. Inferomedial frontal hematomas are usually secondary to anterior communicating artery aneurysms, although occasionally they may be due to internal carotid artery aneurysms. Ruptured posterior inferior cerebellar artery aneurysms can bleed into the cerebellum and brain stem. The cisternal location of SAH is a less specific indicator of aneurysm location. The most useful cisternal localizing sign is blood confined to the anterior interhemispheric fissure, which is indication of an anterior communicating artery aneurysm.[41] Middle cerebral artery bifarction/trifarction aneurysms often fill a sylvian cistern with blood.

The role for CT and MRI in aneurysm screening is somewhat undefined at the present time. CT can be used to screen for aneurysms that are 5 mm or larger if thin slices (1.5 mm) are employed.[42] The CT appearance of an aneurysm is typically that of a rounded area of hyperdensity in close proximity to the circle of Willis on the uncontrasted scan that enhances with contrast (Fig 11–5). At times, only a portion of the aneurysm will enhance. Enhancement can be central due to enhancement of a patent central lumen with peripheral thrombus formation, peripheral due to enhancement of a centrifugally organizing thrombus via peripheral vasa vasorum, or a combination of

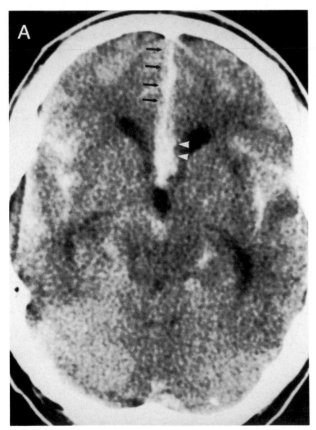

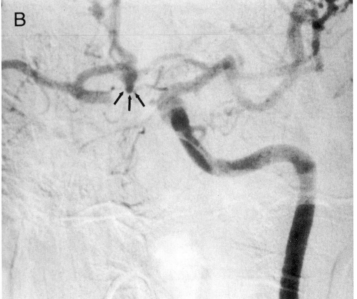

FIG 11–4.
SAH from an anterior communicating artery aneurysm. **A,** uncontrasted CT scan showing a predominance of blood in the interhemispheric fissure *(arrows)* and septum pellucidum *(arrowheads)* due to rupture of an anterior communicating aneurysm. A lesser amount of blood is present in the sylvian fissures and perimesencephalic cistern. **B,** anteroposterior left internal carotid arteriogram demonstrating the anterior communicating aneurysm *(arrows)*.

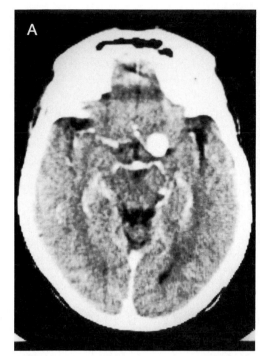

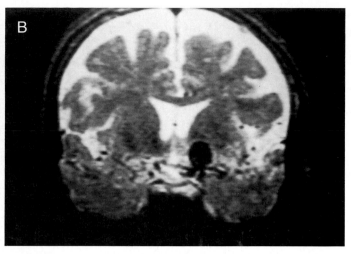

FIG 11–5.
Supraclinoid carotid aneurysm. **A,** contrast-enhanced CT demonstrates a homogeneously enhancing left supraclinoid carotid tip aneurysm. **B,** coronal MRI (SE, 2,000/80) shows signal void due to flowing blood within the aneurysm.

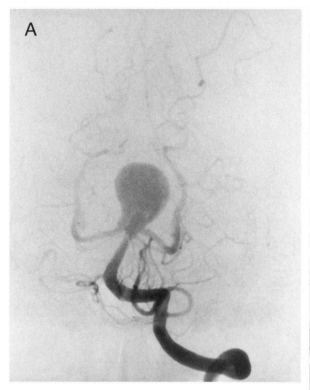

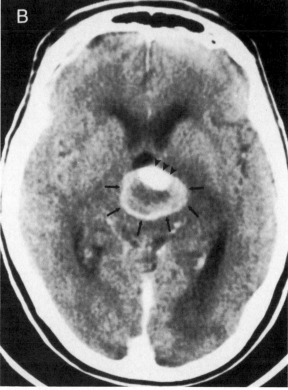

FIG 11–6.
Basilar tip aneurysm with peripheral enhancement. **A,** an antero-posterior left vertebral artery angiogram demonstrates a large aneurysm arising from the distal aspect of the basilar artery. **B,** con-trast-enhanced CT shows enhancement of the lumen of the aneurysm *(arrows).* There is rim enhancement of a peripherally or-ganizing thrombus within the aneurysm *(arrowheads).*

both (Fig 11–6). Occasionally, areas of calcification, typically curvilinear and peripheral, are seen on the uncontrasted scan.[42]

Similarly, MRI can detect aneurysms greater than 5 mm in size as regions of flow void in an area morphologically consistent with a saccular aneurysm (see Fig 11–5). In patients with a known aneurysm or multiple aneurysms, MRI can often pinpoint the site of bleeding by detecting areas of subacute hemorrhage adjacent to the aneurysm.[43]

The inability to visualize a suspected aneurysm on CT or MRI cannot be used to exclude the presence of an aneurysm. Angiography remains the procedure of choice to exclude the presence of aneurysm, to document the presence of multiple aneurysms, and often to confirm the suspicion of an aneurysm detected on CT or MRI. However, re-

cent work with 3DFT MR angiography (MRA) suggests that MRA may become a useful noninvasive method for aneurysm screening and detection.[44]

MRI can accurately differentiate partially thrombosed giant aneurysms (those greater than 2.5 cm in diameter) from intracerebral hematomas and skull base neoplasms. The presence of signal void from flowing blood in the residual patent lumen, a laminated staged thrombus with intervening layers of hemosiderin and methemoglobin, and signal void in the adjacent parent artery allows such differentiation (Fig 11–7).[45] MRI also provides useful information regarding total aneurysm size, the degree and age estimate of the intraaneurysm clot, and the relationship of the aneurysm to and compression of normal brain. Low–flip angle gradient-refocused MRI can provide additional in-

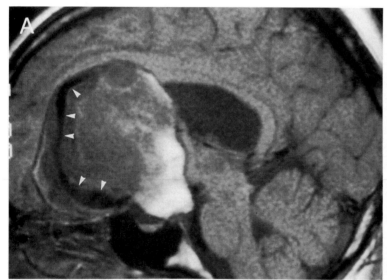

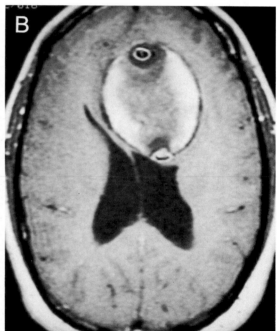

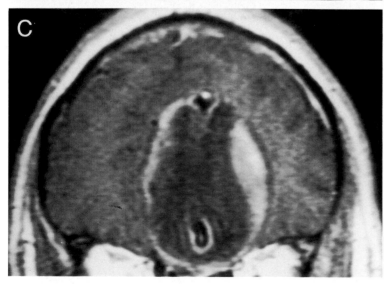

FIG 11–7.
Giant internal carotid artery aneurysm, MRI. **A,** sagittal MRI (SE, 600/20). **B** and **C,** axial **(B)** and coronal **(C)** MRI with gadolinium–diethylenetriamine pentaacetic acid (DTPA) enhancement (SE, 600/20). The images demonstrate a giant aneurysm arising from the supraclinoid portion of the internal carotid artery. The aneurysm is predominantly clotted as evidenced by the laminated signal intensity; however, flow void within the residual lumen of the elevated internal carotid artery is visualized *(arrowheads).* Enhanced images **(B** and **C)** show contrast enhancement at the periphery and center of the patent lumen that is consistent with flow rate variation with the lumen (areas of enhancement within the lumen represent areas of decreased flow rate).

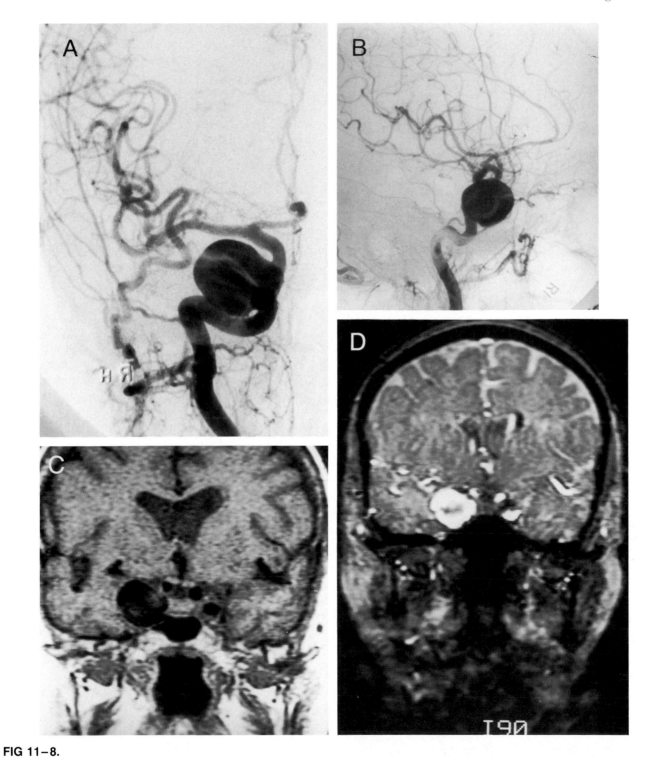

FIG 11–8.
Right cavernous carotid aneurysm with central clot formation. **A** and **B,** anteroposterior **(A)** and lateral **(B)** views of a right common carotid angiogram demonstrate a large right cavernous carotid aneurysm. **C,** coronal MRI (SE, 550/20) demonstrates a signal void within the periphery of the aneurysm that represents flowing blood. Signal intensity within the central portion of the aneurysm may rep-resent either a clot or slowly flowing blood. **D,** gradient-echo coronal MRI (50/15; 45-degree flip angle) demonstrates a high signal intensity in the periphery of the aneurysm that represents flowing blood. The lack of high signal in the center of the aneurysm suggests central clot formation.

formation regarding flow dynamics within the aneurysm (Fig 11–8).[46]

COMPLICATIONS OF ANEURYSM HEMORRHAGE

Hydrocephalus

Most patients who suffer SAH following aneurysm rupture develop hydrocephalus at some time during their recovery. Blood increases CSF protein levels, and the excess CSF protein obstructs microscopic CSF absorptive sites in the pacchionian granulations at the brain surface, thereby causing communicating hydrocephalus.[46]

If intraventricular blood clots, it may occlude the outlet foramina of individual ventricles and cause acute obstructive hydrocephalus. The most common site for obstruction is at the aqueduct of Sylvius because of its small size. Aqueductal obstruction causes enlargement of the lateral and third ventricles, with the fourth ventricle remaining normal in size.

Vasospasm and Infarction

Vasospasm is a common sequela of SAH, especially following aneurysm rupture. Vasospasm is one of the main causes of morbidity and mortality following SAH.[47, 48] Approximately 40% of patients develop vasospasm following aneurysm rupture. Of those who develop vasospasm, about 50% will develop delayed ischemic deficits, half of which will be fatal.[48] The interaction of blood within the subarachnoid space with the adventitia of blood vessel walls is known to induce spasm.[49–54] The exact chemical(s) that causes the spasm is unknown. Serotonin, prostaglandins, and hemoglobin degradation products have been implicated as etiologic agents in vasospasm.[55] Vasospasm rarely manifests itself immediately after SAH. It usually begins about 4 days and resolves by 14 days after SAH. However, there may be delays of up to 10 days before the appearance of vasospasm, and resolution occasionally takes longer than 2 weeks.[56, 57] Angiography shows localized or diffuse narrowing of an artery or arteries. The amount of SAH is usually proportional to the degree of vasospasm in the adjacent arteries. However, vasospasm can be detected remote from and even contralateral to SAH. Spasm can be severe enough to prevent filling of the aneurysm with contrast material and thus give a false-negative angiogram.

Rebleeding and vasospasm are the major causes of late deterioration due to SAH following aneurysm rupture. Repeat CT scanning demonstrates new hemorrhage. If vasospasm is severe enough to cause cerebral or cerebellar infarction, an unenhanced CT scan can depict the infarctions (Fig 11–9). However, negative CT scan findings do not exclude vasospasm. Stable xenon-enhanced CT cerebral blood flow (CBF) mapping is a noninvasive modality that shows decreases in regional brain blood flow due to vasospasm.[58] In the face of negative unenhanced CT results, the finding of focal or multifocal cerebral hypoperfusion on a stable xenon-enhanced CT CBF map (or other blood flow mapping technique) is highly supportive of the diagnosis of vasospasm (see Chapters 6 and 8).

VASCULAR MALFORMATIONS

Numerous schemes have been applied to classifying vascular malformations. Commonly they are divided into four pathologic categories: AVM, venous angioma, cavernous angioma, and capillary hemangioma, also known as capillary telangiectasia.[59] The most common vascular malformation is AVM.

Arteriovenous Malformation

Failure to form a capillary bed during embryonal development results in an AVM. An AVM has high-flow connections between arterioles and venules. While most connections are tortuous and small, an AVM occasionally also contains fistulous components. The brain, dura, and spine may be affected. AVMs are named according to both their anatomic location (frontal, cerebellar, pontine, etc.) and their blood supplies (pial, dural, or mixed). The location of an AVM affects the type of blood supply it receives. A superficial AVM can be pial, dural, or mixed. A pial AVM derives its blood supply from branches of the internal carotid or vertebrobasilar system. A dural AVM is supplied by meningeal, external carotid artery, and muscular vertebral artery branches. A mixed AVM has a combination of the two types of blood supplies. An AVM on the ventricular surface is of the ependymal type. An ependymal AVM may penetrate the brain for a variable distance. It may be small and confined only to the ventricular surface or extend peripherally, even as far as the pial surface.

Approximately 6% of AVMs are multiple.[59]

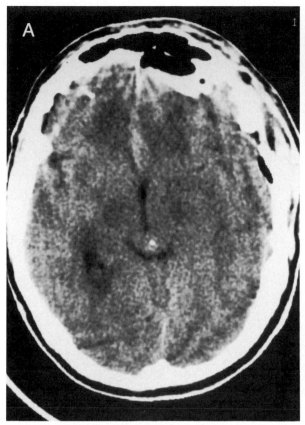

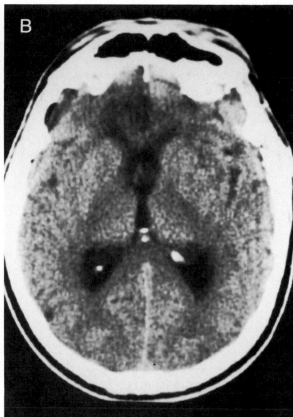

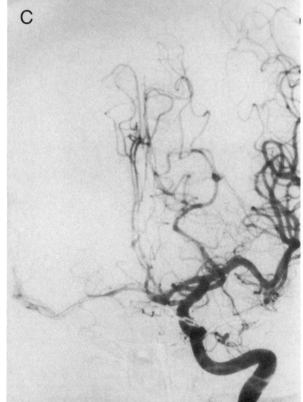

FIG 11–9.
Vasospasm following aneurysm rupture. **A** and **B,** an
uncontrasted CT scan obtained 6 days following
surgical clipping of an acutely ruptured anterior
communicating artery aneurysm demonstrates bifrontal
infarctions. A small amount of residual SAH is seen in
the interhemispheric fissure. **C,** the anteroposterior view
of a left internal carotid angiogram demonstrates diffuse
areas of narrowing of both anterior cerebral arteries that
is consistent with vasospasm. An aneurysm clip is
present inferior to the anterior communicating artery.

The Wyburn-Mason syndrome is a rare association of retinal, orbital, cerebral, and facial AVMs.[60] AVMs in this syndrome commonly involve the optic nerve, optic chiasm, and optic tracts. Intracranial AVMs may also be found in the basifrontal region, the sylvian fissure, and the rostral midbrain. In the Osler-Weber-Rondu syndrome, nervous system angiomas are accompanied by angiomas of the skin, numerous membranes, lungs, and liver.

An AVM commonly causes symptoms by three mechanisms. Frequently an AVM presents with hemorrhage. An AVM that has never bled has approximately a 25% chance of bleeding within 15 years. If an AVM has bled once, the risk rises to 25% in 5 years, and if it has bled more than once, the risk is 25% each year.[61]

The second mechanism by which an AVM can become symptomatic is by stealing of blood from normal brain structures. Blood preferentially flows through the low-resistance pathway provided by the AVM rather than through the higher-resistance pathways of arterial branches serving a capillary bed. The existence of the steal phenomenon has been shown by CBF studies (Fig 11–10).[62, 63] This steal leads to deprivation of metabolites and produces seizures and/or neurologic deficit.

The third mechanism by which an AVM causes symptoms is arterialization of the draining veins.

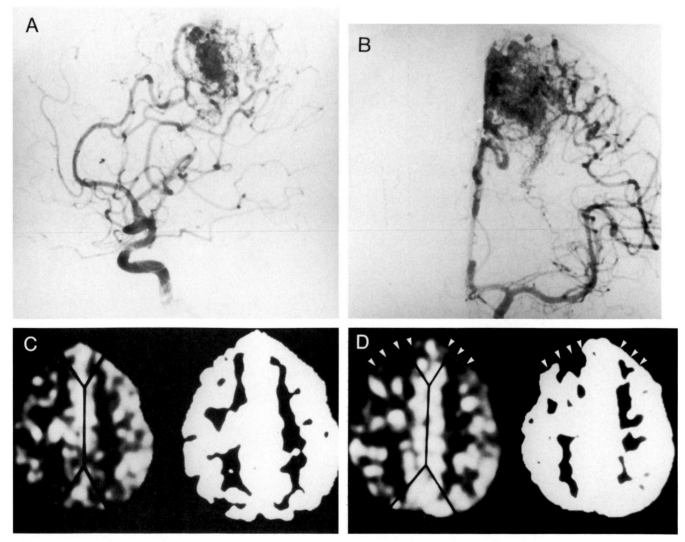

FIG 11–10.
Eighteen-year-old male with a left parietal AVM. Anteroposterior **(A)** and lateral **(B)** views of an internal carotid angiogram depict an AVM with supply from the left pericallosal and left middle cerebral artery branches. **C,** a baseline xenon CT CBF map shows normal flows. **D,** Xe/CT CBF map following acetazolamide administration. Acetazolamide is a generalized cerebral vasodilator. There is a "steal" of blood flow from the anterior cerebral–middle cerebral artery border zones bilaterally *(arrowheads)*.

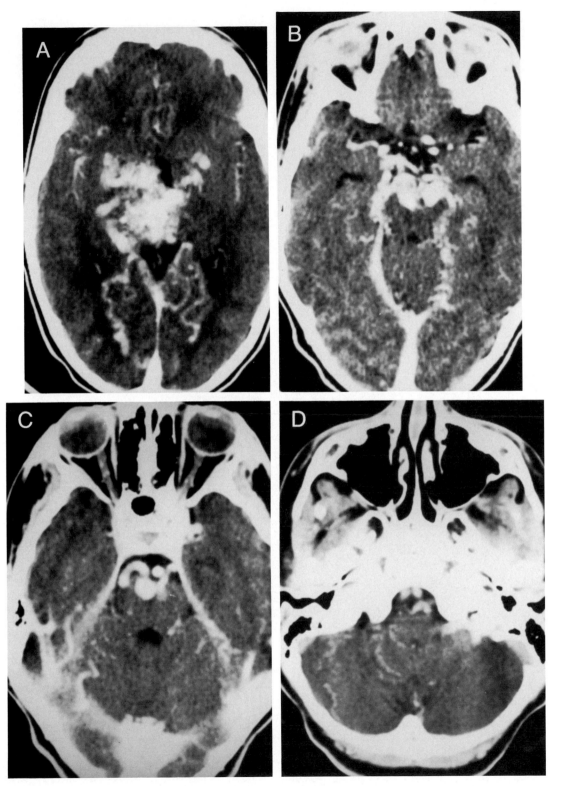

FIG 11–11.
Bithalamic AVM. **A–D,** contrast-enhanced CT scan showing a large bithalamic AVM. The larger enhancing serpiginous structures are dilated draining veins that extend inferiorly along the anterior aspect of the brain stem through the interpeduncular and prepon- tine cisterns to the level of the foramen magnum. There is com- pression of the anterior aspect of the brain stem by the dilated venous drainage.

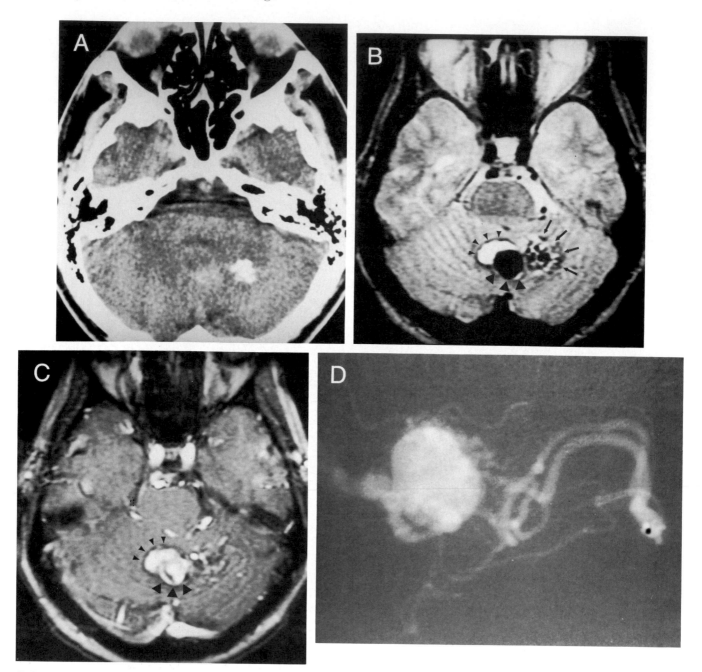

FIG 11–12.
Cerebellar AVM with subacute hemorrhage and venous varix. **A,** an unenhanced CT scan shows calcification within the left cerebellar hemisphere and an area medial to the calcification with heterogeneous attenuation. **B,** axial MRI (SE, 2,500/80) demonstrates several findings: (1) anteriorly in the midline there is an area of increased signal intensity surrounded by a rim of hypointensity representing extracellular methemoglobin and peripheral hemosiderin, respectively, within a subacute hematoma *(small arrowheads);* (2) posterior to the hematoma is an area of signal void representing a venous varix *(large arrowheads);* (3) lateral to the hematoma are multiple areas of signal void representing an AVM nidus and/or calcification *(arrows).* **C,** gradient-echo MRI demonstrates flow within the varix as high signal intensity *(large arrowheads).* The subacute hematoma retains high signal intensity *(small arrowheads).* It is also possible on the gradient-echo image to distinguish an AVM nidus (high signal intensity) from calcification (signal void). **D,** a superselective lateral left superior cerebellar angiogram shows the rapid flow of an AVM nidus into a large varix and draining veins.

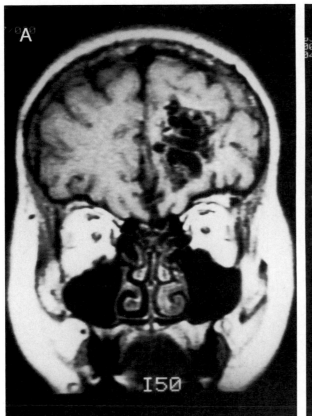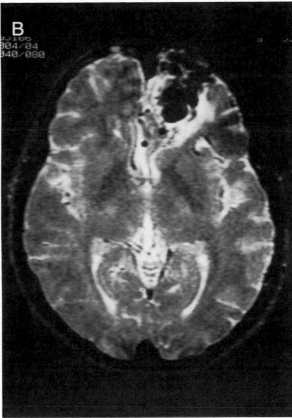

FIG 11-13.
Left frontal AVM. **A,** coronal MRI (SE, 700/30) demonstrates signal void within multiple serpiginous vascular structures compromising the AVM. **B,** an axial image (SE, 2000/80) again shows signal void due to rapidly flowing blood within the AVM. Reactive changes in the adjacent parenchyma are evidenced by the high signal intensity surrounding the AVM.

Normal cerebral veins draining into these arterialized veins experience resistance to drainage that leads to an increased risk of venous infarction and venous hemorrhage in normal brain due to elevated venous backpressure. Enlarged draining veins can also compress adjacent cranial nerves or brain matter and cause seizures, cranial neuropathy, or focal deficit.

When an AVM has bled, CT performed acutely will usually show SAH, IVH, and/or IPH. The location of hemorrhage depends upon both the location and type of the malformation. An ependymal AVM characteristically bleeds into the ventricle, while a pial AVM usually produces SAH with or without IPH.

Whether an AVM has bled, contrast-enhanced CT usually shows serpentine vessels. Larger vessels are usually draining veins, smaller ones feeding arteries (Fig 11-11). Because the arteries that supply an AVM tend to be tortuous, it is difficult with CT alone to determine whether aneurysms are present. Approximately 25% of AVMs have aneurysms on feeding vessels.[39]

Complete evaluation of the morphology and flow characteristics of an AVM requires angiography. Varices of draining veins, also known as "venous aneurysms," are often present (Fig 11-12). Thrombosis of the venous outflow channels of an AVM is suggested when a patient presents with acute deterioration of neurologic status and an unenhanced CT scan demonstrates hyperdense serpentine structures. Venous outflow obstruction is often associated with hemorrhage.

MRI depicts the high-flow vascular channels of an AVM as flow void. MRI surpasses CT in its ability to delineate old microscopic hemorrhage because MRI is extraordinarily sensitive to hemosiderin. MRI also allows more graphic depiction of parenchymal changes adjacent to the AVM (Fig 11-13). In addition, MRI may detect partial or complete nidus thrombosis as areas of hyperintensity within vessels comprising the AVM (Fig 11-14).

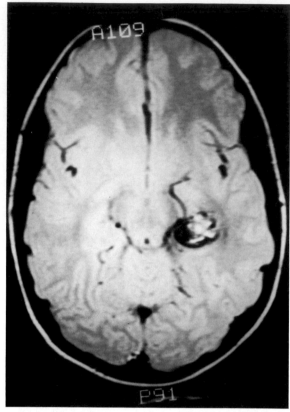

FIG 11–14.
Partially thrombosed left temporal AVM. Axial MRI (SE, 2,000/30) demonstrates areas of high signal that represent thrombosis within a left temporal lobe AVM. Peripheral areas of signal void represent residual patent portions of the AVM.

Venous Angioma

The hallmark of a venous angioma is the presence of a "Medusa's head" appearance, which consists of unusual venules joining to form a larger transparenchymal vein (Figs 11–15 and 11–16). Most occur above the tentorium, but venous angiomas of the posterior fossa have been reported to be more likely to bleed.[64] Increased venous backpressure seems to be the causative event; when the head is dependent and venous pressure is increased, the risk of hemorrhage is increased (Fig 11–15). Venous angiomas may represent anomalous drainage of normal brain, and removal of a venous angioma can result in venous infarction of the normal brain structures it drains.

The most common CT appearance of a venous angioma is an area of faint, punctate or linear hyperdensity on the uncontrasted scan with linear or curvilinear enhancement following contrast administration (Fig 11–16).[65] Other CT appearances of venous angiomas that have been described include a nodular area of hyperdensity on the uncontrasted scan with faint enhancement or an area of nodular enhancement following contrast.[66]

The typical MRI appearance of a venous angioma is an area of linear or globoid signal void on long TR/long TE and short TR/short TE sequences (see Fig 11–15).[67] However, if flow within the angioma is slow, the signal void may be replaced with hyperintensity. In such cases, gradient-echo acquisition sequences may be useful to detect flow within the lesion as areas of hyperintensity. As with AVMs, MRI is extremely sensitive to hemosiderin surrounding the venous angioma from prior hemorrhagic episodes. The relatively slow-flowing venous angioma may also enhance with paramagnetic contrast media (Fig 11–17).

Cavernous Angioma

Cavernous angiomas consist of vascular spaces resembling sinusoids, the walls of which have no muscular or elastic tissue. No neural tissue is interspersed between the vascular spaces.[60] CT shows a dense intraparenchymal lesion that produces no mass effect and enhances with the administration of contrast material. There may be granular calcification radiating from the center of the lesion.[68–70] Cavernous angiomas are characterized by a mixed signal on MRI that represents prior hemorrhage, clot formation, and slowly flowing blood (Fig 11–18). Hemosiderin from prior clotting and subsequent hemolysis often causes a peripheral signal void on long TR/long TE images.[69] Depending on their location, cavernous angiomas may become symptomatic due to hemorrhage within the lesion. Recent reports have also indicated that they are capable of growth.[70] A familial form of cavernous angiomatosis appears to exist.[71] Multiple lesions are common in the familial form (see Chapter 18).

Capillary Hemangiomas/Telangiectasias

Capillary telangiectasias are small vascular spaces lined by a single layer of endothelium. Normal neural tissue can be found interspersed between the small vascular spaces. The feeding arteries and draining vein are typically normal in size.[72] The pons is the most common intra-axial location. They are usually clinically silent but may rarely produce symptoms due to their location or due to bleeding.[73]

The lesions are almost always undetectable on angiography. CT findings are also usually normal,

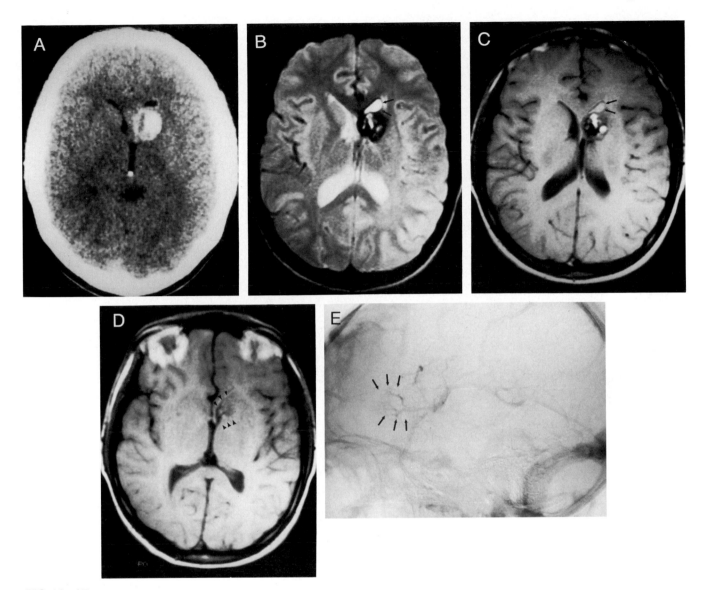

FIG 11–15.
Venous angioma with hemorrhage. **A,** unenhanced CT shows a left caudate nucleus hematoma. A small amount of blood outlines the frontal horn of the left lateral ventricle as well. MRI was performed 3 months later. **B,** SE, 2,000/80; **C** and **D,** SE, 800/26. MRI shows mixed signal intensity characteristics of an evolving left caudal hematoma. The high signal intensity of the CSF within the frontal horn of the left lateral ventricle (**B** and **C,** *arrows*) represents extracellu-lar methemoglobin from associated intraventricular hemorrhage. Flow void within a venous angioma of the septal vein is seen (**D,** *arrowheads*). **E,** venous phase, left internal carotid angiogram, demonstrates a venous angioma of the left septal vein with a typical caput medusae appearance *(arrows)*. (Courtesy of Michael Ku-harik, M.D., Indianapolis.)

and although they may appear as isodense to slightly hyperdense masses, the hyperdensity is due to previous hemorrhage or mineralization. The lesions may occasionally show minimal to moderate contrast enhancement on CT. MRI is usually more useful for detecting capillary telangiectasias since the pons, their most common location, is often poorly visualized on CT due to bone artifact. MRI is also extremely sensitive for detecting evidence of prior hemorrhage.

Angiographically Occult Vascular Malformations

Angiographically occult vascular malformations (AOVM) are slow-flow lesions that are not apparent on routine angiography. The histologic subtype of these malformations is variable. The most common histologic subtype is AVM (44%) followed by cavernous angioma (31%). Venous angioma (10%) and capillary telangiectasias (4%) are least common. Eleven percent are mixed or unclassified angio-

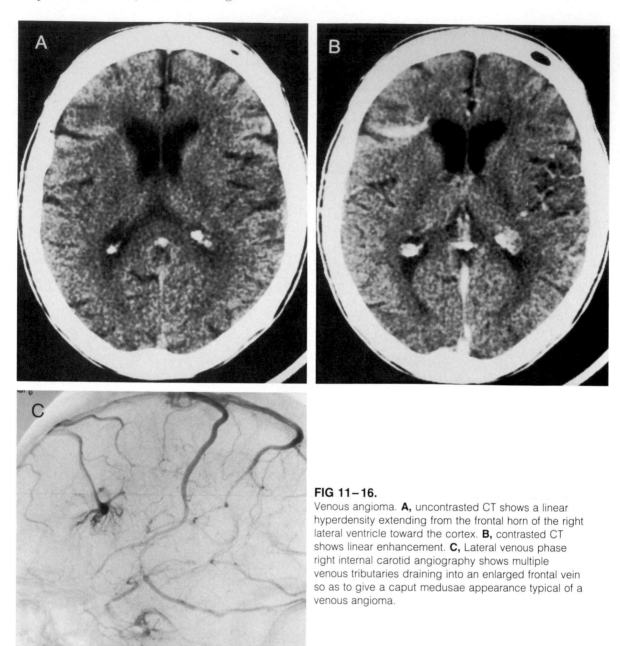

FIG 11–16.
Venous angioma. **A,** uncontrasted CT shows a linear hyperdensity extending from the frontal horn of the right lateral ventricle toward the cortex. **B,** contrasted CT shows linear enhancement. **C,** Lateral venous phase right internal carotid angiography shows multiple venous tributaries draining into an enlarged frontal vein so as to give a caput medusae appearance typical of a venous angioma.

mas.[74] Although subtyping is variable, common histologic features of these malformations include small caliber and thrombosis of the abnormal vessels and evidence of repeated microhemorrhages in the surrounding brain. Symptoms are related to hemorrhage or mass effect from the malformation.

Typically, an AOVM appears hyperdense on the uncontrasted CT scan. The hyperdensity may have a mottled or a homogeneous pattern. Most

AOVMs enhance following contrast administration (Fig 11–19). Those that demonstrate mottled hyperdensity on uncontrasted CT scans enhance more commonly than do those that show homogeneous hyperdensity on the unenhanced scan.[74]

Due to its sensitivity to hemoglobin breakdown products, MRI is the technique of choice to detect an AOVM that has remotely hemor-

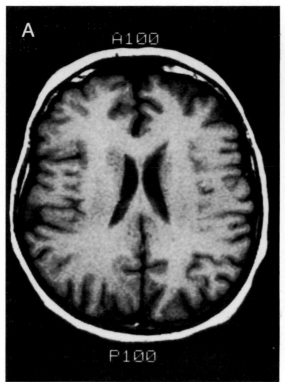
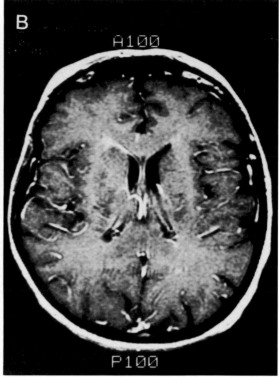

FIG 11–17.
Venous angioma. **A,** noncontrasted MRI (SE, 600/25) shows slight asymmetry of the frontal horns. **B,** MRI (SE, 600/25) contrasted with gadolinium-DTPA demonstrates enhancement of the right frontal venous angioma, which drains into the right septal vein. (Courtesy of Richard E. Latchaw, M.D., Englewood, Colo.)

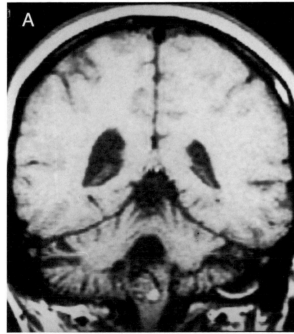
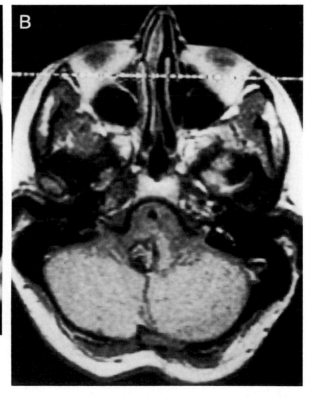

FIG 11–18.
Pontine cavernous angioma. **A,** coronal MRI (SE, 700/30) demonstrates a mulberry appearance of multiple areas of prior hemorrhage surrounded by a hemosiderin rim. **B,** axial MRI (SE, 2,000/30) demonstrates a complete hemosiderin rim surrounding the cavernous angioma.

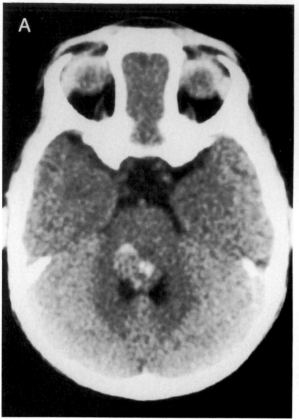 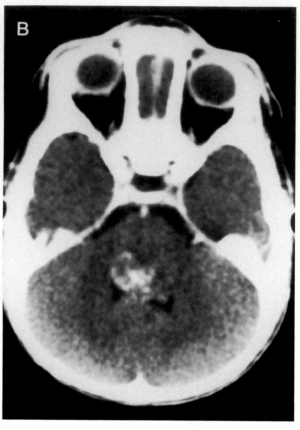

FIG 11–19.
Angiographically occult (thrombosed) AVM. **A,** an uncontrasted CT scan demonstrates a mottled area of hyperdensity arising from the posterior portion of the pons. A portion of the hyperdensity repre- sents calcification. **B,** a contrast-enhanced scan shows inhomoge- neous enhancement of the thrombosed AVM.

rhaged.[75–79] The following MRI characteristics are virtually diagnostic of AOVMs[79]:

1. Focal signal heterogeneity, which corre- sponds to subacute and chronic hemor- rhage.
2. A peripheral circumferential, complete ring of markedly hypointense signal on long TR/ long TE sequences, which represents he- mosiderin deposition.
3. Lack of mass effect or edema.
4. No demonstrable feeding arteries or drain- ing veins.

An AOVM that has acutely hemorrhaged will dem- onstrate edema and mass effect on MRI and may be difficult to distinguish from a hemorrhagic tu- mor. Follow-up examinations showing diminished mass effect and edema and signal characteristics typical of an AOVM are useful in making this dis- tinction (Fig 11–20). An AOVM that has never bled may not have the characteristic MRI appear- ance. In this case, high-resolution uncontrasted CT may be a useful adjunct to detect calcification within the AOVM.[75]

HYPERTENSIVE HEMORRHAGE

Hypertension is a common cause of spontane- ous intracerebral hemorrhage (see Fig 11–3). Hy- pertension induces hyaline fibrinoid degenerative changes in the media of small cerebral arteries. In addition, microaneurysms (Charcot-Bouchard an- eurysms) are found in the walls of small arterioles of hypertensive patients at autopsy.[80] These struc- tural weaknesses predispose to vessel rupture and hemorrhage. The most common location for hyper- tensive hemorrhage is the basal ganglia (64%). Other common locations include hemispheric white matter (13%), the pons and midbrain (12%), the cerebellum (12%), and the thalamus (11%).[81] Hemorrhages associated with hypertension are of- ten large and primarily intraparenchymal in loca-

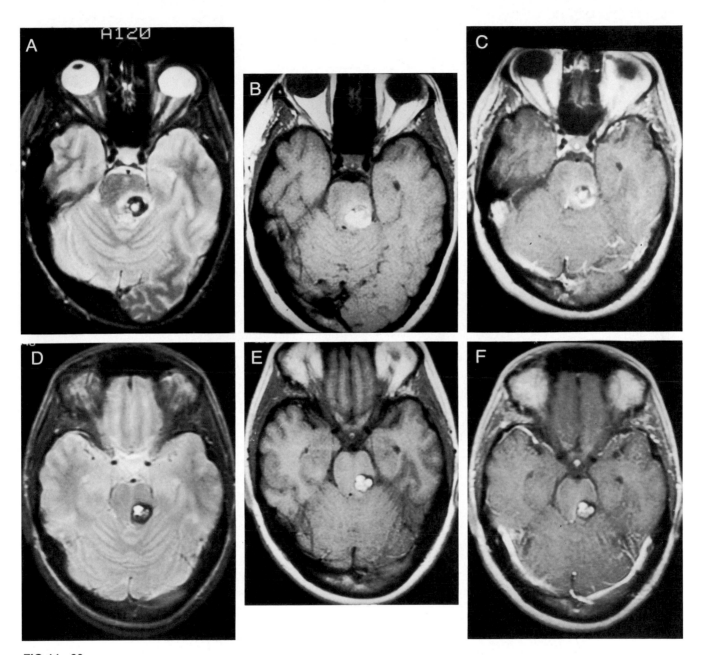

FIG 11–20.
Hemorrhagic angiographically occult vascular malformation, MRI. **A,** SE, 2,500/80. **B,** SE, 600/20. **C,** post–gadolinium-DTPA, SE, 567/30. There is mixed signal intensity consistent with intracellular and extracellular methemoglobin. On the long TR image **(A)** edema and mass effect within the pons is evident. There is enhancement surrounding the hematoma on the post–gadolinium-DTPA image **(C).** At this stage differentiation between hemorrhage into a neoplasm or hemorrhage into an occult AVM cannot be made with certainty. **D–F,** follow-up MRI in 4 months. **D,** SE, 2,500/80. **E,** SE, 600/20. **F,** post–gadolinium-DTPA, SE, 567/30. The scans demonstrate the decreased size of the hematoma. There is a well-defined rim of hypointensity representing hemosiderin on the long TR image **(D).** There is no edema or mass effect. There is no enhancement following contrast **(E and F).** This lesion is an angiographically occult AVM.

tion and often dissect into the ventricular system. The overall mortality rate of hypertensive hemorrhage is approximately 50%, with increasing mortality depending upon the size of the hematoma and the presence and degree of intraventricular extension.[82]

CONGOPHILIC (AMYLOID) ANGIOPATHY

Beginning in the seventh decade of life, congophilic angiopathy becomes the cause of an increasing number of cases of cerebral hemorrhages. Patients with congophilic angiopathy usually present with dementia. In addition, these patients tend to have repeated hemorrhage in unusual locations in that the hemorrhages tend to be lobar and superficial in location in contrast to the typical central location of hypertensive hemorrhages (Fig 11–21). Hemorrhage from congophilic angiopathy is most common in the parieto-occipital region. The basal ganglia, cerebellum, and brain stem are usually spared.[83-85]

Autopsy studies demonstrate congophilic deposits of amyloid protein in the media and adventitia of cortical and leptomeningeal arterioles.

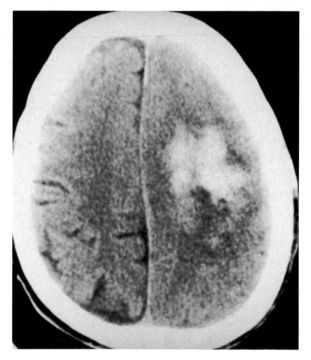

FIG 11–21.
Seventy-one-year-old with amyloid angiopathy. Uncontrasted CT shows a peripheral left parietal hematoma involving both gray and white matter.

There is often segmental fibrinoid degeneration and microaneurysm formation.[86]

TUMORAL HEMORRHAGE

Bleeding into tumors is another cause of intracerebral hemorrhage. It has been reported that 1% to 3% of primary gliomas and 3% to 14% of metastases bleed.[87-90] Glioblastoma multiforme, oligodendroglioma, and ependymoma are the primary brain neoplasms that most commonly hemorrhage (see Chapter 16).[87, 88] Among metastases, melanoma, choriocarcinoma, and renal cell and thyroid carcinomas are the most likely to bleed (Fig 11–22).[89]

Hemorrhagic metastases are often multiple and are located at the gray-white junction. The CT pattern of either primary or metastatic intratumoral hemorrhage may be difficult to distinguish from other causes of hemorrhage (i.e., hemorrhagic infarction). Hemorrhage in an unusual location with an irregular enhancement pattern accompanied by abundant mass effect are features that suggest tumoral hemorrhage.[88] Nonhomogeneous perihemorrhagic enhancement persisting beyond approximately 8 weeks after the ictus is another finding that helps distinguish tumoral hemorrhage from single hypertensive hemorrhage or hemorrhagic infarction.

MRI of hemorrhagic neoplasms often demonstrates marked signal heterogeneity; areas of nonhemorrhagic abnormal signal intensity corresponding to nonhemorrhagic portions of the tumor are often present. When compared with nonneoplastic hematomas, neoplastic hemorrhage has diminished, irregular, or absent hemosiderin deposition; pronounced and persistent edema; and delayed hematoma evolution.[91, 92]

HEMORRHAGIC INFARCTION

Although foci of microscopic petechial hemorrhages occur in approximately 25% of infarction on neuropathologic examination, gross hemorrhage into regions of infarction are uncommon.[93] The mechanism of hemorrhage typically involves reperfusion of areas of ischemic brain. This most commonly occurs when an embolus fragments and migrates distally after occluding an artery for a period of time. Much less commonly, a hemorrhagic component to cerebral infarction is due to luxury per-

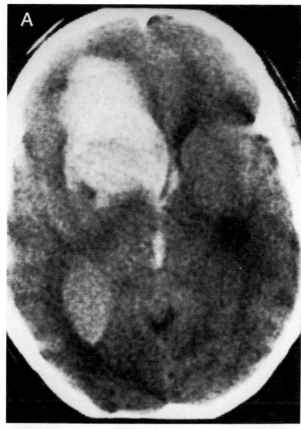

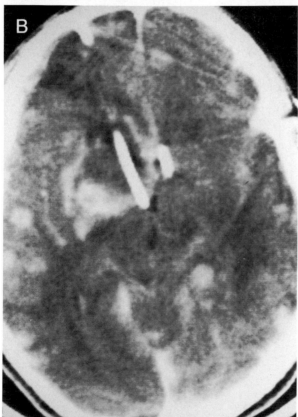

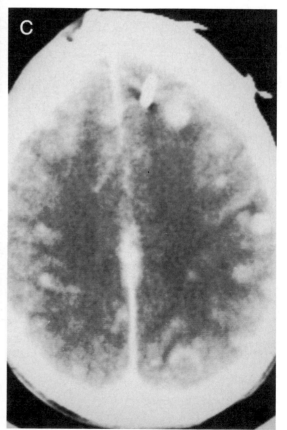

FIG 11–22.
Hemorrhagic metastatic melanoma. **A,** uncontrasted CT demonstrates massive IPH involving the right basal ganglia and right frontal lobe. Blood has dissected into the ventricular system as well. **B** and **C,** contrast-enhanced CT following surgical decompression and biventricular shunt placement demonstrates multiple enhancing metastatic melanoma nodules located primarily at gray-white junctions.

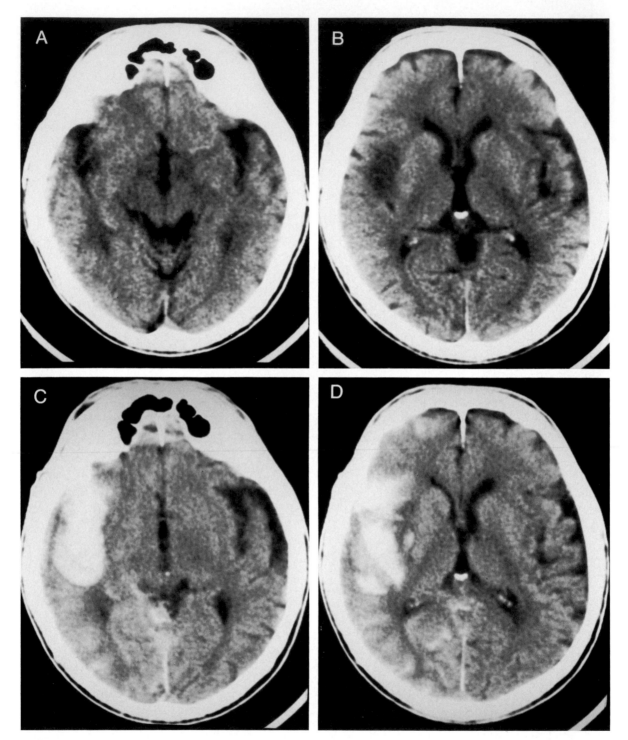

FIG 11–23.
Hemorrhage infarct in a 60-year-old male with an acute onset of left hemiparesis. **A** and **B,** an admission uncontrasted CT scan demonstrates an acute right middle cerebral artery territory infarct.

C and **D,** a CT scan obtained for neurologic deterioration 24 hours following admission shows gross hemorrhage into the area of infarction.

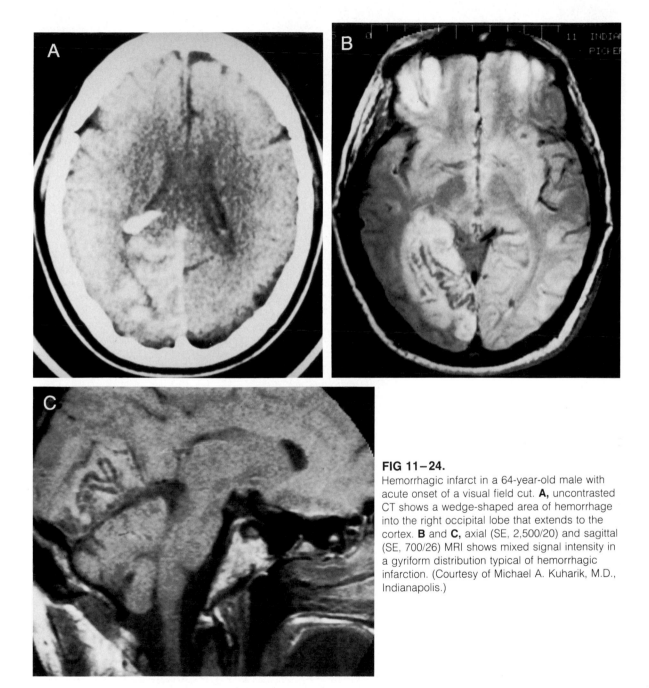

FIG 11–24.
Hemorrhagic infarct in a 64-year-old male with acute onset of a visual field cut. **A,** uncontrasted CT shows a wedge-shaped area of hemorrhage into the right occipital lobe that extends to the cortex. **B** and **C,** axial (SE, 2,500/20) and sagittal (SE, 700/26) MRI shows mixed signal intensity in a gyriform distribution typical of hemorrhagic infarction. (Courtesy of Michael A. Kuharik, M.D., Indianapolis.)

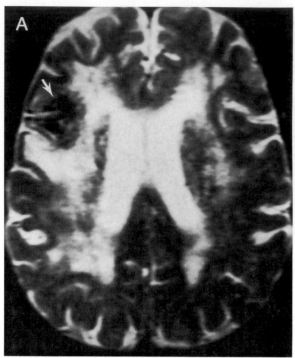 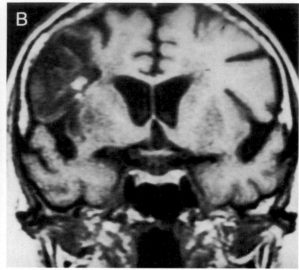

FIG 11–25.
Chronic hemorrhagic cerebral infarction. **A,** axial MRI (SE, 2,500/100). **B,** coronal MRI (SE, 700/20). The scans demonstrate an area of chronic hemorrhagic infarction in the right frontal and parietal lobes with areas of methemoglobin (high signal intensity on short TR/short TE image **(B)** and areas of hemosiderin deposition (low signal intensity on long TR/long TE image [**A,** *arrow*]). Increased signal in the periventricular white matter **(A)** is due to deep white matter ischemic changes.

fusion from leptomeningeal collateral supplies following proximal thrombotic occlusion, restoration of normal blood pressure following a hypotensive episode, or impairment of venous outflow due to developing edema.[94]

Uncontrasted CT scanning is utilized in patients with acute clinical signs of stroke to exclude a hemorrhagic component since the presence of hemorrhage constitutes a contraindication to anticoagulant or thrombolytic therapy. Also, uncontrasted CT is useful in excluding delayed hemorrhage in stroke patients whose neurologic condition deteriorates following the initial event (Fig 11–23).

Petechial hemorrhage into an area of infarction may cause the affected area to become isodense to normal brain parenchyma on an uncontrasted CT scan due to the combined attenuation effects of the blood and the tissue edema. Mass effect due to edema will usually be evident.

If the petechial hemorrhages coalesce to form a gross hemorrhage, unenhanced CT demonstrates a large hematoma surrounded by lucency and located in a vascular distribution. Subacutely, the area about the infarct may enhance, thus making differentiation from a hemorrhagic tumor difficult. Mass effect from the hemorrhagic infarct is usually minimal or decreasing at the time of maximal con-

trast enhancement (2 to 4 weeks), which aids in differentiating between hemorrhagic infarction and tumor.[94] Also, the gyriform pattern of enhancement often seen with hemorrhagic infarcts is not the usual pattern detected with tumoral hemorrhage.

As with other forms of intracranial hemorrhage, the MRI appearance of hemorrhagic infarction varies with the timing of imaging following the ictus.[95] In the acute phase (5 to 18 days) deoxyhemoglobin is present within the cortical hemorrhage, and there is subcortical edema present. On long TR/long TE sequences, this is depicted as slight cortical hypointensity peripheral to subcortical hyperintensity. On short TR/short TE sequences, cortical hemorrhage is isointense to gray matter at this stage. Subacutely (18 to 24 days) there is methemoglobin formation within the cortical hemorrhage that causes a hyperintense appearance of the involved cortex on both long TR/long TE and short TR/short TE sequences. Chronically (greater than 24 days) there is marked hypointensity, most readily seen on long TR/long TE sequences, of the enfolded cortical gyri due to hemosiderin deposition (Figs 11–24 and 11–25).

The timing of the MRI signal intensity changes in hemorrhagic cortical infarction differs somewhat from that of other causes of intraparenchymal hem-

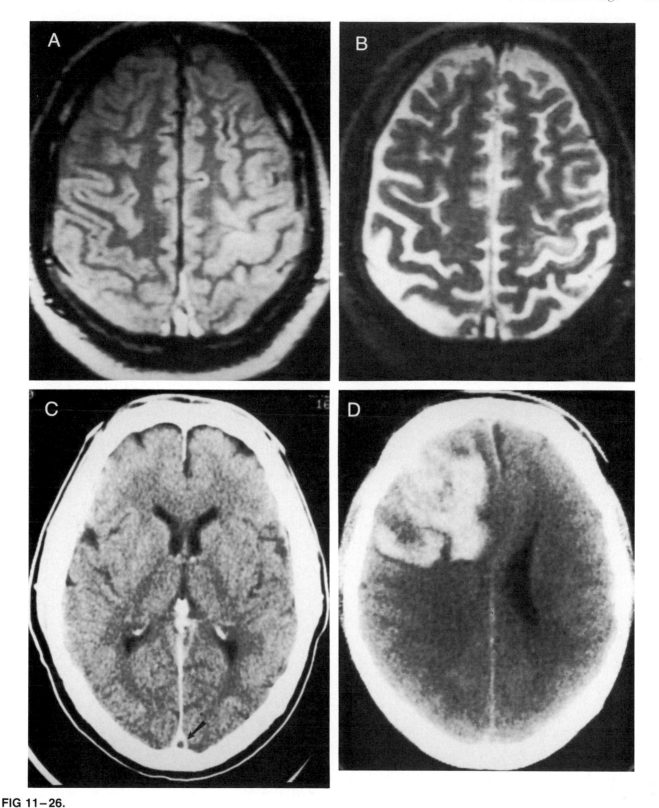

FIG 11–26.
Hemorrhagic infarction secondary to dural sinus thrombosis. Axial MRI (**A:** SE, 2,000/40; **B:** SE, 2,000/80) shows high signal within the sagittal sinus on both even and odd echoes due to sagittal sinus thrombosis. **C,** contrast-enhanced CT demonstrates a triangular area of lack of enhancement (delta sign) in the sagittal sinus *(arrow)* due to thrombosis. **D,** an unenhanced CT scan 4 days later demonstrates a large right frontal hemorrhage secondary to obstruction of venous outflow and venous infarction.

orrhage, which may aid in the differential diagnosis. The difference is thought to be due to a higher local pO_2 in hemorrhagic cortical infarction because of early revascularization and luxury perfusion. The higher pO_2 decreases the percentage of intracellular deoxyhemoglobin and, therefore, diminishes the acute T2 relaxation effect. Also, localization of the hemorrhage to the cortical ribbon in the subacute and chronic stages aids in the diagnosis.

GERMINAL MATRIX HEMORRHAGE

Low–birth weight infants, especially premature babies, are at high risk for the development of GMH. Nearly half of the babies with birth weights of 1,500 g or less develop GMH, although not all manifest clinical disease.[96] In the past the screening examination of choice was CT scanning, but now ultrasonography is the primary imaging modality since it is noninvasive, requires only minimal patient cooperation for an adequate examination, and is almost ideally suited to the newborn whose fontanelles serve as windows for the procedure. Furthermore, ultrasonography can be performed in the neonatal intensive care unit (ICU). Areas of hemorrhage are depicted as echogenic foci on ultrasound.

GMH is graded according to the classification scheme of Papile et al., as follows[96]:

Grade I.—Focal subependymal hemorrhage.
Grade II.—Extension into the lateral ventricle, normal ventricular size.
Grade III.—Extension into the ventricular system with ventriculomegaly.
Grade IV.—Parenchymal extension.

Clinical outcome is dependent upon the grade of hemorrhage. Grades I and II usually resolve without clinical sequelae. The prognosis is worse for grades III and IV. Approximately 33% of neonates with grade III hemorrhage require ventricular shunts for progressive hydrocephalus.[97] Many neonates with grade IV GMH develop large porencephalic cysts in areas of IPH.[98]

MISCELLANEOUS CAUSES OF NONTRAUMATIC INTRACEREBRAL HEMORRHAGE

Venous Hemorrhage

As mentioned previously, increased cerebral venous pressure due to arterialization of venous drainage from an AVM or obstruction of venous outflow due to edema resulting from cerebral infarction may induce venous hemorrhage. Other causes of raised venous pressure that predispose to hemorrhage include dural sinus thrombosis and carotid cavernous fistula.[99–101] Parenchymal hemorrhages are seen in approximately 20% of sinovenous thrombosis cases.[100] The hemorrhages are usually peripheral and are usually unilateral (Fig 11–26).

Cortical venous drainage from a carotid cavernous fistula is associated with a high incidence of IPH. The cortical venous drainage may be due to occlusion or an absence of the normal basal venous outflow pathways. SAH associated with carotid cavernous fistulas is usually secondary to the formation of a cavernous sinus varix that extends into the subarachnoid space.[102]

Coagulopathies

One of the more common coagulopathies associated with intracranial hemorrhage is the use of anticoagulation therapy. Intracranial hemorrhage is much more common in patients treated with warfarin sodium (Coumadin) than with heparin.[103] The incidence of intracranial hemorrhage in patients with thrombocytopenia is approximately 1% to 4%. Generally, if the platelet count exceeds 60,000/mm³ the risk of hemorrhage is low. As the platelet count falls below 20,000/mm³ the risk of hemorrhage drastically increases.[104] Other coagulopathies associated with intracranial hemorrhage include von Willebrand disease and hemophilia. Central nervous system bleeding is the leading cause of death among hemophiliacs.[105]

Mycotic Aneurysms

A major cause of peripheral aneurysms is septic emboli secondary to bacterial endocarditis. Approximately 3% to 10% of patients with bacterial endocarditis develop mycotic aneurysms.[106] Parenchymal hemorrhages secondary to rupture of mycotic aneurysms are typically multiple and peripheral in location (Fig 11–27).

Drug Abuse

Amphetamines, cocaine, and phencyclidine are drugs of abuse that may be associated with IPH.[1–3] Amphetamines are thought to induce necrotizing vasculitis associated with microaneurysm formation.[1] IPH from cocaine abuse is thought to be sec-

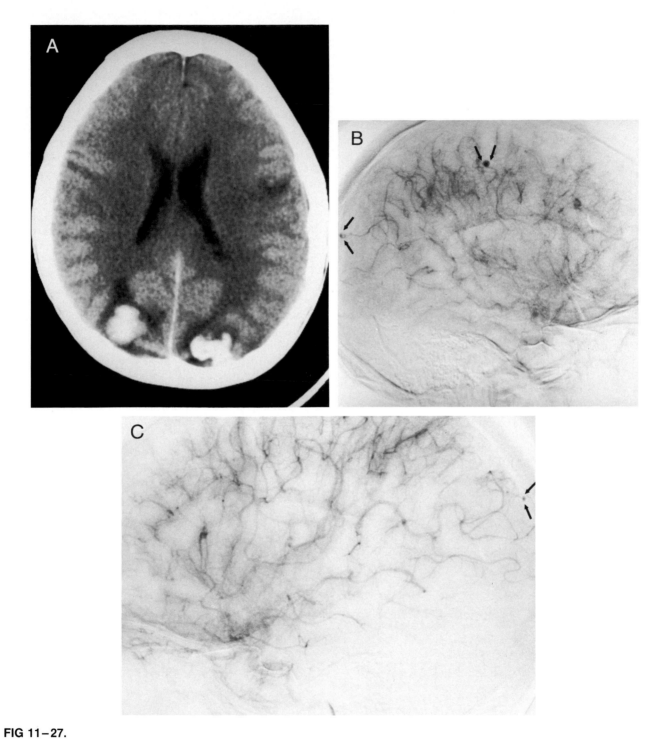

FIG 11–27.
Fourteen-year-old male with acute *Staphylococcus aureus* endocarditis, mycotic aneurysms, and hemorrhage. **A,** an unenhanced CT scan demonstrates peripheral hematomas in the posterior parietal lobes bilaterally. **B** and **C,** capillary phases of right **(B)** and left **(C)** internal carotid artery angiograms demonstrate multiple mycotic aneurysms on the peripheral middle cerebral branches bilaterally *(arrows).*

ondary to the acute rise in systemic blood pressure caused by the drug due to reuptake inhibition of catecholamines at the synaptic level.

REFERENCES

1. Yu YJ, Cooper DR, Wellenstein DE, et al: Cerebral angiitis and intracerebral hemorrhage associated with methamphetamine abuse. *J Neurosurg* 1983; 58:109–111.
2. Lichlenfeld PJ, Rubin DB, Feldman RS: Subarachnoid hemorrhage precipitated by cocaine snorting. *Arch Neurol* 1984; 41:223–224.
3. Bessen HA: Intracranial hemorrhage associated with phenycyclidene abuse. *JAMA* 1982; 248:585–586.
4. Inoui Y, Saiwai S, Miyamato T, et al: Post contrast computed tomography in subarachnoid hemorrhage from rupture aneurysms. *J Comput Assist Tomogr* 1981; 5:341–344.
5. Ghoshhajra K, Scotti L, Marasco J, et al: CT detection of intracranial aneurysm in subarachnoid hemorrhage. *AJR* 1979; 132:613–616.
6. Liliequist B, Lindquist M, Valdimarsson E: Computed tomography and subarachnoid hemorrhage. *Neuroradiology* 1977; 14:21–26.
7. Lim ST, Sage DJ: Detection of subarachnoid blood clot and other thin flat structures by computed tomography. *Radiology* 1977; 123:79–84.
8. Satoh S, Kadoya S: Magnetic resonance imaging of subarachnoid hemorrhage. *Neuroradiology* 1988; 30:361–366.
9. Barkovich AJ, Atlas SW: Magnetic resonance imaging of intracranial hemorrhage. *Radiol Clin North Am* 1988; 26:801–820.
10. Grossman RI, Kemp SS, Yulp C, et al: The importance of oxygenation in the appearance of subarachnoid hemorrhage on high field magnetic resonance imaging. *Acta Radiol*, in press.
11. Neill JM, Hasting AB: The influence of the tension of molecular oxygen upon certain oxidations of hemoglobin. *J Biol Chem* 1925; 63:479–484.
12. Gomori JM, Bilaniuk LT, Zimmerman RA, et al: High field MR imaging of superficial siderosis of the central nervous system. *J Comp Assist Tomogr* 1984; 9:972–976.
13. Gomori JM, Grossman RI, Goldberg HI, et al: High field spin-echo MR imaging of superficial and subependymal siderosis secondary to neonatal intraventricular hemorrhage. *Neuroradiology* 1987; 29:339–343.
14. Davis JM, Ploetz J, Davis KR, et al: Cranial computed tomography in subarachnoid hemorrhages: Relationship between blood detected by CT and lumbar puncture. *J Comput Assist Tomogr* 1980; 4:794–796.
15. Lee Y, Mosei R, Bruner JM, et al: Organized intracerebral hematoma with acute hemorrhage: CT patients and pathological correlations. *AJR* 1986; 147:111–118.
16. Enzmann DR, Britt RH, Lyons BE, et al: Natural history of experimental intracerebral hemorrhage: Sonography, computed tomography, and neuropathology. *AJNR* 1981; 2:517–526.
17. Zimmerman RD, Hein LA, Snow RB, et al: Acute intracranial hemorrhage: Intensity changes on sequential MR scans at 0.5 T. *AJNR* 1988; 9:47–53.
18. Gomori JM, Grossman RI, Goldberg HI, et al: Intracranial hematomas: Imaging by high field MR. *Radiology* 1985; 157:87–93.
19. Zimmerman RD, Deck MF: Intracranial hematomas: Imaging by high field MR. *Radiology* 1986; 159:565–569.
20. Walton JN: Subarachnoid Hemorrhage. London, ES Livingstone, 1956.
21. Jellinger K: Pathology and aetiology of intracranial aneurysms, in Pia HW, Langmaid L, Zierski J (eds): *Advances in Diagnosis and Therapy*. New York, Springer Publishing Co, Inc, 1979, pp 5–19.
22. Bannerman RM, Ingall GB, Graf CJ: The familial occurrence of intracranial aneurysms. *Neurology* 1970; 20:283–292.
23. Chason JL, Hindman WM: Berry aneurysms of the circle of Willis: Results of a planned autopsy study. *Neurology* 1958; 8:41–44.
24. McCormick WF, A Costa-Rua GJ: The size of intracranial saccular aneurysm: An autopsy study. *J Neurosurg* 1970; 33:422–427.
25. Parkarinen S: Incidence, etiology, and prognosis of primary subarachnoid hemorrhage: A study based on 589 cases diagnosed in a defined population during a defined period. *Acta Neurol Scand Suppl* 1967; 29:1–128.
26. Locksly HB: Natural history of subarachnoid hemorrhages, intracranial aneurysms, and arteriovenous malformations: Based on 6,368 cases, in Sahs AL, Perret GF (eds): *Intracranial Aneurysms and Subarachnoid Hemorrhage: A Cooperative Study*. Philadelphia, JB Lippincott, 1969, pp 37–108.
27. Winn HR, Richardson AE, Jane JA: The assessment of the natural history of single cerebral aneurysms that have ruptured, in Hopkins LN, Long DM (eds): *Clinical Management of Intracranial Aneurysms*, New York, Raven Press, 1982, pp 1–10.
28. Kassel NF, Torner JL: Aneurysm bleeding: A preliminary report from the cooperative study. *Neurosurgery* 1983; 13:479–481.
29. Jane JA, Winn HR, Richardson AE: The natural history of intracranial aneurysms rebleeding during the acute and long-term period and implication for surgical management. *Clin Neurosurg* 1977; 24:208–215.
30. McKissock W, Richardson A, Walsh L, et al: Multiple intracranial aneurysms. *Lancet* 1964; 1:623–631.

31. Stehbens WE: Etiology of intracranial berry aneurysms. *J Neurosurg* 1989; 70:823–831.

32. Sekhar LN, Heros RB: Origin, growth, and rupture of saccular aneurysms: A review. *Neurosurgery* 1981; 8:248–260.

33. Ferguson GG: Physical factors in the initiation, growth, and rupture of human intracranial saccular aneurysms. *J Neurosurg* 1972; 37:666–677.

34. Campbell GJ, Roach MR: Fenestrations in the internal elastic lamina at bifarctions of human cerebral arteries. *Stroke* 1981; 12:489–496.

35. Stehbens WE: Experimental arterial loops and arterial atrophy. *Exp Mol Pathol* 1986; 44:177–189.

36. Belber CJ, Hoffman RB: The syndrome of intracranial aneurysms associated with fibromuscular hyperplasia of renal arteries. *J Neurosurg* 1969; 28:556–561.

37. Hatfield PM, Pfister RC: Adult polycystic disease of the kidney (Potter type 3). *JAMA* 1972; 222:1527–1533.

38. McKusik VA: The cardiovascular aspects of Marfan's syndrome: A heritable disorder of connective tissue. *Circulation* 1955; 11:321–328.

39. Newton TH, Troost BT: Arteriovenous malformations and fistulae, in Newton TH, Potts DG (eds): *Radiology of the Skull and Brain.* St Louis, CV Mosby Co, 1974, p 2512.

40. Silver AJ, Pederson ME, Ganti SR, et al: CT of subarachnoid hemorrhage due to ruptured aneurysm. *AJNR* 1981; 2:549–552.

41. Yock OH, Larson DA: Computed tomography on hemorrhage from anterior communicating artery aneurysms, with angiographic correlation. *Radiology* 1980; 134:399–407.

42. Schmid U, Steiger HJ, Huber P: Accuracy of high resolution computed tomography in direct diagnosis of cerebral aneurysms. *Neuroradiology* 1987; 29:152–159.

43. Hackney DB, Lesnick JE, Zimmerman RA, et al: MR identification of bleeding site in subarachnoid hemorrhage with multiple intracranial aneurysm. *J Comput Assist Tomogr* 1986; 10:787–880.

44. Wagle WA, Dumoulin CL, Souza SP, et al: 3DFT MR angiography of carotid and basilar arteries. *AJNR* 1989; 10:911–919.

45. Atlas SW, Grossman RI, Goldberg HI, et al: Partially thrombosed giant intracranial aneurysms: Correlation of MR and pathological findings. *Radiology* 1987; 162:111–114.

46. Tsuruda JS, Halbach VV, Higashida RT: MR evaluation of large intracranial aneurysms using one low flip angle gradient-refocused imaging. *AJNR* 1988; 9:415–424.

47. Griffith HB, Cummings BH, Thompson JG: Cerebral arterial spasm and hydrocephalus in leaking arterial aneurysms. *Neuroradiology* 1972; 4:212–214.

48. Wier BKA: The effect of vasospasm on morbidity and mortality after subarachnoid hemorrhage from ruptured aneurysms, in William RH (ed): *Cerebral Arterial Spasm.* Baltimore, Williams & Wilkins 1980, pp 385–393.

49. Bryan RN, Shah CP, Hilal S: Evaluation of subarachnoid hemorrhage and cerebral spasm by computed tomography. *Comput Tomogr* 1979; 3:144–153.

50. Davis JM, Davis KR, Crowell RM: Subarachnoid hemorrhage secondary to rupture in transcranial aneurysm: Prognostic significance of cranial CT. *AJR* 1980; 134:711–715.

51. Davis KR, New PFJ, Diemann RG, et al: Computed tomographic evaluation of hemorrhage secondary to intracranial aneurysm. *AJR* 1976; 127:143–153.

52. Allcock JM, Drake CG: Ruptured intracranial aneurysms—the role of arterial spasm. *J Neurosurg* 1969; 22:21–29.

53. Wilkins RH, Alexander JA, Odom GL: Intracranial arterial spasm: A clinical analysis. *J Neurosurg* 1968; 29:121–134.

54. Heros RC, Zervas NT, Negoro M: Cerebral vasospasm. *Surg Neurol* 1976; 5:354–362.

55. Wellum GR, Irvine TW, Zervas NT: Cerebral vasoactivity of hemeproteins in vitro: Some mechanistic considerations. *J Neurosurg* 1982; 56:777–783.

56. Weir B, Grace M, Hansen JG, et al: Time course of vasospasm in man. *J Neurosurg* 1978; 48:173–178.

57. Katada K, Kanno T, Sano H, et al: Computed tomography of ruptured intracranial aneurysms in the acute stage. *No Shinkei Geka* 1977; 5:955–963.

58. Yonas H, Good WH, Gur D, et al: Mapping cerebral blood flow by xenon enhanced computed tomography: Clinical experience. *Radiology* 1984; 152:435–442.

59. McCormick WF: The pathology of vascular "arteriovenous" malformations. *J Neurosurg* 1966; 24:807–816.

60. Theron J, Newton TH, Hoyt WF: Unilateral retinocephalic vascular malformations. *Neuroradiology* 1974; 7:185–196.

61. Forster DMC, Steiner L, Hakanson S: Arteriovenous malformation of the brain. A long term clinical study. *J Neurosurg* 1972; 37:562–568.

62. Marks MP, O'Donahue J, Fabricant JI, et al: Cerebral blood flow evaluation of arteriovenous malformations with stable xenon CT. *AJNR* 1988; 9:1169–1175.

63. Tarr RW, Johnson DW, Ritigliano M, et al: Assessment of cerebral blood flow dynamics in patients with arteriovenous malformations using acetazolamide challenge xenon computerized tomography. Presented at the 27th Annual Meeting of the American Society of Neuroradiology. Orlando, Fla, March 1989.

64. Cabanes J, Blasco R, Garcia M, et al: Cerebral venous angiomas. *Surg Neurol* 1979; 11:385–389.

65. Olson E, Gilmor RL, Richmond B: Cerebral venous angiomas. *Radiology* 1984; 151:97–104.

66. Sordet D, Beroud P, Pharaboz C, et al: Angioma veineux cerebral aspects angiographique et tomodenis tometrique. *J Radiol* 1986; 67:285–287.

67. Rigomonti D, Spetzler RF, Drayer BP, et al: Appearance of venous malformations on magnetic resonance imaging. *J Neurosurg* 1988; 69:535–539.

68. Soviardo M, Strata L, Passerini A: Intracranial cavernous hemangiomas: Neuroradiologic review of 36 operated cases. *AJNR* 1983; 4:945–950.

69. Rao KCVG, Lee SH: Cerebrovascular anomalies, in Stark DD, Bradley WG (eds): *Magnetic Resonance Imaging*. St Louis, CV Mosby Co, 1988.

70. Heinz ER: Angiographically occult cerebral vascular malformations and venous angiomas, in Taveras JM, Ferrucci JT (eds): *Radiology: Diagnosis— Imaging—Intervention*. Philadelphia, JB Lippincott, Co, 1988.

71. Rigamonti D, Hadley MN, Drayer BP, et al: Cerebral cavernous angiomas: Incidence and familial occurrence. *N Engl J Med* 1988; 319:343–347.

72. Baker DH, Townsend JJ, Kramer RA, et al: Occult cerebrovascular malformations: A series of 18 histologically verified cases with negative angiography. *Brain* 1979; 102:279–287.

73. Farrell DF, Forno LS: Symptomatic capillary telangiectasis of the brainstem without hemorrhage. *Neurology* 1970; 20:341–346.

74. Lobato RD, Perez C, Rivas JJ, et al: Clinical radiological and pathological spectrum of angiographically occult intracranial vascular malformations: Analysis of 21 cases and review of the literature. *J Neurosurg* 1988; 68:518–531.

75. Griffin C, DeLapaz R, Enzmann DR: Magnetic resonance appearance of slow flow vascular malformations of the brainstem. *Neuroradiology* 1987; 29:506–511.

76. Lemme-Plaghos L, Kucharzykw W, Brant-Zawadski M, et al: MRI of angiographically occult vascular malformations. *AJR* 1986; 146:1223–1225.

77. Schoner W, Bradol GB, Treisch J, et al: Magnetic resonance imaging in the diagnosis of cerebral arteriovenous angiomas. *Neuroradiology* 1986; 28:313–317.

78. New PFJ, Ojeman RG, Davis KR, et al: MR and CT of occult vascular malformations of the brain. *AJNR* 1986; 7:771–779.

79. Gomori JM, Grossman RI, Goldberg HI, et al: Occult cerebral vascular malformations: High-field MR. *Radiology* 1986; 158:707–713.

80. Cole FM, Yates PO: Pseudoaneurysms in relationship to massive cerebral hemorrhage. *J Neurol Neurosurg Psychiatry* 1967; 30:61–66.

81. Pia HW, Langmaid C, Zierski J (eds): Spontaneous intracerebral hematomas. In *Advances in Diagnosis and Therapy*. Berlin, Springer-Verlag, 1980.

82. Cahill DW, Ducker TB: Spontaneous intracerebral hemorrhage. *Clin Neurosurg* 1982; 29:722–779.

83. Loes DJ, Smoker WRK, Biller J, et al: Nontraumatic intracerebral hemorrhage: CT/angiographic correlation. *AJNR* 1987; 8:1027–1030.

84. Patel DV, Hier DB, Thomas CM, et al: Intracerebral hemorrhage secondary to amyloid angiopathy. *Radiology* 1984; 151:397–400.

85. Tucker WS, Bilbao JM, Klodowsky H: Cerebral amyloid angiopathy and multiple intracerebral hematoma. *Neurosurg* 1980; 7:611–614.

86. Wagle WA, Smith TW, Weiner M: Intracerebral hemorrhage caused by cerebral amyloid angiopathy: Radiographic-pathologic correlation. *AJNR* 1984; 5:171–176.

87. Leeds NE, Elkin CM, Zimmerman RD: Glioma of the brain. *Semin Roentgenol* 1984; 19:27–43.

88. Zimmerman RA, Bilanicik LT: Computed tomography of intratumoral hemorrhage. *Radiology* 1980; 135:355–359.

89. Manybur TI: Intracranial hemorrhage caused by metastatic tumors. *Neuroradiology* 1977; 27:650–655.

90. Russell DS, Rubenstein LJ: *Pathology of Tumors of the Nervous System*. Baltimore, Williams & Wilkins, 1977.

91. Atlas SW, Grossman RI, Gomori JM, et al: Hemorrhagic intracranial malignant neoplasms: Spin echo MR imaging. *Radiology* 1987; 164:71–77.

92. Sze G, Krol G, Olsen WL, et al: Hemorrhagic neoplasms: MR mimics of occult vascular malformations. *AJNR* 1987; 8:795–802.

93. Fisher CM, Adams RD: Observations on brain embolism with special reference to the mechanism of hemorrhagic infarction. *J Neuropathol Exp Neurol* 1951; 10:92–94.

94. Davis KR, Ackerman RH, Kistler JP, et al: Computed tomography of cerebral infarction: Hemorrhagic, contrast enhancement, and time of appearance. *Comput Tomogr* 1977; 1:71–76.

95. Hecht-Leavitt C, Gomori JM, Grossman RI, et al: High-field MRI of hemorrhagic cortical infarction. *AJNR* 1986; 7:581–585.

96. Papile LA, Burstein J, Burstein R, et al: Incidence and evolution of subependymal and intraventricular hemorrhage: A study of infants with birth weights less than 1500 gm. *J Pediatr* 1978; 92:529–534.

97. Fleischer AC, Hutchison AA, Bundy AL, et al. Serial sonography of post-hemorrhagic ventricular dilatation and porencephaly after intracranial hemorrhage in the protein neonate. *AJR* 1983; 141:451–455.

98. Grant EG, Kerner M, Schellinger D, et al: Evolution of porencephalic intraparenchymal hemorrhage in the neonate: Sonographic evidence. *AJR* 1982; 138:467–470.

99. Bauser MG, Chiras J, Bories J, et al: Cerebral venous thrombosis—A review of 38 cases. *Stroke* 1987; 16:199–213.

100. Buonamo FS, Moody DM, Ball RM: CT scan find-

ings in cerebral sinovenous occlusion. *J Comput Assist Tomogr* 1978; 2:281–290.

101. Rao CVK, Knipp HC, Wagner EJ: Computed tomographic findings in cerebral sinus and venous thrombosis. *Radiology* 1981; 140:391–398.

102. Halbach VV, Hieshima GM, Higashida RT, et al: Carotid-cavernous fistulae: Indication for urgent treatment. *AJNR* 1987; 4:627–631.

103. Snyder M, Renaudin J: Intracranial hemorrhage associated with anticoagulation therapy. *Surg Neurol* 1977; 7:31–34.

104. Renaudin J, George RP: Coagulopathies causing intracranial hemorrhage, in Wilkins RH, Rengochany SS (eds): *Neurosurgery*. New York, McGraw-Hill International Book Co, 1985.

105. Eyster ME, Gill FM, Blatt PM, et al: Central nervous system bleeding in hemophiliac. *Blood* 1978; 51:1179–1188.

106. Olmsted WW, McGee TP: The pathogenesis of peripheral aneurysms of the central nervous system: A subject review from AFIP. *Radiology* 1977; 123:661–666.

PART V

Inflammatory Diseases of the Brain

12

Intracranial Infections and Inflammatory Diseases

Charles A. Jungreis, M.D.

Robert I. Grossman, M.D.

Innumerable inflammatory and infectious diseases affect the intracranial contents. Nevertheless, the affected tissues can respond in only a limited number of ways. Thus, many diseases appear similar in an imaging examination. Differentiating the possibilities at times will be impossible when based solely on the examination. Often, a comparison with previous examinations or follow-up examinations are required to identify a trend or progression. Furthermore, the clinical history is extremely important, and the imaging examination must be interpreted in the appropriate context to be meaningful.

Infections and inflammation have a tendency to localize in one of several compartments that conceptually and pathophysiologically are limited by the membranes (meninges) surrounding the brain. However, diseases frequently cross from meninges to parenchyma and vice versa. Thus, while this discussion will be organized by location, understand that such localization is artificial and that disease processes may involve both meninges and parenchyma at the same time, often spreading from one to the other.

Both magnetic resonance imaging (MRI) and computed tomography (CT) are exquisitely sensitive examinations, and much has been written on which examination is more appropriate in a particular disease state. Comparisons will not be attempted in this chapter. Also, we will not attempt to demonstrate all forms of infection and inflammation but will demonstrate exemplary cases (Fig 12–1).

EXTRAPARENCHYMAL DISEASE

Anatomy

The meninges surround the brain and separate it from the surrounding calvarium and skull base (Fig 12–2). The meninges are composed of three layers. The dura mater is the outermost layer and is composed microscopically of two distinct layers of fibrous tissue, which give the dura great strength.[1] The outer layer of dura is the periosteum of the inner table of the skull and is relatively adherent to the inner table, particularly at the suture lines where it is continuous with the periosteum of the outer table. The inner layer of the dura and the outer layer of the dura are adherent except where they part to form the venous sinuses. In these same locations, the inner layer of dura frequently extends for some distance away from the outer layer and reflects back on itself to form a very strong double layer of dura. The largest of these dural reflections are known as the falx cerebri, tentorium cerebelli, diaphragma sellae, and falx cerebelli.

The second and middle layer of the meninges, the arachnoid mater, is just under the dura mater and separated from the dura mater by a potential space called the subdural space. The arachnoid is a more delicate tissue than the dura and has a fine network of tissue strands that extend to the surface of the brain and the pia mater. The pia mater is the innermost layer of the meninges, lies on the surface of the brain, and conforms to the surface of the brain by insinuating itself into the many sulci. In addition, the pia intimately surrounds the blood

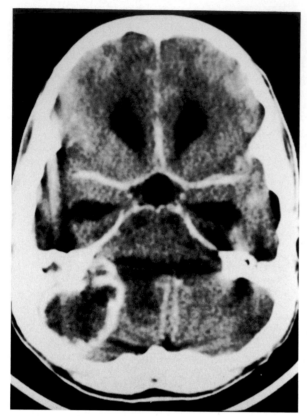

FIG 12–1.
Cerebellar abscess secondary to mastoiditis. On contrast CT, notice the rim enhancement in the right cerebellar hemisphere. The right mastoid air cells are opacified, which is consistent with the known mastoiditis. Secondary hydrocephalus has resulted, and portions of the dilated ventricular system are apparent.

vessels that supply the brain and may even extend a variable distance into the parenchyma with the small perforating vessels.[2] In such areas (particularly the corpus striatum) this investment of pia forms a perivascular space (of Virchow-Robin), is continuous with the subarachnoid space, and is a known route for spread of infection[3, 4] (Fig 12–3).

Together the arachnoid and pia are called the leptomeninges. Between the arachnoid and pia is a fluid-filled space called the subarachnoid space. The fluid in this space is cerebrospinal fluid (CSF); this fluid envelops not only the brain but is continuous with that within the subarachnoid space surrounding the spinal cord as well.

In some locations, especially near the superior sagittal sinus, the arachnoid projects into the inner layer of the dura. In these locations the arachnoid takes a frondlike appearance and forms the arachnoid villi. The dura over these villi becomes very thin, often one cell thick. Thus, at the villi, the subarachnoid space is separated from the deep venous system by a very thin layer of cells. This approximation of the CSF with the blood in the sinuses is very important in CSF dynamics. For example, leptomeningitis that has caused adhesions in the subarachnoid space near the villi obstructs CSF resorption and would be likely to cause hydrocephalus.

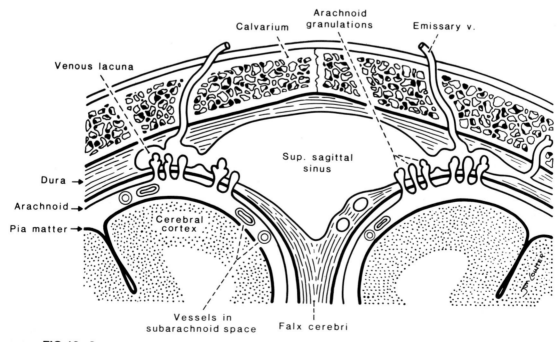

FIG 12–2.
A coronal section through the superior sagittal sinus shows the relation of the brain to the meninges.

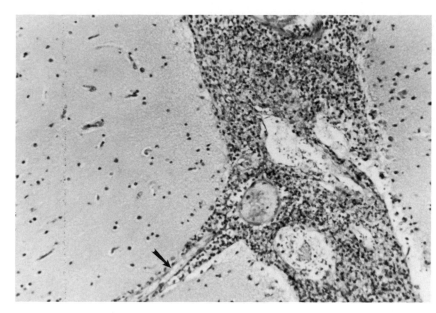

FIG 12–3.
Purulent amoebic meningoencephalitis secondary to infection by *Naegleria fowleri* (photomicrograph, ×60). Numerous leukocytes fill the subarachnoid space between two gyri and extend into the perivascular space around a small arteriole *(arrow)*. (Courtesy of A. Julio Martinez, M.D., University of Pittsburgh.)

Epidural Abscess

Epidural abscess refers to an infection between the inner table of the skull and the dura mater. Epidural abscess most often is secondary to an infection extending from the middle ear, paranasal sinuses, or cranium into the epidural space (Fig 12–4). Syphilis is one of the few causes of a primary epidural abscess (pachymeningitis externa).[5, 6] The CT findings of epidural abscess are

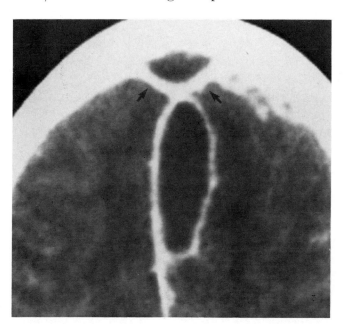

FIG 12–4.
Epidural abscess *(arrows)* in a patient who also has a subdural empyema along the falx. Notice that the epidural abscess crosses the midline to displace the anterior attachment of the falx. This intracranial infection was secondary to frontal sinusitis.

those of an extra-axial low-attenuation area with mass effect. The periphery of the abscess frequently enhances with intravenous contrast. On MRI, the location adjacent to the inner table with mass effect on the adjacent brain structures can also be identified. Signal characteristics within the abscess will vary. Epidural abscesses can cross the midline, a finding that helps distinguish epidural disease from subdural disease.

Extension of an epidural abscess to the subgaleal space, when it occurs, is usually a complication of surgery.[7] Venous sinus thrombosis may also be a consequence of epidural abscess (Fig 12–5) and can be detected by several modalities. For example, in infants with open fontanelles neurosonography can demonstrate an abnormally echogenic torcula and sagittal sinus indicative of thrombus.[8] In patients of any age contrast CT may show enhancement of the dura that is forming the sinus while the thrombosed lumen remains lower in attenuation ("delta sign").[9] Venous sinus thrombosis on MRI may have several appearances depending on the age of the thrombus. Acutely, the sinus may be isointense on T1-weighted (short repetition time [TR], short echo time [TE]) images and hypointense on T2-weighted (long TR, long TE) images.[10] Later, the sinus may become high in signal on both T1- and T2-weighted images.[11] However, we have also seen an acute thrombus as isosignal on both T1- and T2-weighted images, with intense enhancement (signal increase) on T1-weighted images after the administration of intravenous (IV) contrast agents containing gadolinium. In any case, the expected signal void of flowing blood in the si-

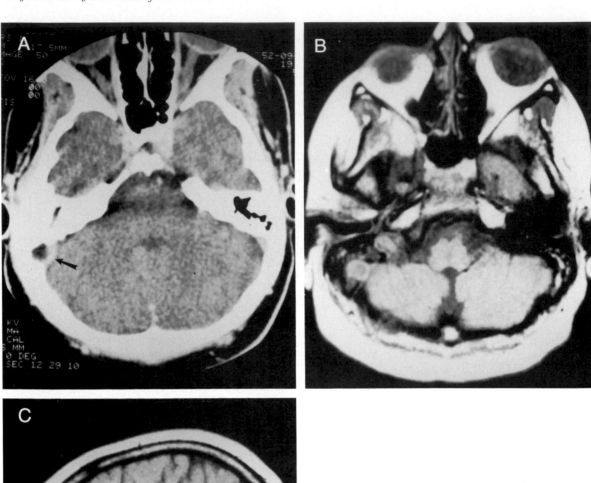

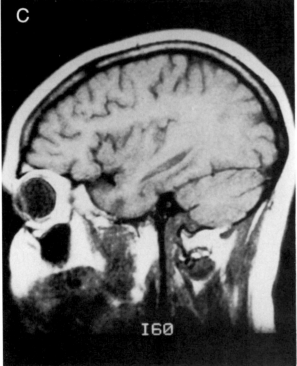

FIG 12–5.
Sinus thrombosis secondary to mastoiditis. **A,** CT after contrast. The periphery of the right sigmoid sinus enhances *(arrow),* but the lumen does not. **B,** MRI at a similar level (short TR). **C,** sagittal MRI (short TR). Notice the relative isosignal in the sigmoid and jugular vein—consistent with thrombosis. Flow void in internal carotid can be identified just anterior to the occluded jugular vein.

nus is not appreciated. Of course, the usual caveats regarding flow must be kept in mind, namely, that flow-related enhancement could be misinterpreted as sinus thrombosis. All bright sinuses are not thrombosed sinuses, and additional or special sequences might be required to be definitive.[12]

Subdural Empyema

Infection within the subdural space may form a subdural empyema, the term for a purulent collection in this potential space. Table 12–1 lists some etiologies for subdural empyema. Clinical signs

TABLE 12–1.

Etiologies of Subdural Empyema

Purulent bacterial meningitis
Postcraniotomy infection
Paranasal sinusitis
Otitis media
Osteomyelitis of the calvarium
Post-traumatic
Hematogenous dissemination

and symptoms include fever, vomiting, meningismus, seizures, and hemiparesis. The mortality from subdural empyema has been reported to range from 25% to 40%. Prompt treatment with appropriate antibiotics and extensive craniotomy can result in a favorable outcome, however.[13–15]

CT features of a subdural empyema are those of a low-attenuation collection in the extra-axial space, usually over the convexities or within the interhemispheric fissure (Fig 12–6). Enhancing margins may be apparent with intravenous contrast. Mass effect on the adjacent parenchyma may efface the cortical sulci and cause a midline shift to the opposite side.

On MRI, the morphologic features are the same as CT. Signal characteristics within the empyema will vary. MRI is more sensitive, however,

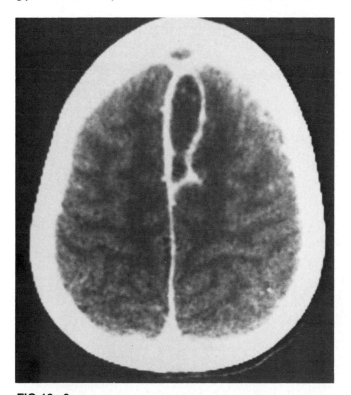

FIG 12–6.
Subdural empyema. Contrast-enhanced CT demonstrates this interhemispheric collection.

to subtle changes in the adjacent brain parenchyma, and this may represent a reaction to the mass effect or an associated cerebritis. Coronal images (with MRI or CT) are sometimes particularly useful in visualizing thin collections in the subdural space.

Leptomeningitis

Infection of the leptomeninges, that is, of the pia and the arachnoid, most often occurs following hematogenous dissemination from a distant infectious focus. Direct extension from an infected site such as a sinus or the middle ear appears to be less common. Following septicemia for any reason, infection of the leptomeninges can occur. Early in the course of infection, the pial vessels become congested. An exudate that covers the brain may form later, especially in the sulci and basal cisterns, and the leptomeninges become thickened.[16] Infection of the parenchymal blood supply may occur since these vessels course through the infected leptomeninges; secondary infarction of the parenchyma may then result from vascular occlusion.[17, 18] If the leptomeninges near the arachnoid villi are involved or if adhesions develop in the subarachnoid space, the CSF flow may be inhibited and result in hydrocephalus.

Clinical features are related to patient age (Table 12–2). Infants and particularly neonates may have a perplexing clinical picture lacking clear signs of meningeal irritation.

The CT appearance in many cases of meningitis is within normal limits.[19] However, intense meningeal enhancement may occur after IV contrast administration (Fig 12–7). If CSF flow is inhibited, hydrocephalus may be apparent. If the brain parenchyma is also involved, enhancement and swelling of that parenchyma may be apparent. In children, in particular, *Haemophilus influenzae* is frequently associated with extra-axial collections

TABLE 12–2.

Clinical Features of Leptomeningitis

Infants	Adults
Fever	Fever
Vomiting	Headache
Irritability	Photophobia
Anorexia	Pain and stiffness of the neck
Constipation	Kernig's sign
Altered state of consciousness	
Seizures	
Bulging fontanelle	
Kernig's sign	

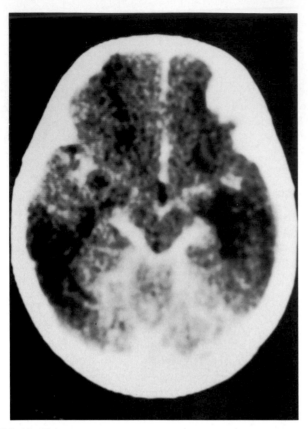

FIG 12–7.
Pneumococcal meningitis. Contrast CT demonstrates intense enhancement of the tentorium, especially along the incisura.

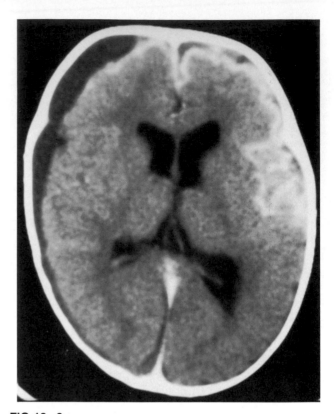

FIG 12–8.
Haemophilus influenzae infection in a child. Contrast CT demonstrates cortical/pial enhancement greater in the left frontal and temporal lobes than on the right. An extra-axial collection can be seen over the right frontal lobe.

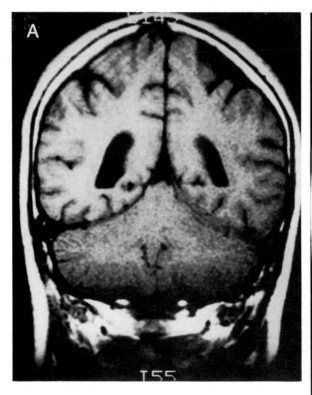 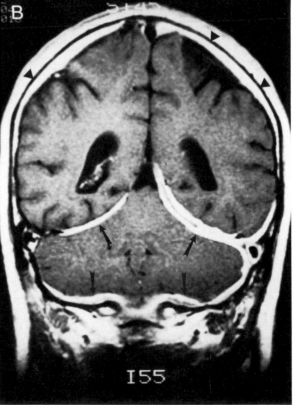

FIG 12–9.
Meningitis secondary to Wegener's granulomatosis: short TR images before **(A)** and after **(B)** the administration of IV gadolinium. The meninges along the tentorium are thickened and enhance intensely all the way around the cerebellum. Do not confuse the enhancing meninges *(arrows)* with the normal diploic space *(arrowheads).*

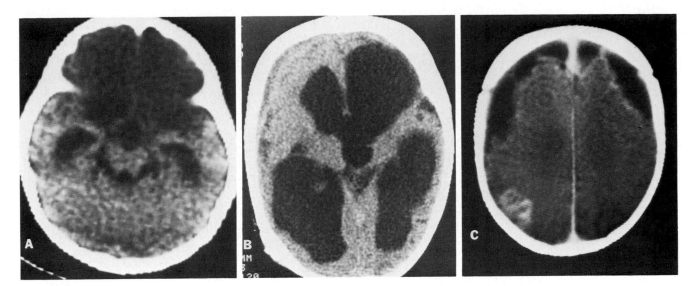

FIG 12–10.
Complications of leptomeningitis. **A,** bifrontal infarction following gram-negative leptomeningitis. **B,** different patient showing significant parenchymal loss with ventricular enlargement. This appearance would be difficult to differentiate from obstructive hydrocephalus, also a potential complication of leptomeningitis.

having low-attenuation characteristics that represent distended subarachnoid spaces (Fig 12–8).

The MRI appearance may also be normal but may serve to demonstrate associated parenchymal signal abnormalities and swelling or exclude such associated abnormalities. Gadolinium-enhanced images may show thickened enhancing membranes and is probably the most sensitive imaging examination for meningitis (Fig 12–9).[20] Extra-axial collections are well demonstrated and may be similar in signal to CSF.

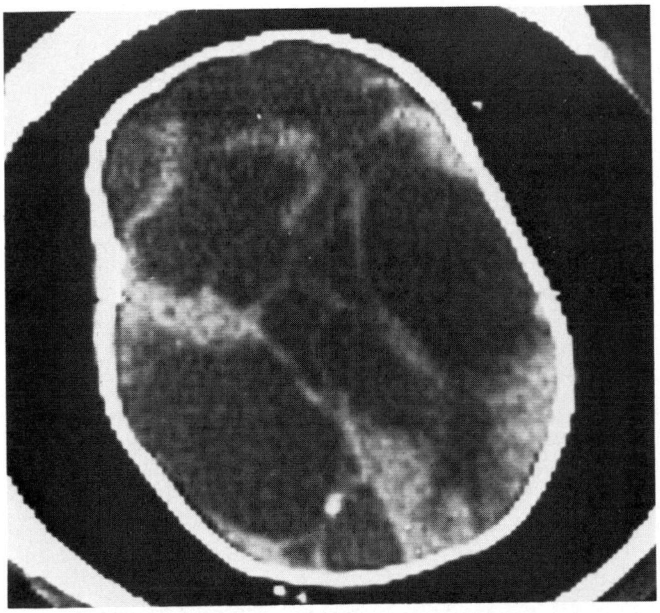

Neonates represent a special case with respect to the cerebral sequelae of leptomeningitis (Fig 12–10). Gram-negative rods such *Escherichia coli* are the chief offenders. Neonatal meningitides are believed to be acquired as a result of the delivery process. The lack of a developed immune system at birth makes the neonates susceptible to these organisms, which are normally innocuous. These children frequently suffer severe parenchymal brain damage that ultimately produces a multicystic brain (Fig 12–11).[21] Multifocal encephalomalacia is the final unfortunate result.

PARENCHYMAL DISEASE

The advent of CT radically altered both the diagnosis and management of parenchymal infection. Mortality from cerebral abscesses in the pre-CT era ranged between 30% and 60%. This has been drastically reduced in the post-CT years, with some centers reporting no mortality with purulent abscesses.[22, 23] CT, and now MRI also, serve as very sensitive examinations for demonstrating the presence of intraparenchymal infection (Fig 12–12). Furthermore, sequential scans, whether CT or MRI, provide a simple means by which results of surgery and/or antibiotic therapy can be monitored.

FIG 12–11.
Polycystic brain from a prior neonatal leptomeningitis and ventriculitis.

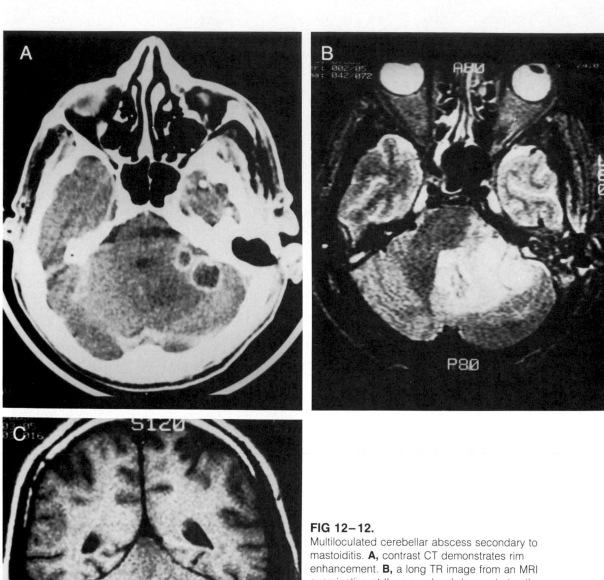

FIG 12–12.
Multiloculated cerebellar abscess secondary to mastoiditis. **A,** contrast CT demonstrates rim enhancement. **B,** a long TR image from an MRI examination at the same level demonstrates the loculations with a large area of surrounding edema that even crosses the midline. Perhaps the CT scan also shows some lucency in the comparable area. **C,** short TR coronal MRI demonstrates the intraparenchymal location and the associated mastoid disease. Notice that the rim is slightly increased in signal intensity, a sign often seen in association with the inflammatory process in the capsule of an abscess.

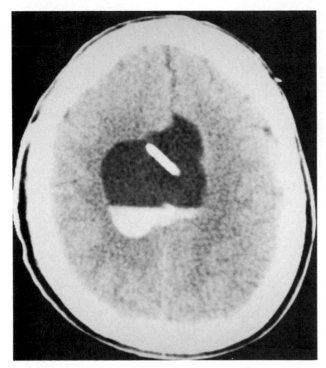

FIG 12–13.
Infected arachnoid cyst. This CT scan was performed following replacement of a drainage tube through which water-soluble contrast had been administered. The fluid level is indicative of a cavity.

Proper imaging of parenchymal disease not only must identify the lesion but must evaluate the surrounding parenchyma and adjacent structures. The characteristics of a lesion demonstrated by CT can usually be divided into solid enhancing types of masses and lesions with ringlike enhancing characteristics. However, the significance of the enhancement pattern may be less important than whether or not a particular area of interest enhances at all. MRI often shows areas of different signal within an abnormal area. Both imaging techniques easily show mass effects. CT is superb at identifying calcification and acute hemorrhages. MRI is particularly sensitive to early parenchymal changes such as edema. MRI is also very sensitive to subacute and chronic areas of previous hemorrhage.

Both MRI and CT are very important in distinguishing whether the disease is multifocal or single. Any individual abscess might be unilocular or multilocular. A fluid-fluid level seen by any technique indicates cavitation (Fig 12–13).

Pyogenic Infections

Cerebral abscess most often is the result of hematogenous dissemination from a primary extracranial infectious site. Some etiologies of cerebral abscess are listed in Table 12–3. The most frequent location for an abscess is the frontal and parietal lobes[24] (Fig 12–14). Intracranial abscesses affect predominantly the preadolescent and middle-aged groups. This is related, in part, to the incidence of congenital heart disease, drug abuse, and otitic and paranasal sinus infections (Fig 12–15). In most series, there is a male predominance. Many causative organisms have been identified, but the common ones are summarized in Table 12–4. No imaging examination can distinguish organisms.

There have been several animal models of cerebral abscess. Wood and coworkers[25] injected infected spheres through the internal carotid artery in monkeys. They concluded that abscess formation was dependent upon stasis of bacteria as well as on a focus of ischemic or necrotic brain. Enzmann and colleagues[26, 27] established brain abscesses in dogs by direct inoculation of bacteria into the brain parenchyma. They divided abscess formation into four stages: (1) early cerebritis (1 to 3 days), (2) late cerebritis (4 to 9 days), (3) early capsule formation (10 to 13 days), and (4) late capsule formation (14 days and later). The cerebritis

TABLE 12–3.
Etiologies of Cerebral Abscess

Hematogenous dissemination
  Pulmonary
  Cardiac
  Drug abuse
  Other
Direct extension
  Otitic
  Paranasal sinus
Trauma
  Penetrating injury
  Postsurgical

TABLE 12–4.
Common Bacteria Causing Cerebral Abscess

Aerobic Bacteria	Anaerobic Bacteria
Staphylococcus aureus	*Streptococcus*
Streptococcus viridans	*Bacteroides*
Hemolytic streptococci	
Pneumococcus	
Gram-negative*	

*E. coli, Proteus, Pseudomonas, H. influenzae.

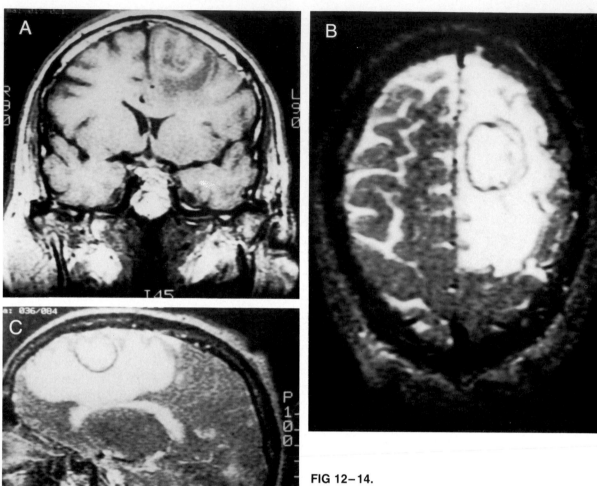

FIG 12–14.
Frontal abscess with surrounding edema. **A,** a coronal
short TR image shows mass effect with compression of
the left lateral ventricle and effacement of the overlying
cortical sulci. **B** and **C,** axial and sagittal long TR
images show an abscess cavity delineated by a thin rim
of low signal and the extensive surrounding edema.

phase of abscess formation was described as an inflammatory infiltrate of polymorphonuclear leukocytes, lymphocytes, and plasma cells. By the third
day, a necrotic center was forming. Surrounding
the necrotic center was a rim of inflammatory cells,
new blood vessels, and hyperplastic fibroblasts. In
the late cerebritis phase, extracellular edema and
hyperplastic astrocytes were seen. Thus the cerebritis phase of abscess formation started as a suppu-
rative focus, which then broke down and began to
become encapsulated by collagen at 10 to 13 days.
The process continued in the late capsule phase
with increasing capsule thickness.

The deposition of collagen is important because collagen appears to limit the spread of the
infection. Factors that affect collagen deposition
include host resistance, duration of infection, characteristics of the organism, and drug therapy. Corticosteroids may decrease the formation of a fibrous capsule and may decrease the effectiveness
of antibiotic therapy in the cerebritis phase as well
as reduce antibiotic penetration into the brain abscess. Corticosteroids also inhibit enhancement
with IV contrast.

Abscesses that are hematogenous in origin
have a predilection to occur at the junction of the
gray and white matter, although virtually all locations may be involved. If the abscess capsule extends to a ventricular surface, associated ventriculitis may occur. Furthermore, rupture into the

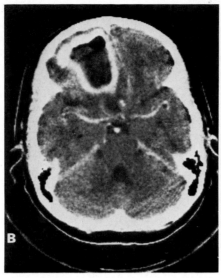

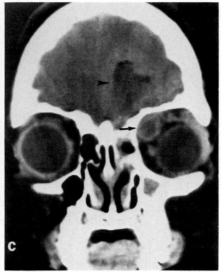

FIG 12–15.
Abscess secondary to sinusitis. **A,** enhanced axial CT shows a right frontal abscess with some gas in the anterior portion of the cavity. **B,** coronal CT demonstrates not only the frontal abscess *(arrowhead)* but also an abscess in the orbit *(arrow),* both of which developed from ethmoidal infection. Note the soft-tissue density in the ethmoids on this side.

ventricular system may disseminate the abscess with grave consequences.

Death from cerebral abscess may occur from extensive infection or from the mass effect generated by the abscess. Surgical drainage is usually required for adequate treatment, but occasionally conservative therapy using antibiotics alone has been utilized successfully in patients with multiple abscesses or in those who are poor surgical candidates.[28–30]

The characteristics of a cerebral abscess depend upon the pathologic phase during which the abscess is being examined. In the cerebritis phase, mass effect may be evident with both CT and MRI. IV contrast on CT may demonstrate "ring enhancement." However, the presence of ring enhancement should not unequivocally be interpreted as implying a capsule formation.[26] Britt and coworkers[27] suggest that the ring lesion of the cerebritis phase may be distinguished from an encapsulated abscess by delayed scanning. In the cerebritis phase, contrast was observed to have diffused into the necrotic center, while this did not occur in the well-formed encapsulated brain abscess.

MRI also reflects these pathologic findings and frequently demonstrates a ringlike area that differs in signal from a central area as well as from the surrounding parenchyma. MRI is more sensitive to associated surrounding edema than is CT. Nevertheless, surrounding edema is usually evident with both modalities.

The morphology of the ring as seen by either MRI or CT may be important. Usually, the ring of an abscess is relatively thin and smooth and sometimes may appear to "point" toward a nearby ventricle. If irregularity or nodularity in the ring is apparent, one must consider that a neoplasm or an unusual infection (fungus) is present. However, many exceptions to this rule occur, and nodular irregular pyogenic abscesses are not that infrequent.[31–33] Some of these represent subacute and chronic abscesses, while others are the result of adjacent daughter abscess formation (Fig 12–16). Thus, the appearance of an abscess can vary and is difficult to distinguish from other etiologies of brain mass. Table 12–5 is a partial differential diagnosis of such lesions.

A properly treated brain abscess may demonstrate areas of abnormal signal by MRI indefinitely and on CT may show areas of enhancement for

TABLE 12–5.

Differential Diagnosis of Ring Enhancement

Pyogenic brain abscess
Fungal infection
Infarction
Primary brain tumor
Metastatic brain tumor
Granuloma
Multiple sclerosis
Subacute hematoma

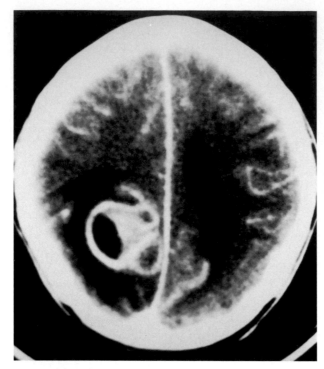

FIG 12–16.
Multilocular abscess in the right parietal lobe: contrast-enhanced CT.

many months without indicating that recurrent disease is present.

Nonpyogenic Inflammatory Disease

Nonpyogenic inflammation may be divided into granulomatous diseases, viral infections, and parasitic infections.

Granulomatous Disease

Tuberculosis.—Intracranial infection with tuberculosis usually has two forms that may be present with or without each other. The first is tuberculous meningitis, and the second form is intraparenchymal tuberculoma. A true tuberculous abscess is an extremely rare event in the central nervous system (CNS)[34] and is essentially indistinguishable from an abscess of any other etiology. Also rare is a tuberculous cerebritis that localizes in the cortical gyri.[35] Although the incidence of intracranial tuberculosis has declined considerably in the past 40 years, it has not been eradicated.

The pathophysiology of tuberculous meningitis begins with an initial focus that is usually pulmonic but may be in the abdomen or genitourinary tract. There is hematogenous dissemination of the bacilli to seed the leptomeninges and brain parenchyma. Granulomas may then be formed and may remain dormant for many years. Alternatively, the infection may completely resolve. If granulomas persist and coalesce, they may form a large lesion. Rupture of such a lesion into the subarachnoid space discharges necrotic debris that appears to affect the basal cisterns preferentially. The reaction of the meninges to the infection may result in vascular occlusions and infarcts as well as in obstruction to the flow of CSF with resulting hydrocephalus. Cranial nerve palsies also occur secondary to the basilar meningitis.

Clinical features of tuberculous meningitis include confusion, headache, lethargy, and meningismus. Progression into a stupor or a coma may occur and may be associated with decerebrate rigidity, cranial nerve palsies, and infarctions. It is interesting to note that 19% of patients with tuberculous meningitis had no evidence of extrameningeal active disease at the time of the diagnosis.[36, 37] Patients have low-grade fevers, with lumbar puncture revealing hypoglycorrhachia, increased protein levels, pleocytosis (predominantly lymphocytes), and negative smears.[38] The tuberculin skin test is often negative early in the disease.[39]

The intracerebral tuberculoma may produce symptoms from its mass effect and associated edema. The symptoms are related to location of the lesion. Tuberculomas may be solitary or multiple.[40] They can occur in both the supratentorial and infratentorial regions. Calcification in tuberculomas is reported to be between 1% and 6%.[41–45] Thus, most tuberculomas are not calcified. An unusual manifestation of a tuberculoma is that occasionally it may cause hyperostosis of the calvarium as it enlarges and becomes adherent to overlying dura, a characteristic simulating the bone changes usually associated with a meningioma.[46]

CT features of tuberculous meningitis are not specific but include enhancement of the meninges, particularly in the basal cisterns (Fig 12–17). CT features of tuberculoma formation usually appear as a nodule that may have low- to high-attenuation values and typically enhances with IV contrast. Some may show a characteristic punctate lucent center representing the central area of caseous necrosis[45] (Fig 12–18). As noted above, only a small percentage will have a calcified center. The CT findings of CNS tuberculosis are summarized in Table 12–6. A very rare manifestation of tuberculous infection is persistent cortical enhancement

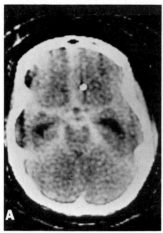
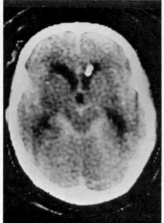
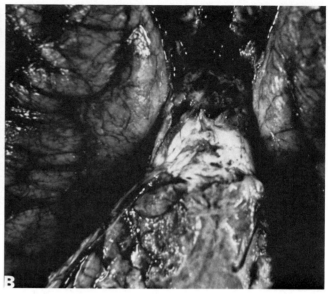

FIG 12–17.
Tuberculous meningitis. **A,** dense enhancement around the basal *(left)* and perimesencephalic *(right)* cisterns with hydrocephalus.

B, specimen in the same patient. Note the purulent exudate around the brain stem.

on CT. This has been seen with large underlying areas of white matter edema[35] but has also been associated with large underlying parenchymal areas of lucency not having mass effect.[47]

MRI features of tuberculoma are a relatively massless area of decreased signal on T1-weighted images and increased signal on T2-weighted images, not a particularly specific characterization.[48, 49]

Rarely, tuberculomas may occur intraventricularly.[50] While this location is unusual, the imaging characteristics of the granuloma are the same as already described. Evidence of ependymal tuberculous infection may also be manifested by asymmetrical hydrocephalus or traction (displacement) of the septum pellucidum, findings supporting a tu-

TABLE 12–6.
CT of Intracranial Tuberculosis

Tuberculoma Nodules (Solitary or Multiple)	Meningitis
Plain scan	Plain scan
Low-high absorption	Obliteration of basal and sylvian cisterns
Mass effect	Calcification in basilar cisterns
Hydrocephalus	Hydrocephalus†
Calcification (1%–6%)*	Infarction
Hyperostosis (rare)	
Contrast scan	Contrast scan
Uniform enhancement	Uniform enhancement of leptomeninges
Small lucent center	Tuberculoma (occasionally)
Low absorption around nodule	
Meningeal enhancement	

* Nodules may decrease in size and show calcification following therapy.
† Ventricular dilatation usually remains in treated tuberculous meningitis.

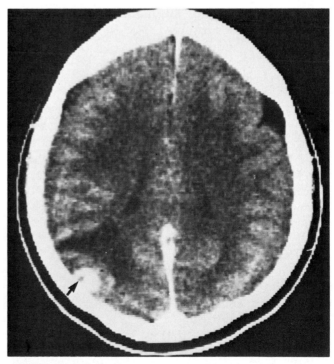

FIG 12–18.
Tuberculoma. Enhanced CT shows a nodule with a small central region of caseous necrosis *(arrow)* surrounded by edema.

berculous etiology, which typically is an adhesive process.

After appropriate antibiotic therapy, tuberculous nodules may decrease in size and show areas of calcification.[45] At times, the tuberculoma may be transformed into a calcified nodule that does not enhance on CT with IV contrast. Complete resorption of a tuberculoma has been reported.[51] Atrophic or porencephalic areas may be the residua of previous parenchymal infection.[35] The dense adhesions that may have formed in the basal cisterns can result in persistent hydrocephalus.

Sarcoidosis.—Sarcoid is a systemic granulomatous disease of unknown etiology that is characterized by noncaseating granulomas (in contrast to the caseating granulomas of tuberculosis). The peak incidence is in the third and fourth decades. Neurologic manifestations occur in approximately 5% of patients,[52] although brain and meningeal involvement has been reported in 14% of autopsies from sarcoid patients.[53] Intracranial sarcoidosis may be the initial manifestation of the systemic disease or may occur in a patient with already documented systemic disease. Only a very small percentage of patients have only neurosarcoid without systemic manifestations.[54–56] The diagnosis of neurosarcoid is an exclusionary one because positive biopsy findings only demonstrate a nonspecific reaction that can be caused by a variety of diseases.

Neurosarcoid has two patterns similar to the patterns seen in tuberculosis. The first pattern is the more common and is that of a chronic basilar leptomeningitis with involvement of the hypothalamus, pituitary gland, and optic chiasm. Patients with this type may present with unilateral or bilateral cranial nerve palsies and endocrine or electrolyte disturbances. These patients may develop obstructive hydrocephalus and may have signs and symptoms of meningeal irritation. The granulomatous process frequently spreads along the perivascular spaces (Virchow-Robin spaces)[57] and causes thrombosis of the perforating blood vessels.[58, 59]

The second pattern is that of parenchymal nodules. These masses are usually associated with extensive arachnoiditis. Microscopically, granulomas are present throughout the brain parenchyma. They have been reported to cause obstructive hydrocephalus when located in the periaqueductal region.[60] These masses may be calcified and are avascular. The sarcoid nodules produce signs and symptoms of an intracranial mass. The CSF abnor-

malities are those of elevated lymphocyte and protein levels with hypoglycorrhachia. Such findings are nonspecific and not diagnostic for this disease.[61]

A granulomatous mass may also develop in an extra-axial location over the convexity or in the interhemispheric fissure and simulate a subdural collection.[62]

The imaging findings will depend on the form and extent of the disease. Calcified nodules or masses of isodense or increased attenuation may be evident on CT. IV contrast generally produces a homogeneous enhancement pattern on CT (Fig 12–19).[63] Meningeal enhancement is also common, although not specific, and has a predilection for the base of the skull (optic pathways, pituitary, and hypothalamus). Intraparenchymal nodules are not usually associated with edema. In contrast to tuberculous granulomas, sarcoid nodules do not usually have lucent centers.

On MRI, variability in the appearance of intra-

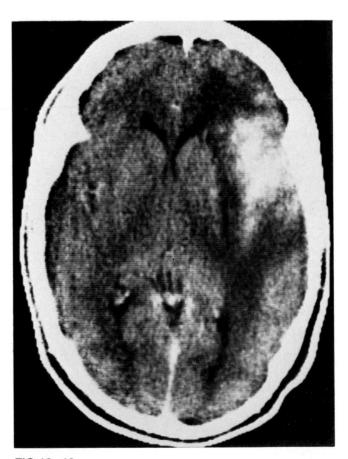

FIG 12–19.
Sarcoid. Contrast CT shows homogeneous enhancement in the sylvian region. (Courtesy of David Norman, M.D., University of California at San Francisco.)

cranial sarcoid has been reported.[62, 64] Usually, parenchymal involvement appears hyperintense on T2-weighted images, although isointense and hypointense lesions have occurred. The periventricular parenchymal involvement is better identified on MRI than on CT.[65] T1-weighted images of parenchymal involvement demonstrate areas that are isointense to hypointense relative to the cerebral cortex.

Both CT and MRI demonstrate mass effects from parenchymal disease very well. Similarly, both imaging techniques can show evidence of obstructive hydrocephalus.

Intracranial sarcoid has occasionally been difficult to distinguish from a brain tumor, pituitary mass, and meningioma and has even simulated a subdural hematoma.[61, 66-68] Corticosteroid therapy remains a major constituent of treatment and in some cases produces a dramatic response with disappearance of the lesions.[52, 69]

Fungal Disease.—Coccidioidomycosis is endemic in the southwestern United States and northern Mexico. The spore is inhaled and then forms a primary pulmonary focus. Hematogenous dissemination to the CNS occurs within a few weeks or months, but dissemination years later has been reported.[70] The intracranial infection may be manifested pathologically by a thick basilar meningitis with meningeal and parenchymal granulomas. The intra-axial granulomas have been reported to have a propensity for the cerebellum.[71] Vasculitis producing vascular occlusion has also been reported.[72] A disseminated cerebral form of coccidioidomycosis predominately occurs in white males, and the diagnosis is confirmed by CSF serology or culture.[71]

The imaging examinations show changes similar to those of other granulomatous disease. Specifically, a basal arachnoiditis may be apparent, particularly on contrasted CT and MRI scans. The sulci and cisterns may be obliterated. Associated with arachnoiditis may be obstructive hydrocephalus. If the disease spreads to the ependyma, the ventricular walls may enhance on CT. Areas of parenchymal abnormality may be secondary to either infarction from the associated vasculitis or to parenchymal infection. An area of low attenuation that may enhance would be expected on CT, while on T2-weighted MRI, such an area would likely have a high signal.

Other CNS fungal diseases also occur but are usually only pathogenic in the immunocompromised patient, which is discussed below.

Viral Infection

Herpes Simplex.—Herpes simplex virus is the most common cause of fatal endemic encephalitis.[73] The survivors of this virus suffer severe memory and personality problems. Supposedly, early diagnosis and speedy therapy with antiviral agents can favorably affect the outcome.[74] Both the oral strain (type I) and the genital strain (type II) may produce encephalitis in humans. Type II is responsible for infection in the neonatal period, presumably acquired either transplacentally or during birth from mothers with genital herpes.[75, 76] This strain may cause a variety of teratogenic problems, including intracranial calcifications, microcephaly, microphthalmos, and retinal dysplasia.[77] Sequelae from neonatal herpes also include multicystic encephalomalacia, porencephalia, seizures, motor deficits, and mental and motor retardation.[78, 79]

The type I virus produces the fulminant, necrotizing encephalitis seen typically in adults. The clinical picture is one of acute confusion and disorientation followed rapidly by stupor and coma. Seizures, viral prodrome, fever, and headache are also common presentations. Those patients with left temporal disease may be symptomatic earlier because of their language impairment and thus may have less obvious changes on imaging studies at the time of their presentation.

The pathologic findings are quite stereotyped. The virus asymmetrically attacks the brain and has a predilection for the temporal lobes, insula, and orbital frontal region. A suggested explanation for the focality of type I herpes simplex may depend on its known latency in the trigeminal ganglia. This latent virus under certain circumstances becomes reactivated and spreads along the trigeminal nerve fibers that innervate the meninges of the anterior and middle cranial fossae.[80] A diffuse meningoencephalitis with a predominantly lymphocytic infiltration is seen. Extensive necrosis with hemorrhage may occur with loss of all neural and glial elements. The end result, if the patient survives, is an atrophic cystic parenchyma. Laboratory diagnosis is dependent on culturing the virus or on fluorescent antibody staining.[81, 82]

In adult type I herpes encephalitis, imaging studies may show normal structures or may demonstrate only minimal findings very early in the

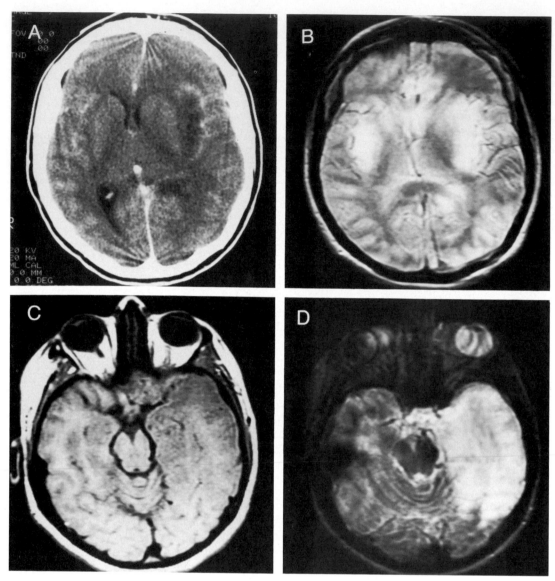

FIG 12–20.
Herpes encephalitis. **A,** contrast CT shows an abnormal lucency in the left insula and in deep white matter lateral to the atrium of the left lateral ventricle. A mass effect is apparent with a midline shift to the right. **B,** axial T2-weighted MRI at a slightly higher level shows abnormal high signal in both the left and right insulae. **C,** axial T1-weighted MRI at a lower level shows decreased signal in the left temporal lobe and compression of the midbrain by the uncus. **D,** axial T2-weighted MRI at the same level as **C** shows abnormal increased signal in the left temporal lobe.

course of the infection.[83] By CT, low-absorption areas in the temporal lobe and insular cortex are typical (Fig 12–20) when they eventually develop. On T2-weighted MRI, these areas are high in signal, are usually detected earlier than with CT, and may appear more extensive on MRI than by CT.[84] Mass effect from these areas may be quite remarkable and show ventricular compression. Hemorrhage into the parenchyma has been reported although is not usual.[83, 85] IV contrast–enhanced CT may demonstrate gyriform enhancement, and after 7 days almost all patients demonstrate enhancement. The mass effect may persist for a considerable period (39 days in one case).[86] Residual imaged abnormalities include areas of parenchymal loss at the site of previous infection.

The features of neonatal herpes encephalitis are quite different from those in adults and are summarized in Table 12–7.[77, 87] Diffuse cortical calcification in an infant has been described.[85] Ependymal calcification is also possible (Fig 12–21).

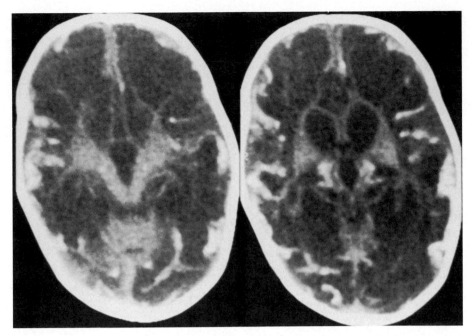

FIG 12–21.
Late features of neonatal herpes encephalitis. Extensive parenchymal loss and abnormal lucency in the remaining parenchyma are evident. Cortical calcifications are present (noncontrast CT).

Subacute Sclerosing Panencephalitis.—Subacute sclerosing panencephalitis (SSPE) is classified as a slow viral infection and usually occurs in children and young adolescents 3 to 9 years following an apparently innocent measles infection (Fig 12–22,A). The CNS infection progresses through stages. Initially, it starts with difficulty in language and behavioral changes.[88, 89] This is followed by intellectual deterioration, ataxia, chorea, dystonic rigidity, seizures, myoclonus, and ocular problems (optic atrophy, cortical blindness, chorioretinitis). In the final stages, the child is unresponsive, displays severe autonomic dysfunction, and progresses to coma and death within months to years.[90, 91] Occasionally the course is prolonged and associated with one or more remissions.

Supportive laboratory evidence of SSPE includes marked elevation of the CSF γ-globulin content. Electroencephalography is characterized by periodic, high-voltage, slow and sharp waves. Elevated levels of neutralizing antibody to measles (rubeola) virus are found in the CSF and serum.[92, 93] It is rare to isolate rubeola from the brain tissue. Pathologic changes include eosinophilic intranuclear inclusions, demyelination, and perivascular lymphocytic infiltrations.

In patients with a rapidly progressive form of the disease, CT usually does not reveal significant abnormality. However, cerebral swelling with compression of the lateral ventricles has been reported as an early finding in SSPE.[94] Children with a prolonged course have extensive central and cortical parenchymal loss. Imaging reflects these changes as areas of decreased attenuation in the subcortical and periventricular white matter on CT. Similar abnormal regions in the caudate nuclei have also been reported and may account for the movement problems (chorea, dystonia, rigidity).[95] No demonstrable contrast enhancement has been reported. The long-term effect of slow virus infection in the brain is profound parenchymal loss.

Other Viruses.—Progressive multifocal leukoencephalopathy (PML) is a papovavirus that typically infects immunocompromised hosts and will be further discussed in that section.

The arthropod-borne viral encephalitides, or arboviruses (i.e., Eastern equine, Western equine), are a group of antigenically related diseases that

TABLE 12–7.
CT Features of Neonatal Herpes Simplex

Multiple cysts
Intracranial calcification (periventricular)
Hydrocephalus
Atrophy

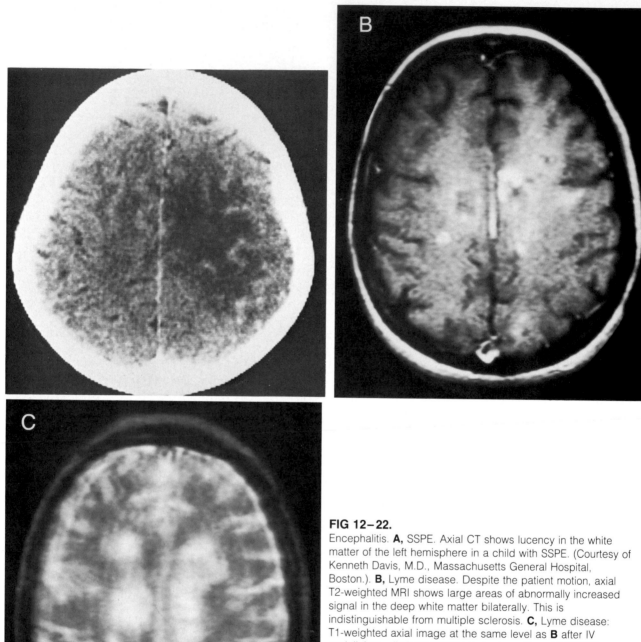

FIG 12–22.
Encephalitis. **A,** SSPE. Axial CT shows lucency in the white matter of the left hemisphere in a child with SSPE. (Courtesy of Kenneth Davis, M.D., Massachusetts General Hospital, Boston.). **B,** Lyme disease. Despite the patient motion, axial T2-weighted MRI shows large areas of abnormally increased signal in the deep white matter bilaterally. This is indistinguishable from multiple sclerosis. **C,** Lyme disease: T1-weighted axial image at the same level as **B** after IV gadolinium–diethylenetriamine pentaacetic acid (DTPA). Again, the varying enhancement and areas of low signal mimic multiple sclerosis.

have slight regional differences.[96] Mosquitoes and ticks are the usual vectors. Diagnosis is based on clinical history and serology. Lesions have appeared on MRI as poorly defined areas of increased signal on spin-density and T2-weighted images in the thalamus, cerebellum, brain stem, and corona radiata. By CT, an area of hypodensity occurs. MRI appears more sensitive than CT to this group of disorders.[84]

Several other encephalitides that are not viral are also transmitted by ticks and will therefore be mentioned here. These include the rickettsias (typhus, Rocky Mountain spotted fever) and the spirochete *Borrelia burgdorferi* (Lyme disease). These pathogens can infect the brain.[97-99] Lyme disease, in particular, may be difficult to distinguish from multiple sclerosis by imaging characteristics alone (Fig 12–22,B).[100] Diagnosis is based on clinical and serologic investigations.

Parasitic Infections

Cysticercosis.—This parasite is endemic in parts of Latin America, Asia, Africa, and Europe. Humans are the only known definitive host for both the adult tapeworm *Taenia solium* as well as for the intermediate host in the larval form *(Cysticercus cellulosae)*, the form that grows in the CNS.[101] The cestode is usually acquired by ingestion of insufficiently cooked pork containing the encysted larvae. The larvae develop into adult tapeworms in the human intestinal tract where they may live for up to 25 years, grow to many meters in length, and produce thousands and thousands of ova.[102] Some ova may be regurgitated into the stomach by reverse peristalsis. Gastric digestion can then release the larvae (oncospheres) from the ova, whereupon the larvae may burrow through the intestinal tract to reach the blood stream. The blood stream disseminates the larvae throughout the body, including the CNS, where the larvae form cysticerci (the cystic form of larvae). Humans may also become infected by directly ingesting the eggs (as an intermediate host) in contaminated food or water and via self-contamination by the anus-hand-mouth route. After several weeks, the embryo that has lodged in the CNS develops a cystic covering and a scolex. The interval between the probable date of infection and the first distinctive symptoms ranges from less than 1 year to 30 years, the average being approximately 4.8 years.[103] The cysticerci vary in size from minuscule to 6 cm in diameter.[104] They may be located in the brain parenchyma and the meninges, intraventricularly, and rarely intraspinally. The cysts may develop anywhere within the subarachnoid space. Symptoms are related to the location and size of the parasite (Table 12–8).[103, 105, 106] Obstructive hydrocephalus may result either from the meningeal/subarachnoid involvement or from a strategically placed cyst.[107, 108]

The plain-films findings of cysticercosis are quite characteristic. Multiple round or oval calcifications may be apparent within the brain parenchyma. The calcifications are usually 1 to 2 mm in diameter and represent the calcified scolex. Sometimes a partially or totally calcified sphere can be demonstrated around the scolex (7 to 12 mm in diameter) and represents the wall of the cyst that has calcified. Only dead larvae calcify.[109] These findings are essentially the same as the familiar plain-film findings typically seen in extracranial locations.

The findings on imaging studies will vary depending on the extent and form of the disease but form a mainstay for the diagnosis of cysticercosis, especially when used in conjunction with serologic testing.[110] The acute encephalitic phase of the infection is more common in children and is characterized by multiple diffuse nodular lesions (85%) with surrounding edema. Sometimes (15%) the lesions are relatively localized to one lobe.[111] Parenchymal cysticercosis occurs in the white matter, cerebral cortex, and basal ganglia.[112]

On CT, the lesions usually appear as areas of decreased attenuation that typically enhance with IV contrast in either a nodular or ringlike fashion. Noncalcified nodules of increased attenuation have also been reported.[112] Generally these also enhance. The encephalitic phase of the disease lasts from 2 to 6 months, with edema persisting after enhancement disappears. The brain parenchyma may contain calcified dead larvae and cysts simultaneously, the cysts appearing similar to CSF (Fig 12–23). Small calcifications may develop as early as 8 months after the acute phase.[111]

TABLE 12–8.

Neurologic Sequelae of Cysticercosis Cerebri

Seizures
Hydrocephalus
Headache
Dementia
Vertigo
Psychological disturbances
Paresthesias, paresis, paralysis
Visual disturbances

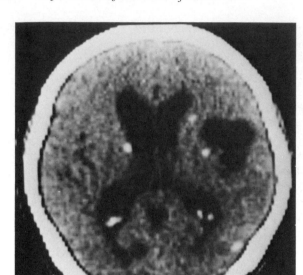

FIG 12–23.
Cysticercosis. Multiple cysts and multiple calcifications are present simultaneously.

Unusual CT features of intracranial cysticercosis have been described and include basal meningeal enhancement, positional cyst alteration, evidence of cortical enhancement with vasculitis, and mycotic aneurysm formation.[111, 113]

Calcification demonstrated by MRI may be more difficult to appreciate, although the areas of cyst formation regardless of whether or not calcification is present are more easily seen with MRI, especially when in the cisternal spaces.[114] MRI shows an oval or round area (usually about 1 cm in diameter) of signal that is similar to although not necessarily identical to CSF. That is, T1-weighted images are low in signal, and T2-weighted images are high in signal. The margins are sharp. The tissue at the interface is higher in signal on the T1-weighted and spin-density images than cortex is and represents the reactive capsule. An edematous zone of several centimeters may surround the cyst. The actual scolex sometimes may be identified as a 2 to 3-mm mural nodule of high signal along the cyst wall.[114] Gadolinium usually enhances the rim of the capsule in the same pattern as seen with iodinated contrast on CT (Fig 12–24).

Larvae can occasionally have a grapelike form in the subarachnoid space and may simulate a tumor in the sellar or cerebellopontine angle regions.[112, 115] The subarachnoid and intraventricular cysts typically do not calcify.[116] Intrathecal metrizamide has been shown on CT not only to outline the cysts but also to be taken up by intraventricular cysts on delayed CT scans.[117]

Toxoplasmosis.—The protozoan *Toxoplasma gondii* is usually associated with the immunocompromised host and will be discussed in that section.

Other Parasites.—Many other parasites have been described in the CNS and present as lesions either within the parenchyma or within the subarachnoid spaces. For example, *Entamoeba histolytica* may cause a severe leptomeningitis and vasculitis. Infestations with *Echinococcus* (hydatid cyst) and *Coenurus cerebralis* have been reported.[113, 118] The latter is the larva of the dog tapeworm, *Multiceps multiceps*, an infection that usually occurs following ingestion of meat contaminated with the larvae. This unusual parasite infects the subarachnoid space and ventricular system to produce hydrocephalus (Fig 12–25).[118–120] Diagnosis requires surgical recovery of the larva. Prevention is based on eliminating contamination of food and hands by dog feces.[121]

Cerebral sparganosis is a rare infestation with the tapeworm larvae of the genus *Spirometra*. Cases have been reported worldwide but are most common in the Far Eastern and Southeast Asian countries. Acutely, lesions may appear indistinguishable from other infections, that is, as a small possibly calcified enhancing mass with surrounding edema. However, in the chronic phase, extensive white matter lucency on CT that is associated with volume loss (as opposed to edema) may develop and appears to be a relatively unique manifestation of this rare infestation.[122]

Opportunistic Infections in the Immunocompromised Host

Table 12–9 lists the pathogens we shall consider. In general, the imaging features of these pathogens are not specific and often cannot be differentiated from the usual pathogens.

As noted in Table 12–10, many factors can produce immunosuppression. However, there are several groups of patients in whom immunocompromise with resultant CNS infection is seen more frequently. Immunocompromise is likely in patients undergoing chemotherapy for malignancy. Another group of immunocompromised patients is those in whom organ transplants have been performed and maintainence is by immunosuppres-

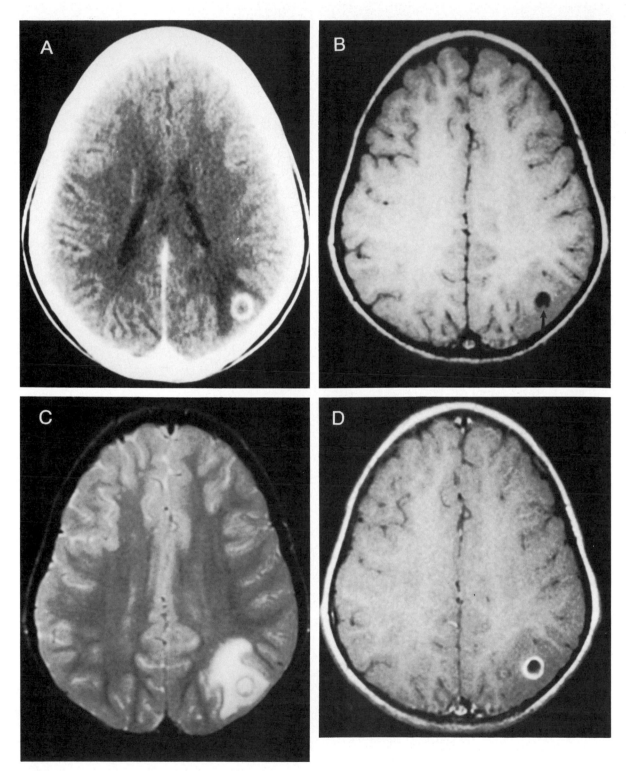

FIG 12–24.
Cysticercosis. **A,** contrast CT shows a ringlike enhancing mass in the left parietal lobe with surrounding edema. **B,** MRI (short TR) shows the same lesion. Notice that a small mural nodule is apparent *(arrow).* **C,** MRI (long TR, long TE) shows the surrounding edema to better advantage. **D,** gadolinium-enhanced MRI (short TR) parallels the CT appearance.

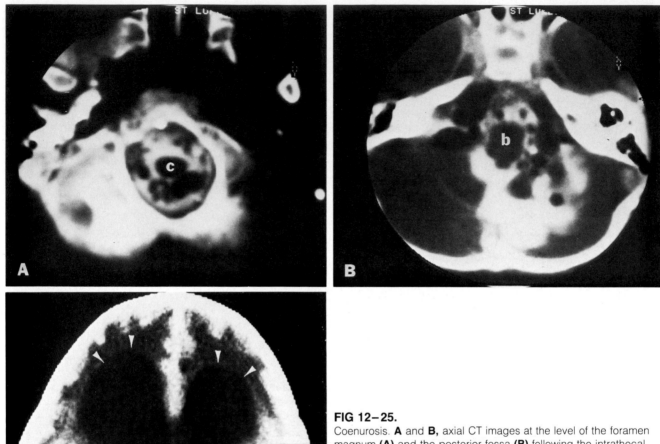

FIG 12–25.
Coenurosis. **A** and **B,** axial CT images at the level of the foramen
magnum **(A)** and the posterior fossa **(B)** following the intrathecal
administration of water-soluble contrast. Multiple cysts (filling
defects) are present within the subarachnoid space. The cysts
are of varying size and configuration and have densities between
20 and 35 Hounsfield units (C = cervicomedullary junction; B =
brain stem). **C,** a supratentorial CT section shows pronounced
dilatation of the third and lateral ventricles. It is difficult to
distinguish between the ventricular margins *(arrowheads)* and the
periventricular transependymal CSF flow. (Courtesy of G. A.
Norris, M.D., St Lukes Hospital, Duluth, Minn.)

sive therapy (Fig 12–26). Finally, human immunodeficiency virus (HIV) has caused the acquired immunodeficiency syndrome (AIDS) epidemic[123, 124]
and is an increasingly frequent cause of opportunistic infection.

AIDS

AIDS is caused by the HIV retrovirus and is
projected to kill as many as 54,000 Americans in
1991.[125] Homosexuals and IV drug abusers have

been especially at risk. Neurologic manifestations
and complications of this disease are common.
Thirty-nine percent of AIDS patients have neurologic symptoms, and 10% have these symptoms as
their initial complaint.[126] The opportunistic pathogens implicated in CNS infection in the AIDS patient are not unique to these patients but are being
seen with increasing frequency as the AIDS population increases.

AIDS patients evaluated with neuroimaging

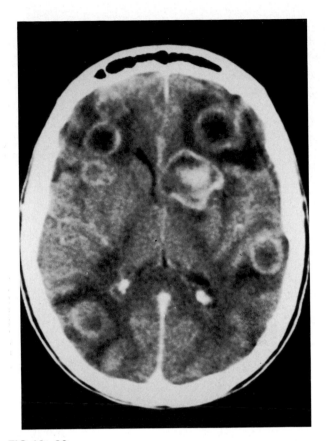

FIG 12–26.
Multiple abscesses in the immunocompromised patient. Contrast CT demonstrates multiple ringlike enhancing lesions, one of which is hemorrhagic. The patient was receiving immunosuppressive therapy following liver transplantation.

TABLE 12–9.
Common Pathogens in the Immunocompromised Host

Bacteria
    Listeria
Fungi
    Candida
    Cryptococcus
    Nocardia
    Aspergillus
    Mucor
Protozoa
    Toxoplasma gondii
Viruses
    AIDS (HIV)*
    PML†
    Herpes

* May not only cause immunocompromise making the host susceptible to other infections but may also cause deficits in its own right.
† PML = progressive multifocal leukoencephalopathy.

TABLE 12–10.
Factors Producing the Immunosuppressed State

Postoperative
Post-traumatic
Foreign body in CNS
Host defense problems
    Humoral dysfunction
    Cell-mediated dysfunction
    Phagocytic dysfunction
Drug therapy
    Antibiotics
    Corticosteroids
    Chemotherapy
    Immunotherapy
Radiation therapy
Transplantation
Vascular dysfunction
    Diabetes mellitus
    Atherosclerosis
    Dehydration
Other
    Malnutrition
    Malignant disease
    Chronic alcoholism
    Metabolic disease

may have no obvious focal areas of abnormality despite clinically apparent deficits. Nevertheless, such patients often appear to have a diffuse generalized atrophy with enlarged cortical sulci, ventricles, and cisterns. Volume loss is not pathognomonic for AIDS, but in the correct clinical setting it does correlate with HIV infection of the CNS. Such a nonspecific pattern of atrophy without focal deficits has been termed "AIDS brain" (Fig 12–27) and may be the most common imaging appearance in this population.

The protozoan *Toxoplasma gondii* has been the most frequent opportunistic organism to infect the AIDS brain in our experience as well as in the experience of others.[126–128] Toxoplasmosis may appear as a single mass or as multiple masses. On enhanced CT, ringlike enhancement patterns are typical, but more nodular patterns are also seen. "Double doses" of contrast often help to better visualize lesions (Fig 12–28). Surrounding edema is usually present. Symptoms are related to the location of the infection. Nodular areas of increased signal on T2-weighted images, particularly in the deep white matter, characterize the MRI appearance.[84]

Also common in the AIDS population is CNS lymphoma. Lymphoma will not be discussed in this section except to emphasize that not only might the appearance be indistinguishable from toxoplasmosis but that both can coexist in a patient.

PML is infection with a papovavirus. PML infection is characterized by abnormal white matter

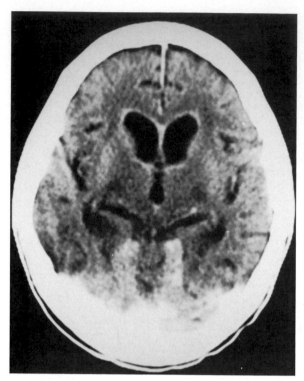

FIG 12–27.
"AIDS brain." Contrast CT shows the generalized volume loss indicated by the large sulci, cisterns, and ventricles in this young male homosexual. Also notice some ependymal enhancement around the frontal horns of the lateral ventricles that is consistent with a secondary ventriculitis.

with no appreciable mass effect (Fig 12–29). Most commonly the cerebral hemispheres are affected. Cerebellar involvement occurs frequently, and the brain stem may also be involved. A single site may be apparent on the initial imaging examination, but progression is the rule. By MRI, this infection appears as an area of increased signal in the white matter on T2-weighted images without mass effect.[129] The differential diagnosis solely based on MRI includes demyelinating disease, from which it may be difficult to distinguish. On CT, the area of cerebritis appears decreased in attenuation, again without mass effect. On CT, PML typically does not enhance with contrast, a feature often helpful in differentiating this disease from toxoplasmosis, lymphoma, and demyelinating disease.

Fungi also constitute organisms frequently implicated in AIDS patients. *Candida* typically appears as an intraparenchymal mass or multiple masses with surrounding edema. IV contrast CT usually produces ringlike enhancement similar to the picture of *Toxoplasma gondii*. Conversely, cryptococcal infection usually develops a leptom-

eningitis that is not easily detected by imaging examinations.[128] Occasionally, however, meningeal enhancement is evident after IV contrast administration. Examination of the CSF is usually required for diagnosis.

An important point to remember in evaluating the AIDS patient is that often more than one organism or neoplasm will be present simultaneously. Imaging characteristics of each pathogen will be apparent but perhaps not easily separated from one another. A brain biopsy for diagnosis of an isolated lesion is feasible. However, when many areas of abnormality coexist, biopsy of each is not reasonable, and empirical medical treatment may be instituted. Such treatment is usually directed toward the most common pathogen, *Toxoplasma gondii*. In these cases, serial scans will help demonstrate the response to therapy. Favorable responses can be considered diagnostic. Nonresponding lesions can then be reconsidered for biopsy.

Other Opportunistic Infections

Listeriosis.—Infection with *Listeria monocytogenes*, a short gram-positive rod, pathologically elicits meningitis, meningoencephalitis, and rarely, brain abscess. *L. monocytogenes* does not present with a distinctive radiologic picture. Laboratory diagnosis may be difficult since the specimens of CSF often contain only a few *Listeria* organisms that are easily mistaken for diphtheroids (gram-positive rods) and are then dismissed as a contaminant.[130] Early in the course, the CT appearance has been described as poorly marginated areas of low attenuation with regions of curvilinear or "gyral" enhancement.[131] Later in the course of the disease, ring enhancement may occur that is consistent with actual abscess formation. If meningitis is present, meningeal enhancement may occur. The encephalitis may be seen on MRI as an abnormal intraparenchymal focus (Fig 12–30). The diagnosis of *Listeria* infection should be considered in patients with impaired cellular immunity and a suspicion of bacterial meningitis and/or cerebritis with imaging findings of meningeal or parenchymal pathology when the bacteriologic studies of the CSF are negative.[132]

Nocardiosis.—*Nocardia*, an aerobic fungus resembling *Actinomyces*, does not produce the sulphur granules seen with *Actinomyces*. *Nocardia* characteristically is associated with a state of com-

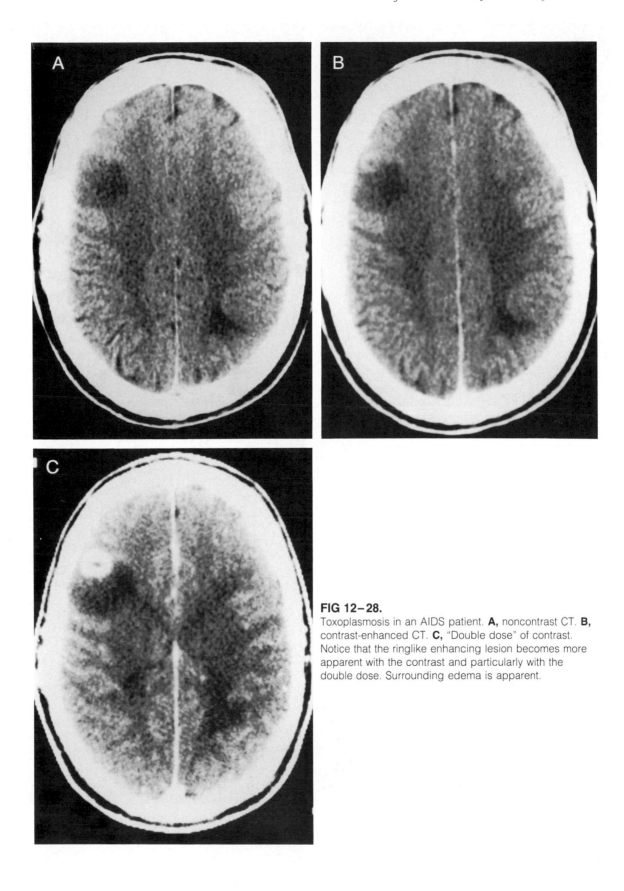

FIG 12–28.
Toxoplasmosis in an AIDS patient. **A,** noncontrast CT. **B,** contrast-enhanced CT. **C,** "Double dose" of contrast. Notice that the ringlike enhancing lesion becomes more apparent with the contrast and particularly with the double dose. Surrounding edema is apparent.

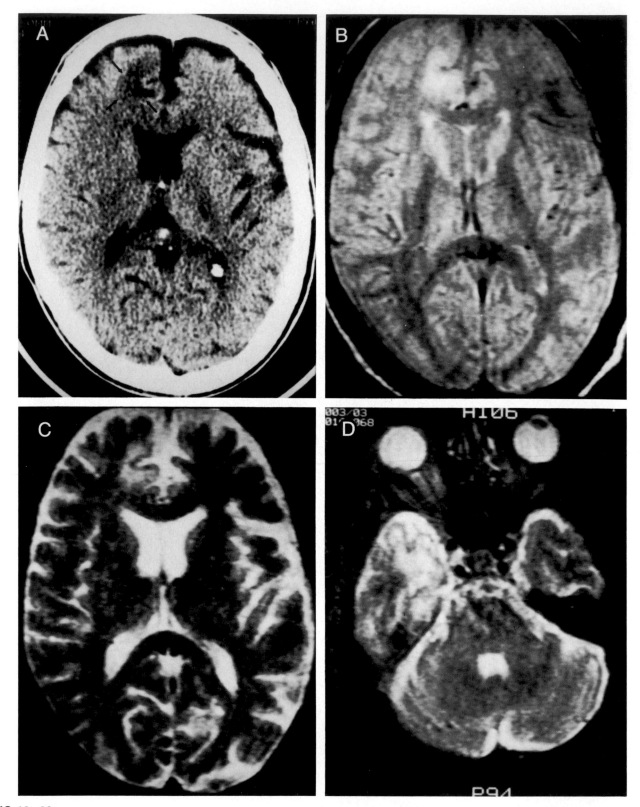

FIG 12–29.
PML infection. **A,** CT shows some lucency in the right frontal lobe *(arrows).* **B** and **C,** long TR images (**B,** short TE; **C,** long TE) shows the same area as abnormally increased in signal but without significant mass effect. **D,** same patient. A lower section shows that the right temporal lobe is also involved.

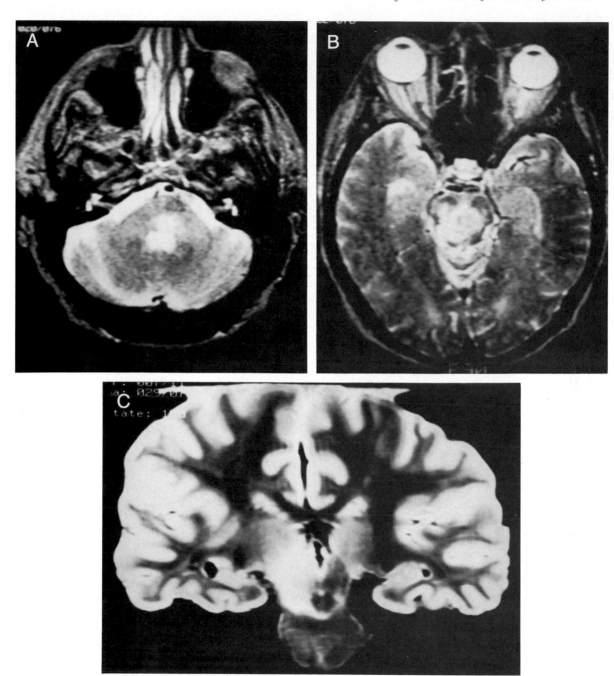

FIG 12–30.
Listeria encephalitis in a renal transplant patient. **A** and **B,** long TR (T2-weighted) images show abnormally high signal in the pons and midbrain. **C,** a coronal section obtained postmortem demonstrates the disease spreading from the midbrain into the right cerebral peduncle.

promised immunity, especially in the setting of corticosteroid therapy.[133] However, it may also infect patients with normal immunity. *Nocardia* complicates a spectrum of diseases that includes pulmonary alveolar proteinosis, sarcoidosis, ulcerative colitis, and intestinal lipodystrophy.[134] Hematogenous dissemination occurs from a pulmonary focus

into the CNS. This usually results in brain abscess formation, with meningitis being rare. The onset of symptoms is often insidious.

Nocardial lesions on imaging studies, while not specific, may contain multiple loculations. Ringlike enhancement on contrast CT occurs (Fig 12–31).[135] The diagnosis should be considered in

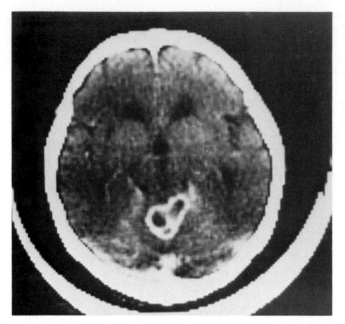

FIG 12–31.
Nocardia asteroides infection. Contrast CT shows a multiloculated enhancing cerebellar abscess in a 79-year-old immunosuppressed patient with chronic lymphocytic leukemia.

the appropriate clinical setting since *Nocardia* is sensitive to sulfonamides.

Aspergillosis.—In contradistinction to *Nocardia* infection where a well-formed capsule is usually apparent, intracranial *Aspergillus* infestation rarely presents with ring enhancement on CT but rather has a more lobular enhancement pattern (Fig 12–32).[136] This ubiquitous fungus may gain entry into the CNS by inoculation, hematogenous dissemination, or direct extension from the paranasal sinuses or, as is most common, from a pulmonary focus. Pathologically, aspergillosis produces meningitis and meningoencephalitis with subsequent hemorrhagic infarction from vascular invasion with secondary thrombosis. Less aggressive presentations include solitary cerebral abscess formation or isolated granulomas.

Abnormalities on CT may be subtle and include areas of low attenuation within the parenchyma with minimal mass effect. The presence of true ring enhancement militates against the aggressive meningoencephalitic variety of aspergillosis. Hemorrhagic areas are more common from this pathogen than most. The relatively benign CT picture may contrast sharply with the clinically apparent consumptive nature of the infection (Fig 12–33). The lack of correlation between the CT and pathologic findings is related to the rapidity of

the destructive process (inability to form an effective capsule). In addition, suppression of enhancement may occur by corticosteroid therapy. The CT findings, within the clinical setting of immunosuppression, corticosteroid therapy, fever, pulmonary infection, and neurologic findings (including a decreased level of consciousness), suggest the aggressive form of intracranial aspergillosis, which implies an extremely poor prognosis.[137]

MRI is very sensitive to the parenchymal infection[136] and shows the nonspecific changes of any inflammation. MRI would be expected to demonstrate hemorrhagic foci with ease.

Candidiasis.—*Candida* is the most common etiology of autopsy-proven cerebral mycosis. It has a propensity for neutropenic patients who are receiving corticosteroids. *Candida* reaches the CNS by hematogenous dissemination from the respiratory or gastrointestinal tract. Microscopic pathology includes vascular inflammation, thrombosis, infarction, and intraparenchymal microabscess for-

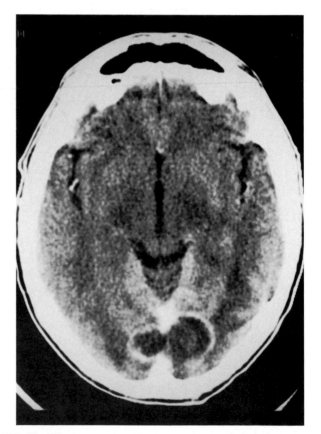

FIG 12–32.
Aspergillosis. Contrast CT demonstrates a multilobulated abscess cavity extending between the two occipital lobes through the falx cerebri that is indicative of the aggressive nature of this infection.

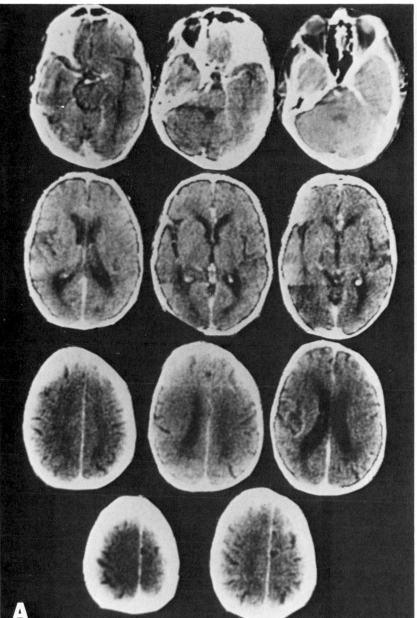

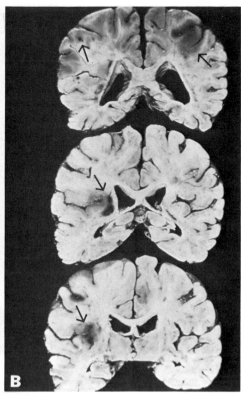

FIG 12–33.
Aspergillosis. **A,** enhanced CT in a renal transplant patient was performed the day prior to expiration and is unremarkable. **B,** a pathologic specimen from the same patient exhibits multiple areas of septic infarction *(arrows)*. The cerebellum was also involved.

mation typically in the middle cerebral artery distribution. Noncaseating granulomas have also been observed.[138, 139] The gross pathologic findings induced by this yeastlike fungus include meningitis, pachymeningitis, septic infarction, abscess, or granuloma.[140, 141] These various pathologic presentations consequently generate different appearances when neuroimaging. Nodules may enhance and have surrounding edema (Fig 12–34). Calcified granuloma, infarction, frank abscess formation, and hydrocephalus may be present.[140, 141] The infectious presentation depends on the state of the host's natural defenses. The inability to mount an effective localizing cell-mediated immune response when challenged favors an aggressive infection rather than granuloma formation. Endophthalmitis is a complication of *Candida* septicemia.[143] This finding in the face of intracranial lesions in the suppressed host strongly supports the diagnosis of CNS candidiasis.

Cryptococcusis.—*Cryptococcus* is a nonmycelial yeast with a polysaccharide capsule that distinctively stains with India ink. Sensitive immunologic diagnosis can also be made by detecting crytococcal antigen or anticryptoccal antibody in

hancement in those cases with meningoencephalitis.[163]

There is some evidence that links herpes zoster with cerebral granulomatous angiitis.[164] Granulomatous angiitis has also been reported in immunosuppressed patients, particularly those with lymphoproliferative disorders.[164–166] There is diffuse infiltration of small cerebral arteries and veins (<200 μm in diameter) by lymphocytes, giant cells, and mononuclear cells.[167] Clinical manifestations include disorientation and impaired intellectual function, usually progressing to death within 1 year. Multiple low-absorption regions are shown on CT scans, and may or may not enhance with contrast administration (Fig 12–37).[168, 169] These areas correspond to segmental abnormalities in the blood-brain barrier secondary to vasculitis. Thus, herpes zoster represents one etiology with two unique manifestations (large-vessel infarction and cerebral granulomatous angiitis), each with discrete CT features.

Miscellaneous

Radiation/Chemotherapy

The most frequent finding in patients treated with radiation therapy for primary brain tumors, skull lesions, and intracranial metastases is generalized parenchymal loss.[170, 171] Localized areas of atrophy may be present if smaller volumes have been irradiated. The effects of irradiation have been separated into those occurring early (within weeks) and late (4 months to many years later).[172] The early changes are transient and may not be associated with any imaging abnormality. However, the late effects of radiation are those of a vasculitis that may progress to actual small-vessel occlusion. Vascular occlusion with infarction may not be distinguishable from vascular occlusion of other etiologies unless the area of abnormality appears to conform to a radiation portal (Fig 12–38). Radiation changes without actual necrosis may result in abnormal white matter, particularly in the periventricular locations around the lateral ventricles.[173] This is evident as abnormally lucent white matter on CT or as areas of high signal on T2-weighted images of MRI (Fig 12–39). The presence of actual necrosis is usually difficult to differentiate from nonnecrotic radiation changes since edema and enhancement can occur in either.

At times mass effect and enhancement (on CT or MRI) may be present in an irradiated area of parenchyma and will be indistinguishable from per-

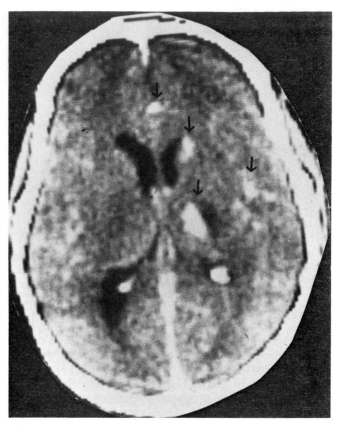

FIG 12–37.
Granulomatous angiitis. Enhanced CT shows multiple areas of involvement *(arrows)*. This patient had an acute personality change.

sistent or recurrent tumor. In fact, a difficulty with neuroimaging is in separating the presence of residual or recurrent tumor from radiation-induced changes including frank radionecrosis. The signs and symptoms of radiation necrosis are nonspecific and do not differentiate it from recurrent tumor. Comparison with previous scans or, alternatively, follow-up scans often are required for differentiation.

Dystrophic Calcification

Calcification in the gray matter and basal ganglia may be demonstrated in patients who have received radiation therapy and/or methotrexate months to years after cessation of therapy (Fig 12–40).[174–178] A microangiopathy is produced that is characterized histologically by noninflammatory small-vessel degeneration associated with dystrophic calcification in adjacent gray matter. The most susceptible areas are the putamen and globus pallidus, the gray-white junction, and the cerebellar cortex.[179] Mineralizing angiopathy relates directly to the length of survival following cessation of ra-

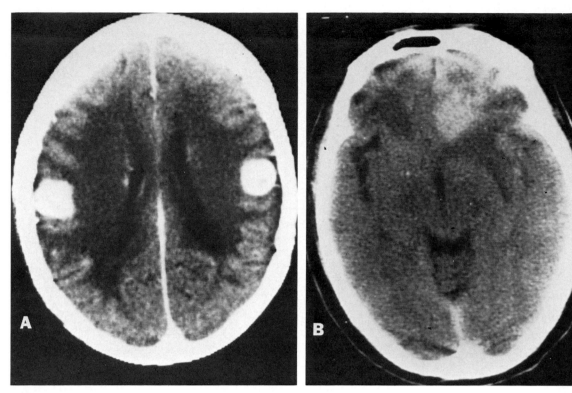

FIG 12–38.
Radiation changes. **A,** enhanced CT demonstrates bilateral enhancing masses in a patient treated with opposing radiation ports 2 years prior to this scan for a low-grade temporal lobe glioma. The surrounding white matter is abnormally lucent bilaterally as well. **B,** an enhancing left frontal mass is present in a patient previously irradiated for a basal cell carcinoma of the forehead.

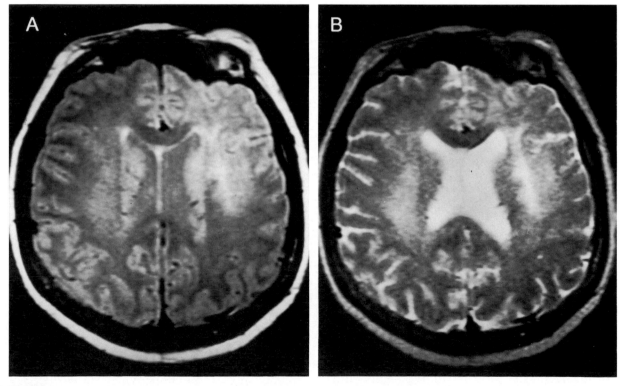

FIG 12–39.
Radiation changes detected by MRI of a patient who previously received whole-brain irradiation. **A,** Spin-density image (long TR, short TE). **B,** T2-weighted image (long TR, long TE). The deep white matter bilaterally is abnormal in signal on both images, more pronounced in the left hemisphere. Notice on the T2-weighted image that the signal is similar to that of the CSF in the ventricles but does not remain the same signal as CSF on the spin-density image.

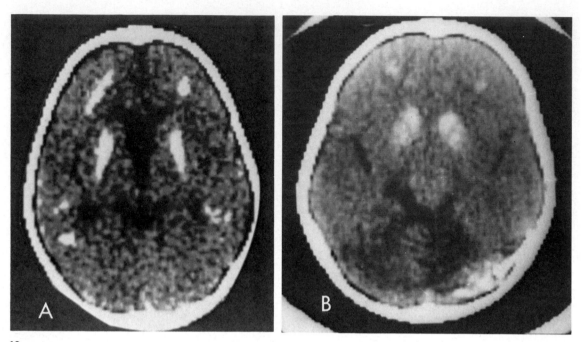

FIG 12–40.
Dystrophic calcification. **A,** in the lenticular nucleus and vascular watershed zones in a young leukemic patient treated with intrathecal methotrexate and irradiation. **B,** calcification in the basal ganglia and parenchymal loss in the cerebellum are secondary to intrathecal methotrexate and radiation therapy for leukemia.

diation therapy and the number of CNS relapses that occur.

The patients most commonly affected are children treated for a variety of neoplasms including acute lymphocytic leukemia, medulloblastoma, and glioblastoma. Subtle neurologic findings are associated and include memory loss, abnormal electroencephalographic (EEG) features, seizures, and personality changes.[180]

The calcification is best appreciated on CT since it may not be dense enough to be clear on MRI. Areas of abnormal signal, especially within the white matter from the previous chemotherapy and/or radiation therapy, may be more apparent on MRI (increased T2-weighted signal). On any neuroimaging, these children may demonstrate generalized volume loss with resultant increased ventricular and cortical sulcal size.[181]

Disseminated Necrotizing Leukoencephalopathy

Disseminated necrotizing leukoencephalopathy (DNL) is a syndrome that affects patients who have been treated with CNS radiation and chemotherapy, particularly intrathecal or IV methotrexate. Its onset occurs shortly after completion of therapy and is characterized clinically by a subacute course, the initial symptoms of which are confusion, ataxia, seizures, slurred speech, spasticity, dysphagia, and lethargy. Progression to dementia, coma, and death may occur.[182] Pathologic characteristics of this lesion include extensive areas of white matter demyelination and necrosis, astrocytosis, and a lack of inflammatory cellular response.[183]

The major CT finding in DNL is white matter areas of low attenuation (Fig 12–41).[184] The areas of white matter abnormality rarely exhibit contrast enhancement.[185] Direct installation of methotrexate into the ventricle may also produce a necrotizing leukoencephalopathy with the finding of a focal low-attenuation mass that may enhance with contrast material (Fig 12–42).[186]

Lupus Cerebritis

Patients with systemic lupus erythematosus (SLE) frequently have cerebral involvement. While the disorder begins as an arteriolitis, the parenchymal consequences can be considerable and are a leading cause of death in such patients.[187] The usual imaging abnormalities reflect the perivascular inflammation with small vessel occlusions and ruptures.[188] Cortical atrophy, lacunar infarcts, and intraparenchymal hemorrhages are usual. Recently, one report documented a pattern of generalized white matter lucency on CT without

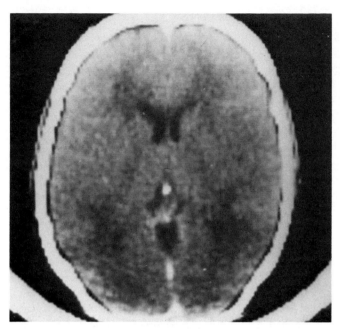

FIG 12–41.
DNL: CT of a 10-year-old patient with acute lymphocytic leukemia treated with irradiation and IV and intrathecal methotrexate. Note the periventricular lucency in the white matter that appeared just after cessation of therapy.

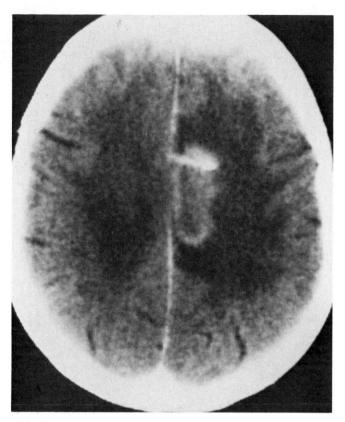

FIG 12–42.
Focal necrotizing leukoencephalopathy in a patient receiving intraventricular methotrexate. Note the enhancing mass (contrast CT) at the site of the ventricular canula. Also note the abnormal lucency in the surrounding white matter.

mass effect or enhancement in an SLE patient that is indistinguishable from the findings that may be seen from infection with PML[189] or from the changes seen secondary to small-vessel disease of any etiology. The authors suggested that brain biopsy might be required to distinguish whether such changes were secondary to the disease process or to an opportunistic PML infection (Fig 12–43). Clinically this translates into determining whether the neurologic changes (including psychosis) are related to the primary disease, a secondary infection, or even a steroid-induced psychosis.

The appearance of lupus cerebritis may also simulate multiple sclerosis on both CT and MRI. For example, on T2-weighted (long TR, long TE) MRI the periventricular white matter in the cerebral hemispheres may be high in signal in both diseases, thus making the imaging distinction difficult.

Postimmunization Encephalitis

Very rarely, following a routine childhood immunization, a transient parenchymal reaction may occur with signs and symptoms of cerebral encephalitis. Extensive parenchymal abnormalities are seen on MRI (Fig 12–44) that are not distinguish-able from other etiologies of encephalitis. Diagnosis depends on the clinical history of recent immunization and spontaneous resolution.

Congenital Infections

Neonates are susceptible to maternal infections. These are acquired either transplacentally in utero or during birth as the baby descends through the vaginal canal. This group of infectious agents has gone by the "TORCH" syndrome, an acronym for toxoplasmosis, other, rubella, cytomegalovirus (CMV), and herpes, which in the past have been the usual offending agents. Recently, syphilis *(Treponema pallidum)* has had a resurgence, and HIV (AIDS virus) has also begun to appear with alarmingly increasing frequency (Fig 12–45).

These disorders may cause areas of calcification, cerebritis, infarction, porencephalia, hydrocephalus, and generalized atrophy. A clue to the specific organism may be found by observing the combination of abnormalities. For example, calcifications are often present in association with CMV

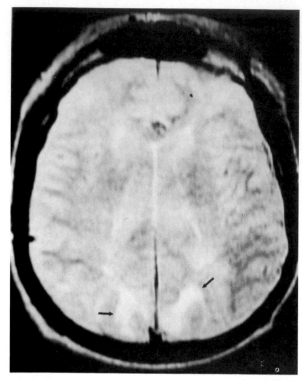

FIG 12–43.
Lupus cerebritis. MRI (spin-density image) demonstrates abnormal signal in the posterior white matter bilaterally *(arrows).*

and toxoplasmosis. CMV typically causes periventricular calcifications. Toxoplasmosis may also cause periventricular calcifications but often has more peripheral calcific foci as well. Furthermore, toxoplasmosis very frequently causes aqueductal obstruction with obstructive hydrocephalus, while CMV usually does not. Whether or not hydrocephalus is present therefore may be a helpful differential point. Ocular changes may also be helpful. Clinical retinitis almost invariably accompanies cerebral toxoplasmosis. The other congenital infection usually associated with ocular changes is rubella, where microphthalmos in addition to destructive parenchymal changes of the brain is often present.

Infants are also particularly susceptible to bacterial infections that are acquired by a route unrelated to birth. These are not true congenital infections but present in infancy and should therefore be considered in the appropriate age group. The common pathogens are included in Table 12–11. The imaging characteristics are similar to the appearance of pyogenic infection in the adult. A mass or masses with rim enhancement and surrounding edema may be demonstrated. Extension to an ependymal surface with secondary ventriculitis

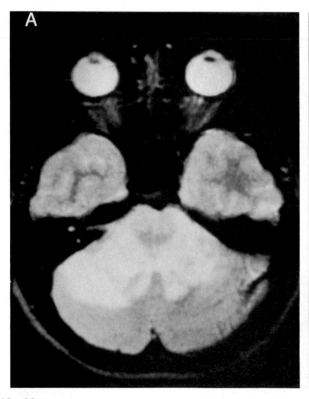

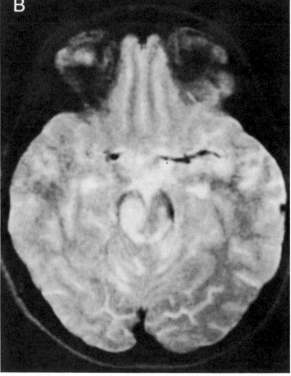

FIG 12–44.
Postimmunization encephalitis. Two T2-weighted axial images demonstrate extensive abnormal signal throughout much of the cerebellum and brain stem following a childhood immunization.

The clinical symptoms and MRI abnormalities resolved spontaneously over several months.

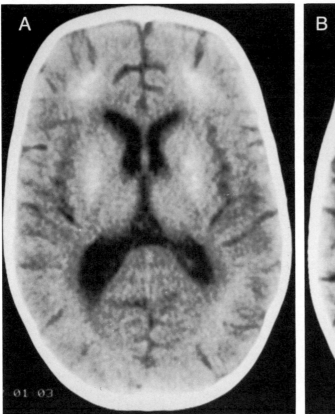

FIG 12–45.
Congenital AIDS. **A,** noncontrast CT demonstrates calcification in the basal ganglia and frontal white matter. **B,** 5 months later the calcification is denser, and significant parenchymal loss has occurred.

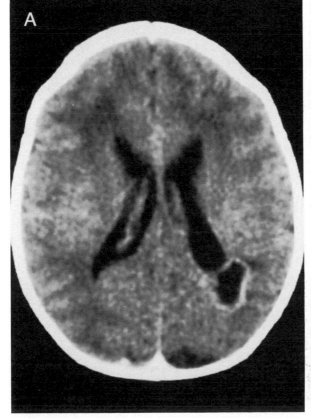
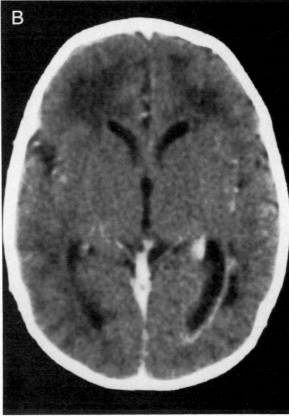

FIG 12–46.
Citrobacter abscess and ventriculitis in a young child (contrast CT). **A,** periventricular abscess with rim enhancement. **B,** ependymal enhancement in the atrium and occipital horn of adjacent lateral ventricle.

TABLE 12–11.

Common CNS Infections in Neonates and Infants

Congenital (TORCH)
  Toxoplasmosis
  Rubella
  CMV
  Herpes
  Syphilis *(T. pallidum)*
  Aids (HIV)
Citrobacter
Enterobacter
E. coli
Haemophilus influenzae
Group B streptococci

may occur (Fig 12–46). While rim enhancement is characteristic of abscess formation, *Citrobacter* meningitis may lead to vasculitis, infarction, and rim enhancement mimicking a true abscess.[190] Late sequelae include parenchymal loss, gliosis, and hydrocephalus.

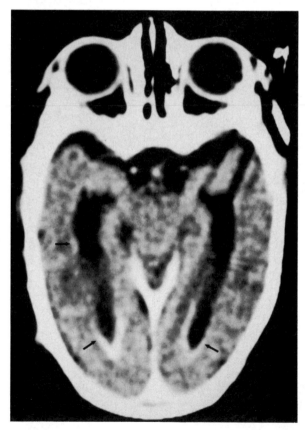

FIG 12–47.
Neonatal ventriculitis. Contrast CT demonstrates ependymal enhancement *(arrows)* in the lateral ventricles secondary to *Enterobacter* infection.

Ventriculitis

Infection of the ependyma lining and ventricles may occur secondary to rupture of a parenchymal abscess into the ventricles (Fig 12–46), extension from a meningeal infection, or following ventricular shunting. In neonates, ventriculitis may be the only manifestation of diffuse leptomeningitis (Fig 12–47). Chronic ventriculitis results in synechiae within the ventricles that may cause obstruction to the flow of CSF and hydrocephalus.

Neuroimaging may demonstrate enlarged ventricles and septations. On CT, periventricular areas of low attenuation may be demonstrated with enhancement of the ependymal surface. MRI may demonstrate periventricular abnormal white matter with abnormal increased signal on T2-weighted images. Occasionally, noninfectious ependymal irritations such as subarachnoid blood can cause ependymal enhancement on CT.

Acknowledgments

Many thanks must go to Ms. Kelly Morris and Mrs. Betsy Cervone for their preparation of this manuscript.

REFERENCES

1. Gray H: *Anatomy of the Human Body*, ed 30. Philadelphia, Lea & Febiger, 1985, pp 1122–1123.
2. Jungreis CA, Kanal E, Hirsch WL, et al: MR appearance of normal perivascular spaces mimicking lacunar infarction. *Radiology* 1988; 169:101–104.
3. Martinez AJ, Nelson EC, Jones MM, et al: Experimental *Naegleria* meningoencephalitis in mice: An electron microscope study. *Lab Invest* 1971; 25:465.
4. Martinez AJ, Duma RJ, Nelson EC, et al: Experimental *Naegleria* meningoencephalitis in mice: Penetration of the olfactory mucosal epithelium by *Naegleria* and pathologic changes produced: A light and electron microscope study. *Lab Invest* 1973, 29:121
5. Galbraith JG, Barr VW: Epidural abscess and subdural empyema. *Adv Neurol* 1974; 6:257–267.
6. Segall HD, Rumbaugh CL, Bergeron RT, et al: Brain and meningeal infections in children: Radiological considerations. *Neuroradiology* 1973; 6:8–16.
7. Sandu VK, Handel SF, Pinto RS, et al: Neuroradiolgic diagnosis of subdural empyema and CT limitations. *AJNR* 1980; 1:39–44.
8. Edwards MK, Kuharik MA, Cohen MD: Sonographic demonstration of cerebral sinus thrombosis. *AJNR* 1987; 8:1153–1155.

9. Rao KCVG, Knipp HC, Wagner MD: Computed tomographic findings in cerebral sinus and venous thrombosis. *Radiology* 1981; 140:391–398.

10. Macchi PJ, Grossman RI, Gomori JM, et al: High field MR imaging of cerebral venous thrombosis. *J Comput Assist Tomogr* 1986; 10:10–15.

11. McMurdo SK Jr, Brant-Zawadzki M, Bradley WG Jr: Dural sinus thrombosis: Study using intermediate field strength MR imaging. *Radiology* 1986; 161:83–86.

12. Sze G, Simmons B, Krol G, et al: Dural sinus thrombosis: Verification with spin-echo techniques. *AJNR* 1988; 9:679–686.

13. Hitchcock E, Andreadis A: Subdural empyema: A review of 29 cases. *J Neurol Neurosurg Psychiatry* 1964; 27:422–450.

14. Bannister G, Williams B, Smith S: Treatment of subdural empyema. *J Neurosurg* 1981; 55:82–88.

15. Jacobson PL, Farmer TW: Subdural empyema complicating meningitis in infants: Improved prognosis. *Neurology* 1981; 31:190–193.

16. Adams RD, Sidman RL: Meningeal infections, abscess and granulomas of the brain, in *Introduction to Neuropathology*. New York, McGraw-Hill International Book Co, 1968.

17. Headings DL, Glasgow LA: Occlusion of the internal carotid artery complicating haemophilus influenzae meningitis. *Am J Dis Child* 1977; 131:854–856.

18. Taft TA, Chusid MJ, Sty JR: Cerebral infarction in hemophilus influenzae type B meningitis. *Clin Pediatr (Phila)* 1986; 26:177–180.

19. Zimmerman RA, Patel S, Bilaniuk L: Demonstration of purulent bacterial intracranial infections by computed tomography. *AJR* 1976; 127:155–165.

20. Matthews VP, Kuharik MA, Edwards MK, et al: Gd-DTPA enhanced MR imaging of experimental bacterial meningitis: Evaluation and comparison with CT. *AJNR* 1988; 9:1045–1050.

21. Packer RJ, Bilaniuk LT, Zimmerman RA: CT parenchymal abnormalities in bacterial meningitis: Clinical significance. *J Comput Assist Tomogr* 1982; 6:1064–1068.

22. Carey ME, Chou SN, French LA: Experience with brain abscesses. *J Neurosurg* 1972; 36:1–9.

23. Beller AJ, Sahar A, Praissi I: Brain abscess: Review of 89 cases over a period of 30 years. *J Neurol Neurosurg Psychiatry* 1973; 36:757–768.

24. Chun CH, Johnson JD, Hofstetter M, et al: Brain abscess: A study of 45 consecutive cases. *Medicine (Baltimore)* 1986; 65:415–431.

25. Wood JH, Lightfoote WE II, Ommaya AK: Cerebral abscesses produced by bacterial implantation and septic embolization in primates. *J Neurol Neurosurg Psychiatry* 1979; 42:63–69.

26. Enzmann DR, Britt RH, Yeager AS: Experimental brain abscess evolution: Computed tomographic and neuropathologic correlation. *Radiology* 1979; 133:113–122.

27. Britt RH, Enzmann DR, Yeager AS: Neuropathological and computerized tomographic findings in experimental brain abscess. *J Neurosurg* 1981; 55:590–603.

28. Whelan MA, Hillal SK: Computed tomography as a guide in the diagnosis and follow-up of brain abscesses. *Radiology* 1980; 135:663–671.

29. Rosenblum ML, Hoff JT, Norman D, et al: Decreased mortality from brain abscesses since the advent of computerized tomography. *J Neurosurg* 1978; 49:658–668.

30. Rosenblum ML, Hoff JT, Norman D, et al: Nonoperative treatment of brain abscesses in selected high-risk patients. *J Neurosurg* 1980; 52:217–225.

31. New PFJ, David KR, Ballantine HT: Computed tomography in cerebral abscess. *Radiology* 1976; 121:641–646.

32. Stevens TA, Norman D, Kramer RA, et al: Computed tomographic brain scanning in intraparenchymal pyogenic abscesses. *AJR* 1978; 130:111–114.

33. Joubert MJ, Stephanov S: Computerized tomography and surgical treatment in intracranial suppuration. *J Neurosurg* 1977; 47:73–78.

34. Yang PJ, Reger KM, Seeger JF, et al: Brain abscess: An atypical CT appearance of CNS tuberculosis. *AJNR* 1987; 8:919–920.

35. Jinkins JR: Focal tuberculous cerebritis. *AJNR* 1988; 9:121–124.

36. Falk A: U.S. Veterans Administration Armed Forces cooperative study on the chemotherapy of tuberculosis: XII. Tuberculous meningitis in adults, with special reference to survival, neurologic residuals, and work status. *Am Rev Respir Dis* 1965; 91:823–831.

37. Mayers MM, Kaufman DM, Miller MH: Recent cases in intracranial tuberculomas. *Neurology* 1978; 28:256–260.

38. Kennedy DH, Fallon RJ: Tuberculous meningitis. *JAMA* 1979; 241:264–268.

39. Barrett-Connor E: Tuberculous meningitis in adults. *South Med J* 1967; 60:1061–1067.

40. Castio M, Lepe A: Cerebral tuberculoma. *Acta Radiol* 1963; 1:821–827.

41. Dastur HM: Tuberculoma, in Vinken PJ, Bruyn GW (eds): *Handbook of Clinical Neurology*, vol 19. Amsterdam, North Holland Publishing Co, 1975, pp 413–426.

42. Sibley WA, O'Brien JL: Intracranial tuberculomas: A review of clinical features and treatment. *Neurology* 1956; 6:157–165.

43. Gonzalez PRM, Herrero CV, Joachim GF, et al: Tuberculous brain abscess: Case report. *J Neurosurg* 1980; 52:419–422.

44. Centeno RS, Winter J, Bentson JR: Central ner-

vous system tuberculosis related to pregnancy. *Comput Tomogr* 1982; 6:141–145.

45. Whelan MA, Stern J: Intracranial tuberculomas. *Radiology* 1981; 138:75–81.

46. Elisevich K, Arpin EJ: Tuberculoma masquerading as a meningioma. *J Neurosurg* 1982; 56:435–438.

47. Suss RA, Resta S, Diehl JT: Persistent cortical enhancement in tuberculous meningitis. *AJNR* 1987; 8:716–720.

48. Venger BH, Dion FM, Rouah E, et al: MR imaging of pontine tuberculoma. *AJNR* 1987; 8:1149–1150.

49. Winkler ML, Olsen WL, Mills TC, et al: Hemorrhagic and nonhemorrhagic brain lesions: Evaluation with 0.35-T fast MR imaging. *Radiology* 1987; 165:203–207.

50. Berthier M, Sierra J, Leiguarda R: Intraventricular tuberculoma. *Neuroradiology* 1987; 29:163–167.

51. Peatfied RC, Shawdon HH: Five cases of intracranial tuberculoma followed by serial computerized tomography. *J Neurol Neurosurg Psychiatry* 1979; 42:373–379.

52. Delaney P: Neurologic manifestations in sarcoidosis: Review of the literature with a report of 23 cases. *Ann Intern Med* 1977; 87:336–345.

53. Ricker W, Clark M: Sarcoidosis—a clinicopathologic review of three hundred cases, including twenty-two autopsies. *Am J Clin Pathol* 1949; 19:725–749.

54. Wierderholt WC, Siebert RG: Neurological manifestations of sarcoidosis. *Neurology (Minneapolis)* 1965; 15:1147–1154.

55. Silverstein A, Feuer MM, Siltzback LE: Neurologic sarcoidosis. *Arch Neurol* 1965; 12:1–11.

56. Jefferson M: Sarcoidosis of the nervous system. *Brain* 1957; 80:540–555.

57. Mirfakhraee M, Crofford MJ, Guinto FC Jr, et al: Virchow-Robin space: A path of spread in neurosarcoidosis. *Radiology* 1986; 158:715–720.

58. Meyer JS, Foley JM, Compagna-Pinto D: Granulomatous angitis of the meninges in sarcoidosis. *Arch Neurol Psychiatry* 1953; 69:587–600.

59. Herring AB, Urich H: Sarcoidosis of the central nervous system. *J Neurol Sci* 1969; 9:405–422.

60. Kumpe DA, Rao CVGK, Garcia JH, et al: Intracranial neurosarcoidosis. *J Comput Assist Tomogr* 1979; 3:324–330.

61. Cahill DW, Saleman M: Neurosarcoidosis: A review of the rarer manifestations. *Surg Neurol* 1981; 15:204–211.

62. Hayes WS, Sherman JL, Stern BJ: MR and CT evaluation of intracranial sarcoidosis. *AJNR* 1987; 8:841–847.

63. Babu VS, Eisen H, Pataki K: Sarcoidosis of the central nervous system. *J Comput Assist Tomogr* 1979; 3:396–397.

64. Kwan ESK, Wolpert SM, Hedges TR III: Tolosa-

Hunt syndrome revisited: Not necessarily a diagnosis of exclusion. *AJNR* 1987; 8:1067–1072.

65. Ketonen L, Oksanen V, Kuuliala I: Preliminary experience of magnetic resonance imaging in neurosarcoidosis. *Neuroradiology* 1987; 29:127–129.

66. Decker RE, Mardayat M, Mare J, et al: Neurosarcoidosis with computerized tomographic visualization and transsphenoidal excision of a supra- and intrasellar granuloma. *J Neurosurg* 1979; 51:814–816.

67. Goodman SS, Margulies ME: Boeck's sarcoid simulating a brain tumor. *Arch Neurol* 1959; 81:419–423.

68. deTribolet N, Zander E: Intracranial sarcoidosis presenting angiographically as a subdural hematoma. *Surg Neurol* 1978; 9:169–171.

69. Brooks JJR, Stuckland MC, Williams JP, et al: Computed tomography changes in neurosarcoidosis clearing with steroid treatment. *J Comput Assist Tomogr* 1979; 3:398–399.

70. Einstein H: Coccidioidomycosis of the central nervous system, in Thompson RA, Green JR (eds): *Advances in Neurology*, vol 6. New York, Rosen Richards Press, Inc, 1974, pp 101–105.

71. Dublin AB, Phillips HE: Computed tomography of disseminated cerebral coccidioidomycosis. *Radiology* 1980; 135:361–368.

72. Ferris EJ: Arteritis, in Newton TH, Potts DG (eds): *Radiology of the Skull and Brain*, vol 2, book 4. St Louis, CV Mosby Co, 1974, pp 2566–2597.

73. Meyer HM Jr, Johnson RT, Crawford IP, et al: Central nervous system syndromes of "viral" etiology: A study of 713 cases. *Am J Med* 1960; 29:334–347.

74. Whitley RJ, Soong SJ, Dolin R, et al: Adenine arabinoside therapy of biopsy proven herpes simplex encephalitis. *N Engl J Med* 1977; 297:289–294.

75. South MA, Tompkins WA, Morris CR, et al: Congenital malformation of the central nervous system associated with genital type (type 2) herpes virus. *J Pediatr* 1969; 75:13–18.

76. Tuffli GA, Mahmias AJ: Neonatal herpetic infection: Report of two premature infants treated with systemic use of indoxuridine. *Am J Dis Child* 1969; 118:909–914.

77. Dublin AB, Merten DF: Computed tomography in the evaluation of herpes simplex encephalitis. *Radiology* 1977; 125:133–134.

78. Haynes RF, Amixi PH, Cramblett GH: Fatal herpes virus hominis (herpes simplex virus) infections in children. *JAMA* 1978; 206:312–319.

79. Smith JB, Groover RV, Klass DW, et al: Multicystic cerebral degeneration in neonatal herpes simplex virus encephalitis. *Am J Dis Child* 1977; 131:568–572.

80. Davis LE, Johnson RT: An explanation for the lo-

calization of herpes simplex encephalitis. *Ann Neurol* 1979; 5:2–5.

81. Taber LH, Brasier F, Couch RB, et al: Diagnosis of herpes simplex virus infection by immunofluorescence. *J Clin Microbiol* 1976; 3:309–312.

82. Tomlinson AH, Chinn IJ, MacCallum FO: Immunofluorescence staining for the diagnosis of herpes encephalitis. *J Clin Pathol* 1974; 27:495–499.

83. Zimmerman RD, Russell EJ, Leeds NE, et al: CT in the early diagnosis of herpes simplex encephalitis. *AJR* 1980; 134:61–66.

84. Schroth G, Kretzschmar K, Gawehn J, et al: Advantage of magnetic resonance imaging in the diagnosis of cerebral infections. *Neuroradiology* 1987; 29:120–126.

85. Enzmann DR, Ranson B, Norman D, et al: Computed tomography of herpes simplex encephalitis. *Radiology* 1978; 129:419–425.

86. Davis JM, Davis KR, Kleinman GM, et al: Computed tomography of herpes simplex encephalitis, with clinical pathological correlation. *Radiology* 1978; 129:409–417.

87. Sage MR, Dubois PJ, Oakes J, et al: Rapid development of cerebral atrophy due to perinatal herpes simplex encephalitis. *J Comput Assist Tomogr* 1981; 5:763–766.

88. Wilson D: Measles—quick and slow (editorial). *Lancet* 1971; 2:27.

89. Rish WS, Haddad FS: The variable natural history of subacute sclerosing panencephalitis. *Arch Neurol* 1979; 36:610–614.

90. Jabbour JT, Garcia JH, Lemmi H, et al: SSPE: A multidisciplinary study of eight cases. *JAMA* 1969; 207:2248–2254.

91. Zeman W, Kolar O: Reflections on the etiology and pathogenesis of subacute sclerosing panencephalitits. *Neurology* 1968; 18:1–7.

92. Sever JL, Zeman W: Serological studies of measles and subacute sclerosing panencephalitis. *Neurology* 1968; 18:95–97.

93. Connely JH: Additional data on measles virus antibody and antigen in subacute sclerosing panencephalitis. *Neurology* 1968; 18:87–89.

94. Pedersen H, Wulff CH: Computed tomographic findings of early subacute sclerosing panencephalitis. *Neuroradiology* 1982; 23:31–32.

95. Duda EE, Huttenlocker PR, Patronas NJ: CT of subacute sclerosing panencephalitis. *AJNR* 1980; 1:35–38.

96. Jawetz E, Melnick JL, Adelberg EA: *Review of Medical Microbiology*, ed 11. Los Altos, Calif, Lange Medical Publications, 1974, pp 357–358.

97. Steere AC, Malawista SE, Hardin JA, et al: Erythema chronicum migrans and Lyme arthritis. *Ann Intern Med* 1977; 86:685–698.

98. Reik L, Steere AC, Bartenhagen NH, et al: Neuro-

logic abnormalities of Lyme disease. *Medicine (Baltimore)* 1979; 58:281–294.

99. Steere AC, Grodzicki RL, Kornblatt AN, et al: The spirochetal etiology of Lyme disease. *N Engl J Med* 1983; 308:733–740.

100. Peterman SB, Hoffman JC: Lyme disease simulating multiple sclerosis. Presented at the 27th Annual Meeting of the ASNR, Orlando, Fla, March 20–24, 1989.

101. Haining RB, Haining RG: Cysticercosis cerebri. *JAMA* 1960; 172:2036–2039.

102. Brown HW: *Basic Clinical Parasitology*, ed 4. New York, Appleton-Century-Crofts, 1975, pp 191–193.

103. Dixon HBF, Lipscomb FM: Cysticercosis: An analysis and followup of 450 cases, in *Privy Council, Medical Research Council Special Report*, No. 229. London, Her Majesty's Stationery Office, 1961, pp 1–59.

104. Labato RD, Lamas E, Portallo JM: Hydrocephalus iu cerebral cysticercosis. *J Neurosurg* 1981; 55:786–793.

105. Simms NM, Maxwell RE, Christenson PC, et al: Internal hydrocephalus secondary to cysticercosis cerebri: Treatment with a ventriculoatrial shunt. *J Neurosurg* 1969; 30:305–309.

106. Stepien L: Cerebral cysticercosis in Poland: Clinical symptoms and operative results in 132 cases. *J Neurosurg* 1962; 19:505–531.

107. Dublin AB, French BN: Cysticercotic cyst of the septum pellucidum. *AJNR* 1980; 1:205–206.

108. Jankowski R, Zimmerman RD, Leeds NE: Cysticercosis presenting as a mass lesion at foramen of Monro. *J Comput Assist Tomogr* 1979; 3:694–696.

109. Santin G, Vargas J: Roentgen study of cysticercosis of central nervous system. *Radiology* 1966; 86:520–527.

110. Chang KH, Kim WS, Cho SY, et al: Comparative evaluation of brain CT and ELISA in the diagnosis of neurocysticercosis. *AJNR* 1988; 9:125–130.

111. Rodriquez-Carbajal J, Salgado P, Gutierrez-Olvarado R, et al: The acute encephalitic phase of neurocysticercosis: Computed tomographic manifestations. *AJNR* 1983; 4:51–55.

112. Carabajal JS, Palacious E, Azar-Kia B, et al: Radiology of cysticercosis of the central nervous system including computed tomography. *Radiology* 1977; 125:127–131.

113. Zee C, Segall HD, Miller C, et al: Unusual neuroradiological features of intracranial cysticercosis. *Radiology* 1980; 137:397–407.

114. Suss RA, Maravilla KR, Thompson J: MR imaging of intracranial cysticercosis: Comparison with CT and anatomopathologic features. *AJNR* 1986; 7:235–242.

115. Stern WE: Neurosurgical considerations of cys-

ticercosis of the central nervous system. *J Neurosurg* 1981; 55:382–389.

116. Bentson JR, Wilson GH, Helmer E, et al: Computed tomography in intracranial cysticercosis. *J Comput Assist Tomogr* 1977; 1:464–471.

117. Zee CS, Tsai FY, Segall HD, et al: Entrance of metrizamide into an intraventricular cysticercosis cyst. *AJNR* 1981; 2:189–191.

118. Danziger J, Bloch S: Tapeworm cyst infestations of the brain. *Clin Radiol* 1975; 26:141–148.

119. Hoermos JA, Healy GR, Schultz MG, et al: Fatal human cerebral coenurosis. *JAMA* 1970; 213:1461–1464.

120. Schellhas KS, Norris GA, Loken T: Disseminated subarachnoid coenurosis. Submitted for publication.

121. Brown HW: *Basic Clinical Parasitology*, ed 4. New York, Appleton-Century-Crofts, 1975, pp 208.

122. Chang KH, Cho SY, Chi JG, et al: Cerebral sparganosis: CT characteristics. *Radiology* 1987; 165:505–510.

123. Ho DD, Rota TR, Schooley RT, et al: Isolation of HTLV-III from cerebrospinal fluid and neural tissues of patients with neurologic syndromes related to the acquired immunodeficiency syndrome. *N Engl J Med* 1985; 313:1493–1497.

124. Koenig S, Gendelman HE, Orenstein JM: Detection of AIDS virus in macrophages in brain tissue from AIDS patients with encephalopathy. *Science* 1986; 233:1089–1093.

125. Jenness D: Scientist's roles in AIDS control. *Science* 1986; 233:825.

126. Levy RM, Rosenbloom S, Perrett LV: Neuroradiologic findings in AIDS: A review of 200 cases. *AJNR* 1986; 7:833–839.

127. Kelly WM, Brant-Zawadzki M: Acquired immunodeficiency syndrome: Neuroradiologic findings. *Radiology* 1983; 149:485–491.

128. Whelan MA, Kricheff II, Handler M, et al: Acquired immunodeficiency syndrome: Cerebral computed tomographic manifestations. *Radiology* 1983; 149:477–484.

129. Guilleux MH, Steiner RE, Young IR: MR imaging in progressive multifocal leukoencephalopathy. *AJNR* 1986; 7:1033–1035.

130. Buchner LH, Schneierson SS: Clinical and laboratory aspects of *Listeria monocytogenes* infections. *Am J Med* 1968; 45:904–921.

131. Haykal H, Zamani A, Wang AM: CT features of early *Listeria monocytogenes* cerebritis. *AJNR* 1987; 8:279–282.

132. Lechtenberg R, Sierra MF, Pringle GF, et al: *Listeria monocytogenes*: Brain abscess or meningoencephalitis. *Neurology* 1979; 29:86–90.

133. Smith PW, Steinkraus GE, Henricks BW, et al: CNS nocardiosis. *Arch Neurol* 1980; 37:729–730.

134. Case 20-1980: Case records of the Massachusetts General Hospital. *N Engl J Med* 1980; 302:1194–1199.

135. Tyson GW, Welch JE, Butler AB, et al: Primary cerebellar nocardiosis. *J Neurosurg* 1979; 51:408–414.

136. Jinkins JR, Siqueira E, Zuheir Al-Kawi M: Cranial manifestations of aspergillosis. *Neuroradiology* 1987; 29:181–185.

137. Grossman RI, Davis KR, Taveras JM, et al: Computed tomography of intracranial aspergillosis. *J Comput Assist Tomogr* 1981; 5:646–650.

138. Parker JC, McCloskey JJ, Lee RS: The emergence of candidiasis: The dominant postmortem cerebral mycosis. *Am J Clin Pathol* 1978; 70:31–36.

139. Black JT: Cerebral candidiasis: Case report of brain abscess secondary to *Candida albicans*, and review of literature. *J Neurol Neurosurg Psychiatry* 1970; 33:864–870.

140. Case 45-1981: Case records of the Massachusetts General Hospital. *N Engl J Med* 1981; 305:1135–1146.

141. Gorell JM, Palutkas WA, Chason JL: *Candida* pachymeningitis with multiple cranial nerve pareses. *Arch Neurol* 1979; 36:719–720.

142. Whelan MA, Stern J, deNapoli RA: The computed tomographic spectrum of intracranial mycosis: Correlation with histopathology. *Radiology* 1981; 141:703–707.

143. Fishman LS, Griffin JR, Spico FL, et al: Hematogenous *Candida* endophthalmitis—a complication of candidemia. *N Engl J Med* 1972; 286:675–681.

144. Bindschadler DD, Bennett JE: Serology of human cryptococcosis. *Ann Intern Med* 1968; 68:45–52.

145. Harper CG, Wright DM, Perry G, et al: Cryptococcal granuloma presenting as an intracranial mass. *Surg Neurol* 1979; 11:425–429.

146. Everett BA, Kusske JA, Rush JL, et al: Cryptococcal infection of the central nervous system. *Surg Neurol* 1978; 9:157–163.

147. Blitzer A, Lawson W, Meyers BR, et al: Patient survival factors in paranasal sinus mucormycosis. *Laryngoscope* 1980; 90:635–648.

148. Long EL, Weiss DL: Cerebral mucormycosis. *Am J Med* 1980; 26:625–635.

149. Ginsberg F, Peyster RG, Hoover ED, et al: Isolated cerebral mucormycosis: Case report with CT and pathologic correlation. *AJNR* 1987; 8:558–560.

150. Succar MB, Nichols RD, Burch KH: Rhinocerebral mucormycosis. *Arch Otolaryngol* 1979; 105:212–214.

151. Masucci EF, Fabara JA, Saini N, et al: Cerebral mucormycosis (phycomycosis) in a heroin addict. *Arch Neurol* 1982; 39:304–306.

152. Hameroff SB, Eckholdt JW, Lindenberg R: Cerebral phycomycosis in a heroin addict. *Neurology* 1970; 20:261–265.

153. Chmel H, Grieco MH: Cerebral mucormycosis and

renal aspergillosis in heroin addicts without endocarditis. *Am J Med Sci* 1973; 266:225–231.

154. Adelman LS, Aronson SM: The neuropathologic complications of narcotic addiction. *Bull NY Acad Med* 1969; 45:225–233.

155. Price DL, Wolpow ER, Richardson EP Sr: Intracranial phycomycosis: A clinicopathological and radiological study. *J Comput Assist Tomogr* 1971; 14:359–375.

156. Raji MR, Agha FP, Gabriele OF: Nasopharyngeal mucormycosis. *J Comput Assist Tomogr* 1981; 5:767–770.

157. Lazo A, Wilner HI, Metes JJ: Craniofacial mucormycosis: Computed tomographic and angiographic findings in two cases. *Radiology* 1981; 139:623–626.

158. Wilson WB, Grotta JC, Schold C, et al: Cerebral mucormycosis: An unusual case. *Arch Neurol* 1979; 36:725–726.

159. Dolin R, Reichman RC, Mazur MH, et al: Herpeszoster-varicella infections in immunosuppressed patients. *Ann Intern Med* 1978; 89:375–388.

160. Gallagher JG, Merigan TC: Prolonged herpeszoster infection associated with immunosuppressive therapy. *Ann Intern Med* 1979; 91:842–846.

161. Hedges TR III, Albert DM: The progression of the ocular abnormalities of herpes zoster. *Ophthalmology* 1982; 39:165–177.

162. Mackenzie RA, Forbes GS, Karnes WE: Angiographic findings in herpes zoster arteritis. *Ann Neurol* 1981; 10:458–464.

163. Enzmann DR, Brant-Zawadzki M, Britt RH: CT of central nervous system infections in immunocompromised patients. *AJNR* 1980; 1:239–243.

164. Rosenblum WI, Hadfield MG: Granulomatous angiitis of the nervous system in cases of herpes zoster and lymphosarcoma. *Neurology* 1972; 22:348–354.

165. Greco FA, Kolins J, Rajjoub RK, et al: Hodgkin's disease and granulomatous angiitis of the central nervous system. *Cancer* 1976; 38:2027–2032.

166. Newcastle NB, Tom NI: Noninfectious angiitis of the nervous system associated with Hodgkin's disease. *J Neurol Neurosurg Psychiatry* 1962; 25:51–58.

167. Kolodny EH, Rebeiz JJ, Caviness VS, et al: Granulomatous angiitis of the central nervous system. *Arch Neurol* 1968; 19:510–524.

168. Valavanis A, Friede R, Schubiger O, et al: Cerebral granulomatous angiitis simulating brain tumor. *J Comput Assist Tomogr* 1979; 3:536–538.

169. Faer MJ, Mead JH, Lynch RD: Cerebral granulomatous angiitis: Case report and literature. *AJR* 1977; 129:463–467.

170. Carella RS, Pay N, Newall J, et al: Computerized (axial) tomography in the serial study of cerebral tumors treated by radiation. *Cancer* 1976; 37:2719–2728.

171. Wilson GH, Byfield J, Hanafee WN: Atrophy following radiation therapy for central nervous system neoplasms. *Acta Radiol* 1972; 11:361–368.

172. Lampert PW, Davis RL: Delayed effects of radiation on the human central nervous system: "Early and late" delayed reactions. *Neurology* 1964; 14:912–917.

173. Tsuruda JS, Kortman KE, Bradley WG, et al: Radiation effects on cerebral white matter: MR evaluation. *AJNR* 1987; 8:431–437.

174. Flament-Durand J, Ketelbant-Balasse P, Maurus R, et al: Intracerebral calcifications appearing during the course of acute lymphocytic leukemia treated with methotrexate and x-rays. *Cancer* 1975; 35:319–325.

175. Lee KI, Suh JH: CT evidence of gray matter calcification secondary to radiation therapy. *Comput Tomogr* 1977; 1:103–110.

176. McIntosh S, Fischer DB, Rothman SG, et al: Intracranial calcifications in childhood leukemia. *J Pediatr* 1977; 91:909–913.

177. Numaguchi Y, Hoffman JC, Sones PJ: Basal ganglia calcification as a late radiation effect. *AJR* 1975; 123:27–30.

178. Davis PC, Hoffman JC Jr, Pearl GS, et al: CT evaluation of effects of cranial radiation therapy in children. *AJNR* 1986; 7:639–644.

179. Price RA: Pathology of central-nervous-system diseases in childhood leukemia, in Ongerboer de Visser BW, Basch DA, van Woerkrom JL, et al (eds): *Neuro-Oncology.* The Hague, Martinus Nijhoff Publishers, 1980, pp 186–205.

180. Price RA, Birdwell DA: The central nervous system in childhood leukemia. *Cancer* 1978; 42:717–728.

181. Peylan-Ramu N, Poplack DG, Pizzo PA, et al: Abnormal CT scans of the brain in asymptomatic children with acute lymphocytic leukemia after prophylatic treatment of the central nervous system with radiation and intrathecal chemotherapy. *N Engl J Med* 1978; 298:815–818.

182. Rubinstein LJ, Herman MM, Song TF, et al: Disseminated necrotizing leukoencephalopathy: A complication of treated central nervous system leukemia and lymphoma. *Cancer* 1975; 35:291–305.

183. Price RA, Jamieson PA: The central nervous system in childhood leukemia. *Cancer* 1975; 35:306–318.

184. Lane B, Carroll BA, Pedley TA: Computerized cranial tomography in cerebral diseases of white matter. *Neurology* 1978; 28:534–544.

185. Shalen PR, Ostrow PT, Glass PJ: Enhancement of the white matter following prophylactic therapy of the central nervous system for leukemia. *Radiology* 1981; 140:409–412.

186. Bjorgen JE, Gold LHA: Computed tomographic appearance of methotrexate-induced necrotizing leukoencephalopathy. *Radiology* 1977; 140:409–412.

187. Adelman DC, Saltiel E, Klinenberg JR; The neuropsychiatric manifestations of systemic lupus erythematosus: An overview. *Semin Arthritis Rheum* 1986; 15:185–199.

188. Blaniuk LT, Patel S, Zimmerman RA: Computed tomography of systemic lupus erythematosus. *Radiology* 1977; 124:119–121.

189. Marsteller LP, Marsteller HB, Braun A, et al: An unusual CT appearance of lupus cerebritis. *AJNR* 1987; 8:737–739.

190. Foreman SD, Smith EE, Ryan NJ, et al: Neonatal *Citrobacter* meningitis: Pathogenesis of cerebral abscess formation. *Ann Neurol* 1984; 16:655–659.

13

Diseases of the White Matter

Meredith A. Weinstein, M.D.

Sylvester Chuang, M.D.

Poser[1] has divided the demyelinating diseases into two groups: the myelinoclastic (demyelinating) group, where myelin is normally formed and is subsequently injured or destroyed by either endogenous or exogenous agents or a combination of both; and the dysmyelinating diseases, in which some enzymatic disturbance interferes either with the formation of myelin or with its maintenance. The following classification of diseases of the white matter is primarily based on the classifications of Poser[1] and of Gilroy and Meyer.[2]

I. Myelinoclastic diseases
  A. Primary idiopathic (?acquired allergies and infections)
    1. Multiple sclerosis (MS)
    2. Diffuse sclerosis (Schilder's disease, 1912 type)
    3. Optic neuromyelitis (Devic's disease)
    4. Concentric sclerosis (Baló's disease)
    5. Transitional sclerosis
  B. Acquired allergic and infectious diseases resulting in breakdown of myelin
    1. Postvaccinal encephalomyelitis
    2. Postinfectious encephalomyelitis (acute disseminated encephalomyelitis)
    3. Acute hemorrhagic leukoencephalitis
    4. Postinfectious polyneuritis (Landry-Guillain-Barré syndrome)
  C. Viral-induced
    1. Subacute sclerosing panencephalitis (SSPE)
    2. Subacute rubella syndrome
    3. Progressive multifocal leukoencephalopathy (PML)
  D. Degenerative-toxic
    1. Central pontine myelinolysis (CPM)
    2. Marchiafava-Bignami disease
    3. Carbon monoxide encephalopathy
    4. Anoxic encephalopathy
  E. Vascular
    1. Binswanger's disease
    2. Maladie de Schilder-Foix
  F. Posttherapy
    1. Methotrexate leukoencephalopathy
    2. Disseminated necrotizing leukodystrophy (DNL)
II. Dysmyelinating diseases
  A. Leukodystrophies (genetically determined metabolic disorders with primary involvement of myelin)
    1. Metachromatic leukodystrophy
    2. Globoid cell leukodystrophy (Krabbe's disease)
    3. Spongy degeneration (Canavan's disease)
    4. Adrenoleukodystrophy
    5. Alexander's disease
    6. Pelizaeus-Merzbacher disease
  B. Lipid storage diseases with neuronal involvement (genetically determined metabolic disorders with secondary involvement of myelin)
    1. GM_2 gangliosidosis (Tay-Sachs disease)
    2. GM_1 gangliosidosis

TABLE 13–1.
Myelinoclastic Diseases

Disease	Age at Onset	Etiology	Computed Tomography
Multiple sclerosis	Any age Peak 15–45 yr Median 33 yr	Unknown	Sharply marginated plaques 0.6–1.4 cm in diameter, predominantly periventricular, others elsewhere in white matter A. Decreased attenuation without contrast, increased with contrast (acute and subacute lesions) B. Isodense without contrast, increased with contrast (acute and subacute lesions) C. Decreased without and with contrast (chronic lesions) D. Atrophy E. Mass effect (very rare)
Diffuse sclerosis	50% under 10 yr	Unknown; same as multiple sclerosis?	Extensive bilateral areas of decreased attenuation with extensive enhancement in acute stage; margins may be sharply or poorly defined
Acute hemorrhagic leukoencephalitis	Young adults	Allergic response to virus	Decreased attenuation coefficients, focal or diffuse, unilateral or bilateral
Subacute sclerosing panencephalitis	Most 5–15 yr	Measles	Rapidly progressive disease, normal-to-minimal abnormalities Chronic course, decreased attenuation coefficients of white matter, caudate nuclei, or other basal ganglia without enhancement
Subacute rubella syndrome	Congenital infection	German measles	Diffuse decreased attenuation of white matter, basal ganglia, and centrum semiovale; may calcify
Progressive multifocal leukoencephalopathy	See Chapter 12		
Central pontine myelinolysis	Any	Rapid increase in serum sodium	Variable-sized areas of decreased attenuation in pons; may have slight enhancement at periphery
Marchiafava-Bignami disease	Adults	A. Alcoholism B. Nutritional deficiency?	A. Acute, decreased attenuation of the corpus callosum B. Subacute, enhancement of the corpus callosum C. Chronic, atrophy of the corpus callosum and cortical atrophy, predominantly frontal
Carbon monoxide and anoxic encephalopathy	All		Enlarged sulci and cortical atrophy; less commonly decreased attenuation of entire white matter, cerebral hemispheres
Binswanger's disease	Elderly	Arteriosclerosis	Decreased attenuation of white matter without enhancement
Methotrexate leukoencephalopathy	See Chapter 21		
Disseminated necrotizing leukodystrophy	See Chapter 21		

TABLE 13–2.

Dysmyelinating Diseases (Leukodystrophies)

Disease	Age of Onset	Etiology	Computed Tomography
Metachromatic leukodystrophy A. Late infantile B. Juvenile C. Adult	12–18 mo 5–10 yr Adulthood	Decreased arylsulfatase A Autosomal recessive	Extensive, diffuse symmetric decreased attenuation coefficients of white matter without enhancement with mild-to-moderate ventricular dilatation
Globoid cell leukodystrophy (Krabbe's disease)	3–5 mo	Decreased galactocerebroside β-galactosidase Autosomal recessive	Ventricular or cortical atrophy; may have decreased attenuation of white matter
Spongy degeneration (Canavan's disease)	2–3 mo	Unknown Autosomal recessive	Megalencephaly, symmetric decreased attenuation of white matter
Adrenoleukodystrophy	School-aged boys	Abnormal, long-chain fatty acid metabolism Sex-linked recessive	Type 1: early phase: irregular areas of decreased attenuation in occipital lobes; subsequent involvement of parietal, temporal, and frontal lobes; enhancement along leading edge of lesion Type 2: enhancement of internal capsule, corona radiata, forceps major, and cerebral peduncles
Alexander's disease	0–12 mo	Unknown Usually sporadic	Megalencephaly, decreased attenuation coefficient of white matter, predominantly frontal lobes and anterior limbs of internal capsule; may be decreased attenuation coefficient of basal ganglia, which may enhance
Pelizaeus-Merzbacher disease	Early infancy	Unknown Sex-linked recessive	Decreased attenuation of white matter

3. Ceroid lipofuscinoses
4. Niemann-Pick disease (sphingomyelin lipidosis)
5. Gaucher's disease (cerebroside lipoidosis)
6. Cerebrotendinous xanthomatosis
7. Fabry's disease
C. Aminoacidopathy

Brief synopses of the clinical and computed tomographic (CT) findings of each of these diseases are given in Tables 13–1 and 13–2. Table 13–3 correlates CT findings with magnetic resonance imaging (MRI) findings.

TABLE 13–3.

Magnetic Resonance Imaging Findings in Myelinoclastic and Dysmyelinating Diseases

1. All CT lesions described in Tables 13–1 and 13–2 will be increased in signal intensity on spin-density and T2-weighted MR images. If visualized on T1-weighted MR images, they will be decreased in signal intensity.
2. All lesions that enhance on CT with iodinated contrast material will enhance on MRI with gadolinium diethylenetriamine pentaacetic acid (DTPA).

MYELIN

Abnormalities of the myelin sheath in the central nervous system (CNS) are the subject of this chapter. All axons with a diameter greater than 1 μm in the central and peripheral nervous systems of vertebrates are surrounded by a myelin sheath.[3] The ratio of the diameter of the axon to the thickness of the myelin sheath varies from 5:1 to 25:1. Myelin is almost entirely absent in the cerebrum of the newborn, gradually increases during the first 3 months, and increases more rapidly between the 3rd and 13th month. From the 13th month to the age of 10 to 12 years, when the brain reaches its full adult size, there is a constant increase in myelin in relation to the lipids contained in the nerve cells and axons.[4] Five infant baboons were serially studied with CT during the first year of their lives to determine the rate and degree of normal white matter maturation in the frontal, occipital, and parietal areas. Frontal white matter was the most immature in the immediate postnatal period, but it became equal in attenuation to the other regions by 4 weeks of age.[5]

Myelin is a part of the cell wall membrane of the oligodendroglia in the CNS and of the Schwann cell in the peripheral nervous system. The formation and maintenance of myelin is dependent on both the oligodendroglia (or Schwann cell) and the axon; myelin is not formed by either axons grown alone or by oligodendroglia (or Schwann cells) grown alone in tissue culture. If an axon is interrupted, both the axon and its myelin sheath undergo degeneration even though the oligodendroglia is not injured. The process is known as wallerian degeneration after Waller, who in 1850 cut the hypoglossal or glossopharyngeal nerves of frogs and showed degeneration of myelin.[6] To form and maintain myelin, an intact blood supply is also necessary.

Almost any injury or disease of the CNS can cause destruction of myelin. Trauma, infection, neoplasm, metabolic disease, and vascular lesions can cause demyelination associated with damage to neurons. Demyelinating disease is a condition in which there is an injury to myelin sheaths with relative preservation of axons, nerve cells, and supporting structures (periaxial degeneration). In most of the demyelinating diseases, degeneration of the axons and tissue necrosis may occur.[7]

MYELINOCLASTIC DISEASES

Primary Myelinoclastic Diseases

Multiple Sclerosis
History.—In 1838 Carswell[8], and from 1839 to 1842 Cruveilhier,[9] recognized and described the lesions of MS. In 1849 Frerichs,[10] a German internist, used the term *Hirnsklerose* ("brain sclerosis"), and in 1866 a French neurologist, Vulpian,[11] described clinical and pathologic findings of patients with MS. In 1879, Charcot[12] recognized the essential pathologic feature of MS: demyelination with relative preservation of axons.

Epidemiology.—The most common demyelinating disease, MS is relatively uncommon, with a prevalence rate of 58/100,000 in the United States (0.058%). On Jan 1, 1976, there were 123,000 MS patients in the mainland United States. The age of the person at the first symptom was less than 20 years in 13%, 20 to 29 years in 30%, 30 to 39 years in 28%, 40 to 49 years in 14%, and 50-plus years in 15%, for a median age of onset of 33 years. The average age of onset for females is 2 to 3 years earlier than for males. Females have a prevalence rate of 72/100,000, males of 42/100,000. Sixty-three percent of MS cases occur in females and 37% in males. Whites have a prevalence rate of 62/100,000; nonwhites have a rate of 31/100,000.[13]

There is ever-increasing evidence that MS is a disease acquired years before clinical onset. There is a marked variation in the incidence of MS that is related to latitude. Different races have markedly different susceptibilities to MS.

The compilation of nearly 200 studies has shown that MS is distributed throughout the world in three zones of high, medium, and low frequencies. The prevalence rates are over 30/100,000 in high-frequency areas, which include Europe between 45 and 65 degrees latitude, southern Canada, northern United States, New Zealand, and southern Australia.[14]

Medium-frequency areas with prevalence rates of 5 to 25 (and mostly 10–15)/100,000 are adjacent to high-frequency areas and include southern Europe, southern United States, and most of Australia. In the United States, 37 degrees latitude is the approximate border between the northern high-frequency areas and the southern medium-frequency regions. Incidence rates per 100,000 population (followed by latitude) for some representative United States and Canadian cities are Winnipeg, 40 (50 degrees); Rochester, Minn., 64 (44 degrees); Boston, 51 (42 degrees); Denver, 37 (40 degrees); San Francisco, 30 (37 degrees); New Orleans, 12 (30 degrees); Houston, 7 (30 degrees); and Hawaii, 10 (20 degrees).[15] Except for one white group in South Africa, all studied areas of Asia and Africa have low prevalence rates of MS (under 5/100,000).

White populations inhabit all the high- and medium-risk areas. In America, blacks, Orientals, and possibly Indians have much lower rates of MS than whites, but the incidence of each group parallels the geographic gradient found for whites.[14] The incidence of MS is very low in Japan, India, and Korea, with prevalence rates of 2/100,000 in Fukuoka (34 degrees latitude), Sapporo (43 degrees), Bombay (18 degrees), and Seoul (38 degrees).[15] No well-documented case of MS has been reported in African blacks.

While the etiology of MS is unknown, there is

evidence suggesting an infectious (slow virus) etiology. Migration studies have shown that those migrating after 15 years of age retain the MS risk of their birthplace and that those migrating before 15 years of age acquire the risk of their new residence.[14] In the Faeroe Islands, a group of small islands between Norway and Iceland at 62 degrees latitude, an epidemic of MS occurred. Between 1920 and 1977, 25 cases of MS occurred among native-born Faroese, excluding those with prolonged foreign residence. Twenty-four of these cases occurred between 1943 and 1960; one occurred in 1970. Before 1943, the prevalence rate was 0/100,000. After 1943, the prevalence rate was 87/100,000. All 14 early-onset cases (1943–1949) were in persons 11 to 45 years of age in 1940. All but two late-onset cases (1952–1960) were in persons up to 10 years of age in 1940. For 5 years beginning in April 1940, British troops occupied the Faeroes in large numbers. All but three of the Faeroese who had MS lived in locations where the British troops were stationed, and these three had direct contact with the British.[16] It is therefore probable that the British troops, or something brought along with the British troops, such as dogs, caused an epidemic on the Faeroes.

It is noteworthy that canine distemper was pandemic in the islands during World War II. Canine distemper was absent before the British occupation, and since 1956 or 1957 there have been no further cases of canine distemper among dogs on the Faeroe Islands. Other studies have shown an association between dogs with distemper and neurologic illnesses with symptoms of MS.[17–19]

In addition to the apparent association with dogs having distemper, other indications that MS may have an infectious etiology are similarities between the epidemiology of MS and poliomyelitis. A person has a 1.7 times greater chance of acquiring MS if he or she has had a tonsillectomy. This increased risk is similar to the increased risk of acquiring poliomyelitis after tonsillectomy.[20] Prior to immunization, the incidence of poliomyelitis had a variation with latitude that was similar to MS. It has been postulated that in equatorial regions where sanitation is poor, infection with the poliomyelitis virus and with the MS etiologic agent is universal early in life. It is further postulated that poliomyelitis does not cause paralytic disease and the MS etiologic agent does not cause clinical manifestations of MS in this young age group. With improvement in the level of sanitation, there is a rising incidence in the level of paralytic poliomyelitis. There is an increased incidence of MS in people of a higher socioeconomic group who have grown up with a higher level of sanitation.[21] This was also true of paralytic poliomyelitis prior to immunization. It has therefore been postulated that MS may be an unusual manifestation of a common enteric virus in those people who have had less contact with this viral agent during early life and have failed to develop immunity by late childhood.[22]

The epidemiology of MS suggests a genetic or familial predisposition. Siblings of MS patients have a 20 times greater probability of acquiring MS, and children of MS patients have a 12 times greater probability of acquiring the disease.[23] Ten percent of patients with MS have a positive family history of MS. Identical twins of MS patients have a 20% to 25% chance of developing the disease, and fraternal twins have less than a 15% chance. The twin that is affected is more likely to have been exposed to tonsillectomies, infections, and animals.[24, 25]

Histocompatibility antigens (HLA) have been extensively studied because of their importance in organ transplantation. Several closely linked genes on chromosome 6 determine HLA types. The major human histocompatibility complex is called HLA, and several diseases are associated with particular HLA antigens. Among patients with MS, HLA-3 and HLA-7 have consistently been found to be increased in the range of 40% as compared with 25% in the normal population.[26] It is noteworthy that only 1 person in 100 infected with the virus of poliomyelitis develops a paralytic illness. It has been reported that there is an increase in HLA-3 and HLA-7 in patients with paralytic poliomyelitis.[27] In summary, there is much evidence, but no proof, that MS is caused by a slow virus in a genetically susceptible group of people.[28, 29]

Magnetic Resonance Imaging.—*Comparison With CT and Clinical Findings.*—MRI is much more sensitive than CT for the detection of MS plaques (Fig 13–1). In 65 patients with definite MS, MRI was positive in 55 (85%), CT in 16 (25%), cerebrospinal fluid (CSF) analysis in 48 (74%), and paraclinical tests (visual evoked response, auditory evoked response, somatosensory evoked response, and urodynamic assessment) in 51 (79%). There was no correlation of the paraclinical and MRI findings.[30]

In another study, 95% of 136 patients with MS had MS plaques demonstrated with MRI. CSF

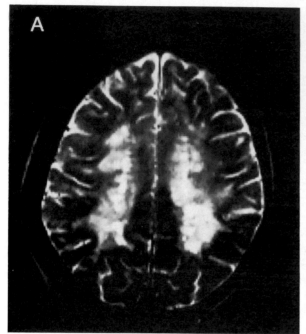
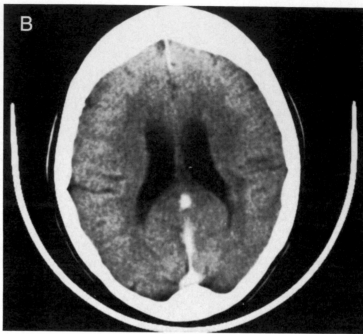

FIG 13–1.
Multiple sclerosis. **A,** extensive multiple confluent periventricular plaques on a T2-weighted MR image. **B,** normal CT with contrast in the same patient illustrating increased sensitivity of MRI compared with CT to detect MS plaques.

studies were positive in 90% and visual evoked potentials (VEP) were positive in 83%. Negative CSF and VEP occurred with positive MRI and negative MRI with positive CSF or VEP.[31]

"Magnetic Resonance (MR) imaging is the strongest single complementary test to help assure that the diagnosis of MS is assigned correctly. MR imaging also affords an easy, quantifiable means for continued evaluation of the patient's disease and appears to provide a similar means to follow the disease activity."[32]

Distribution of Lesions With Autopsy Correlation.—The lesions of MS are most frequently observed in the periventricular white matter but may occur anywhere in the white matter (Fig 13–2). Although 10% of MS lesions are found on pathologic examination in the gray matter,[33] these lesions are not visualized with MRI. With MRI, MS plaques are frequently found in the brain stem and cerebellum. With high-resolution MRI, MS plaques are visualized in the cervical cord (Figs 13–3, 13–4).

The distribution of MS lesions is highly variable. A case with extensive lesions in the spinal cord and optic nerves may show only a few small lesions in the cerebral hemispheres. In the brain, the lesions are roughly symmetric. Lesions are very commonly periventricular, in particular around the angles of the ventricles (frontal horns, atrium, posterior and temporal horns). These periventricular plaques may appear small in coronal sections, but they are often continuous from the tips of the occipital horns to the tips of the frontal and temporal horns.[34]

Myelin sheath stains show that lesions in the brain are frequently around the lateral and third ventricles. The lesions vary in size from that of a pinhole to almost an entire hemisphere. Plaques of varying size may be found in the optic nerves, chiasm, or tracts. The lesions are most numerous in the white matter of the cerebrum, brain stem, cerebellum, and spinal cord. Lesions involving the gray matter of the brain and roots of the spinal and cranial nerves are unusual.[1]

Plaques numbering 1,594 were found on autopsy examinations of the brains of 22 patients with MS. Seventy-four percent of the plaques were in the white matter, 17% were in the junction of the cortex and white matter, 5% in the gray matter of the cortex, and 4% in the central gray matter. Forty percent of the lesions occurred in the periventricular regions. Large plaques were almost always periventricular, the largest occurring around the posterior and anterior horns. The gray

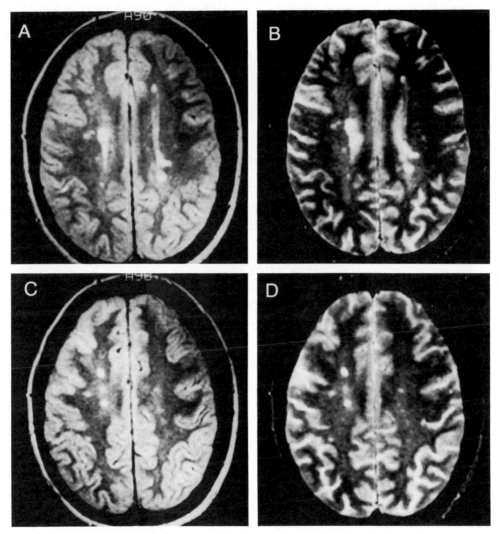

FIG 13–2.
Forty-two-year-old woman with MS. **A,** periventricular MS plaques are clearly visualized on spin-density–weighted MR image. **B,** the same lesions are visualized with T2-weighted image. **C,** more superior section in same patient demonstrates plaques in periventricular and subcortical white matter. **D,** the same lesions are visualized with T2-weighted image.

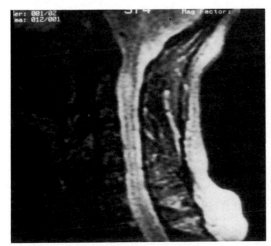

FIG 13–3.
Twenty-nine-year-old woman with MS plaque in the cervical spinal cord at the level of the C2 vertebral body. The lesion is increased in signal intensity on this T2-weighted MR image and on the spin-density–weighted image (not shown).

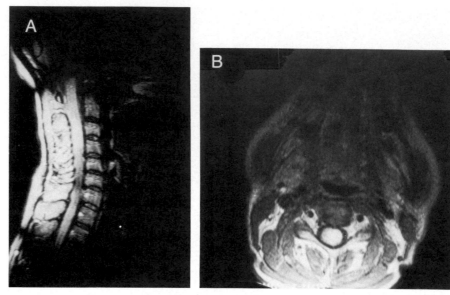

FIG 13–4.
MS plaque in the cervical spinal cord, upper level of the C3 and C4 vertebral bodies. This patient presented with recurrent spinal cord symptoms. Examination of the brain showed asymptomatic MS plaque. Plaque is seen on **(A)** sagittal, and **(B)** axial MR images.

matter cortical plaques were difficult to see microscopically. Almost all of the cortical plaques were found in only 2 of the 22 cases.[35]

Radiofrequency Pulse Sequences.—MS plaque are visualized as areas of increased signal on spin-density– and T2-weighted images. Most frequently, the T1-weighted image is normal in patients with MS.[36] Some of the lesions visualized on the spin-density– and T2-weighted images may be seen on the T1-weighted images as areas of decreased signal (Fig 13–5). Lesions are most fre-

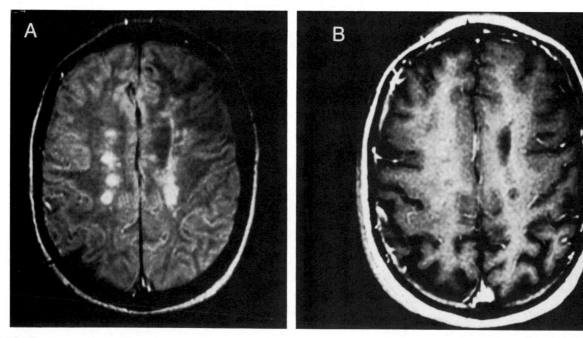

FIG 13–5.
Multiple sclerosis. **A,** spin-density–weighted image demonstrates classic periventricular MS lesions. **B,** most of the lesions detected on the T2-weighted image are not visualized on this T1-weighted MR image.

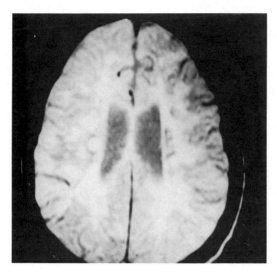

FIG 13–6.
Twenty-five-year-old man with clinically severe MS. There are confluent areas of increased MR signal in the periventricular white matter. Without knowledge of the patient's age and history, it would be difficult to determine if these findings represented an "aged brain" or postradiation changes.

quently observed on the T1-weighted image in patients with extensive lesions on the spin-density– and T2-weighted image (Fig 13–6).

Atrophy.—The incidence of atrophy in reported series ranges from 21% to 78%.[37, 38] The atrophy may be visualized as enlargement of the lateral ventricles, of the cortical sulci, of the basal cisterns, or of a combination of these. The atrophy

is found both in patients with plaques and in those without plaques. Shrinkage of white matter secondary to sclerosis and tissue loss secondary to demyelination contribute to the atrophy found in MS (Fig 13–7). The longer the duration of MS signs and symptoms, the more likely is atrophy to be found. Patients with atrophy are more severely affected by dementia and diffuse hyperreflexia.[37, 39]

Mass Effect.—Very rarely, an MS plaque will present with mass effect.[40–43] Most of the reported cases with mass effect have shown contrast enhancement. In the majority of these cases, the contrast enhancement has been around the periphery of the lesion, but in some cases the enhancement has occurred throughout the lesion. All of these lesions have been large in size. It has frequently been impossible to differentiate such lesions from primary and metastatic brain tumors on the original scan (Figs 13–8 through 13–11). Interval follow-up scans and clinical correlation may enable the correct diagnosis to be made in these cases, but several of these cases have been biopsied[40, 42] because they could not be differentiated from tumors. The results of the biopsies in these cases may be equivocal.

Specificity of Lesions.—Under 40 years of age, areas of increased signal in the periventricular and subcortical white matter on spin-density– and T2-weighted images are almost always associated with clinically significant disease. There are a large

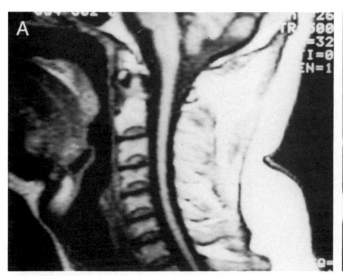
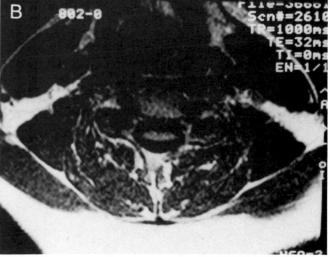

FIG 13–7.
Patient with history of severe MS showing atrophy of the spinal cord on **(A)** sagittal and **(B)** axial views.

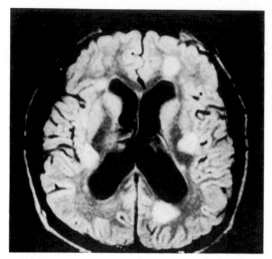

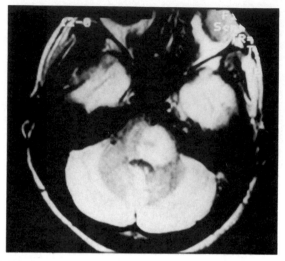

FIG 13–8.
Large periventricular and subcortical white matter MS plaques.

FIG 13–9.
MS plaque in the brain stem with mass effect. The lesion mimics a brain stem tumor. A single small supratentorial periventricular area of increased MR signal was the only imaging indication that this brain stem lesion was an MS plaque.

number of diseases which may have periventricular and subcortical areas of increased signal on T2-weighted images. Most of these diseases can be differentiated from MS on the basis of history and physical, or MRI findings. Sarcoidosis may have MRI and clinical findings which closely mimic MS.[44] When sarcoidosis presents with optic neuritis, it may be difficult to differentiate from MS.[45] Other diseases which may have periventricular and subcortical areas of increased signal are Sjögren's syndrome,[46] Binswanger's disease, moyamoya disease,[47] postradiation changes, acquired immunodeficiency syndrome (AIDS), and other brain infections.

With increasing age, areas of increased signal in the periventricular or subcortical white matter,

or both, are frequently observed. These lesions have been facetiously called "UBOs" or unidentified bright objects. They are virtually never observed below age 40, infrequently observed between the age of 40 and 50, and observed with increasing frequency and increasing severity over the age of 50 years. Predominantly in the basal ganglia, but also in other parts of the brain, some of these lesions may represent dilated Virchow-Robin spaces.[48] The lesions which do not represent dilated Virchow-Robin spaces probably represent areas of brain edema, ischemia, or infarction which may result in secondary degeneration, gliosis, or

FIG 13–10.
Large MS plaque in the left hemisphere. MS plaques may exhibit mass effect and be difficult to differentiate from tumors. A careful search should be made for additional lesions demonstrated with MRI.

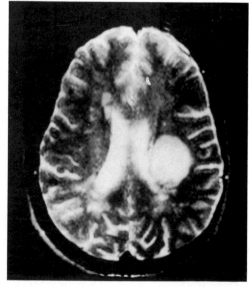

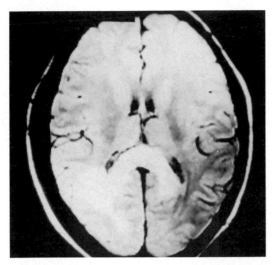

FIG 13–11.
MS plaque primarily involving the splenium of the corpus callosum and right parietal white matter. This lesion was interpreted as a lymphoma. Biopsy showed demyelination without tumor.

demyelination. The term "aged brain" has been used to describe these lesions in older persons.[49]

In patients over the age of 50 years, it can be difficult to differentiate MS plaques from the lesions seen with aging. With appropriate clinical findings, the more the lesions are periventricular in location, the more likely are the lesions to be MS plaques in those over the age of 50. It must be emphasized that virtually identical MR images represent "aged brain" in the elderly and "classic

findings of multiple sclerosis" in those under 50 years of age.

Fazekas et al.[50] have found that in those over 50 years of age, specificity for MS differentiated from "aged brain" is significantly improved if at least two of the following three criteria are found:

1. Lesions over 6 mm in diameter
2. Lesions abutting ventricular body
3. Infratentorial lesions

Increased Iron Deposition in Thalamus and Putamen.—The visualization of iron (ferritin) deposited within the basal ganglia of the brain with spin-echo technique is dependent upon the square of the magnetic field strength. The relaxation mechanism for the visualization of this iron is preferential T2 proton relaxation enhancement (PT2-PRE). The usual relaxation mechanism for MRI is dipole-dipole interaction. PT2-PRE can be visualized with low- and medium-field-strength magnets if gradient recall images are used.

Using a 1.5T magnet, Drayer et al.[51] found "relative decreased signal intensity most evident in the putamen and thalamus on T2 weighted images" in patients with MS (Fig 13–12). They postulated that decreased signal may be related to abnormally increased iron accumulation in those locales, with the underlying mechanism remaining speculative. They found that these areas of de-

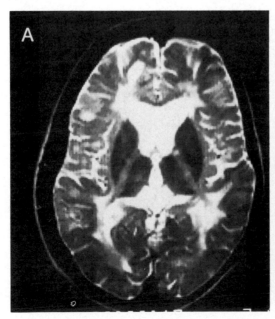
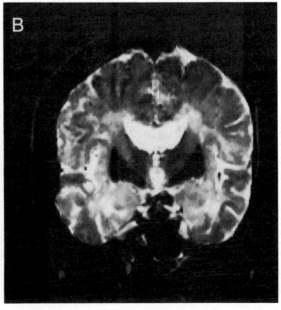

FIG 13–12.
Iron deposition. **A,** patient with severe multiple sclerosis shows increased iron deposition in the putamen and thalamus on axial T2-weighted MR image obtained with a 1.4T system. **B,** coronal T2-weighted image shows increased iron deposition in the putamen.

creased signal intensity correlated with the severity of lesions of MS but not with the patient's age or duration of disease.

Because of the normal variability of iron deposition in the brain, increased iron deposition in the basal ganglia is easily recognizable only in severe cases of MS.

Enhancement With Gadolinium DTPA.—MR using gadolinium DTPA is more sensitive than contrast-enhanced CT to diagnose active MS plaques with breakdown of the blood-brain barrier (BBB) (Figs 13–13, 13–14). In 13 of 14 cases, in which clinical activity had changed within 4 weeks of one study, there was enhancement of MS

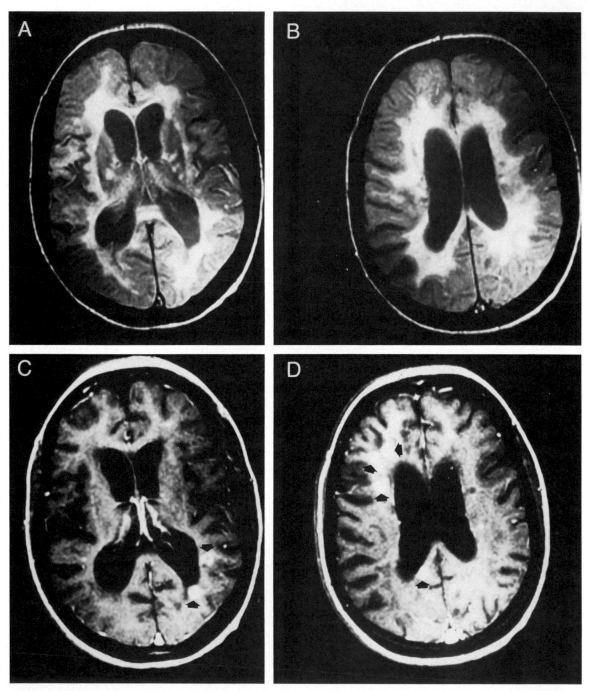

FIG 13–13.
Forty-three-year-old woman with clinically active multiple sclerosis. **A** and **B,** spin-density–weighted MR images show confluent areas of increased signal in the periventricular regions. **C** and **D,** T1- weighted images after the administration of gadolinium DTPA show focal areas of periventricular and subcortical enhancement *(arrows)* indicating active MS plaque.

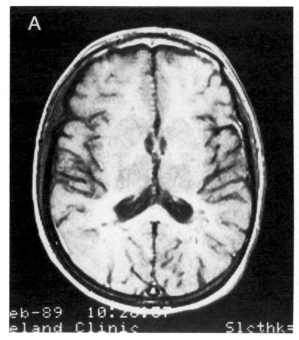

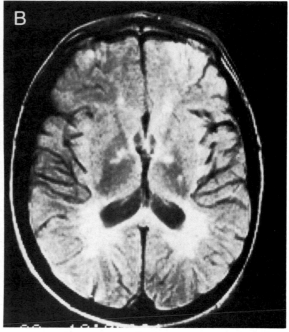

FIG 13–14.
Active MS. **A,** spin-density–weighted MR image shows confluent areas of increased signal without associated mass effect adjacent to the atria of the lateral ventricles. **B,** after the administration of gadolinium DTPA, there is enhancement of these confluent areas of increased signal in the periventricular region indicating break-down of the blood-brain barrier.

plaques.[52] Enhancement was found in 20 patients, only 14 of whom were considered to have clinically active lesions. MRI was more sensitive to detect activity of MS than was clinical examination. It was further concluded that this is not surprising since many lesions occur in clinically silent areas of the brain and that "some lesions may be so subtle that clinical signs and symptoms are virtually undetectable."

Grossman et al.[53] found that T1-weighted images obtained 3 minutes after the injection of gadolinium DTPA were better than 30-minute and 55-minute postinjection studies to detect enhancement. Five of 29 lesions identified on the 3-minute scan were no longer identified on the scans obtained 55 minutes after the injection of gadolinium.

Computed Tomography.—Patients with clinically evident MS may have a normal CT scan. The abnormalities found with CT scanning in MS patients are plaques of decreased attenuation that do not enhance with contrast material in older lesions; plaques of decreased or isodense attenuation coefficients that enhance with contrast material in the acute phase; atrophy, both periventricular and cortical[54]; and much more rarely, large areas of decreased attenuation coefficients that en-

hance after the administration of contrast material and usually have mass effect.[41–43] Hemorrhagic complications of MS have also been rarely reported.[55]

Sensitivity of CT.—Two cadaver brains from patients with MS were studied using a high-resolution CT scanner.[56] Plaques smaller than 0.6 cm were not detected with CT. Some larger plaques were misinterpreted as normal structures. In the first brain, 31 demyelinated plaques were found by pathologic examination. Five of these plaques, all larger than 1 cm, were detected with CT. Six additional lesions 1.6 to 3.2 cm in greatest diameter, located immediately adjacent to the lateral ventricles, were detected only after the anatomic specimens and CT images were compared. The remaining 20 lesions, ranging from 0.6 to 1.2 cm in diameter, were not detected prospectively or retrospectively. All lesions in this brain were periventricular.

Thirty-nine demyelinated plaques were found in the second brain. Only three of these plaques, 0.6 to 1.4 cm in greatest diameter, were detected with CT. The other 36 lesions, all less than 1 cm in diameter, were missed with CT both prospectively and retrospectively.

Although contrast enhancement may have

aided in the detection of additional lesions, most of the small plaques undetected without contrast material would probably not have been detected after contrast enhancement. The incidence of low-attenuation areas visualized with CT has a very high correlation with autopsy series.

Plaques With Decreased Attenuation Coefficients.

—Most of the plaques visualized with CT are periventricular, frequently near the anterior and posterior horns, but the plaques are visualized in all parts of the white matter. Plaques of decreased attenuation coefficient have not been observed in the cortical gray matter. This correlates with the autopsy material, which showed that cortical plaques were difficult to see microscopically. Most of the plaques seen with CT are 2 cm or less in size, although the low-attenuation coefficient areas in reported series vary in diameter from 0.3 to 7.2 cm.[37, 39]

The number of visualized plaques varies from one to eight per patient. The number of MS patients with visualization of plaques also varies in reported series from 18%[57] to 47%[58] of cases. In approximately 25% of the overall reported series, the plaques can be visualized using the CT image only (without an analysis of the CT number printout). The plaques have attenuation coefficients that vary from 10 to 27 Hounsfield units (HU), with normal white matter having an average attenuation coefficient of 30 HU.

Plaques visualized as areas of decreased attenuation coefficient in patients with an exacerbation of active disease may increase in size and number, may become isodense with the surrounding brain, or may remain stable (Figs 13–15 through 13–17).[55]

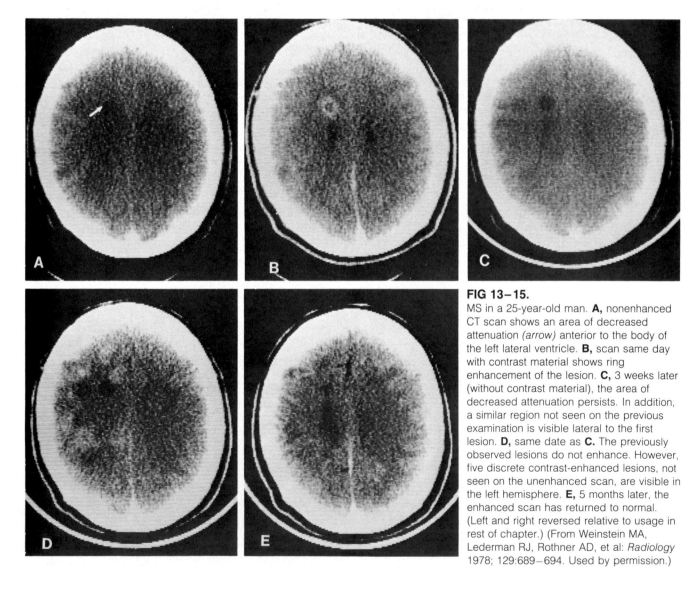

FIG 13–15.

MS in a 25-year-old man. **A,** nonenhanced CT scan shows an area of decreased attenuation *(arrow)* anterior to the body of the left lateral ventricle. **B,** scan same day with contrast material shows ring enhancement of the lesion. **C,** 3 weeks later (without contrast material), the area of decreased attenuation persists. In addition, a similar region not seen on the previous examination is visible lateral to the first lesion. **D,** same date as **C.** The previously observed lesions do not enhance. However, five discrete contrast-enhanced lesions, not seen on the unenhanced scan, are visible in the left hemisphere. **E,** 5 months later, the enhanced scan has returned to normal. (Left and right reversed relative to usage in rest of chapter.) (From Weinstein MA, Lederman RJ, Rothner AD, et al: *Radiology* 1978; 129:689–694. Used by permission.)

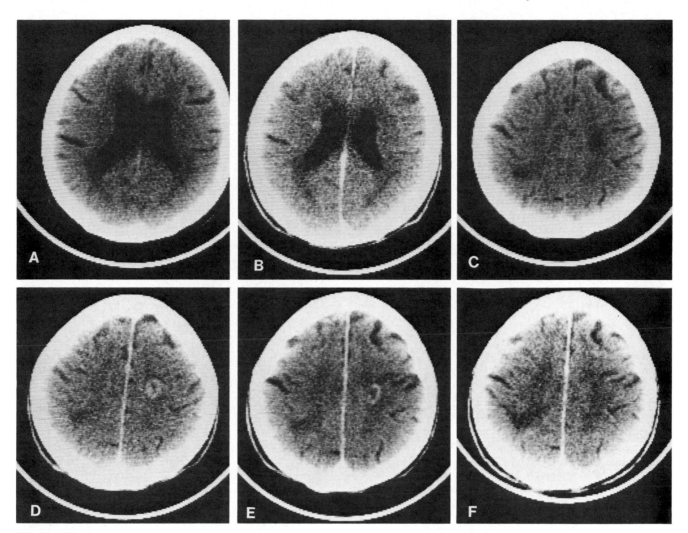

FIG 13–16.
MS in a 59-year-old man. Scans **A** through **E** were obtained on the same date. **A,** CT without contrast material. This scan and the scan taken at this level 7 months previously show mild dilatation of the sulci and ventricles. No lesions are seen. **B,** CT with contrast material. A periventricular lesion is shown on the left. On other sections, three other enhanced periventricular lesions were present, but were not seen on the unenhanced scans. CT scans with and without enhancement 8 days later showed no change. **C,** CT without contrast material. There is an area of decreased attenuation in each hemisphere. **D,** CT with contrast material. The lesion in the left hemisphere remains decreased in attenuation, while the one on the right exhibits ring enhancement. **E,** CT with contrast material. There is less enhancement of the ring lesion, but the left lesion is unchanged. **F,** 3 months later (with contrast material), the left lesion remains unchanged. The right lesion can no longer be seen, either without or with contrast material. (Left and right reversed relative to usage in rest of chapter.) (From Weinstein MA, Lederman RJ, Rothner AD, et al: *Radiology* 1978; 129:689–694. Used by permission.)

Although the CT visualization of MS plaques has been reported in the spinal cord,[59] brain stem, and optic nerves,[58] it is highly probable that some, if not most or all, of the reported lesions are artifacts and not true lesions. Many of these abnormalities were reported on early-generation CT scanners, which produced a large number of artifactual densities.

Because MS plaques are small, more plaques should be detected in thin sections of the brain (approximately 4 or 5 mm) by minimizing overlap of plaque and normal brain tissue (partial volume effect). Because some plaques have almost the same attenuation coefficient as normal brain tissue, scanners with greater contrast resolution detect more of these plaques than earlier-generation scanners.

Plaques With Contrast Enhancement.—In one report, 14 of 57 patients with moderate or severe signs and symptoms of an acute exacerbation of MS demonstrated a total of 48 well-delineated

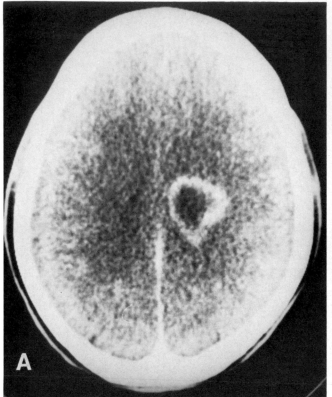

FIG 13–17.
Multiple sclerosis. **A,** CT with contrast material. Scan obtained during acute clinical exacerbation of MS shows an enhancing ring lesion in the parietal lobe. **B,** CT 6 weeks later (with contrast material). The previously visualized lesion is no longer enhanced, although a smaller area of decreased attenuation coefficient is again seen. (Courtesy of Lawrence H.A. Gold, M.D., University of Minnesota, Minneapolis.)

plaques on CT.[55] Twenty-two lesions were periventricular, and the remainder were elsewhere in the white matter. When they were first seen, 17 were decreased in attenuation coefficient both without and with contrast material, 16 were decreased in attenuation coefficient without contrast material and enhanced with it, and 15 could not be identified without contrast material and were seen well after enhancement (see Figs 13–15 and 13–16). Of the nine MS plaques that were not seen on the original nonenhanced CT scan but were seen on a follow-up scan, eight showed contrast enhancement.

Over time, lesions that initially exhibited decreased attenuation coefficients without contrast material but showed contrast enhancement subsequently became decreased in attenuation coefficient both with and without contrast material. None of the lesions that failed to demonstrate contrast enhancement initially enhanced on follow-up scans. The lesions that did enhance initially showed decreased attenuation coefficients on both the preinfusion and postinfusion follow-up examinations. Some remained decreased in attenuation coefficient, and some became normal, both with and without contrast material. These data demonstrate that only acute MS lesions enhance with contrast material. It is likely that the enhancement usually clears after a period of weeks, but the enhancement may last or even increase over a period of several months, suggesting continuing active demyelination of the lesion (see Fig 14–17).[41, 60]

Contrast enhancement in MS plaques represents a breakdown in the BBB, which results in extravasation of contrast material.[61] Many substances that would readily enter other tissue and organs of the body are only selectively permeable to the vascular endothelium in the CNS. In general, the molecular size and polarity are inversely proportional to vascular permeability in the CNS. Liquids are highly permeable. Water, even though it is a dipolar substance, is highly permeable and follows the osmotic gradient. There are specific active transport mechanisms for certain sugars, biogenic amines, amino acids, and ions. Outside the CNS, endothelial cells contain fenestrations and pinocytotic vesicles. The CNS endothelium does not contain these structures, but consists of continuous belts of tight junctions. The capillaries are completely enclosed by astrocytic perivascular foot processes, which are unique to the CNS. All of these features constitute the BBB.[62] Compromise of the BBB increases vascular permeability to the extravasation of plasma constituents into the extracellular space. The edema in MS is vasogenic, predominantly white matter edema. This is in distinction to cytotoxic edema, where the BBB is intact and the edema due to influx of a plasma ultrafiltrate causing generalized intracellular overhydration; to ischemic edema, which affects both the white and gray matter and is secondary to infarction of the blood vessels; and to interstitial edema, which is secondary to hydrocephalus.

Experience with radionuclide brain scans in MS is confirmatory that the enhancement of MS plaques is due to breakdown of the BBB. In one reported series, 5 of 28 patients with a clinical diagnosis of MS had abnormal radionuclide images.[63] None of the 14 patients with inactive disease had an abnormal brain scan. In another series, 3 of 160 patients (1.8%) had abnormal radionuclide images representing a breakdown of the BBB.[64] The radionuclide image will be abnormal only during the period when the CT scan shows contrast enhancement. Because smaller lesions can be better resolved with CT than with radionuclide imaging, and because plaques can be shown by CT but not by the radionuclide image when the BBB is intact, more MS plaques are shown by CT than by radionuclide imaging.

Additional evidence that the enhancement of MS plaques is due to the breakdown of the BBB is found in multiple reports that corticosteroids that reestablish the BBB in vasogenic edema have been reported to suppress contrast enhancement of MS lesions.[62] Histologic and pathologic material, both in MS and in experimental allergic encephalomyelitis, also confirm the breakdown of the BBB in MS.

Atrophy.—See previous discussion of Atrophy under Magnetic Resonance Imaging.

Mass Effect.—See previous discussion of Mass Effect under Magnetic Resonance Imaging and also Figure 13–18.

High Volume of Contrast Medium and Delayed Scanning.—In most CT examinations, 37 to 40 g of iodine are used for contrast enhancement (100 mg of 76% methylglucamine diatrizoate equals 37 g iodine). Studies have shown that if this dosage is doubled (74 to 82 g iodine) and/or delayed scans (1 hour after contrast injection) are obtained, lesions may be seen that are not visualized on the regular contrast-enhanced scan: more metastases are visualized, areas of equivocal enhancement are more definitively defined, lesions are more distinct, the shape and size of the lesions are better seen, and macrocystic lesions can be differentiated from microcystic ones.[65-67]

Reports have shown that more MS plaques can be visualized with high doses and/or delayed scans.[68-70] Seventy consecutive patients with known MS or with signs or symptoms highly suspicious of acute or relapsing MS were studied in the largest of these reports.[70] The patients were examined before contrast medium infusion, immediately after 40 g of iodine, and 1 hour after an additional rapid drip of 42 g of iodine. The patients were divided into three groups: group 1, definite MS; group 2, suspected MS; group 3, MS eventually excluded. In the 39 cases in group 1, the conventional enhanced scan was positive in 25 cases and the high-volume delayed scan in 32 cases. The high-volume delayed scan added the following information in 23 of these 32 cases: (1) better visualization of equivocal areas in 17 cases, (2) enhancement of low-attenuation coefficient plaques not enhanced on the standard CT in 13 cases, (3) enhancement of isodense plaques not enhanced on the standard CT in 9 cases, and (4) visualization of low-attenuation plaques not seen on the standard CT in 4 cases. In 21 of the suspected MS cases, the conventional CT scan was positive in 2 cases and the high-volume delayed scan in 5 cases. Using a combination of high volumes of contrast media and 1-hour delayed scans, this study demonstrated previously unreported enhancing plaques in the cortical gray matter and in the gray-white matter junction areas.

CT: Clinical Correlation.—Patients with definite MS may have normal CT scans. Plaques may not be visualized because they are small, because they are isodense with the brain, because corticosteroids may mask the lesions, or because the lesions may be located in the brain stem, optic nerves, and spinal cord where they cannot be visualized because of CT artifacts from the surrounding bone.

Multiple reports have shown that in patients with abnormal CT scans, the location and activity of the clinically determined lesions may not corre-

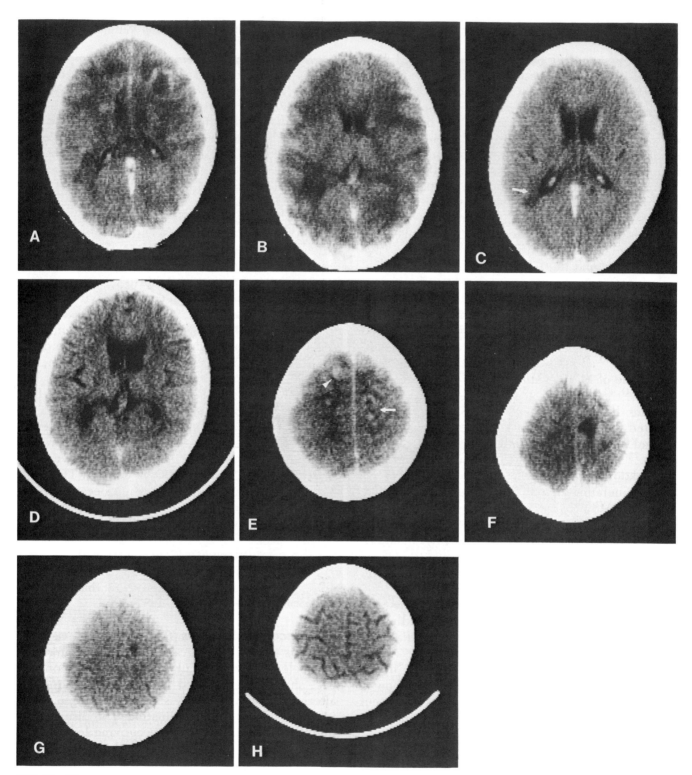

FIG 13–19.

Diffuse sclerosis in a 14-year-old girl. **A,** CT with contrast material. Diffuse, patchy areas of decreased attenuation can be seen in the white matter, together with focal areas of enhancement. **B,** CT 6 days later (with contrast material), the areas of decreased attenuation persist. There is no enhancement of the lesions. **C,** CT 2 months later (with contrast material), there is a residual area of decreased attenuation (arrow) lateral to the atrium of the left lateral ventricle. **D,** 6 months later (with contrast material), the scan has returned to normal. **E,** scan obtained at same time as **A** (with contrast material). There is a lesion (arrow) in the right parietal lobe. Without contrast material, it exhibited decreased attenuation. A second enhanced lesion (arrowhead) can be seen in the anterior part of the section on the left. **F,** scan obtained at the same time as **B** (with contrast material). The lesion on the right is no longer enhanced by contrast material. The lesion on the left cannot be seen. **G,** scan obtained at the same time as **C.** The lesion persists, but has decreased in size. **H,** scan obtained at the same time as **D.** The lesion can no longer be seen. The sulci have increased in size. (Left and right reversed relative to usage in rest of chapter.) (From Weinstein MA, Lederman RJ, Rothner AD, et al: *Radiology* 1978; 129:689–694. Used by permission.)

sclerosis is that of MS, but with large plaques in the subcortical white matter.

Acquired, Allergic, and Infectious Diseases Resulting in Myelin Breakdown

Postvaccinal Encephalomyelitis

The recommended schedule for childhood immunization is diphtheria, pertussis, tetanus, and trivalent polio vaccine at age 2, 4, 6, and 15 months, respectively, with measles, mumps, and rubella immunization at 15 months, and an additional diphtheria, pertussis, and tetanus immunization (DPT) at 48 months. Pertussis and possibly influenza, which are prepared from whole killed organisms, may cause allergic reactions producing encephalopathy (Figs 13–20 and 13–21). These reactions, occurring in less than 1 in 100,000 vaccine recipients, are characterized by demyelination occurring within 4 days of immunization. Recovery is usually complete. Guillain-Barré syndrome appears to have followed influenza immunization only after the 1976 swine flu immunizations.

Measles, mumps, rubella, and trivalent oral poliovirus vaccines, which are prepared from live attenuated viruses, can cause symptomatic viral

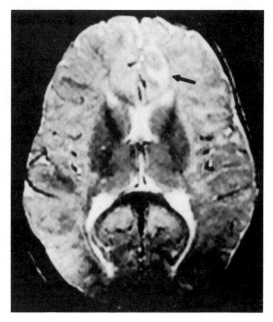

FIG 13–21.
Postvaccination encephalomyelitis. After diphtheria-pertussis-tetanus vaccination, patient shows area of increased signal of T2-weighted MR images in the subcortical white matter of the medial aspect of the left frontal lobe *(arrow)*.

infections of the nervous system. Measles encephalitis occurs in 1 in 1 million vaccine recipients; rubella neuritis occurs in less than 1 in 10,000 recipients; and paralytic poliomyelitis occurs in 1 in 3 million vaccine recipients or close contacts of recipients.[77]

Until recently, rabies vaccine consisted of killed rabies virus produced in rabbit brain tissue. One in 750 patients receiving this vaccine developed encephalomyelitis, which was fatal 20% of the time. A duck embryo vaccine now used for rabies does not contain nerve tissue and causes fewer and less severe reactions.[78] After rabies, the most common postvaccinal encephalomyelitis had occurred after smallpox vaccination. The disease occurred in 1 in 4,000 vaccinations and about 20 times more frequently after primary vaccination than after revaccination.[78] Now that smallpox vaccinations have been eliminated, this common cause of postvaccinal encephalitis is no longer seen.

Postinfectious Encephalomyelitis (Disseminated Encephalomyelitis)

Most cases of disseminated encephalomyelitis begin 1 to 3 weeks after a viral illness or vaccination. One third of all encephalitides reported in the United States are believed to be disseminated

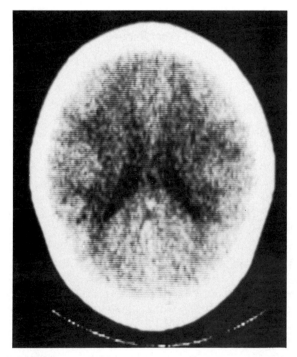

FIG 13–20.
Postvaccination encephalomyelitis. Decreased attenuation of the white matter is seen bilaterally on this axial CT scan in a child who had recent diphtheria-pertussis-tetanus vaccination. The white matter edema resolved after several weeks.

encephalomyelitis. Immune-mediated encephalomyelitis (IME), acute disseminated encephalomyelitis, postinfectious demyelination, postinfectious multifocal leukoencephalopathy, and post- or parainfectious encephalomyelitis probably refer to the same disease. Acute hemorrhagic leukoencephalitis may be a more severe form of disseminated encephalomyelitis.[79, 80]

Neurologic complications used to occur most frequently after measles. One in 800 to 1 in 1,000 measles patients developed encephalomyelitis with a 10% to 20% mortality rate and an equal rate of permanent neurologic damage.[78] With the widespread use of measles vaccine, measles encephalitis is becoming rarer. Influenza virus, Epstein-Barr virus, and the viruses of the childhood exanthems such as chickenpox and rubella (German measles) have been associated with this disease but in many cases no specific cause can be identified. The latent period differentiates this disease from viral encephalitis; there is no direct viral infection of the brain. Most patients with disseminated encephalomyelitis respond to corticosteroid therapy and do not have residual neurologic deficits.

The CT[81, 82] and MRI findings in disseminated encephalomyelitis are multiple bilateral poorly marginated lesions in the cerebral white matter. Lesions may be present in the basal ganglia.[79] There is no decrease in the volume of the cerebral white matter and there is sparing of the subarcuate white matter[80] (Fig 13–22). MRI is more sensitive

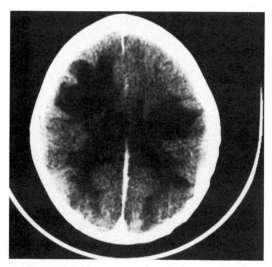

FIG 13–22.
CT examination of a 5-year-old child with acute disseminated encephalomyelitis. The scan shows multiple areas of decreased attenuation coefficient within the subcortical white matter without associated mass effect and without evidence of hemorrhage. (Courtesy of Richard E. Latchaw, M.D., University of Pittsburgh.)

than CT for the detection of lesions. With corticosteroid therapy, disseminated encephalomyelitis is frequently self-limited and usually resolves in 2 to 4 weeks with the MRI examination showing minimal or no residual abnormalities.[79]

Acute hemorrhagic leukoencephalitis is the most rapidly progressive demyelinating disease. It mainly affects young adults, but may also involve children. The patient may present with headache, fever, stiff neck, hemiplegia, confusion, aphasia, and seizures. Invariably, peripheral leukocytosis is present, with counts ranging from 20,000 to 40,000 cells per cubic millimeter. The CSF is often under increased pressure, with polymorphonuclear pleocytosis up to 3,000/mm^3. Most patients used to die within 2 to 4 days, but some patients recovered with almost no residual symptoms. CT scanning shows diffuse low density of the white matter (Fig 13–23), while T2-weighted MRI shows diffuse white matter hyperintensity.

Postinfectious Polyneuritis (Landry-Guillain-Barré Syndrome)

This is a distinctive neuropathy characterized by inflammatory lesions scattered throughout the peripheral nervous system. The lesions consist of circumscribed areas in which myelin is lost, combined with an infiltrate of lymphocytes and macrophages.[83] Because this disease is predominantly one of the peripheral nervous system, it will not be discussed further in this chapter.

Viral-Induced Myelinoclastic Diseases

Subacute Sclerosing Panencephalitis

Subacute sclerosing panencephalitis is a slow-virus measles infection of the brain with an incidence of 1 in 1 million in the United States. Acute measles encephalitis, which is a different, much more benign disease, occurs in approximately 1 in 800 to 1 in 1,000 measles patients. While SSPE is progressive and fatal, spontaneous remissions occur that may last for several years. One half of the patients have clinical measles after the age of 2 years. The latent period after the measles infection is approximately 6 years,[84] with most cases presenting between 5 and 15 years of age. One study demonstrated that SSPE patients lack antibodies to one of the viral proteins (M protein) despite high antibody titers to other viral proteins.[85]

The disease has been divided into four stages.[86] Stage 1 patients have decreased mental proficiency and behavior abnormalities. In stage 2, there is

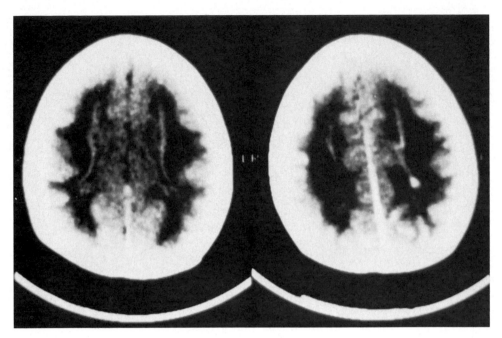

FIG 13–23.
Acute hemorrhagic leukoencephalopathy. The unenhanced CT shows decreased attenuation of the white matter. Differentiation from other leukodystrophies cannot be made on the basis of CT alone.

progressive intellectual deterioration, myoclonic seizures, ataxia, and choreiform movements. One half of the patients have ocular signs, including cortical blindness, optic atrophy, and chorioretinitis. Coma, opisthotonos, and decerebrate rigidity occur in stage 3. Stage 4 patients have loss of cortical function. The disease is diagnosed by elevated titers of measles antibody in both the serum and CSF and by electroencephalogram (EEG) with characteristic synchronous periodic high-voltage complexes.

The cerebral cortex and white matter of both hemispheres and the brain stem are involved in SSPE. The cerebellum is usually spared. Patients with rapidly progressive clinical courses and in whom the pathologic changes are primarily cortical have normal or minimally abnormal CT scans. In patients with a chronic course, the CT shows diffuse and extensive atrophy, decreased attenuation in the white matter, and areas of decreased attenuation in the caudate nucleus or other basal ganglia (Fig 13–24). There is no contrast enhancement of the lesions.[87, 88]

MRI is more sensitive than CT for demonstrating lesions in the white matter, basal ganglia, and cerebellum[89] (Fig 13–25).

Subacute Rubella Syndrome
Usually, the defects associated with congenital German measles are nonprogressive after the second or third year of life, although progression may occur after stable periods of 8 to 19 years. It appears that the German measles virus acquired in utero persists in the nervous system of these latter patients and may become active again, resembling SSPE.

The CT examination shows decreased attenuation coefficients of the white matter, which are believed to represent retardation of myelination (Fig 13–26). Calcifications may occur in the basal ganglia and centrum semiovale.[90]

Progressive Multifocal Leukoencephalopathy
See Chapter 12.

Degenerative-Toxic Myelinoclastic Diseases

Central Pontine Myelinolysis
This is a disease characterized by areas of demyelination of the pons, which may be only a few millimeters in diameter or may occupy the entire pons. There is always a rim of intact myelin between the lesions and the surface of the pons. In extensive cases, the lesion may extend posteriorly into the medial lemnisci and rarely into the midbrain. Large lesions may be associated with demyelinating disease of the thalamus, internal capsule, lateral geniculate bodies, and cerebral cortex.[91]

The disease was originally considered to be secondary to chronic alcoholism, but subsequently

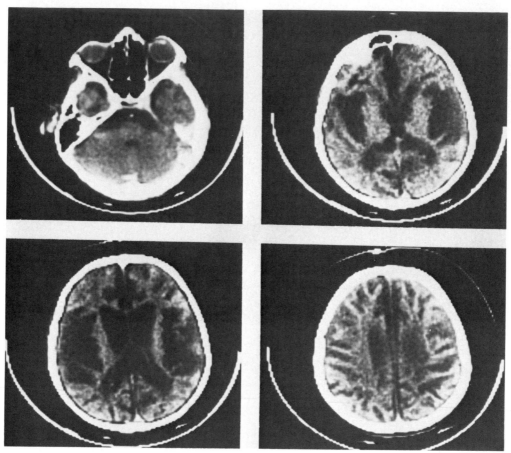

FIG 13–24.
Subacute sclerosing panencephalitis in a 14-year-old boy. Note extensive atrophy affecting both white and gray matter of cerebral hemispheres, especially of the temporal lobes. Pontine atrophy is visualized. (From Duda EE, Huttenlocher PR, Patronas NJ, et al: *AJNR* 1980; 1:35–36. Used by permission.)

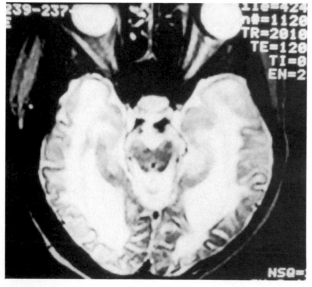

FIG 13–25.
MRI examination in patient with subacute sclerosing panencephalitis shows confluent areas of increased signal in the subcortical white matter without associated mass effect.

has been found in children and other patients without a history of alcohol abuse. The disease is now thought to be associated with a rapid rise in the serum sodium (greater than 20 mEq/L in 1 to 3 days) in previously hyponatremic patients.[92] Almost always associated with some other severe, frequently life-threatening disease, CPM is difficult to diagnose during life, because the patients frequently are comatose from metabolic or other causes. The clinical syndrome of CPM is a sudden disturbance in mental status and flaccid quadriparesis occasionally associated with abnormal conjugate eye movements and pseudobulbar palsy.[91]

The CT in CPM shows a variable-sized area of decreased attenuation in the pons, which may have slight contrast enhancement at the periphery (Fig 13–27).[93, 94]

CPM is clearly visualized with MRI as areas of decreased signal intensity within the pons on T1-weighted images, frequently triangular in shape with sparing of the descending corticospinal

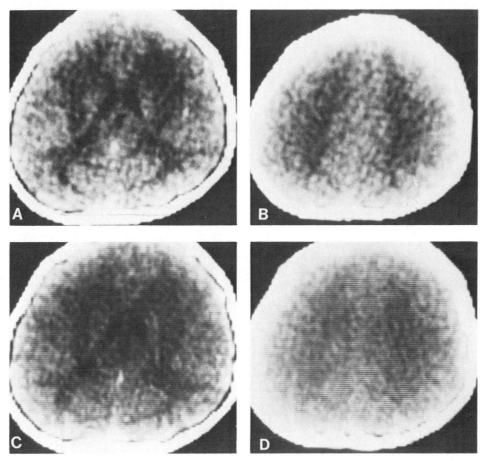

FIG 13–26.
Congenital rubella syndrome in a young female. **A** and **B,** CT scan at 19 months of age. **C** and **D,** CT scan at 3 years, 7 months of age. There is decreased attenuation of white matter in the earlier scan, somewhat improved in the later examination. (From Ishikawa A, Murayama T, Sakuma N, et al: *Arch Neurol* 1982, 39:420–421. Used by permission.)

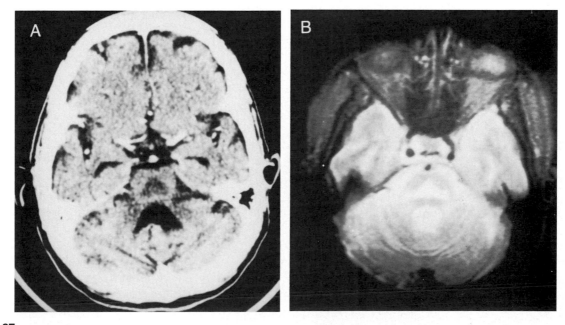

FIG 13–27.
Central pontine myelinolysis. **A,** CT examination shows triangular area of decreased attenuation coefficient within the pons. **B,** T2-weighted axial MRI examination shows similar area of increased signal intensity within the pons. (Courtesy of Drs. Hans Newton and David Norman, University of California, San Francisco.)

tracts.[95] There is increased signal intensity on spin-density– and T2-weighted images within the pons, extending into the thalami (Figs 13–27 and 13–28).[95] Lesions which mimic CPM with MR examination have been described in "aged brain," normal-pressure hydrocephalus, brain stem infarct, and brain stem encephalitis.[96]

Marchiafava-Bignami Disease

This is a disease of necrosis of the corpus callosum in patients who usually have a long history of drinking red wines, but probably also occurs from ingesting other forms of alcohol. The disease has been reported in nonalcoholics and may represent a nutritional deficiency. The patients have clinical signs of acute and subacute severe intellectual impairment, with callosal disconnection on psychometric testing. They may undergo spontaneous improvement to a more chronic stage.[91, 97]

During the acute stage, there is on CT decreased attenuation of the corpus callosum (Fig 13–29). During the subacute stage, there may be

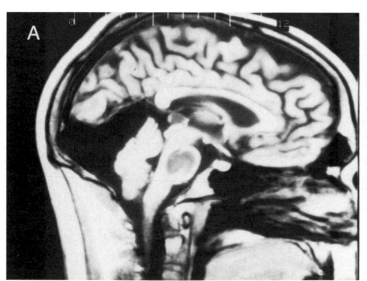

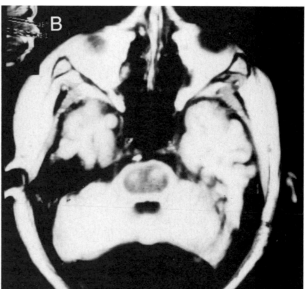

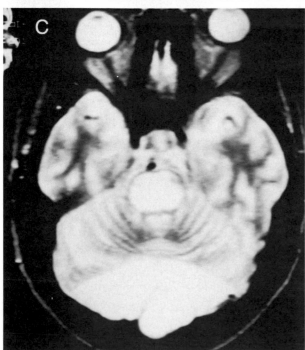

FIG 13–28.
Central pontine myelinolysis. **A,** T1-weighted sagittal MR image shows extensive area of decreased signal intensity within the pons. **B,** axial T1-weighted image shows decreased signal within the pons. **C,** T2-weighted axial image shows extensive area of increased signal within the pons. (Courtesy of Alison Smith, M.D., Metropolitan General Hospital, Cleveland)

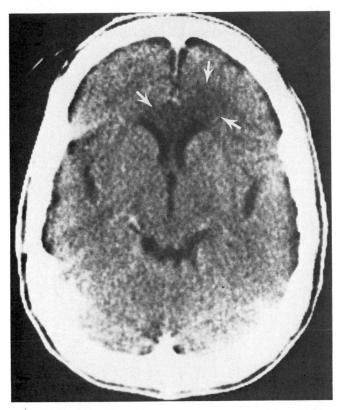

FIG 13–29.
Marchiafava-Bignami disease. Areas of decreased CT attenuation *(arrows)* are in the corpus callosum. (Courtesy of John C. Morris, M.D., Washington University, St. Louis)

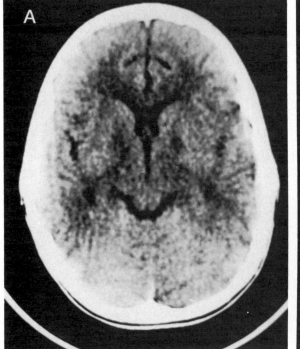
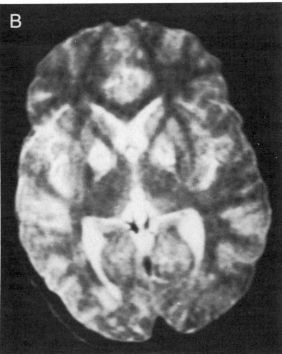

FIG 13–30.
Carbon monoxide poisoning. **A,** unenhanced axial CT scan. Areas of decreased attenuation are seen bilaterally within the globus pallidus. **B,** T2-weighted axial MR scan. Increased signal intensity is present in the same locations as the CT scan demonstrating the damage to the basal ganglia from anoxia.

contrast enhancement in the corpus callosum. In the chronic stage, there is atrophy of the corpus callosum and cortical atrophy, predominantly frontal.[97]

Carbon Monoxide Encephalopathy

Carbon monoxide encephalopathy usually effects the basal ganglia. The areas most affected are the globus pallidus and putamen, which on CT are shown as areas of decreased attenuation (Fig 13–30,A). MR scanning shows these areas to have decreased signal intensity on the T1-weighted image and increased signal intensity on the T2-weighted image (Fig 13–30,B). Similar findings are present throughout the white matter. These areas of signal abnormality probably represent hypoxic regions with secondary gliosis.

Hypoxic and Ischemic Encephalopathy

The classic pathologic changes of hypoxic encephalopathy in the adult are in the cortical and subcortical neurons, with relative sparing of the white matter. However, in both acute and chronic hypoxic encephalopathy, the white matter may show demyelination.[98] The most common CT findings of adult posthypoxic encephalopathy are enlarged sulci from cortical atrophy. In some patients, there is decreased attenuation of part or all of the cerebral hemispheric white matter.[98]

Hypoxic or ischemic encephalopathy in neonates is different from that seen in adults. In the neonate, periventricular leukomalacia, as described by Virchow in 1867, is seen. In a full-term infant the watershed regions are between the central and peripheral vascular territories in the periventricular area. An episode(s) of low blood pressure results in hypoxia or ischemia in these periventricular regions, possibly leading to infarction. Hemorrhage may occur secondarily.[99, 100]

In the full-term infant the white matter has a greater water content than is present in the premature infant. Hence, there is relatively good correlation between the decreased attentuation seen on CT scan and the pathologic changes following hypoxia and ischemia (Fig 13–31). The marked decrease in the attenuation of both gray and white matter in these patients suggests severe edema (Fig 13–32). The CT scan allows relatively good

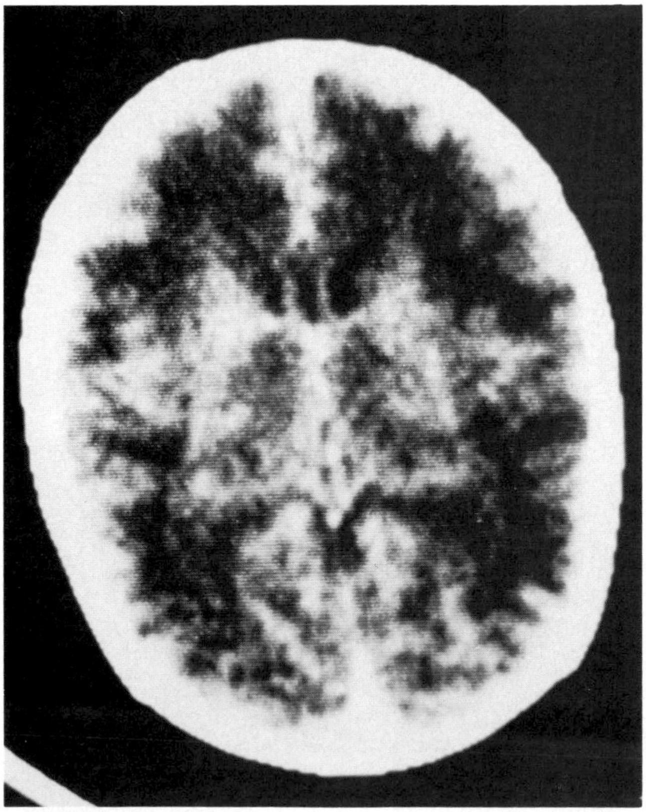

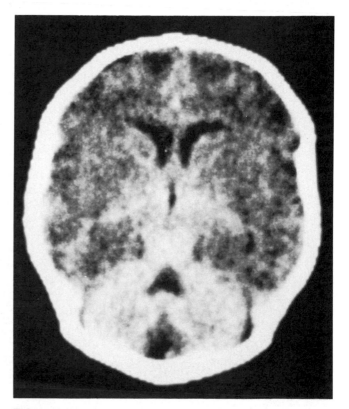

FIG 13–31.
Severe anoxia. Multiple areas of decreased attenuation on this unenhanced CT scan are seen in the gray and white matter as well as the basal ganglia from severe hypoxic-ischemic insult.

FIG 13–32.
Severe brain edema from anoxia. There is global supratentorial decreased attenuation, sparing the basal ganglia. Note the low density as compared with the infratentorial region which has normal density.

predictability of the degree of brain damage of these full-term infants.[101]

However, the premature infant's brain has a relatively high water content, producing a relatively low attenuation on the normal premature infant's CT scan. Hence, the correlation between the CT scan attenuation coefficients and the degree of brain damage is relatively poor.[101] In these premature infants, ultrasound has proved to be the method of choice for the diagnosis of periventricular leukomalacia (PVL). These areas of PVL are shown to be echogenic on the initial ultrasound scan (Fig 13–33,A). A few days after the insult, however, the areas of PVL become cystic on ultrasonography (Fig 13–33,B). It is only at this stage that high-resolution CT scanning demonstrates the typical findings (Fig 13–33,C).

Myelinoclastic Diseases of Vascular Etiology

Binswanger's Disease

Binswanger's disease, or subcortical arteriosclerotic encephalopathy, is a slowly progressive disorder caused by cerebral arteriosclerosis, in which the small arteries and arterioles of the white matter and basal ganglia are predominantly affected. The disease is characterized clinically by hypertension, dementia, spasticity, syncope, and seizures. Pathologically, there is diffuse demyelination or foci of necrosis.

Many elderly patients demonstrate confluent areas of abnormal signal in the periventricular regions. Recent reports state that subcortical arteriosclerotic encephalopathy may be more common than was previously realized.[102, 103] There is con-

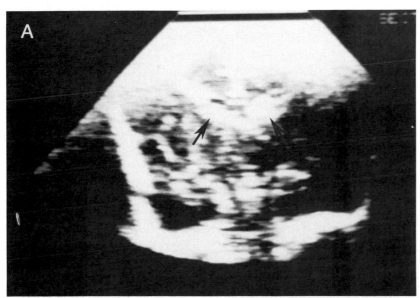
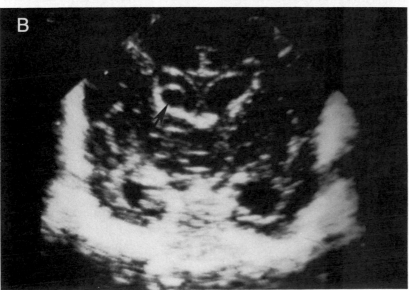
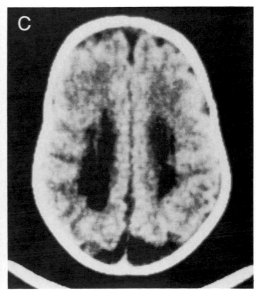

FIG 13–33.
Periventricular leukomalacia. **A,** coronal ultrasound of early periventricular leukomalacia. The hypoxic-ischemia areas are shown as increased echogenicity *(arrows)* in the regions of the heads of the caudate bilaterally. **B,** follow-up coronal ultrasound shows the damaged areas as cystic areas of decreased echogenicity *(arrow).* **C,** axial CT—late finding of periventricular cysts which show up much better than the ultrasound finding.

troversy as to the prevalence of subcortical arteriosclerotic encephalopathy. The CT examination shows areas of decreased attenuation in the white matter without enhancement.[104, 105] On MR examination there is decreased signal in the periventricular regions on T1-weighted images, and increased signal on T2-weighted images (Fig 13–34).

Maladie de Schilder-Foix

This disease is characterized by nonprogressive demyelinating lesions of the white matter secondary to vascular disease.

Posttherapy Myelinoclastic Diseases

Methotrexate Leukoencephalopathy
See Chapter 21.

Disseminated Necrotizing Leukodystrophy
See Chapter 21.

DYSMYELINATING DISEASES

These are diseases in which an enzymatic disturbance interferes either with the formation of myelin or with its maintenance. The specific metabolic abnormalities remain unknown for some of these diseases.

Leukodystrophies

The leukodystrophies (Gr. *leuko-*, white + L. *dystrophia*, defective nutrition) are a group of genetically determined metabolic disorders with primary involvement of myelin, but in which the metabolic abnormalities were originally unknown. Subsequently, some of the metabolic abnormalities of these diseases have been determined.

In the past, different classification systems of the leukodystrophies were based on histopathologic findings, staining properties, clinical findings, and age of onset. This has resulted in a large number of eponyms for the same disease and probably in different metabolic abnormalities being labeled as the same disease. Metachromatic and globoid cell leukodystrophy are now known to be lipid storage diseases; spongy sclerosis is found in many aminoacidopathies; and adrenoleukodystrophy is a fatty acid metabolic defect.

The leukodystrophies will be discussed as a category of dysmyelinating disease because the term is widely used in the literature, with the real-

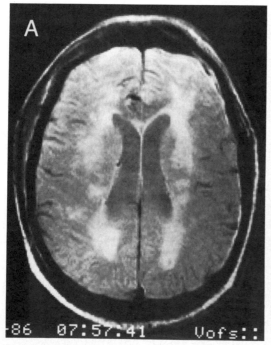
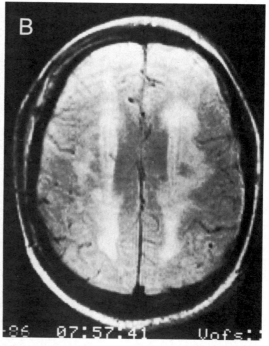

FIG 13–34.
A and **B,** subcortical arteriosclerotic encephalopathy in patient with a history of hypertension and dementia shows periventricular areas of increased signal without associated mass effect on spin-density–weighted MR images.

ization that the term "leukodystrophy" should eventually be abandoned. The diseases currently classified as leukodystrophies should be recategorized by their metabolic abnormality when the enzymatic defect responsible for each disease becomes known. In some of the leukodystrophies, enzyme deficiencies result in defective catabolism of the lipid components of myelin. This leads to the accumulation of complex lipids that are weakly sudanophilic and of cholesterol esters that are strongly sudanophilic. Sudanophilic tissues are those readily stained with Sudan, which is a group of azo compounds used as stains for fats. The terms *sudanophilic leukodystrophy* or *orthochromatic leukodystrophy* (Gr. *ortho*, straight, correct + Gr. *chroma*, color = normally colored or stained) refer to a classification based on histologic staining and comprise a heterogeneous group of diseases, including phenylketonuria, maple syrup urine disease, oasthouse urine disease, Cockayne's syndrome, adrenoleukodystrophy, and Pelizaeus-Merzbacher disease.[106] These staining classifications are differentiated from the metachromatic leukodystrophies. In metachromatic staining, different elements of a tissue take on different colors with the same dye.

Metachromatic Leukodystrophy

Metachromatic leukodystrophy, the most common leukodystrophy with at least 200 reported

cases,[106] is due to a lack of the enzyme arylsulfatase A, which is a lysosomal enzyme that hydrolizes the sulfate group from sulfatite in cell membranes.[107] The disease is diagnosed by low-to-absent arylsulfatase A in the urine, leukocytes, or cultured fibroblasts. There are three distinct forms of this disease: late infantile, juvenile, and adult. Each probably represents an independent autosomal recessive disorder.[2]

The most common type is the late infantile variety, in which symptoms develop between 12 and 18 months of age. The first symptom is clumsiness in walking as a result of weakness in the legs. Weakness and hypotonia of the lower extremities with reduction or absence of tendon reflexes are more common, but there may be spasticity. Upper limb involvement follows. There is progressive dementia, and 50% of those afflicted develop seizures. Death occurs between 2 and 10 years after the onset of the disease.[2, 108]

In the juvenile type, the age of onset is between 5 and 10 years, with progressive dementia and ataxia. The disease is more difficult to recognize in the adult and frequently presents as psychiatric illness with eventual progressive dementia.

The CT findings in all reported cases of metachromatic leukodystrophy are extensive, diffuse, symmetrically decreased attenuation of the white matter without enhancement (Fig 13–35,A). There is mild-to-moderate ventricular enlargement.[108–110]

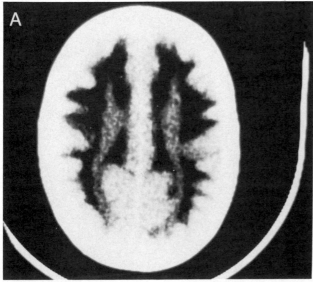
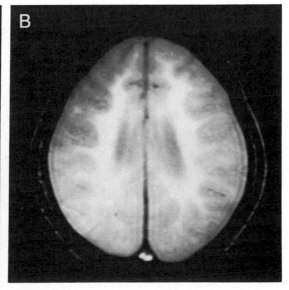

FIG 13–35.
Metachromatic leukodystrophy. **A,** unenhanced axial CT scan. Diffuse decreased attenuation is seen bilaterally in the periventricular white matter. **B,** spin-density–weighted axial MR scan. The same areas seen on the CT scan are viewed as areas of increased signal intensity.

The low attenuation of the white matter may be due to a loss of myelin rather than the accumulation of lipids.[107]

The MRI findings in metachromatic leukodystrophy are diffuse areas of increased signal in the periventricular white matter on the spin-density– and T2-weighted images (Fig 13–35,B).[111, 112]

Globoid Cell Leukodystrophy (Krabbe's Disease)

This is an autosomal recessive disease with approximately 100 reported cases, secondary to a deficiency of galactocerebroside β-galactosidase. The disease is diagnosed by demonstrating a deficiency of this enzyme in serum, leukocytes, fibroblasts, or cultured amniotic fluid. There are distended epithelioid (globoid) cells and collections of multinucleated bodies (globoid bodies throughout the white matter), along with punctate calcifications. The brain is small with diffuse loss of white matter.

The disease occurs almost entirely in infants of 3 to 5 months of age. Rarely, globoid cell leukodystrophy starts in the late infantile or juvenile period. The disease begins with increased irritability and crying and with extreme sensitivity to light and noise, which causes myoclonic jerks. The infant rapidly deteriorates and usually dies within 1 year of the onset of symptoms.[2, 106]

Description of the CT findings in this disease are sparse.[110, 113, 114] Periventricular areas of increased attenuation (Fig 13–36) correlate with the fine calcification seen pathologically. While not every case demonstrates this calcification, when present it presents a unique appearance among the leukodystrophies. Certainly, the lack of decreased attenuation should suggest the possibility of Krabbe's disease, given the correct history.

The MRI findings in Krabbe's disease are areas of increased signal in the periventricular and subcortical white matter on the spin-density– and T2-weighted images. The arcuate white matter is also involved (Fig 13–37).[112, 113]

Spongy Degeneration (Canavan's Disease)

This is an autosomal recessive disease of unknown etiology that occurs most often in Jewish families from eastern Europe. Approximately 90 cases of this disease have been reported. It begins in the first 2 or 3 months of life and usually leads to death within a few years. The infant develops flaccidity, apathy, blindness, and decorticate rigidity.[106, 115]

Spongy degeneration of the brain has also been found in a number of inborn errors of amino acid metabolism, including maple syrup urine disease, homocystinuria, phenylketonuria, argininosuccinicaciduria, and nonketonic hyperglycemia. It has also been seen in a case of 3-hydroxy-3-methyl-glutaryl-CoA-lyase deficiency, an extremely rare

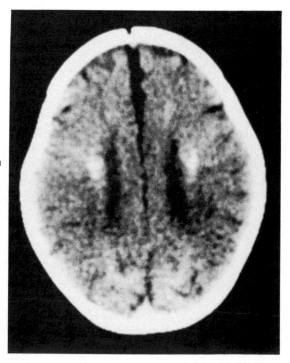

FIG 13–36.
Krabbe's disease. Unenhanced axial CT scan demonstrates calcifications in the periventricular white matter. Combined with the history, the findings are highly suggestive of Krabbe's disease. Krabbe's disease has never demonstrated decreased attenuation of periventricular white matter on CT scan.

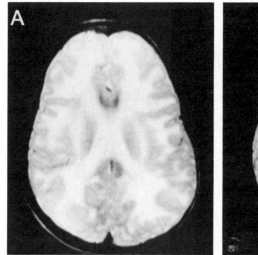
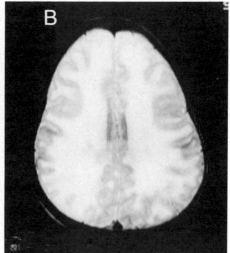

FIG 13–37.
Krabbe's disease. **A,** diffuse areas of increased MR signal in the subcortical white matter without associated mass effect. **B,** more

superior section shows involvement of the subarcuate white matter.

enzymatic defect of leucine metabolism.[116] Thus, spongy degeneration of the brain may be a nonspecific response of the brain to various abnormal metabolites. Serum arylsulfatase A hexosaminisidose (metachromatic leukodystrophy) and galactocerebroside β-galactosidase (Krabbe's disease) are normal.

Spongy degeneration and Alexander's disease are the only leukodystrophies that cause megalen-

cephaly. Symmetric diffuse decrease in the attenuation of the white matter is demonstrated by CT in Canavan's but not in Alexander's disease (Figs 13–38, 13–39, 13–40).[115, 118] Also in contradistinction to Alexander's disease, there is no enhancement of the white matter. On MRI, there is decreased signal throughout the white matter on T1-weighted images, and increased signal on T2-weighted sequences (see Fig 13–40).

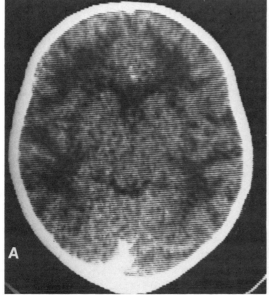
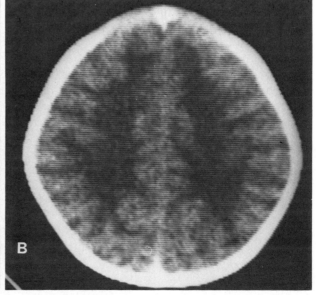

FIG 13–38.
Canavan's disease in a 7-month-old boy with increasing head circumference. **A,** there is decreased CT attenuation of the white matter with normal ventricles. **B,** a more cephalad section shows

decreased attenuation of the centrum semiovale. (From Rushton AR, Shaywitz BA, Duncan CC, et al: *Ann Neurol* 1981; 10:57–60. Used by permission.)

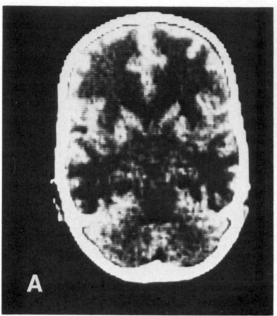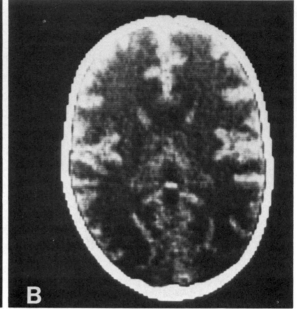

FIG 13–39.
Canavan's disease. **A** and **B,** there is a marked symmetric diffuse decrease in the CT attenuation of the white matter in this patient with megalencephaly. (Courtesy of David Weslowski, M.D., William Beaumont Hospital, Detroit.)

Adrenoleukodystrophy

This is a sex-linked recessive disease in which the exact inborn error of metabolism is unknown, but in which there is an abnormality of long-chain fatty acid metabolism resulting in lipid storage. There is an accumulation of lipid-filled, *p*-aminosalicylic acid–positive inclusions within macrophages of the CNS, adrenal cortex, testes, and peripheral nerves. The adrenal glands are atrophic.

The disease occurs in school-aged boys, with an insidious change in personality, mental deterioration, visual impairment, spasticity, and ataxia. The disease progresses rapidly, and most patients are demented, blind, deaf, and quadriparetic within several years.

Signs and symptoms of adrenal insufficiency usually precede the neurologic abnormalities. However, the adrenal insufficiency is variable in this disease, ranging from overt Addison's disease with abnormal skin pigmentation to normal adrenals by clinical and laboratory examination, but with a family history of Addison's disease. The diagnosis can be confirmed by finding elevated C_{26} fatty acid in cultured skin fibroblasts.[119]

Three histopathologic zones of destruction of the CNS white matter have been described in this disease, primarily in parieto-occipital and posterotemporal regions. Zone 1, along the leading edge of the lesion, shows myelin destruction with axonal sparing and little or no inflammatory response. Zone 2 shows increased demyelination with some axonal loss and many lipid-containing macrophages; there is a marked perivascular mononuclear inflammatory cell response. Zone 3 is inactive, central in location, and gliotic.[120]

The CT findings correlate with the histopathologic zones of destruction as described above. The earliest changes occur in the posterior cerebral regions (Figs 13–41, 13–42). Irregular areas of decreased attenuation subsequently involve the parietal, temporal, and frontal lobes. Occasionally, the frontal lobes will be involved initially, simulating a "butterfly glioma."[121] These bilateral changes are not necessarily symmetric. Enhancement occurs along the leading edge of the lesion corresponding to zones 1 and 2. With progression of the disease, the areas of enhancement are located more anteriorly. Generalized central and cortical atrophy develop later as rim enhancement fades.[122–126]

There is another CT pattern in adrenoleukodystrophy that is called type 2 and is characterized by the absence of posterior periventricular areas of decreased attenuation. With contrast infusion, there is marked enhancement of various white matter tracts or fiber systems such as the internal capsule, corona radiata, forceps major, and cerebral

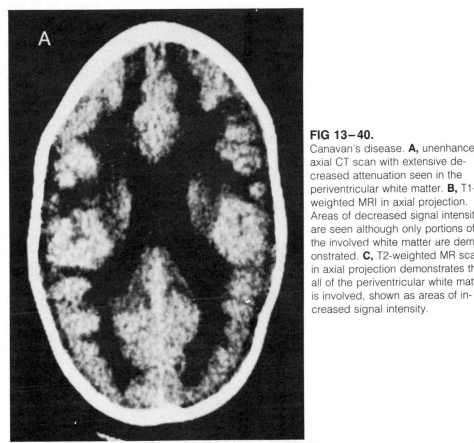

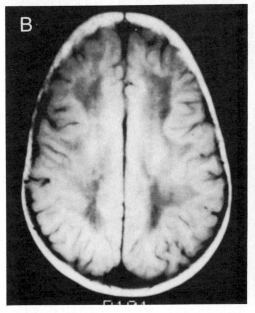

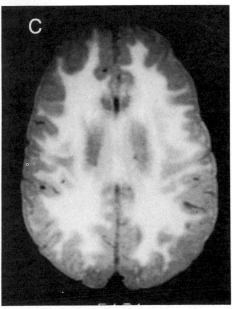

FIG 13–40.
Canavan's disease. **A,** unenhanced axial CT scan with extensive decreased attenuation seen in the periventricular white matter. **B,** T1-weighted MRI in axial projection. Areas of decreased signal intensity are seen although only portions of the involved white matter are demonstrated. **C,** T2-weighted MR scan in axial projection demonstrates that all of the periventricular white matter is involved, shown as areas of increased signal intensity.

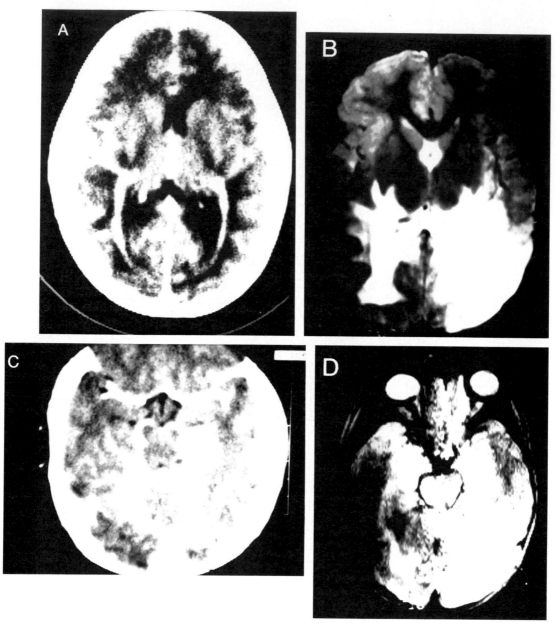

FIG 13–41.
Adrenoleukodystrophy. **A,** CT examination shows areas of decreased attenuation coefficient in occipital white matter. **B,** T2-weighted MRI examination shows areas of increased attenuation coefficient in occipital white matter. **C,** CT examination with contrast enhancement was originally interpreted as normal. Areas of decreased signal intensity can be visualized in the cerebral peduncles. **D,** areas of increased signal intensity are clearly visualized in the spinothalamic tracts within the midbrain on this T2-weighted axial image.

peduncles (Figs 13–43, 13–44). This pattern is believed to be specific for a phenotypic variant or an evolving stage of adrenoleukodystrophy.[127] Cases with both type 1 and 2 findings and with calcification have been reported.[128, 129]

The areas of dysmyelination in adrenoleukodystrophy are more clearly visualized with MRI than with CT (Figs 13–41, 13–42, 13–45).[130] Le-

sions extending into the corticospinal tracts can be better visualized with MRI than with CT (see Fig 14–41).

Alexander's Disease

This is the rarest of the leukodystrophies and is of uncertain pathogenesis. All proven cases have been sporadic except for one in which the family

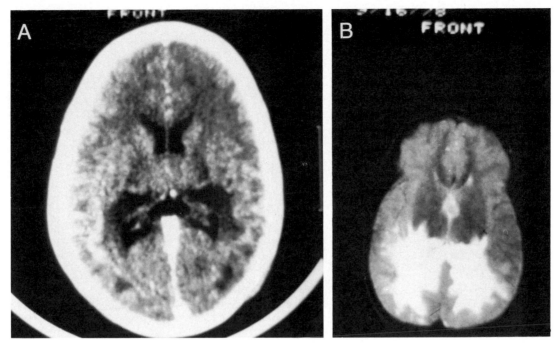

FIG 13–42.
Adrenoleukodystrophy. **A,** this enhanced axial CT scan shows the classic appearance with decreased attenuation of the white matter, mostly in the trigone regions. There are more peripheral areas of enhancement as well. **B,** T2-weighted MR scan in axial projection demonstrates involved areas in the region of trigones as areas of increased intensity.

history strongly suggested that three siblings of an autopsy-proven case were affected. The disease is usually manifest during the first year of life, with progressive retardation, symmetric spastic weakness, and convulsions in an infant with a rapidly enlarging head. Death occurs in months to years.

The brain is characterized by diffuse demyelination combined with Rosenthal fibers, which are believed to represent inert metabolic products from degeneration of astrocytes. These Rosenthal

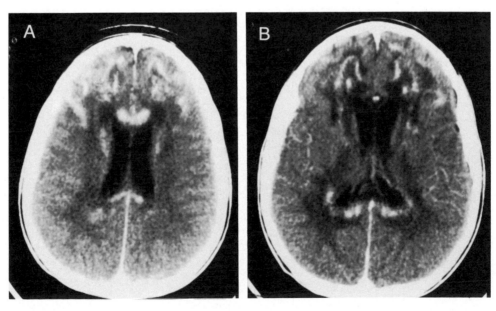

FIG 13–43.
Adrenoleukodystrophy. **A,** CT examination shows contrast enhancement in the splenium and genu of the corpus callosum and in the white matter of both frontal lobes. **B,** more inferior CT section shows areas of enhancement in the periventricular white matter and in both frontal lobes. (Courtesy of Richard E. Latchaw, M.D., University of Pittsburgh.)

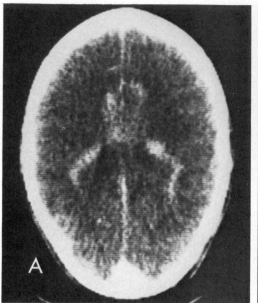
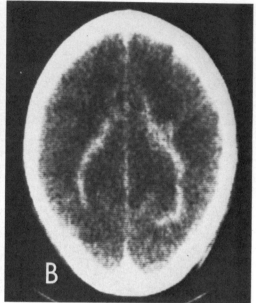

FIG 13–44.
An 11-year-old boy with adrenoleukodystrophy type 2 (with contrast). **A** and **B,** axial CT scans show enhancement of the corpus callosum and corona radiata. (From DiChiro G, Eiben EM, Manz HJ, et al: *Radiology* 1980; 137:687–692. Used by permission.)

fibers are most prominent in the frontal white matter, basal ganglia, thalami, and hypothalamus (Fig 13–46). The abnormal astrocytic deposits occur mainly in the footplate, which is an integral part of the BBB. Breakdown of these footplates allows for contrast enhancement.[131]

All cases of Alexander's disease have demonstrated megalencephaly. This is one of two leukodystrophies presenting with megalencephaly, the other being Canavan's disease. Alexander's differs from Canavan's in that lesions may enhance with contrast. Alexander's is one of two leukodystrophies showing such enhancement, the other being adrenoleukodystrophy. Hence, Alexander's disease

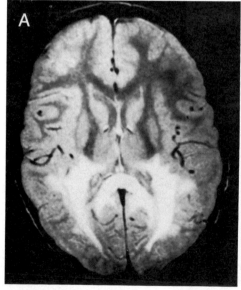
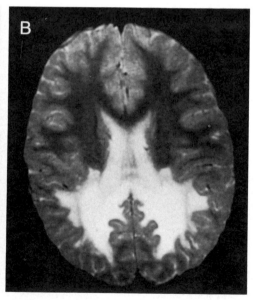

FIG 13–45.
Adrenoleukodystrophy. **A,** confluent areas of increased MR signal are visualized in the white matter of the occipital lobes and in the splenium of the corpus callosum. **B,** more superior axial T2-weighted section shows areas of increased signal in the occipital and parietal white matter without association mass effect. (Courtesy of Richard E. Latchaw, M.D., University of Pittsburgh.)

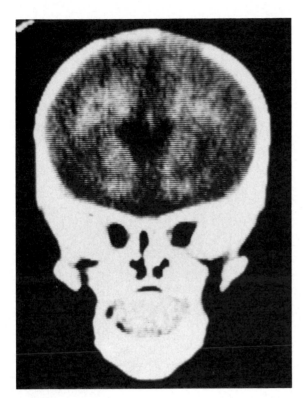

FIG 13–46.
Alexander's disease. The enhanced coronal CT scan shows increased attenuation in the periventricular white matter as well as basal ganglia. This is one of the two leukodystrophies that shows contrast enhancement and the only one with megalencephaly that enhances.

is the only leukodystrophy with megalencephaly and contrast enhancement.

In one reported case of Alexander's disease, there were symmetric, well-demarcated lesions in the deep cerebral white matter on CT, sparing the subependymal regions and considerably more extensive in the frontal lobes than elsewhere. The lateral ventricles were moderately dilated. There was symmetric contrast enhancement of the caudate nuclei, the anterior columns of the fornices, the periventricular brain substance, the central portion of the forceps minor, and the region of the optic radiations (Fig 13–47). A second case in the same report showed symmetric decreased attenuation of the white matter of both frontal lobes, of the caudate and lenticular nuclei, and of the anterior limbs of the internal capsules without abnormal enhancement (Fig 13–48).[132] A third case has been described with decreased attenuation of the white matter in the frontal lobes.[133]

MR scanning demonstrates decreased intensity of the white matter on T1-weighted sequences and increased intensity on the T2-weighted images

(see Fig 13–48). The T1-weighted sequence may also demonstrate the increased attenuation of the basal ganglia representing the Rosenthal fibers (Fig 13–49,B).

Pelizaeus-Merzbacher Disease

This is an extremely rare condition with several rarer subtypes. The classic disease is sex-linked recessive and manifests in early infancy. There are characteristic areas of preserved myelin. There is a slow progression of the disease characterized by speech abnormalities, grimacing, ataxia, choreiform movements, rotatory nystagmus, spasticity, and mental deterioration. Pathologically, there is sclerosis of the white matter of the cerebrum and cerebellum. The deficient enzyme has not been identified.

In one 14-year-old patient with marked clinical symptoms, the CT was normal. However, CT examination of his 25-year-old uncle demonstrated cerebellar atrophy, periventricular areas of decreased absorption coefficients, and cortical atrophy.[134] A report of a 10-year-old patient with far-advanced disease discusses a subtle decrease in the CT attenuation of the frontal white matter.[110] A fourth reported case in an 18-month-old child described diffuse decrease in the CT attenuation of the white matter in the cerebrum and cerebellum.[109] MRI demonstrates nonspecific hyperintensity throughout the white matter on T2-weighted images (Fig 13–50), even when the CT is normal (Fig 13–51).[135, 136]

Lipid Storage Diseases With Neuronal Involvement

Mucopolysaccharidoses are inborn errors of metabolism in which mucopolysaccharides are not normally degraded. They collect in lysosomes, causing abnormality of metabolism of other large molecules. Watts and colleagues provide a good summary of the subject and associated CT findings.[137]

CT demonstrates decreased density throughout the white matter, with or without hydrocephalus (Figs 13–52 and 13–53).[137] MRI provides an unusual appearance that appears to be highly specific. On the T1-weighted images there are multiple tiny areas of decreased intensity within the white matter (Fig 13–54,B). Pathologically these are accumulations of foam cells ("gargoyle cells") within dilated Virchow-Robin spaces. T2-weighted

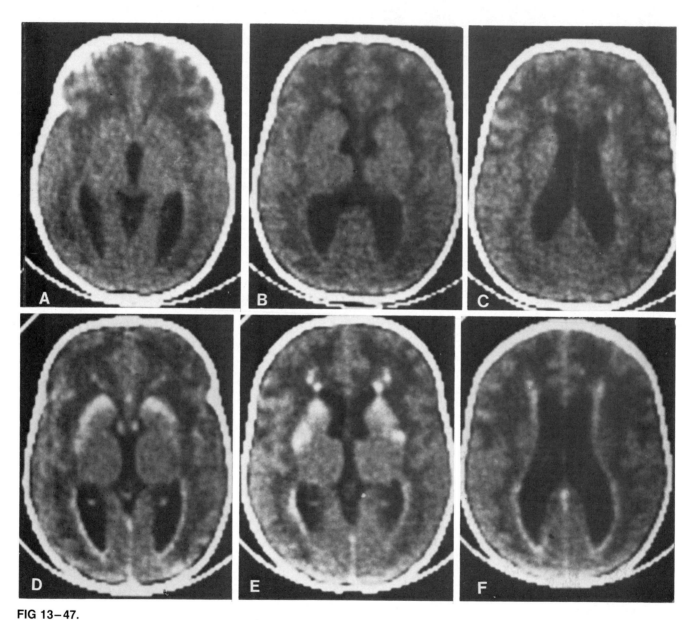

FIG 13–47.
Alexander's disease in a 7-month-old boy. **A–C,** unenhanced CT shows symmetric low-attenuation areas in white matter. **D–F,** enhanced CT reveals increased attenuation in the caudate nuclei, the periventricular areas, and the optic radiations. (From Holland IM, Kendall BE: *Neuroradiology* 1980; 20:103–106. Used by permission.)

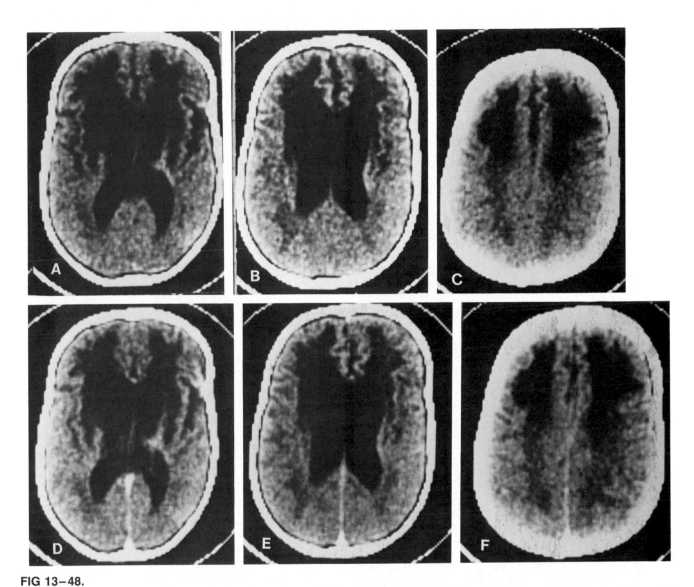

FIG 13–48.
Alexander's disease in a 6-year-old girl. **A–C,** unenhanced CT shows marked bilateral decreased attenuation of white matter in the frontal lobes, caudate nuclei, anterior limb of the internal capsules, and periependymal regions in parietal and occipital lobes. **D–F,** enhanced CT shows no unusual enhancement. (From Holland IM, Kendall BE: *Neuroradiology* 1980; 20:103–106. Used by permission.)

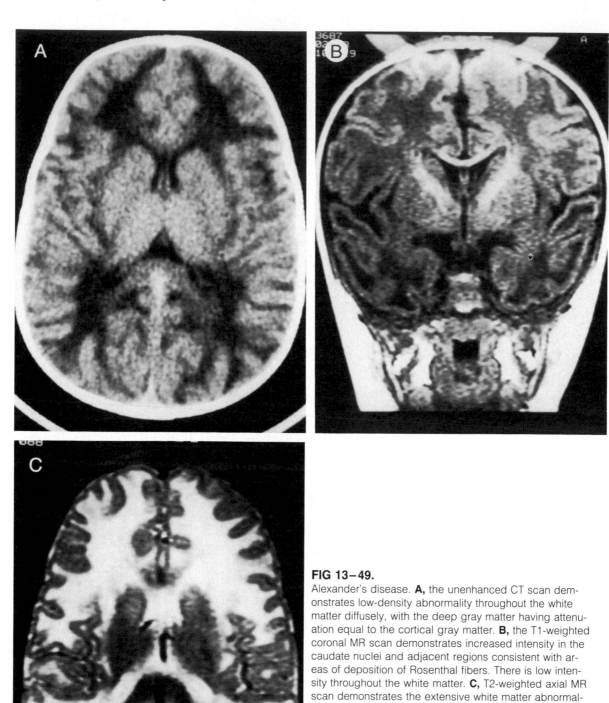

FIG 13–49.
Alexander's disease. **A,** the unenhanced CT scan demonstrates low-density abnormality throughout the white matter diffusely, with the deep gray matter having attenuation equal to the cortical gray matter. **B,** the T1-weighted coronal MR scan demonstrates increased intensity in the caudate nuclei and adjacent regions consistent with areas of deposition of Rosenthal fibers. There is low intensity throughout the white matter. **C,** T2-weighted axial MR scan demonstrates the extensive white matter abnormality as denoted by the diffuse hyperintensity. (Courtesy of Richard E. Latchaw, M.D., University of Pittsburgh.)

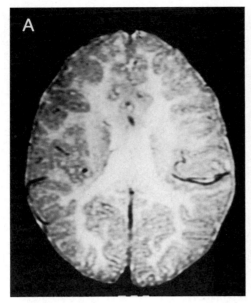
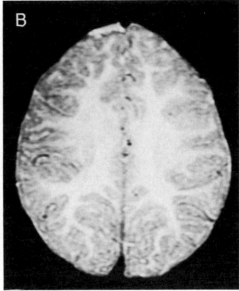

FIG 13–50.
Pelizaeus-Merzbacher disease. **A,** there are confluent areas of increased signal in the subcortical white matter without associated mass effect on this T2-weighted axial MR image. **B,** T2-weighted image obtained more superiorly shows confluent areas of increased signal in the subcortical white matter superior to the lateral ventricles. (Courtesy of Richard E. Latchaw, M.D., University of Pittsburgh.)

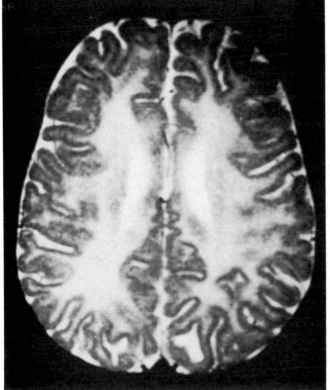

FIG 13–51.
Pelizaeus-Merzbacher disease: T2-weighted axial MR scan. Areas of dysmyelination are shown as increased signal intensity. The CT scan in the same patient was normal.

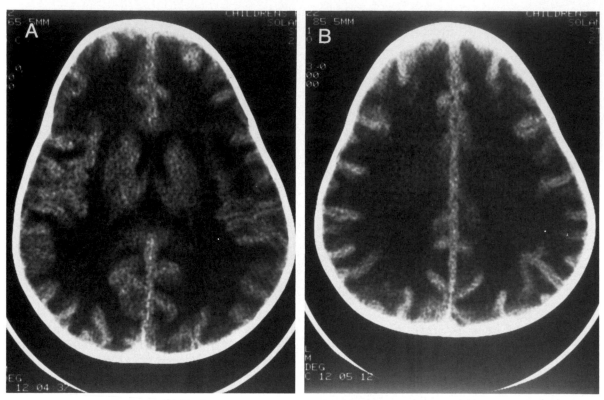

FIG 13-52.
Sphingolipidosis. There are very extensive areas of decreased attenuation coefficient within the white matter with sparing of the gray matter. There is no associated hydrocephalus. (Courtesy of Richard E. Latchaw, M.D., University of Pittsburgh.)

FIG 13-53.
Hurler's disease. There are confluent areas of decreased attenuation coefficient within the white matter with associated mild hydrocephalus. (Courtesy of Richard E. Latchaw, M.D., University of Pittsburgh.)

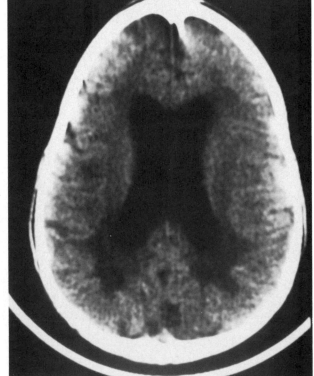

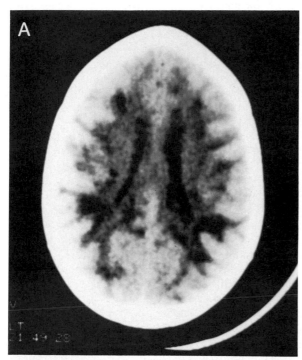

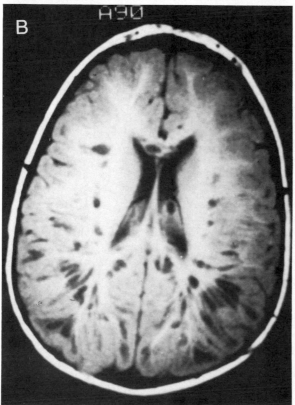

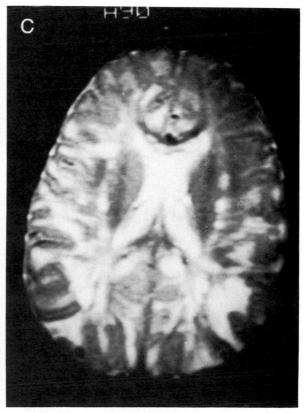

FIG 13–54.
Mucopolysaccharidosis. **A,** enhanced axial CT scan. Areas of decreased attenuation are seen in the periventricular white matter. Unlike other leukodystrophies, the decreased attenuation is uneven in different regions. **B,** T1-weighted MR scan in axial projection shows multiple small areas of decreased signal intensity in the white matter representing areas of deposits of mucopolysaccharides. This is pathognomonic of the disease. **C,** T2-weighted MR scan in axial projection demonstrates more extensive involvement than could be appreciated on the T1-weighted scan. While diffuse hyperintensity masks the degree of pathognomonic focality of the mucopolysaccharide deposits as seen on the T1-weighted study **(B),** much of the hyperintensity on this T2-weighted image still appears quite focal.

images demonstrate focal areas of pronounced hyperintensity, representing the accumulations of mucopolysaccharide-containing cells, interspersed throughout the areas of lesser hyperintensity (Fig 13–54,C).[138]

REFERENCES

1. Poser CM: Diseases of the myelin sheath, in Baker AB (ed): *Clinical Neurology*, vol 2. Philadelphia, Harper & Row, 1981, pp 1–3,7.

2. Gilroy J, Meyer JS: Demyelinating diseases of the nervous system, in Gilroy J, Meyer JS (eds): *Medical Neurology*, ed 3. New York, MacMillan Publishing Co, 1979, pp 137–144.

3. Duncan D: A relation between axone diameter and myelination determined by measurement of myelinated spinal root fibres. *J Comp Neurol* 1934; 60:437–471.

4. Blackwood W: Normal structure and general pathology of the nerve cell and neuroglia, in Blackwood W (ed): *Greenfield's Neuropathology*, vol 1. Chicago, Year Book Medical Publishers, Inc, 1976, p 10.

5. Quencer RM: Maturation of normal primate white matter: Computed tomographic correlation. *AJNR* 1982; 3:365–372.

6. Waller A: Experiments on the section of the glossopharyngeal and hypoglossal nerves of the frog, and observations of the alterations produced thereby in the structure of their primitive fibers. *Philos Trans R Soc Lond Biol* 1850; 140:423–429.

7. Adams RE, Kubic CS: The morbid anatomy of the demyelinative diseases. *Am J Med* 1952; 12:510–546.

8. Carswell R: *Atrophy, in Pathological Anatomy: Illustrations of the Elementary Forms of Disease.* London, Longman, 1838, plate 4.

9. Cruveilhier J: *Anatomie Pathologique du Corps Humains*, vol 2, part 52. Paris, Baillier, 1839–1842, plate 2.

10. Frerichs F: Über Hirnsklerose. *Haeser Arch* 1849; 10:334.

11. Vulpian E: Notes sur la sclérose en plaque. *L' Union Med* 1866; 30:475.

12. Charcot JM: Lectures on the diseases of the nervous system. Delivered at La Salpêtrière (trans from ed 2 by Sigerson G). Philadelphia, Lea & Febiger, 1879.

13. Baum HM, Rothschild BB: The incidence and prevalence of reported multiple sclerosis. *Ann Neurol* 1981; 10:420–428.

14. Kurtzke JF: Epidemiologic contributions to multiple sclerosis: An overview. *Neurology* 1980; 30:61–79.

15. Alter M, Loewenson R, Harshe M: The geographic distribution of multiple sclerosis: An examination of mathematical models. *J Chron Dis* 1973; 26:755–767.

16. Kurtzke JF, Hyllested K: Multiple sclerosis in the Faroe Islands. I. Clinical and epidemiological features. *Ann Neurol* 1979; 5:6–31.

17. Chan WWC: Multiple sclerosis and dogs. *Lancet* 1977; 1:487–488.

18. Cook SD, Natelson BH, Levine BE, et al: Further evidence of a possible association between house dogs and multiple sclerosis. *Ann Neurol* 1978; 3:141–143.

19. Cook SD, Dowling PC: Distemper and multiple sclerosis in Sitka, Alaska. *Ann Neurol* 1982; 11:192–194.

20. Poskanzer DC: Tonsillectomy and multiple sclerosis. *Lancet* 1965; 2:1264.

21. Poskanzer DC, Schapira K, Miller H: Multiple sclerosis and poliomyelitis. *Lancet* 1963; 1:917.

22. Poskanzer DC: Etiology of multiple sclerosis: Analogy suggesting infection in early life, in Alter M, Kurtzke JF (eds): *The Epidemiology of MS.* Springfield, Ill, Charles C Thomas Publisher, 1968, pp 62–74.

23. Berry RJ: Genetical factors in the aetiology of multiple sclerosis. *Acta Neurol Scand* 1969; 45:459–483.

24. Schapira K, Poskanzer DC, Miller H: Familial and conjugal multiple sclerosis. *Brain* 1963; 86:315.

25. Kurtzke JF, Bobowisk AR, Brody JA: Twin studies of multiple sclerosis: An epidemiologic inquiry. *Neurology* (Minn) 1977; 27:341.

26. Naito S, Namerow N, Mickey MR, et al: Multiple sclerosis: Association with HL-A 3. *Tissue Antigens* 1972; 2:1–4.

27. Pietsch MC, Morris PJ: An association of HL-A 3 and HL-A 7 with paralytic poliomyelitis. *Tissue Antigens* 1974; 4:50–55.

28. Weiner HL, Hauser SL: Neuroimmunology: I. Immunoregulation in neurological disease. *Ann Neurol* 1982; 1:437–449.

29. Lisak RP: Multiple sclerosis: Evidence for immunopathogenesis. *Neurology (NY)* 1980; 30:99–105.

30. Sheldon JJ, Siddharthan R, Tobias J, et al: MR imaging of multiple sclerosis: Comparison with clinical and CT examinations in 74 patients. *AJR* 1985; 145:957–964.

31. Uhlenbrock D, Seidel D, Gehlen W, et al: MR imaging in multiple sclerosis: Comparison with clinical, CSF, and visual evoked potential findings. *AJNR* 1988; 9:59–67.

32. Gebarski SS: The passionate man plays his part: Neuroimaging and multiple sclerosis. *Radiology* 1988; 169:275–276.

33. Drayer BP: Magnetic resonance imaging of multiple sclerosis. *BNI Quarterly* 3(4):1987.

34. Oppenheimer DR: Demyelinating diseases, in Blackwood W (ed): *Greenfields' Neuropathology*, vol 2. Chicago, Year Book Medical Publishers, Inc, 1976, pp 470–499.

35. Brownell B, Hughes JT: The distribution of plaques in the cerebrum in multiple sclerosis. *J Neurol Neurosurg Psychiatry* 1962; 25:315–320.

36. Smith AS, Weinstein MA, Modic MT, et al: Magnetic resonance with marked T_2 weighted images: Improved demonstration of brain lesions, tumor, and edema. *AJNR* 1985; 6:691–697.

37. Hershey LA, Gado MH, Trotter JL: Computerized tomography in the diagnostic evaluation of multiple sclerosis. *Ann Neurol* 1979; 5:32–39.

38. Gyldensted C: Computed tomography of the cerebrum in multiple sclerosis. *Neuroradiology* 1976; 12:33–42.

39. Aita JF: Cranial CT as an aid in diagnosis of multiple sclerosis. *Appl Radiol* 1981; 33–37.

40. Rieth KG, DiChiro G, Cromwell LD, et al: Primary demyelinating disease simulating glioma of the corpus callosum. *J Neurosurg* 1981; 55:620–624.

41. van der Velden M, Bots GTAM, Endtz LJ: Cranial CT in multiple sclerosis showing a mass effect. *Surg Neurol* 1979; 12:307–310.

42. Marano GD, Goodwin CA, Ko JP: Atypical contrast enhancement in computerized tomography of demyelinating disease. *Arch Neurol* 1980; 37:523–524.

43. Weisberg L: Contrast enhancement visualized by computerized tomography in acute multiple sclerosis. *Comput Tomogr* 1981; 5:293–300.

44. Miller DH, Kendall BT, Barter S, et al: Magnetic resonance imaging in central nervous system sarcoidosis. *Neurology (NY)* 1988; 38:378–383.

45. Meisler DM, Tomsak RL, Weinstein MA, et al: Magnetic resonance imaging (MRI) and HLA typing in patients with peripheral retinal perivasculitis and intermediate uveitis (ARVO abstract). *Invest Opthalmol Vis Sci* 1986; 18:121.

46. Alexander EL, Malinow K, Lejewski BS, et al: Primary Sjögren's syndrome with central nervous system disease mimicking multiple sclerosis. *Ann Intern Med* 1986; 104:323–330.

47. Rudick RA, Schiffer RB, Schewtz KM, et al: Multiple sclerosis. The problem of incorrect diagnosis. *Arch Neurol* 1986; 43:578–583.

48. Braffman BH, Zimmerman RA, Trojanowski JQ, et al: Brain MR: Pathologic correlation with gross and histopathology. 1. Lacunar infarction and Virchow-Robin spaces. *AJNR* 1988; 9:621–628.

49. Drayer BP: Imaging of the aging brain. Part I. Normal findings. *Radiology* 1988; 166:785–796.

50. Fazekas F, Offenbacher H, Fuchs S, et al: Criteria for an increased specificity of MRI interpretation in elderly subjects with suspected multiple sclerosis. *Neurology (NY)* 1988; 38:1822–1825.

51. Drayer BP, Burger P, Hurwitz B, et al: Reduced signal intensity of MR images of thalamus and putamen in multiple sclerosis: Increased iron content? *AJNR* 1987; 8:413–419.

52. Grossman RJ, Braffman BH, Brorson JR, et al: Multiple sclerosis: Serial study of gadolinium-enhanced MR imaging. *Radiology* 1988; 169:117–122.

53. Grossman RJ, Gonzalez-Scarano F, Atlas SW, et al: Multiple sclerosis: Gadolinium enhancement study in MR imaging. *Radiology* 1986; 161:721–725.

54. Weinstein MA, Lederman RJ, Rothner AD, et al: Interval computed tomography in multiple sclerosis. *Radiology* 1978; 129:689–694.

55. Jankovic J, Derman H, Armstrong D: Haemorrhagic complications of multiple sclerosis. *J Neurol Neurosurg Psychiatry* 1980; 43:76–81.

56. Haughton VM, Ho KC, Williams AL, et al: CT detection of demyelinated plaques in multiple sclerosis. *AJR* 1979; 132:213–215.

57. Jacobs L, Kinkel WR: Computerized axial transverse tomography in multiple sclerosis. *Neurology (NY)* 1976; 26:390–391.

58. Cala LA, Mastaglia FL, Black JL: Computerized tomography of brain and optic nerve in multiple sclerosis. *J Neurol Sci* 1978; 36:411–426.

59. Coin CG, Hucks-Folliss A: Cervical computed tomography in multiple sclerosis with spinal cord involvement. *J Comput Assist Tomogr* 1979; 3:421–422.

60. Nelson MJ, Miller SL, McLain W, et al: Multiple sclerosis: Large plaque causing mass effect and ring sign. *J Comput Assist Tomogr* 1981; 5:892–894.

61. Aita JF, Bennett DR, Anderson RE, et al: Cranial CT appearance of acute multiple sclerosis. *Neurology (NY)* 1978; 28:251–255.

62. Sears ES, Tindall RSA, Zarnow H: Active multiple sclerosis. *Arch Neurol* 1978; 35:426–434.

63. Gize RW, Mishkin FS: Brain scans in multiple sclerosis. *Radiology* 1970; 97:297–299.

64. Antunes JL, Schlesinger EB, Michelsen WJ: The abnormal brain scan in demyelinating diseases. *Arch Neurol* 1974; 30:269–271.

65. Davis J, Davis KR, Newhouse J, et al: Expanded high iodine dose in computed cranial tomography: A preliminary report. *Radiology* 1979; 131:373–380.

66. Raininko R, Majurin ML, Virtama P, et al: Value of high contrast medium dose in brain CT. *J Comput Assist Tomogr* 1982; 6:54–57.

67. Hayman LA, Evans RA, Hinck VC: Delayed high iodine dose contrast computed tomography. *Radiology* 1980; 136:677–684.

68. Morariu MA, Wilkins DE, Patel A: Multiple sclerosis and serial computerized tomography: Delayed contrast enhancement of acute and early lesions. *Arch Neurol* 1980; 37:189–190.

69. Predes JL: Contrast dose in CT scanning. *Arch Neurol* 1981; 38:67–68.

70. Vinuela FV, Fox AJ, Debrun GM, et al: New perspectives in computed tomography of multiple sclerosis. *AJR* 1982; 139:123–127.

71. Reisner T, Maida E: Computerized tomography in multiple sclerosis. *Arch Neurol* 1980; 37:475–477.

72. Robertson WC, Gomez MR, Reese DF, et al: Computerized tomography in demyelinating disease of the young. *Neurology (NY)* 1977; 27:838–842.

73. Lebow S, Anderson DC, Mastri A, et al: Acute multiple sclerosis with contrast-enhancing plaques. *Arch Neurol* 1978; 35:435–439.

74. Feigin I, Popoff N: Regeneration of myelin in multiple sclerosis. *Neurology (NY)* 1966; 16:364–372.

75. Prineas JW, Connell F: Remyelination in multiple sclerosis. *Ann Neurol* 1979; 5:22–31.

76. Perier O, Gregoire A: Electron microscopic features of multiple sclerosis lesions. *Brain* 1965; 88:937–952.

77. Fenichel GM: Neurological complications of immunization. *Ann Neurol* 1982; 12:119–128.

78. Adams RD, Victor M (eds): *Principles of Neurology*, ed 2. New York, McGraw-Hill Book Co, 1981, pp 658–662.

79. Dunn V, Bale JF, Zimmerman RA, et al: MRI in children with postinfectious disseminated encephalomyelitis. *Magn Reson Imaging* 1986; 4:25–32.

80. Bird CR, Hedberg MC, Drayer BP: Magnetic resonance imaging of white matter in infants and children. *BNI Quarterly* 5(1):1989.

81. Valentine AR, Kendall BE, Harding BN: Computed tomography in acute haemorrhagic leukoencephalitis. *Neuroradiology* 1982; 22:215–219.

82. Reich H, Shu-Ren L, Goldblatt D: Computerized tomography in acute leukoencephalopathy: A case report. *Neurology* 1979; 29:255–258.

83. Pineas JW: Pathology of the Guillain-Barré syndrome. *Ann Neurol* 1981; 9(suppl):6–19.

84. Choppin PW: Measles virus and chronic neurological diseases. *Ann Neurol* 1981; 9:17–20.

85. Adams RD, Victor M (eds): *Principles of Neurology*, ed 2. New York, McGraw-Hill Book Co, 1981, p 527.

86. Jabbour JT, Garcia JH, Lammi H, et al: SSPE: A multidisciplinary study of eight cases. *JAMA* 1969; 207:2248–2254.

87. Duda EE, Huttenlocher PR, Patronas NJ: CT of subacute sclerosing panencephalitis. *AJNR* 1980; 1:35–38.

88. Pederson H, Wulff CH: Computed tomographic findings of early subacute sclerosing panencephalitis. *Neuroradiology* 1982; 23;31–32.

89. Tsuchiya K, Yamauchi T, Furui S, et al: MR imaging vs CT in subacute sclerosing panencephalitis. *AJNR* 1988; 9:943–946.

90. Ishikawa A, Murayama T, Sakuma N, et al: Computed cranial tomography in congenital rubella syndrome. *Arch Neurol* 1982; 39:420–421.

91. Adams RD, Victor M (eds): *Principles of Neurology*, ed 2. New York, McGraw-Hill Book Co, 1981, pp 720–723.

92. Norenberg MD, Leslie KO, Robertson AS: Association between rise in serum sodium and central pontine myelinolysis. *Ann Neurol* 1982; 11:128–135.

93. Telfer RB, Miller EM: Central pontine myelinolysis following hyponatremia, demonstrated by computerized tomography. *Ann Neurol* 1979; 6:455–456.

94. Anderson TL, Moore RA, Grinnell VS, et al: Computerized tomography in central pontine myelinolysis. *Neurology (NY)* 1979; 29:1527–1530.

95. Rippe D, Edwards M, D'Amour P, et al: MR imaging of central pontine myelinolysis. *J Comput Tomogr* 1987; 11:724–726.

96. Miller GM, Baker HL Jr, Okazaki H, et al: Central pontine myelinolysis and its imitators: MR findings. *Radiology* 1988; 168:795–802.

97. Rancurel G, Gardeur D, Thibierge M, et al: Computed tomography of Marchiafava-Bignami disease. Presented at the Twelfth Neuroradiologicum Symposium, Washington, DC, Oct 10–16, 1982.

98. Yagnik P, Gonzalez C: White matter involvement in anoxic encephalopathy in adults. *J Comput Assist Tomogr* 1980; 4:788–790.

99. Hambleton G, Wigglesworth JS: Origin of intraventricular hemorrhage in the pre-term infant. *Arch Dis Child* 1976; 5:651–659.

100. Pape KE, Wigglesworth JS: *Hemorrhage, Ischemia and the Perinatal Brain*. Philadelphia, JB Lippincott Co, 1979, p 105.

101. Flodmark O, Becker LE, Harwood-Nash DC, et al: Correlation between computed tomography and autopsy in premature and full-term neonates that have suffered perinatal asphyxia. *Radiology* 1980; 137:93–103.

102. Lotz PR, Ballinger WE, Quisling RG: Subcortical arteriosclerotic encephalopathy: CT spectrum and pathologic correlation. *AJNR* 1986; 7:817–822.

103. Roman GC: Senile dementia of the Binswanger type. A vascular form of dementia in the elderly. *JAMA* 1987; 258:1782–1788.

104. Rosenberg GA, Kornfeld M, Stovring J, et al: Subcortical arteriosclerotic encephalopathy (Binswanger): Computerized tomography. *Neurology* 1979; 29:1102–1106.

105. Rosenberg GA, Kornfeld M, Stovring J, et al: CT scan in subcortical arteriosclerotic encephalopathy. *Neurology* 1980; 30:791–792.

106. Poster CM: Diseases of the myelin sheath, in Baker AB (ed): *Clinical Neurology*, vol 2, rev ed. Philadelphia, Harper & Row, 1981, pp 104–107.

107. Robinson WC, Gomez MR, Reese DG, et al: Computed tomography in demyelinating disease. *Neuroradiology* 1977; 27:828–842.

108. Buonanno FS, Fall MR, Laster W, et al: Computed tomography in late-infantile metachromatic leukodystrophy. *Ann Neurol* 1978; 4:43–46.

109. Robertson WC, Gomez MR, Reese DF, et al: Com-

puterized tomography in demyelinating disease of the young. *Neurology (NY)* 1977; 27:838–842.

110. Heinz ER, Drayer BP, Haenggell CA, et al: Computed tomography in white-matter disease. *Radiology* 1979; 130:371–378.

111. Waltz G, Harik SI, Kaufman B: Adult metachromatic leukodystrophy. Value of computed tomographic scanning and magnetic resonance imaging of the brain. *Arch Neurol* 1987; 44:225–227.

112. Nowell MA, Grossman RI, Hackney DB, et al: MR imaging of white matter disease in children. *AJNR* 1988; 9:503–509.

113. Tallie Z, Baram AM, Goldman AKP: Krabbe disease: MRI and CT findings. *Neurology (NY)* 1986; 36:111–115.

114. Barnes DM, Enzmann DR: The evolution of white matter disease as seen on computed tomography. *Radiology* 1981; 138:379–383.

115. Lane B, Carroll BA, Pedley TA: Computerized cranial tomography in cerebral diseases of white matter. *Neurology (NY)* 1978; 28:534–544.

116. Lisson G, Leupold D, Bechinger D, et al: CT findings in a case of deficiency of 3-hydroxy-3-methylglutaryl-CoA-lyase. *Neuroradiology* 1981; 22:99–101.

117. Rushton AR, Shaywitz BA, Duncan CC, et al: Computed tomography in the diagnosis of Canavan's disease. *Ann Neurol* 1981; 10:57–60.

118. Andriola MR: Computed tomography in the diagnosis of Canavan's disease. *Ann Neurol* 1982; 11:323.

119. O'Neill BP, Moser HW, Marmion LC: The adrenoleukomyeloneuropathy (ALMN) complex: Elevated C_{26} fatty acid in cultured skin fibroblasts and correlation with disease expression in three generations of a kindred, abstracted. *Neurology (NY)* 1980; 30:352.

120. Schaumburg HH, Powers JM, Raine CS, et al: Adrenoleukodystrophy: A clinical and pathological study of 17 cases. *Arch Neurol* 1975; 32:577–591.

121. Reith KG, DiChiro G, Cromwell LD, et al: Primary dymyelinating disease simulating glioma of the corpus callosum. *J Neurosurg* 1981; 55:620–624.

122. Quisling RG, Andriola MR: Computed tomographic evaluation of the early phase of adrenoleukodystrophy. *Neuroradiology* 1979; 17:285–288.

123. O'Neill BP, Forbes GS: Computerized tomography and adrenoleukodystrophy: Differential appearance in disease subtypes. *Arch Neurol* 1981; 38:293–296.

124. Eiben RM, DiChiro G: Computer assisted tomography in adrenoleukodystrophy. *J Comput Assist Tomogr* 1977; 13:308–314.

125. Furuse M, Obayashi T, Tsugi S, et al: Adrenoleukodystrophy. *Radiology* 1978; 126:707–710.

126. Duda EE, Huttenlocher PR: Computed tomography in adrenoleukodystrophy: Correlation of radiological and histological findings. *Radiology* 1976; 120:349–350.

127. DiChiro G, Eiben EM, Manz HJ, et al: A new CT pattern in adrenoleukodystrophy. *Radiology* 1980; 137:687–692.

128. Dubois PJ, Lewis FD, Drayer BP, et al: Atypical findings in adrenoleukodystrophy. *J Comput Assist Tomogr* 1981; 5:888–891.

129. Brooks BS, El Gammal T: An additional case of adrenoleukodystrophy with both type I and type II CT features. *J Comput Assist Tomogr* 1982; 6:385–388.

130. Kumar AJ, Rosenbaum AE, Naidu S, et al: Adrenoleukodystrophy: Correlating MR imaging with CT. *Radiology* 1987; 165:497–504.

131. Farrell K, Chuang S, Becher L: Computed tomography in Alexander's disease. *Ann Neurol* 1984; 15:605–607.

132. Holland IM, Kendall BE: Computed tomography in Alexander's disease. *Neuroradiology* 1980; 20:103–106.

133. Boltshauser E, Spiess H, Isler J: Computed tomography in neurodegenerative disorders in childhood. *Neuroradiology* 1978; 16:41–43.

134. Statz A, Boltshauser E, Schinzel A, et al: Computed tomography in Pelizaeus-Merzbacher disease. *Neuroradiology* 1981; 22:103–105.

135. Penner MW, Li KC, Gebarski SS, et al: MR imaging of Pelizaeus-Merzbacher disease. *J Comput Assist Tomogr* 1987; 11:591–593.

136. Journel H, Roussen M, Gandon Y, et al: Magnetic resonance imaging in Pelizaeus-Merzbacher disease. *Neuroradiology* 1987; 29:403–405.

137. Watts RWE, Spellacy E, Kendall BE, et al: Computed tomography studies on patients with mucopolysaccharidoses. *Neuroradiology* 1981; 21:9–23.

138. Johnson MA, Desai S, Hugh-Jones K, et al: Magnetic resonance imaging of the brain in Hurler's syndrome. *AJNR* 1984; 5:816–819.

PART VI

Degenerative Disorders and Dementia

14

Brain Iron and Movement Disorders

Burton P. Drayer, M.D.

BASIC PRINCIPLES

Brain Iron

High–field strength magnetic resonance imaging (MRI) is a unique, in vivo technique for mapping the distribution of brain iron.[15] Discrete areas of decreased signal intensity on T2-weighted images are noted in the globus pallidus, red nucleus, reticular substantia nigra, and dentate nucleus of the cerebellum (Table 14–1) (Figs 14–1 and 14–2). These findings on MRI coincide with previous histochemical and Perls' stain (for ferric iron) postmortem studies for sites of maximal brain iron distribution (Fig 14–3).[9, 10, 15, 21, 23, 24, 35, 42] Ferritin (storage iron) has a crystalline ferricohydroxide core with 4,000 ferric ions per molecule encased by a protein shell (25 A; molecular weight [mol wt], 480,000) that prevents traditional paramagnetic relaxation effects.[15] Slow statistical fluctuations in the magnetization of each ferritin core created by intracellular iron result in local magnetic field gradients, inhomogeneities, and subsequent decline in the transverse (T2) relaxation time.[7, 30, 32] This accounts for the excellent visualization of iron on high–field strength MRI units using a T2-weighted spin-echo pulse sequence.[15, 44] The effects of ferritin (decreased signal intensity) are even better seen on gradient-refocused, limited–flip angle pulse sequences because they are extremely sensitive to the effects of magnetic susceptibility.[18, 48]

Iron and copper are the two key trace metals involved in brain function.[9] Iron enzymes play an important role in oxidative reactions. DPNH–cytochrome C reductase has a high iron content, and iron-containing flavoproteins play an important role in cellular respiration.[40] Nonheme iron is a required *cofactor for monoamine synthetic degradative* enzymes, helps maintain monoamine oxidase levels, and regulates the dopamine receptor.[49] Chronic administration of chlorpromazine, an iron-chelating agent, will increase the concentration of iron in the caudate nucleus. Iron may also play an important role in normal aging. The combination of hydrogen peroxide and ferrous iron produces highly reactive, hydroxyl-free radicals and ferric iron.[20] In humans and nonhuman primates, only negligible brain iron is present at birth, with a progressive increase in granular iron to adult levels by 15 to 25 years of age.[10, 15, 23, 24] In the elderly, the iron concentration in the putamen increases preferentially until it approaches that of the globus pallidus.[15, 23]

An abnormal concentration of brain pigments that contain iron or other elements that exhibit magnetic susceptibility may be delineated in various neurodegenerative movement disorders by MRI (Table 14–2). Relatively distinct patterns of abnormally increased or decreased signal intensities on T2-weighted images correspond to findings on neuropathologic studies. For simplicity and classification, these disorders were separated into three groups with relatively distinct dominant clinical symptomatology—parkinsonian, choreiform, and dystonic.

PARKINSONIAN DISORDERS

The clinical presentation of bradykinesia, rigidity, and resting tremor characterize the most common disorder in this group, *idiopathic Parkinson's disease.* The accurate diagnosis of this disorder is of great importance because dopamine re-

TABLE 14–1.

Normal Distribution of Brain Iron*

Location	Amount (mg Fe/100 g)
Globus pallidus	≈20
Red nucleus	
Pars reticulata of the substantia nigra	
Dentate nucleus of the cerebellum	≈10–15
Putamen	
Caudate	
Subthalamic nucleus of Luys	
Arcuate "U" fibers	
Mammillary bodies	
Thalamus	≈5
Cerebral cortex	
Frontal white matter	
Optic radiations	≈2

*Data from Hallgren B, Sourander P: *J Neurochem* 1958; 3:41–51; Diezel PB: Iron in the brain: A chemical and histochemical examination, in Waelsch H (ed): *Biochemistry of the Developing Nervous System.* New York, Academic Press, Inc, 1955, pp 145–152; and confirmed in terms of relative concentration by Drayer BP, et al.

placement therapy has been highly successful in alleviating the progressively devastating symptoms. Parkinson's disease primarily involves the pars compacta of the substantia nigra and thus the neurons of origin of the striatonigral dopaminergic system. Various studies have described an excessive accumulation of iron in Parkinson's disease and early investigators—prior to the dopamine revolution—studied the possibility that iron may play a similar role in Parkinson's disease to that of copper in Wilson's disease. A variety of etiologies have been implicated in the genesis of parkinsonian syndromes including manganese, carbon monoxide, 1-methyl-4-phenyl-1,2,3,6-tetrahydropyridine (MPTP), virus, and hypertension.[1, 4, 17, 31, 37] Patients with parkinsonian features who respond poorly to antiparkinsonian medications *(Parkinson's-plus syndrome)* can be divided into two major groups: (1) multiple-system atrophies (striatonigral degeneration [SND],[1, 6] Shy-Drager orthostatic hypotension,[4, 43] olivopontocerebellar atrophy [OPCA][4, 43]) and (2) progressive supranuclear palsy (Steele-Richardson-Olszewski syndrome).[5, 45]

The dominant MRI finding in the Parkinson's-plus group (especially with multiple-system atrophies) is an abnormally prominent hypointensity in the putamen—equal or more hypointense than the globus pallidus—best seen on T2-weighted images in a high–field strength MRI system.[11, 14, 34] (Figs 14–4 to 14–6). Recent advances in gradient-echo imaging should ameliorate the sensitivity of lower–field strength MRI units because these pulse sequences greatly improve the detection of magnetic susceptibility effects.[18, 48] A similar finding, putaminal hypointensity, is seen more in drug-responsive parkinsonians as compared with normal adult controls, but normal signal intensity is also common, which makes the finding less useful. Abnormal signal hypointensity was noted in the puta-

TABLE 14–2.

Parkinson Syndromes: Pathologic Localization

Condition	RS	SN	CN	PUT	GP	DN	Luys	OPC	RAS	PAq	CG	CW	ILC*
Parkinson's disease													
Idiopathic	++		±		+						±	±	
MPTP	++												
Postencephalitic	++								+				
Manganese					++								
Carbon monoxide					++						+	+	
Vascular			±	±								++	
Multiple system atrophy													
Striatonigral degeneration	++	+		++	+	±	±	±			±	±	
Shy-Drager	++			++	+			+			±	±	++
Olivopontocerebellar atrophy	+			++	+	±	±	++			+	±	
Progressive supranuclear palsy	+	++			++	++	++		+	++	±		
Amyotrophic lateral sclerosis	±		±								±	±	

*RN = red nucleus; SN = substantia nigra; CN = caudate nucleus; PUT = putamen; GP = globus pallidus; DN = dentate nucleus of cerebellum; Luys = subthalamic nucleus of Luys; OPC = olivopontocerebellar atrophy; RAS = reticular activating system; PAq = periaqueductal gray/colliculi; CG = cerebral gray; CW = cerebral white; ILC = intermediolateral (sympathetic) cell column of spinal cord.

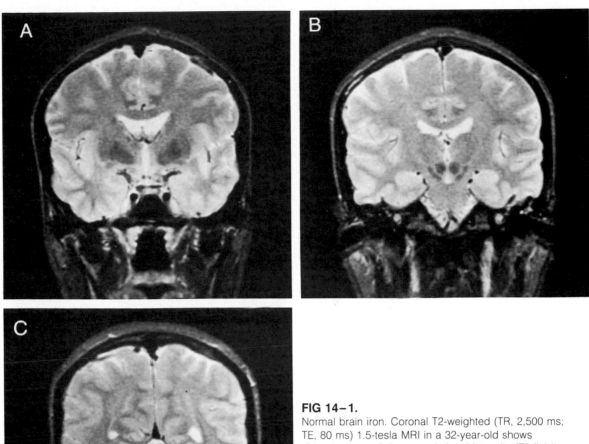

FIG 14–1.
Normal brain iron. Coronal T2-weighted (TR, 2,500 ms; TE, 80 ms) 1.5-tesla MRI in a 32-year-old shows discrete areas of decreased signal intensity (T2 field heterogeneity effect due to iron) in the globus pallidus, red nucleus, substantia nigra, and dentate nucleus of the cerebellum.

men in six teenagers from two families with olivo-pontocerebellar atrophy.[14]

A smudging of the normally sharply defined hypointensity in the substantia nigra[11] and a decreased distance between the substantia nigra and red nucleus[16] have been reported (Fig 14–5). These findings may be due to atrophic changes in the pars compacta of the substantia nigra that bring the pars reticulata and red nucleus into closer proximity or due to increased iron or pigmentary deposition in the degenerating pars compacta. There is controversy concerning the chemical composition of the hypointensity on the T2-weighted images. Although it may be due to excessive iron accumulation[11, 15, 17, 37]—possibly related to accel-erated hydroxyl-free, radical formation[20] or declining dopamine concentration—other metals (e.g., cobalt, manganese, chromium) may exhibit magnetic susceptibility properties.[11, 14, 34] Abnormal accumulation of the pigments hematin, neuromelanin, and lipofuscin have been reported in the putamen with striatonigral degeneration.[6]

Generalized cortical and posterior fossa *atrophy* is a nonspecific finding that is common in all parkinsonian patients[46] and best evaluated by using heavily T1- or T2-weighted images. With increasing longevity due to antiparkinsonian therapy, clinical and neuropathologic abnormalities (i.e., dementia, senile plaques, neurofibrillary tangles, and granulovacuolar degeneration) that indi-

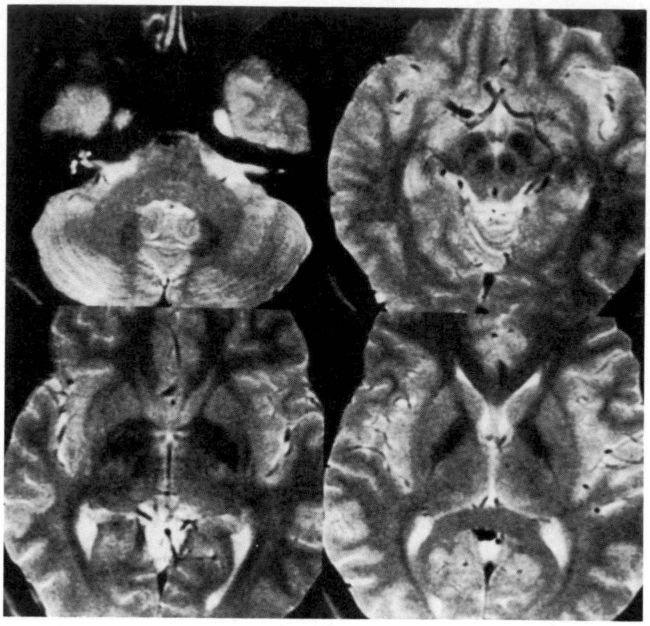

FIG 14–2.
Normal brain iron. Axial T2-weighted (TR, 2,500 ms; TE, 80 ms) 1.5-tesla MRI in a 43-year-old highlights the preferential distribution of iron (decreased signal intensity) in γ-aminobutyric acid (GABA) efferent basal ganglia nuclei: dentate nucleus, red nucleus, pars reticulata of the substantia nigra, and globus pallidus.

cate Alzheimer's disease are becoming more common. Punctate or more confluent areas of signal hyperintensity in the cerebral white matter, capsular, and basal ganglia regions on intermediate or T2-weighted images are somewhat more common in parkinsonian patients when compared with age-matched controls. The relationship of white matter hyperintensities to the progressive dementia is uncertain. These hyperintensities in the distribution of noncollateralizing, perforating, medullary, and lenticulostriate arteries most likely represent an often subclinical manifestation of a combination of one or more of the following factors:

1. Hypoperfusion (secondary to cardiac dysfunction, hypotensive episodes, etc.)
2. Arteriolar disease (secondary to hypertension, other vascular risk factors, etc.)
3. Aging (secondary to vascular or metabolic events)[2, 3, 8, 27, 31, 36]

The final result of any of the above factors involves a spectrum of brain alterations including dilated perivascular spaces (état criblé)[2, 3] and commonly associated myelin pallor or atrophic perivascular demyelination,[27] gliosis, ischemia, small infarctions (état lacunaire),[19, 47] or bilaterally symmetrical confluent diffuse white matter infarction and demyelination[12, 13, 26] (Binswanger's microangiopathic leukoencephalopathy [BML]). Unfortunately, all of these changes are associated with increased mobile protons and thus an increased T2-

relaxation time.[12, 13] État criblé is frequently noted in the basal ganglia region with Parkinson's disease and in healthy normal elderly adults, but the finding does not seem related to parkinsonian symptoms.[31] The thalamus and pons do not exhibit changes of état criblé.[19]

CHOREIFORM DISORDERS

The most common choreiform disorder, *Huntington's disease*, occurs with a prevalence of 5 to 10 per 100,000 population and is characterized by progressive, purposeless, abrupt, involuntary choreic movements; personality disorder; and dementia. There is dense fibrillary gliosis, atrophy involving the striatum and cerebral cortex (frontal and parietal), and a loss of small neurons. Preferential atrophic changes involve the head of the caudate nucleus with subsequent dilatation of the frontal horns of the lateral ventricle and the anterosuperior putamen. Histochemical analyses of postmortem brains have defined an increase in iron accumulation in the head of the caudate and anterior putamen.[29] Apparently the amount of iron and the duration of illness or brain weight are not correlated, and serum and iron concentrations in other organs are normal. Klintworth[29] suggested that premature neuronal cell loss with lipofuscin and iron accumulation may be related to accelerated autophagocytosis in Huntington's disease and iron

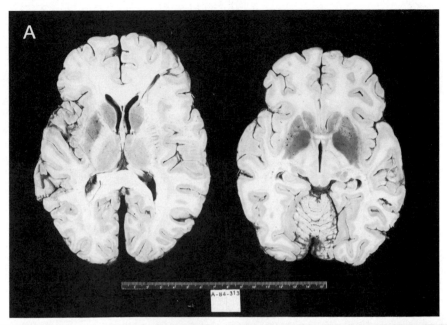

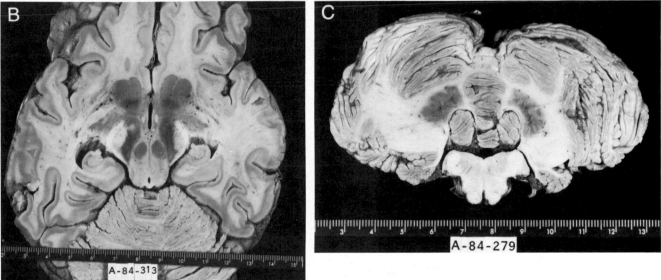

FIG 14–3.
Normal brain iron. Perls' stain for ferric iron depicts maximal staining in the globus pallidus, red nucleus, substantia nigra, and dentate nucleus; this coincides with the MRI findings.

deposition may be a nonspecific although important marker of the disease. Neurotransmitter abnormalities include a decrease in striatonigral GABA and striatal choline acetyltransferase levels. Molecular genetic studies have suggested that a locus on chromosome 4 may control the genetic expression of Huntington's disease and thus provide a method for early detection.[22]

In ten patients with Huntington's disease studied by MRI we confirmed that caudate atrophy with frontal horn enlargement was always present.[14, 41]

An abnormally decreased signal intensity (equivalent to the globus pallidus), best defined on T2-weighted images, was seen in the caudate nucleus of five of ten and in the putamen in four of ten patients. Subtle hyperintensity on the T2-weighted images was suggested in four of ten patients in the striatum. Cerebral atrophy with frontal dominance was apparent in eight of ten patients (Fig 14–7). Because the diagnosis of Huntington's disease is often apparent from the clinical examination and family history, the real need is to determine

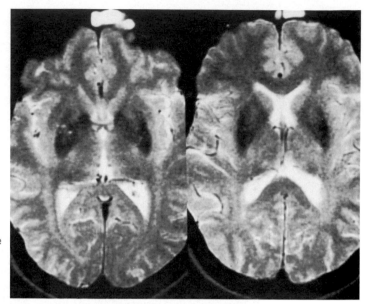

FIG 14–4.
Drug-unresponsive Parkinson's disease (striatonigral degeneration) in a 60-year-old individual with bradykinesia, rigidity, and resting tremor who is responding poorly to antiparkinsonian medications. There is abnormally prominent signal hypointensity in the putamen that represents excessive iron or other magnetically susceptible pigment (T2-weighted MRI: TR, 2,500 ms; TE, 80 ms). The subtle *white dots* scattered throughout the globus pallidus and putamen likely represent état criblé.

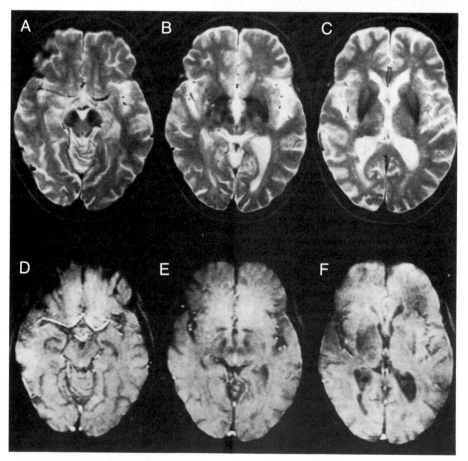

FIG 14–5.
Striatonigral degeneration. **A–C,** T2-weighted (TR, 2,500 ms; TE, 80 ms) 1.5-tesla MRI in a patient with parkinsonian symptoms and poor drug response illustrates abnormal signal hypointensity in the putamen and smudging and spreading of the substantia nigra hypointensity extending into the pars compacta (decreased distance between the red nucleus and substantia nigra); this suggests increased iron or pigment accumulation in these two important dopaminergic brain sites or degenerative atrophic changes in the pars compacta. **D–F,** gradient-echo images (TR, 300 ms; TE, 12; flip angle, 60 degrees) are extremely sensitive to iron, even when T1 weighted, and highlight the putaminal and substantia nigra abnormalities.

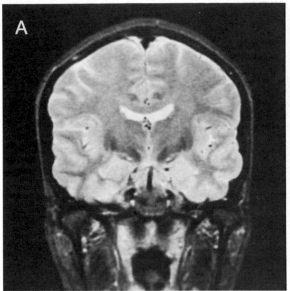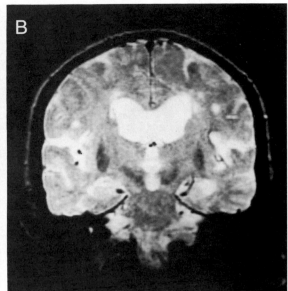

FIG 14–6.
Normal **(A)** vs. striatonigral degeneration **(B)** with severe parkinsonian symptoms: coronal T2-weighted (TR, 2,500 ms; TE, 80 ms) 1.5-tesla MRI. **A,** normal. Hypointensity is maximal in the globus pallidus and substantia nigra. **B,** striatonigral degeneration. The hypointensity in the putamen is more pronounced than in the glo-bus pallidus. Although straightforward in this 82-year-old patient, the distinction of normal aging from parkinsonian syndromes may be difficult because the hypointensity in the putamen normally decreases with age to almost equal the hypointensity in the globus pallidus.

whether MRI can presymptomatically screen for this autosomal dominant disorder.

Choreic movements may be the major symptom in a variety of disorders: the self-limited *Sydenham's chorea, systemic lupus erythematosus (SLE),* and *tardive dyskinesia* secondary to chronic neuroleptic therapy. *Chorea acanthocytosis* presents with mild chorea, tongue biting, tics, peripheral neuropathy, and red blood cell acanthocytes. *Hyperthyroidism* may result in chorea, and it has been hypothesized that thyroid hormone may enhance the dopamine receptor sensitivity to endogenous neurotransmitters.[28] Recent cases from our institution suggest that *hypothyroidism* is associated with a marked increase in iron accumulation (signal hypointensity on T2-weighted images) in the normal brain sites.[13] Isolated, mild, nonprogressive choreiform movements of the limbs without emotional disturbances or a family history may occur in the elderly *(senile chorea).* Aside from senile chorea where mild neuronal loss may be found in the striatum, no specific neuropathologic finding has been described for the other choreiform disorders. A small *infarction* or *hemorrhagic lesion* in the subthalamic nucleus of Luys often accompanies a more violent, flinging form of hemichorea (i.e., hemiballismus). A childhood *(Westphal variant)* form of Huntington's disease presents with akinesia, rigidity, emotional disturbances, and seizure.

DYSTONIAS

Dystonic movements are rapid, repetitive, and twisting; cause unusual postures; and appear with action. The major idiopathic childhood form of dystonia is called torsion dystonia, or *dystonia musculorum deformans.* Primary adult-onset dystonia generally remains in a limited location and mainly involves the arms *(writer's cramp),* the neck *(torticollis),* the vocal cords *(spastic dysphonia),* or the face and mandible with oromandibular dystonia and blepharospasm *(Meige's syndrome).* Despite profound abnormalities of movement, a morphologic localization, neuropathologic substrate, or neurotransmitter deficiency has not been elucidated. Not surprisingly, no MRI abnormality has yet been defined in these idiopathic torsion dystonias.

The dominant clinical feature of dystonia may result from a variety of pathologic processes. The characteristic MRI abnormality in most of these secondary dystonias is a well-circumscribed, relatively bilaterally symmetrical area of prominently increased signal intensity on the T2-weighted im-

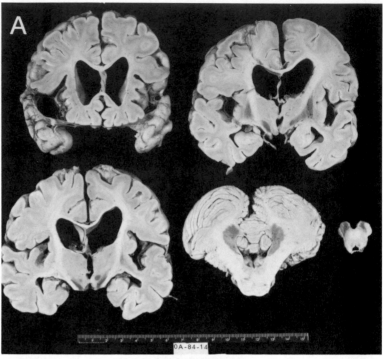

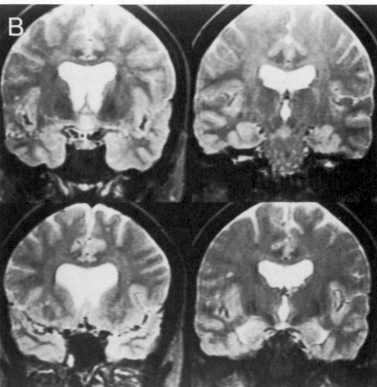

FIG 14–7.
Huntington's disease. **A,** Perls' stain for ferric iron of an autopsied brain suggests mildly increased iron levels in the putamen. The caudate is severely atrophic, resulting in prominent enlargement of the frontal horns of the lateral ventricles. **B,** T2-weighted (TR, 2,500 ms; TE, 80 ms) 1.5-tesla MRI in a 33-year-old woman with no overt symptomatology but a strong family history of Huntington's disease. There is no definite caudate atrophy or abnormal iron accumulation. Mild enlargement of the frontal horns for age is visible.

ages in the putamen and often the caudate nucleus (striatum), with some extension into the adjacent lateral globus pallidus (Table 14–3). Severe *diffuse anoxic injury* commonly results from cardiac arrest that causes sudden hypotension, which is followed by a prolonged period of reduced cerebral blood flow. This course of events causes hemorrhagic infarction in the border zones between the major cerebral arteries (e.g., parieto-occipital region) and/or cortical laminar necrosis and hip-

TABLE 14–3.

Dystonias: MRI Approach

Condition	Striatum		Pallidum		PAq* Gray		SN/RN*	
	↑ SI*	SI ↓	↑ SI	SI ↓	↑ SI	SI ↓	↑ SI	SI ↓
Dystonia musculorum deformans	–	–	–	–	–	–	–	–
Hallervorden-Spatz	+	–	–	+	–	–	–	+
Wilson's	+	+	–	–	–	–	–	–
Leigh's	+	–	–	–	+	–	–	–
Inherited	+	–	–	–	–	–	–	–
Anoxia	+	–	+	–	–	–	–	–

*PAq = periaqueductal; SN = substantia nigra; RN = red nucleus; SI = signal intensity.

pocampal (Sommer's sector) ischemia. In the putamen and lateral globus pallidus, cavitary necrosis causes increased signal intensity on T2-weighted images and decreased (or increased if microhemorrhages present) signal intensity on T1-weighted images. The localization of pathologic and MRI abnormalities is extremely similar in *acquired non-wilsonian hepatocerebral degeneration* secondary to portal-systemic encephalopathy. *Hepatic failure* exhibits a characteristic signal hyperintensity on T1-weighted images that is localized to the globus pallidus. A variety of mechanisms may account for this hyperintensity—Alzheimer's type II glia, manganese, nitroxide stable-free radicals, or protein accumulation. Head trauma, encephalitis, and kernicterus may all cause dystonic symptoms.

Hallervorden-Spatz disease is an autosomal recessive disorder of childhood that is typified by stiffness of gait, frozen facial expression, spasticity, and dystonic postures. The characteristic neuropathologic findings include axonal spheroids and a golden brown discoloration of the medial globus pallidus due to iron-containing lipopigments inside and outside neurons and astrocytes.[33] Iron

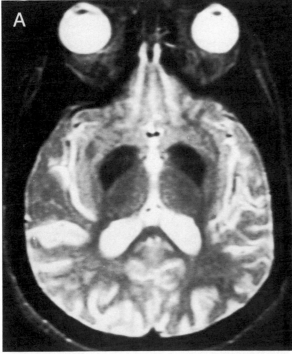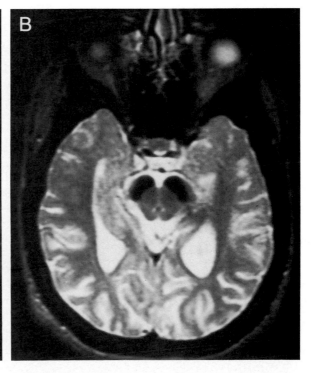

FIG 14–8.
Hallervorden-Spatz disease. T2-weighted, coronal, gradient-echo, 1.5-tesla MRI (TR, 600 ms; TE, 40 ms; flip angle, 20 degrees) in a 16-year-old patient with characteristic clinical presentation. The hy-pointensity in the globus pallidus **(A)** and substantia nigra **(B)** are prominently accentuated for a child of this age and consistent with marked iron accumulation.

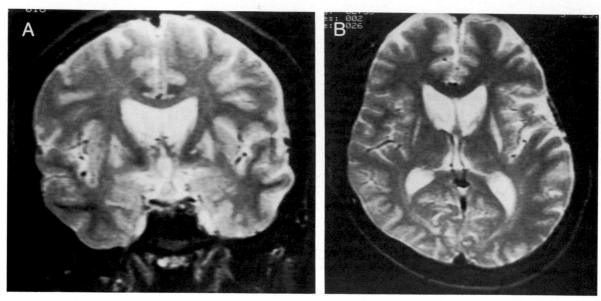

FIG 14–9.
Inherited striatal degeneration. This 32-year-old patient and two other family members have a chronic, slowly progressive, dystonic movement disorder. As opposed to the parkinsonian patients, these dystonic patients exhibited symmetrical signal hyperintensity in the putamina on T2-weighted (TR, 2,500 ms; TE, 80 ms) images.

pigmentation in the pars reticulata of the substantia nigra and red nucleus is less striking. With T2-weighted spin-echo or gradient-echo MRI, these abnormalities are readily detected as prominent foci of decreased signal intensity reflecting the effects of magnetic susceptibility from the increased iron deposition[38] (Fig 14–8). As stated above, iron in these locations is minimal in normal children less than 10 years old.[10, 15]

Dystonia may also be seen with *Wilson's disease.* The pathology involves brick red pigmentation and microcavitation in the putamen with less

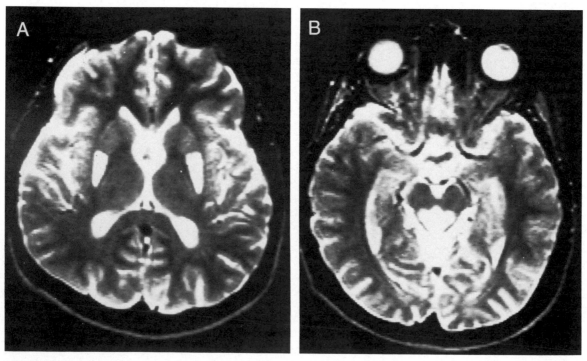

FIG 14–10.
Leigh's disease. T2-weighted (TR, 2,000 ms; TE, 100 ms) images define prominent signal hyperintensity in the putamen and periaqueductal gray matter that is characteristic of Leigh's disease.

severe changes in the frontal cortex, dentate nucleus, globus pallidus, and substantia nigra. In addition to accumulation of nonceruloplasmin-bound copper, there may also be associated abnormalities in iron-binding globulin and iron transfer from cells to plasma transferrin. The major MRI abnormalities, which reflect the dominant effect of cavitation in the striatum, are an increased signal intensity on T2-weighted images and decreased signal intensity on T1-weighted images.[25] Because iron often accumulates at sites of copper deposition,[9] future studies with high–field strength MRI systems should concentrate on whether this abnormal copper and iron can be localized as a region of decreased signal intensity. Signal hyperintensity in the putamen is also seen with *cytoplasmically inherited striatal degeneration* (Fig 14–9) with associated Leber's optic atrophy and *Kearn-Sayre ophthalmoplegia plus* mitochondrial cytopathy (of-

ten associated with cerebral white matter demyelination).[38] *Leigh's disease* (subacute necrotizing encephalomyelopathy [SNE]) often involves the putamen (increased signal intensity on T2-weighted images) but is clearly distinguished by additional involvement of the periaqueductal gray matter, substantia nigra, pons, and medial thalamus (Fig 14–10).

CONCLUSIONS

MRI is a powerful technique that uniquely provides functional information in a high-resolution anatomic format. This capability for delineating in vivo pathochemistry is highlighted by the diagnostic evaluation of movement disorders (Table 14–4 and Fig 14–11). Specific regions of the

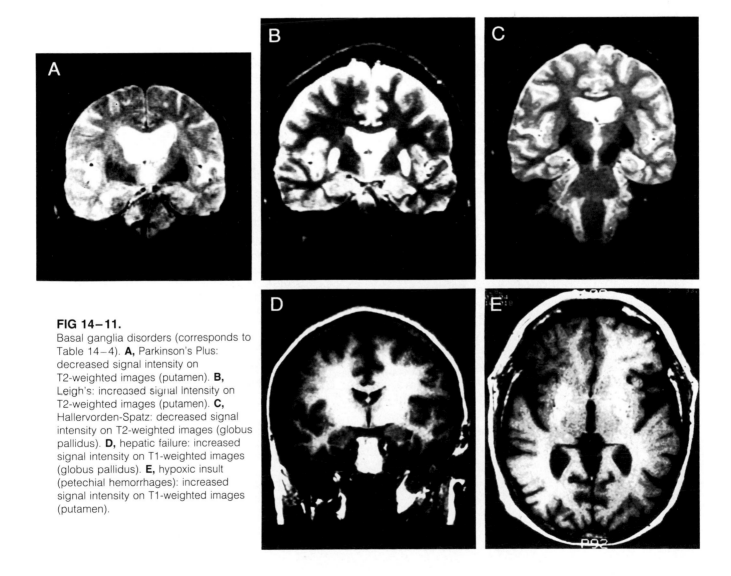

FIG 14–11.
Basal ganglia disorders (corresponds to Table 14–4). **A,** Parkinson's Plus: decreased signal intensity on T2-weighted images (putamen). **B,** Leigh's: increased signal intensity on T2-weighted images (putamen). **C,** Hallervorden-Spatz: decreased signal intensity on T2-weighted images (globus pallidus). **D,** hepatic failure: increased signal intensity on T1-weighted images (globus pallidus). **E,** hypoxic insult (petechial hemorrhages): increased signal intensity on T1-weighted images (putamen).

TABLE 14-4.

Basal Ganglia Disorders: Summary

Putamen—"T2," Hypointense	Putamen—"T2," Hyperintense	Globus Pallidus—"T2," Hypointense	Globus Pallidus—"T1," Hyperintense
Parkinson's plus	Hypoxic injury	Hallervorden-Spatz	Hepatic failure
SND	Wilson's	Hypothyroidism	Neurofibromatosis
Shy-Drager	Inherited		Hypoxic injury (subacute
OPCA	Striatal		petechial hemorrhages;
Cerebral white matter	Degeneration		includes putamen)
disease (severe)	Leigh's (SNE)		
Hypothyroidism	Ophthalmoplegia plus		

brain have areased T2 relaxation time (effects of magnetic susceptibility) closely correlating with the distribution and concentration of nonheme iron on postmortem examination. T1-weighted MRI clearly delineated enlargement of the ventricles and subarachnoid spaces. Hyperintensity on T2-weighted images is a highly sensitive marker of increased mobile protons, i.e., seen with infarction, edema, gliosis, or demyelination.

Movement disorders predominantly characterized by bradykinesia and rigidity (e.g., Parkinson's disease, multiple system atrophies) display abnormalities in the putamen and substantia nigra (decreased signal intensity on T2-weighted images). Conversely, disorders with predominant dystonic symptomatology have increased signal intensity in the putamen on T2-weighted images. Signal hyperintensity on T1-weighted images in the globus pallidus favors hepatic disease, but in the putamen and caudate it favors hypoxic microhemorrhages. Iron pigment deposition in the globus pallidus decreases the T2 relaxation time in the globus pallidus in children with Hallervorden-Spatz disease. Caudate atrophy, frontal horn enlargement, and variable striatal signal intensity typify Huntington's disease. Finally, small or confluent hyperintensities may be found in the cerebral white matter and basal ganglia, either with or without clinical symptomatology. These changes are probably markers of arteriolar disease secondary to hypertension, hypoperfusion, and/or aging and may reflect état criblé, atrophic perivascular demyelination, gliosis, demyelination, ischemia, infarction, or BML.[12, 13] A knowledge of neuropathology and MRI principles should thus permit not only the improved diagnosis but also an expanded understanding of the nature, course, mechanism, and response to therapy of neurodegenerative movement disorders.

REFERENCES

1. Adams RD, Bogaert LV, Lecken HV: Striato-nigral degeneration. *J Neuropathol Exp Neurol* 1964; 23:584–608.
2. Awad IA, Johnson PC, Spetzler RF, et al: Incidental subcortical lesions identified on magnetic resonance imaging in the elderly. *Stroke* 1986; 17:1909–1917.
3. Awad IA, Spetzler RF, Hodak JA, et al: Incidental subcortical lesions identified on magnetic resonance imaging in the elderly. I. Correlations with age and cerebrovascular risk factors. *Stroke* 1986; 17:1084–1089.
4. Bannister R, Oppenheimer DR: Degenerative diseases of the nervous system associated with autonomic failure. *Brain* 1972; 95:457–474.
5. Behrman S, Carroll JD, Janota I, et al: Progressive supranuclear palsy. *Brain* 1969; 92:663–678.
6. Borit A, Rubinstein LJ, Urich H: The striatonigral degenerations: Putaminal pigments and nosology. *Brain* 1975; 98:101–112.
7. Brittenham GM, Farrell DE, Harris JW, et al: Magnetic susceptibility measurement of human iron stores. *N Engl J Med* 1982; 307:1671–1675.
8. Brun A, England E: A white matter disorder in dementia of the Alzheimer type: A pathoanatomical study. *Ann Neurol* 1986; 19:253–262.
9. Cumings JN: The copper iron content of brain and liver in the normal and hepatolenticular degeneration. *Brain* 1948; 71:410–415.
10. Diezel PB: Iron in the brain: A chemical and histochemical examination, in Waelsch H (ed): *Biochemistry of the Developing Nervous System.* New York, Academic Press, Inc, 1955, pp 145–152.
11. Drayer BP, Olanow W, Burger P, et al: Parkinson plus syndrome: Diagnosis using high-field MR imaging of brain iron. *Radiology* 1986; 159:493–498.
12. Drayer BP: Imaging of the aging brain. I. Normal findings. *Radiology* 1988; 166:785–796.
13. Drayer BP: Imaging of the aging brain. II. Pathologic conditions. *Radiology* 1988; 166:797–806.

14. Drayer BP: Neurometabolic applications of magnetic resonance, in *American College of Radiology Categorical Course on Magnetic Resonance: Syllabus*, Bethesda, MD, ACR, 1985, pp 185–211.

15. Drayer B, Burger P, Darwin R, et al: Magnetic resonance imaging of brain iron. *AJNR* 1986; 7:373–380.

16. Duguid JR, De La Paz R, DeGroot I: Magnetic resonance imaging of the midbrain in Parkinson's disease. *Ann Neurol* 1986; 20:744–747.

17. Earle KM: Studies on Parkinson's disease including x-ray, fluorescent spectroscopy of formalin-fixed brain tissue. *J Neuropathol Exp Neurol* 1968; 27:1–14.

18. Edelman RR, Johnson K, Buxton R, et al: MR of hemorrhage: A new approach. *AJNR* 1986; 7:751–756.

19. Fisher CM: Lacunes: Small deep cerebral infarcts. *Neurology* 1965; 15:774–784.

20. Floyd RA, Zaleska MM, Harmon JH: Possible involvement or iron and oxygen free radicals in aspects of aging brain, in Armstrong D (ed): *Free Radicals in Molecular Biology, Aging and Disease* New York, Raven Press, 1984, pp 143–161.

21. Francois C, Hguyen-Legros J, Percheron G: Topographical and cytological localization of iron in the rat brain. *Neuroscience* 1984; 11:595–603.

22. Grisella JF, Wexler NS, Conneally PM, et al: A polymorphic DNA marker genetically linked to Huntington's disease. *Nature* 1983; 306:234–238.

23. Hallgren B, Sourander P: The effect of age on the nonhaemin iron in the human brain. *J Neurochem* 1958; 3:41–51.

24. Hill JM, Switzer RC III: The regional distribution and cellular localization of iron in the rat brain. *Neuroscience* 1984; 11:595–603.

25. Johnson MA, Pennock JM, Bydder GM, et al: Clinical NMR imaging of the brain in children: Normal and neurological disease. *AJNR* 1983; 4:1013–1026.

26. Kinkel WR, Jacobs L, Polachini I, et al: Subcortical arteriosclerotic encephalopathy (Binswanger's disease). Computed tomographic, nuclear magnetic resonance, and clinical correlations. *Arch Neurol* 1985; 42:951–959.

27. Kirkpatrick JB, Hayman LA: White matter lesions in MR imaging of clinically healthy brains of elderly subjects: Possible pathologic basis. *Radiology* 1982; 162:509–511.

28. Klawans HL, Shenker DM: Observations on the dopaminergic nature of hyperthyroid chorea. *J Neural Transm* 1972; 33:73–81.

29. Klintworth GK: Huntington's chorea—morphologic contributions of a century. *Advances in Neurology.* New York, Raven Press, 1973, pp 353–368.

30. Koenig SH: A theory of solvent relaxation by solute clusters of noninteracting paramagnetic ions, as ex-

emplified by ferritin (abstract). *Soc Magn Reson Med* 1985; 2:873–874.

31. Okazaki H: Hypertensive vascular disease of the CNS, in Okazaki H (ed): *Fundamentals of Neuropathology*, Tokyo, Igaku-Shoin, 1983, pp 55–57.

32. Packet KJ: The effects of diffusion through locally inhomogeneous magnetic fields on transverse nuclear spin relaxation in heterogeneous systems: Proton transverse relaxation in striated muscle tissue. *J Magn Reson* 1973; 9:438–443.

33. Park BE, Netsky MG, Betsill WL: Pathogenesis of pigment and spheroid formation in Hallervorden-Spatz syndrome and related disorders. *Neurology* 1975; 25:1172–1178.

34. Pastakia B, Polinsky R, Chiro GD, et al: Multiple system atrophy (Shy-Drager syndrome): MR imaging. *Radiology* 1986; 159:499–502.

35. Perls M: Nachweis von Eisenokyd in gewissen pigmenten. *Virchows Arch [A]* 1867; 39A:42–48.

36. Rezek DL, Morris IC, Fulling KH, et al: Periventricular white matter lucencies in senile dementia of the Alzheimer type and in normal aging. *Neurology* 1987; 37:1365–1368.

37. Rojas G, Asenjo A, Chiorino R, et al: Cellular and subcellular structure of the ventrolateral nucleus of the thalamus in Parkinson disease: Deposits of iron. *Confin Neurol* 1965; 26:362–376.

38. Schaffert DA, Johnsen SD, Johnson PC, et al: Magnetic resonance imaging in pathologically proven Hallervorden-Spatz disease. *Neurology* 1989; 39:400–442.

39. Seidenwurm D, Novotny E, Marshall W: MR and CT in cytoplasmically inherited striatal degeneration. *AJNR* 1986; 7:629–632.

40. Seitelberger F: Pigmentary disorders, in Minckler J (ed): *Pathology of the Nervous System*, New York, McGraw-Hill International Book Co, 1972, pp 1324–1338.

41. Simmons JT, Pastakia B, Chase TN, et al: Magnetic resonance imaging in Huntington's disease. *AJNR* 1986; 7:25–28.

42. Spatz H: Uber den Eisennachweis im Gehirn, besonders in Zentren des extrapyramidal-motorischen Systems. *Z Gesante Neurol Psychiatr* 1922; 77:261–290.

43. Spokes EGS, Bannister R, Oppenheimer DR: Multiple system atrophy with autonomic failure. *J Neurol Sci* 1979; 43:59–82.

44. Stark DD, Moseley ME, Bacon BR, et al: Magnetic resonance imaging and spectroscopy of hepatic iron overload. *Radiology* 1985; 154:137–142.

45. Steele JC, Richardson JC, Olszewski J: Progressive supranuclear palsy. *Arch Neurol* 1964; 10:333–359.

46. Steiner I, Gomori JM, Melamed E: Features of brain atrophy in Parkinson's disease: A CT scan study. *Neuroradiology* 1985; 27:158–160.

47. Tomlinson BE, Blessed G, Roth M: Observations

on the brains of nondemented old people. *J Neurol Sci* 1968; 7:331–356.

48. Wehrli FW, Drayer BP: Introduction to fast-scan magnetic resonance. *Banon Neurological Institute Quarterly* 1987; 3:2–14.

49. Youdim MBH, Yehuda S, Ben-Schachar D, et al: Behavioral and brain biochemical changes in iron deficient rats: The involvement of iron and dopamine receptor function, in Pollitt E, Leibel RL (eds): *Iron Deficiency: Brain Biochemistry and Behavior.* New York, Raven Press, 1982, pp 39–56.

15

Computed Tomography, Magnetic Resonance Imaging, and Positron Emission Tomography in Aging and Dementing Disorders

Ajax E. George, M.D.

Mony J. DeLeon, Ed.D.

It is an ancient belief that specific areas of the brain have specific functions.[1] As early as 1870, Fritsch[2] produced movement of body parts by electrically stimulating the motor cortex of the brain. Today, the motor homunculus is accepted as an accurate representation of specific motor functions of the cerebral cortex. Cognitive functions, however, such as memory, awareness, personality, and intelligence continue to baffle and challenge us to identify their site and mechanism of function. Such knowledge would permit us to evaluate the significance of structural and functional changes demonstrated by computed tomography (CT), magnetic resonance imaging (MRI), and positron emission tomography (PET).

Popular and scientific belief assumes that the cortex is the essential organ of thinking and consciousness. After all, there is extraordinary enlargement of the human cortex, especially in the temporal, parietal, and frontal regions, when compared with that of lower animals.[3] If the cerebral cortex is the site of cognition, then the cognitive impairment and memory loss phenomena seen in aging and dementia must have a counterpart in the cerebral cortex.

Today, Alzheimer's disease[4] (AD) (also known as senile dementia of the Alzheimer type [SDAT] and primary degenerative dementia [PDD]) is rec-ognized as the most common cause of dementia in the elderly and accounts for more than 50% of cases. Other dementing disorders include multi-infarct or vascular dementia, Parkinson's disease (PD), Pick's disease, and Huntington's chorea. AD was originally described in 1907[4] as a presenile dementing disorder. AD both in the presenile and elderly population is manifested initially as a loss of recent memory and progresses eventually to disorientation, loss of affect and personality, urinary and fecal incontinence, and ultimately death.[5] Neuropathologic studies have shown an increased incidence of cortical atrophy as well as ventricular enlargement in patients who died suffering from AD[6] when compared with the brains of normal control groups[7] (see below for recent neuropathologic studies).

Imaging studies using pneumoencephalography (PEG) and early CT studies[8] also found broad and weak correlations between cerebral atrophy and dementia. Recently with the use of CT and MRI specific temporal lobe changes have been identified that hold promise not only as correlates but as potential diagnostic markers of AD.[9-12] In addition, MRI using specially designed sequences has provided us for the first time with the ability to quantitate gray and white matter[13] in AD as well as a variety of other diseases. Initial studies have shown[14] that the cerebral atrophy seen in AD is indeed due to preferential loss of gray matter over white. These results corroborating the more recent neuropathology literature are described in greater detail below.

PD is another disease that prior to MRI had no known imaging diagnostic features. Ongoing work in this area is attempting to identify changes in the brain stem and basal ganglia that may be useful as diagnostic markers and as monitors of treatment strategies including adrenal brain implants.

NEUROPSYCHOLOGICAL LITERATURE

Specific temporal lobe structural changes have been identified in AD. However, memory deficits and cognitive defects may result from a wide variety of pathologies other than PDD. It may be worthwhile to review the literature on experimental brain lesions in order to identify brain behavioral relationships; these relationships help reveal the sites that control memory and cognition.

First of all, unilateral removal of a large part of the frontal lobe produces no loss of memory and no obvious disability.[1] The patient, however, does to a variable degree lose the ability to take initiative and plan activities. According to Bricken,[15] bilateral removal of the frontal lobes results in personality change and memory impairment for recent events. Penfield and Rasmussen[3] also noted that removal of the frontal lobe anterior to the precentral gyrus resulted in an "amazing" lack of obvious defect. In a series of bilateral frontal gyrectomies, however, Penfield and Rasmussen found increasing impairment of mental performance as bilateral removals were carried further back into the intermediate frontal cortex. Stimulation of the temporal cortex in an epileptic discharge may produce complex psychological phenomena and hallucinations. The patient may feel that a present experience suddenly becomes a familiar one. Electrode stimulation of the temporal cortex may bring to consciousness life experiences from dreaming or from previous readings.[3] Ablation of the temporal cortex limited to the anterior 5 cm is apparently associated with no memory impairment. Bilateral lobectomy was described by Kluver and Bucy[16] in an animal model. A lobectomized monkey was no longer afraid of a snake that he had previously been terrified of, apparently having a loss of memory of previous experiences. Babkin (cited by Pavlov[17]) also showed that a dog that has lost both

temporal lobes no longer responds to his name. Bilateral temporal lobectomies in humans have been associated with severe anterograde amnesia.[18]

Ojemann and co-workers[19, 20] have shown that electrical stimulation of the ventrolateral aspect of the thalamus improved short-term memory performance, but only with stimulation of the *left* portion of the thalamus. These experiments were performed during thalamotomy for dyskinesia. Left thalamic insult by stroke or hemorrhage may result in *thalamic aphasia* and short-term verbal memory disturbance. It is clear that bilateral thalamic infarcts are associated with profound memory loss and dementia,[21] and this has been termed "thalamic dementia." This condition is exemplified by the following case history: a 44-year-old mildly hypertensive male engineer (Fig 15–1) while working outdoors suddenly became mute, staring without expression into the distance. The patient slowly regained speech over the next few weeks but was left with a profound and incapacitating loss of memory for recent events, although he did

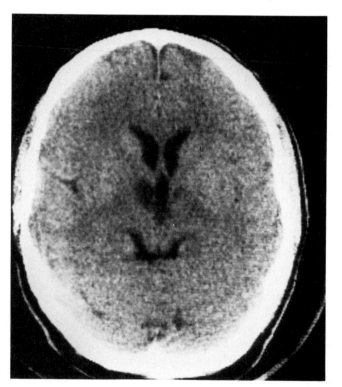

FIG 15–1.
Thalamic dementia in a 44-year-old man with bilateral thalamic infarcts of sudden onset. A 2-cm-diameter radiolucency involves the dorsomedial and anterior aspects of the right thalamus consistent with infarction. There is no associated mass effect. The third ventricle is somewhat dilated for age. A smaller left thalamic infarct is also present in the same region. The study is otherwise unremarkable. (Courtesy of C. Anayiotos, M.D., Long Branch, NJ.)

retain certain memories of events in the distant past. A CT scan revealed bilateral thalamic infarcts (Fig 15–1). Thorough subsequent evaluation of his metabolic, cardiac, and vascular status including cerebrovascular angiography produced negative results. The infarcts at this point are presumed to be of hypertensive origin, and the case has been classified as an example of thalamic dementia.

The concept of thalamic dementia has also received attention in the lay literature. The *Los Angeles Times* in 1979 reported the story of a 20-year-old man who sustained a freak accident when a fencing foil entered his nostril and the tip lodged in the thalamus. The patient had severe loss of recent memory. Since then he has been able to function at the level required to take care of himself. A CT scan confirmed the presence of thalamic injury as a consequence of the previous trauma (Kuhl, D.E., personal communication, 1981). Further evidence of the importance of the thalami and subcortal nuclei is suggested by the well-known selective involvement of the mammillary bodies, thalami, and hypothalami in Korsakoff's disease.[22] Selective loss of recent memory characterizes this condition, common in alcoholics. In a study of 82 brains of patients with Wernicke-Korsakoff syndrome, Victor and colleagues[22] found a high degree of correlation between the memory defect and involvement, primarily neuronal loss, of the mammillary bodies, the medial dorsal nucleus of the thalamus, and the medial part of the pulvinar. In 5 patients with attacks of Wernicke's disease consisting of ophthalmoparesis, ataxia, and confusional apathetic state and in whom the memory defects completely cleared, the medial dorsal nucleus was normal. These were the only 5 cases in the series in which the nucleus was spared. Involvement to a lesser degree (minimal to moderate) was also noted in the midbrain, pons, and medulla.

In view of the experimental literature, Penfield and Rasmussen[3] proposed the intriguing hypothesis that memories are stored in either or both temporal cortices, that the frontal cortex is utilized in the elaboration of thought but that the important coordinator of these functions actually exists in subcortical centers, notably the mesencephalon and diencephalon, and that the diencephalon is in fact the "seat of consciousness" and the center that summons and coordinates memory. In this hypothesis, the mesencephalon and diencephalon in effect represent the central processing unit, and the temporal cortices represent memory banks, with right or left being used interchangeably. Removal of both leaves the central processing unit with no memory storage capacity. Recent neuropathologic evidence[23–25] (see below) suggests that AD-specific lesions in the hippocampus disconnect central nuclei from their cortical projections and result in memory loss.

NORMAL AGING

In the first in vivo studies, correlations between cerebral atrophy as seen by PEG and normal and pathologic aging produced inconsistent results. This was in part due to the difficulty in acquiring normative data and is underscored by the following policy statement made in 1929 by the American Roentgen Ray Society: "It was realized that we cannot expect encephalographic procedures to be carried out on normal individuals and the best that we can do is declare our judgment as to what is approximately normal from a large number of negative encephalographic studies."[26]

In an early PEG study using planimetry, Heinrich[27] found that ventricular area increased with age, especially after 65 years of age. The subarachnoid spaces were also noted to enlarge. Andersen and coworkers[28] (cited by Jacobsen and Melchior[29]), reviewing the results of PEG performed on healthy male criminals, found that only 1 of 43 studies demonstrated moderate "internal" atrophy. Iivanainen[30] noted cortical atrophy increasing with age but found no correlation between ventricular size and age. Thus a consistent relation between ventricular or sulcal enlargement and aging had not been established in the PEG literature.

Studies of normal aging by CT, MRI, and PET have shown that the normal brain undergoes significant atrophic changes (Figs 15–2 to 15–5) without significant metabolic changes (Fig 15–6). When using the glucose analogue ^{18}F-deoxyglucose or ^{11}C-2-deoxyglucose and PET, no significant[31–33] or small differences[34] have been shown between the glucose utilization of young and elderly normals.

Studies of normal subjects by several methods of CT scan evaluation (Figs 15–7 and 15–8) have consistently found that the size of both ventricles (Fig 15–9) and cortical sulci increase with age.[32, 35–43] Ventricular size roughly doubles between the third and seventh decades. Preliminary quantification studies of sulci by using MRI (Fig

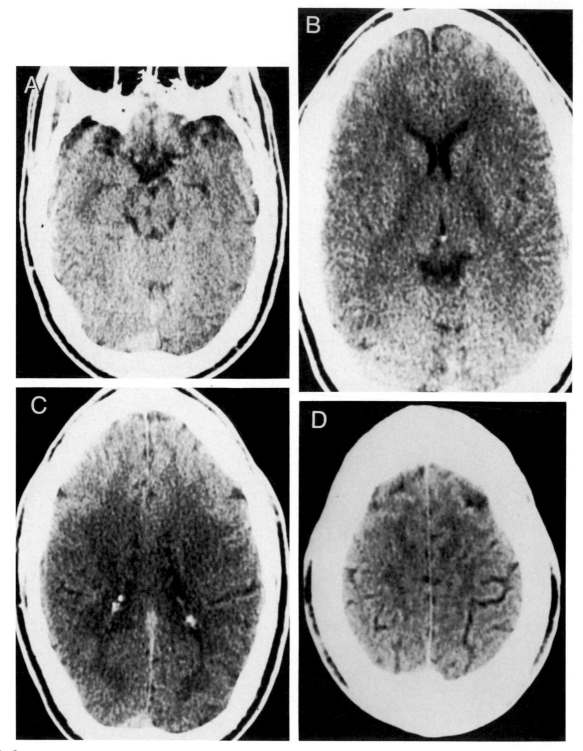

FIG 15–2.
CT of a normal 29-year-old male with the composite ventricular volume representing 5% of the brain. **A,** temporal lobe level. The temporal horns are of normal size. A hippocampal lucency is not present. **B,** basal ganglia level. The third ventricle is less than 5 mm in diameter. The internal capsule is clearly visualized bilaterally. Compare with the MRI of a young normal control in Figure 15–9,A. **C,** ventricular body level. **D,** high convexity. There is normal differentiation of gray and white structures. Sulci are approximately 3 to 4 mm in width.

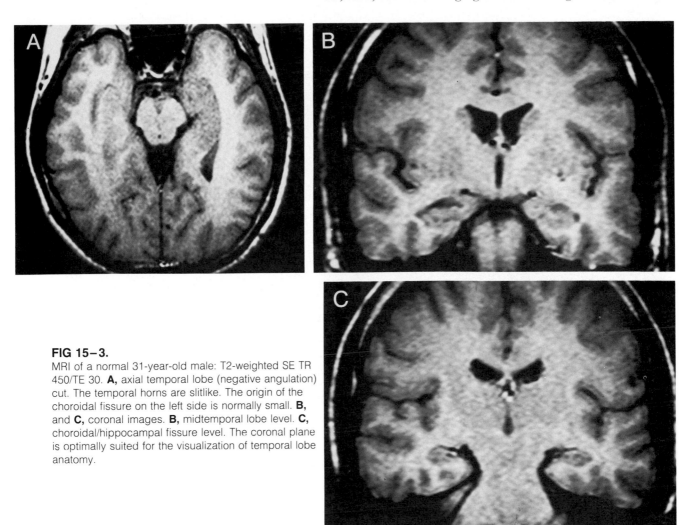

FIG 15–3.
MRI of a normal 31-year-old male: T2-weighted SE TR
450/TE 30. **A,** axial temporal lobe (negative angulation)
cut. The temporal horns are slitlike. The origin of the
choroidal fissure on the left side is normally small. **B,**
and **C,** coronal images. **B,** midtemporal lobe level. **C,**
choroidal/hippocampal fissure level. The coronal plane
is optimally suited for the visualization of temporal lobe
anatomy.

15–10) suggest a comparable or less severe enlargement during the life span. Many normal elderly individuals show no evidence or minimal evidence of ventricular enlargement while typically
showing evidence of cortical atrophy. Very rarely
"supernormal" elderly individuals show neither
ventricular nor sulcal atrophy. Occasionally, this is
seen even in great age.

Zatz and coworkers[44] studied CT attenuation
values in normal volunteers and found a decrease
with age in subjects over the age of 54 years. Cala
and coworkers[10] found no change in the attenuation of either white or gray matter in volunteers
under the age of 40 years. In our studies of normal
volunteers, we found no differences in the attenuation values of white matter (in the absence of leukoencephalopathy) of young normals when compared with old normals over the age of 65 years.
The results of gray matter assessments have not
been conclusive because of the technical difficul-

ties inherent in the derivation of reliable gray matter attenuation values. These difficulties are due in
part to the increase in attenuation values that occurs adjacent to the calvarium secondary to beam
hardening.[45]

In a recent MRI study of T2 relaxation values
of normal volunteers derived from a 6 echo spin
echo study using the 1.5-Tesla Philips supercon-
ducting magnet, we found a significant prolongation of T2 relaxation values in elderly normal individuals when compared with young normals.[46]
This is apparently due to an increase in water occurring in the normal aging brain. MRI will also
frequently show small foci of high signal on T2-
weighted images at the anterolateral aspects of the
frontal horns. This finding, attributed to a normal
variant, "ependymitis granularis,"[47] is very common in patients over the age of 60 years. In normal
individuals MRI will also often demonstrate on
T2-weighted images small (3 to 5 mm) high-signal

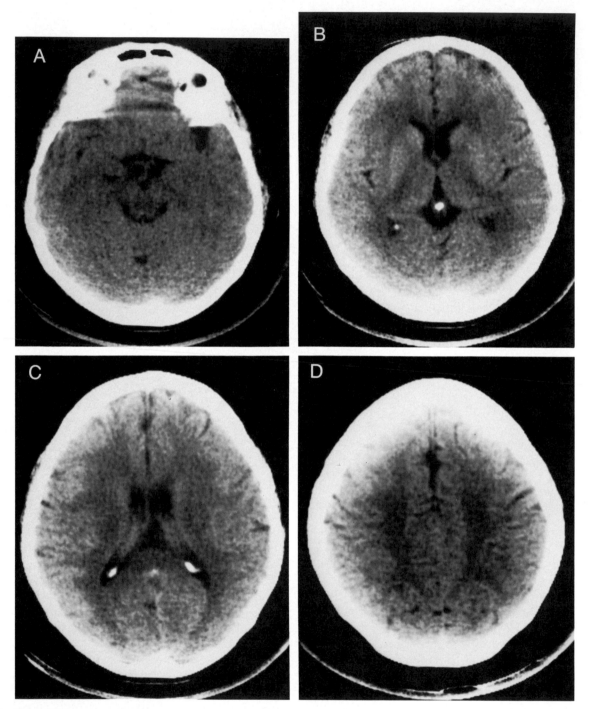

FIG 15–4.
CT of normal 65-year-old female control. The ventricular system shows only mild enlargement when compared with a young normal. There is mild sulcal prominence. **A,** temporal lobe level. **B,** basal ganglia. **C,** ventricular body level. **D,** centrum. Gray-white discrimination is excellent.

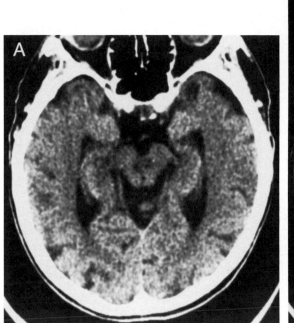
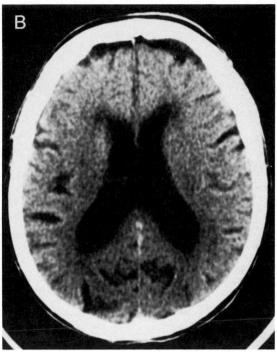

FIG 15–5.

CT of an 83-year-old female normal volunteer with leukoencephalopathy. Moderate to severe cortical and central atrophy is noted. Patchy periventricular lucencies are due to microvascular disease.

A, at the temporal lobe level (negative angle cut), hippocampal lucencies of moderate severity are present. **B,** ventricular body level.

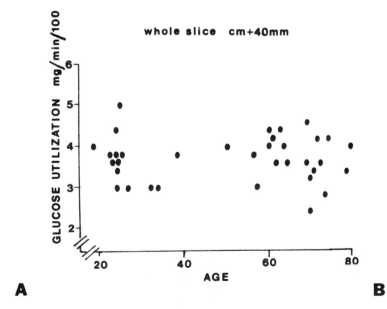
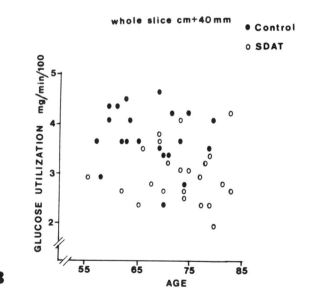

FIG 15–6.

Scattergrams. **A,** PET metabolic values, young vs. old normals. No difference is noted in the glucose utilization values for young vs. old. **B,** PET metabolic values, Alzheimer patients vs. normal control spouses. A significant difference is present in the two groups: $P <$ .01 of 7% to 25%.

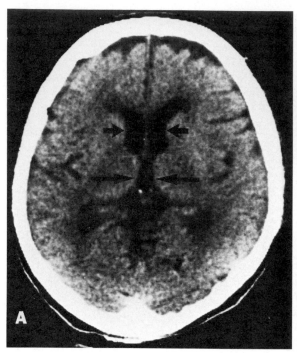
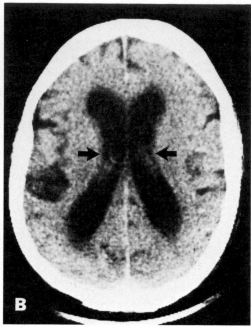

FIG 15–7.
Linear ventricular measurements utilized for CT analyses. **A,** basal ganglia level. The width of the third ventricle *(long arrows)*, bicaudate diameters *(short arrows)*, bifrontal span, and diagonal widths of the frontal horns were derived from this level. The maximal width of the cranium as measured from inner table to inner table was used for brain correction. **B,** ventricular body level. The cut showing the largest representations of the lateral ventricles was utilized. The waist of the two ventricles was measured at their narrowest point *(arrows)*. The width of the cranium from inner table to inner table was utilized for brain correction.

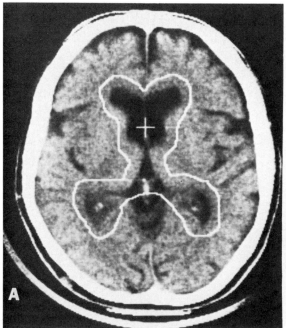
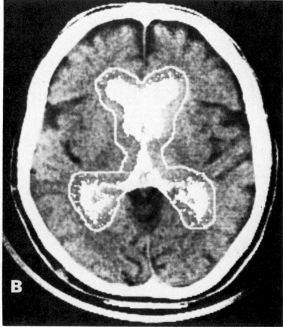

FIG 15–8.
Software derivation of ventricular volume. This procedure was utilized at every level to show ventricular structures, and summations of the ventricular volumes were obtained and corrected for brain size by dividing by the sum of the five greatest brain volumes. **A,** the region of interest is operator defined to include the ventricular structures of interest. A CSF range is then indicated by the operator. For these analyses, the range −11 to +25 Hounsfield units was utilized. **B,** computer-generated highlighting of the pixels falling within the range designated in **A.**

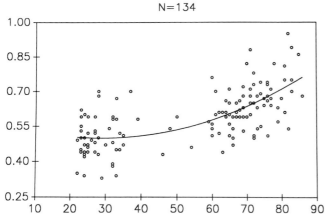

LINEAR VENTRICULAR SIZE AS A FUNCTION OF AGE
N=134

FIG 15–9.
Scattergram ventricular size as a function of age: CT cross-sectional study of normal volunteers. Ventricular size was determined by using a composite of linear measurements. Regression curve of the second order.

foci in the periventricular white matter. These sub-cortical hyperintensities (SCHs) or unidentified bright objects (UBOs) may be very extensive in entirely normal individuals (Fig 15–11) (see "Leukoencephalopathy of Aging" below).

In summary, structural changes as shown by

CT or MRI clearly occur with aging and most typically appear as progressive cortical atrophy and ventricular enlargement; it appears that glucose metabolism does not change significantly with the aging process.

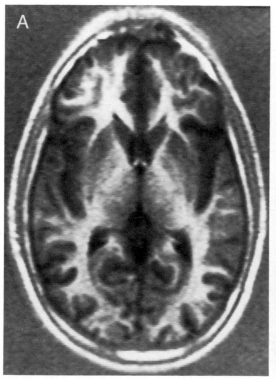

FIG 15–10.
MRI "dual-sequence scanning" of a normal control 35-year-old male. **A,** gray-white sequence (inversion-recovery, TR 1,400/TI 420/TE 30). There is excellent discrimination of gray and white structures. The globus pallidus can be differentiated into internal and external segments and is clearly differentiated from the putamen. **B,** CSF sequence (inversion-recovery, TR 5,000/TI 500/TE 100). This sequence nullifies signal from brain parenchyma while highlighting the signal from CSF.

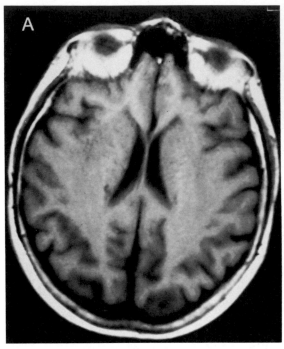

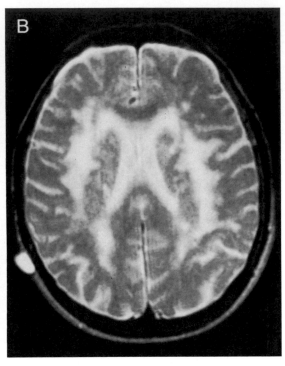

FIG 15–11.
MRI of a normal 79-year-old female control with severe leukoencephalopathy but without atrophy ("supernormal") and without cognitive or motor impairment. **A,** T1-weighted image (TR 566/TE 19) at the ventricular body level. **B,** a T2-weighted image at the same level (TR 2,088/TE 80) shows diffuse high-signal patchy lesions involving virtually the entire visualized white matter.

ALZHEIMER'S DISEASE

Neuropathologic Features

In addition to the presence of increased cerebral atrophy, senile plaques, neurofibrillary tangles, and granulovacuolar degeneration have been described as the histologic features of AD. These histologic features are also seen in normal aging but are much more common in the brains of Alzheimer patients who demonstrate extensive involvement of the cortex, especially of the temporal, parietal, and frontal lobes.[6, 48] *Plaque counts have been found to correlate with cortical atrophy but not ventricular dilatation.* This lack of correlation may be due to the distortion of the ventricular system that occurs in the brain after death due to postmortem changes, especially brain swelling. Marked temporal lobe atrophy was observed in the group with the highest plaque count. Furthermore, Blessed and colleagues[49] demonstrated a correlation between plaque counts and the severity of dementia.

More recent studies, however, have specifically implicated the medial temporal lobes in the pathogenesis of AD. In a quantitative neuropathologic study, Ball reported[23] that neuronal loss was much more severe in the hippocampi of Alzheimer brains when compared with normals and that both tangles and granulovacuoles were more common in the *posterior half of the hippocampus* in AD brains. Shefer[50] (cited by Ball[23]) found that neurons in seven brain regions including the subiculum showed a 20% loss in normal aging as compared with a 50% loss in AD. Hyman et al.[24, 25] reported marked cell loss in the subiculum and entorhinal cortex in Alzheimer brains as well as large numbers of neurofibrillary tangles in the subiculum and hippocampus. These affected structures normally interconnect the hippocampal formation with the cortex, the thalamus, and the hypothalamus, structures that are integral to memory. In effect, the hippocampus becomes isolated in Alzheimer patients. Therefore, since the earliest pathologic changes in AD may involve the medial temporal lobe, it follows that CT, MRI, and PET evaluations, whether for diagnostic or research purposes, should be tailored to optimally visualize the temporal lobes (see below).

Several neurotransmitter deficits have also been demonstrated in AD. It is, however, unclear whether these are the cause or the result of the disease. Loss of cortical acetylcholine transferase has been shown in the brains of senile dementia patients[51-54] and is apparently secondary to a loss of subcortical neurons of the basal nucleus of Meynert located below the ventral globus pallidus; the axons of this nucleus provide cholinergic innervation to the frontal and hippocampal cortex.[55] This connection has been confirmed in animal models.[56] Whitehouse and associates[57] showed a profound (>75%) loss of neurons of the basal nucleus of Meynert in the brains of patients with AD.

Significant reduction of norepinephrine concentration has also been shown in the gyrus frontalis and putamen of senile dementia patients.[58] Mann and coworkers[59] found reduced norepinephrine levels in several regions of the cerebral cortex that they attributed to a failure of the nucleus locus coeruleus in the brain stem. Bondareff and colleagues[60] found a loss of more than 80% of the locus coeruleus neurons in a subgroup of patients with high dementia scores, thus indicating a deficit of adrenergic innervation to the cortex.

The aforementioned studies suggest that the disintegration of cortical functions may result from the degeneration of brain stem and basal ganglia nuclei that project to the cortex.

Pneumoencephalographic Literature

Studies of dementia by PEG led to differing conclusions. Engeset and Lonnum[61] as well as Nielsen and colleagues[62, 63] found a correlation between ventricular size at PEG and intellectual impairment but with marked scatter. The width of the third ventricle and height of the left lateral ventricle appeared to be the individual measurements that corresponded best with intellectual impairment. The same authors found that cognitive impairment showed a closer correlation with sulcal than ventricular dilatation. On the other hand, Huber[64, 65] found that PEG brain atrophy associated with organic personality changes was usually central and presumably involved the white matter and the nuclei.

Gosling[66] reported that generalized cerebral atrophy was occasionally found in patients without impairment of intellectual functions. Mann[67] also showed that radiologic cortical atrophy at PEG could not be equated with dementia and that a third of the patients with demonstrable radiologic cortical atrophy were free of any evidence of dementia at 5- and 10-year follow-ups.

In summary, the PEG studies seemed to confirm that a relationship exists between dementia and sulcal as well as ventricular enlargement, with some studies supporting a closer correlation with cortical atrophy.

Review of Early CT Literature

The advent of CT promised the realization of a heretofore impossible task, the noninvasive visualization of the brain in vivo. It was assumed on the basis of the pathology and PEG literature that cortical atrophy and ventricular enlargement would represent the in vivo anatomic correlates of dementia. Confidence in this preconceived notion was so strong that early CT interpretations, despite the lack of established norms, frequently included the diagnosis of "cerebral atrophy." It soon became apparent that there were problems with this basic concept as previously noted in the PEG literature: (1) many patients with cerebral atrophy were not demented, and (2) many patients with dementia did not demonstrate obvious atrophy. Consequently, early CT studies of dementia produced inconsistent results. In these early CT studies, measures of CT structural change represented attempts to quantitate cerebral atrophy by estimating the amount of cerebrospinal fluid (CSF) within the cranial cavity. Several investigators[68-70] found no significant correlation between psychometric scores and CT assessment of cerebral atrophy. Nathan and Frumkin[70] studied community-residing persons over 65 years of age with CT and subtests of the Wexler Adult Intelligence Scale (WAIS). For CT groups rated as showing minimal, moderate, or advanced atrophy, no differences were found for any of the cognitive measures except one, the Mental Health Rating Scale. (The authors do not specify whether sulci were evaluated in the atrophy rating.) Similarly, Claveria and associates[69] tested 81 patients diagnosed on the basis of CT as having cerebral atrophy and found no correlation between ventricular and sulcal atrophic changes seen on CT and psychometric test performance. Hughes and Gado[68] found no significant correlation between psychometric scores (the Clinical Dementia Rating) and CT measurements of ventricular and sulcal enlargement in a group of 100 hospital patients over the age of 65 years.

Other studies including our own[71-79] (Figs 15-8 and 15-12) found significant relationships between ventricular size and cognitive deficit. The correlations, however, were relatively weak. Measuring ventricular area by planimeter, Roberts and Caird[77] demonstrated a "broad" relation between increasing ventricular dilatation and intellectual impairment as measured by the Chricton Behav-

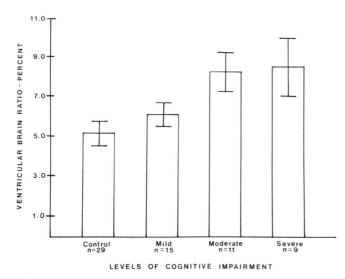

FIG 15–12.
Bar graphs of mean ventricular volume (ventricular brain ratio percentage) and standard error of the mean for different levels of cognitive impairment. Global Deterioration Scale (GDS) scores of 1 and 2 = control group; GDS of 3 = mild impairment group; GDS of 4 = moderate impairment; GDS of 5, 6, and 7 = severe group. The largest increment in ventricular volume is noted between the mild group (*n* = 15) and the moderate group (*n* = 11).

ioral Rating Scale and the 30-point memory test. No relationship was demonstrated between measures of cortical atrophy and the psychometrics. Earnest and coworkers[78] concluded that CT evidence of atrophy only weakly predicted impaired mental function. Jacoby and Levy[79] found that demented subjects showed significantly more CT evidence of atrophy than did normal controls, but with considerable overlap.

In our initial studies, we derived a large number of linear and subjective measures in search of the best descriptors of structural change in AD.[72–75, 80] We found consistent relationships between ventricular as well as sulcal enlargement and cognitive impairment, but the correlations were relatively weak ($p < .03$, $r = .42$). Contrary to expectations, ventricular dilatation was a significantly better correlate of dementia than was cortical atrophy. In these early studies, these results were most likely due to the poor resolution of cortical changes by CT due to beam hardening by the adjacent calvarium. Subsequent work with thin-section CT and with MRI (see below) has shown that the earliest changes are indeed cortical and probably localized to the temporal lobes. Of the linear measures obtained in the early studies, the width of the third ventricle was the strongest cor-

relate with dementia, thereby lending support to the hypothesis that significant alterations occur at the level of the basal ganglia and the base of the brain in dementia.

These findings therefore reaffirm that relationships do exist between structural changes as demonstrated by CT and cognitive impairment and that the structural changes of AD are superimposed and overlap with the structural changes of normal aging. Ventricular volume determinations using algorithm summation of pixels falling within a specified range (see Fig 15–8) and corrected for brain size (ventricular-brain ratio) was significantly larger (44%) in the Alzheimer patients than in normal controls ($p < .01$) but with considerable overlap (see Fig 15–12).[72] The mean for the normal elderly group was 5.2 ± 3, and for the Alzheimer group it was 7.5 ± 3. Furthermore, ventricular volume increased with increasing cognitive deficit ($p < .05$, $r = 4.2$). Thus the strength of the correlations with psychometrics remained weak despite the use of more precise estimates of ventricular size. Gado and coworkers[71] in an earlier report used a similar method to study the ventricular and sulcal size of community-residing volunteers. Highly significant ($p < .0001$) differences were found between the normal and impaired groups. Ventricular volume corrected for brain size was 5.3% ($\pm$ 1.9%) in controls and 10.5% ($\pm$ 4.8%) in the impaired group. Sulcal size was 6.1% $\pm$ 2.5% and 10.6% $\pm$ 3.3%, respectively. Linear measures showed less pronounced differences between the normal and impaired groups. The authors concluded that the conflicting results in the literature concerning variations in ventricular and sulcal size in dementia and normal aging were in part a reflection of the insensitivity of linear measures. Subsequent evidence (see below) indicates that ventricular and diffuse cortical changes are late and insensitive indicators of AD.

Parenchymal Measures

Gray-White Matter Discriminability
Impressed by the variability that exists in the density differences between gray and white matter structures in different patients, we tested a variable that we called gray-white matter discriminability[80] to assess its relationship to cognitive impairment. Gray-white matter discriminability, defined as the subjective contrast between central

white matter and cortical gray matter, was rated in a group of Alzheimer patients studied with an early Philips 200 translation-rotation scanner. Loss of gray-white matter discriminability was significantly ($P < .05$) related to the severity of cognitive impairment and to ventricular size. No correlation was found between loss of discriminability and age. This study suggested the presence of parenchymal CT changes in AD that were more pronounced at the cortical level. Subsequent neuropathologic and MRI evidence indicates that the loss of gray-white discriminability most likely re-

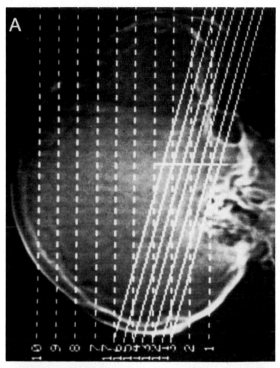

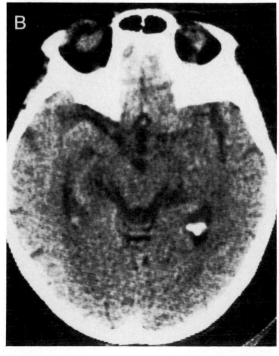

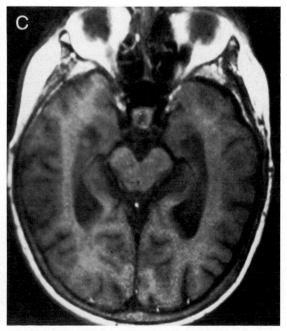

FIG 15–13.
Negative-angle scanning for optimal visualization of the temporal lobes. **A,** CT scannogram with temporal lobe cuts (20 degrees negative to the canthomeatal line) superimposed on routine 10-mm cuts parallel to the CM line. **B,** CT scan with a negative-angle cut of the temporal lobe in a 71-year-old female with mild dementia. There is moderate right temporal lobe atrophy with enlargement of the temporal horns and moderate hippocampal lucencies bilaterally. **C,** same patient 2 years later: T1-weighted negative-angle MRI (TR 450/TE 30, 5-mm cut). The hippocampal lucencies are moderate. Medial and lateral cortical atrophy is of moderate severity.

flects attenuation of the cortical ribbon due to a loss of gray matter.[13, 14]

CT Attenuation Values in Dementia

Studies of CT attenuation values in normal aging[40, 44] have shown a decrease in white matter attenuation values after the age of 56 years. Naeser et al[81] found decreasing attenuation values with increasing dementia. Because all of the dementia patients also demonstrated atrophy, it is possible that the decrease in attenuation values reflected in part a sampling of increasing sulcal CSF. Gado and as-

sociates[82] found no difference between dementia patients and controls. Gray-white matter difference scores did not correlate with cognitive scores but were significantly related to ventricular size. This result was in agreement with our previous finding that subjective gray-white matter discriminability was related to ventricular enlargement and especially the width of the third ventricle.[80] Several other studies have addressed the question of attenuation changes in dementia[83, 84] with variable results. It appears from the above that in the absence of leukoencephalopathy (see below) normal aging is not associated with changes in attenuation val-

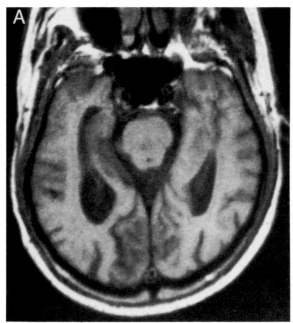

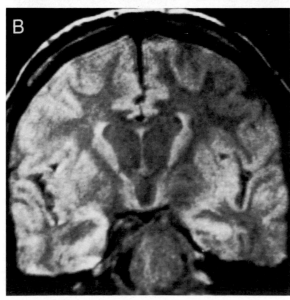

FIG 15–14.
MRI features of AD in a 63-year-old male. **A,** negative-angle temporal lobe T1-weighted cuts (TR 450/TE 30) show bilateral temporal horn dilatation right more than left and a right-sided hippocampal "lucency." **B,** coronal mixed-sequence spin-echo MRI (TR 2,100/TE 30) shows severe atrophy of the right temporal lobe with dilatation of the right temporal horn. Left-sided atrophic changes are moderate. An increased band of abnormal signal involves the medial and inferior temporal cortex, more so on the right. **C,** a ventricular body-level T1-weighted image shows the ventricular and sulcal enlargement to be moderate and within normal limits for age.

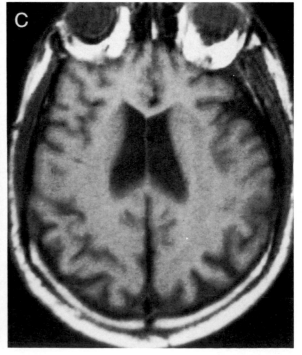

ues, at least of white matter, nor is there convincing evidence of a difference in the attenuation values of Alzheimer and normal subjects.

Radiologic Features (CT, MRI, PET) of Alzheimer's Disease

Supported by the neuropathology studies described above, recent radiologic studies[9–13] have shown that focal structural changes of the temporal lobes may be the earliest manifestations of AD. The use of "negative-angle" thin-section cuts with CT or MRI, i.e., a plane parallel with the temporal lobe (Fig 15–13) will visualize the temporal lobe changes to best advantage. MRI studies, in addition to showing improved contrast resolution, are also able to demonstrate the brain and temporal lobes in the coronal plane (Fig 15–14). The temporal lobe changes are often asymmetrical, involving one temporal lobe more than the other. These changes include dilatation of the temporal horns, medial and lateral atrophy and the presence of a hippocampal "lucency" (Figs 15–13,B and C; 15–14,A; 15–15,A; 15–16,A; and 15–17,A and F). Neuropathologic correlations with CT and MRI indicate that the hippocampal lucency represents dilatation of the choroidal-hippocampal fissure complex (Figs 15–15 and 15–18). Dilatation of these spaces indicates atrophy of the adjacent subiculum and hippocampus, and this has been specifically implicated in the neuropathologic studies described above. Hippocampal lucency shows the highest accuracy in the identification of AD.[9, 13] *Temporal lobe atrophy is present in virtually all patients with the diagnosis of AD;* however, as many as 45% of normal elderly individuals may show a mild to moderate degree of temporal lobe atrophy. Therefore, the absence of temporal lobe atrophy is a sign of very high specificity, i.e., identifies true normals. Dual-sequence MRI[14] (see Fig 15–10,A and B) has for the first time permitted the in vivo quantitation of gray matter, white matter, and CSF within the cranial cavity. The first study (see Fig 15–10,A) is an inversion-recovery sequence (TR 5,000/TI 490/TE 100) that highlights the signal from CSF while virtually eliminating the signal from brain. The second sequence (see Fig 15–10,B) (inversion-recovery, TR 1,400/TI 420/TE 30) highlights parenchymal white matter signal while dampening the signal from gray matter. By coregistering the regions of interest (ROI) and doing a pixel-by-pixel analysis that includes subtracting the CSF measurement of the first sequence from the second sequence the amounts of gray and white matter can be quantitated. Initial studies have shown that there is a selective loss of gray matter in the temporal lobes and cerebral hemispheres of AD patients when compared with normal controls.[14]

Temporal lobe atrophic changes are progressive when studied in a longitudinal manner.[85] Our work has demonstrated different rates of clinical

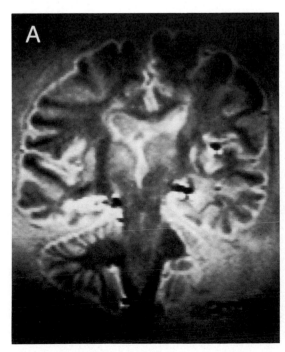
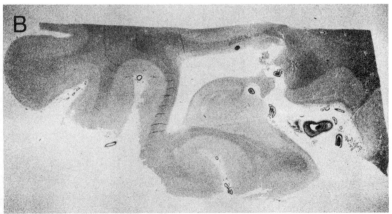

FIG 15–15.
Radiologic pathologic correlation of a severe hippocampal lucency in a 74-year-old male with severe dementia due to AD. **A,** postmortem coronal MRI (TR 2,100/TE 30) shows dilated hippocampal/choroidal fissures bilaterally with trapped air. **B,** a coronal histopathologic specimen with Luxol fast blue/periodic acid–Schiff (PAS) stain shows marked atrophy of the parahippocampal gyrus and of the hippocampal formation and severe dilatation of the choroidal fissure.

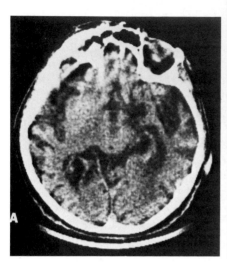
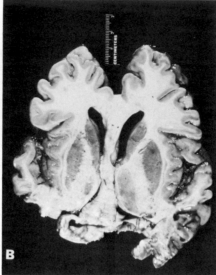
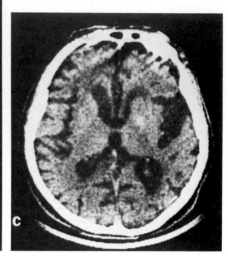

FIG 15–16.
Alzheimer brain CT neuropathologic correlation in an 83-year-old woman with severe AD. The patient was only able to utter unintelligible sounds. **A,** a basal CT cut shows marked shrinkage of the temporal lobes and dilatation of the sylvian fissures. The temporal horns are also enlarged, and the anterior third ventricle is dilated. **B,** a pathologic section through the basal ganglia shows marked shrinkage of the temporal gyri bilaterally. The cortical ribbon of gray matter is markedly shrunken. A large number of plaques and tangles was shown histologically to involve the entire temporal and frontal cortex. **C,** basal ganglia CT cut with moderate enlargement of the ventricular system and moderately severe dilatation of the sulci. The gaping sylvian fissures, especially on the left side, are again demonstrated.

deterioration over a 2- to 3-year interval. The rapidly deteriorating patients will show progressive structural changes, typically with increasing atrophy of the temporal lobes (see Fig 15–17) and to a lesser extent progressive involvement of the parietal lobes as well as the rest of the cerebral cortex. AD and dementia, however, may be associated with severe temporal lobe atrophy in the absence of otherwise marked ventricular or generalized cortical atrophy (see Figs 15–14 and 15–16). These findings are shown in Figure 15–16, which depicts the antemortem CT and postmortem neuropathologic correlation in an 83-year-old woman with severe AD. Severe atrophic temporal lobe changes are present, but there is only moderate dilatation of the lateral ventricle bodies. Notice the marked enlargement of the left choroidal/hippocampal fissure complex in Figure 15–16,A.

Naguib and Levy[86] re-evaluated ten AD patients after 2 years by CT assessments of ventricular areas and psychometric testing. The results indicated that the five patients who were more impaired at follow-up showed a significantly greater increase in ventricular size than did the five stable patients. Initial ventricular measurements did not predict further decline. Gado et al.[87] studied 21 mild AD patients and 21 controls on two occasions separated by a 1-year interval. Using linear measurements they found that the AD group had a greater longitudinal rate of ventricular change. Brinkman and Largen[88] followed up five significantly demented patients with a second CT after 15 to 35 months. The results indicated that the patients had rates of linear ventricular change that exceeded those predicted from published cross-sectional normative data. Our longitudinal studies using CT (and CT in conjunction with MRI) on 45 AD patients and 50 controls showed a rate of ventricular enlargement that was four times greater than normal in the Alzheimer patients.[85] We also found a small subgroup that demonstrated intellectual decline in the absence of ventricular or cortical change.

In metabolic imaging with PET the glucose analogue 2-deoxyglucose (2-DG) is labeled with a positron emitter such as ^{11}C or ^{18}F. During a 30- to 40-minute uptake period following intravenous or intra-arterial injection the ^{11}C-2-DG is phosphorylated and trapped by the cells. No further metabolism of the glucose analogue occurs in contradiction to glucose, which is normally metabolized by the cells. This permits imaging of the distribution of trapped ^{11}C-DG-6-PO$_4$ in the brain by the PET scanner. Each positron emitted travels a very short

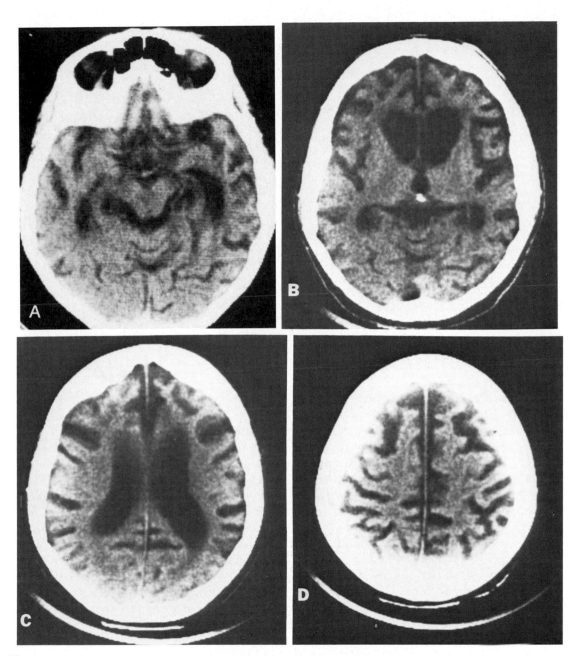

FIG 15–17.
A, temporal cut. There is atrophy of the temporal lobes with enlargement of the sylvian fissures and temporal horns. Bilateral hippocampal lucencies are present. **B,** a basal ganglia cut shows marked dilatation of the sulci and fissures, especially frontally, with marked enlargement of the frontal horns. This pattern is essentially indistinguishable from Huntington's disease and Pick's disease. Visualization of gray and white structures is very poor. **C,** ventricular body level. Note the asymmetrical enlargement of the ventricular system, with the left lateral ventricle somewhat larger than the right accentuating this frequently seen normal variation. **D,** high convexity level. The frontal as well as parietal and central sulci are markedly dilated. The frontal fissures and sulci, however, are involved to a somewhat greater degree than the remaining sulci.

(Continued.)

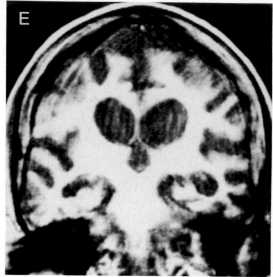

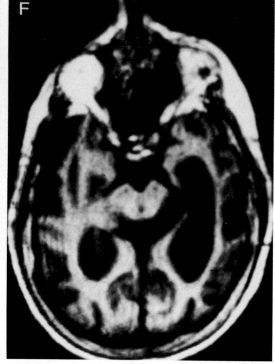

FIG 15–17 (cont.).
E and **F,** MRI obtained 3 years following the CT scan shows marked progression of diffuse cerebral as well as temporal lobe atrophy. **E,** a coronal T1-weighted image shows bilateral temporal lobe atrophy on the left more than the right. **F,** axial T1-weighted image with a marked hippocampal lucency on the left and extremely severe dilatation of both temporal horns, the left more than the right.

distance in brain matter and collides with an electron, and the two are annihilated, thereby producing two high-energy photons (511 keV) traveling in diametrically opposite directions. It is these coincident x-rays that are detected by the PET scanner. The actual metabolic values are then derived with the use of an operational equation[89] in conjunction with ^{11}C-DG values derived from serial blood samples, the published average measured lumped constant,[90] and the average gray matter kinetic constants for k1, k2, and k3.[89]

PET scanning using labeled glucose analogues has shown diffuse metabolic brain deficits in AD, but with the most severe changes involving the temporal (approximately 28% deficit)[91–93] (Figs 15–6,B, and 15–19) and parietal lobes.[94, 95] These changes are in keeping with the structural atrophy shown by CT and MRI. Similar results are being shown by single-photon–emission computed tomography (SPECT) with the use of ^{123}I-iodoamphetamine or other markers of cerebral perfusion.[96, 97] These neuroimaging changes shown by CT, MRI, PET, and SPECT parallel the distribution of neuropathologic changes, i.e., plaques and tangles seen in AD.

It is unclear from the work to date whether the metabolic reductions seen in AD secondarily reflect the disease process and resulting atrophy or whether the metabolic derangement represents part of the primary pathology. In these PET studies measures of glucose metabolism will be depressed both in atrophy as well as in the presence of metabolic dysfunction. In an effort to address this question, recent in vitro studies of brain microvessel transport activity in our laboratory[98] have shown that glucose uptake as well as phosphorylation are decreased in tissue derived from AD brains. These results suggest that the decreased glucose utilization in AD that is shown by PET is due to pathologic metabolism rather than a reflection of cerebral atrophy.

In summary, contrary to the previously widely held belief that the role of structural studies in the diagnosis of AD is one of exclusion, recent studies have shown strong evidence that AD may be diagnosed in life by neuroimaging techniques. Focal temporal lobe atrophic changes are highly sensitive and early markers of AD. In addition, the importance of temporal lobe metabolic and blood flow changes has been shown in the PET literature by several groups including our own. Typically, PET studies of glucose metabolism show a prefer-

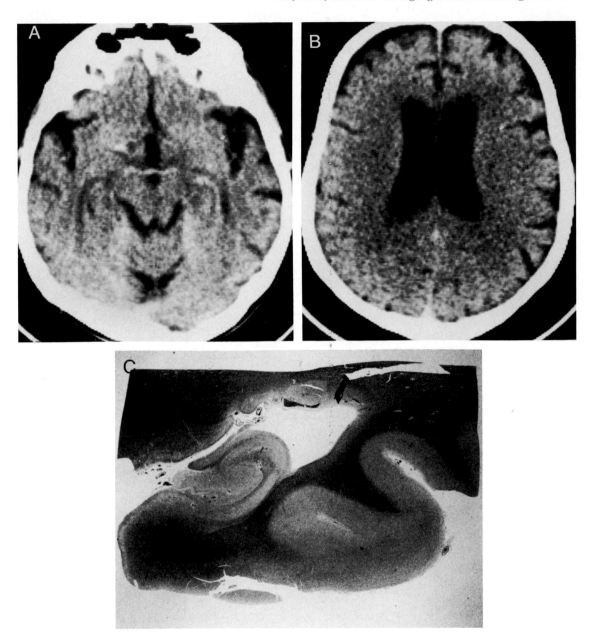

FIG 15–18.
Radiologic pathologic correlation of a 64-year-old male patient with cerebral atrophy and a normal hippocampal lucency. There is no pathologic evidence of AD. **A** and **B,** premortem CT shows only mild enlargement of the temporal horns and minimal hippocampal lucencies. The ventricles are moderately enlarged. **C,** a coronal postmortem histopathologic specimen (Luxol fast blue/PAS) shows an enlarged temporal horn. The choroidal fissure is present but not enlarged. The parahippocampal gyrus and the hippocampal formation are intact. Compare with Figure 15–15,B.

ential metabolic reduction, and SPECT studies show a perfusion deficit[97] in the temporal and parietal lobes of Alzheimer patients when compared with normals and patients with (normal-pressure) hydrocephalus.[99]

CT and MRI temporal lobe changes are much more evident in patients under the age of 60 years because of the absence of the normally expected age-related atrophy. These Alzheimer changes include dilatation of the subarachnoid spaces as well as widening of the temporal horn and the presence of a characteristic hippocampal lesion presenting on CT as a lucency and on MRI as a low signal focus on T1- and a high signal focus on T2-weighted images. These changes are progressive in patients who show clinical decline; however, approxi-

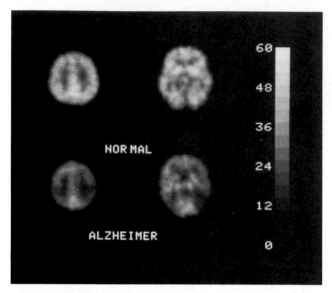

FIG 15–19.
PET scanning of AD *(bottom row)* vs. an elderly spouse control *(upper row):* PET VI study using ^{11}C-DG. Glucose utilization is expressed in micromoles per 100 g of tissue per minute (gray scale). The AD patient shows lower metabolic activity for the temporal and parietal lobes. *Right,* basal ganglia level; *left,* centrum level 7 cm above CM line. Overall (global) metabolic values are also reduced in the AD patient.

mately 50% of subjects with the diagnosis of AD remain stable at 2- to 3-year follow-up and show no evidence of progression of temporal lobe or cerebral atrophy. Progression of the disease results in diffuse ventricular as well as cortical atrophy, although the temporal lobe changes tend to be more advanced in all stages of the disease.

LEUKOENCEPHALOPATHY IN NORMAL AND PATHOLOGIC AGING

Thirty percent of atrophy (presumed AD) patients and 16% of normal controls demonstrate periventricular white matter lucencies (leukoencephalopathy) on CT (see Fig 15–5).[100, 101] The prevalence of white matter regions is much higher when using MRI (see Fig 15–11).[102] Originally described as "mysterious white matter lucencies in the elderly" on early CT scans, these lesions came to be known as "UBOs," or unidentified bright objects on MRI. This leukoencephalopathy is age dependent and shows increasing prevalence over the age of 60 years.[100] Hachinski et al. have proposed the term "leuko-araiosis," or white matter thinning, to describe these lesions.[103, 104]

Autopsy work including our own[100, 105–108] has shown hypertensive-type changes in the white matter that consist of patches of demyelination associated with hyalinosis of the arterioles and rarefaction of the white matter. Brun and Englund[109] have suggested that these lesions are associated with hypotension rather than hypertension. Bradley et al.[110] identified these changes as an incidental finding in sequential MRI scans of elderly patients. We have found that these brain changes are related to impairment of the motor activity, gait disturbances, hypertension, and as noted above, increasing age.[100, 111] An increased incidence of falls in the elderly has also been reported in the presence of leukoencephalopathy.[112] Although MRI is highly sensitive to the identification of these lesions, its specificity is poor.[113] It should be stressed that the presence of leukoencephalopathy in the elderly can be a normal finding (see Fig 15–11) and should not be interpreted as an indication of dementia.

The presence of leukoencephalopathy in patients who have AD may in fact potentiate the severity of the dementia as shown by autopsy studies (Fig 15–20).[100] This increased patient burden (AD plus leukoencephalopathy) is supported by PET studies showing that AD patients with leukoencephalopathy have milder reductions in glucose metabolism in the temporal and parietal lobes (i.e., less severe evidence of AD) than equally impaired patients without leukoencephalopathy.[93, 114]

Multi-infarct Dementia, Vascular Dementia, and Binswanger's Disease

There is considerable confusion with regard to these terms. Multiple infarcts, whether cortical or subcortical, especially when bilateral, may result in dementia (Figs 15–21 and 15–22).[115–118] Functional disability and dementia, however, may be surprisingly limited despite the presence of severe multiple subcortical lesions when these lesions are limited to the white matter. Gray matter lesions, whether cortical or deep, may be associated with profound intellectual and memory deficits. Binswanger[119] described a slowly progressive disease characterized by a loss of memory and intellectual impairment associated with recurrent neurologic deficits. What Binswanger described was apparently a multi-infarct dementia with hypertensive small-vessel changes and multiple cortical infarcts. The presence of periventricular lucencies on CT or high-intensity lesions on T2-weighted MRI should not be interpreted as "Binswanger disease" or multi-infarct dementia unless first it can be established (by T1-weighted MRI images, CT,

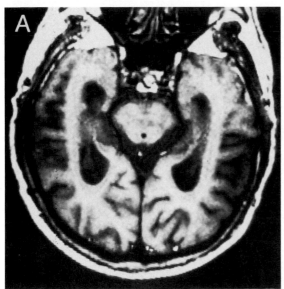

FIG 15–20.
AD with superimposed leukoencephalopathy: MRI of a 70-year-old male. **A,** negative-angle T1-weighted temporal lobe cuts show advanced Alzheimer-type changes with dilatation of the temporal horns, cortical atrophy, and bilateral severe hippocampal lucencies. **B,** in a coronal T1-weighted image the temporal lobe atrophic changes are more severe on the right side. **C,** intermediate-weighted coronal cuts show marked atrophy of both temporal lobes with abnormally increased signal of the atrophic temporal cortices bilaterally. In addition, there are diffuse high-signal patches involving the periventricular white matter.

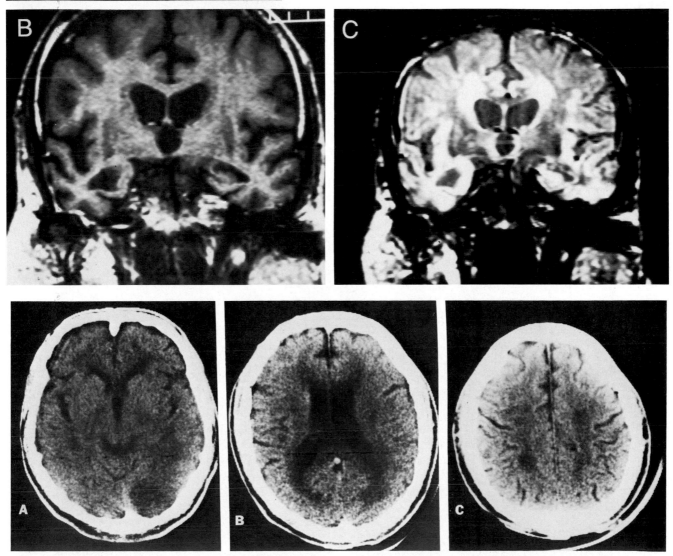

FIG 15–21.
Multi-infarct dementia: enlarged ventricles in an elderly man. **A,** basal ganglia level. A left occipital infarct is present. There are also lucencies in the frontal white matter bilaterally. **B,** ventricular body level. Patchy radiolucencies throughout the white matter are con-sistent with the demyelinated patches of subcortical microvascular disease. Note the more discrete lucencies indicating the presence of lacunar infarcts. **C,** high centrum semiovale cut. Scattered white matter lucencies are again seen as well as lacunar infarcts.

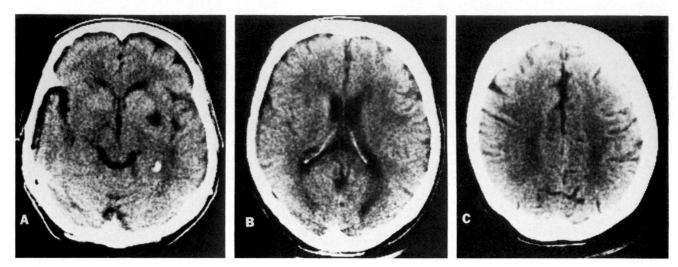

FIG 15–22.

Multi-infarct dementia (normal ventricular system) in an elderly man. **A,** basal ganglia level. A large lacunar infarct is situated in the left striate region. **B,** ventricular body level. Findings are similar to Figure 15–21,B. Patchy radiolucencies are scattered throughout the white matter, but the ventricular system is not enlarged. **C,** centrum semiovale level. Multiple lucencies indicate the presence of demyelinated patches.

SPECT, or PET) that multiple infarcts are present and second that the patient is indeed demented.

PICK'S DISEASE

This is a rare cause of dementia originally described in 1892.[120] The diagnosis is usually made at autopsy. The onset of Pick's disease is often in the presenile age group. A familial occurrence has been reported, and the course of the disease is more rapid than AD. Both on CT and at neuropathology[121] frontal and temporal lobe atrophy are typically present with dilatation of the frontal and temporal horns (Fig 15–23).[122, 123] Pathologically, there is severe nerve cell loss, and intracytoplas-

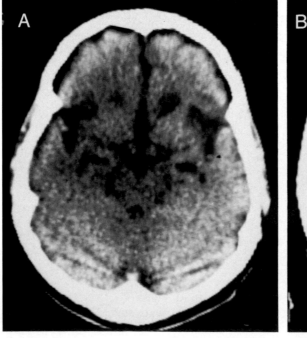
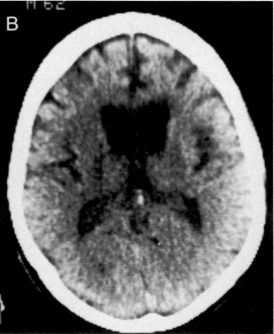

FIG 15–23.

Autopsy-proven Pick's disease in a 62-year-old male. The frontal horns are dilated, and there is evidence of frontal lobe and tempo-ral atrophy. These radiologic features are not sufficiently character-istic to differentiate from AD.

mic argentophilic bodies (Pick's bodies), eosinophilic inclusions (Hirano bodies), and granulovacuolar degeneration are present. By CT or MRI the diagnosis of Pick's disease can be suggested in the presence of advanced atrophy of both the frontal and temporal lobes. However, AD may also present with this type of pattern.

COMMUNICATING HYDROCEPHALUS

Hydrocephalus can be defined as increased intracranial CSF due either to an obstruction of the normal flow and absorption of CSF or rarely due to the overproduction of CSF. Hydrocephalus is intially associated with increased intracranial pressure but may later reach a state of equilibrium known as arrested or normal-pressure hydrocephalus (NPH). An increased intracranial CSF volume also occurs in cerebral atrophy, in which case CSF

simply occupies the space of the degenerated brain. Atrophy is sometimes referred to as "hydrocephalus ex vacuo." The latter term should be avoided in order not to create confusion between hydrocephalus and atrophy.

Hakim and Adams[124] described an idiopathic form of communicating hydrocephalus known as normal-pressure hydrocephalus. The classic clinical triad includes gait impairment, described originally as magnetic gait, dementia, and urinary incontinence. In diagnostically unequivocal cases of NPH symptoms are relieved by shunting. The most dramatic improvement is shown in the gait impairment associated with the hydrocephalus. Dementia may or may not improve after shunting.

The differentiation between hydrocephalus and atrophy can be very difficult in the elderly. The cardinal CT features of (communicating) hydrocephalus (Fig 15–24) are early dilatation and rounding of the temporal horns in the absence of

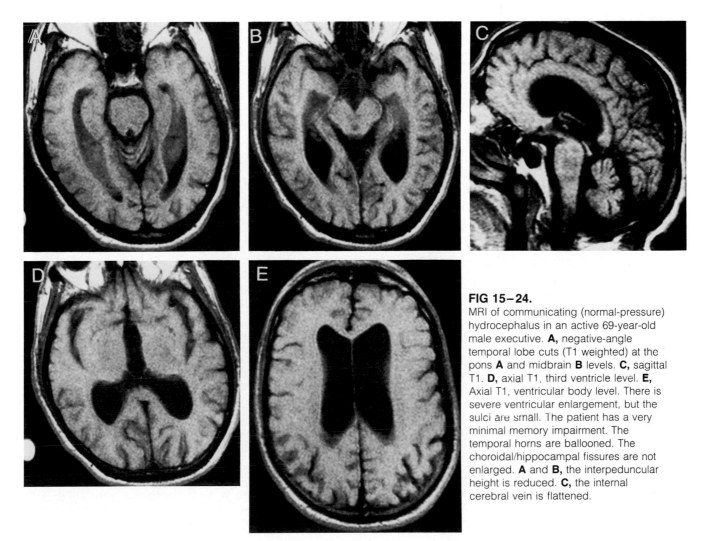

FIG 15–24.
MRI of communicating (normal-pressure) hydrocephalus in an active 69-year-old male executive. **A,** negative-angle temporal lobe cuts (T1 weighted) at the pons **A** and midbrain **B** levels. **C,** sagittal T1. **D,** axial T1, third ventricle level. **E,** Axial T1, ventricular body level. There is severe ventricular enlargement, but the sulci are small. The patient has a very minimal memory impairment. The temporal horns are ballooned. The choroidal/hippocampal fissures are not enlarged. **A** and **B,** the interpeduncular height is reduced. **C,** the internal cerebral vein is flattened.

temporal lobe cortical atrophy and in the absence of a hippocampal lucency, rounding and enlargement of the frontal horns, ballooning and rounding of the third ventricle, dilatation of the bodies of the lateral ventricles, and enlargement of the fourth ventricle. Typically patients are only minimally impaired (see Fig 15–24) by comparison with atrophy patients with comparable ventricular size. Discriminability of gray and white structures is preserved or accentuated in hydrocephalus. The presence of sulcal effacement is strongly supportive of the diagnosis of hydrocephalus. The presence of sulcal dilatation, however, does not rule out hydrocephalus. The height of the interpeduncular fossa as shown by sagittal MRI is decreased in hydrocephalus.[125] MRI may also demonstrate a periventricular T2 halo even in chronic hydrocephalus. A signal void in the aqueduct and third ventricle indicates that these channels are patent but does not help differentiate hydrocephalus from atrophy.[126]

Reports in the literature including our own have shown deficits in cerebral blood flow[127–131]

and glucose metabolism[99, 132] when using PET and deoxyglucose in association with hydrocephalus. The characteristic focal temporal lobe metabolic and perfusion deficits seen in AD are often absent in hydrocephalus.[99] This difference may permit differentiation of hydrocephalus from atrophy in difficult cases. Metabolic deficits may be reversed by shunting procedures. However, glucose metabolism *depression* even in the face of marked clinical improvement has also been reported after shunting of NPH.[132] This finding suggests that in NPH the brain is hypermetabolic prior to ventricular shunting, presumably as a response to the hydrocephalus.

PARKINSON'S DISEASE

Parkinson's disease (PD) is a subcortical degenerative disease of the extrapyramidal system

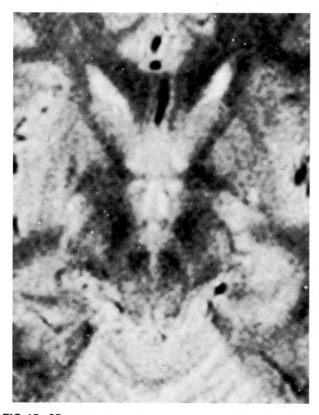

FIG 15–25.
Normal visualization of the brain stem nuclei of a 64-year-old male: spin-echo, 1.5 tesla (TR 2,100/TE 60). The substantia nigra and red nuclei are clearly visualized. They are separated by a normal pars compacta.

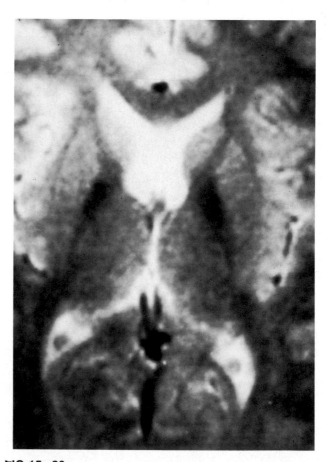

FIG 15–26.
Normal visualization of the globus pallidus of a 47-year-old male on a T2-weighted image: 1.5-tesla scan, spin-echo (TR 2,100/TE 60, 6-mm cut). The globus pallidus shows normally decreased signal when compared with the putamen.

that is characterized by neuronal loss of the pars compacta (Fig 15–25 for normal anatomy) of the substantia nigra, depigmentation, and the presence of intracytoplasmic Lewy bodies.[133]

Patients exhibit bradykinesia, cogwheel rigidity, and resting tremor. Midbrain MRI changes, specifically thinning of the pars compacta, has been suggested as a possible diagnostic feature of PD.[134, 135] CT and MRI studies otherwise may only show age-related atrophy.

There is a group of neurologic entities that mimic PD but do not respond to antiparkinsonian drug therapy. These conditions have similar and overlapping features and have been lumped into the category "Parkinson-plus syndrome"; these include Shy-Drager syndrome, or multiple-system atrophy, olivopontocerebellar atrophy, and striatonigral degeneration. A characteristic decrease in signal intensity of the putamen has been described in Parkinson's-plus[136, 137] due to abnormally increased concentration of iron in the putamen and to a lesser degree the caudate neuclus and the pars compacta of the substantia nigra. Conse-

quently, these structures show lower signal intensity than the globus pallidus. Normally, especially with high–field strength MRI, the globus pallidus shows the most marked signal decrease in the basal ganglia (Fig 15–26). The neuropathologic features of AD and associated dementia are also seen in at least one third of parkinsonian patients.[138, 139] These similarities raise interesting and as yet unanswered questions about a possible relationship between AD and PD.

PET studies of PD have produced some very exciting results. The DOPA analogue 6-fluoro-L-DPOA (6-FD) labeled with ^{18}F accumulates in brain areas with high dopamine content.[140] In PD a marked decrease in 6-FD concentration is demonstrated in the striate bodies. The putamen shows more severe deficits than the caudate nucleus does.[141] More specifically, the dopamine (D2) receptors themselves can be imaged by using the ^{11}C-labeled dopamine receptor ligand 2-methylspiperone.[142] Initial studies have shown significant D2 binding impairment in PD.[143]

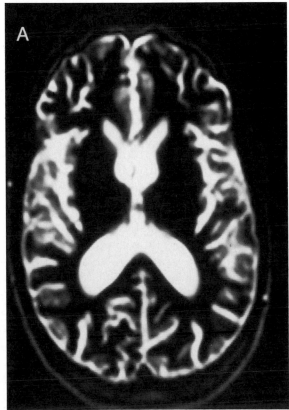
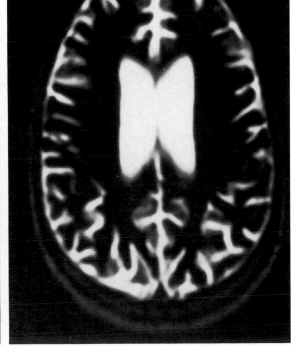

FIG 15–27.

Advanced cerebral atrophy in a 33-year-old male with AIDS and dementia: inversion-recovery "CSF" sequence (TR 5,000/TI 500/TE 100). There is generalized enlargement of the ventricles and sulci.

This type of diffuse cerebral atrophy in AIDS patients is presumed to be the result of infiltration of brain parenchyma by the human immunodeficiency virus (HIV).

HUNTINGTON'S CHOREA

This hereditary movement disorder is characterized pathologically by severe degeneration of the caudate nuclei.[144] Consequently, the frontal horns and especially the bicaudate diameter show progressive enlargement.[145] Patients develop progressive choreiform movements and dementia in adult life. Decreased levels of γ-aminobutyric acid (GABA) have been reported in the CSF. When using PET, a marked decrease in striated glucose consumption has been demonstrated in Huntington's disease; however, striatal 6-fluoro-L-DOPA concentrations are normal, in contradistinction to PD.[146]

OTHER DEMENTING DISORDERS

There are multiple other diseases associated with dementia.[5] These include arteritis and postirradiation leukoencephalopathy[147]; dementia pugilistica; and infectious diseases including progressive multifocal leukoencephalopathy (PML), acquired immunodeficiency syndrome (AIDS) dementia (Fig 15–27),[148] Jacob-Creutzfeldt disease, kuru and lues, multiple sclerosis, and muscular dystrophy.[5]

REFERENCES

1. Ranson SW, Clark SL: The anatomy of the nervous system: Its development and function, in *The Cerebral Cortex*, ed 8. Philadelphia, WB Saunders Co, 1947, p 291.
2. Fritsch G: Uber die elektrische erregbarkeit des girns. *Arch F Anat Physiol* 1870; 3000.
3. Penfield W, Rasmussen T: The cerebral cortex of man, in *Cortex and Diencephalon*. New York, Macmillan Publishing Co, Inc, 1950, pp 204–206.
4. Alzheimer A: Uber eine eigenartige Erkrankung der Hirninde. *Alleg Z Psychiatr* 1907; 64:146.
5. Haase GR: Disease presenting as dementia, in Wells CE (ed): *Dementia*, ed 2. Philadelphia, FA Davis Co Publishers 1977, p 27.
6. Tomlinson BE, Blessed G, Roth M: Observations on the brains of demented old people. *J Neurol Sci* 1970; 11:205–242.
7. Tomlinson BE, Blessed G, Roth M: Observations on the brains of non-demented old people. *J Neurol Sci* 1968; 7:331–356.
8. Huckman MS, Fox J, Topel J: The validity of criteria for the evaluation of cerebral atrophy by computed tomography. *Radiology* 1975; 116:85–92.
9. George AE, de Leon MJ, Stylopoulos LA, et al: CT diagnostic features of Alzheimer disease: Importance of the choroidal/hippocampal fissure complex. *AJNR* 1990; 11:101–107.
10. LeMay M, Stafford JL, Sandor T: Statistical assessment of perceptual CT scan ratings in patients with Alzheimer type dementia. *J Comp Assist Tomogr* 1986; 10:802–809.
11. LeMay M: CT changes in dementing diseases: A review. *AJNR* 1986; 7:841–853.
12. Kido DK, Caine ED, Booth HA: Temporal lobe atrophy in patients with Alzheimer's disease (abstract). *AJNR* 1987; 8:931.
13. de Leon MJ, George AE, Stylopoulos LA, et al: Early marker for Alzheimer's disease: The atrophic hippocampus. *Lancet* 1989; 672–673.
14. George AE, Stylopoulos LA, de Leon MJ, et al: MR imaging quantification of selective temporal lobe gray matter loss in Alzheimer disease (abstract). *Radiology* 1988; 169:127. In review.
15. Bricken RM: *The Intellectual Functions of the Frontal Lobe*. New York, Macmillan Publishing Co Inc, 1936.
16. Kluver H, Bucy PC: Preliminary analysis of functions of the temporal lobes of monkeys. *Arch Neurol Psychiatry* 1939; 42:979–1000.
17. Pavlov IP: *Conditioned Reflexes*. Oxford, England, Oxford University Press, 1927, p 430.
18. Scoville WB, Milner B: Loss of recent memory after bilateral hippocampal lesions. *J Neurol Neurosurg Psychiatry* 1957; 20:11–21.
19. Ojemann GA, Blick K, Ward A Jr: Improvement and disturbances of short term verbal memory with human ventrolateral thalamic stimulation. *Brain* 1971; 94:240–255.
20. Ojemann GA: Mental arithmetic during human thalamic stimulation. *Neuropsychologia* 1974; 12:1–10.
21. Tomlinson BE: The pathology of dementia, in Wells CE (ed): *Dementia*, ed 2, Philadelphia, FA Davis Co Publishers, 1977, p 117.
22. Victor M, Adams RD, Collins GH: The *Wernicke-Korsakoff* Syndrome. Philadelphia, FA Davis Co Publishers, 1971, pp 88–132.
23. Ball MJ: Neuronal loss, neurofibrillary tangles and granulovacuolar degeneration in the hippocampus with aging and dementia. *Acta Neuropathol (Berl)* 1977; 37:111–118.
24. Hyman BT, Van Hoesen GW, Damasio AR: Alzheimer's disease: Cell-specific pathology isolates the hippocampal formation. *Science* 1984; 225:1168–1170.
25. Hyman BT, Van Hoesen GW, Kromer LG, et al: Perforant pathway changes and the memory impairment of Alzheimer's disease. *Ann Neurol* 1986; 20:472–481.
26. American Roentgen Ray Society: Report of committee on standardization of encephalography. *AJR* 1929; 22:474–480.
27. Heinrich A: Das normale enzephalogramm in

seiner abhagigkeit vom lebersalter. *Z Alterns-forsch* 1939; 1:345–354.

28. Andersen E, Vive Larsen J, Jacobsen HH: Atrophia cerebri. *Ugeskr Laeger* 1963; 125:86–91.

29. Jacobsen HH, Melchior JC: On pneumoencephalographic measuring methods in children. *AJR* 1967; 101:188–194.

30. Iivanainen M: Pneumoencephalographic and clinical characteristics of diffuse cerebral atrophy. *Acta Neurol Scand* 1975; 51:310–327.

31. de Leon MJ, Ferris SH, George AE: Computed tomography and positron emission transaxial tomography evaluations of normal aging and Alzheimer's disease. *J Cereb Blood Flow Metab* 1983; 3:391–394.

32. de Leon MJ, George AE, Ferris SH, et al: Positron emission tomography and computed tomography assessment of the aging human brain. *J Comput Assist Tomogr* 1984; 8:88–94.

33. de Leon MJ, George AE, Tomanelli J, et al: Positron emission tomography studies of normal aging: A replication of PET III and 18-FDG using PET VI and 11-C-2DG. *Neurobiol Aging* 1987; 8:319–323.

34. Kuhl DE, Metter EJ, Riege WH, et al: Effects of human aging on patterns of local cerebral glucose utilization determined by the [18-F] fluorodeoxyglucose method. *J Cereb Blood Flow Metab* 1982; 2:163–171.

35. Glydensted C, Kosteljanetz M: Measurements of the normal ventricular system with computed tomography: A preliminary study of 44 adults. *Neurology* 1976; 10:205–215.

36. Hahn FJY, Rim K: Frontal ventricular dimensions on normal computed tomography. *AJR* 1976; 126:593–596.

37. Haug G: Age and sex dependence of the size of normal ventricles on computed tomography. *Neuroradiology* 1977; 14:201–204.

38. Jacoby RJ, Levy R, Dawson JM: Computed tomography in the elderly: I. The normal population. *Br J Psychiatry* 1980; 136:249.

39. Yamamura H, Ito M, Kubota K, et al: Brain atrophy during aging: A quantitative study with computed tomography. *J Gerontol* 1980; 4:492–498.

40. Cala LA, Thickbroom GW, Black JI, et al: Brain density and cerebrospinal fluid space size: CT of normal volunteers. *AJNR* 1981; 2:41–47.

41. Barron SA, Jacobs L, Kindel W: Changes in size of normal lateral ventricles during aging determined by computerized tomography. *Neurology* 1976; 26:1011–1013.

42. Hatazawa J, Ito M, Yamamura H, et al: Sex differences in brain atrophy during aging: A quantitative study with computed tomography. *J Am Geriatr Soc* 1982; 3:1–11.

43. Zatz LM, Jernigan TL, Ahbumada AJ Jr: Changes on computed cranial tomography with aging: Intracranial fluid volume. *AJNR* 1982; 3:1–11.

44. Zatz LM, Jernigan TL, Ahumada AJ Jr: White matter changes in cerebral computed tomography related to aging. *J Comput Assist Tomogr* 1982; 6:19–23.

45. DiChiro G, Brooks RA, Dubal L, et al: The apical artifact: elevated attenuation values toward the apex of the skull. *J Comput Assist Tomogr* 1978; 2:65–70.

46. Kowalski H, George AE, de Leon MJ, et al: Regional cerebral MRI T2 values: Effects of normal aging. *Presented at the 40th Annual Meeting of the American Academy of Neurology*, Cincinnati, April 1988.

47. Sze G, DeArmond S, Brant-Zawadzki M, et al: Foci of MRI signal (pseudolesions) anterior to the frontal horns: Histologic correlations of a normal finding. *AJNR* 1986; 7:381–387.

48. Brun A, Englund E: Regional pattern of degeneration in Alzheimer's disease: Neuronal loss and histopathological grading. *Histopathology* 1981; 5:549–564.

49. Blessed G, Roth M, Tomlinson BE: The association between quantitative measures of dementia and of senile change in the cerebral grey matter of elderly subjects. *Br J Psychiatry* 1968; 114:797.

50. Shefer VF (cited in Ball, 1977): Absolute number of neurons and thickness of the cerebral cortex during aging, senile and vascular dementia and Pick's and Alzheimer's diseases. *Zh Nevropatol Psikhiat* 1972; 72:1024–1029. Translated in *Neurosci Behav Psychol* 1973; 6:319–324.

51. Bowen DM, Smith CB, White P, et al: Neurotransmitter-related enzymes and indices of hypoxia in senile dementia and other abiotrophies. *Brain* 1976; 99:459–496.

52. Davis P, Maloney AJR: Selective loss of central cholinergic neurons in Alzheimer's disease. *Lancet* 1976; 2:1403.

53. Perry RD, Pena C: Experimental production of neurofibrillary regeneration: II. Electron microscopy, phosphatase histochemistry and electron probe analysis. *J Neuropathol Exp Neurol* 1965; 24:200–210.

54. White P, Goodhart MJ, Keet SP, et al: Neocortical cholinergic neurons in elderly people. *Lancet* 1977; 1:668–670.

55. Emson PC, Lindvall O: Distribution of putative neurotransmitters in the neocortex. *Neuroscience* 1979; 1:1–30.

56. Johnston MV, McKinney M, Coyle J: Evidence for a cholinergic projection to neocortex from neurons in basal forebrain. *Neurobiology* 1979; 76:5392–5396.

57. Whitehouse PJ, Price DL, Struble RG, et al: Alzheimer's disease and senile dementia: Loss of neurons in the basal forebrain. *Science* 1982; 215:1237–1239.

58. Adolfsson R, Gottfries CG, Roos BE, et al: Changes in the brain catecholamines in patients

with dementia of Alzheimer's type. *Br J Psychiatry* 1979; 135:216–223.

59. Mann DMA, Lincoln J, Yates PO, et al: Changes in the monoamine containing neurones of the human CNS in senile dementia. *Br J Psychiatry* 1980; 136:533–541.

60. Bondareff W, Mountjoy CQ, Roth M: Loss of neurons of origin of the adrenergic projection to the cerebral cortex (nucleus locus coeruleus) in senile dementia. *Neurology* 1982; 32:164–168.

61. Engeset A, Lonnum A: Third ventricles of 12 mm width or more: A preliminary report. *Acta Radiol* 1958; 50:5–11.

62. Nielsen R, Peterson O, Thygesen P, et al: Encephalographic cortical atrophy: Relationships to ventricular atrophy and intellectual impairment. *Acta Radiol* 1966; 4:437–448.

63. Nielsen R, Peterson O, Thygesen P, et al: Encephalographic ventricular atrophy. *Acta Radiol* 1966; 4:240–256.

64. Huber G: Die bedentung der neuroradiologic für die psychiatrie. *Fortsch Med* 1963; 81:705.

65. Huber G: Zur diagnose, prognose und typologic hirnatrophischer syndrome. *Radiology* 1965; 5:456.

66. Gosling RH: The association of dementia with radiologically demonstrated cerebral atrophy. *J Neurol Neurosurg Psychiatry* 1955; 18:129–133.

67. Mann AH: Cortical atrophy and air encephalography: Clinical and radiological study. *Psychol Med* 1973; 3:374–378.

68. Hughes CP, Gado M: Computed tomography and aging of the brain. *Radiology* 1981; 139:391–396.

69. Claveria LE, Moseley IF, Stevenson JF: The clinical significance of cerebral atrophy as shown by CAT, in DuBoulay FG, Moseley IF (eds): *The First European Seminar on Computerized Tomography in Clinical Practice.* Berlin, Springer-Verlag, 1977, pp 213–217.

70. Nathan RJ, Frumkin K: Cerebral atrophy and independence in the elderly. Presented at the Annual Meeting of the American Psychiatric Association, Atlanta, May 8–12, 1978.

71. Gado MH, Hughes CP, Danziger W, et al: Volumetric measurements of the cerebrospinal fluid spaces in objects with dementia and in controls. *Radiology* 1982; 144:535–538.

72. George AE, de Leon MJ, Rosenbloom S, et al: Ventricular volume and cognitive deficit: A computed tomographic study. *Radiology* 1983; 149:493–498.

73. de Leon MJ, Ferris SH, George AE, et al: A new method for the CT evaluation of brain atrophy in senile dementia. *IRCS Med Sci* 1979; 7:404.

74. de Leon MJ, Ferris SH, Blau I, et al: Correlations between computerized tomographic changes and behavioral deficits. *Lancet* 1979; 2:538.

75. de Leon MJ, Ferris SH, George AE, et al: Computed tomography evaluations of brain-behavior relationships in senile dementia of the Alzheimer's type. *Neurobiol Aging* 1980; 1:69–79.

76. Mersky H, Ball MJ, Blume WT, et al: Relationships between psychological measurements and cerebral organic changes in Alzheimer's disease. *Can J Neurol Sci* 1980; 7:45–49.

77. Roberts MA, Caird FI: Computerized tomography and intellectual impairment in the elderly. *J Neurol Neurosurg Psychiatry* 1976; 39:986–989.

78. Earnest MP, Heaton RK, Wilkenson WE, et al: Cortical atrophy, ventricular enlargement and intellectual impairment in the aged. *Neurology* 1979; 29:1138–1143.

79. Jacoby RJ, Levy R: Computed tomography in the elderly: II. Diagnosis and functional impairment. *Br J Psychiatry* 1980; 136:256–269.

80. George AE, de Leon MJ, Ferris SH, et al: Parenchymal CT correlates of senile dementia: Loss of gray-white discriminability. *AJNR* 1981; 2:205–213.

81. Naeser MA, Gebhardt C, Levine HL: Decreased computerized tomography numbers in patients with senile dementia. *Arch Neurol* 1980; 37:401–407.

82. Gado M, Danziger WL, Chi D, et al: Brain parenchymal density measurements by CT in demented subjects and normal controls. *Radiology* 1983; 147:703–710.

83. Bondareff W, Baldy R, Levy R: Quantitative computed tomography in senile dementia. *Arch Gen Psychiatry* 1981; 38:1365–1368.

84. Wilson RS, Fox JH, Huckman MS, et al: Computed tomography in dementia. *Neurology* 1982; 32:1054–1057.

85. de Leon MJ, George AE, Reisberg B, et al: Alzheimer's disease: Longitudinal CT studies of ventricular change. *AJNR* 1989; 10:371–376.

86. Naguib M, Levy R: CT Scanning in senile dementia: A follow-up of survivors. *Br J Psychiatry* 1982; 141:618–620.

87. Gado M, Hughes CP, Danziger W, et al: Aging, dementia, and brain atrophy: A longitudinal computed tomographic study. *AJNR* 1983; 4:699–702.

88. Brinkman SD, Largen JW Jr: Changes in brain ventricular size with repeated CAT scans in suspected Alzheimer's disease. *Am J Psychiatry* 1984; 141:81–83.

89. Phelps ME, Huang SC, Hoffman EJ, et al: Tomographic measurement of local cerebral glucose metabolic rate in humans with [18F] 2-fluoro-2-deoxy-D-glucose: validation of method. *Ann Neurol* 1979; 6:371–388.

90. Reivich M, Alavi A, Wolf A, et al: Glucose metabolic rate kinetic model parameter determination in humans: The lumped constants and rate constants for [18F] fluorodeoxyglucose and [11C] deoxyglucose. *J Cereb Blood Flow Metab* 1985; 5:179–192.

91. Ferris SH, de Leon MJ, Wolf AP, et al: Positron emission tomography in the study of aging and senile dementia. *Neurobiol Aging* 1980; 1:127–131.

92. de Leon MJ, Ferris SH, George AE, et al: Positron emission tomography (PET) and computed tomography (CT) evaluations combined in the study of senile dementia. *AJNR* 1983; 4:568–571.

93. Miller JD, de Leon MJ, Ferris SH, et al: Abnormal temporal lobe response in Alzheimer's disease during cognitive processing as measured by ^{11}C-2-deoxyglucose (^{11}C-2DG) and PET. *J Cereb Blood Flow Metab* 1987; 7:248–251.

94. Chase TN, Foster NL, Mansi I: Alzheimer's disease and the parietal lobe. *Lancet* 1983; 2:225.

95. Friedland RP, Brun A, Budinger TF: Pathological and positron emission tomographic correlations in Alzheimer's disease. *Lancet* 1985; 1:228.

96. Holman BL: Perfusion and receptor SPECT in the dementias. *J Nucl Med* 1986; 27:855–860.

97. Kramer EL, Sanger JJ, Smith GS, et al: Temporal lobe deficits and basal ganglia preservation on semiquantitative I-123 IMP brain SPECT in Alzheimer's dementia (abstract). *Radiology* 1988; 169:265.

98. Marcus DM, de Leon MJ, Tsai J, et al: Altered glucose metabolism in microvessels from patients with Alzheimer's disease (abstract). *Gerontologist* 1987; 27:120.

99. George AE, de Leon MJ, Klinger A, et al: Positron emission tomography (PET) of communicating hydrocephalus: Differential diagnosis from Alzheimer disease. Presented at the 40th Annual Meeting of the American Academy of Neurology, Cincinnati, April 1988. Submitted for publication.

100. George AE, de Leon MJ, Gentes CI, et al: Leukoencephalopathy in normal and pathologic aging: 1. CT of brain lucencies. *AJNR* 1986; 7:561–566.

101. London E, de Leon MJ, George AE, et al: Periventricular lucencies in the CT scans of aged and demented patients. *Biol Psychiatry* 1986; 21:960–962.

102. George AE, de Leon MJ, Kalnin A, et al: Leukoencephalopathy in normal and pathologic aging: 2. MRI of brain lucencies. *AJNR* 1986; 7:567–570.

103. Hachinski VC, Potter P, Merskey H: Leukoaraiosis. *Arch Neurol* 1987; 44:21–23.

104. Steingart A, Hachinski VC, Lau C, et al: Cognitive and neurologic findings in demented patients with diffuse white matter lucencies on computed tomographic scan (leuko-araiosis). *Arch Neurol* 1987; 44:36–39.

105. Goto K, Ishii N, Fukasaw H: Diffuse white matter disease in the geriatric population. A clinical neuropathological and CT study. *Radiology* 1981; 141:687–695.

106. Kirkpatrick JB, Hayman LA: White matter lesions in MR imaging of clinical healthy brains of elderly subjects: Possible pathologic basis. *Radiology* 1987; 162:509–511.

107. Lotz PR, Ballinger WE Jr, Quisling RG: Subcortical arteriosclerotic encephalopathy: CT spectrum and pathologic correlation. *AJNR* 1986; 7:817–822.

108. Braffman BH, Zimmerman RA, Trojanowski JQ, et al: Brain MR: Pathologic correlation with gross and histopathology. (1) Lacunar infarction and Virchow-Robin spaces. *AJNR* 1988; 9:621–628. (2) Hypertense white matter foci in the elderly. *AJNR* 1988; 9:629–636.

109. Brun A, Englund E: A white matter disorder in dementia of the Alzheimer type: A pathoanatomical study. *Ann Neurol* 1986; 19:253–262.

110. Bradley WG Jr, Waluch V, Brant-Zawadzki M, et al: Patchy, periventricular white matter lesions in the elderly: A common observation during NMR imaging. *Noninvasive Med Imag* 1984; 1:35–41.

111. Kluger A, Gianutsos J, de Leon MJ, et al: Significance of age-related white matter lesions. *Stroke* 1988; 19:1054–1055.

112. Masdeau J, Lantos G, Wolfson L: Hemispheric white matter lesions in the elderly prone to falling. *Acta Radiol Suppl* 1986; 369:392.

113. Zimmerman RD, Fleming CA, Lee BCP, et al: Periventricular hyperintensity as seen by magnetic resonance: Prevalence and significance. *AJNR* 1986; 7:13–20.

114. de Leon MJ, George AE, Miller JD, et al: Altered patterns of positron emission tomography glucose metabolism in Alzheimer patients with microvascular white matter disease (abstract). *Am J Physiol Imag* 1988; 3:52–53.

115. Janota I: Dementia, deep white matter damage and hypertension: "Binswanger disease." *Psychol Med* 1981; 11:39–48.

116. Rosenberg GA, Kornfeld M, Stovring J, et al: Subcortical arteriosclerotic encephalopathy (Binswanger): Computerized tomography. *Neurology* 1979; 29:1102–1106.

117. Tomongaga M, Hiroski Y, Tohgi H: Clinicopathologic study of progressive subcortical vascular encephalopathy (Binswanger type) in the elderly. *J Am Geriatr Soc* 1982; 30:524–529.

118. Burger PC, Burch JG, Kunze U: Subcortical arteriosclerlotic encephalopathy (Binswanger's disease). A vascular etiology of dementia. *Stroke* 1976; 7:626–631.

119. Binswanger O: Die abrengzung der allgemeinen progressiven paralyse. *Berl Klin Wochenschr* 1894; 31:1103–1105, 1137–1139, 1180–1196.

120. Pick A: Ueber die Benziehungen der senilen Hirnatrophiel zur Aphasie. *Prager Med Wochenschr* 1892; 17:165.

121. Corsellis JAN: In Blackwood W, Corsellis JAN (eds): *Greenfield's Neuropathology*, ed 3. Chicago, Edward Arnold Publishing Co, 1976, pp 817–821.

122. McGeachie RF, Fleming JO, Sharer LR, et al: Di-

agnosis of Pick's disease by computed tomography. *J Comput Assist Tomogr* 1979; 3:113.

123. Groen JJ, Hekster RFM: Computed tomography in Pick's disease. *J Comput Assist Tomogr* 1982; 6:907.

124. Hakim S, Adams RD: The special clinical problem of symptomatic hydrocephalus with normal cerebrospinal fluid pressure. *J Neurol Sci* 1965; 2:307–327.

125. El Gammal T, Allen MB, Brooks BS, et al: MR evaluation of hydrocephalus. *AJNR* 1987; 8:591–597.

126. Stollman AL, George AE, Pinto RS, et al: Periventricular high signal lesions and signal void on magnetic resonance imaging in hydrocephalus. *Acta Radiol Suppl* 1986; 369:388–391.

127. Greitz T: Cerebral circulation in adult hydrocephalus studied with angiography and the 133 xenon method. *Scand J Lab Clin Invest* 1968; suppl 102:XIIC.

128. Greitz T, Crepe A, Kalmer M, et al: Pre and post-op evaluations of cerebral blood flow in low pressure hydrocephalus. *J Neurosurg* 1969; 31:644–651.

129. Grubb RL, Raichle MC, Gado M, et al: Cerebral blood flow oxygen utilization of blood volume in dementia. *Neurology* 1977; 27:905–910.

130. Ingvar DH, Gustafson L: Regional cerebral blood flow in organic dementia with early onset. *Acta Neurol Scand* 1970; 43(suppl 46):42–73.

131. Raichle ME, Eichling TO, Gado M, et al: Cerebral blood volume in dementia. *Neurology* 1974; 24:415.

132. George AE, de Leon MJ, Miller J, et al: Positron emission tomography of hydrocephalus: Metabolic effects of shunt procedures. *Acta Radiol Suppl* 1986; 369:435–439.

133. Oppenheimer DR: Diseases of the basal ganglia, cerebellum and motor neurons, in Adams JH, Corsellis JAN, Duchen LW (eds): *2. Greenfield's Neuropathology*, New York, John Wiley & Sons, Inc, 1984; pp 699–747.

134. Duguid JR, De La Paz R, De Groot J: Magnetic resonance imaging of the midbrain in Parkinson's disease. *Ann Neurol* 1986; 20:744–747.

135. Braffman BH, Grossman RI, Goldberg HI, et al: MR imaging of Parkinson disease with spin-echo and gradient-echo sequences. *AJNR* 1988; 9:1093–1099.

136. Drayer BP, Olanow W, Burger P, et al: Parkinson plus syndrome: Diagnosis using high field MR imaging of brain iron. *Radiology* 1986; 159:493–498.

137. Pastakia B, Polinsky R, Di Chiro G, et al: Multiple system atrophy (Shy-Drager syndrome): MR imaging. *Radiology* 1986; 159:499–502.

138. Lieberman A, Dziatolowski M, Kupersmith M, et al: Dementia in Parkinson's disease. *Ann Neurol* 1979; 6:355–359.

139. Hakim AM, Mathieson G: Dementia in Parkinson disease: A neuropathologic study. *Neurology* 1979; 29:1209–1214.

140. Garnett ES, Firnau G, Nahmias C: Dopamine visualized in the basal ganglia of living man. *Nature* 1983; 305:137–138.

141. Martin WRW, Adam MJ, Bergstrom M, et al: In vivo study of DOPA metabolism in Parkinson's disease, in Fahn S, et al (eds): *Recent Developments in Parkinson's Disease*. New York, Raven Press, 1986, pp 97–102.

142. Wagner HN, Burns HD, Dannals RF, et al: Imaging dopamine receptors in the human brain by positron emission tomography. *Science* 1983; 221:1264–1266.

143. Leenders K, Palmer A, Turton D, et al: DOPA uptake and dopamine receptors binding visualized, in *The Human Brain in Vivo*, in Fahn S, et al (eds): *Recent Developments in Parkinson's Disease*. New York, Raven Press, 1986.

144. Neophytides AN, Di Chiro G, Barron SA, et al: Computed axial tomography in Huntington's disease. *Adv Neurol* 1979; 23:185–191.

145. Terrence CF, Delaney JF, Alberts MC: Computed tomography for Huntington's disease. *Neuroradiology* 1977; 13:173–175.

146. Garnett ES, Firnau G, Nahmias C, et al: Reduced striatal glucose consumption, and prolonged reaction times are early features in Huntington's disease. *J Neurol Sci* 1984; 65:321–327.

147. Stylopoulos LA, George AE, de Leon MJ, et al: Longitudinal CT study of parenchymal brain changes in glioma survivors. *AJNR* 1988; 9:517–522.

148. Navia BA, Price RW: The acquired immunodeficiency syndrome dementia complex as the presenting or sole manifestation of human immunodeficiency virus infection. *Arch Neurol* 1987; 44:65–69.

PART VII

Cranial and Intracranial Neoplasms

Introduction

Richard E. Latchaw, M.D.

David W. Johnson, M.D.

Emanuel Kanal, M.D.

There have been numerous attempts to classify the many neoplasms involving the intracranial contents and the surrounding bony structures. Specifically, there have been a number of classifications of the neuroepithelial tumors beginning with Bailey and Cushing in 1926.[1] These authors identified 20 separate cell types within the developing central nervous system (CNS) and proposed a classification of tumors based on 14 main groups. In 1952, Kernohan and Sayre[2] produced a grading of gliomas based on histologic criteria of an increasing degree of malignancy. In their scheme, benign astrocytoma was grade I, while glioblastoma multiforme represented grade IV. Ependymomas and oligodendrogliomas were similarly graded. Russell and Rubenstein[3] have classified neuroepithelial tumors according to their apparent cell line, similar to Bailey and Cushing, with categories including tumors of neuroglial origin, those of neuronal cell origin, and those arising from central neuroepithelium (retina, neurohypophysis, pineal gland, and choroid plexus). Rorke[4] has suggested that neoplasms occurring primarily in infancy and childhood and composed primarily of undifferentiated neuroepithelial cells, including medulloblastoma, cerebral neuroblastoma, and pineal parenchymal tumors, be classified together as various forms of primitive neuroectodermal tumor (PNET). The International Classification of Central Nervous System Tumors was drafted under the auspices of the World Health Organization in 1979 and represents a consensus.[5] It is based on concepts of cell line differentiation similar to those of Bailey and Cushing, and Russell and Rubenstein.

No one classification of intracranial tumors is agreeable to all parties concerned, nor can it satisfy all requirements made upon it. Any classification should have as its goal the organization of the components into a system that can be rationally considered at the time of differential diagnosis and that proves to be useful for treatment and prognosis. For the purpose of this presentation of the radiologic appearances of the various cranial and intracranial neoplasms, the following classification is utilized:

I. Neuroepithelial neoplasms
   A. Tumors of glial origin
      1. Astrocytoma, benign and malignant
      2. Glioblastoma multiforme
      3. Oligodendroglioma
      4. Tumors of ependymal origin
         a. Ependymoma
         b. Subependymoma
   B. Tumors of choroid plexus epithelium
      1. Choroid plexus papilloma
      2. Choroid plexus carcinoma
   C. Primitive neuroectodermal tumors (PNET)
      1. Medulloblastoma
      2. Cerebral neuroblastoma
      3. Pineal parenchymal tumors

D. Tumors of central ganglion cell origin
  1. Gangliocytoma (ganglioneuroma)
  2. Ganglioglioma
E. Tumors of the retina: retinoblastoma
II. Primary cerebral sarcomas
  A. Fibrosarcoma
  B. Gliosarcoma
III. Primary cerebral lymphoma
IV. Tumors of the meninges
  A. Meningioma
  B. Malignant meningioma
  C. Hemangiopericytoma
  D. Primary sarcomas
V. Nerve sheath tumors
  A. Schwannoma
  B. Neurofibroma
VI. Chemodectomas
VII. Tumors and tumorlike lesions of maldevelopmental origin
  A. Teratoma
  B. Germinoma
  C. Epidermoid
  D. Dermoid
  E. Lipoma
  F. Craniopharyngioma
  G. Neuroepithelial cyst (including colloid cyst)
  H. Arachnoid cyst
  I. Hamartomas
  J. Vascular malformations
    1. Arteriovenous malformation
    2. Capillary telangiectasia
    3. Cavernous angioma
    4. Venous angioma
VIII. Tumors of vascular origin
  A. Hemangioblastoma
  B. Hemangioendothelioma
  C. Angiosarcoma
IX. Pituitary neoplasms
X. Metastatic tumors
XI. Tumors of bone
  A. Calvarium
    1. Benign
      a. Epidermoid
      b. Hemangioma
    2. Aggressive/malignant
      a. Eosinophilic granuloma
      b. Sarcomas
  B. Skull base
    1. Osteoma, osteochondroma, osteogenic sarcoma
    2. Chondroma, chondrosarcoma
    3. Chordoma

The clinical and radiologic diagnosis of a specific intracranial neoplasm depends upon many factors, one of which is location. Therefore, Chapter 16 deals with tumors of the cerebral parenchyma, including the neuroepithelial tumors, primary sarcoma, and primary cerebral lymphoma. Chapter 17 discusses extra-axial masses (meningeal neoplasms, tumors of nerve sheath origin, and chemodectomas) and tumors of the skull base and calvarium. The various maldevelopmental tumors, pineal region tumors, and tumors of blood vessel origin have multiple interrelationships and are therefore considered together in Chapter 18. The phakomatoses are those hereditary syndromes having skin lesions and CNS tumors of maldevelopmental origin and are therefore discussed in Chapter 18. Craniopharyngioma and pituitary tumors represent specific diagnostic problems and are therefore considered together elsewhere in this book. Finally, a separate chapter in this section is devoted to the various manifestations of metastatic disease involving the cerebral parenchyma and meninges (Chapter 19).

While a relatively short presentation could have been devoted to generalities on the typical appearances of the most common cranial and intracranial tumors, there is an attempt in this section to discuss in depth the magnetic resonance (MR) and computed tomography (CT) scan appearances of many tumors. It has become apparent that the radiologist is frequently able to make a preoperative histologic diagnosis in a large percentage of cases or to give a short and accurate differential diagnosis. Such accuracy stems from the pattern of radiographic findings in any given neoplasm, including the site of occurrence, CT density or MR intensity, pattern of contrast enhancement, sharpness of margins, multiplicity, and a wealth of other radiographic findings. It is thus important to discuss the salient radiographic findings for both the more common cranial and intracranial neoplasms and the less common but significant differential diagnostic possibilities.

An effort has been made to discuss some of the more important neuropathologic concepts for a number of the tumor categories. An understanding of the pathology of these tumors is mandatory when attempting to explain the particular pattern of radiologic findings for any given neoplasm. Some physiologic concepts regarding contrast enhancement and the blood-brain barrier will also be discussed, although a more complete discussion of the mechanisms of enhancement will be found in Chapters 5 and 6. Differential diagnosis is strongly emphasized throughout this section. Such differential diagnosis includes not only tumors that simulate the one under discussion, but non-neoplastic conditions as well. Chapter 20 of this section is devoted entirely to important points of differential diagnosis.

Evaluation of the brain following treatment for an intracranial neoplasm can be difficult, and is presented in Chapter 21. Symptoms may suggest recurrence of the tumor or a complication of therapy, and it is therefore necessary to understand the variety of often confusing appearances that follow surgery, irradiation, or chemotherapy.

Magnetic resonance imaging (MRI) is preferred over CT as the diagnostic modality for the majority of intracranial diseases, and for the evaluation of an intracranial tumor in particular. MRI surpasses CT in the following ways:

1. Better delineation of soft tissue anatomy: Because of tissue intensity differences, such as the difference between gray and white matter and the contrast between the optic chiasm and surrounding structures, MRI defines parenchymal anatomy much better than does CT. CT is better for the spatial resolution of small structures having high CT contrast and/or low MR signal, such as the bony ossicles.

2. Sensitivity to abnormality: MRI is far superior to CT in the sensitivity to an abnormality of tissue composition. Because of MRI's ability to detect small changes in the water content of tissues, MRI may define an abnormality, or the extent of that abnormality, much earlier than CT.

3. Sensitivity to contrast agents: Only a small amount of a paramagnetic contrast agent is necessary to change sufficiently the relaxation parameters of a tissue to be detected with MRI. In contradistinction, enhancement on CT depends upon the physical presence of enough contrast agent within a tissue to alter the attenuation of the x-ray beam. These small amounts of paramagnetic agents are associated with a pronounced decrease in adverse reactions relative to the iodinated compounds used in CT.

4. The specificity of tumor characterization is better in many conditions with MRI than with CT. For example, MRI has the ability to define subacute and chronic collections of blood or vascular lesions much better than does CT, and is superior in the evaluation of the contents of a cystic lesion.

CT is superior to MRI in the evaluation of fine bony or calcific structures.

5. Multiple projections are obtained with ease. Direct coronal imaging with CT is cumbersome, and sagittal imaging is impossible except with small infants. Image reformations using mathematical techniques are generally necessary for many coronal and all sagittal CT presentations. MRI, on the other hand, gives both the coronal and sagittal projections with ease, allowing better appreciation of the relationships of a lesion to surrounding anatomic structures.

6. Lack of CT beam-hardening artifact near bony structures: Bony structures absorb lower energy portions of the x-ray beam, producing a higher energy beam that produces streak artifacts around and between the bony structures. This makes evaluation of tissues at the skull base or near the surface of the cerebral convexities more difficult with CT than with MRI. MRI is therefore better than CT for the evaluation of skull base tumors, meningeal tumors, and infections, etc.

7. There is no ionizing radiation with MRI. While the amount of radiation to a specific point is relatively low with the CT scanning technique relative to other x-ray procedures for the diagnosis of neurologic disease, and while the brain is relatively resistant to the effects of radiation, it is obviously preferable not to have any ionizing radiation. Not only is tissue irradiation avoided with MRI, but there has been no demonstration that MRI produces any prolonged deleterious physiologic effects.

CT is better than MRI in a number of clinical situations. The demonstration of acute intracranial hemorrhage is more rapid and more reliable with CT than with MRI. Small calcifications are detectable with CT, whereas larger areas of homogeneous calcification are required for MR detection. A tissue matrix with less homogeneous calcification will still give an MR signal and therefore will be detected as soft tissue, not the signal void of calcification. Currently MR imaging sequences are relatively long compared with CT, so that CT is a better modality if a rapid study is desired. The MR imager is a long tube and most of our current physiologic monitoring devices are sensitive to magnetic flux, making the monitoring of an acutely ill patient much more difficult with MRI than with CT.

Because of these relative advantages and disadvantages, MRI is preferred over CT for the following neurologic presentations which suggest the presence of a possible intracranial mass lesion: focal motor or sensory changes; seizures; symptoms suggesting demyelinating disease vs. tumor; known systemic tumor with possible intracranial metastasis. CT is the preferred imaging modality if there is an acute change in neurologic status suggesting the possibility of acute intracranial hemorrhage. The role of MRI vs. CT as a screening examination for nonspecific symptoms such as headache without neurologic signs is controversial.

Because MRI is the imaging modality of choice for the evaluation of an intracranial mass lesion, the MRI appearances of a variety of intracranial neoplasms is emphasized in the following chapters. However, we must not underemphasize the role of CT in the diagnosis of intracranial neoplasm. There are far more CT scanners than MR imagers both in this country and around the world. We have much more experience with the variety of appearances of intracranial tumors on CT than on MRI. Paramagnetic contrast agents have only recently been approved for general use, so that experience with enhancement patterns of MRI is less than with CT. Therefore, while MRI appearances are emphasized, we build upon our experiences with CT and discuss both the similarities and differences between MRI and CT.

Finally, an explanation is in order regarding the terminology for MR sequences as utilized in the six chapters in this section. Saying that an image is "T1-weighted" or "T2-weighted" can be misleading. Utilizing magnets with field strengths between 0.06T and 1.95T, which are the overwhelming majority in clinical use, and utilizing the spin-echo technique, all images have some degree of T1 and T2 weighting within them. Furthermore, every MR image has a fixed amount of relative proton-density weighting. The field strength with which a patient is examined will differ from institution to institution, as will the specific values for TR, TE, and flip angle assigned for a given procedure. It is more appropriate to discuss pulsing sequences in a more generic fashion, which should also be more acceptable to the MRI purist.

Utilizing the spin-echo MR technique, we have the following three major categories of pulsing sequences in most frequent clinical use:

1. Short TR, short TE sequence: TR of approximately 500 to 700 ms, TE of approximately 10 to 20 ms on a 1.5T system. This produces a relatively heavy T1-weighting to the image. This image will be called the *short TR image.*

2. Long TR, short TE sequence: TR of 2,000 to 3,500 ms or greater, TE less than 30 ms on a 1.5T system. This gives a relative "balance" to the T1 and T2 components with neither being especially emphasized for most biologic tissues so that the appearance relies primarily on the density of the spins. This image, the first echo of a multiecho long TR spin-echo sequence, is often called the spin density or balanced image. In these chapters, it is called the *long TR, short TE image.*

3. Long TR, long TE sequence: TR of 2,000 to 3,500 ms or greater, TE greater than 60 ms on a 1.5T system. This produces a relatively heavy T2 weighting, although there may still be some T1 present in tissues such as cerebrospinal fluid (CSF) with a long T1. This is called the *long TR/ TE image.*

Other types of pulsing sequences are described as necessary, including gradient-echo imaging and inversion-recovery sequences. Relative proton-density differentials, of course, are constantly present between tissues imaged by MR, regardless of the sequence utilized.

REFERENCES

1. Bailey O, Cushing H: *A Classification of Tumors of the Glioma Group.* Philadelphia, JB Lippincott Co, 1926.
2. Kernohan JW, Sayre GP: *Tumors of the Central Nervous System* in *Atlas of Tumor Pathology,* section 10, fasc 35. Washington, DC, Armed Forces Institute of Pathology, 1952.
3. Russell DS, Rubenstein LJ: *Pathology of Tumours of the Nervous System.* Baltimore, Williams & Wilkins Co, 1989.
4. Rorke LB: Cerebellar medulloblastoma and its relationship to primitive neuroectodermal neoplasms. *J Neuropathol Exp Neurol* 1983; 42:1–15.
5. Zulch KJ: *Histological Typing of Tumors of the Central Nervous System.* Geneva, World Health Organization, 1979.

16

Primary Intracranial Tumors: Neuroepithelial Tumors, Sarcomas, and Lymphomas

Richard E. Latchaw, M.D.

David W. Johnson, M.D.

Emanuel Kanal, M.D.

NEUROEPITHELIAL TUMORS

The more common neuroepithelial tumors are listed in the classification found in the introduction to this section. While some of these tumors are relatively site-specific, such as the medulloblastoma (PNET) to the cerebellum, many of them can be found in a variety of locations. The incidence and age of onset of any particular tumor will vary according to its location. For example, the cerebellar astrocytoma is a tumor of childhood whereas cerebral hemispheric astrocytoma is more commonly found in adults. The appearance of the neoplasm may likewise differ according to location, even though the tumors are of the same histologic types. For example, cerebellar astrocytoma, even of low grade, usually enhances dramatically whereas most brain stem astrocytomas, even if malignant, show little, if any, enhancement. Therefore, it is advantageous to discuss neuroepithelial tumors in terms of location. The differential diagnosis of the neuroepithelial tumors (excluding other types of neoplasms), according to location, is as follows:

A. Cerebral hemispheres
1. Astrocytoma, benign and malignant
2. Glioblastoma multiforme
3. Oligodendroglioma
4. Primitive neuroectodermal tumors (PNET)
5. Ganglioglioma, gangliocytoma
6. Ependymoma
7. Neuroepithelial cyst
B. Brain stem
1. Astrocytoma, benign and malignant
2. Glioblastoma multiforme
C. Cerebellum and fourth ventricle
1. Astrocytoma, benign and malignant
2. Glioblastoma multiforme
3. Medulloblastoma (PNET)
4. Ependymoma; subependymoma
5. Choroid plexus papilloma and carcinoma
D. Intraventricular tumors
1. Ependymoma; subependymoma
2. Astrocytoma, benign and malignant
3. Choroid plexus papilloma and carcinoma
4. Colloid cyst (neuroepithelial cyst)
E. Pineal parenchymal tumors: pineocytoma and pineoblastoma

Neuroepithelial cysts (including colloid cyst) are not true neoplasms, but are cysts of maldevelopmental origin. They are discussed in this chapter, however, because they are important additions to the differential diagnosis of mass lesions in the given area. Other tumors of non-neuroepithelial origin (such as intraventricular meningioma) are sufficiently rare within the cerebral parenchyma or ventricular system that their radiographic appearance will be discussed elsewhere, particularly in Chapters 17 or 18.

Neuroepithelial Tumors of the Cerebral Hemispheres

Astrocytoma and Glioblastoma Multiforme

The histologic characterization of glial tumors, which is based upon the predominating cell type and grading into benign and malignant forms relative to the degree of anaplasia, has undergone a great deal of change over the years, resulting in overlapping terms for the same neoplasm. In 1952, Kernohan and Sayre[1] divided astrocytic tumors into grades I through IV, with grade I being the most benign and grade IV being the most malignant (glioblastoma multiforme). A simplified system is in more widespread use today. The term *astrocytoma* (old astrocytoma I and II) refers to a neoplasm with a relatively benign appearance, having a homogeneous grouping of cells with little atypia or anaplasia. The terms *malignant astrocytoma* or *anaplastic astrocytoma* (old astrocytoma III) refer to a neoplasm with a greater degree of anaplasia than the more benign form, but not containing all of the necessary malignant features to be called *glioblastoma*. The term *glioblastoma multiforme* (old astrocytoma IV) is reserved for a malignant neoplasm having abundant glial pleomorphism, numerous mitotic figures and giant cells, pseudopalisading of cells, vascular hyperplasia, and focal areas of necrosis. These histologic characteristics, particularly the presence of necrosis, correlate with a significantly poorer postoperative survival.[2-4] The premortem classification of a particular astrocytic tumor is difficult, with many neuropathologists emphasizing that true classification can only be made at autopsy. The actual grade or classification of an astrocytic neoplasm is based upon the most malignant portion present, and it is impossible to adequately sample a tumor at the time of either tumor resection or needle biopsy, particularly the latter. Therefore, most studies that have attempted to correlate the radiographic appearance of the tumor on the magnetic resonance (MR) or computed tomography (CT) scans with the morphologic characteristics and pathologic grade of the tumor have inherent error in tumor sampling. For this reason alone, statements regarding the MR and CT scan characteristics found with a particular degree of malignancy must be looked upon with some degree of skepticism. There are numerous physical and physiologic factors involved in tissue characterization by MR and CT, making correlation of appearance and histologic grading tenuous at best.

Density and Intensity on Nonenhanced Scans.—There are multiple factors that are responsible for the change in the attenuation of the CT x-ray beam or that effect the proton density and MR relaxation characteristics of tissues. These multiple factors result in the density of a tissue or lesion as seen on the CT scan or the intensity of these tissues as seen on the MR image. An increase in the water content of a lesion and the surrounding tissue relative to the normal brain results in decreased CT density, decreased intensity on short TR images, and increased intensity on long TR/TE images (Figs 16–1 and 16–2). The increased water concentration is predominantly free in the extracellular space. Interstitial microcysts are characteristic of some tumors, while others have a greater degree of intracellular water. The degree of cellular compactness effects density and intensity, with the more compact tumors appearing more dense on the unenhanced CT scan (Fig 16–3) and brighter on the short TR MR image respectively. Central necrosis produces decreased CT density, decreased intensity on the short TR MR image, and increased MR intensity on long TR/TE studies. MR imaging (MRI) is much more sensitive to the protein content of a cystic structure than is CT. In general, the higher the protein content, the shorter the T1 relaxation time, resulting in increased intensity of the cyst compared with cerebrospinal fluid (CSF) on a T1 basis on the short TR image (Fig 16–4,A).[5] This may even yield increased signal compared to CSF on long TR spin-echo images due to the short T1 of the cyst as compared with CSF (Fig 16–4,B). Pure CSF and water have very long T2 relaxation times, longer than most other biologic fluids, and certainly longer than highly proteinaceous cysts. If a very long TR/TE MR sequence were performed, and if sufficient signal were present, the proteinaceous cyst would be found to be less bright than CSF. Conversely, the protein content of a cyst must be very high to effect the CT appearance.

The presence of fat is much easier to see on MR than with CT. Fat has a characteristic appearance, being bright on short TR MR images due to its short T1 compared to white matter, gray matter,

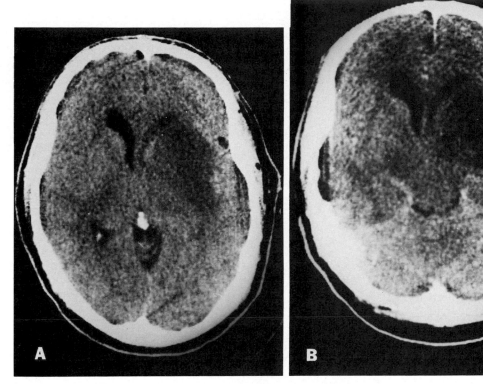

FIG 16–1.
Well-differentiated astrocytoma. Nonenhanced **(A)** and enhanced **(B)** scans demonstrated low density within the inferior left frontal and left temporal lobes. Only minimal enhancement along the lat-eral margin of the low density tumor is present **(B)**. Although the margins are relatively sharp and the neoplasm is quite low-dense, no macroscopic or microscopic cysts were present.

CSF, air, or bone. The moderate-to-short T2 of fat results in decreased signal intensity on long TR/TE images. A larger, homogeneous collection of fat must be present to demonstrate the characteristic low attenuation on CT, with values of −50 to −100 Hounsfield units (HU). Finally, a variety of paramagnetic and ferromagnetic substances may be present which might effect the MR appearance but have no effect on the CT scan.

On the unenhanced CT scan, the majority of astrocytomas present either with areas of decreased density (see Fig 16–1) or with patchy areas of low density mixed with regions of isodensity. The findings may be quite subtle, and a normal unenhanced CT scan is not infrequent. The rim so commonly seen with a malignant tumor on the enhanced scan may appear to be of slightly increased density relative to normal brain on the unenhanced views (Fig 16–5). This increased density may be more apparent than real because of the decreased density of peritumoral edema combined with the low density of central necrosis or cyst formation. The borders of the lesion are usually poorly defined on the unenhanced scan, with those margins melding imperceptibly into areas of surrounding cerebral edema or into areas of more normal-appearing brain. Contrast enhancement is required for a better definition of the lesion and its margins. Various authors in the past have suggested that if a brain tumor is suspected, the nonenhanced CT scan is of little differential diagnostic value.[6, 7] More importantly, some small tumors that are isodense on the unenhanced scan would be missed if the radiographic findings on the preinfusion scan were to be used as the basis for administering contrast material. The CT scanners in use today have significantly better contrast and spatial resolution than those of the 1970s and early 1980s. Most medium-to-large tumors show focal mass effect on the sulci or ventricular system, or alteration of the gray or white matter densities, either from the tumor itself or the peritumoral edema. All of those findings are usually apparent on the unenhanced CT scan performed on the current high-quality CT systems. However, small tumors could be missed without contrast administration. As a general rule, therefore, we continue to urge the use of contrast enhancement if an intracranial mass

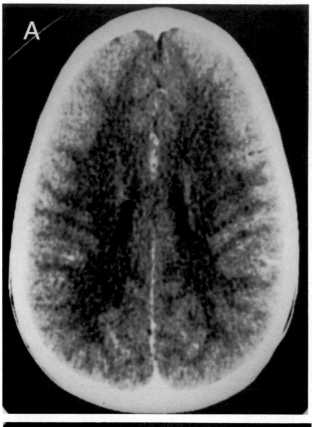

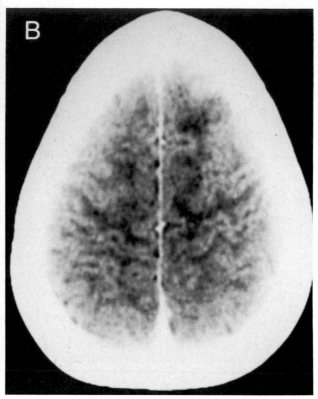

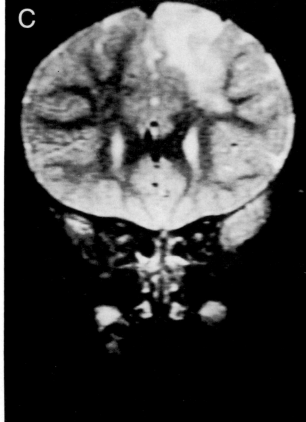

FIG 16–2.
Low-grade astrocytoma. **A,** an enhanced CT scan at the level of the top of the lateral ventricles does not demonstrate any significant mass effect on either the ventricular system or the cortex in the left frontal region. **B,** a higher cut demonstrates some poorly marginated low density in the high convexity left frontal lobe. **C,** the heavily T2-weighted coronal MR scan with a long TR/TE (TR 3,200, TE 120) demonstrates the extensive hyperintensity throughout the left frontal lobe. Hyperintensity extends through white matter tracks inferiorly to the supraventricular region and then laterally toward the frontoparietal junction. There is also hyperintensity of the overlying high-convexity cortex. This case illustrates the pronounced sensitivity of MR in evaluating the presence and extent of neoplasm which may be quite subtle on CT.

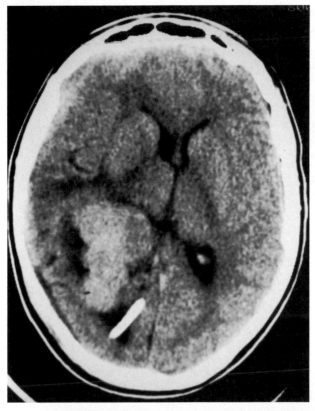

FIG 16–3.
Compact astrocytoma. This unenhanced CT scan shows relatively high density of nonhemorrhagic recurrent astrocytoma in the posterior right cerebral hemisphere. Relatively dense cellularity with little interstitial water accounts for this appearance. The patient has had previous surgery and a portion of an intraventricular shunt is seen in the right occipital region.

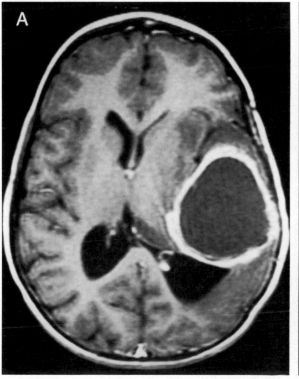

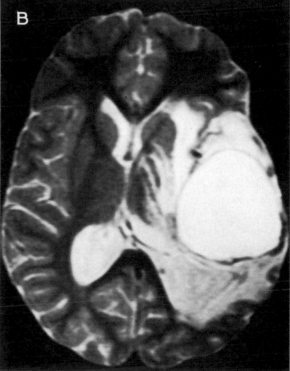

FIG 16–4.
Cystic glioblastoma. **A,** the short TR (TR 400, TE 20) sequence was performed following enhancement with gadolinium DTPA and demonstrates dense enhancement on the periphery of the large cystic lesion representing viable neoplasm and abnormal blood-brain barrier. There is sharp margination between the enhancing tumor and the central fluid, indicative of a true cyst. The intensity of the fluid is greater than ventricular CSF, indicating a higher protein content. Enhancement extends to the hypointense *(black)* calvarial cortex, so that there may well be dural invasion. **B,** the long TR/TE sequence (TR 2,750, TE 80) shows the hyperintensity of the cyst fluid relative to CSF, again indicative of the higher protein content. Fingers of edema extend along white matter tracks between deep gray nuclei, with extensive homogeneous edema involving both white and gray matter more superficially.

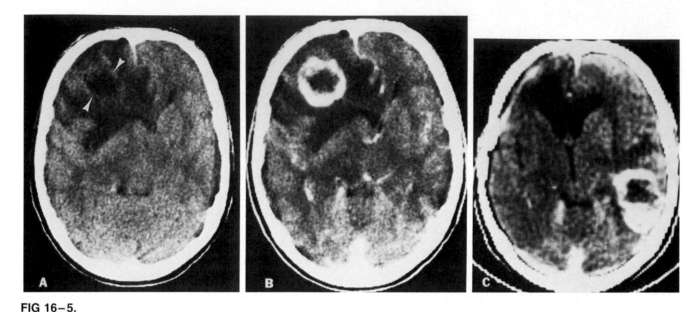

FIG 16−5.

Glioblastoma multiforme with intracranial metastasis via CSF. **A,** the unenhanced scan demonstrates the rim of tumor tissue *(arrowheads)* surrounding a more central necrotic portion of the tumor. The ring is made more prominent by the central necrosis and surrounding peritumoral edema. **B,** the enhanced scan demonstrates the shaggy ring of enhancing tumor. Note that there is no evidence of tumor in the left temporal region at this time. **C,** 5 months later, following surgery and irradiation of the right frontal glioblastoma multiforme, the patient presents with a left posterior temporal enhancing centrally necrotic mass. The contiguity of the temporal mass to the surface of the brain suggests that this second lesion represents metastasis via the CSF pathways.

is suspected from symptoms or signs, and not rely on the appearance of the unenhanced scan.

The appearance of the unenhanced short TR MR scan is similar to the unenhanced CT scan, in that most astrocytomas present as low intensity of the entire region of tumor and "edema," relative to normal white matter (Fig 16−6). As will be discussed later, the boundaries between the tumor and the edematous but otherwise normal brain are poorly defined. There are tongues of tumor within the edematous tissue, so that the separation of tumor from edema is not possible.[8−13] The midportion of the tumor may have even lower intensity due to necrosis, particularly if it is a malignant tumor. The presence of debris and high protein content makes the central portion of a cystic or necrotic tumor more intense than CSF on the short TR images due to the shorter T1 of the proteinaceous fluid and debris (see Fig 16−4). More compact portions of the tumor, or those with less water content, will be closer to isointensity with normal brain, or even of slightly higher intensity (Fig 16−6,A).

The unenhanced long TR study demonstrates high intensity from the entire region owing to the increased water content within both the tumor and the edematous surrounding brain as compared with normal white and gray matter (Figs 16−2,

16−4, 16−6, and 16−7). The pronounced sensitivity of this sequence to changes in tissue water content makes MRI the preferred imaging technique over CT for the detection of glioma (see Fig 16−2). More compact tumor may appear to be less intense (Fig 16−8). The boundaries between tumor and edematous but nonneoplastic brain cannot be defined because the tumor itself is hyperintense owing to an increased amount of free water (interstitial, intracellular), as is the edematous nonneoplastic surrounding tissue (see Fig 16−7). In addition, there is histologically a lack of sharp demarcation between the infiltrating neoplasm and the normal brain.[8−13]

Edema.—An understanding of the formation of peritumoral edema and of contrast enhancement of a neoplastic lesion requires knowledge of the blood-brain barrier (BBB). The normal BBB regulates the passage of water, nutrients, and macromolecules from the capillaries into the cerebral parenchyma. The BBB consists of tight junctions between the capillary endothelial cells, the capillary basement membrane, the glial footplate that wraps around the capillary, and various transport mechanisms in both the capillary endothelial and glial cells. Disruption of the BBB may occur from a variety of insults, including neoplastic invasion, in-

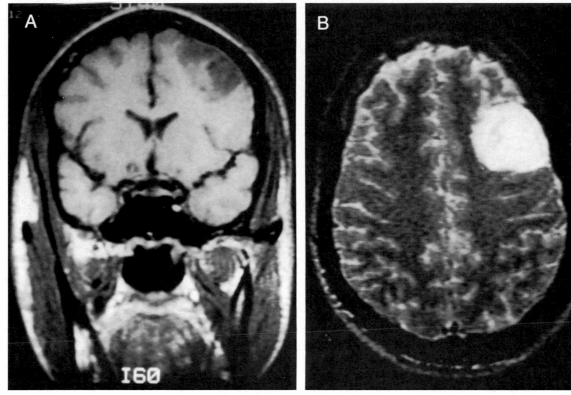

FIG 16–6.
Left frontal astrocytoma. **A,** the coronal short TR MR scan (TR 800, TE 25) demonstrates relatively well-circumscribed hypointensity of the left frontal cortex and underlying white matter. There is an area of isointensity within the deeper portion of the tumor. **B,** the long TR/TE sequence (TR 2,500, TE 75) demonstrates the relatively well-circumscribed hyperintense tumor.

farction, and inflammatory disease to name a few examples. Disruption of the BBB allows excessive fluid to pass from the capillaries into the extracellular space. Macromolecules may also pass through the disrupted BBB, setting up an osmotic gradient that further attracts water molecules. This process is termed *vasogenic edema,* and is a typical response of neoplastic growth.

Tumor vessels have an abnormal BBB. There is disagreement as to whether there is a decreased number of tight junctions, widening of existing junctions, fenestrations, or focal irregularities of the basement membrane.[14] There is more extracellular space between the cells in white matter than gray matter, so that vasogenic edema occurs more readily in white matter. Because neoplasms induce vasogenic edema, and because of the propensity for vasogenic edema to involve white matter, peritumoral edema is most prominent in the white matter.

Cytotoxic edema, on the other hand, begins as intracellular swelling secondary to any type of insult to the cell membrane. Ischemia, a decreased concentration of nutrients such as glucose, and cellular poisons result in an insult to basic cellular function including maintenance of normal cell membrane activity, with resultant cellular inhibition of water. Damage to the BBB then follows, leading to vasogenic edema. Edema such as that from ischemia is found in both gray and white matter. Radiographically, infarction involves both gray and white matter, and low density on CT, low intensity on short TR, and hyperintensity on long TR/TE MR scans involving both gray and white matter are characteristic.

The CT scan appearance of vasogenic edema is that of low density, particularly in the white matter, extending like fingers along white matter tracts (see Fig 16–7,A). On MRI, the same areas are of iso- to low intensity on short TR images and are bright on long TR sequences (see Figs 16–2,C, 16–4, 16–7). These are nonspecific findings. In particular, areas of abnormal brightness on long TR sequences can be seen in areas of gliosis, demyelination, and other non-neoplastic etiologies. The edema produces mass effect on local structures, with compression of the ventricular system, and effacement of cortical sulci (see Figs 16–4, 16–7).

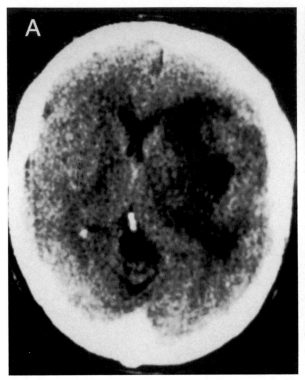 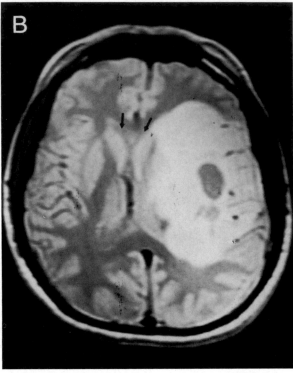

FIG 16−7.
Left hemispheric astrocytoma. **A,** the enhanced CT scan shows low density extending throughout white matter tracks in the left frontal, temporal, and parietal lobes, with a more circumscribed focus at the frontoparietal junction with a density equal to CSF. **B,** the proton-density image (TR 2,500, TE 25) demonstrates even more tumor and edema than does the CT scan. It is impossible to separate tumor from edema. The intensity of the cyst remains equal or even slightly lower in intensity relative to CSF within the displaced frontal horns *(arrows),* indicative of a low protein concentration.

Astrocytomas and glioblastomas are infiltrating tumors. As such the definition between the neoplasm, edematous white matter, and normal brain cannot be defined with accuracy either at gross pathologic examination or with any type of imaging study yet devised for evaluation of the brain, including CT and MRI.[8−13] Tumor may extend through normal tissue and not produce a change in the peritumoral water content to a degree that can be detected with even so sensitive a methodology as high-field MRI. High-field MR scanning, including MRI of postmortem brain slices, in a patient with known gliomatosis cerebri demonstrated areas of "edema" containing fingers of tumor, and normal MR signals in areas with histologic evidence of tumor invasion (Fig 16−9). Tumor invasion, in fact, extended from the frontal lobes to the upper cervical spinal cord, with most areas not showing the hyperintensity characteristic of edema as a first sign of tumor invasion. It cannot be stressed too strongly that even high-field MRI may only show the "tip of the iceberg" with infiltrating gliomas of even advanced and aggressive stages.

Contrast Enhancement.—The use of contrast enhancement for neurologic imaging is discussed much more fully in Chapters 5 and 6. Briefly, iodine is excellent at attenuating the CT x-ray beam, while gadolinium is a very effective paramagnetic agent, with its imaging effect being primarily the shortening of the T1 relaxation time. Both iodine and gadolinium are attached to macromolecules. In CT scanning, the presence and degree of enhancement is proportional to the amount of the iodinated macromolecules that pass into a lesion. For an intraaxial lesion such as neoplasm, infarction, inflammation, etc., there is disruption of the BBB and movement of macromolecules, including the contrast agent, into the extravascular spaces, including the interstices of the neoplasm. Extraaxial neoplasms, such as acoustic neuroma and pituitary adenoma which are outside of the BBB, enhance because of the accumulation of contrast material within sinusoids and other vascular and extravascular pools within the lesion. Vascular lesions, such as aneurysm or arteriovenous malformation (AVM) and some highly vascular intraaxial tumors,

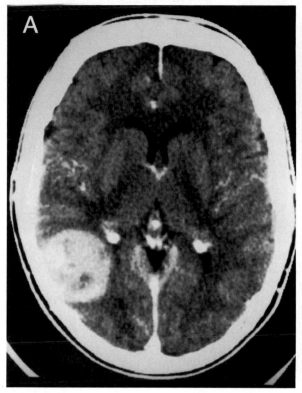 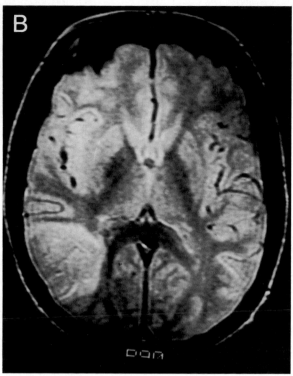

FIG 16–8.
Well-circumscribed anaplastic astrocytoma. **A,** the well-circumscribed anaplastic astrocytoma enhances intensely on the CT scan. **B,** the proton-density MR sequence (TR 2,750, TE 30) shows the intensity of the tumor to be similar to gray matter, indicative of a relatively compact tumor with less free water than other tumors illustrated.

enhance in part or in total because of the presence of the contrast agent within the vascular pool of the lesion.

Enhancement with MRI is more complicated, with multiple factors involved in the presence and degree of enhancement. The proton density and the relaxation parameters, T1 and T2, are a function of the structure of the lesion, the amount of bound water, and other physiologic properties that represent the environment of the lesion. Like CT, the disruption of the BBB is an integral factor, as are the type of agent injected (including the size of the macromolecule), the time after administration, and the route of administration. MR enhancement of an intraaxial lesion such as a neoplasm depends primarily upon the disruption of the BBB and movement of the paramagnetic macromolecules into the extravascular spaces, analogous to CT, to produce shortening of T1 relaxation times. Extraaxial neoplasms outside of the BBB depend upon movement of the MR contrast agent into extravascular pools, again analogous to CT. The presence and speed of intravascular flow determines whether vascular structures will enhance. Vascular lesions having rapid flow may not enhance because of dephasing or because of the rapid exit of the contrast agent from the slice. Slower-flowing vessels such as medium and small veins and capillary beds usually enhance. Finally, multiple scanning parameters may be altered including the TR, TE, and flip angle. In general, MRI is much more sensitive at detecting contrast enhancement of a lesion with small amounts of administered paramagnetic contrast agent than is CT, which requires iodinated agents to attenuate the beam.

As previously explained, higher degrees of malignancy of intraaxial neoplasms are generally correlated with a greater abnormality of the BBB. Therefore, more contrast material escapes and the more malignant lesion demonstrates more contrast enhancement (see Figs 16–4, 16–5) than does the more benign lesion with a more intact BBB (see Fig 16–9). There are, however, many exceptions to this rule, as will be discussed. In addition, a minimally impaired BBB or a lesion with little extracellular space may not allow the passage of many macromolecules containing either iodine or gadolinium out of the capillaries, but may allow some

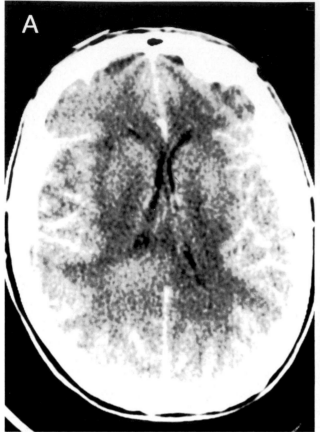

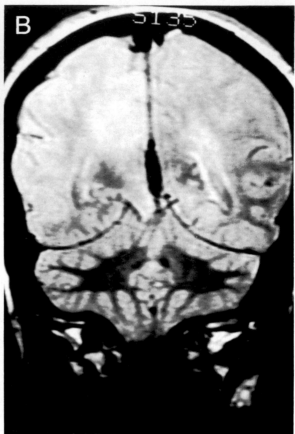

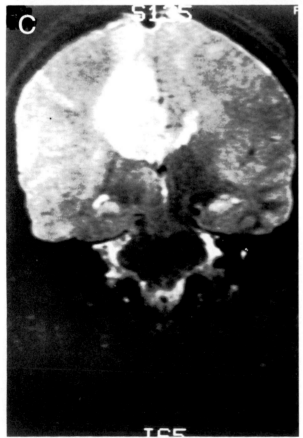

FIG 16–9.
Gliomatosis cerebri. **A,** the enhanced axial CT scan demonstrates slight enhancement within the right side of the splenium of the corpus callosum, and mass effect on the posterior right lateral ventricle. **B,** the coronal proton-density MR image (TR 3,000, TE 25) shows hyperintensity throughout the medial right parietal lobe, and loss of definition of corticomedullary junctions throughout the right hemisphere. Note the unremarkable appearance of the cerebellum. **C,** the heavily T2-weighted sequence (TR 3,000, TE 75) demonstrates the extensive high intensity throughout the medial right parietal lobe, extension to the high-convexity cortex, effacement of corticomedullary junctions and sulci throughout the right hemisphere, extension through the splenium of the corpus callosum into the left hemisphere, and effacement of sulci and corticomedullary junctions of the high left parietal lobe. Note the unremarkable appearance of the pons. The basal ganglia bilaterally, and the left temporal and left frontal lobes all appeared normal (not shown), as did the cerebellum and brain stem. The patient died 13 days after this MR scan. In vitro postmortem MRI of the formalin-fixed brain showed similar findings to those seen in the in vivo study. Histopathologic examination demonstrated infiltrative anaplastic astrocytoma involving both the gray and white matter of both cerebral hemispheres diffusely, the cerebellum, and the brain stem. While the regions of poor gray-white differentiation identified on the antemortem MRI were infiltrated by neoplastic astrocytes, there were also areas of neoplastic infiltration which appeared normal by both in vivo and in vitro MRI, particularly the thalami and basal ganglia, cerebellum, and brain stem. (From Koslow S, Hirsch WL, Classen D, et al: Gliomatosis cerebri: MR-pathologic correlation. To be published. Used by permission.)

small water molecules to pass. Therefore, one can have an abnormal attenuation on CT or abnormal intensity on MRI from a tumor and yet not have much or any enhancement after contrast administration (Fig 16–10).

On CT, increased attenuation of the x-ray beam produces increased density of the lesion or a whiter appearance on the x-ray film (see Fig 16–8). On MRI, the paramagnetic effect of gadolinium-diethylenetriamine pentaacetic acid (DTPA) at approved doses is primarily by shortening the T1 relaxation time, producing a brighter signal on short TR images (see Fig 16–4). There is relatively little effect by gadolinium on the T2 relaxation time and essentially no effect on the proton density of the tissues per se.

Between 100 and 150 cc of iodinated contrast media, commonly 60% concentration, is administered as an intravenous bolus, a drip, or a combination of the two. The use of an ionic vs. a nonionic agent is discussed in Chapter 5. In the past, some authors advocated a double dose of iodinated contrast material administered over 15 minutes and followed by a delay in scanning of 1 to 2 hours in order to visualize a subtle tumor(s).[15, 16] This delayed high-dose (DHD) technique produces high blood levels of iodine and allows time for the movement of the contrast material across a relatively intact BBB. They found this technique to be superior to either immediate scanning following a double dose of contrast material or to delayed scanning following a conventional dose. They found that the DHD technique allowed the visualization of single or multiple tumors not otherwise seen in 11.5% of cases in which the conventional dose was first utilized. There was no significant change in serum electrolyte values in those patients who had normal renal function before the DHD scan.[15, 16] Much of this work, however, was performed before or just at the time of the advent of the newest high-resolution CT scanners, which have given much better contrast resolution for the detection of subtle neoplasms. In addition, MRI has relegated this technique to one of historical interest. Subtle tumors and the possibility of multiple metastases are far better evaluated with MRI, particularly enhanced MRI, than with CT, even using the DHD technique. The possibility of adverse reactions to such a high dose of contrast material is obviated with the use of MRI.

Relative "healing" of the BBB occurs with use of corticosteroids.[17, 18] In some patients it is difficult clinically to withdraw those corticosteroids in order to obtain a definitive CT scan, and high vol-

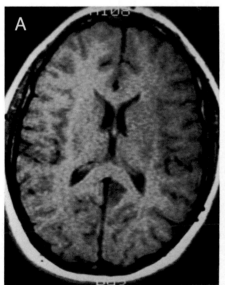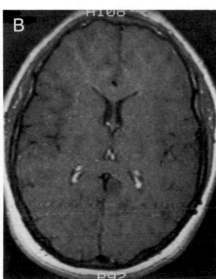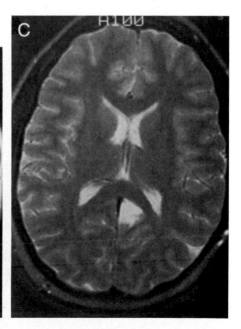

FIG 16–10.
Mixed glioma with hyperintensity on long TR/TE sequence but no enhancement. **A,** the nonenhanced short TR image (TR 500, TE 20) demonstrates a low-intensity abnormality involving the medial left parietal lobe just behind the splenium of the corpus callosum. **B,** the enhanced short TR image (same TR and TE) does not dem-onstrate any enhancement within the lesion. However, there is hyperintensity throughout the lesion on the long TR/TE sequence (**C,** TR 2,867, TE 80). This sequence indicates the increased free water content within the low-grade mixed glioma, but a relatively intact blood-brain barrier.

umes of iodinated contrast material can be used to overcome the "steroid effect." In these cases, again, MRI is the technique of choice.

The only approved paramagnetic contrast agent at the present time is gadolinium DTPA, which is commonly administered as a 0.1 mmol concentration at 0.2 mg/kg. Other paramagnetic contrast agents will be forthcoming in the future (see Chapter 6). Studies with MR scans at varying time intervals following contrast administration have demonstrated the maximum effect on the T1 relaxation time to be quite variable, but generally within the first 15 minutes. Delayed scans have shown a broadening of the borders of the enhancing area with time as a manifestation of the diffusion of the contrast agent through the tissues. In fact, there may be a relative thickening of the rim

of enhancement over time (Fig 16–11). That is, there is both diffusion of contrast material into central areas of necrosis and tumor, and movement of contrast material across tissues where the BBB is damaged but still relatively intact relative to other areas. The use of delayed MR scanning following contrast infusion for the detection of lesions with a relatively intact BBB has yet to be studied in depth.

Generally speaking, we prefer to obtain only a contrast-enhanced CT scan in a patient with a suspected intracranial mass lesion. We and others have found little efficacy in the use of a preceding nonenhanced scan in the majority of patients. There is little help in the differential diagnosis on the nonenhanced scan.[6, 7] Usually, intratumoral calcification, which may help in the differential

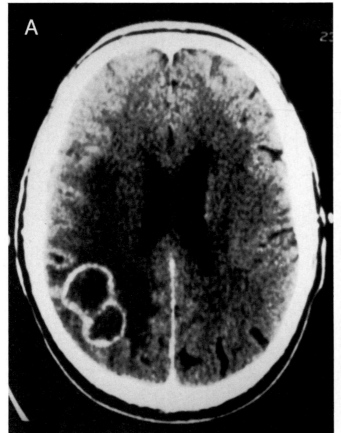

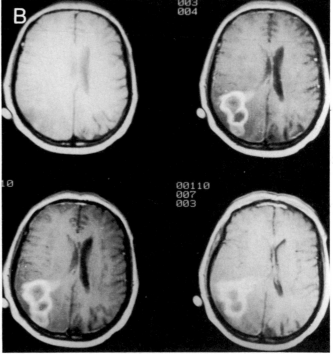

FIG 16–11.
Centrally necrotic glioblastoma with progressive internal and peripheral MR enhancement over time. **A,** the patient has a known recurrent centrally necrotic right parietal glioblastoma multiforme that has a relatively thin peripheral ring of enhancement on the CT scan. **B,** a sequential short TR MR study was performed over time following the injection of gadolinium DTPA (TR 500, TE 20). The top left image is before enhancement. The top right is 3 minutes after contrast injection, the bottom left 30 minutes after contrast injec-

tion, and the bottom right 55 minutes after contrast injection. There is progressive enhancement internal to the original ring, indicating either diffusion of contrast material into the central area of necrosis or enhancement of tumor with less blood supply. There is progressive enhancement external to the ring, with extension toward the atrium of the right lateral ventricle. This indicates a more extensive abnormality of the blood-brain barrier and indicates the difficulties in defining precisely the boundaries of the neoplasm.

evaluation, can be detected with contrast enhancement present. Retrospective evaluation of over 5,000 CT scanning procedures demonstrated that in less than 0.3% of cases did the patient have to return for an evaluation of possible calcification for differential diagnosis.[6] The obviation of many nonessential unenhanced CT scans, requiring only a few patients to return for a nonenhanced scan, makes this a reasonable and financially prudent policy. Acute neurologic change, on the other hand, may signal the presence of intracranial hemorrhage. In such a case, we always obtain a nonenhanced scan before contrast infusion.

With MR scanning, it is currently our belief that we should obtain both nonenhanced long and short TR sequences before contrast infusion, followed by short TR imaging after contrast infusion. The long TR sequence may occasionally demonstrate areas of abnormal water content but no or minimal enhancement and, therefore, would be missed on an enhanced short TR sequence alone (see Fig 16–10). In addition, the bright signal of an enhancing area on the short TR sequence has the same signal as fat or certain phases of hemorrhage

on a short TR series. It is, therefore, our current policy that all patients receiving contrast material have a preceding nonenhanced short TR sequence to assist in this differentiation.

The enhancement patterns of astrocytomas are similar on both MRI and CT, although MRI seems to be more sensitive to the presence of enhancement. With low-grade astrocytomas there is generally a relatively intact BBB, so that there is only patchy enhancement or no enhancement (see Figs 16–1, 16–2, and 16–10). There is poor definition of tumor boundaries (see Fig 16–9), as previously discussed. More malignant lesions usually have more exuberant enhancement[19] (see Figs 16–4, 16–5, and 16–8), although there are many significant exceptions. Relatively benign cystic astrocytomas of childhood often have a markedly enhancing nodule or vivid rim enhancement (see Figs 16–39 to 16–42), and solid cerebellar astrocytomas of childhood frequently enhance to a marked degree even with a relatively benign histology.[20–22] Conversely, there may be minimal or no enhancement of malignant astrocytomas (Figs 16–12 and 16–13) and occasionally glioblastoma multiforme.[8, 22]

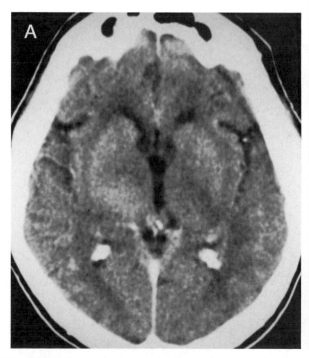 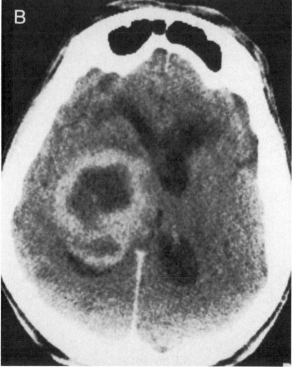

FIG 16–12.
Rapid progression of glioblastoma. This 75-year-old woman initially presented with left-sided weakness, and an enhanced CT scan demonstrating poorly marginated enhancement of moderate degree involving the right thalamus and posterior limb of the internal capsule **(A).** Nine months later, there is a large ring-enhancing lesion of the deep right cerebral hemisphere, with two areas of central ecrosis **(B).**

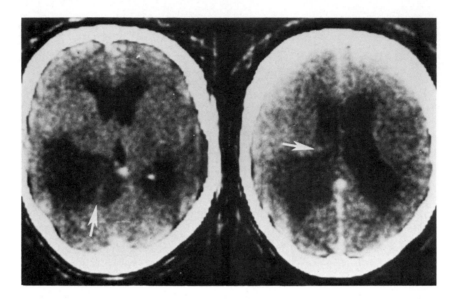

FIG 16–13.

High-grade astrocytoma with microcystic components. A large low-density parietal lobe mass is present with absorption coefficients close to those of the CSF within the ventricular system. The mass does not represent a dilated ventricular atrium, but is separated from the lateral ventricle *(arrows),* which is compressed and distorted. A grossly solid lesion was found at the time of surgery, not a grossly cystic lesion, although intracellular microcysts were found on pathologic examination, accounting for the low density of this lesion. (From Latchaw RE, Gold HLA, Moore JS, et al: *Radiology* 1977; 125:141–144. Used by permission.)

Brain stem gliomas are frequently malignant but do not always demonstrate significant enhancement.[23, 24]

Malignant astrocytomas and glioblastoma multiforme frequently enhance as a rim around a central area of necrosis.[12] This pattern of ring enhancement is nonspecific, and has also been seen with metastases, resolving hematomas, abscesses, and occasionally infarctions. While it has been stated that an abscess generally has a thin rim of enhancement while the shaggy rim is characteristic of malignant neoplasm (see Fig 16–12), there have been many examples of thick-rimmed abscesses, particularly those that are in the early stages of evolution from cerebritis.[18] Relatively thin-rimmed malignant neoplasms are also demonstrated (see Fig 18–11,A). Infarctions generally demonstrate areas of peripheral enhancement at the junction of viable and nonviable tissue, and generally do not form a perfect ring of enhancement. There may be progressive enhancement of the central portion of the neoplastic ring lesion over time. Contrast material may diffuse into either a cystic cavity or an area of necrosis. There may also be an admixture of necrotic tumor and viable tumor with decreased blood supply and therefore delayed enhancement (see Fig 16–11).[16, 25] MRI has demonstrated progressive enhancement of the tissue outside the early enhancing rim,[26] giving further evidence for the inability to perfectly define tumor boundaries (see Fig 16–11). There is also progressive enhancement of the central hypointense zone, representing either delayed enhancement in the mixture of necrotic and viable tumor or diffusion into necrotic tissue (see Fig 16–11).

While the ring lesion is characteristic of glioblastoma multiforme, malignant astrocytoma and glioblastoma may have a pattern of nodular enhancement like more benign tumors or metastases (Fig 16–14).[27] Occasionally, it may be difficult to distinguish a peripherally located malignant primary tumor or metastasis from an extraaxial tumor such as meningioma that invaginates into the cerebral parenchyma (Fig 16–15). Multiple projections, such as those easily obtained with MRI, help in this differentiation. Displacement or "buckling" of the gray-white junction has been described on CT with extraaxial lesions to help in differentiation from an intraaxial lesion, which produces edema of the white matter, loss of the normally sharp corticomedullary junction, and flattening of sulci.[28] The MR relaxation characteristics of the typical meningioma, which is usually isointense to brain parenchyma on nonenhanced scans, also aids in differentiation.

The differentiation of a true macroscopic cyst from an area of necrosis may be important, in that a

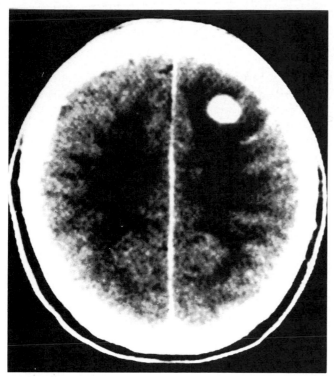

FIG 16–14.
Anaplastic astrocytoma having the appearance of a metastasis. This solid well-circumscribed neoplasm with abundant surrounding cerebral edema has an appearance more typical of solitary metastasis.

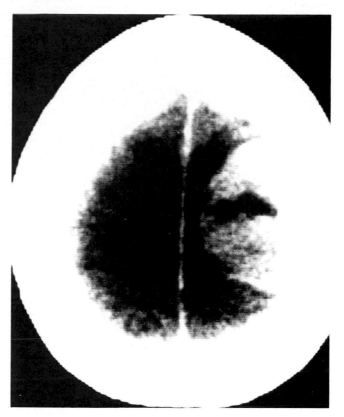

FIG 16–15.
Well-circumscribed high-convexity glioblastoma multiforme. The enhanced scan demonstrates a sharply marginated mass high over the left cerebral convexity and based along the inner table of the skull. Many of the features suggest a benign tumor such as meningioma. There is a central area of necrosis and/or cyst formation.

cystic component can be surgically drained (Fig 16–16). On CT, the diagnosis of a true cyst requires the visualization of sharp margins of the cystic cavity. A fluid-fluid level from diffusion of contrast material may also be seen. On MRI, both the increased protein of a neoplastic cyst and necrotic debris will shorten the T1 relaxation time relative to CSF, making it more intense than CSF on short TR images (see Fig 16–4).[5, 29] Occasionally, the rim of neoplasm may be very thin or there may be lack of enhancement, making it difficult to differentiate a neoplastic and non-neoplastic cyst such as arachnoid cyst on CT. MRI can aid in this differentiation. A non-neoplastic cyst should have a T1 relaxation time close to that of CSF. If not, with a grayer appearance than CSF on short TR images secondary to the presence of a higher protein content, one must be suspicious of neoplasm.

Some astrocytomas, both benign and malignant, present as low-density lesions without evidence of contrast enhancement and with absorption coefficients on CT that are close to CSF (see Fig 16–13).[8, 30, 31] Such an appearance suggests a cystic tumor or possibly a non-neoplastic process

such as porencephaly, arachnoid cyst, or infarct. Indeed, these authors have seen such mistakes in CT diagnosis made not infrequently. The margins of such a low-density tumor are usually not as sharp and smooth as a grossly cystic lesion. The low density on CT, and the low intensity on short TR and hyperintensity on long TR/TE MR sequences, is accounted for by the presence of a relatively high water content within the neoplasm, either interstitial microcysts or high intracellular water content. It must again be emphasized that the diagnosis of neoplasia in such a case does not rest upon the presence of contrast enhancement, nor upon specific absorption coefficients[8] or relaxation values. The morphologic characteristics, such as the margins of the lesion, generally lead to the correct diagnosis. On MRI, a lesion that has a shorter T1 than CSF should give suspicion that this may result because of the presence of a higher protein content, and thus the lesion may be neoplastic.[5, 29]

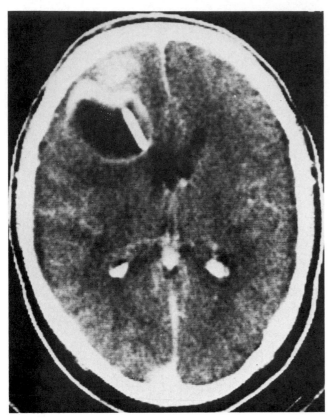

FIG 16–16.
Cystic astrocytoma with shunt. The right frontal lobe neoplasm is cystic as indicated by the sharp margins of the internal lucency. A shunt has been placed into the cyst cavity for decompression.

Lilja and co-workers[32] studied a group of high-grade gliomas by CT in patients immediately before death, followed by extensive postmortem sectioning and radiologic-pathologic correlation. They found that areas of little or no enhancement that are either isodense or of low density contain fingers of viable neoplasm throughout the region. Areas of nonenhancing low-density tumor with histologic characteristics of malignancy have a CT or MR appearance similar to that of edematous peritumoral normal brain (see Fig 16–7).[8–13, 32] MR scanning of postmortem slices has shown normal-appearing brain in areas with histologic evidence of malignancy (see Fig 16–9). Therefore, in summary, while it can be said that the greater degree of enhancement generally parallels a higher degree of malignancy, the lack of enhancement does not rule out malignancy.[8] In general, minimal-to-moderate patchy enhancement is characteristic of lower-grade astrocytomas, while intense enhancement in a ring pattern is characteristic of malignant astrocytoma and glioblastoma. When such a ring lesion is present on the MR or CT scan, the odds are strong that a malignant astrocytoma is present. The lack of such a pattern, however, does not exclude malignancy.

Mass Effect and Herniations.—The amount of mass effect with any given astrocytic tumor is dependent to a large degree upon the amount of surrounding "edema" (see Figs 16–1, 16–6). Infiltrating neoplasms with little surrounding edema may produce little or no apparent mass effect on the ventricular system, the structure upon which mass effect is most apparent (see Fig 16–9). A lack of apparent mass effect does not exclude a diagnosis of neoplasm. Temporal and occipital lobe masses and high-convexity tumors may produce little distortion of the distant ventricular system, although effacement of the cortical sulci may be present with the masses close to the convexity (see Figs 16–6 and 16–8). Multiple projections may be necessary to see such distortions. Sagittal and coronal reformatted CT images are significant additions to the axial views. These multiple projections are easily available with MR (see Figs 16–2 and 16–6). In addition, there is a lack of the beam-hardening artifact from the calvarium present on CT scans. This allows for better visualization of sulcal effacement. Finally, MRI has inherently greater ability to differentiate gray and white matter, and to detect distortion of these structures from subtle local mass effect. For all of these reasons, MRI is favored over CT for the evaluation of subtle mass effect.

The inner table of the skull prevents the brain from moving laterally because of a focal cerebral hemispheric mass. Rather, the brain shifts medially toward the opposite hemisphere. The midline structures of the brain shift relative to the rigid falx, producing subfalcine herniation. The falx descends closer to the splenium of the corpus callosum than it does to the rostral corpus, allowing more shift anteriorly than posteriorly. A mass in the temporal lobe or middle cranial fossa may push the medial aspect of the temporal lobe medially and inferiorly through an available site of decompression, the tentorial incisura. Displacement of the uncus of the temporal lobe medially toward the suprasellar cistern and inferiorly over the edge of the tentorium, producing a crease in the uncus, is termed *uncal herniation*. Medial displacement of the hippocampal gyrus over the more posterior edge of the tentorium is termed *hippocampal herniation*. Both are variations of transtentorial herniation. Diffuse supratentorial pressure or a focal infratentorial mass may exert sufficient pressure to force the cerebellar tonsils inferiorly through the foramen magnum, compressing the medulla. This downward cerebellar herniation commonly follows a great deal of mass effect and increased intracranial pressure producing subfalcine and transtentorial herniation, with cerebellar herniation the final death-producing event. Far less common is upward cerebellar herniation through the tentorial notch from an inferiorly located posterior fossa mass. This upward cerebellar herniation forces the superior cerebellar vermis through the tentorial notch, obliterating the superior cerebellar and/or quadrigeminal cisterns.

Hemorrhage.—Hemorrhage into an astrocytoma or glioblastoma is more common with the higher grades of malignancy, although hemorrhage into lower-grade gliomas does occur. Such hemorrhage generally results as the tumor outgrows its blood supply, producing areas of necrosis and secondary hemorrhage. Hemorrhage may also occur

because tumor vessels have relatively weak walls that rupture easily, or because of growth of the neoplasm into normal cerebral vessels.[33]

On the CT scan, acute hemorrhage has a high density (white) (Fig 16–17), and is easier to detect than the often subtle low MR intensity of acute hemorrhage. CT is therefore preferred in the evaluation of acute neurologic change to exclude acute hemorrhage. With the dissolution of the clot and phagocytosis of the blood products, the high density of acute blood becomes low density over time. The low density of an old hematoma cavity cannot be differentiated from an area of necrosis, cyst formation, or edema on the CT scan. MRI is much better at identifying these subacute and chronic hemorrhagic collections (Fig 16–18), as discussed in Chapter 9. Briefly, acute hemorrhage is initially isointense and then becomes hypointense on long TR/TE sequences. Subacute blood is of high intensity on both short and long TR sequences. Chronic hemorrhage with hemosiderin is markedly hypointense, particularly on long TR or gradient-refo-

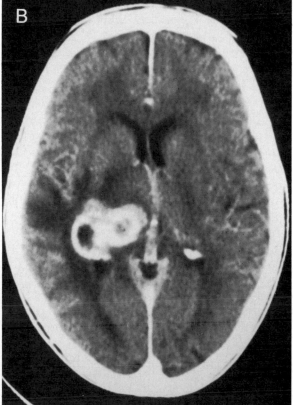
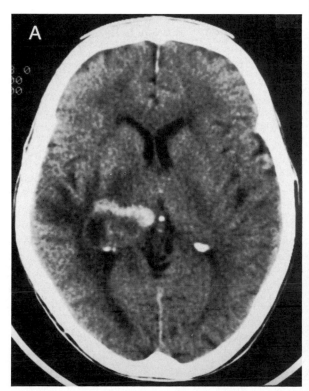

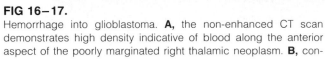

FIG 16–17.
Hemorrhage into glioblastoma. **A,** the non-enhanced CT scan demonstrates high density indicative of blood along the anterior aspect of the poorly marginated right thalamic neoplasm. **B,** con-trast enhancement masks the presence of hemorrhage, and demonstrates central areas of necrosis.

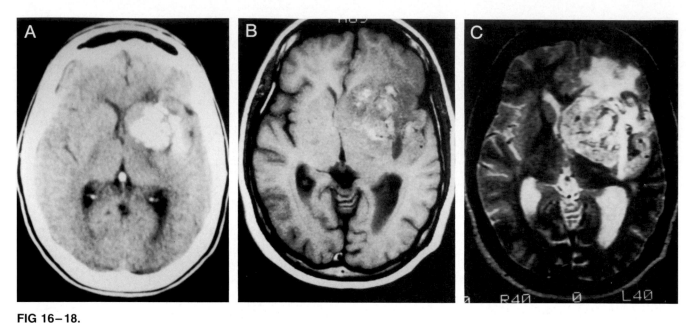

FIG 16–18.
Subacute and chronic hemorrhage into calcified anaplastic astrocytoma. **A,** the nonenhanced CT scan demonstrates extensive calcification throughout the deep posterior left frontal anaplastic astrocytoma. **B,** the majority of this calcification is not seen on the MR scan, but multiple areas of hyperintensity are seen throughout the tumor on the short TR image (TR 600, TE 20). **C,** the long TR/TE sequence (TR 2,500, TE 75) demonstrates similar areas of hyperintensity indicative of subacute blood, and also an area of marked hypointensity posteriorly and laterally indicative of hemosiderin of chronic hemorrhage. Small round areas of hypointensity represent either blood vessels or other areas of hemosiderin deposition. Extensive white matter edema is seen.

cused sequences. Blood products may exist for quite some time, and will be detected by MRI. The intensity of the intratumoral clot may not change as rapidly as nontumorous hemorrhage because of an impaired vascular supply to the necrotic portion of the tumor. The MR signal may be very complex and heterogeneous, indicating recurrent bleeding.[34]

Areas of hypointensity, particularly around the periphery of a tumor (see Fig 16–4), have frequently been called hemosiderin collections without definite pathologic proof. Not all areas of hypointensity in an area of neoplasm represent hemosiderin. Ferric iron deposits are known to occur in areas of glioma and also produce a marked hypointensity. Further radiographic-pathologic correlation is obviously necessary.

Hemorrhage may be the initial neurologic event in a patient without known cerebral tumor. The diagnosis of tumorous rather than nontumorous hemorrhage frequently depends upon a high degree of suspicion with a hemorrhage in an unusual location, with a dispersed distribution of the blood unlike the usual consolidated traumatic or hypertensive hematoma, or with an unusual history such as progressive neurologic deficit preceding the sudden event. In such a case, contrast enhancement at the periphery of the acute hemorrhage

may suggest underlying neoplasm (see Fig 16–17). In the subacute stage, however, a resolving spontaneous hematoma will have an abnormal BBB, allowing marginal enhancement.[17] MRI may show areas of abnormal tissue intensity at the periphery of the hematoma, even without enhancement, again suggesting neoplasm. MRI may also show multiple lesions suggesting metastases.

Calcification.—Calcification within an astrocytoma is indicative of slow growth and therefore is usually found in low-grade astrocytoma. However, such a tumor may undergo malignant degeneration (see Fig 16–18). CT easily demonstrates even punctate calcification (Fig 16–19). With MRI, relatively large and dense areas of homogeneous calcification must be present to produce the pronounced hypointense signal characteristic of calcification (Fig 16–19,C). If there is an admixture of calcified and noncalcified tissue, the noncalcified matrix will provide a signal and the calcification will not be detected. CT is more sensitive to the presence of calcification than is MRI, regardless of the pulsing sequence used.[35]

Tumor Spread.—Astrocytomas and glioblastomas infiltrate into the surrounding parenchyma by coursing along white matter tracts. Infiltration into

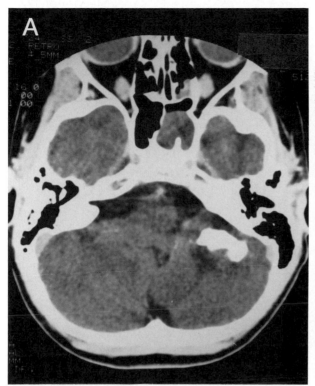

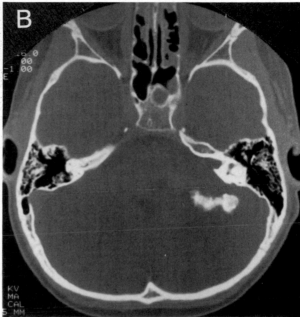

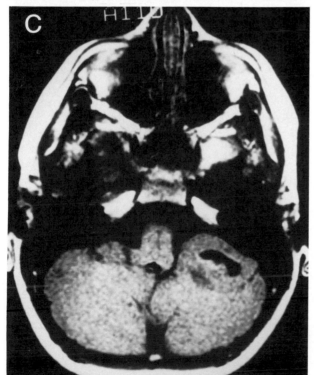

FIG 16–19.
Heavily calcified low-grade cerebellar astrocytoma. **A,** this 7-year-old child has dense calcification within the anterior left cerebellar hemisphere on the enhanced CT scan. **B,** there is a low-density abnormality surrounding the calcification which is confirmed with a "bone window." **C,** the short TR MR scan (TR 600, TE 20) demonstrates the marked hypointensity of the confluent calcification and the lesser hypointensity of the cerebellar neoplasm.

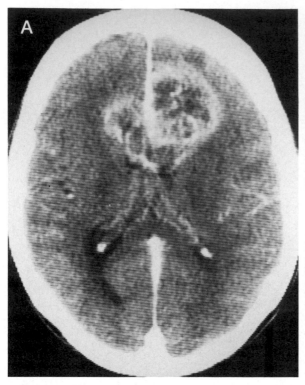

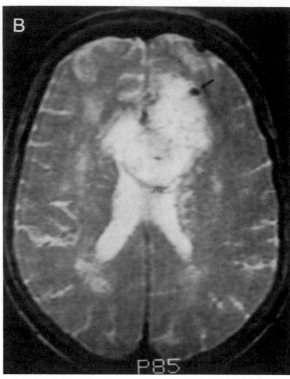

FIG 16–20.

Spread of glioblastoma through the anterior corpus callosum. **A,** the enhanced CT scan shows a ring-enhancing glioblastoma with central necrosis involving the medial left frontal lobe with extension through the corpus callosum into the medial right frontal lobe. **B,** the long TR/TE MR scan (TR 2,500, TE 75) shows a similar distribution of the tumor, although there is more abnormality involving the right frontal lobe white matter than seen on the CT scan. The low-intensity focus *(arrow)* in the left frontal lobe may represent focal hemosiderin deposition from previous hemorrhage.

the corpus callosum (Figs 16–9, 16–20, and 16–21) or the anterior or posterior commissures allows spread to the opposite hemisphere. Infiltration into the brain stem may also occur (Fig 16–22), allowing extension into the posterior fossa. Infiltration into subependymal tissues produces a periventricular mode of spread (Fig 16–23). This is generally an ominous sign for the patient's prognosis; even when the neurologic condition appears stable, periventricular spread is usually indicative of a rapid downhill course.[36]

The extension of neoplasm to a ventricular or cortical surface allows seeding of tumor cells via CSF pathways (see Fig 16–5). This may occur with many intracranial neoplasms, but is most common with malignant astrocytoma and glioblastoma.[37] Occasionally one sees multiple foci of glioma that represent separate sites of primary tumor (multifocal glioma) rather than metastases via CSF pathways.[38, 39] The necessary pathologic criteria for a diagnosis of multifocal glioma include the lack of linkage between the tumor masses along white matter tracts and the lack of contiguity of the tumor to cortical or ependymal surfaces.[38] If both lesions presented simultaneously, the imaging diagnosis could be metastases or lymphoma rather than multifocal glioma, and there would be no way to make the distinction without biopsy.

Astrocytomas and glioblastomas may grow into the dural coverings of the brain, but usually do not completely penetrate the dural structures. Rarely will these tumors destroy the overlying calvarium.[40] Dural invasion can be demonstrated angiographically, with tumor vessels to the glioma being supplied by the meningeal vascular system, but it is not usually seen on CT, since both the falx and dura normally enhance vividly with iodinated contrast material, as does the tumor. The falx and dura normally enhance only mildly with gadolinium, however, so that enhanced MRI might demonstrate dural invasion as a hyperintense tumor infiltrating the dural structures (see Fig 16–4). Rather than penetration of the falx, infiltration of the opposite hemisphere usually requires parenchymal extension such as through the corpus callosum (see

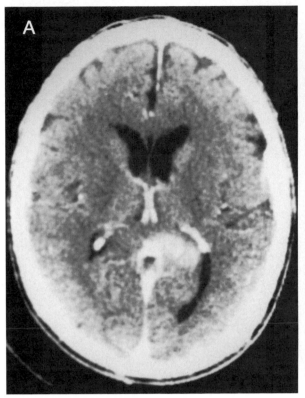

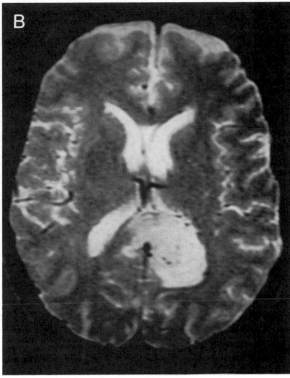

FIG 16–21.
Extension of malignant glioma through the splenium of the corpus callosum, better shown on MRI. **A,** the enhanced CT scan demonstrates enhancement involving the left side of the splenium. The enhancement terminates at the midline, although the right side of the splenium is thicker than normal. **B,** the MR sequence (TR 2,500, TE 75) demonstrates hyperintensity indicative of tumor and edema extending more deeply into the medial left parietal lobe and further across the midline into the right side of the splenium than appreciated on CT.

Figs 16–20 and 16–21) or seeding of tumor cells via CSF pathways (see Fig 16–5).

Nonenhanced MRI is better than CT for demonstrating this tumor spread wherever it occurs owing to the alteration of the water content of invaded tissues (see Figs 16–9 and 16–21). When the spread is contiguous to CSF-containing spaces, however, it may be impossible to perceive. Enhanced MRI is significantly better than nonenhanced MRI for determination of tumor extension. However, it must again be emphasized that not all of the tumor spread can be seen with even the best quality MR study with or without enhancement. Infiltrating tumor can be seen histologically when premortem enhanced MR and postmortem MR imaging of thin brain sections fail to show tissue changes (see Fig 16–9).

Grading of Malignancy and Pathologic-Radiographic Correlation.—The difficulty in grading the degree of malignancy by the radiographic appearance,[19, 22, 41–44] and the lack of accuracy in defin-

ing tumor boundaries by imaging techniques relative to those demonstrated histologically,[8–13] have been repeatedly emphasized in this chapter. Theoretically, the brighter a lesion on a T2 basis, or the more hypointense a lesion on a T1 basis, the more water should be present, indicative of a greater degree of disruption of the BBB and therefore malignancy. However, there may be microcystic change within lower-grade tumors, increasing the water content. Cellular compactness leaves less room for water, producing a more isointense lesion (see Fig 16–3). Theoretically, the more intense the degree of enhancement, the more disruption there is of the BBB and therefore a greater degree of malignancy. Histologic evidence of malignancy may be present without corresponding imaging evidence of leaking of the BBB, either with water accumulation or contrast enhancement (see Fig 16–13).

We and other authors have attempted to correlate histology with a variety of CT scan numeric parameters including attenuation coefficients, electron density, and atomic number following contrast

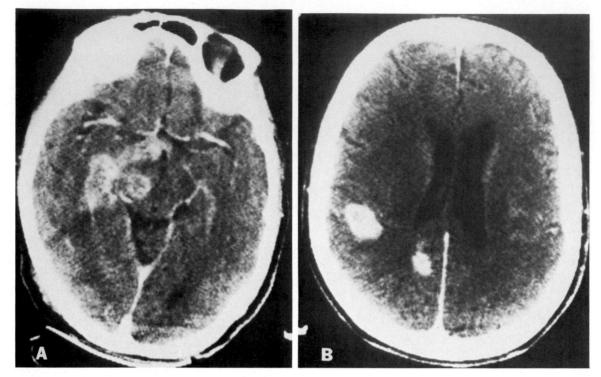

FIG 16–22.
Glioblastoma multiforme with both invasion of the brain stem and nodular fingers of tumor extension. **A,** a low-enhanced scan demonstrates the malignant glioma within the right temporal lobe. Extension of tumor is into the brain stem and hypothalamus-optic chiasm. Fingers of tumor extended more superiorly, so that a higher cut **(B)** discloses separate nodules simulating hematogenous metastases.

FIG 16–23.
Periventricular spread of glioblastoma. The enhanced CT scan demonstrates dense enhancement of a right hemispheric glioblastoma. There is enhancement at the anterior tips of both frontal horns, with extension along the horns into the interventricular septum. Spread of neoplasm is along subependymal pathways.

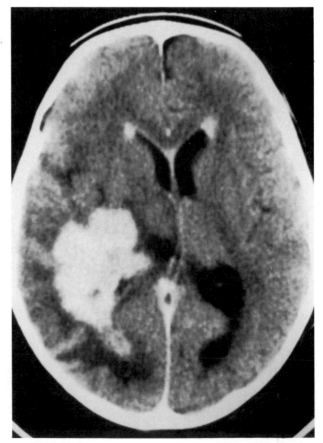

enhancement.[45, 46] While attenuation coefficients themselves did not correlate with a prediction of neoplasm or the degree of malignancy of that neoplasm, it appeared in early work that electron density or change of atomic number or both correlated with the degree of malignancy. In selected cases, the greater the degree of BBB disruption, the greater the degree of enhancement and therefore the greater change of atomic number. While these studies initially demonstrated an ability to separate benign neoplasms from gliomas from metastases,[45, 46] the correlations were not consistent. Likewise, correlations of histology with the time of enhancement using time-density curves[47] or histograms[48] were inconsistent.

There is a great deal of overlap of MR relaxation times among neoplastic and non-neoplastic lesions. The use of specific T1, T2, and spin-density parameters has not resulted in any greater ability to diagnose neoplastic from non-neoplastic disease or to predict the degree of malignancy relative to the use of morphologic characteristics which likewise have a significant degree of error, as repeatedly emphasized in this chapter.

Radiographic-pathologic correlation is further confounded by the difficulty in appropriate sampling at the time of biopsy. A higher-grade focus of tumor may be present and missed with the biopsy needle. Accuracy in correlative studies requires the comparison of images made immediately post mortem with autopsy specimens.[32]

We are left with attempting to make a radiographic diagnosis based on morphologic characteristics, knowing that there will be errors. If the findings are classic for glioblastoma multiforme, with a ring-enhancing lesion on either MRI or CT around an area of central necrosis with abundant surrounding edema, the diagnosis of glioblastoma is likely, with the realization that metastasis and abscess may have similar appearances. Low-grade neoplasm is extremely doubtful with such an appearance. A subtle infiltrating lesion with little edema or mass effect and patchy areas of minimal-to-moderate enhancement are more typical of a low-grade infiltrating astrocytoma. Cerebritis and infarction can have similar appearances, as can a number of other non-neoplastic lesions. While these findings are typical of a low-grade neoplasm, more malignant changes may be demonstrated histologically and the radiographic-histologic correlation is significantly poorer than with the findings of classic glioblastoma.

The problem of tumor boundary identification is a significant one. Surgical removal of the astrocytoma of childhood may be possible since it is relatively well circumscribed,[49] but surgical extirpation of an infiltrating astrocytoma or glioblastoma is usually not possible. The setting of ports for radiation therapy depends upon a presumption of boundaries. Brachytherapy is a technique of irradiation utilizing an isotope such as iodine 125 within metallic seeds which are placed stereotactically into the tumor. The dosimetry is determined by assuming tumor boundaries on an imaging study. The concept of brachytherapy is obviously flawed because those tumor boundaries cannot be accurately determined. Effective treatment for primary infiltrating gliomas may well await different forms of therapy which are not dependent upon an ability to separate tumorous from nontumorous tissue, but rather upon cellular metabolic[50–52] or membrane characteristics.

Oligodendroglioma

Many of the statements made for astrocytoma can be made as well for oligodendroglioma. An oligodendroglioma may be indistinguishable from an astrocytoma on the imaging studies, with this distinction being made only at pathologic examination. However, there are two radiographic features that may give a presurgical indication of oligodendroglioma. The first is that of rather abundant calcification (Fig 16–24). While an astrocytoma may also calcify, an oligodendroglioma appears to have a propensity for rather extensive calcification. This calcification may be either peripheral or central, and while the curvilinear appearance as seen on skull films has been described as typical for oligodendroglioma, a nodular appearance is more common on the CT scan.[53] Peripheral slow-growing tumors may erode the calvarium.[54] Oligodendroglioma may undergo malignant degeneration, with the CT scan demonstrating a combination of heavily calcified tumor contiguous to an infiltrating or obvious necrotic and rapidly growing neoplasm.[53]

The second feature is the relatively frequent appearance of a purely low-density or low-intensity tumor, with little if any enhancement (Fig 16–25).[30, 54] The attenuation coefficients on CT may be very low, simulating a non-neoplastic cyst or an area of encephalomalacia. Such a low density may not be associated with a true cyst, but a relatively high interstitial water content or microcystic change may be present to account for the low density. The presence of irregular margins on at least

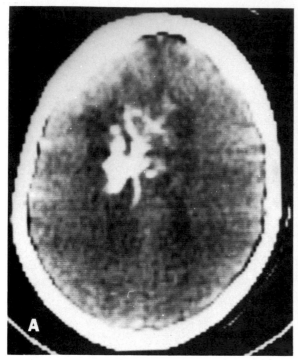

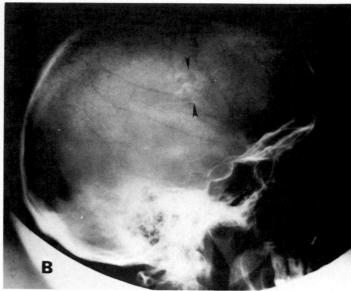

FIG 16–24.
Oligodendroglioma with curvilinear calcifications. **A,** the axial CT scan demonstrates clumpy, confluent, and curvilinear calcifications involving the medial right frontal and parietal lobes and adjoining the corpus callosum. An enhanced scan (not shown) dem-onstrated extensive enhancing neoplasm throughout the same regions. The curvilinear calcifications *(arrowheads)* seen on the lateral skull film **(B)** are characteristic of oligodendroglioma.

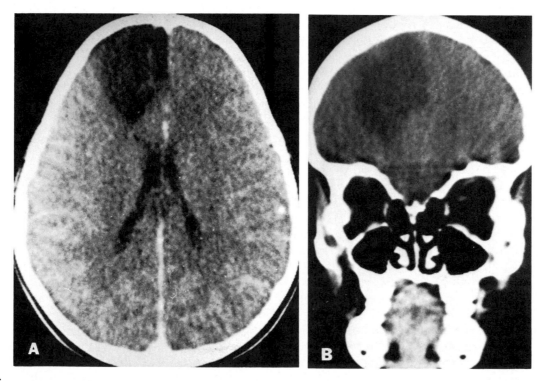

FIG 16–25.
Low-dense, nonenhancing oligodendroglioma. **A,** the axial enhanced scan demonstrates a low-density lesion in the right frontal tip without definite mass effect and with sharp margination, suggesting the possibility of a longstanding cyst or other nonneoplastic process. **B,** the coronal scan better demonstrates the irregular margination of the lesion, indicative of neoplasm. At surgery, this was a noncystic low-grade glioma. (From Varma RR, Crumrine PK, Bergman I, et al: *Neurology* 1983; 33:806–808. Used by permission.)

one projection rules out the diagnosis of arachnoid cyst, which should be smoothly marginated in all projections. Multiple projections (see Fig 16–25,B) may be necessary in order to visualize the irregular margination.[30] Rarely, oligodendroglioma may present as an intraventricular mass,[55] with its low

CT density and low MR intensity (short TR sequence) blending with the CSF (Fig 16–26).

MRI is better than CT at differentiating such a low-intensity, nonenhancing tumor from a nonneoplastic cyst or focal volume loss. MRI easily provides the multiple projections for margin evalu-

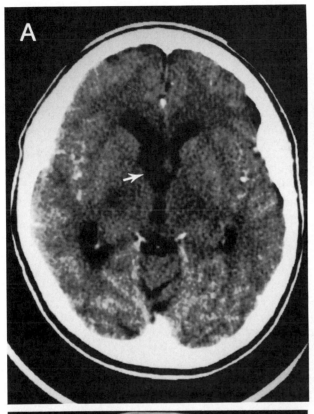

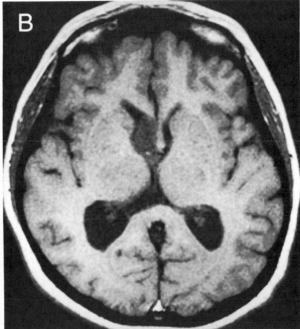

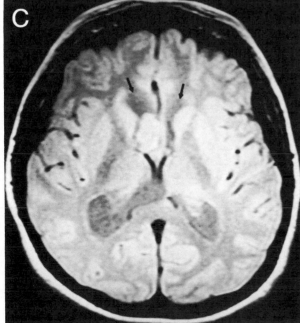

FIG 16–26.
Intraventricular oligodendroglioma. **A,** the enhanced CT scan demonstrates asymmetry of the frontal horns, and apparent enlargement of the right foramen of Monro *(arrow)*. The low-density neoplasm blends with the CSF. **B,** the short TR MR scan (TR 600, TE 20) demonstrates the tumor within the right frontal horn with extension through the right foramen of Monro into the third ventricle. The intensity of the tumor is greater than the CSF, indicating a higher protein content. **C,** the higher protein content is further illustrated on the proton-density study (TR 2,500, TE 25) where the tumor is hyperintense relative to the CSF within the frontal horns *(arrows)* which is similar to the intensity of the internal capsules. Note the hyperintensity of the heads of the caudate nuclei relative to the frontal horns *(arrows)*.

tion (Fig 16–27). It also allows an evalution of the cyst contents. If the lesion does not appear exactly like CSF, as does an arachnoid cyst, a neoplasm may be present with a high protein content (see Figs 16–26 and 16–27) and biopsy is required.

Primitive Neuroectodermal Tumor

Primitive neuroectodermal tumor (PNET) is a term for a group of malignant cerebral neoplasms that occur primarily in children and that have similar histologic characteristics.[56] Rorke[57] has subclassified these tumors according to the line of cellular differentiation. The following five subtypes are recognized: glial, ependymal, neuronal, bipotential, and unspecified. The neuronal subtype includes medulloblastoma and primary cerebral neuroblastoma.

Medulloblastoma represents differentiation along neuronal lines by a tumor originating in the cerebellum. Such a classification would explain the occasional diagnosis of "cerebral medulloblastoma," which simply would be a neuronal subtype of PNET located in the supratentorial compartment.

Primary intracranial neuroblastoma represents the differentiation of primitive cells into more mature ganglion-like cells that in the better differenti-

ated tumors form Homer-Wright rosettes as in extracranial neuroblastoma. Less well-differentiated examples may require electron microscopy to identify dendritic processes characteristic of the neoplasm to separate it from the other forms of PNET.[58] This rare neoplasm has probably been called ependymoma or oligodendroglioma in the past.[59] The malignant tumor may invade venous structures, leading to extracranial metastases.[60] Metastases via the CSF pathways are also common. Primary intracranial neuroblastoma is to be differentiated from metastatic neuroblastoma from an extracranial site, in which metastases are generally to the calvarium, base of the skull, and orbits, while metastases to intracranial structures from an extracranial site are extremely rare.[61] The MR and CT scan findings of primary neuroblastoma are nonspecific and consist of a diffusely enhancing, well-circumscribed mass lesion (Fig 16–28) with a variable amount of surrounding cerebral edema, simulating an astrocytoma of childhood.[61–63] However, four radiographic findings singly or in combination may suggest the appropriate diagnosis.[62, 64, 65] First, the lesion is frequently large at resection, with over one half in one series being at least 7.5 cm in size (Fig 16–29). Second, cyst for-

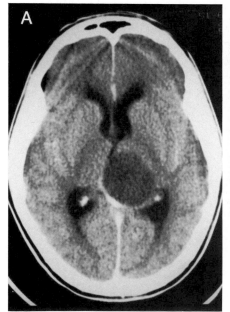 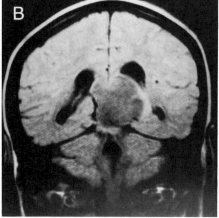 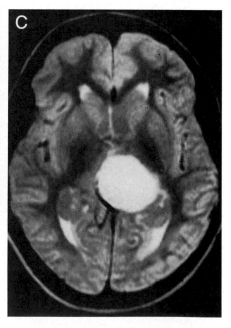

FIG 16–27.
Periventricular oligodendroglioma. **A,** the enhanced CT scan demonstrates a low-density lesion of the left thalamus. The density is greater than CSF. **B,** the coronal MR sequence (TR 600, TE 25) shows the margins superiorly and laterally to be irregular. The neoplastic protein concentration is greater than that in CSF producing less hypointensity. **C,** the proton-density MR sequence (TR 2000, TE 50) shows the pronounced hyperintensity of the tumor relative to the CSF, having an intensity equal to gray matter. There is periventricular hyperintensity representing transependymal egress of fluid from obstructive hydrocephalus. A very long TR/TE sequence would be necessary to demonstrate the decreased hyperintensity of the tumor relative to CSF.

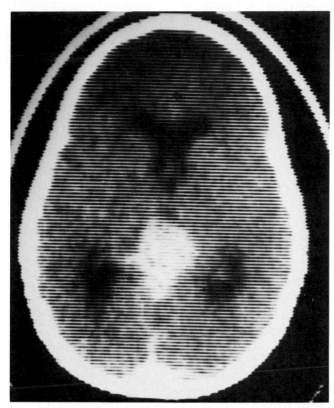

FIG 16–28.
Primary intracranial neuroblastoma. A diffusely enhancing neoplasm behind and above the third ventricle was found in this 6-year-old child. Biopsy revealed neuroblastoma, and there was no site of origin of extracranial neuroblastoma. Metastatic extracranial neuroblastoma rarely involves the cerebral parenchyma. (From Latchaw RE, L'Heureux PR, Young G, et al: *AJNR* 1982; 3:623–630. Used by permission.)

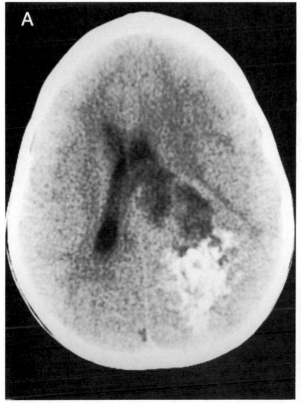 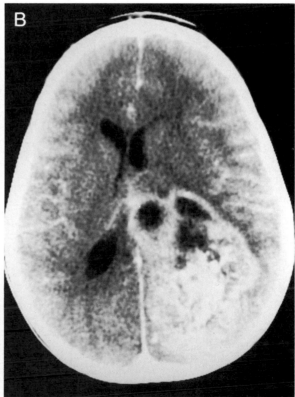

FIG 16–29.
Large calcified primitive neuroectodermal tumor (PNET). **A,** the unenhanced CT scan demonstrates a large area of calcification within the left parietal lobe in this 2-year-old child, with low-density abnormality compressing the posterior portion of the left lateral ventricle. **B,** the enhanced study demonstrates pronounced enhancement surrounding the calcification, with extension anteriorly into periventricular tissues. Multiple central cystic-necrotic areas are present.

mation or necrosis within the tumor is a common finding (see Fig 16–29), with three studies reporting cystic-necrotic change in 40% to 80% of cases. Third, calcification is frequent (50%–70%) (see Fig 16–29). Fourth, approximately one half of neuroblastomas are vascular at angiography.

Ganglioglioma

Ganglioglioma is an uncommon benign neoplasm which may be found in a wide range of age groups, from the young to middle aged. It is made up of a combination of ganglion and glial cells, and the lesion appears to grow slowly as denoted by the frequent presence of calcification and contoural changes in the skull.[66–68] True cyst formation occurs in approximately one half of cases.[69] Enhancement is moderate to marked, even though the lesion has a benign histologic character. This enhancement may either be diffuse and homoge-

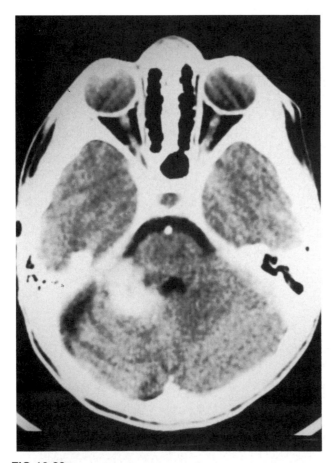

FIG 16-30.
Ganglioglioma. The enhanced CT scan demonstrates confluent and pronounced enhancement of this slow-growing tumor involving the right brachium pontis with little compression or displacement of the fourth ventricle.

neous (Fig 16–30) or peripheral about the margins of the cyst.[66–69]

Neuroepithelial Cyst

The term *neuroepithelial cyst* refers to a group of non-neoplastic cystic lesions lined by neural epithelium. These lesions may be intraparenchymal,[70] intraventricular, extraaxial, or intraspinal. The intraventricular category includes the choroid plexus cyst, present in approximately 50% of autopsied brains and asymptomatic during life,[71] and the colloid cyst of the third ventricle, considered later under intraventricular masses.

An intraparenchymal neuroepithelial cyst may simulate a nonenhancing low-density or cystic astrocytoma on CT scan (Fig 16–31), with the diagnosis requiring cyst wall biopsy. Experience with MRI is limited. CSF-like signal characteristics and sharp margins help confirm the correct diagnosis (Fig 16–32).[72] A lesion with other signal characteristics requires biopsy to exclude neoplasm. Stereotactic aspiration may be necessary for therapy, and cyst wall biopsy may be performed at that time.

The differential diagnosis also includes inflammatory cysts involving the parenchyma, such as echinococcal or cysticercotic cysts. These cysts are usually multiple, calcification is present in cysticercotic cysts, and scolex may be visualized within the echinococcal cysts. Arachnoid and epidermoid cysts are extraaxial in location, but may invaginate into the parenchyma.

Brain Stem Tumors

Brain stem neoplasms most commonly occur in children, with two out of three patients being children in a study of 41 brain stem tumors. In the same series, three out of four brain stem tumors were gliomas, so that 80% of brain stem gliomas occurred in the childhood age group.[23] Histologic evidence of malignancy (malignant astrocytoma, glioblastoma) is common, with close to 50% having pathologic evidence and a clinical course of malignancy.[23, 24]

The appearance of the unenhanced CT scan is that of a diffuse expansion of low density, isodensity, or an admixture of densities. It produces mass effect on the fourth ventricle with anterolateral bulging of the belly of the pons (Fig 16–33). Hemorrhage into the lesion is uncommon (Fig 16–34),

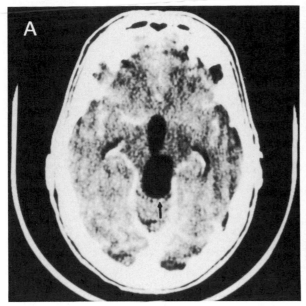 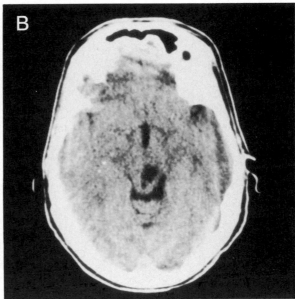

FIG 16–31.

Periaqueductal neuroepithelial cyst. **A,** the enhanced CT scan demonstrates a cystic lesion in the region of the aqueduct, with a density equal to the CSF within the dilated third ventricle. It was difficult to determine whether the lesion was intraaxial, or extraaxial within a subarachnoid cistern, but a rim of the quadrigeminal plate tissues *(arrow)* posterior to the cyst comfirmed its intraaxial location. **B,** the lesion was punctured stereotactically, with the post-drainage CT scan demonstrating the intraaxial location. Biopsy revealed a benign epithelial lining.

as is calcification, while cystic or necrotic changes are relatively common (Figs 16–34 to 16–36).[23] Contrast enhancement varies from no enhancement (see Fig 16–33) to pronounced enhancement (see Fig 16–35). The enhancement pattern does not correlate well with the histologic grade of malignancy.[24, 73] Pathologic findings or a clinical course of malignancy are common with brain stem tumors, particularly those that are diffusely hypodense on the precontrast CT scan.[24] These malignant tumors may or may not enhance, and low-grade tumors may enhance,[73] again pointing to the difficulty of attempting to grade the histologic degree of malignancy on the basis of CT enhancement characteristics.

While the typical brain stem glioma is rather symmetric in location, producing bilateral neurologic findings, there may be an exophytic component to the tumor, with extension posteriorly into the fourth ventricle and cisterna magna,[73] anteriorly into the prepontine subarachnoid cisterns to encase the basilar artery (see Fig 16–34), or laterally toward the cerebellopontine angle. This exophytic component may show a greater degree of contrast enhancement than the typical glioma confined to the brain stem[73] and therefore may mimic an extraaxial mass lesion.[23] Spread of tumor occurs through the cerebellar peduncles into the cerebel-

lum (see Figs 16–33 and 16–34), inferiorly into the medulla and spinal cord (see Fig 16–34), or superiorly through the upper brain stem into the cerebral hemispheres.

MRI is far superior to CT scanning for the evaluation of brain stem tumors.[74] Typically, a brain stem astrocytoma demonstrates low signal intensity on a short TR sequence and high signal on long TR images (Fig 16–37). Enhancement with gadolinium may define the extent of the tumor, or at least the extent of the BBB disruption, even better (Figs 16–36 and 16–38). The midline sagittal MRI view demonstrates both the expansion and the abnormal texture of the tumor in a way not convenient with CT (see Fig 16–34).[75] The cephalic and caudal extensions are well demonstrated. Reformatted sagittal CT images require the initial placement of a water-soluble contrast medium into the thecal sac to delineate the expansion (see Fig 16–33), and then the abnormal texture of the tumorous brain stem cannot be evaluated. MRI is able to evaluate medullary expansions (see Fig 16–38) and to distinguish exophytic brain stem tumors from cerebellar tumors which can be difficult with axial CT. MRI is not plagued by beam-hardening artifacts off the petrous bones (Hounsfield artifact) which makes evaluation of the pons and medulla difficult on CT.

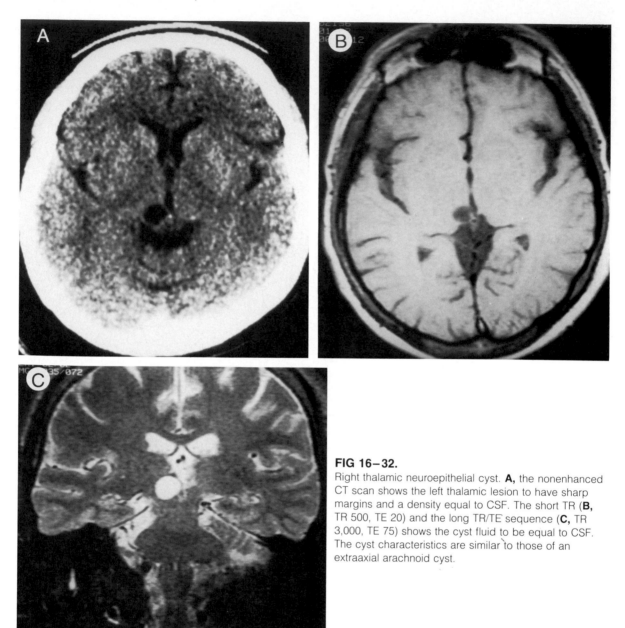

FIG 16–32.
Right thalamic neuroepithelial cyst. **A,** the nonenhanced CT scan shows the left thalamic lesion to have sharp margins and a density equal to CSF. The short TR (**B,** TR 500, TE 20) and the long TR/TE sequence (**C,** TR 3,000, TE 75) shows the cyst fluid to be equal to CSF. The cyst characteristics are similar to those of an extraaxial arachnoid cyst.

MRI is particularly good for ruling out differential diagnostic possibilities, including a cyst of the brain stem, an angiomatous lesion of the brain stem with its characteristic flow-void areas or hemosiderin deposits from previous hemorrhage, and extraaxial tumor or aneurysm.

Tumors of the Cerebellum and Fourth Ventricle

Primary neoplasms involving the cerebellum and fourth ventricle are far more common in chil-

dren than adults. The differential diagnosis of these primary neoplasms in children include astrocytoma, midline medulloblastoma, ependymoma, intraventricular dermoid, and choroid plexus papilloma. Hemangioblastoma is more commonly found in the adult, and is the most common primary cerebellar tumor of adulthood. Other primary tumors in this older age group are primary astrocytoma and glioblastoma, primary lymphoma, medulloblastoma of the lateral cerebellar hemisphere in the young adult, and intraventricular meningioma, all of which are relatively rare. A solitary cerebel-

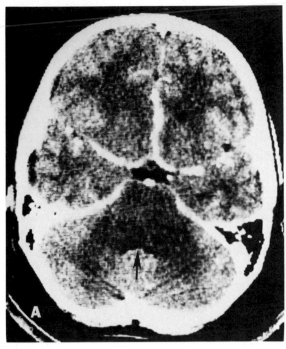
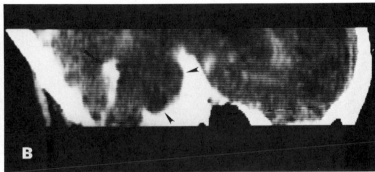

FIG 16–33.

Nonenhancing brain stem glioma. **A,** enhanced axial scan demonstrates diffuse low density throughout the pons, compressing the anterior portion of the fourth ventricle *(arrow)*. There is diffuse spread of nonenhancing neoplasm through the cerebellar pedun-cles into both cerebellar hemispheres. **B,** a reformatted sagittal view performed during metrizamide (Amipaque) cisternography demonstrates the diffuse bulging of the pons *(arrowheads)* and posterior displacement of the fourth ventricle *(arrow)*.

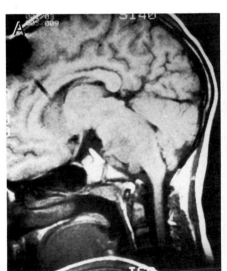
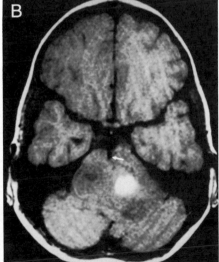
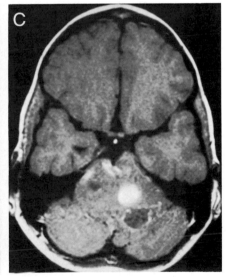

FIG 16–34.

Hemorrhagic enhancing exophytic brain stem tumor. **A,** the short TR sagittal MR image (TR 500, TE 20) demonstrates a diffuse expansion of the pons with extension superiorly into the mesencephalon and inferiorly into the medulla. The tumor is both isointense and hypointense, and there are exophytic components anteriorly and inferiorly. **B,** the axial unenhanced short TR image (TR 700, TE 20) shows a cystic or necrotic area within the right side of the pons, an area of subacute hemorrhage in the left side of the pons with its typical hyperintensity, and tumor extending anteriorly to surround the basilar artery *(arrow)*. **C,** a gadolinium DTPA–enhanced sequence at the same level demonstrates spotty enhancement within the anterior portion of the tumor, better definition of the exophytic components surrounding the hypointense basilar artery, and enhancing tumor extending into the left cerebellar hemisphere.

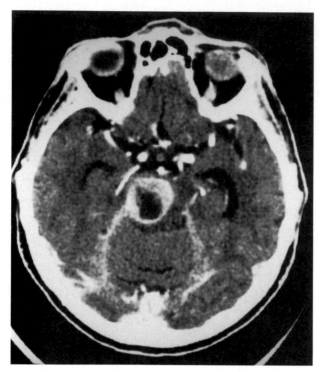

FIG 16–35.
Intense ring enhancement of mesencephalic glioblastoma. The enhanced CT scan through the mesencephalon demonstrates the intense ring enhancement of this malignant tumor.

lar mass lesion in an adult is much more common than a metastatic tumor.

Cerebellar astrocytoma, medulloblastoma, and ependymoma are discussed in this section; choroid plexus papilloma and primary lymphoma are covered later in this chapter. Meningioma is discussed in Chapter 17, and hemangioblastoma and dermoid cyst are discussed in Chapter 18. Obstructive hydrocephalus is a common sequela of these tumors. Before beginning the discussion of individual tumors, a few concepts regarding hydrocephalus are appropriate.

Hydrocephalus

There are two major forms of hydrocephalus: obstructive and communicating. Obstructive hydrocephalus occurs secondary to a block somewhere along the intraventricular CSF pathways, from the lateral ventricles to the foramina of Magendie and Luschka. This produces high pressure within the ventricular system, and secondary dilatation of that part of the ventricular system distal to the block. The point of blockage can usually be determined by the abrupt change in caliber of the ventricular system. For example, an aqueductal block produces enlargement of the third and lat-

eral ventricles, with a small fourth ventricle distal to the block. A block at the foramina of Monro, as from a colloid cyst, produces enlarged lateral ventricles with a small third ventricle. A block at the foramina of Magendie and Lushka, however, produces enlargement of the entire ventricular system, simulating communicating hydrocephalus. The choroid plexus continues to produce fluid until the intraventricular pressure is quite high. This increased fluid production continues to expand the ventricular system. Some compensatory mechanisms to handle the fluid production are available, including transependymal flow of CSF from the ventricular system into the periventricular tissues for local absorption. The increased periventricular tissue fluid content is seen as low density on a CT scan and high intensity on a long TR/TE MR scan. A less common and efficacious compensatory mechanism is absorption of some fluid by the choroid plexus itself.

Communicating hydrocephalus, on the other hand, denotes a lack of a block within the ventricular system. The term *communicating hydrocephalus* arose many years ago when the hydrocephalic patient underwent ventriculostomy of a lateral ventricle, and a dye was placed into that lateral ventricle, only to be recovered in the spinal subarachnoid space. This indicated a lack of obstruction within the ventricular system proper. There are a variety of types of communicating hydrocephalus. The most common is secondary to a block over the cerebral convexity, producing a high pressure within the subarachnoid spaces below the block and within the ventricular system. Theoretically, the entire ventricular system should enlarge, although dilatation of the fourth ventricle only occurs in approximately one third of cases. This convexity block is a common sequela to previous subarachnoid hemorrhage, meningitis, trauma, or other causes of adhesions that block CSF flow. A block just at the superior sagittal sinus or lack of appropriate development of the pacchionian granulations may likewise produce communicating hydrocephalus.

As the ventricles dilate, the intraventricular pressure drops. If it drops into a high-normal range, normal-pressure hydrocephalus results. The syndrome of normal-pressure hydrocephalus includes ataxia, dementia, and urinary incontinence. This is a phenomenon secondary to a convexity block from any cause and is a treatable cause of dementia, although it is probably much less common than originally thought.

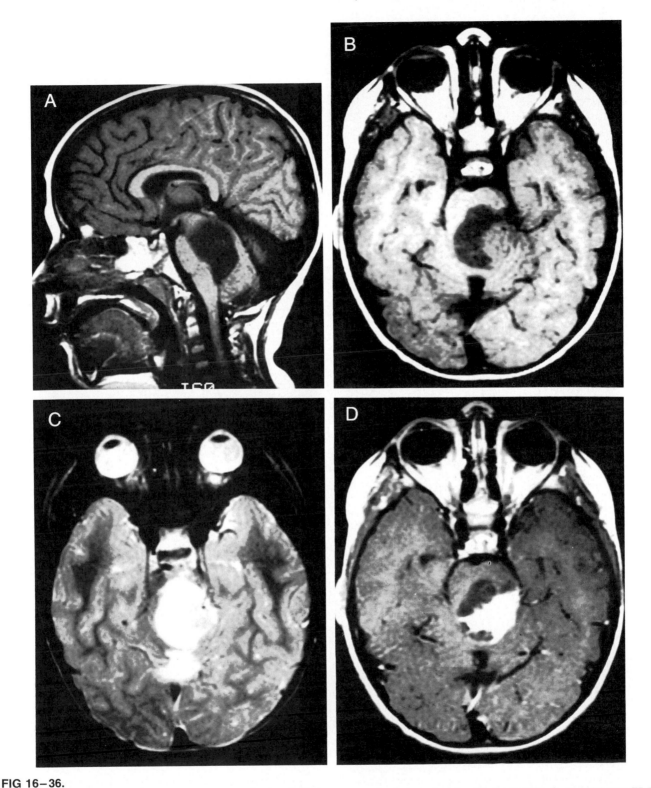

FIG 16–36.
Enhancing cystic glioblastoma of the brain stem. **A,** the sagittal short TR image (TR 500, TE 20) demonstrates a large cystic lesion involving the posterior portion of the brain stem, extending into the cerebellum. **B,** the short TR axial image (TR 650, TE 20) shows an isointense nodular component projecting into the left side of the cystic cavity. The sharp marginations of the low-intensity lesion suggest a true cyst and not just necrosis. **C,** an axial long TR/TE image at a slightly higher level than **B** (TR 2,867, TE 80) demonstrates hyperintensity of the cyst fluid and the left-sided nodule, which is isointense to gray matter. **D,** a gadolinium-enhanced short TR image (TR 600, TE 20) shows the irregularity of the enhancing nodule, which was histologically glioblastoma.

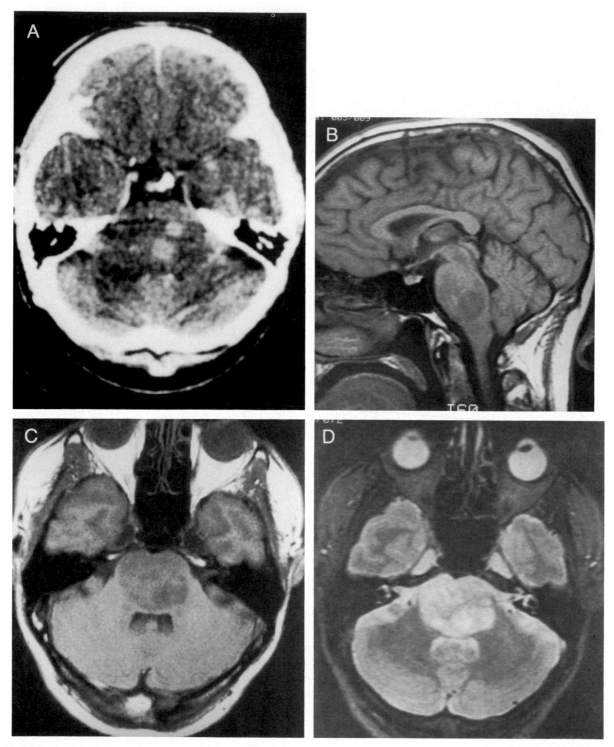

FIG 16–37.

Pontine glioma with extension into mesencephalon and medulla. **A,** the enhanced axial CT scan demonstrates spotty enhancement within the midportion of the pontine glioma. **B,** the sagittal short TR image (TR 600, TE 20) nicely demonstrates the diffuse pontine expansion with hypointense and isointense signals. There is extension superiorly into the mesencephalon and inferiorly into a moder-

ately widened medulla. The short TR (**C,** TR 600, TE 20) and long TR/TE (**D,** TR 2,500, TE 75) axial sequences show the classic MR signals of a relatively low-grade glioma, with essentially all of the pons occupied by a hypointense signal on the short TR study and mixed hyper- and isointense signals on the long TR/TE study.

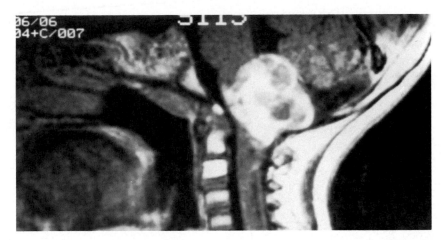

FIG 16–38.
Intensely enhancing astrocytoma of the medulla. The sagittal short TR image (TR 400, TE 20) following the administration of gadolin- ium DTPA demonstrates intense enhancement of multilobular med- ullary glioma which has areas of cyst formation and necrosis.

There are other causes of communicating hydrocephalus. Specifically, overproduction of CSF may occur from a choroid plexus papilloma, with the ventricles dilating secondary to this increased fluid production. High CSF protein from, for example, an intraspinal tumor may produce blockage at the pacchionian granulations and secondary communicating hydrocephalus. Both forms of hydrocephalus are distinguished from increased ventricular size and sulcal size which should be termed *volume loss* but are also called *hydrocephalus ex vacuo* or *atrophy.* Volume loss occurs from any number of conditions that produce shrinkage of the tissues. While the increased ventricular size simulates hydrocephalus, there is also increased sulcal size, usually in equal proportions. Transependymal flow is not present, although there may be increased intensity in the periventricular tissues on MRI secondary to ischemic changes from small-vessel vascular disease that commonly accompanies volume loss in the older population.

Astrocytoma and Glioblastoma

Three out of four cerebellar astrocytomas originate within the cerebellar hemisphere, with the rest beginning in the cerebellar vermis.[20] This tumor is usually large at presentation and has one of two common appearances: either a solid lesion or a cystic tumor, with an equal division between the cystic and solid types.[21] Calcification occurs in approximately 25% of cases, and obstructive hydrocephalus is usually present.

On the unenhanced CT scan, the solid tumor or cyst nodule may be of slight increased density, isodensity (Fig 16–39), or mixed high and low density.[21] Enhancement of a solid tumor is usually homogeneous, with sharply defined margins (Fig 16–40), although a few small cysts may be present. Grossly cystic tumors have either a solid nodule (see Fig 16–39) or a rim of enhancement (Fig 16–41). The degree of enhancement does not correlate with the degree of malignancy, with marked enhancement being seen in benign tumors.[22, 76]

Multiplanar MRI shows the anatomic relationships far better than does CT, including the possible spread into the brain stem and upper spinal cord.[77] Unenhanced short TR images show the isointensity to low intensity of the solid component of the tumor and the low intensity of the cyst (Fig 16–42). The protein content of the cyst usually makes it more intense than the CSF of the fourth ventricle on short TR images. High signal intensity on the long TR/TE sequences is often present in both solid and cystic components (see Fig 16–42). Enhanced short TR images show an enhancement pattern similar to the enhanced CT scan, with pronounced enhancement of the solid components of the tumor, the cyst nodule, and the cyst margin, singly or severally (see Fig 16–42).

Glioblastoma is a tumor primarily of older age groups, and has characteristics similar to those described for cerebral glioblastoma.[78]

Medulloblastoma

Medulloblastoma ranks just below astrocytoma in incidence in some series of pediatric cerebellar masses, and is slightly more common in others. When presenting in childhood, medulloblastoma usually originates in the cerebellar vermis along the roof of the fourth ventricle.[79, 80] However, a

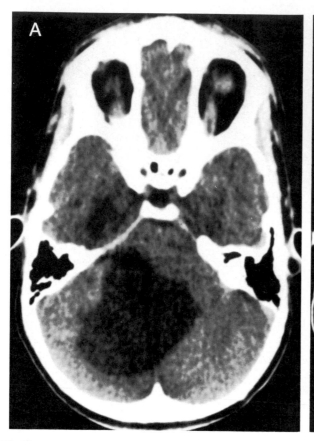
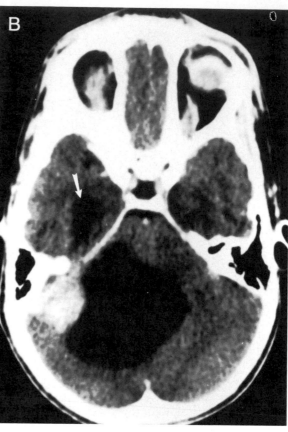

FIG 16–39.

Cystic astrocytoma. **A,** the nonenhanced scan demonstrates a large, well-marginated cyst within the right cerebellar hemisphere and vermis. The nodule is situated more laterally and is isodense to the cerebellum. **B,** this nodule is demonstrated on the enhanced scan with the nodule and cyst contiguous to the right petrous bone and edge of the tentorium. There is obstructive hydrocephalus as denoted by the dilated right temporal horn *(arrow).* The densities of the cyst fluid and the CSF within the dilated right temporal horn are equal.

variant of the medulloblastoma occurs in the adolescent and young adult age groups, originating laterally within a cerebellar hemisphere.[81] This latter tumor is frequently desmoplastic and has been called cerebellar sarcoma.

The vermian medulloblastoma has a CT scan appearance very similar to the solid astrocytoma. This is a large centrally located mass lesion of slight-to-moderate increased density without contrast material, compressing the fourth ventricle and producing obstructive hydrocephalus (Fig 16–43).[20] The mass characteristically enhances markedly and homogeneously, with the margins sharply demarcated from the surrounding brain (see Fig 16–43). There is usually no evidence of cyst formation or calcification, findings which are more typical of astrocytoma and ependymoma, respectively. Occasionally, however, less common features will be present, including small cysts (Figs 16–44, 16–45), areas of calcification, or hemorrhage.[82, 83] The combination of increased density on the preinfusion scan and the marked and homogeneous enhancement in a midline tumor is strongly suggestive of the diagnosis of medulloblastoma. Although the solid astrocytoma may have a similar appearance, the precontrast density is not usually as great as with medulloblastoma, and small cysts and calcification are more common than in medulloblastoma.

MRI with its multiple projections is better at defining the relationships of the medulloblastoma to surrounding structures. It may be able to demonstrate the origin of the tumor from the roof of the fourth ventricle (Figs 16–44 to 16–46), in contradistinction to the origin of the typical ependymoma from the ventricular floor. Nonenhanced short TR images of medulloblastoma show the tumor to be mildly hypointense to isointense to the cerebellum, depending upon the degree of cellular compactness and, therefore, high proton density.

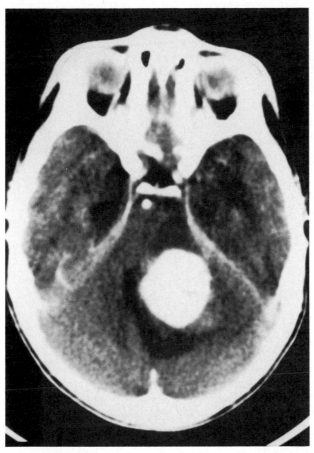

FIG 16–40.
Densely enhancing nodule of a cystic cerebellar astrocytoma. The enhanced CT scan demonstrates an intensely enhancing nodule with sharp marginations located within a lower-density but likewise sharply marginated cystic lesion of the cerebellar vermis with extension into the left brachium pontis and brain stem.

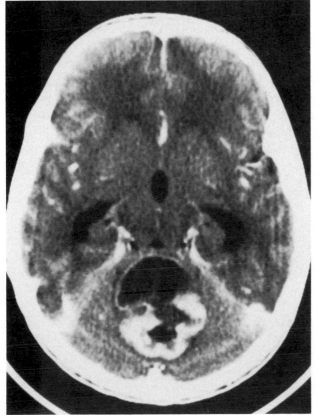

FIG 16–41.
Cystic astrocytoma with enhancing rim. The enhanced CT scan demonstrates a large cystic lesion within the superior cerebellar vermis, with enhancement of the rim. This enhancement is thick and irregular posteriorly and thin along the anterior cyst margin. There is obstructive hydrocephalus.

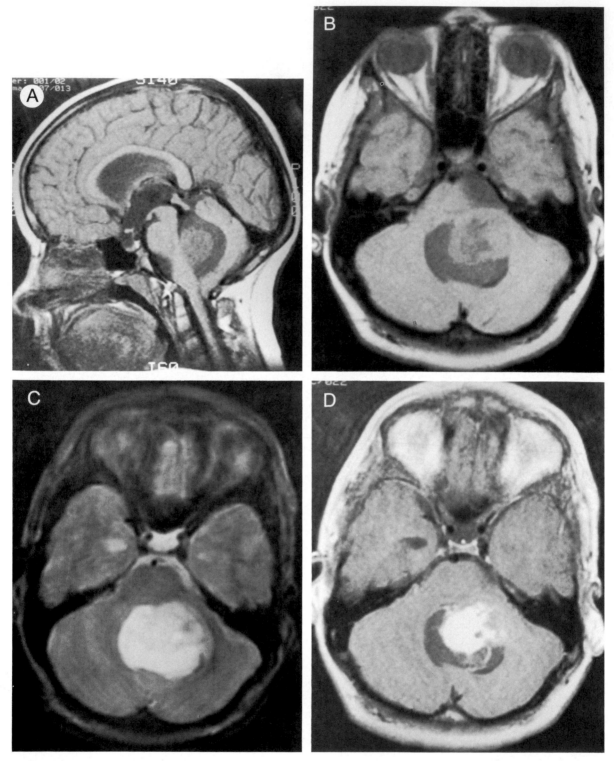

FIG 16–42.
Gadolinium DTPA enhancement of a cystic cerebellar astrocytoma. **A,** the short TR sagittal view (TR 500, TE 20) demonstrates a large cyst within the vermis, with the cyst fluid being more intense than the dilated third ventricle. A central nodule of decreased intensity relative to cerebellum is present. **B,** the axial short TR image (TR 600, TE 20) shows the nodule to be located anteriorly and to the left within the cyst. The periphery of the nodule is slightly less intense than the cerebellum, with even more hypointense central portions. **C,** the cyst fluid is markedly hyperintense on the long TR/TE study (TR 2,824, TE 800) with the nodule being of lesser intensity. **D,** the gadolinium DTPA–enhanced short TR study (TR 600, TE 20) demonstrates marked enhancement of the nodule with rim enhancement of much of the cyst, and irregularity of the anterolateral portion of the nodule as it infiltrates the brachium pontis and posterior brain stem.

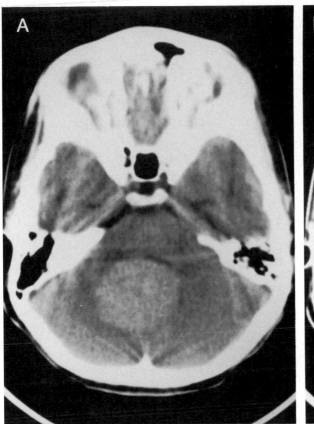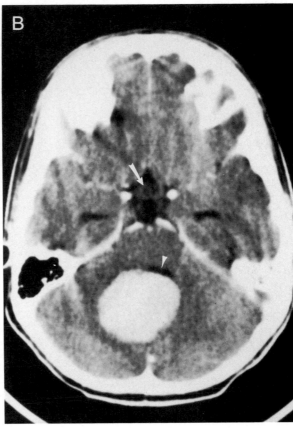

FIG 16–43.

Medulloblastoma. **A,** the unenhanced CT scan shows a solid, sharply marginated lesion of the cerebellar vermis with a density greater than the cerebellum itself. **B,** the enhanced study demonstrates marked homogeneous enhancement of the well-circumscribed mass which compresses the fourth ventricle *(arrowhead)* into a slit and displaces it to the left. There is a poorly defined increased density in the region of the pituitary infundibulum *(arrow)* which may represent metastasis via the CSF pathways.

There is high intensity of tumor and surrounding edema on long TR/TE sequences (see Figs 16–44 and 16–45). Enhanced short TR views demonstrate the marked enhancement seen on CT (see Fig 16–46).

The more laterally originating medulloblastoma in the older age group may simulate astrocytoma. In our limited experience with such lesions, the degree of contrast enhancement has not been as florid (Figs 16–47 and 16–48) as that with the midline childhood medulloblastoma. This is certainly in keeping with the histologic finding of an extensive amount of dense fibrous tissue within the lesion.

Medulloblastoma may invade contiguous parenchymal structures, including the brain stem and spinal cord (see Fig 16–46). These tumors commonly metastasize via CSF pathways to produce a suprasellar mass (see Fig 16–44), multiple enhancing masses on the surface of the brain (Figs 16–49 and 16–50), ependymal implants along the ventricular surface (see Fig 16–50),[84] or "dropped metastases" along the outer surface of the spinal cord (see Fig 16–48). The frequency of finding subfrontal or suprasellar spread has been attributed to shielding of the eyes during radiation therapy.[85] The contrast-enhanced scan demonstrating diffuse cisternal enhancement (Figs 16–49 and 16–51) is indicative of widespread implants throughout the subarachnoid spaces. Systemic metastasis, especially to bone, is unusual and occurs late in the disease process.[86]

Spread of medulloblastoma may be present relatively early, and all patients should undergo either myelography or enhanced MRI following initial surgery to detect spinal canal involvement. Myelography is better than unenhanced MRI for spread to the spinal canal, since unenhanced MRI is poor at detecting small dropped metastases.[87] Enhanced MRI is significantly better at such detection.[88] Myelography has a very high level of spatial resolution for tiny abnormalities, while

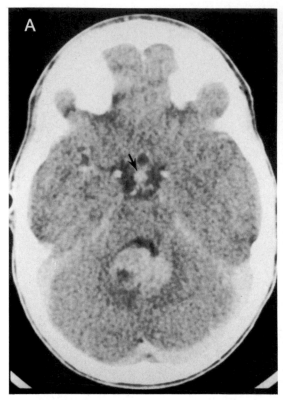

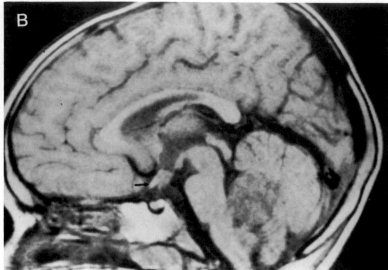

FIG 16–44.
Cystic medulloblastoma with suprasellar metastasis. **A,** the enhanced CT scan demonstrates a moderately enhancing mass lesion compressing the roof of the fourth ventricle. The lesion contains a small cystic or necrotic low-density area posteriorly on the right. There is a mass in the region of the infundibulum *(arrow)* representing a suprasellar metastasis via the CSF pathways. **B,** the sagittal short TR MR image (TR 600, TE 20) shows the typical hypointensity of the vermian medulloblastoma which compresses the roof of the fourth ventricle. The suprasellar metastasis *(arrow)* is isointense to gray matter.

MRI affords better contrast resolution. MRI may be marred, however, by turbulent CSF and respiratory motion, particularly in the thoracic region. Enhanced MRI and myelography may both have a role in evaluating metastatic disease. This is not an insignificant issue; if dropped metastases are found, a boost of radiation is administered to the areas of involvement beyond the level typically given to the entire neuraxis.

Ependymoma

Ependymomas occur more commonly in the posterior fossa, with the less common supratentorial tumors arising either within a ventricle or within the cerebral parenchyma itself.[89–91] While the majority of ependymomas occur in childhood, between 23% and 46% will occur in patients greater than 18 years of age.[89, 92, 93] Of the pediatric posterior fossa masses, ependymoma is much less common than either medulloblastoma or astrocytoma.

Posterior fossa ependymomas generally originate from the floor of the fourth ventricle. While they are frequently isodense on the precontrast scan, 50% of the lesions are calcified (Fig 16–52).[89] Poor enhancement or nonhomogeneous enhancement (see Fig 16–52) is more common than the vivid homogeneous enhancement typical of medulloblastoma or astrocytoma. Calcification is also more frequently seen with ependymoma than with medulloblastoma or astrocytoma. Tumor may extend through the foramen of Luschka into the cerebellopontine angles, or through the foramen of Magendie to lie dorsal to the medulla and upper spinal cord (Fig 16–53). Seeding along CSF pathways is similar to medulloblastoma.

Sagittal MRI is helpful in demonstrating the origin of the tumor from the floor of the fourth ventricle (see Fig 16–53), as opposed to medulloblastoma which arises from the roof. CT is better at demonstrating the tumoral calcification than is MRI.

Supratentorial ependymomas may originate either along the ependymal lining of a ventricle or within the white matter of a cerebral hemisphere. In the latter situation, it is theorized that the ependymoma originates from ependymal rest cells, which are far from the ventricular lining, but are connected to the ventricle by a band of ependymal tissue.[89] These parenchymal ependymomas are frequently large at the time of presentation; one series found that 94% were larger than 4 cm.[94] They commonly (56%) contain true cysts (Fig 16–54), with calcification in 38%.[94] The differen-

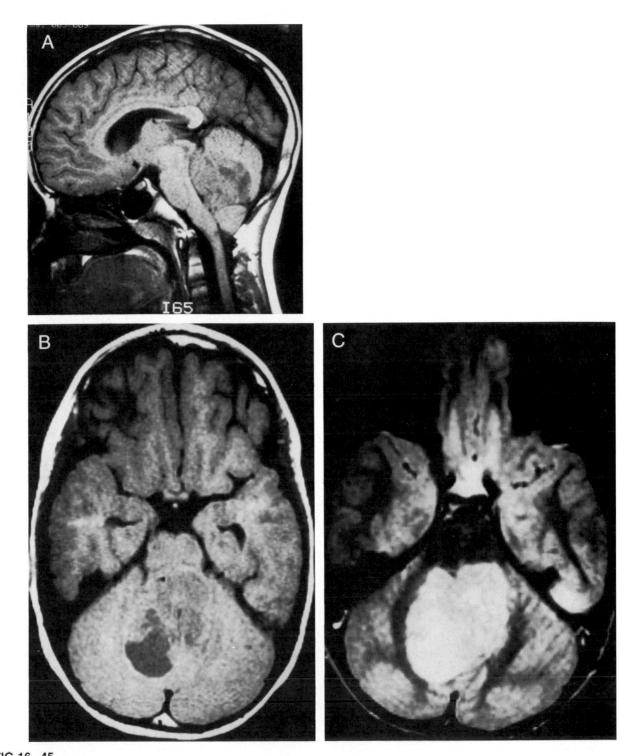

FIG 16–45.

Cystic medulloblastoma. **A,** the sagittal short TR image (TR 500, TE 20) demonstrates the mottled but predominately hypointense cerebellar vermian lesion compressing the roof of the fourth ventricle. **B,** the axial short TR image (TR 700, TE 20) shows a similar appearance for most of the tumor, but a large cystic component extends into the medial right cerebellar hemisphere. **C,** the long TR/TE axial sequence at the same level as **B** (TR 2,609, TE 30) demonstrates the hyperintensity of the solid portion of the tumor, with even more marked hyperintensity of the cystic-necrotic component.

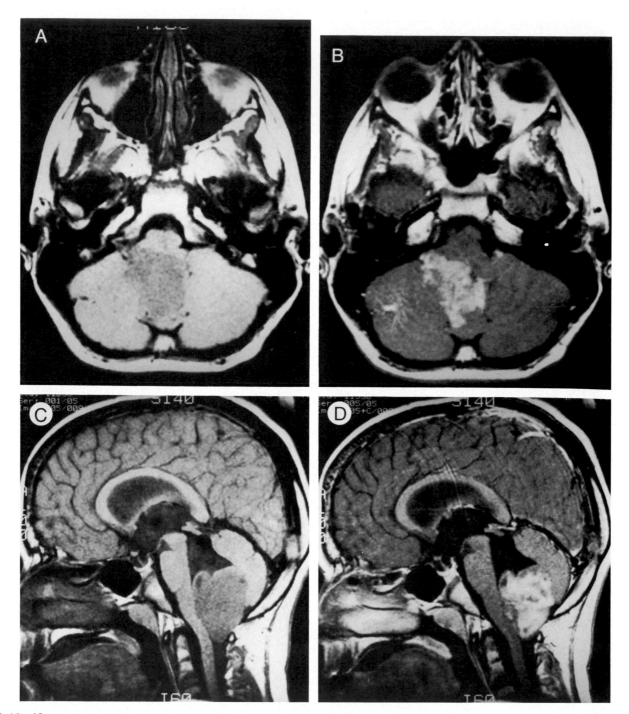

FIG 16–46.

Gadolinium DTPA–enhancing medulloblastoma invading the brainstem. **A,** the short TR image (TR 600, TE 20) demonstrates the hypointense medulloblastoma of the inferior vermis with extension laterally into the inferior cerebellar peduncle and medulla. **B,** a short TR image (TR 600, TE 20) following the injection of gadolinium DTPA shows intense enhancement of the tumor, with some patchy areas. Note is made of the venous angioma within the inferolateral portion of the right cerebellar hemisphere, an incidental finding. **C,** a sagittal nonenhanced short TR image (TR 500, TE 20) nicely demonstrates the sharply marginated tumor of the inferior vermis, compressing the posterior portion of the dilated fourth ventricle. The tumor extends through the foramen of Magendie into the upper cervical subarachnoid space. **D,** a gadolinium-enhanced short TR image (TR 500, TE 20) demonstrates the pronounced enhancement of the tumor which contains multiple necrotic areas.

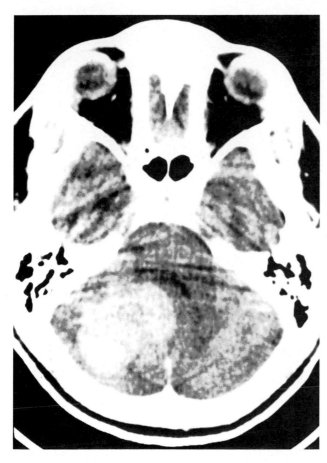

FIG 16–47.
Desmoplastic medulloblastoma. The enhanced CT scan demonstrates homogeneous but mild enhancement of a right cerebellar mass lesion which proved to be a desmoplastic medulloblastoma in this 23-year-old man. Such mild enhancement is typical of the adult form of medulloblastoma.

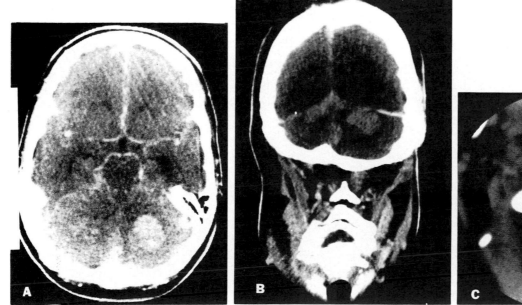

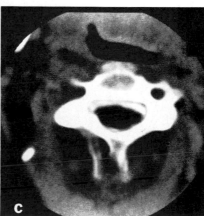

FIG 16–48.
Cerebellar hemispheric medulloblastoma in an adult. **A,** the axial enhanced scan demonstrates a well-circumscribed homogeneous mass within the left cerebellar hemisphere. The degree of enhancement is only moderate, which appears to be typical with adult medulloblastoma. **B,** the coronal view not only demonstrates the primary tumor focus within the superior portion of the left cerebellar hemisphere, just below the tentorium, but diffuse subtento- rial tumor extension and invasion into the vermis. **C,** postoperative metrizamide myelography demonstrates enlargement of the cervical spinal cord, which has an irregular margin. At the time of posterior fossa craniotomy for excisional biopsy of the cerebellar mass, diffuse infiltration both into the cervical spinal cord and along its outer margins was found.

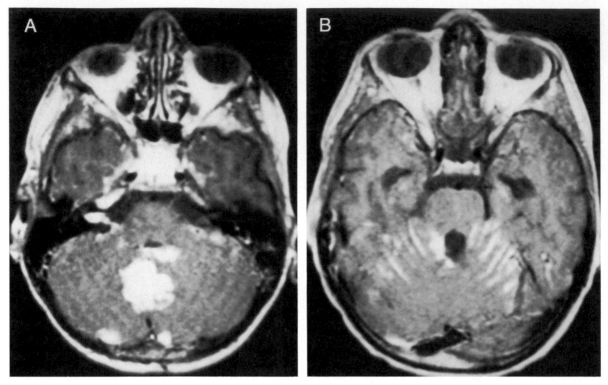

FIG 16–49.
Gadolinium-enhanced medulloblastoma with metastases to the cerebellar surface. **A,** a short TR gadolinium-enhanced axial image (TR 500, TE 20) demonstrates the enhancement of the vermian tumor with less contiguous enhancement behind the fourth ventricle. There are enhancing metastases within the right internal auditory canal and along the cerebellar surfaces of the cerebellopontine angles bilaterally. Enhancement over the posterior cerebellum is also noted. **B,** a higher cut (TR 500, TE 20) shows enhancement within the sulci between the cerebellar folia, some enhancement to the right of the dilated rostral fourth ventricle, and possibly some enhancement over the temporal lobes.

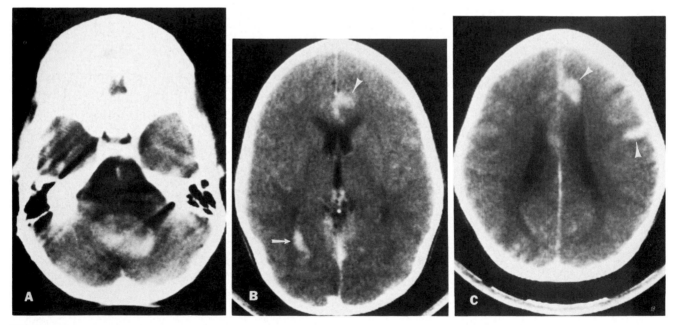

FIG 16–50.
Medulloblastoma with diffuse subarachnoid and intraventricular seeding. **A,** the enhanced scan in the posterior fossa demonstrates a well-marginated midline enhancing neoplasm typical of medulloblastoma. The quality of the scan is marred by motion artifact. **B, C** higher enhanced cuts demonstrate multiple tumor deposits in cerebral sulci *(arrowheads)* and intraventricular spread producing a deposit with the right occipital horn (**B,** *arrow*).

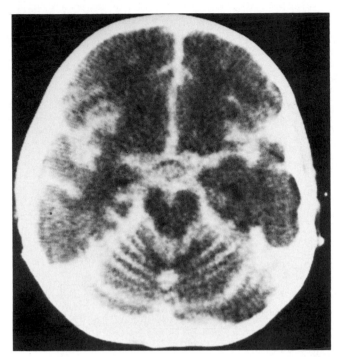

FIG 16–51.
Diffuse meningeal enhancement produced by seeding of medulloblastoma. Diffuse CSF seeding with medulloblastoma has produced such intense enhancement with the intravenous contrast agent that the scan simulates a metrizamide cisternogram.

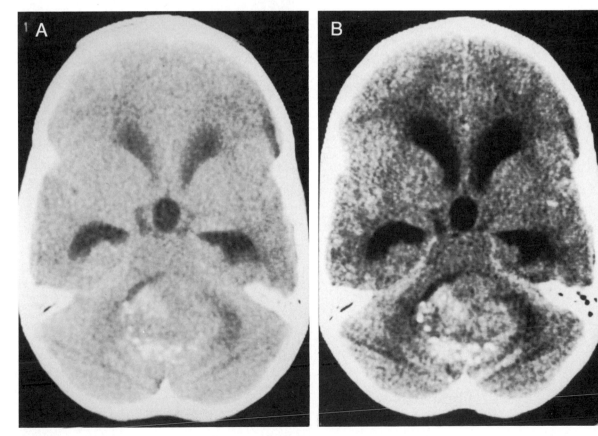

FIG 16–52.
Calcified ependymoma. The unenhanced **(A)** and enhanced **(B)** CT scans demonstrate a large vermian mass lesion with mottled calcification and only mild enhancement, producing obstructive hydrocephalus.

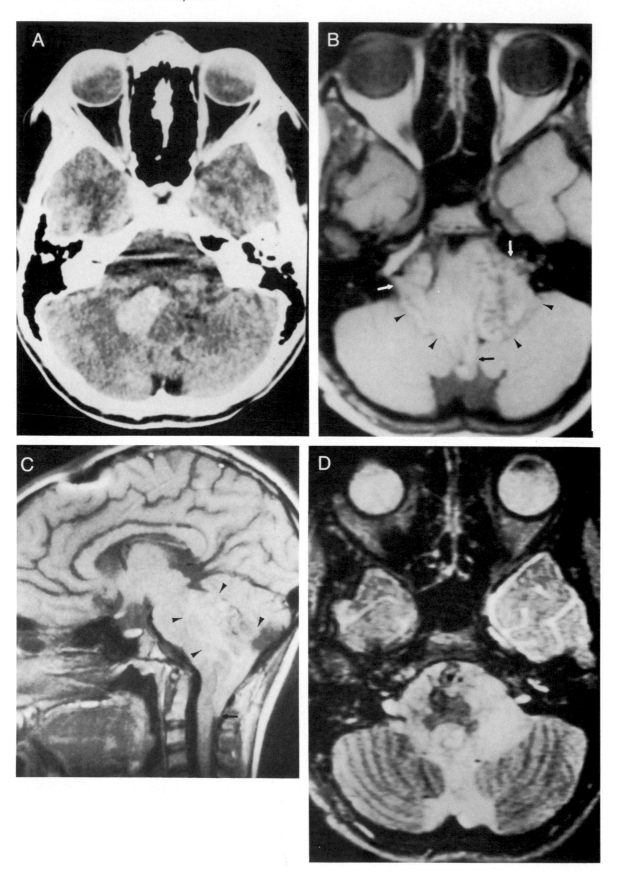

tial diagnosis of supratentorial hemispheric ependymoma includes ganglioglioma, which is a slower-growing, relatively benign lesion; oligodendroglioma; astrocytoma; and PNET. The ependymoma presenting within a lateral ventricle is typically of large size at the time of diagnosis as a result of its decompression into the ventricular system, with parenchymal mass effect and obstructive hydrocephalus occurring as late complications.

Intraventricular Neuroepithelial Tumors

The differential diagnosis of lesions originating or presenting primarily within a ventricle include ependymoma, subependymoma (subependymal astrocytoma), choroid plexus papilloma, colloid cyst, and meningioma. Ependymomas arising within a ventricle or within the cerebral parenchyma have been discussed previously. Meningiomas are considered in greater detail in Chapter 17.

Subependymoma (Subependymal Astrocytoma)

The subependymoma is a variant of ependymoma in which there is a proliferation of subependymal astrocytes.[95] The majority of these tumors occur within the fourth ventricle,[96] although 27% may be supratentorial, located along the walls of the lateral ventricle.[97] The majority of these tumors are asymptomatic, without evidence of active growth or obstruction to the outflow of CSF, and are incidental findings at autopsy in elderly males.[95–97] However, the symptomatic tumors are either strategically located to produce blockage of the CSF flow or are large at the time of presentation, with their intraventricular placement allowing for a large size before symptoms are produced. The septum pellucidum is a common supratentorial intraventricular location[97]; the centripetal growth produces a well-circumscribed mass lesion within the frontal horns (Fig 16–55).

On CT, the intraventricular astrocytoma is usu-

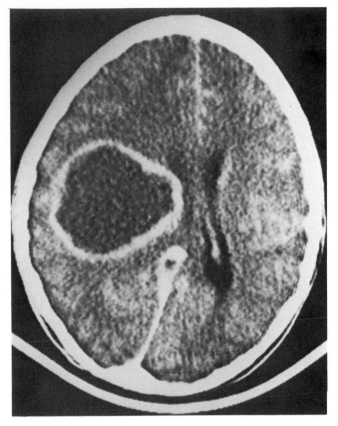

FIG 16–54.
Parietal ependymoma. This 13-year-old child presented with a large mass lesion of the right parietal lobe, compressing the right lateral ventricle. The lesion may have originated from either the ventricular ependyma or from ependymal rest cells within the hemisphere. The lesion is primarily cystic, with a densely enhancing rim.

ally isodense to brain on the unenhanced study, and enhances slightly. The major differential diagnostic possibility, colloid cyst herniating superiorly into the base of the septum pellucidum, is usually hyperdense without contrast but may be isodense, and usually does not enhance or shows only rim enhancement. On MRI, while both astrocytoma and colloid cyst may be hyperintense on long TR/TE images, the astrocytoma is isointense

FIG 16–53.
Fourth ventricular ependymoma extending into cerebellopontine angles and upper cervical subarachnoid space. **A,** the enhanced CT scan demonstrates a homogeneous enhancing tumor behind and to the right of the fourth ventricle. There is less well-circumscribed enhancement extending medially and into the left brachium pontis. The MR scan defines the true extent of this large tumor. **B, C,** the short TR axial and sagittal scans (TR 500, TE 20) show a large mass lesion (outlined by *arrowheads*) contiguous and most likely infiltrating into the posterior portion of the brain stem, occupying and obliterating the fourth ventricle. There is extension bilat-erally through the lateral recesses, out the foramina of Luschka to fill the cerebellopontine angles (**B,** *white arrows*). There is extension posteroinferiorly through the foramen of Magendie (**B,** *black arrow*) to extend into the cisterna magna and down into the retromedullary upper cervical subarachnoid space (**C,** *black arrow*). **D,** the long TR/TE sequence (TR 2,750, TE 75) demonstrates diffuse hyperintensity of the cerebellar vermis, perimedullary subarachnoid spaces, and foramen of Magendie. It is impossible to distinguish tumor from edema or CSF. The left lateral margin of the medulla is irregular, indicating invasion.

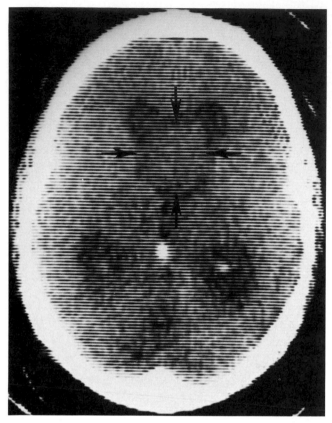

FIG 16–55.
Intraventricular glioma arising from the septum pellucidum. There is a sharply marginated round lesion *(arrows)* that is relatively isodense to the rest of the brain and has its epicenter in the septum pellucidum. The mass obstructs the foramen of Monro, producing dilatation of both frontal horns. Surgery revealed a well-circumscribed low-grade glioma that could be removed in its entirety. (From Latchaw RE, Gold LHA, Tourje EJ: *Minn Med* 1977; 60:554–559. Used by permission.)

to hypointense on short TR sequences while the colloid cyst is very variable, depending upon the cyst contents.

A variant of the subependymal astrocytoma is the subependymal giant cell astrocytoma that is seen in tuberous sclerosis. These tumors most frequently occur in the region of the foramen of Monro, producing obstruction of CSF flow, and are associated with the periventricular calcifications classically seen in tuberous sclerosis. While benign tubers may undergo calcification, the neoplasm occurring from degeneration of a tuber may be isodense on the preinfusion CT scan. It is extremely important to perform an enhanced scan on all patients with tuberous sclerosis in order to detect a breakdown of the BBB indicative of neoplastic degeneration. This entity is described more fully in Chapter 18.

Choroid Plexus Papilloma

Choroid plexus papilloma is a rare benign neoplasm, amounting to 0.5% of all intracranial tumors for all age groups.[98] However, it amounts to 10% of intracranial tumors within the first year of life.[98] The most common point of origin is within the trigone of the lateral ventricle,[99] with the second most common location being the fourth ventricle. Involvement of the third ventricle is uncommon,[98, 100, 101] and origin in the cerebellopontine angle from choroid extending through the foramen of Luschka is rare.[102]

The CT scan appearance is that of a well-marginated lesion with increased density before contrast enhancement due to the large blood pool (Fig 16–56), and calcification is frequent.[103–105] The lesion enhances markedly (see Fig 16–56), generally with a homogeneous texture.[103–105] Intraventricular meningioma has a similar appearance on CT scan, although this tumor is extremely unusual in the pediatric age group, particularly in very young children.

MRI demonstrates an isointense cauliflower-like mass on short TR images (Fig 16–57), hyperintensity on long TR sequences, and marked enhancement with gadolinium. The presence of blood or hemosiderin is evidence of previous hemorrhage. Signal voids represent either blood vessels feeding or draining this vascular lesion (see Fig 16–57), or clumps of calcification or hemosiderin.

Hydrocephalus is typically present with these tumors. While hemorrhage from this vascular tumor producing adhesions and secondary obstruction to CSF flow has been suggested as a cause of the hydrocephalus,[106] the more widely accepted explanation is that of overproduction of CSF. Surgical resection leads to a decrease of CSF production and decrease in ventricular size without ventricular shunting.[99, 107] Thus, as illustrated in Figure 16–56, hydrocephalus associated with an intraventricular lesion that could not produce ventricular obstruction by its position alone is evidence for the preoperative diagnosis of choroid plexus papilloma.

Colloid Cyst

Colloid cyst is included in this chapter because of its neuroepithelial origin, although it could also be included under congenital tumors of maldevelopmental origin.[108] The cyst arises from the roof of the third ventricle, just behind the foramina of Monro. Although this lesion is probably present

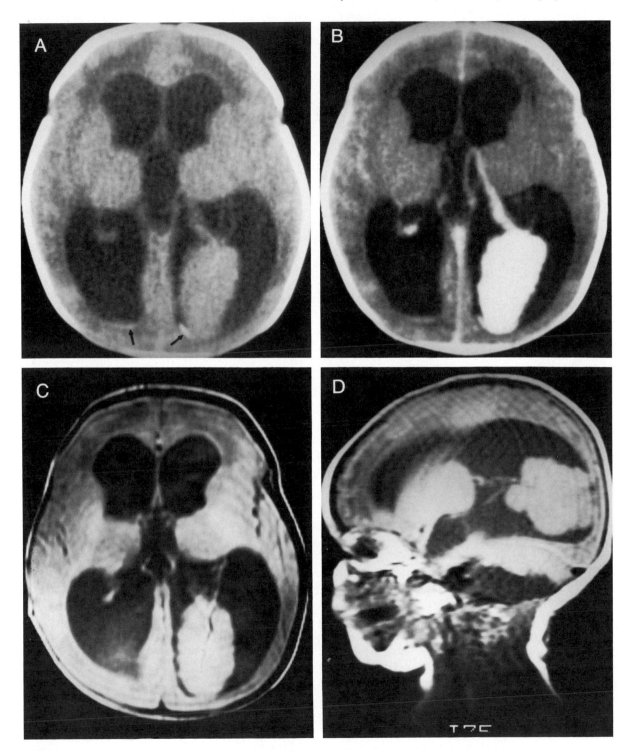

FIG 16–56.
Choroid plexus papilloma with hydrocephalus. **A,** the unenhanced axial CT scan shows a marked degree of dilatation of the third and lateral ventricles, and a mass that is isodense to gray matter located within the atrium of the left lateral ventricle. Linear hyperdense accumulations *(arrows)* within the atria bilaterally probably represent a small amount of hemorrhage from the vascular mass. **B,** the enhanced CT scan demonstrates marked enhancement of the papilloma, and of the choroid plexus extending to the left foramen of Monro. **C, D,** unenhanced axial and sagittal short TR MR images (TR 600, TE 20) demonstrate the lobular papilloma which is of equal intensity to gray matter. The marked hydrocephalus in this 4-day-old female is probably from an overproduction of CSF, although hemorrhage from this vascular tumor could produce adhesions.

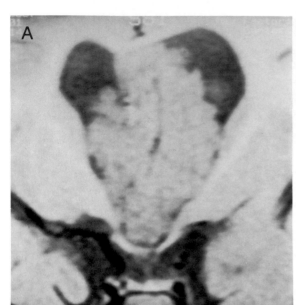
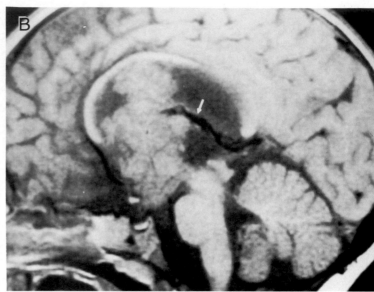

FIG 16–57.
Choroid plexus papilloma of the third ventricle. Coronal **(A)** and sagittal **(B)** short TR MR scans (TR 500, TE 20) demonstrate a cauliflower-like tumor that is less intense than gray matter, occupying a dilated third ventricle in this 1-year-old female. The curvilin- ear hypointense structures leading posteriorly from the lesion **(B,** *arrow)* represent veins draining from the vascular mass lesion into the internal cerebral veins.

from birth, its very slow growth means that it does not generally present until adulthood.[109]

The CT scan appearance is classically that of a lesion located at the foramina of Monro, having a moderate-to-marked density without the use of contrast enhancement (Fig 16–58). This hyperdensity is secondary to a combination of desquamated material within the cyst, hemosiderin, and calcium.[110] However, the colloid cyst is not infrequently isodense (3 of 14 cases in one series[110] and 9 of 18 in another[111]) to only slightly hyperdense (Fig 16–59). Colloid cysts enhanced with contrast material to a mild degree in 10 of 13 cases in one report[110] (Figs 16–60 and 16–61). The enhancement may be secondary to blood vessels in the wall of the cyst or leakage of contrast into the cyst cavity.[110] The enhanced scan may also show separation of the veins at the foramina of Monro by the cyst.

MRI findings are very variable ranging from hypo- to iso- to hyperintensity on all sequences. The signals may be homogeneous or heterogeneous.[112]

The lesion obstructs one or both foramen of Monro, leading to dilatation of one or both of the lateral ventricles and a small or normal-sized third ventricle (see Figs 16–58 and 16–59).[110] Because a foramen of Monro is only a few millimeters in width, a small isodense lesion strategically located at the foramen may produce a marked degree of hydrocephalus, yet may be difficult to visualize because of the marked enlargement of the lateral ventricles.

The major differential diagnostic consideration of a mass in this region is astrocytoma of the septum pellucidum. Typically, a glioma is isodense on the precontrast CT scan and enhances mildly. MRI shows hypointensity to isointensity on the short TR study and hyperintensity on long TR sequences. Other possibilities include ependymoma and intraventricular meningioma which do not necessarily originate from the point of origin of a colloid cyst immediately behind the foramina of Monro; their density characteristics are discussed elsewhere in this section. Craniopharyngioma may be bright or gray on short TR images and therefore may simulate a colloid cyst; the calcification present in 80% of childhood craniopharyngiomas and 20% of adult lesions may not be seen on MRI but is easily detected on CT. Its extension to the

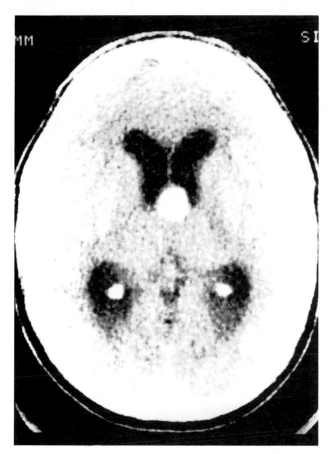

FIG 16–58.
Hyperdense colloid cyst. The unenhanced CT scan demonstrates marked hyperdensity of a lesion at the foramen of Monro, the classic CT appearance of a colloid cyst.

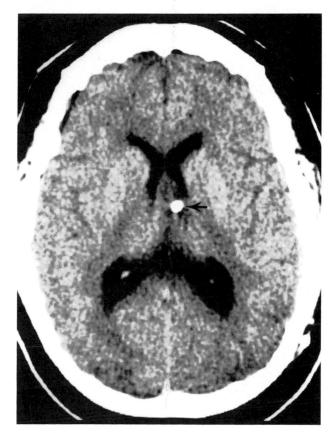

FIG 16–59.
Isodense colloid cyst on CT. The unenhanced axial CT scan demonstrates an isodense mass lesion involving the septum pellucidum and foramen of Monro. A shunt tube *(arrow)* was placed for acute hydrocephalus. Surgically this was a colloid cyst.

suprasellar space on sagittal views, however, is diagnostic. Finally, a thrombosed basilar tip aneurysm is hyperintense on short TR MR images and may project into the third ventricle. Sagittal imaging showing its relationship to the flow void of the basilar artery resolves the confusion.

The colloid cyst may be stereotactically punctured under CT control, with the aspiration of mucoid material and secondary decompression of the ventricular system (see Chapter 44). The growth rate of these cysts is so slow that decompression without complete removal may be sufficient to alleviate symptoms.

Pineal Parenchymal Tumors

The pineal parenchymal tumors, pineocytoma and pineoblastoma, are tumors of neuroepithelial origin. However, they are relatively rare compared with other tumors originating in the pineal region, particularly germinoma and teratoma, which are tumors of congenital origin. The entire group of pineal region tumors is therefore discussed in Chapter 18.

SARCOMAS

Primary sarcomas of the cerebral parenchymal are rare. Primary sarcomas are more common in the meninges,[113, 114] but primary fibrosarcoma has been described, particularly following radiation therapy for lesions such as pituitary tumor.[115, 116]

Feigin originally described a tumor with a mixture of glioblastoma and sarcomatous changes: the gliosarcoma. The prognosis of this tumor is similar to that of glioblastoma, although there may be more remote metastases due to the sarcomatous component.[117] The radiographic appearance is that of multiple foci of nonhomogeneously enhancing and infiltrating masses with irregular borders (Fig

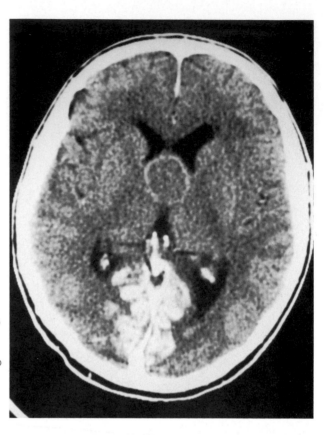

FIG 16–60.
Isodense colloid cyst with peripheral enhancement and bilateral occipital infarcts. This 35-year-old woman presented initially with bilateral cortical blindness. This enhanced CT scan demonstrates gyriform enhancement of the occipital cortex bilaterally. This scan also demonstrates an isodense lesion at the foramen of Monro, with enhancement of its rim. Surgically this was a colloid cyst. While no hydrocephalus is present on this scan, movement of the colloid cyst to block one or both foramina of Monro, producing acute obstructive hydrocephalus, could have produced compression of both posterior cerebral arteries at the tentorial notch, accounting for the occipital infarctions.

16–62). The appearance may simulate the extensive spread throughout a hemisphere seen with some glioblastomas. The unilaterality is against typical hematogenous metastases.

PRIMARY CEREBRAL LYMPHOMA

Primary cerebral lymphoma has also been called *primary reticulum cell sarcoma of the brain, histiocytic lymphoma,* and *microglioma.*[118, 119] This tumor has become of great interest today because of its appearance in those patients undergoing long-term immunosuppression, particularly posttransplantation patients, and in patients with acquired immunodeficiency syndrome (AIDS).[120–122] The appearance of lymphoma associated with AIDS is frequently different from that in patients without AIDS, and the radiologic appearances will be described separately.

Up to one half of the patients with non-AIDS primary malignant lymphoma have multiple cerebral lesions, which are generally located deep within the hemisphere in areas such as the basal ganglia, thalamus, and corpus callosum (Figs 16–63 and 16–64).[119–124] On the preinfusion CT scan, the tumor has been described as varying from isodense to high density,[119–125] with the high-density pattern seen in 48 of 52 cases in one series.[126] The increased density is most likely due to the dense packing of the cells, similar to medulloblastoma.[122, 125] There is generally homogeneous enhancement,[121–126] and the margins are slightly irregular indicating infiltration into the surrounding brain (see Figs 16–63 and 16–64). There is usually little edema,[123] and periventricular spread is common (see Fig 16–63).[121] MR findings are isointensity or hypointensity to gray matter on precontrast short TR scans, isointensity to slight hyperintensity relative to gray matter on long TR/TE sequences,[127] and moderate-to-marked enhancement.

The diagnosis of non-AIDS malignant lymphoma of the brain may be suggested on the basis of the homogeneous enhancement of one or multiple deep lesions which are dense on the precontrast CT scan. Typically, glial tumors are hypodense on the precontrast CT scan and have patchy or mixed enhancement patterns. Hematogenous metastases present with sharper margins and more surrounding edema than the typical lesions of primary malignant lymphoma. The appearance on the

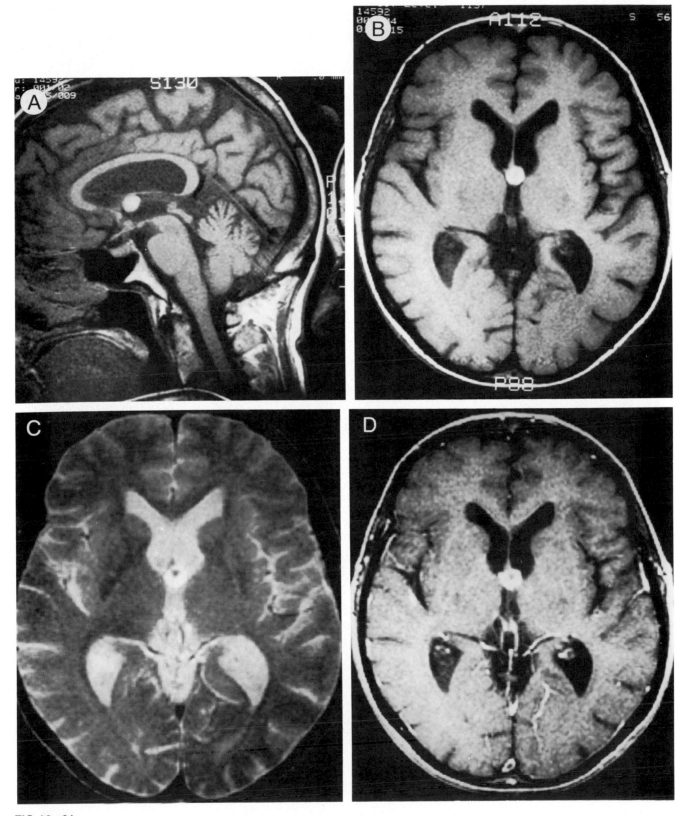

FIG 16–61.
Hyperintense, enhancing colloid cyst on MRI. **A,** the T1-unenhanced short TR sagittal sequence (TR 400, TE 20) demonstrates the classic hyperintense lesion at the foramina of Monro. The unenhanced axial short TR (**B,** TR 600, TE 20) and long TR/TE (**C,** TR 2,500, TE 80) scans demonstrate the hyperintense lesion on both sequences. While subacute hemorrhage classically gives hyperin- tensity on both short TR and long TR/TE sequences, fatty esters are probably responsible in this case. **D,** the gadolinium DTPA–enhanced short TR image (TR 600, TE 30) demonstrates peripheral enhancement blending with the inherent hyperintensity of the lesion.

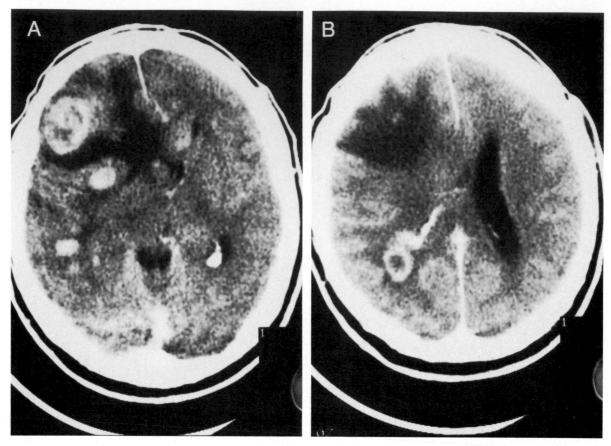

FIG 16–62.
Gliosarcoma (Feigin tumor). **A,** the lower of the two enhanced CT images demonstrates a large nodular lesion in the right frontal lobe having patchy internal characteristics, and abundant surrounding edema. **B,** there are multiple nodules within the more posterior portion of the right hemisphere, with an additional nodular extension seen behind the atrium of the right lateral ventricle.

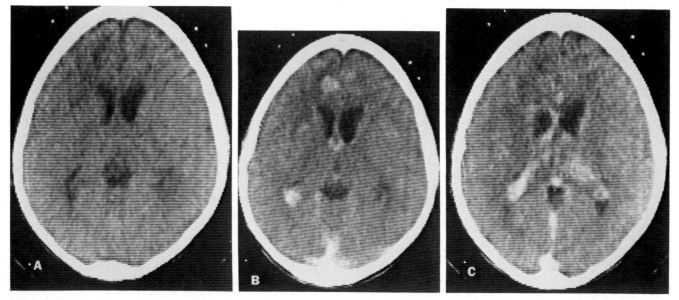

FIG 16–63.
Posttransplant primary lymphoma of the brain. Progressive somnolence occurred while this patient was on immunosuppressive therapy a number of months following renal transplantation. This led to a CT scan. **A,** the unenhanced scan demonstrates some patchy low density within both frontal lobes and distortion of the frontal horns. **B, C,** the enhanced scans demonstrate multiple homogeneously enhancing nodular densities within the parenchyma and diffuse periventricular enhancement producing distortion of the ventricular contour. Infection was considered, but there was little improvement with antibiotics and antifungal agents. At autopsy, diffuse primary lymphoma of the brain was found.

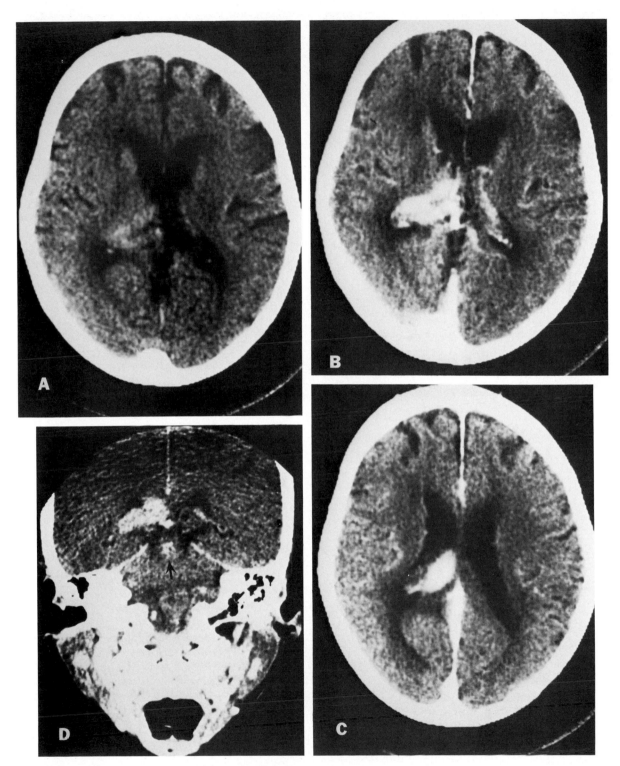

FIG 16–64.
Primary histiocytic lymphoma of the brain. Headache prompted a CT scan, with an unenhanced view **(A)** demonstrating a neoplasm of moderate increased density compressing and distorting the body and atrium of the right lateral ventricle. **B, C,** the enhanced axial views demonstrate diffuse, homogeneously enhancing tumor infiltrating around and through the right lateral ventricle and contiguous parenchyma. **D,** the coronal view demonstrates the relationship of the neoplasm to the ventricular system and infiltration into the quadrigeminal plate *(arrow)*.

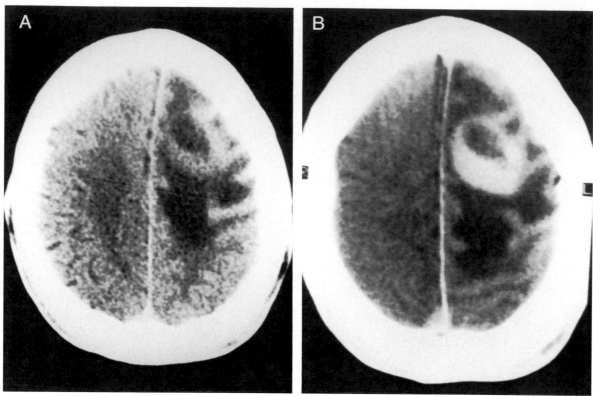

FIG 16–65.

Primary malignant lymphoma of the brain with central necrosis. The unenhanced **(A)** and enhanced **(B)** CT scans demonstrate a dense and homogeneous ring of enhancement around a central area of necrosis in this high-convexity left posterior frontal primary lymphoma. There is abundant surrounding edema.

long TR MR study of only slight hyperintensity or isointensity, along with only slight edema, may be quite helpful in distinguishing lymphoma from metastasis or glial tumor. Infection must always be considered in the immunocompromised patient. Cerebritis enhances slightly on CT, in a patchy fashion, while abscess demonstrates ring enhancement. On MRI, differentiation of lymphoma from infection may be quite difficult if a ring lesion (abscess) is not present.[127] Infarction will be within a vascular distribution.

Ring enhancement of primary cerebral lymphoma (Fig 16–65) is common in patients with AIDS,[122] occurring in 76% in one series.[126] This differs from the non-AIDS appearance of homogeneous enhancement. Pathologic examination of these AIDS-related tumors reveals extensive central necrosis.[122] The ringlike lesion(s) simulates infections that are typically seen in these patients, such as fungal abscess(es) or parasitic infection.[122] The only difference may be the sharpness of the margins seen with toxoplasmosis or with cryptococcal or other fungal abscesses, relative to the shaggy margins of the enhancing rings of AIDS

lymphoma. However, biopsy will usually be necessary to make the differentiation.

REFERENCES

1. Kernohan JW, Sayre GP: *Tumors of the Central Nervous System*, in *Atlas of Tumor Pathology*, section 10, fasciscle 35. Washington, DC, Armed Forces Institute of Pathology, 1952.
2. Nelson JS, Tsukada Y, Schoenfeld DL, et al: Necrosis as a prognostic criterion in malignant supratentorial, astrocytic gliomas. *Cancer* 1983; 52:550.
3. Burger PC, Vogel FS, Green SB, et al: Glioblastoma multiforme and anaplastic astrocytoma. Pathologic criteria and prognostic implications. *Cancer* 1985; 56:1106.
4. Nelson DF, Nelson JS, Davis DR, et al: Survival and prognosis of patients with astrocytoma with atypical or anaplastic features. *J Neuro Oncol* 1985; 3:99.
5. Kjos BO, Brant-Zawadzki M, Kucharczyk W, et al: Cystic intracranial lesions: Magnetic resonance imaging. *Radiology* 1985; 155:363–369.
6. Latchaw RE, Gold LHA, Tourje EJ: A protocol for the use of contrast enhancement in cranial com-

puted tomography. *Radiology* 1978; 126:681–687.

7. Butler AR, Kricheff II: Non-contrast CT scanning: Limited value in suspected brain tumor. *Radiology* 1978; 126:689–693.

8. Latchaw RE, Gold LHA, Moore JS, et al: The non-specificity of absorption coefficients in the differentiation of solid tumors and cystic lesions. *Radiology* 1977; 125:141–144.

9. Lunsford LD, Martinez AJ, Latchaw RE: Magnetic resonance imaging does not define tumor boundaries. *Acta Radiol* 1986; [Suppl] *(Stockh)* 369:370–373.

10. Kelly PJ, Daumas-Duport C, Kispert DB, et al: Imaging-based stereotaxic serial biopsies in untreated intracranial glial neoplasms. *J Neurosurg* 1987; 66:865–874.

11. Earnest F, Kelly PJ, Scheithauer BW, et al: Cerebral astrocytomas: Histopathologic correlation of MR and CT contrast enhancement with stereotactic biopsy. *Radiology* 1988; 166:823–827.

12. Burger PC, Dubois PJ, Schold SC, et al: Computerized tomographic and pathologic studies of the untreated, quiescent, and recurrent glioblastoma multiforme. *J Neurosurg* 1983; 58:159–169.

13. Johnson PC, Hunt SJ, Drayer BP: Human cerebral gliomas: Correlation of postmortem MR findings and neuropathologic findings. *Radiology* 1989; 170:211–217.

14. Russell DS, Rubinstein LJ: Deformations and other structural changes produced by intracranial tumours: Effects of radiation and other forms of therapy on intracranial and spinal tumours and their surrounding tissues, in *Pathology of Tumours of the Nervous System*. Baltimore, Williams & Wilkins Co, 1989, pp 857–861.

15. Hayman LA, Evans RA, Hinch VC: Delayed high iodine dose contrast computed tomography: Cranial neoplasms. *Radiology* 1980; 136:677–684.

16. Shalen PR, Hayman LA, Wallace S, et al: Protocol for delayed contrast enhancement in computed tomography of cerebral neoplasia. *Radiology* 1981; 139:397–402.

17. Laster DW, Moody DM, Ball MR: Resolving intracerebral hematoma: Alteration of the "ring sign" with steroids. *AJR* 1978; 130:935–939.

18. Whelan MA, Hilal SK: Computed tomography as a guide in the diagnosis and follow-up of brain abscesses. *Radiology* 1980; 135:663–671.

19. Tchang S, Scotti G, Terbrugge K, et al: Computerized tomography as a possible aid to histological grading of supratentorial gliomas. *J Neurosurg* 1977; 46:735–739.

20. Naidich TP, Lin JP, Leeds NE, et al: Primary tumors and other masses of the cerebellum and fourth ventricle: differential diagnosis by computed tomography. *Neuroradiology* 1977; 14:153–174.

21. Zimmerman RA, Bilaniuk LT, Bruno L, et al: Computed tomography of cerebellar astrocytoma. *AJR* 1978; 130:929–933.

22. Butler AR, Horii SC, Kricheff II, et al: Computed tomography in astrocytomas. A statistical analysis of the parameters of malignancy and the positive contrast-enhanced CT scan. *Radiology* 1978; 129:433–439.

23. Bilaniuk LT, Zimmerman RA, Littman P, et al: Computed tomography of brain stem gliomas in children. *Radiology* 1980; 134:89–95.

24. Albright AL, Guthkelch AN, Packer RJ, et al: Prognostic factors in pediatric brain-stem gliomas. *J Neurosurg* 1986; 65:751–755.

25. Norman D, Stevens EA, Wing SD, et al: Quantitative aspects of contrast enhancement in cranial computed tomography. *Radiology* 1978; 129:683–688.

26. Schorner W, Laniado M, Niendorf HP, et al: Time-dependent changes in image contrast in brain tumors after gadolinium-DTPA. *AJNR* 1986; 7:1013–1020.

27. Steinhoff H, Grumme TH, Kazner E, et al: Axial transverse computerized tomography in 73 glioblastomas. *Acta Neurochir* 1978; 42:45–56.

28. George AE, Russell EJ, Kricheff II: White matter buckling: CT sign of extraaxial intracranial mass. *AJR* 1980; 135:1031–1036.

29. Jungreis CA, Chandra R, Kricheff II, et al: In vitro magnetic resonance properties of CNS neoplasms and associated cysts. *Invest Radiol* 1988; 23:12–16.

30. Varma RR, Crumrine PK, Bergman I, et al: Childhood oligodendrogliomas presenting with seizure and low density lesion on CT scan. *Neurology (NY)* 1983; 33:806–808.

31. Handa J, Nakaro Y, Handa H: Computed tomography in the differential diagnosis of low-density intracranial lesions. *Surg Neurol* 1978; 10:179–185.

32. Lilja A, Bergstrom K, Spansare B, et al: Reliability of computed tomography in assessing histopathological features of malignant supratentorial gliomas. *J Comput Assist Tomogr* 1981; 5:625–636.

33. Zimmerman RA, Bilaniuk LT: Computed tomography of acute intratumoral hemorrhage. *Radiology* 1980; 135:355–359.

34. Destian S, Sze G, Krol G, et al: MR imaging of hemorrhagic intracranial neoplasms. *AJNR* 1988; 9:1115–1122.

35. Atlas SW, Grossman RI, Gomon JM, et al: Calcified intracranial lesions: Detection with gradient-echo-acquisition rapid MR imaging. *AJNR* 1988; 9:253–259.

36. McGeachie RE, Gold LHA, Latchaw RE: Periventricular spread of tumor demonstrated by computed tomography. *Radiology* 1977; 125:407–410.

37. Erlich SS, David RL: Spinal subarachnoid metastasis from primary intracranial glioblastoma multiforme. *Cancer* 1978; 42:2854–2864.

38. Kieffer SA, Salibi NA, Kim RC, et al: Multifocal glioblastoma: Diagnostic implications. *Radiology* 1982; 143:709–710.

39. Van Tassel P, Lee Y, Bruner JM: Synchronous and metachronous malignant gliomas: CT findings. *AJNR* 1988; 9:725–732.

40. Woodruff WW, Djang WT, Voorhees D, et al: Calvarial destruction: An unusual manifestation of glioblastoma multiforme. *AJNR* 1988; 9:388–389.

41. Joyce P, Bentson J, Takehasin M, et al: The accuracy of predicting histologic grades of supratentorial astrocytomas on the basis of computerized tomography and cerebral angiography. *Neuroradiology* 1978; 16:346–348.

42. Marks TE, Gado M: Serial computed tomography of primary brain tumors following surgery, irradiation and chemotherapy. *Radiology* 1977; 125:119–125.

43. Steinhoff H, Lanksch W, Kazner E, et al: Computed tomography in the diagnosis and differential diagnosis of glioblastomas: A qualitative study of 295 cases. *Neuroradiology* 1977; 14:193–200.

44. Silverman C, Marks JE: Prognostic significance of contrast enhancement in low-grade astrocytomas of the adult cerebrum. *Radiology* 1981; 139:211–213.

45. Latchaw RE, Payne JT, Gold LHA: Effective atomic number and electron density as measured with a computed tomography scanner: Computation and correlation with brain tumor histology. *J Comput Assist Tomogr* 1978; 2:199–208.

46. Latchaw RE, Payne JT, Loewenson RB: Predicting brain tumor histology: Change of effective atomic number with contrast enhancement. *AJNR* 1980; 1:289–294.

47. Lewander R: Contrast enhancement with time in gliomas. Stereotactic computer tomography following contrast medium infusion. *Acta Radiol* 1979; 20:689.

48. Naidich TP, Pinto RS, Kushner MJ, et al: Evaluation of sellar and parasellar masses by computed tomography. *Radiology* 1976; 120:91–99.

49. Tomita T, McLone DG, Naidich TP: Mural tumors with cysts in the cerebral hemispheres of children. *Neurosurgery* 1986; 19:998–1005.

50. Lilja A, Lundqvist H, Olsson Y, et al: Positron emission tomography and computed tomography in differential diagnosis between recurrent or residual glioma and treatment-induced brain lesions. *Acta Radiol* 1989; 30:121–128.

51. Mosskin M, von Holst H, Ericson K, et al: The blood tumour barrier in intracranial tumours studied with x-ray computed tomography and positron emission tomography using 68-Ga-EDTA. *Neuroradiology* 1986; 28:259–263.

52. Ericson K, Lilja A, Bergstrom M, et al: Positron emission tomography with ([^{11}C]methyl)-L-methionine, [^{11}C]D-glucose, and [^{68}Ga] EDTA in supratentorial tumors. *J Comput Assist Tomogr* 1985; 9:683–689.

53. Vonofakos D, Barcu H, Hacker H: Oligodendrogliomas: CT patterns and emphasis on features indicating malignancy. *J Comput Assist Tomogr* 1979; 3:783–788.

54. Lee Y-Y, Tassel PV: Intracranial oligodendrogliomas: Imaging findings in 35 untreated cases. *AJNR* 1989; 10:119–127.

55. Garza-Mercado R, Campa H, Grajeda J: Primary oligodendroglioma of the septum pellucidum. *Neurosurgery* 1987; 21:78–80.

56. Hart MN, Earle KM: Primitive neuroectodermal tumors of the brain in children. *Cancer* 1973; 32:890–897.

57. Rorke LB: Cerebellar medulloblastoma and its relationship to primitive neuroectodermal neoplasms. *J Neuropathol Exp Neurol* 1983; 42:1–15.

58. Priest J, Dehner LP, Sung JH, et al: Primitive neuroectodermal tumors (embryonal gliomas) of childhood: A clinicopathologic study of 12 cases, in Humphrey GB, Benner G (eds): *Pediatric Oncology*, Boston, Martinua Nijhoff Publishers, 1981, pp 247–264.

59. Horten BC, Rubinstein LJ: Primary cerebral neuroblastoma: A clinicopathological study of 35 cases. *Brain* 1976; 99:735–756.

60. Sakaki S, Mori Y, Motozaki T, et al: A cerebral neuroblastoma with extracranial metastases. *Surg Neurol* 1981; 16:53–59.

61. Latchaw RE, L'Heureux PR, Young G, et al: Neuroblastoma presenting as central nervous system disease. *AJNR* 1982; 3:623–630.

62. Ganti SR, Silver AJ, Diefenbach P, et al: Computed tomography of primitive neuroectodermal tumors. *AJNR* 1983; 4:819–821.

63. Davis PC, Wichman RD, Takei Y, et al: Primary cerebral neuroblastoma: CT and MR findings in 12 cases. *AJNR* 1990; 11:115–120.

64. Chambers EF, Turski PA, Sobel D, et al: Radiologic characteristics of primary cerebral neuroblastomas. *Radiology* 1981; 139:101–104.

65. Zimmerman RA, Bilaniuk LT: CT of primary and secondary craniocerebral neuroblastoma. *AJNR* 1980; 1:431–434.

66. Zimmerman RA, Bilaniuk LT: Computed tomography of intracranial ganglioglioma. *CT* 1979; 3:24–30.

67. Nass R, Whelan MA: Gangliogliomas. *Neuroradiology* 1981; 22:67–71.

68. Castillo M, Davis PC, Takei Y, et al: Intracranial ganglioglioma: MR, CT, and clinical findings in 18 patients. *AJNR* 1990; 11:109–114.

69. Demierre B, Stichnoth FA, Hori A, et al: Intracerebral ganglioglioma. *J Neurosurg* 1986; 65:177–182.

70. Palma L: Supratentorial neuroepithelial cysts. Re-

port of two cases. *J Neurosurg* 1975; 42:353–357.

71. Czervionke LF, Daniels DL, Meyer GA, et al: Neuroepithelial cysts of the lateral ventricles: MR appearance. *AJNR* 1987; 8:609–613.

72. Numaguchi Y, Connolly ES, Kumra AK, et al: Computed tomography and MR imaging of thalamic neuroepithelial cysts. *J Comput Assist Tomogr* 1987; 11:583–585.

73. Stroink AR, Hoffman HJ, Hendrick EB, et al: Transependymal benign dorsally exophytic brain stem gliomas in childhood: Diagnosis and treatment recommendations. *Neurosurgery* 1987; 20:439.

74. Packer RJ, Zimmerman RA, Luerssen TG, et al: Brainstem gliomas of childhood: Magnetic resonance imaging. *Neurology (NY)* 1985; 35:397–401.

75. Koehler PR, Haughton VM, Daniels DL, et al: MR measurement of normal and pathologic brainstem diameters. *AJNR* 1985; 6:425–427.

76. Tadmor R, Harwood-Nash DCF, Savoiardo M, et al: Brain tumors in the first two years of life: CT diagnosis. *AJNR* 1980; 1:411–417.

77. Lee BCP, Kneeland JB, Deck MDF, et al: Posterior fossa lesions: Magnetic resonance imaging. *Radiology* 1984; 153:137–143.

78. Tibbs PA, Mortara RH: Primary glioblastoma multiforme of the cerebellum. A case report. *Acta Neurochir (Wien)* 1980; 52:13–18.

79. Zimmerman RA, Bilaniuk LT, Pahlajani H: Spectrum of medulloblastoma demonstrated by computed tomography. *Radiology* 1978; 126:137–141.

80. Enzmann DR, Domar D, Levin V, et al: Computed tomography in the follow-up of medulloblastomas and ependymomas. *Radiology* 1978; 144:57–63.

81. Hughes PG: Cerebellar medulloblastoma in adults. *J Neurosurg* 1984; 60:994–997.

82. Zee C-S, Segall HD, Miller C, et al: Less common CT features of medulloblastoma. *Radiology* 1982; 144:92–102.

83. Weinstein ZR, Downey EF: Spontaneous hemorrhage in medulloblastomas. *AJNR* 1983; 4:986–988.

84. North C, Segall HD, Stanley P, et al: Early CT detection of intracranial seeding from medulloblastoma. *AJNR* 1985; 6:11–13.

85. Jereb B, Sundaresan N, Horten B, et al: Supratentorial recurrences in medulloblastoma. *Cancer* 1981; 47:806–809.

86. Kleinman GM, Hochberg FH, Richardson EP: Systemic metastases from medulloblastoma: Report of two cases and review of the literature. *Cancer* 1981; 48:2296–2309.

87. Krol G, Sze G, Malkin M, et al: MR of cranial and spinal meningeal carcinomatosis: Comparison with CT and myelography. *AJNR* 1988; 9:709–714.

88. Sze G, Abramson A, Krol G, et al: Gadolinium-DTPA in the evaluation of intradural extramedullary spinal disease. *AJNR* 1988; 9:153–163.

89. Swartz JD, Zimmerman RA, Bilaniuk LT: Computed tomography of intracranial ependymomas. *Radiology* 1982; 143:97–101.

90. Barone BM, Elvidge AR: Ependymomas. A clinical survey. *J Neurosurg* 1970; 33:428.

91. Fokes EC, Earle KM: Ependymomas: Clinical and pathological aspects. *J Neurosurg* 1968; 30:585.

92. Kricheff II, Becker M, Schneck SA, et al: Intracranial ependymomas: Factors influencing prognosis. *J Neurosurg* 1964; 21:7–14.

93. Dohrmann GJ, Farwell JR, Flannery JT: Ependymomas and ependymoblastomas in children. *J Neurosurg* 1976; 45:273–283.

94. Armington WG, Osborn AG, Cubberley DA, et al: Supratentorial ependymoma: CT appearance. *Radiology* 1985; 157:367–372.

95. Russell DS, Rubinstein LJ: Primary tumors of neuroectodermal origin, in Russell DS, Rubinstein LJ (eds): *Pathology of Tumors of the Nervous System.* Baltimore, Williams & Wilkins Co, 1977, pp 146–282.

96. Stevens JM, Kendall BE, Love S: Radiological features of subependymoma with emphasis on computed tomography. *Neuroradiology* 1984; 26:223–228.

97. Sheithauer BW: Symptomatic subependymoma: Report of 21 cases with review of the literature. *J Neurosurg* 1978; 29:689–696.

98. Jooma R, Grant DN: Third ventricle choroid plexus papillomas. *Childs Brain* 1983; 10:242–250.

99. Turcotte JF, Copty M, Bedard F, et al: Lateral ventricle choroid plexus papilloma and communicating hydrocephalus. *Surg Neurol* 1980; 13:313.

100. Schellhas KP, Siebert RC, Heithoff KB, et al: Congenital choroid plexus papilloma of the third ventricle: Diagnosis with real-time sonography and MR imaging. *AJNR* 1988; 9:797–798.

101. Tomasello F, Albanese V, Beinini F, et al: Choroid plexus papilloma of the third ventricle. *Surg Neurol* 1981; 16:69–71.

102. Chan RC, Thompson GB, Durity FA: Primary choroid plexus papilloma of the cerebellopontine angle. *Neurosurgery* 1983; 12:334.

103. Hawkins JC III: Treatment of choroid plexus papilloma in children: A brief analysis of twenty years' experience. *Neurosurgery* 1980; 6:380–384.

104. Coin CG, Coin JW, Glover MB: Vascular tumors of the choroid plexus: Diagnosis by computed tomography. *J Comput Assist Tomogr* 1977; 1:146–148.

105. Tomita T, Naidich TP: Successful resection of choroid plexus papillomas diagnosed at birth: Report of two cases. *Neurosurgery* 1987; 20:774.

106. Milhorat TH: Choroid plexus and cerebrospinal fluid production. *Science* 1969; 166:1514–1516.

107. Gudeman SK, Sullivan HG, Rosver MJ, et al: Surgical removal of bilateral papillomas of the choroid plexus of the lateral ventricles with resolution of hydrocephalus: Case report. *J Neurosurg* 1979; 50:677–681.

108. Russell DS, Rubenstein LJ: Tumours and tumour-like lesions of maldevelopmental origin, in *Pathology of Tumours of the Nervous System*. Williams & Wilkins, Baltimore, 1989, pp 721–727.

109. Wilson CB, Moossy J, Boldrey EB, et al: Pathology of intracranial tumors, in Newton TH, Potts GD (eds): *Radiology of the Skull and Brain*, vol 3. St Louis, CV Mosby Co, 1977, pp 3016–3018.

110. Ganti SR, Antunes JL, Louis KM, et al: Computed tomography in the diagnosis of colloid cysts of the third ventricle. *Radiology* 1981; 138:388–391.

111. Powell MP, Torrens MJ, Phil M, et al: Isodense colloid cysts of the third ventricle: A diagnostic and therapeutic problem resolved by ventriculoscopy. *Neurosurgery* 1983; 13:234.

112. Waggenspack GA, Guinto FC: MR and CT of masses of the anterosuperior third ventricle. *AJNR* 1989; 10:105–110.

113. Russell DS, Rubinstein LJ: Tumors of meninges and of related tissues, in *Pathology of Tumors of the Nervous System*. Baltimore, Williams & Wilkins Co, 1989, pp 507–517.

114. Latchaw RE, Gabrielsen TO, Seeger JF: Cerebral angiography in meningeal sarcomatosis and carcinomatosis. *Neuroradiology* 1974; 8:131–139.

115. Kingsley DPE, Kendall BE: CT of the adverse effects of therapeutic radiation of the central nervous system. *AJNR* 1981; 2:453–460.

116. Martin WH, Cail WS, Morris JL, et al: Fibrosarcoma after high energy radiation therapy for pituitary adenoma. *AJNR* 1980; 1:469–472.

117. Russell DS, Rubenstein LJ: Tumours of central neuroepithelial origin, in *Pathology of Tumours of the Nervous System*, Williams & Wilkins, Baltimore, 1989, pp 233–237.

118. Whelan MA, Kricheff II: Intracranial lymphoma. *Semin Roentgenol* 1984; 19:91.

119. Mendenhall NP, Thar TL, Agee OF, et al: Primary lymphoma of the central nervous system. Computerized tomography scan characteristics and treatment results for 12 cases. *Cancer* 1983; 52:1993–2000.

120. Tadmor R, Davis KR, Roberson GH, et al: Computed tomography in primary malignant lymphoma of the brain. *J Comput Assist Tomogr* 1978; 2:135–140.

121. Enzmann DR, Kirkorian J, Norman D, et al: Computed tomography in primary reticulum cell sarcoma of brain. *Radiology* 1979; 130:165–170.

122. Lee Y-Y, Bruner JM, Van Tassel P, et al: Primary central nervous system lymphoma: CT and pathologic correlation. *AJNR* 1986; 7:599–604.

123. Holtas S, Nyman U, Cronqvist S: Computed tomography of malignant lymphoma of the brain. *Neuroradiology* 1984; 26:33–38.

124. Jack CR Jr, O'Neill BP, Banks PM, et al: Central nervous system lymphoma: Histologic types and CT appearance. *Radiology* 1988; 167:211–215.

125. Kasner E, Wilske J, Steinhoff H, et al: Computer assisted tomography in primary malignant lymphomas of the brain. *J Comput Assist Tomogr* 1978; 2:125–134.

126. Smirniotopoulos JG, Murphy FM: Radiology of CNS lymphoma. Presented at the 27th Annual Meeting of the American Society of Neuroradiology, Orlando, Fla, March 1989.

127. Schwaighofer BW, Hesselink JR, Press GA, et al: Primary intracranial CNS lymphoma: MR manifestations. *AJNR* 1989; 10:725–729.

17

Primary Intracranial Tumors: Extra-axial Masses and Tumors of the Skull Base and Calvarium

Richard E. Latchaw, M.D.

David W. Johnson, M.D.

Emanuel Kanal, M.D.

This chapter is devoted to tumors that arise from the meninges and other extra-axial soft tissues including nerve sheaths and chemoreceptor tissue at the base of the brain, from the bones of the skull base, and from the calvarium. The differential diagnosis of skull base tumors and tumors involving the cerebellopontine angle (CPA) is given in Table 17–1.

MASS LESIONS OF THE MENINGES

Meningioma

Meningiomas constitute 15% to 18% of all intracranial neoplasms, second in incidence only to neuroepithelial tumors. The most common sites are over the cerebral convexity, with the majority in this location adjoining the falx and superior sagittal sinus. Most of these favor the middle third of the dural sinus, with the anterior third the next most common.[1] Less common are convexity meningiomas situated more laterally. Second to convexity meningiomas are those at the skull base involving the sphenoid ridge, parasellar region, tuberculum and/or diaphragma sellae, planum

sphenoidale, and olfactory grooves. Meningiomas of the tentorial notch and posterior fossa, including the clivus and foramen magnum, constitute approximately 10% of cases. Intraventricular meningioma is rare and is thought to be secondary to an infolding of meningeal tissue during formation of the stroma of the choroid plexus.[1, 2] Meningioma in the pineal and third ventricular region most commonly is attached to the falx-tentorial junction ("carrefour falcotentorial meningioma"), but may also arise from the meningeal tissue within the velum interpositum.[3] Finally, meningioma may arise from the sheath of a cranial nerve, particularly the optic nerve, to give a meningioma located at the optic foramen or within the orbit.[2]

The magnetic resonance imaging (MRI) and computed tomographic (CT) scan characteristics of meningiomas in these various locations are the same, and all the lesions will be considered together. Meningiomas have been divided into numerous histologic varieties ranging from meningothelial to angioblastic subtypes. The rapidity of growth and propensity to recur may differ among the various types, but imaging studies generally cannot differentiate one from the other, although

TABLE 17–1.

Differential Diagnosis of Skull Base Tumors

I. Cribriform plate and planum sphenoidale
  A. Esthesioneuroblastoma
  B. Meningioma
  C. Chondroid tumors (chondroma, chondrosarcoma)
  D. Ethmoid tumors: adenocystic carcinoma
  E. Encephalocele
II. Sphenoid and parasphenoid
  A. Body
    1. Chordoma
    2. Chondroid tumors
      a. Chondroma
      b. Condrosarcoma
      c. Osteochondroma
    3. Hematopoietic Tumors
      a. Plasmacytoma
      b. Lymphoma
      c. Leukemia
    4. Carcinoma
    5. Metastasis
      a. Direct extension
        1. Nasopharyngeal carcinoma
        2. Rhabdomyosarcoma
      b. Hematogenous spread
        1. Neuroblastoma
        2. Carcinoma
    6. Mucocele
  B. Nasopharynx
    1. Squamous cell carcinoma
    2. Lymphoma
  C. Cavernous sinus
    1. Meningioma
    2. Schwannoma
    3. Aneurysm
    4. Metastasis, e.g., adenocystic carcinoma
  D. Sella
    1. Pituitary adenoma
    2. Craniopharyngioma
    3. Metastasis
    4. Cyst, e.g., Rathke's pouch cyst
III. Clivus and foramen magnum
  A. Chordoma
  B. Meningioma
  C. Chondrosarcoma
  D. Direct extension of malignant neoplasm
    1. Nasopharyngeal carcinoma
    2. Rhabdomyosarcoma
IV. Cerebellopontine angle
  A. Schwannoma
  B. Meningioma
  C. Epidermoid cyst
  D. Arachnoid cyst
  E. Vascular lesion: aneurysm, venous varix, arterial loop
  F. Metastasis
V. Jugular foramen
  A. Glomus jugulare tumor (chemodectoma)
  B. Schwannoma
  C. Meningioma

one report suggests T2-weighted MRI may distinguish fibroblastic/transitional types from angioblastic or syncytial forms.[4]

The nonenhanced CT scan usually demonstrates a homogeneous mass that is isodense or of slightly increased density relative to normal brain (Fig 17–1). The presence and appearance of calcification is variable and may be nodular or very fine and punctate (psammomatous) (Fig 17–2). Occasionally, the entire meningioma will be densely calcified with no enhancement visible through the calcification (Figs 17–3 and 17–4).

Beam hardening artifacts on CT from contiguous bony structures may obscure a small meningioma. In addition, because meningiomas are located along the margins of the brain, away from anatomic structures that denote mass effect such as the ventricular system, it may be extremely difficult to visualize these tumors without the use of contrast material. Characteristically, there is intense enhancement of a homogeneous nature, and the margins are sharply demarcated in all projections (see Figs 17–1 and 17–2). A meningioma is typically broad based and borders a bony structure or free dural margin. Depending upon location, coronal views are very helpful in evaluating the relationship to the bony and dural structures and to the brain (Figs 17–5 and 17–6).

The typical meningioma on unenhanced short repetition time (TR) MRI is isointense to slightly hypointense relative to the contiguous gray matter (Figs 17–5 to 17–7).[4, 5] It is more commonly isointense to mildly hyperintense to gray matter on long TR sequences (Figs 17–6 to 17–9).[5] Therefore, it may be difficult to distinguish a meningioma from contiguous brain parenchyma, particularly if the mass is small and there is little or no mass effect. Occasionally, a small mass may displace or indent vascular structures that have signal void because of rapidly flowing blood. Larger masses may be seen by their mass effect or because of the presence of parenchymal edema (Fig 17–8).[6] Some meningiomas have relaxation parameters sufficiently different from cortex to allow easy visualization. Occasionally, meningiomas are quite hypointense to cortex on short TR images (see Fig 17–3). Others are hypointense or hyperintense to cortex on long TR images. Meningiomas that are hypointense to cortex on T2-weighted sequences tend to be composed primarily of fibroblastic or transitional elements, while those that are hyperintense (see Fig 17–5) contain a predominance of syncytial or angioblastic elements.[4]

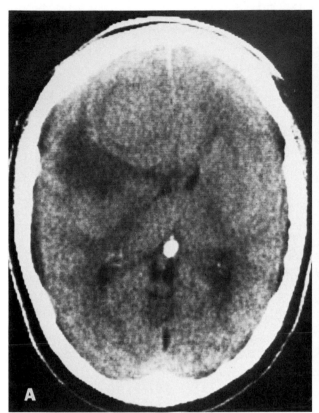
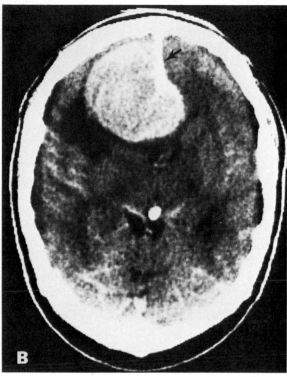

FIG 17–1.

Falx meningioma. The unenhanced scan **(A)** demonstrates a large mass lesion of slightly increased density relative to the normal brain that is located in the right frontal region. There is a moderate amount of surrounding edema and compression of the frontal horns. The enhanced scan **(B)** demonstrates intense homogeneous enhancement of this lesion with sharp margination. The mass is based along the falx *(arrow)* and has all the characteristics of a falx meningioma.

Because of the problem of conspicuity on unenhanced MRI, the use of a contrast agent is extremely important. One of the major advantages of enhanced MRI over unenhanced scanning is the ability to detect meningeal disease. Meningiomas demonstrate intense enhancement with gadolinium–diethylenetriamine pentaacetic acid (DTPA) (see Figs 17–4 and 17–7).[7–10] There is usually only mild enhancement of the dura and falx with paramagnetic contrast agents, as opposed to the vivid enhancement of these structures with iodinated contrast agents for CT scanning. Therefore, enhanced MRI may distinguish between the enhancing meningioma and the normal dura. If the meninges enhance markedly or assymetrically, this may indicate spread of tumor along the meninges (see Fig 17–7). However, dural enhancement may also be indicative of meningeal hyperemia without tumor invasion.

A thin rim of rather low signal on the short TR images may separate the meningioma from the contiguous brain. In most cases this is probably a vascular capsule around the meningioma (see Fig 17–7).[6] Compressed, ischemic, and/or edematous parenchyma may also give a low signal on short TR sequences. Cerebrospinal fluid (CSF) containing space between the tumor and meninges or parenchyma may also play a role.[5] Nodular or punctate calcification within the meningioma, easily seen with CT, may not be visualized on MRI.[6] There is usually tissue matrix giving signal and obscuring the presence of calcification, even when the meningioma appears densely calcified on CT (see Fig 17–3). Larger clumps of calcification may be seen as MRI signal voids (see Fig 17–4). Such signal voids may also represent large blood vessels within the tumor (see Fig 17–9). MRI exquisitely demonstrates the flow void of larger blood vessels such as the internal carotid arteries, which may be encased by parasellar meningioma (Fig 17–10).[6] MRI is the procedure of choice for evaluating parasellar meningiomas, in part by its ability to demonstrate this relationship to the vascular structures and in part because of its ability to exclude para-

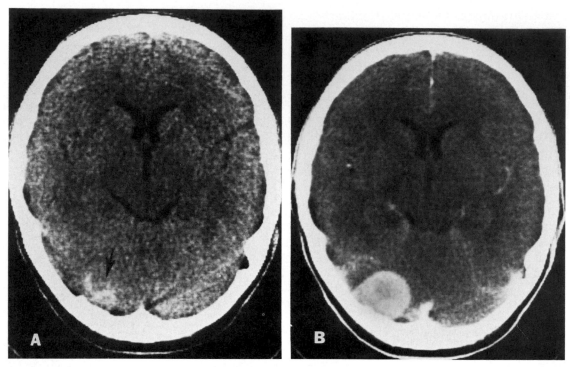

FIG 17–2.
Meningioma with psammomatous calcification. The unenhanced scan **(A)** shows punctate calcification in the right occipital region *(arrow)*. The enhanced scan **(B)** demonstrates homogeneous enhancement of the calcified mass with sharp margination. The mass is based along the inner table of the right occipital bone and has all the characteristics of a meningioma containing psammomatous calcification.

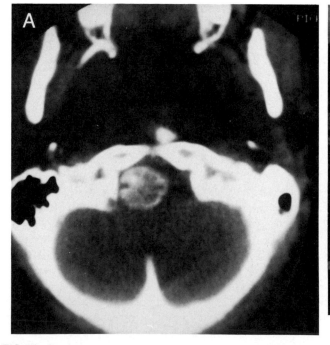

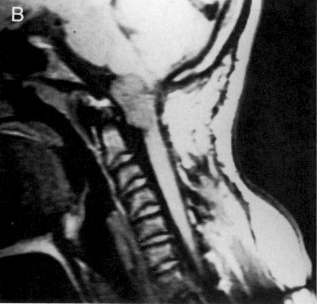

FIG 17–3.
Foramen magnum meningioma. The unenhanced axial CT scan **(A)** demonstrates a heavily calcified, well-circumscribed meningioma of the foramen magnum. The sagittal short TR MRI scan **(B,** TR = 600, echo time [TE] = 25) shows that the calcification is not apparent on MRI but rather that the tumor matrix is seen through the calcification. The lesion is quite hypointense relative to the brain stem that is displaced.

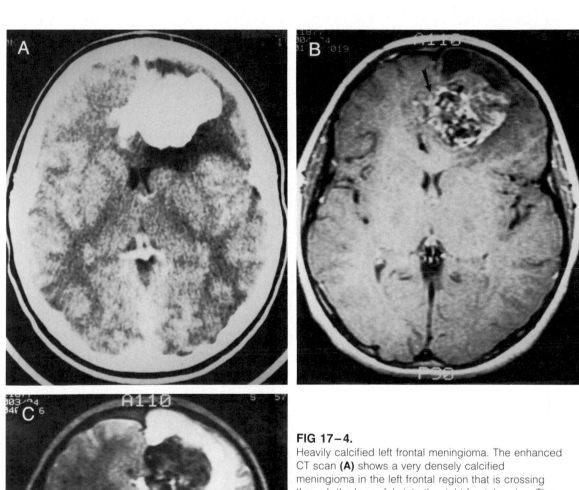

FIG 17–4.
Heavily calcified left frontal meningioma. The enhanced CT scan **(A)** shows a very densely calcified meningioma in the left frontal region that is crossing through the lower falx into the right frontal region. There is a moderate amount of surrounding cerebral edema with mass effect on the left frontal horn. Enhancement was not apparent, with the density being similar between the unenhanced (not shown) and enhanced studies. The heavily T2-weighted MRI study (**B,** TR = 2,500, TE = 100) demonstrates the presence of calcification as hypointensity. The calcification is seen because it is so confluent. The hyperintensity represents surrounding cerebral edema. The gadolinium-enhanced short TR image (**C,** TR = 800, TE = 20) demonstrates enhancement of the lesion, not apparent on the enhanced CT scan because of the calcium, and extension through the falx into the right frontal region.

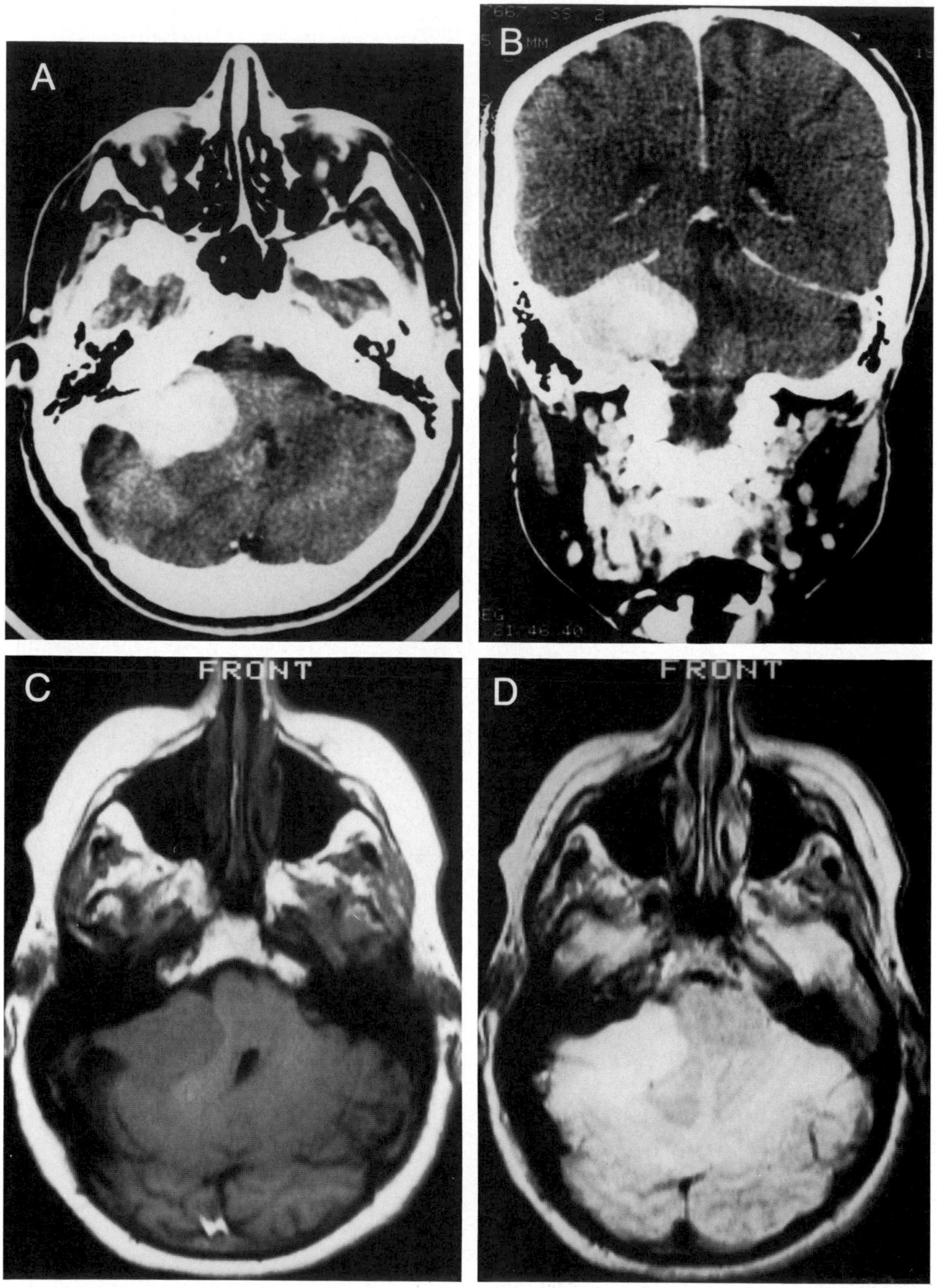

FIG 17–5.
Petrous/tentorial meningioma. Enhanced CT scans in the axial **(A)** and coronal **(B)** projections demonstrate the homogeneously and densely enhancing sharply circumscribed mass lesion with a broad base against both the petrous bone and the tentorium; the coronal study nicely shows the relationship to the tentorium. The short TR MR scan (**C,** TR = 600, TE = 20) shows the tumor to be hypointense relative to brain stem and cerebellum, with the lesion becoming hyperintense to these other tissues on the long TR, short TE proton-density study (**D,** TR = 2,000, TE = 25). This "turning" from hypointensity/isointensity to hyperintensity is less common for meningioma than is persistence of isointensity on the multiple sequences.

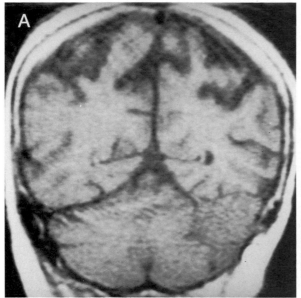 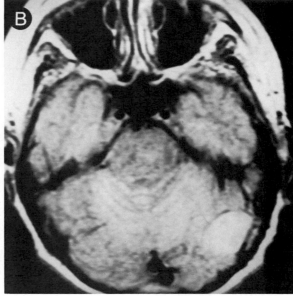

FIG 17–6.
Coronal MRI is useful for defining relationships of meningioma to the tentorium. The T1-weighted study (**A,** TR = 600, TE = 20) demonstrates the slightly hypointense meningioma and its relationship to the tentorium, the cerebellum, and the temporal lobe. This rela- tionship is not as apparent on the axial projection (**B,** TR = 2,500, TE = 25). The meningioma becomes slightly hyperintense on this proton-density image.

sellar aneurysm in the differential diagnosis.

The amount of cerebral edema surrounding a meningioma is quite variable. While there is frequently little if any edema surrounding these slow-growing benign lesions (see Figs 17–2, 17–5, and 17–7), moderate-to-marked edema may be present in up to 42% of meningiomas (see Figs 17–1, 17–4, and 17–8).[11] The presence of abundant edema may falsely suggest the presence of a parenchymal lesion such as a metastatic tumor. The amount of cerebral edema is not proportional to the size of the tumor, nor to the location, type of meningioma, presence of bony invasion, or evidence of malignant degeneration. There is also no correlation between the amount of edema and the presence of obstruction of cerebral veins and dural sinuses.[11, 12]

Benign meningiomas may invade the surrounding tissues, including the dura (Figs 17–4, 17–8, and 17–11) and contiguous bony structures (Figs 17–9 and 17–12 to 17–14). As mentioned, MRI may be far more sensitive at demonstrating dural invasion than CT is. Bony invasion frequently produces an osteoblastic response, with hyperostosis seen in up to 27% of meningioma cases, especially those located in the planum sphenoidale/parasellar regions.[11] By CT, hyperostosis is

dense (see Figs 17–9 and 17–12 to 17–14). On MRI, since cortical bone normally produces a signal void, it is harder to appreciate the presence of hyperostosis than with CT in subtle cases. More overt cases demonstrate thickening of the signal void or a decrease in the hyperintense marrow signal relative to the contralateral normal side.

Hyperostotic bone may be produced with both metastatic carcinoma of the prostate and fibrous dysplasia. Usually fibrous dysplasia produces a homogeneous bony expansion characterized as "ground glass" (Fig 17–15) rather than the more patchy bony thickening with meningioma. Fibrous dysplasia may also affect an entire bone and extend beyond the structures contiguous to the intracranial cavity. For example, fibrous dysplasia may involve not only the sphenoid ridge but also the body of the sphenoid and pterygoid process. Fibrous dysplasia may also extend into the facial bones. Another appearance of fibrous dysplasia is that of "blistering" of the calvarium, which is a focal expansion of bone with a relatively lucent center. Blistering is a response of the calvarium and not the skull base in fibrous dysplasia, whereas hyperostosis can be present at either the base or the calvarium. Meningioma does not produce this blistered appearance, but may produce bony erosion.

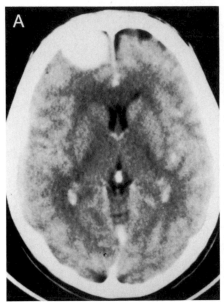

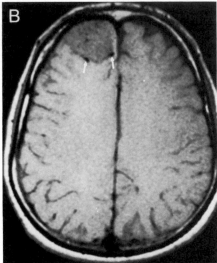

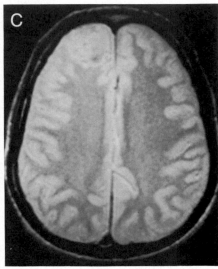

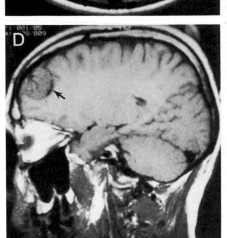

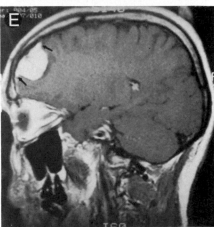

FIG 17–7.
Gadolinium-enhancing right frontal meningioma with a vascular capsule. The enhanced CT scan **(A)** demonstrates the classic appearance of a densely enhancing, sharply marginated right frontal meningioma based against the dura. The short TR MRI sequence **(B,** TR = 683, TE = 20) shows the meningioma to be slightly hypointense relative to gray matter and to have blood vessels characterized by their hypointensity along the posterior and medial margins *(arrows)*. On the long TR, short TE study **(C,** TR = 2,687, TE = 30), the meningioma is isointense to gray matter. The sagittal unenhanced short TR image **(D,** TR = 500, TE = 20) nicely demonstrates the relationship of the hypointense tumor to the skull and shows the vascular capsule posteriorly *(arrow)*. The gadolinium-DTPA–enhanced short TR image **(E,** TR = 500, TE = 20) in the same projection as **D** not only demonstrates homogeneous enhancement, but there is enhancement spreading along the dura *(arrows)*. This latter enhancement is thick, which suggests tumor rather than simply hyperemic dura.

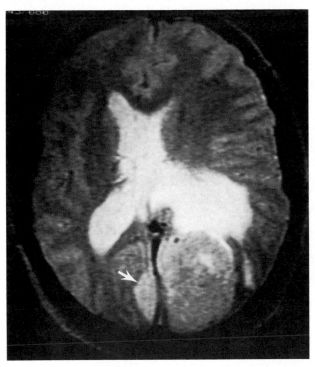

FIG 17–8.
Isointense meningioma with abundant edema. This long TR/TE study (TR = 2,500, TE = 75) shows the left parafalcine meningioma to be isointense to cortex. There is abundant cerebral edema surrounding the displaced left ventricular atrium. Tumor courses through the hypointense falx into the right parieto-occipital region *(arrow)*.

On CT, the bony erosion is easy to visualize, particularly if "bone windows" are used (Fig 17–13). On MRI, the erosion of cortical bone is more difficult to perceive and is denoted by a thinning of the normal signal void or interruption of the normal marrow signal.

Meningioma may completely penetrate the calvarium to invade the scalp (see Fig 17–13). Rarely, there is extension through and destruction of the bones at the base of the skull, with spread of meningioma into the parapharyngeal and facial regions (Fig 17–16). Such extensive invasion and spread is not necessarily indicative of malignant degeneration. Intracranial tumors may spread along the optic nerve to be both intracranial and intraorbital (see Fig 17–9),[13] and primary intraorbital meningiomas may spread posteriorly to produce an intracranial component.

In one series, 15% of benign meningiomas reviewed had atypical features on CT scan.[14] Necrosis, scarring, old hemorrhage, and fat deposition produced irregularity of the tumor margins and nonhomogeneous enhancement (Fig 17–17) and occasionally resulted in a "ring sign." The necrosis was thought to be due to rapid growth with secondary tumor ischemia. Focal high-density areas were found to be due to acute hemorrhage within the tumor. Such tumors were not necessarily of the angioblastic variety, but the hemorrhage was considered secondary to rupture of thin tumor vessels.

Old hemorrhage produced areas of low density, as did regions of lipomatous degeneration. Finally, low-density zones contiguous to typical meningiomas represented trapped CSF within arachnoid cysts. All of the posterior fossa meningiomas in this series were typical in CT appearance; if cystic changes were found in a posterior fossa mass, the lesion was not a meningioma but another tumor type such as schwannoma. However, the authors of this chapter have occasionally seen necrotic or cystic change in large posterior fossa meningiomas. These atypical intratumoral components, including fat, blood, necrosis, and cyst formation, have characteristic MRI appearances and are easier to evaluate on MRI than on CT.[4] Fat is hyperintense on short TR images, necrosis and cyst formation are hypointense on short TR and hyperintense on long TR sequences, and peritumoral nonneoplastic arachnoid cyst formation has the appearance of CSF. Blood has its typical MRI appearance, depending upon its stage of evolution. Methemoglobin and hemosiderin are easy to visualize with MRI, and chronic hemorrhage can be appreciated on MRI whereas it may not be appreciated by CT.

The majority of convexity meningiomas are easily recognized on enhanced MRI or CT scans, and there is usually only a limited differential diagnosis. A primary glioma originating in the high convexity may appear to be based along the inner table of the skull and simulate meningioma (see

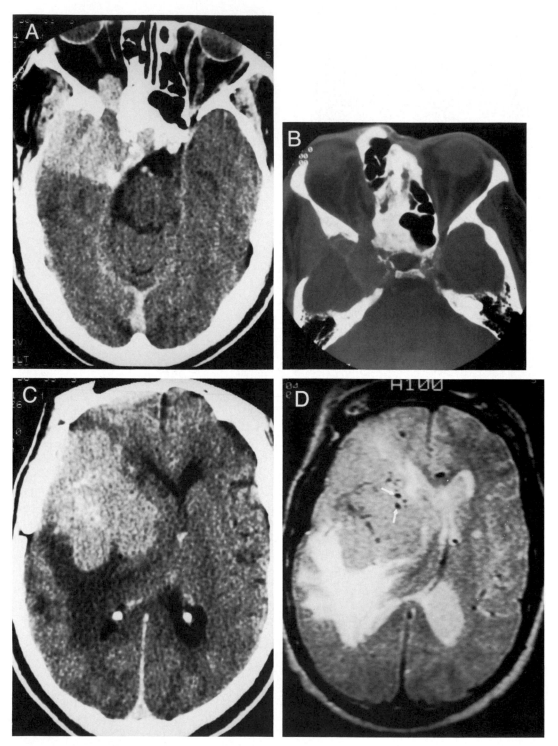

FIG 17–9.
Right sphenoid and orbital meningioma producing hyperostosis. The enhanced CT scan **(A)** shows that the homogeneously enhancing meningioma of the right sphenoid ridge and temporal fossa extends through the superior orbital fissure into the orbit and medially into the suprasellar space. The "bone window" **(B)** nicely shows the hyperostotic bone, which is nonhomogeneous. There is extension of the tumor superiorly to invaginate into the right frontal and parietal lobes **(C)** and produce abundant edema and ventricular displacement. The long TR/TE MRI scan **(D,** TR = 2,500, TE = 75) shows the superior extension to be isointense to gray matter. The surrounding edema is markedly hyperintense. There are multiple hypointense bleed vessels within the tumor *(arrows).*

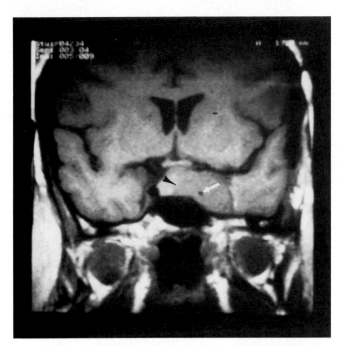

FIG 17–10.
Parasellar meningioma encasing the left internal carotid artery. This short TR coronal image (TR = 500, TE = 200) demonstrates a parasagittal meningioma isointense to cortex that is extending into the sella turcica, with its medial margin *(arrowhead)* abutting the more intense pituitary gland. There is encasement of the hypointense and narrowed left internal carotid artery *(arrow)*.

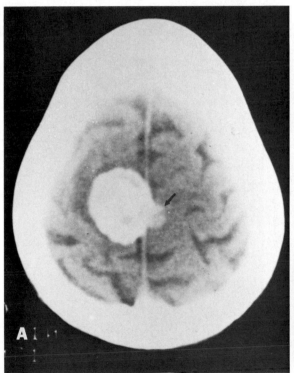

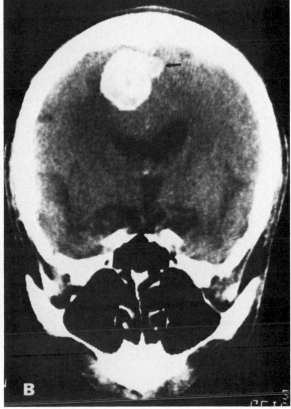

FIG 17–11.
Heavily calcified parafalcine meningioma with extension through the falx. Nonenhanced axial **(A)** and coronal **(B)** scans demonstrate a heavily calcified parafalcine meningioma with extension of calcified tumor through the falx *(arrows)*.

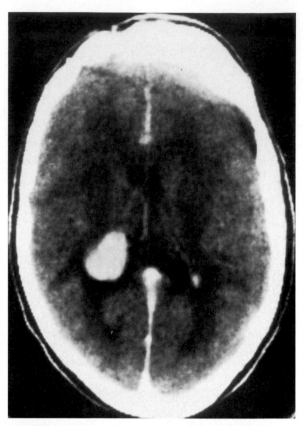

FIG 17–12.
Bifrontal meningioma with hyperostosis and intraventricular meningioma.
This enhanced CT scan demonstrates the sharply marginated right atrial
intraventricular meningioma and the *en plaque* bifrontal meningioma, larger
on the left. There is marked hyperostosis as the tumor has not only invaded
and crossed the falx and dura but has also extended into the calvarium.

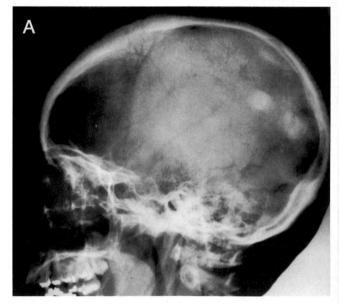

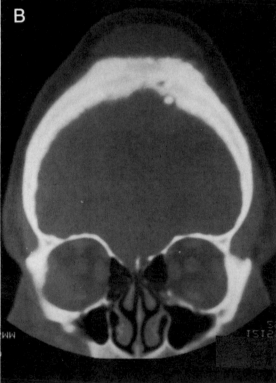

FIG 17–13.
Intraosseous and extraosseous extension of meningioma. The
lateral skull film **(A)** demonstrates two areas of
well-circumscribed hyperostosis in the parietal regions and
less well defined increased bony density more superiorly. The
coronal CT scan with "bone windows" **(B)** demonstrates the
marked hyperostosis of the parietal bones and the large
soft-tissue mass in the scalp. The studies are indicative of an
intracranial meningioma with spread through the dura into the
bone and subsequent spread into the scalp.

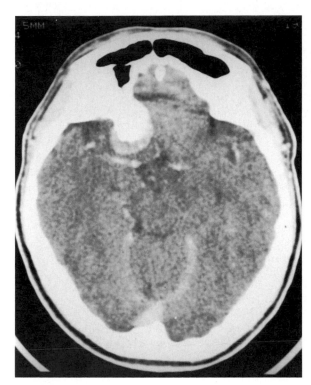

FIG 17–14.

En plaque meningioma of the right anterior clinoid process. This enhanced CT scan demonstrates a thin rim of tumor surrounding a markedly hyperostotic right anterior clinoid process.

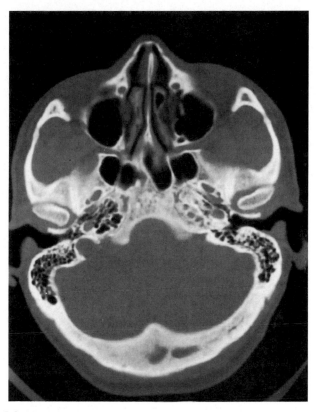

FIG 17–15.

Fibrous dysplasia of the occipital bones. This axial CT scan with "bone windows" demonstrates the homogeneous hypodensity of the diploic space of the occipital bones relative to the more normal diploic density laterally. This homogeneous "ground-glass" appearance is characteristic of fibrous dysplasia.

Fig 16–15). A large exophytic mass originating within the bony calvarium may project into the intracranial space. If the mass is sharply marginated and enhances homogeneously on CT, as can be seen with many metastatic tumors such as carcinoma of the prostate or breast or with myeloma, the appearance may simulate meningioma (see Fig 19–7). MRI may be able to define the relatively nonenhancing dura relative to the enhancing metastasis, thereby demonstrating its extradural origin. If there is a large amount of surrounding cerebral edema, it may be difficult to distinguish between an intra-axial mass such as glioma or metastasis and an extra-axial mass such as meniogioma (see Fig 17–8). While a peripheral intra-axial mass may destroy the gray matter/white matter junction (Fig 17–18), an extra-axial benign mass typically leaves this junction intact, displaces the cortex from the inner table of the skull, and buckles the underlying white matter.[15]

A meningioma is a vascular lesion, and metastatic deposits tend to go to highly vascular regions. It is not surprising, therefore, that a metastasis may be found within a meningioma on rare occasions. The rapidity of growth of a meningioma

or the invasion of contiguous structures may indicate such a process. Rarely, meningioma and glioma (usually glioblastoma) may occur in close juxtaposition and result in "collision tumors" (Fig 17–19). While both tumors are relatively common and may occur together by chance, it is interesting to speculate on the role of the glioma in stimulating the proliferation of arachnoid cells to produce the meningioma.[16]

It may be impossible to distinguish between parasellar schwannoma, meningioma, and aneurysm on CT (see Chapter 23). All three typically have a homogeneous CT enhancement pattern and sharp margination. Facial pain is more common with a fifth nerve schwannoma than with meningioma. Dynamic CT may be necessary for a diagnosis of aneurysm in order to demonstrate its rapid filling after a bolus of contrast material, but a partially or totally thrombosed aneurysm may not fill rapidly. Angiography is usually definitive for a diagnosis of aneurysm, although, again, total thrombosis may make diagnosis difficult. MRI is excel-

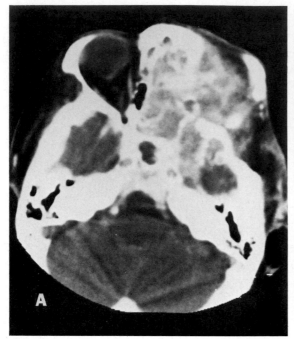
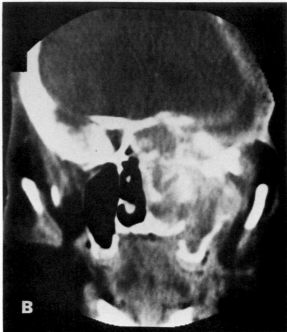

FIG 17–16.
Meningioma with extension into the face. The axial **(A)** and coronal **(B)** scans demonstrate a massive, enhancing neoplasm involving the left temporal fossa, sphenoid, left orbit and nose, left maxillary antrum, and contiguous facial structures. Histologically, this was a benign meningioma. Long-standing meningiomas of the temporal fossae and/or orbit may invade the facial structures and produce extensive bony destruction mimicking a malignant neoplasm. Such extensive spread is not necessarily indicative of malignant degeneration of the meningioma.

FIG 17–17.
Partially cystic/necrotic meningioma. There is a well-marginated mass based along the inner table of the skull of the high left cerebral convexity. While the majority of this mass enhances in a homogeneous fashion typical of meningioma, there is a cystic and/or necrotic component anteriorly. Histologically, this was a typical meningioma. Fourteen percent of meningiomas have atypical features such as necrosis and cyst formation.

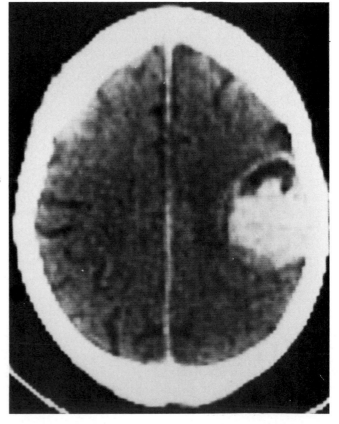

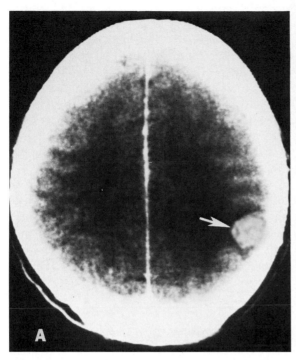
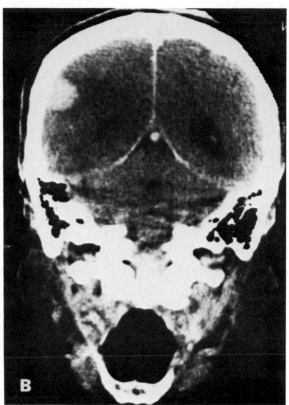

FIG 17–18.
Right parietal metastasis simulating meningioma. The axial **(A)** and coronal **(B)** projections demonstrate solitary metastatic lesion **(A, arrow)** from carcinoma of the lung. The metastasis was to the corticomedullary junction and destroyed the interface between the gray and white matter. This latter characteristic confirms the intra-parenchymal location of the lesion, even though the extension of the mass to the inner table of the skull suggests a diagnosis such as meningioma.

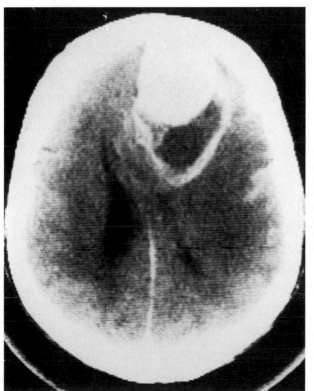

FIG 17–19.
Contiguous meningioma and glioblastoma multiforme ("collision tumors"). Left frontal lobe surgical exploration resolved the difficult diagnosis presented by this enhanced CT scan. More anteriorly, based against the inner table and the falx, there is a homogeneously enhancing meningothelioma and more posteriorly there is ring enhancement of a glioblastoma multiforme with a necrotic center. Interestingly, there is little surrounding cerebral edema.

lent in distinguishing these three lesions. Typically, schwannoma is isointense with respect to gray matter on short TR images but becomes quite hyperintense on long TR sequences. Meningiomas generally stay isointense or become mildly hyperintense relative to gray matter when comparing short and long TR scans. A patent aneurysm shows the signal void of rapidly moving blood, whereas partial or total thrombosis generally shows a characteristic admixture of hypointensity and hyperintensity with hemosiderin deposition. All three lesions may exhibit exuberant contrast enhancement on MRI. If both short and long TR sequences are obtained before contrast infusion, there should be no problem in differentiation in most cases.

The distinction between schwannoma and meningioma may also be difficult on CT when the lesion is located in the CPA. The findings of increased density on the preinfusion CT scan, calci-

fication, a broad base against the petrous bone, an eccentric relationship to the internal auditory canal, and the lack of necrosis and cyst formation all favor meningioma. The meningioma may extend through the tentorial notch to the middle cranial fossa and produce a "comma" shape (Fig 17–20); we have rarely seen this configuration with acoustic schwannoma. MRI makes this distinction in most cases, with long TR images demonstrating the hyperintensity of the schwannoma and the isointensity to mild hyperintensity of the meningioma relative to cerebellar cortex.

Finally, the differential diagnosis of a clival meningioma includes chordoma, chondrosarcoma, and nasopharyngeal carcinoma extending superiorly. All three of the latter lesions are malignant and produce bone destruction, whereas the meningioma generally produces only mild bone erosion, possibly accompanied by hyperostosis. Chondrosarcoma typically contains calcification, but this is

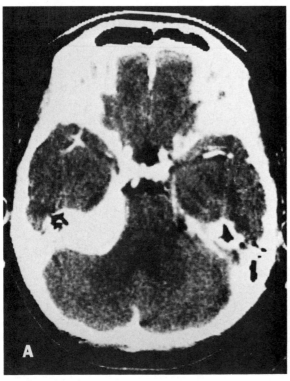 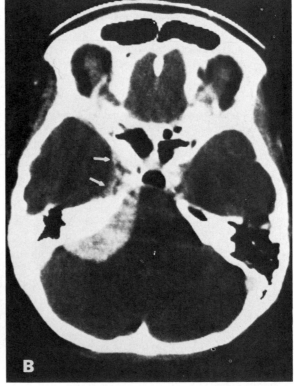

FIG 17–20.
Cerebellopontine meningioma extending to the middle cranial fossa. The enhanced axial scans demonstrate a large homogeneously enhancing, well-marginated tumor involving the right CPA and producing mild compression of the lateral aspect of the fourth ventricle **(A)**. The lesion is centered along the ridge of the right petrous bone, typical of meningioma and unusual for acoustic schwannoma. Image **B** was taken with a wide window (bone win-

dow) to allow separation of the enhancing tumor from the underlying petrous bone. There is extension of tumor into the medial aspect of the right middle cranial fossa that is producing displacement of the lateral margin of the right cavernous sinus *(arrows)*. Extension into the middle cranial fossa to produce a "comma shape" is characteristic for meningioma.

less common with either clival chordoma or meningioma. Chordoma exhibits two patterns, one of which is characterized by patches of marked hyperintensity within a background of isointensity on short TR images, while the second pattern is of isointensity on short TR and hyperintensity on long TR images, similar to chondrosarcoma. Both patterns differ from the relative isointensity of most meningiomas when both short and long TR sequences are considered.

Multiple Meningiomas and Meningosarcoma

Multiple meningiomas (Fig 17–21) may occur in neurofibromatosis, in which there are not only meningiomas but also schwannomas, neurofibromas, and various gliomas. Multiple meningiomas may also occur without the syndrome.

The diagnosis of malignant meningioma depends upon the histologic characteristics of a highly cellular tumor with more mitoses, and more atypicality of those mitoses relative to benign meningiomas, as well as poor cellular differentiation. The malignant meningioma (meningosarcoma) generally shows rapid recurrence, with spreading along the dura and/or tentorium (Fig 17–22).

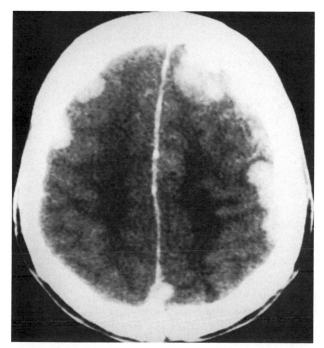

FIG 17–21.
Multiple meningiomas in a patient with neurofibromatosis. Multiple enhancing meningiomas are present along the inner table of the skull laterally, and there is also a posterior falx meningioma.

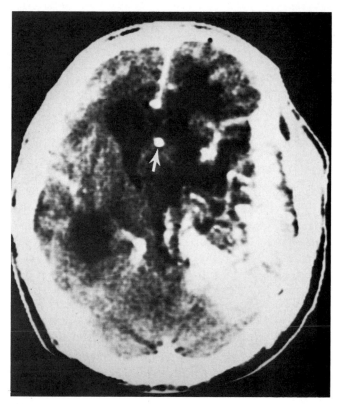

FIG 17–22.
Meningosarcoma. There is extensive homogenously enhancing neoplasm along the inner table of the left frontal, temporal, and parietal bones, with extension medially along the left side of the tentorium. The patient has undergone previous left-sided craniotomy for attempted resection. There is a shunt *(arrow)* within the compressed and displaced left frontal horn. The mass quickly recurred and spread along the meninges within a 6-month period of time, consistent with the histologic diagnosis of meningosarcoma.

There are irregular margins of the tumor, with fringes of tumor interdigitating with cerebral parenchyma. While benign meningiomas commonly parasitize the pial vasculature, the malignant meningioma actually invades cerebral parenchyma. This may produce early drainage into deep cerebral veins. There is usually abundant edema, microscopic or macroscopic necroses are commonly present, and there may be pronounced bone destruction.[17-20] In one series, the best correlative finding with malignancy was the presence of a significant accumulation of tumor extending well away from the more circumscribed focus of meningioma, termed "mushrooming."[18] Benign meningiomas may demonstrate some of these changes, such as cystic or necrotic change as the tumor outgrows its blood supply. Previous reference has been made to the fact that 15% of benign meningiomas had atypical CT features.[14]

Hemangiopericytoma

Debate continues regarding the relationship of hemangiopericytoma to angioblastic meningioma as originally defined by Bailey, Cushing, and Eisenhardt; whether an angioblastic meningioma should be considered a hemangiopericytoma; whether the angioblastic meningioma is a form of sarcoma; and whether intracranial hemangiopericytoma is a distinct entity or a form of meningioma.[21] Some argue for the existence of the pericyte in the blood vessel walls of the central nervous system (CNS). There is morphologic similarity of the CNS tumor to hemangiopericytomas originating in other parts of the body. However, Russell and Rubenstein cite examples of transitional forms between meningiomas (especially the meningothelial and fibroblastic types) and both angioblastic meningiomas and hemangiopericytomas. They argue that the pericyte is a form of mesenchymal cell whose identity is determined by its relationship to a capillary blood vessel and, like the arachnoid cell from which come meningiomas, is polyblastic in potential. Therefore, Russell and Rubenstein favor keeping hemangiopericytoma within the family of meningiomas.[21] Whatever their histogenesis, there is total agreement that hemangiopericytoma exhibits more malignant clinical behavior than do other forms of meningioma. The tumor has a high recurrence rate and may metastasize to extracranial locations.[21] From an imaging standpoint, the tumor has the characteristics of a meningioma.

Typically, the tumor is isodense or hyperdense on the preinfusion CT scan and enhances homogeneously in a fashion similar to meningioma (Figs 17–23 and 17–24).[22] Calcification and bony sclerosis found with many meningiomas are not typically seen. MRI experience is limited, but an appearance simulating meningioma is usual. The angiographic demonstration of meningeal blood supply and a persistent homogeneous stain (Fig 17–24) makes distinction from meningioma difficult or impossible.

A peripherally located hemangiopericytoma based along the inner table of the skull may be indistinguishable from a meningioma on imaging studies. The appropriate diagnosis may be suggested by the presence of a meningioma-like lesion in a location not common for meningioma. The history of rapid recurrence after previous surgery or the presence of metastases (Fig 17–24) may likewise suggest the appropriate diagnosis.

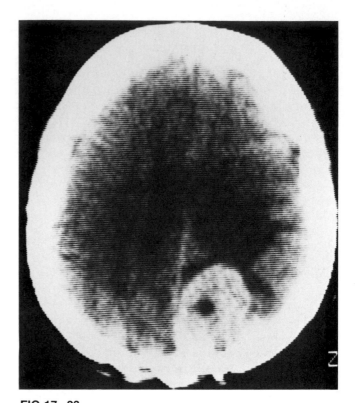

FIG 17–23.
Hemangiopericytoma. This well-circumscribed, intensely enhancing mass based along the inner table of the skull has an appearance similar to many meningiomas. The internal area of cyst formation or necrosis can be seen with some meningiomas, as can edema as extensive as in this case. (Courtesy of Richard Kasdan, M.D., CT Scan Associates, Inc., Pittsburgh.)

Other Solid Neoplasms

Other lesions of the meninges include diffuse primary meningeal sarcomatosis,[22–24] primary leptomeningeal melanoma,[25] and neurocutaneous melanosis,[26, 27] which is a malignant condition closely related to the other phakomatoses, particularly neurofibromatosis, with the presence of café au lait spots.[28]

Arachnoid Cyst

An arachnoid cyst is an extraparenchymal non-neoplastic fluid accumulation having a density equal to CSF. The most frequent location is the temporal fossa, with other common sites being the CPA, the circumcerebellar spaces, the ambient and quadrigeminal plate cisterns, the suprasellar cisterns, and the interhemispheric fissure. While some arachnoid cysts are most likely secondary to trauma[29] or infection, the majority appear to be congenital in nature. Controversy exists as to the pathogenesis of the congenital lesions. One theory

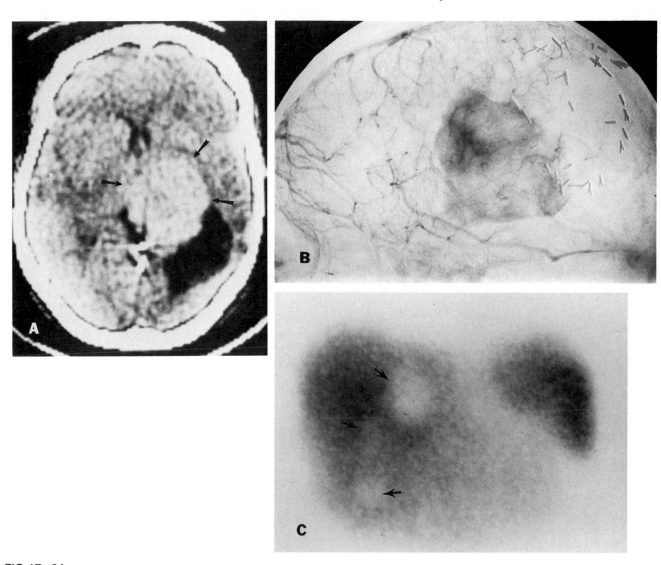

FIG 17–24.
Metastatic hemangiopericytoma. The axial enhanced CT scan **(A)** demonstrates a large, homogeneously enhancing and relatively well circumscribed mass lesion located deep within the left cerebral hemisphere and midline *(arrows)*. The patient has had previous surgery, as denoted by metallic clips posterior to the lesion in the midline, with the diagnosis of hemangiopericytoma. The lateral view of the left carotid angiogram **(B)** showed persistence of the intense stain of the well-demarcated lesion into the venous phase. Metastases have occurred, as denoted on the anteroposterior view of the liver/spleen radionuclide scan **(C),** with multiple metastatic lesions in the right lobe of the liver *(arrows)*.

presumes the accumulation of fluid between leaves of arachnoid during cerebral development as a cause of secondary hypoplasia of the contiguous brain tissue.[30] The contrasting theory advocates primary hypoplasia of the cerebral tissue with secondary cystic accumulation of fluid.[31] In either case, the slowly growing lesion present during skull maturation produces bony deformity (Fig 17–25).

CT scanning demonstrates that arachnoid cysts are sharply marginated, nonenhancing lesions of a density equal to CSF. An arachnoid cyst located in the temporal region frequently has a straight posterior margin that represents the interface between the cyst and the deformed temporal lobe (Fig 17–26).[32] An arachnoid cyst located in the posterior frontal region and/or frontotemporal junction has characteristic angular margins where it adjoins the hypoplastic frontal operculum and temporal lobe.

The differential diagnosis of these low-density lesions include epidermoid cyst, dermoid cyst, and cystic or microcystic glioma. The epidermoid has attenuation coefficients on CT between −10 and

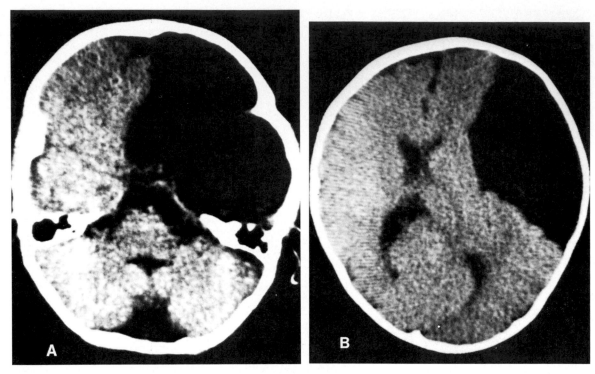

FIG 17–25.
Left frontotemporal arachnoid cyst. This is a large cystic expansion in the left frontotemporal region **(A)** with a density of CSF. The extra-axial expansion has produced thinning and deformity of the overlying calvarium. There is hypoplasia of much of the left frontal and temporal lobes, but not enough to prevent a pronounced midline shift **(B).** The sharp margins, including the relatively "square" margin along the left basal ganglia, represent the interfaces between the cyst and the deformed frontal and temporal lobes.

FIG 17–26.
Left temporal arachnoid cyst. The low-density, well-marginated cyst in the left temporal region has a classic appearance for an arachnoid cyst. The "square" or slightly inwardly convexed posterior margin of the cyst is the interface between the cyst and the deformed residual temporal lobe.

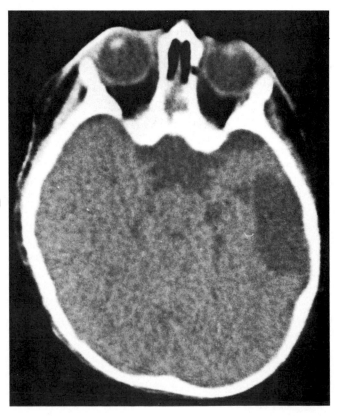

+20 Hounsfield units (HU). If the lesion has ruptured, the margins may be irregular as opposed to the sharp margination of an arachnoid cyst. A dermoid has CT values of fat (as low as −80 to −100 HU) and sebaceous debris and hair in portions of the cyst, with focal areas of intensity as high as +50 HU. Low-density, nonenhancing glial neoplasms have been diagnosed as arachnoid, epidermoid, or porencephalic cysts. The distinction between a low-density glial tumor and a cyst such as an arachnoid cyst does not depend upon CT absorption coefficients, which may be similar in either case.[33] Rather, the distinction can be made by an evaluation of the margins of the lesion. While low-density glial tumors frequently have relatively sharp contours in many areas, some degree of irregularity is usually present (see Figs 16–13 and 16–25). An arachnoid cyst, on the other hand, is sharply marginated in all projections; evaluation using CT requires multiple scanning projections and/or reformatted images.

MRI is even better than CT for a definite diagnosis of arachnoid cyst. The MRI intensity of an arachnoid cyst is equal to CSF (Fig 17–27), while grossly cystic or microcystic neoplasms have a higher protein content than CSF does and, therefore, have shorter T1 and T2 relaxation parameters than the CSF-like arachnoid cyst.[34] Most epidermoid cysts also differ from CSF, although they may occasionally have relaxation parameters very similar to CSF (see Chapter 18). Any intensity pattern different from CSF should raise suspicion of a lesion other than an arachnoid cyst. MRI is also better able than CT to evaluate margins because any plane can be directly imaged, which precludes reconstruction algorithms (Fig 17–28). Therefore, MRI is preferable over CT for the evaluation of these lesions.

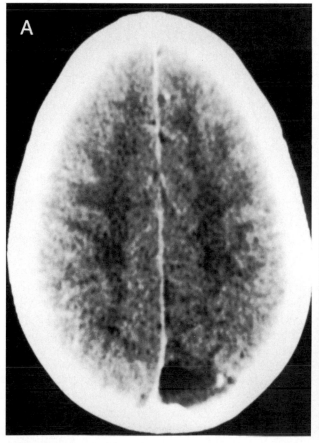

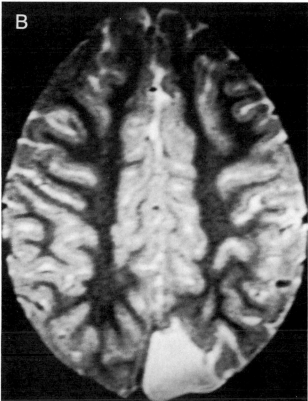

FIG 17–27.
Arachnoid cyst well characterized on MRI. The enhanced CT scan **(A)** is confusing in that the margins of the posterior left parietal low-density lesion are less well defined and are less sharp than desirable for a diagnosis of arachnoid cyst. The possibility of low-density, nonenhancing oligodendroglioma cannot be excluded. The long TR/TE MRI scan (**B,** TR = 2,500, TE = 75) demonstrates the sharp margination of the lesion, the hypoplasia of the underlying gyri rather than mass effect, and an intensity equal to CSF. These are all characteristics of arachnoid cyst. Neoplasm with a higher protein content would be less intense, the margins would be more irregular, and mass effect on a developed brain would be apparent.

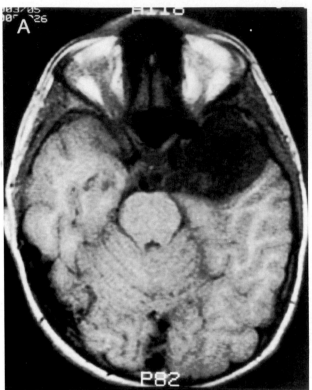 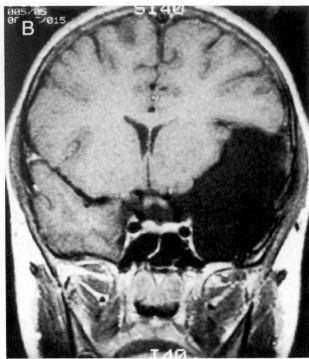

FIG 17–28.
Value of multiple MRI projections in evaluating a low-density lesion. The unenhanced short TR axial sequence (**A,** TR = 550, TE = 20) demonstrates a large, low-intensity lesion in the anterior left temporal fossa. While there must be some hypoplasia of the underlying temporal lobe in view of the lack of more apparent mass effect for the size of the lesion, some mass effect is present as denoted by the compressed white matter. The short TR coronal image with gadolinium-DTPA enhancement (**B,** TR = 600, TE = 20) nicely defines the hypoplasia of portions of the frontal and temporal lobes and the minimal mass effect on the ventricular system for a lesion of this size, characteristic of arachnoid cyst.

The margins of an arachnoid cyst may be difficult to separate from adjoining ventricular structures. For example, an arachnoid cyst in the quadrigeminal and superior cerebellar cisterns may produce compression of the aqueduct that leads to obstructive hydrocephalus (Fig 17–29). This appearance may be indistinguishable, however, from obstructive hydrocephalus from any other cause such as congenital aqueductal stenosis producing ventricular enlargement and a dilated suprapineal recess of the third ventricle or a ventricular diverticulum (Fig 17–30). Likewise, an arachnoid cyst in the intrasellar/suprasellar cisterns may be difficult to separate from a dilated third ventricle.[35] Sagittal and coronal projections are invaluable additions to axial views when evaluating the complex anatomy of these cysts and their relationships to contiguous parenchymal and ventricular structures. MRI more easily provides the three orthogonal views than does CT, and the thin membrane between the arachnoid cyst and the contiguous

CSF-containing structures may be more apparent with MRI than with CT (Fig 17–31).

Intraventricular, intracisternal, or intracystic water-soluble contrast studies with CT may be necessary to separate the cyst from contiguous portions of a CSF-containing structure (see Fig 17–29). They may also aid in the presurgical evaluation of CSF and cyst fluid dynamics in order to determine the need for a cystoperitoneal shunt. Theories for fluid accumulation in cysts that are relatively noncommunicating with CSF include secretion by the cyst wall, osmotic differences between cyst fluid and CSF, and a ball-valve mechanism of slits in the cyst wall that allows the slow entry of CSF but no egress of fluid from the cyst.[36] The slow accumulation of contrast over a matter of hours, as detected by CT scanning (see Fig 17–29), gives support to the ball-valve theory.[36, 37]

Hydrocephalus is generally thought to be a result of compression of intraventricular CSF pathways. However, communicating hydrocephalus

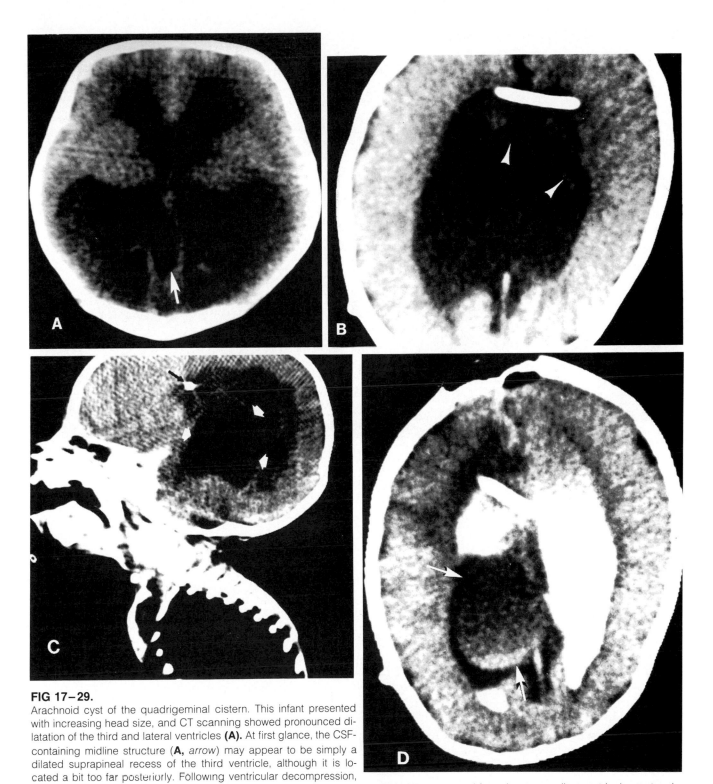

FIG 17–29.
Arachnoid cyst of the quadrigeminal cistern. This infant presented with increasing head size, and CT scanning showed pronounced dilatation of the third and lateral ventricles **(A).** At first glance, the CSF-containing midline structure (**A,** *arrow*) may appear to be simply a dilated suprapineal recess of the third ventricle, although it is located a bit too far posteriorly. Following ventricular decompression, there has been marked enlargement of the cystic structure in the midline, which is separated from the surrounding ventricular system by a membrane (**B,** *arrowheads*). A direct sagittal scan **(C)** nicely demonstrates the relationship of the cyst (*white arrows*) separated from the surrounding ventricular system by a membrane. The shunt within the lateral ventricles is noted (*black arrow*). To further evaluate the anatomy of the cyst and the degree of communication with the ventricular system, metrizamide was instilled through the intraventricular shunt **(D).** There is slow accumulation of contrast material in the dependent posterior portion of the cyst (*arrows*) over a number of hours. This poor communication indicated the need for resection or decompressive shunting of the cyst itself. The cyst most likely originated within the quadrigeminal cistern and produced compression of the aqueduct. Surrounding ventricular enlargement kept its apparent size small, but ventricular decompression allowed it to expand rapidly. Its deep periventricular position and its density equal to CSF made it difficult to separate from the surrounding ventricular system.

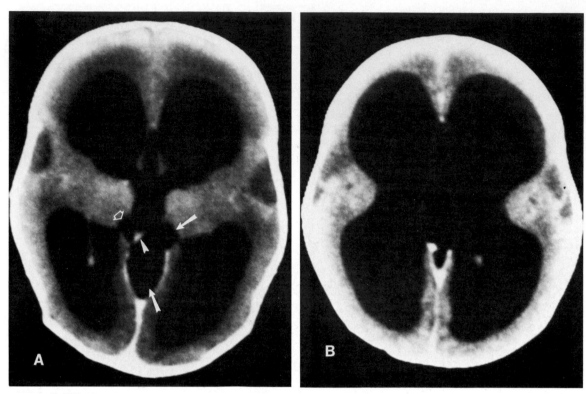

FIG 17–30.
Obstructive hydrocephalus with ventricular diverticula. There is marked dilatation of the third and lateral ventricles **(A** and **B),** most likely from aqueductal obstruction. A diverticulum from the medial aspect of the left ventricular atrium **(A,** *closed arrows)* extends medially and posteriorly through the tentorial incisura to lie in the superior cerebellar cistern. A smaller diverticulum is seen on the right **(A,** *open arrow).* An enhancing vascular structure *(arrowhead)* separates both the smaller right ventricular diverticulum and the posterior portion of the third ventricle from the larger left ventricular diverticulum. No separation is seen between the left ventricular di- verticulum and the lucency in the superior cerebellar cistern, which suggests that the lucencies are in contiguity and are all a larger diverticulum. An arachnoid cyst in the quadrigeminal cistern, analogous to that seen in Figure 17–29, cannot be absolutely excluded. The easiest method of confirmation is to repeat the scan following ventricular shunting to see whether the posterior and medial cystic lucencies are decompressed. A water-soluble contrast agent could also be placed through the shunt to look for communication.

may result from abnormalities of CSF flow over the convexities and an absorption block secondary to a more diffuse manifestation of the arachnoidal congenital anomaly. The presence of hydrocephalus may be the reason to undertake surgical drainage or cystoperitoneal shunting of the cyst. If decompression of the cyst does not relieve the hydrocephalus, however, ventricular shunting may also be necessary.[37] The presence of symptoms from compression of pericystic tissues may also lead to treatment. It should be emphasized that because of the long-standing presence of the lesion and/or the underlying parenchymal hypoplasia, cyst shunting may not produce much apparent decrease in the size of the lesion or change in the contour of the underlying brain on follow-up scans.

The concept of a "communicating arachnoid cyst" makes no sense. This terminology has been used specifically for prominent arachnoid-like spaces in the retrocerebellar region. Arachnoid pouches have been discussed under "Posterior Fossa Cysts" in Chapter 24. Briefly, a cystic retrocerebellar space may occur from evagination of the tela choroidea of the fourth ventricle. In some patients there is communication between this space and the perimedullary and/or supracerebellar cisterns, and this has led to use of the term "mega cisterna magna." In others, there is limited or no communication between the arachnoid pouch and the perimedullary cisterns, but there is communication with the ventricular system. Communicating hydrocephalus results and requires shunting. This type of arachnoid pouch should not be confused with an arachnoid cyst of the classic variety in which there is no or poor communication with any CSF-containing space.

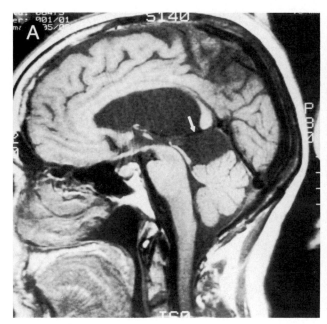

FIG 17–31.
Quadrigeminal plate arachnoid cyst with demarcation between the cyst and the third ventricle as demonstrated on sagittal MRI. Short TR midline sagittal MRI (**A,** TR = 600, TE = 20) demonstrates a low-intensity lesion of the quadrigeminal plate cistern that has an intensity equal to but separated from the third ventricle by a thin hypointense membrane *(arrow)*. The long TR/TE axial study (**B,** TR = 2,500, TE = 100) demonstrates the cyst to have an intensity equal to CSF of the subarachnoid cisterns.

PRIMARY LESIONS OF THE CEREBELLOPONTINE ANGLE AND INTERNAL AUDITORY CANAL

Schwannoma and Neurofibroma (Nerve Sheath Tumors)

Tumors originating from cranial nerves are either schwannomas or neurofibromas. The term *schwannoma* refers to the origin of the neoplasm from the Schwann cell, the cell that lines the axon beyond the pia. "Neuroma," "neurinoma," and "neurilemoma" are all imprecise terms for nerve sheath tumors and should be discarded.[38] Neurofibromas are also tumors that originate from cranial nerves but are generally found in patients with neurofibromatosis (von Recklinghausen's disease). Although a neurofibroma is similar to a schwannoma, it has a looser texture and is usually in continuity with a thickened displastic nerve root,[39] while the schwannoma is a more focal tumor attached to the nerve sheath. From an imager's point of view, it is logical to incorporate both under the term *nerve sheath tumor.*

The most common nerve sheath tumor is that of the eighth cranial nerve ("acoustic neuroma") and generally arises from the superior division of the vestibular portion, while the second most common is of the fifth cranial nerve ("trigeminal neuroma") and originates anywhere along the course of the nerve. Schwannomas of the seventh nerve are less common, and rarely, a nerve sheath tumor may originate from cranial nerves IX, X, or XI passing through the jugular foramen or from the 12th cranial nerve.[40–42]

Typically, nerve sheath tumors are of low density or isodensity on unenhanced CT. The degree of contrast enhancement is moderate to marked and may be homogeneous (Fig 17–32) or nonhomogeneous in character as a result of cystic change (Fig 17–33). A tumor of cranial nerves IX, X, or XI has a similar appearance to an eighth nerve schwannoma, with the only difference being the location of the lesion. Involvement of cranial nerves IX, X, or XI produces erosion of the jugular foramen (Fig 17–34), while an eighth nerve tumor produces erosion of the internal auditory canal (IAC) (see Fig 17–32). A seventh nerve sheath tumor produces erosion anywhere along the course of the facial nerve, including the IAC, the region of the geniculate ganglion, the middle ear promon-

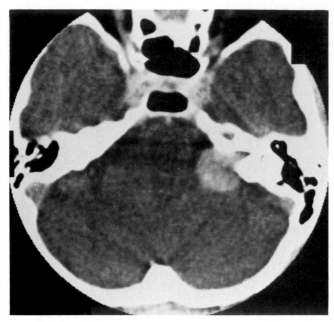

FIG 17–32.
Classic acoustic schwannoma. The neoplasm in the left CPA enhances homogeneously, and there is extension of tumor into an enlarged left IAC. These are classic findings of an eighth nerve schwannoma.

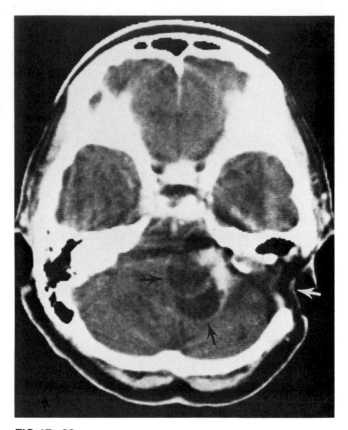

FIG 17–33.
Cystic acoustic schwannoma mimicking an intracerebellar tumor. There is a large neoplasm *(black arrows)* with both cystic and solid components involving the left CPA and cerebellar hemisphere with extension to the midline. The patient has had a previous retromastoid craniotomy *(white arrow).* The combination of solid and cystic components is common with schwannomas. The deep invagination into the cerebellar hemisphere mimics a primary intracerebellar tumor such as cystic astrocytoma.

tory, and/or the canal for the descending portion of the nerve.

A major differential diagnostic consideration of an enhancing mass on CT in the CPA is meningioma. A meningioma is almost always homogeneous in its contrast enhancement (very rarely will posterior fossa meningiomas have a cystic or necrotic component), frequently has a broad base of attachment to the petrous bone, is somewhat eccentric from the IAC, and may extend in "comma" fashion through the tentorial incisura to lie partially within the middle cranial fossa (see Fig 17–20), a finding these authors have only very rarely seen with an acoustic tumor. An acoustic nerve sheath tumor, on the other hand, is generally located at or in the IAC and produces erosion of that structure, is frequently inhomogeneous or cystic in its enhancement pattern, and stays below the tentorium. CSF loculations ("arachnoid cysts") are common near acoustic tumors but not meningiomas.

Enhanced CT scanning is adequate for large lesions but inadequate for smaller lesions. In the middle and late 1970s, CT scanners with relatively low resolution demonstrated a high rate of false-negative diagnosis of nerve sheath tumors less than 2 cm in size.[43–45] With the newer high-resolution scanners, CPA lesions of less than 1 cm, or purely intracannicular lesions, may still be missed, primarily secondary to artifact from contiguous bony structures. Beginning in the later 1970s, CT scanning following either positive-contrast or air cisternography was utilized in an attempt to demonstrate these small tumors. Four to 5 cc of a water-soluble contrast material is injected intrathecally, the patient placed in a Trendelenberg position with the side of interest down, which allows collection of the contrast into the CPA and IAC for subsequent multidirectional tomography and/or CT scanning.[46,47] For air cisternography, 4 to 10 cc of air, carbon dioxide, or oxygen is injected intrathecally via lumbar puncture, with the patient placed in a lateral decubitus position, side of interest up. Slices of 1.5-mm thickness are obtained, followed by reversal of the superior side and

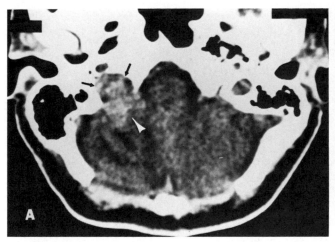 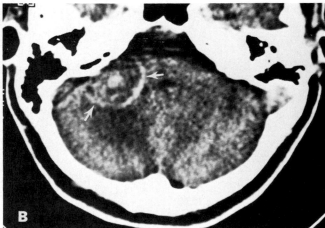

FIG 17–34.
Schwannoma originating in the jugular fossa. The enhanced axial scan seen in **A** demonstrates an enhancing neoplasm *(arrowhead)* within and extending beyond an enlarged right jugular fossa *(arrows)*. A slightly higher cut **(B)** demonstrates the more superior portion of the tumor, which has the appearance of a "target." There is a peripheral rim of enhancement *(arrows)* with a central collection of enhancement and nonenhancing, partially necrotic tumor between the areas of enhancement. An acoustic schwannoma may have an identical appearance to that seen in **B.** The enlargement of the jugular fossa by tumor is evidence for the origin of the schwannoma from a cranial nerve within the fossa. At the time of surgery, it was believed that the schwannoma originated from the right 11th cranial nerve.

reinjection of air in order to study the contralateral structures.[48–50] While both of these CT cisternographic techniques may demonstrate small lesions within the CPA or IAC, they are invasive and have been almost totally replaced by MRI scanning,[51–53] particularly that utilizing an intravenously injected paramagnetic contrast agent such as gadolinium-DTPA.[54, 55]

MRI characteristics of nerve sheath tumors include isointensity to slight hypointensity on short TR images relative to the pons, areas of even more hypointensity representing cystic change, and hyperintensity on long TR images when compared with the brain stem for both the solid and cystic components (Figs 17–35 to 17–38). The contrast to noise ratio (CNR) between the tumor and surrounding CSF or bone allows detection of relatively small tumors when compared with CT (Figs 17–35 and 17–39). Nerve sheath tumors demonstrate marked enhancement with gadolinium-DTPA (see Fig 17–36). Intracanalicular tumors only a few millimeters in size may now be easily diagnosed with enhanced MRI (Figs 17–40 and 17–41), which makes this the procedure of choice for evaluating the CPA and IAC for possible tumor and replaces enhanced CT or CT following either air or positive-contrast cisternography.

One of the major differential diagnostic possibilities for a mass lesion in the CPA is meningi-

oma. Meningiomas are usually isointense on short TR MRI sequences and isointense to mildly hyperintense on the long TR study. While they also enhance markedly, that enhancement is usually homogeneous as opposed to the inhomogeneity of medium to large nerve sheath tumors (see Fig 17–36). One author reports greater enhancement of nerve sheath tumors than meningiomas, possibly due to more patent endothelial gap junctions and a larger extracellular space in schwannomas than meningiomas that allows more accumulation of contrast agent in the schwannoma.[10] Other distinguishing features, including the broad base of the meningioma away from the IAC and neurovascular complex, have been discussed earlier.

Occasionally, it can be difficult to distinguish an extra-axial posterior fossa lesion from an intra-axial lesion of the cerebellar hemisphere.[56] A slowly growing extra-axial mass may invaginate into the cerebellar parenchyma and simulate a cerebellar mass lesion, or there may be abundant cerebellar edema associated with invagination that suggests a primary or secondary cerebellar mass (see Fig 17–38). Likewise, a cerebellar mass may have an exophytic component projecting into the CPA. MRI is better than CT at making this distinction because of its better soft-tissue characterization and the ease of obtaining multiple projections.

Other CPA masses include arachnoid cyst, epi-

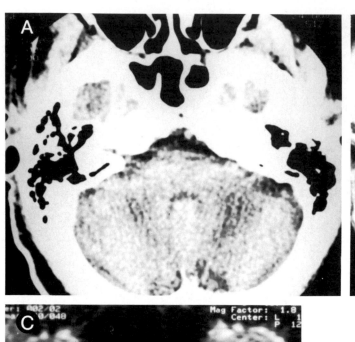

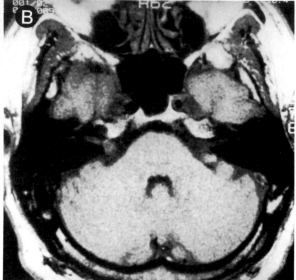

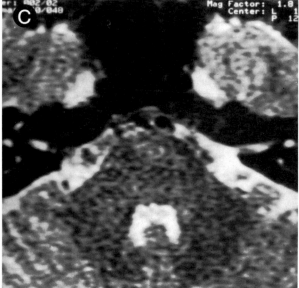

FIG 17–35.
Small intracannicular and extracannicular acoustic schwannoma missed on CT scan but apparent on MRI. The enhanced CT scan **(A)** does not demonstrate the mass lesion within the right CPA or IAC. The short TR MRI scan (**B,** TR = 600, TE = 20) demonstrates the schwannoma, which is slightly hypointense relative to the pons and involves both the right CPA and IAC. The long TR/TE study (**C,** TR = 4,000, TE = 120) was performed with a very long TR and TE in order to differentiate tumor from CSF.

dermoid cyst, and metatasis. The first two lesions differ from meningioma and nerve sheath tumor in their CT density and MRI intensity patterns, which mimic CSF, and their lack of enhancement. It may be difficult or impossible to separate the arachnoid cyst from surrounding CSF unless there is mass effect or unless the cyst membrane can be seen on MRI. Epidermoid cyst may have a calcified wall. The presence of desquamated epithelium and cholesterol crystals within the cyst may allow differentiation from surrounding CSF on short and/or very long TR/TE images and/or on gradient-echo sequences using a low flip angle and long TE. Metastases usually produce bone destruction and grow rapidly.

A nerve sheath tumor of the trigeminal nerve located at the petrous apex may have an identical appearance to an acoustic tumor, with the only difference being presentation of pain in the fifth nerve distribution and the relatively high position of the lesion on the scan relative to the CPA. A nerve sheath tumor located in the middle cranial fossa presents on CT as an enhancing mass lesion with either a homogeneous or inhomogeneous character[57] that produces erosion of the lateral wall of the sella and the base of the skull; multiple projections are of great value in defining the extent of the mass and involvement of the cavernous sinus and contiguous sella (Fig 17–42). The major differential diagnostic considerations for this parasellar

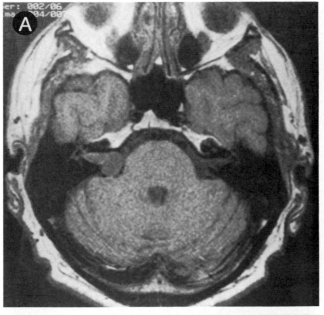

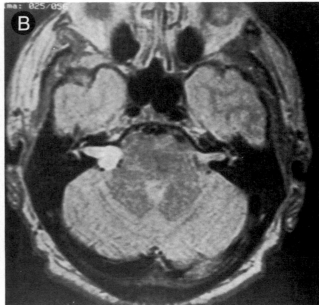

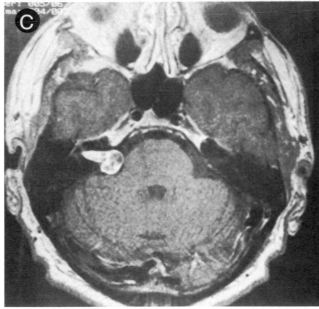

FIG 17–36.
Acoustic schwannoma demonstrated on multiple sequences. The unenhanced short TR sequence (**A,** TR = 600, TE = 25), the long TR, short TE sequence (**B,** TR = 3,000, TE = 30), and the enhanced short TR study (**C,** TR = 600, TE = 25) all are equally efficacious at demonstrating the CPA and IAC mass lesion. The enhanced study (**C**) is better at demonstrating the nonhomogeneity of the tumor, so characteristic of schwannoma.

location are meningioma and carotid artery aneurysm. The differentiation may be extremely difficult on the CT scan but is easily made with MRI, as discussed earlier. Rarely, schwannoma may extend into the parapharyngeal or other extracranial soft tissues (Fig 17–43), similar to meningioma (see Fig 17–16).

Meningioma

The MRI and CT characteristics of meningioma have been presented earlier in the chapter.

Arachnoid Cyst

The CT and MRI characteristics of arachnoid cyst have been discussed earlier in this chapter. Briefly, the MRI signal intensities on both short and long TR sequences and the density on CT match those of CSF; any deviation from this rule indicates that the lesion is not an arachnoid cyst. There is no calcification in the wall and no enhancement of the lesion. It may not be perceived unless there is mass effect on surrounding structures. See Chapter 26 regarding the differential imaging characteristics of arachnoid cyst from the

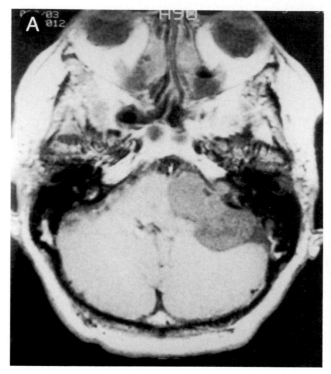

FIG 17–37.
Large broad-based cystic acoustic schwannoma. The short TR sequence (**A,** TR = 700, TE = 20) demonstrates a large lesion broad based against the petrous bone that is hypointense relative to the cerebellum. There is an extension into the left IAC. The long TR/TE

image (**B,** TR = 2,600, TE = 100) demonstrates the nonhomogeneity of the lesion and better defines the more solid portion extending into the left IAC.

Dandy-Walker syndrome and other pericerebellar cystic lesions.

Epidermoid Cyst

This lesion is discussed in more depth in Chapter 18. Briefly, this is a congenital tumor of ectodermal origin containing variable amounts of desquamated epithelium and cholesterol crystals. Its CT density varies from being close to CSF to mildly hyperdense when compared with CSF. It fails to enhance, and it occasionally has calcification in its walls.[58–60] It may be impossible to perceive the lesion on CT in relation to CSF unless there is mass effect on surrounding structures. Depending upon the cyst contents, it may be distinguished from CSF on short TR MRI by being slightly more intense and from CSF on long TR images by its decreased intensity relative to CSF. However, it may very closely mimic CSF on routine MRI studies, which require very long TR and TE values to demonstrate the decreased signal intensity relative to CSF. It may be indistinguishable from an arachnoid cyst if its density and/or intensity are equal to CSF and if its margins are

intact. It may have irregular margins if rupture has occurred or if it invaginates into crevices between normal tissues.[60]

SKULL BASE TUMORS

The differential diagnosis of skull base tumors is given in Table 17–1 and is dependent upon the location of the lesion. Esthesioneuroblastoma is presented in this section, as are chordoma, chondroma, chondrosarcoma, and other tumors involving the sphenoid bone. Chemodectoma of the petrous bone is discussed. Meningiomas were presented earlier in this chapter. Paranasal sinus and nasopharyngeal tumors secondarily affecting the skull base are presented in Chapters 30 and 32. Lesions involving the CPA have been discussed earlier, while petrous bone tumors other than chemodectomas are presented in Chapter 29.

Esthesioneuroblastoma

Esthesioneuroblastoma is a rare tumor arising from the sensory neuroepithelium of the olfactory

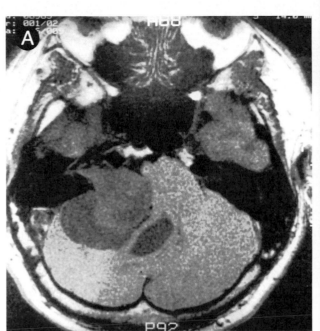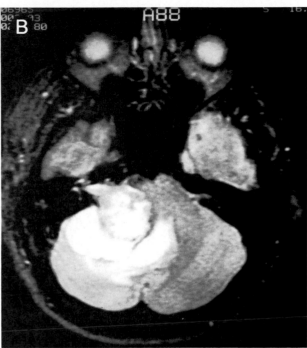

FIG 17–38.
Acoustic schwannoma with extensive cerebellar edema and a possible arachnoid cyst. The short TR study (**A,** TR = 600, TE = 20) demonstrates a large mass lesion in the right CPA that is invaginating into the right IAC and indenting the pons and cerebellum. There is extensive low-density abnormality surrounding the lesion. The long TR/TE study (**B,** TR = 4,000, TE = 75) shows the nonhomogeneity of the more solid tumor mass and the peripheral high-intensity "cystic" lesion(s) surrounding the solid tumor mass. More peripheral still is less well demarcated tissue of less hyperintensity, probably representing edema. In all probability the findings are that of a nonhomogeneous CPA and IAC schwannoma, a cyst of the tumor or possibly a separate arachnoid cyst, and an edematous cerebellum. So much intrinsic cerebellar abnormality may mistakenly suggest the presence of a primary or secondary cerebellar neoplasm. Such an error may be made more easily on CT, with MRI making the differentiation in most cases.

mucosa. It generally arises within the superior and lateral aspects of the nasal cavity, near the ethmoid sinuses and cribriform plate. The most common ages of presentation are adolescence and adults in the sixth decade or greater.[61]

The tumor exhibits slow growth[61] and nonspecific symptoms of local pain, nasal obstruction, and epistaxis, which give this tumor the name "the great imposter."[62] The differential diagnosis of a mass lesion in this region includes encephalocele, meningioma, schwannoma, carcinoma, and malignant lymphoma.[62] The tumor demonstrates either local invasion or, less commonly (approximately 20%), systemic metastases. Aggressive surgery and radiation therapy have produced long survival times.[61]

Radiographic evaluation demonstrates extensive bone destruction in the region of the nasal cavity, ethmoid and other paranasal sinuses, and medial walls of the orbits as well as destruction of the cribriform plate and base of the skull, with intracranial extension. Angiography demonstrates a mild degree of hypervascularity.[63] Intracranial extension may be extensive, with a large amount of tumor occupying the basal portion of the frontal and, rarely, middle cranial fossae.[62, 63] MRI reports are rare, but one case report shows a tumor of low intensity to white matter and isointensity to gray matter on a short TR sequence and spotty areas of intratumoral hyperintensity on the long TR/TE sequence.[62]

Figure 17–44 demonstrates the classic CT appearance of a large bulky tumor occupying the nasal cavity and paranasal sinuses, with nonhomogeneous enhancement and extensive bone destruction. There is apparent elevation of the enhancing dura. MRI scanning in a different patient (Fig 17–45) shows a large bulky tumor destroying the hypointense bone of the cribriform plate and extending intracranially to elevate the hypointense dura. The tumor mass is slightly hypointense to cerebral cortex on the short TR image but markedly hyperintense on the long TR/TE sequence. Cyst formation is present (Fig 17–44,C).

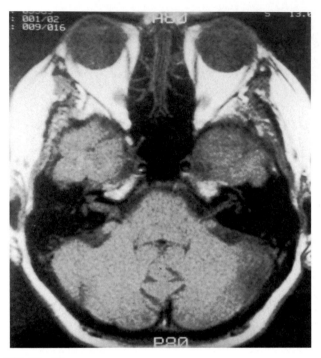

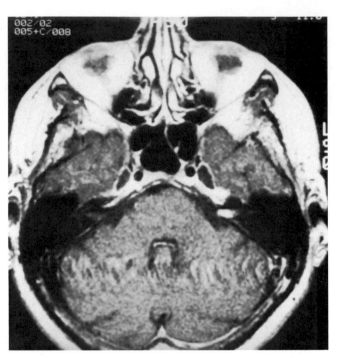

FIG 17–39.
Intracannilicular acoustic schwannoma demonstrated on a short TR MRI sequence. The short TR sequence (TR = 600, TE = 20) demonstrates the primarily intracannilicular tumor of the right IAC to be minimally hypointense relative to the pons but more intense than the contents of the left IAC. There is slight widening of the right IAC.

FIG 17–41.
Enhanced MRI demonstration of a small acoustic schwannoma. A tiny acoustic schwannoma involves the left IAC, with minimal projection into the left CPA, on this short TR (TR = 600, TE = 25) enhanced study.

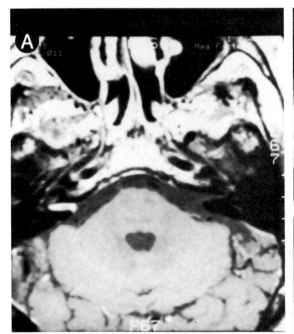

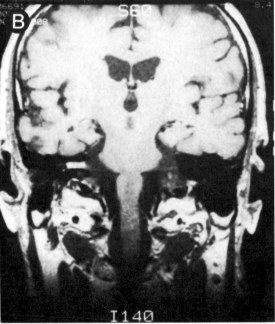

FIG 17–40.
Enhanced MRI demonstration of a small intracannilicular acoustic schwannoma. The gadolinium-DTPA–enhanced short TR (TR = 600, TE = 25) images in the axial **(A)** and coronal **(B)** projections nicely demonstrate the purely intracannilicular schwannoma, which enhances intensely. This tiny tumor has not caused canal enlargement.

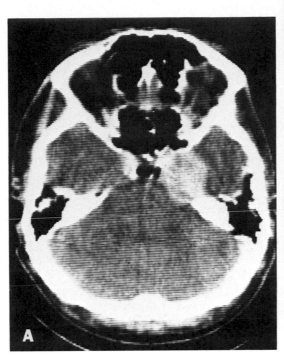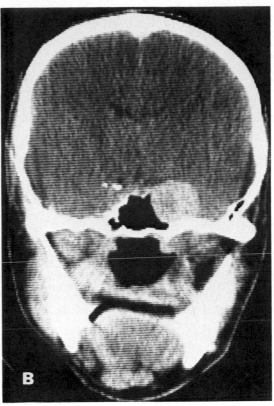

FIG 17–42.

Trigeminal schwannoma. Enhanced axial **(A)** and coronal **(B)** scans demonstrate a homogeneously enhancing, round, well-marginated mass in the medial aspect of the middle cranial fossa. The long-standing presence of this tumor is denoted by the concave deformity of the lateral wall of the sphenoid sinus. Differential diag-nosis includes aneurysm, schwannoma, and meningioma. No hy-perostosis can be seen to suggest meningioma, and the patient presented with facial pain. Left carotid angiography demonstrated a subtle stain.

Esthesioneuroblastoma must be differentiated from meningioma originating along the olfactory grooves (Fig 17–46). Meningioma in this region generally has homogeneous enhancement, as do most intracranial meningiomas. While facial extension rarely occurs with meningioma (see Fig 17–16), differentiation is usually easy. Most esthesioneuroblastomas present as a large intranasal/paranasal sinus mass that elevates the dura (see Figs 17–44 and 17–45), with the dural relationship indicative of the extracranial origin, whereas meningioma without paranasal sinus/facial extension is an intradural lesion without dural elevation.

Chordoma

Chordoma originates from notochordal remnants and therefore may be found anywhere along the craniospinal axis from the sphenoid bone to the sacrum, with the two ends of the axis favored in location.[1, 64] Approximately 35% to 40% occur intrac-

ranially, with the most common locations being the body of the sphenoid bone and the clivus. The chordoma is a slowly growing neoplasm with a long latent period but is locally invasive and tends to recur following any but the most radical surgical procedures. Two types of chordoma are identified by some.[65] The "typical chordoma" has cords of cells within a gelatinous matrix. The "chondroid chordoma" has variable amounts of cartilaginous tissue interspersed in tumor matrix. Others argue effectively that the chondroid type is simply chondrosarcoma and should not be considered a variant of chordoma.[64] The prognosis is significantly better with the "chondroid type", with longevity proportional to the amount of cartilaginous tissue present.[65, 66]

Calcification is common and occurs in approximately two thirds of cases (Fig 17–47).[67] Bone destruction is almost always present and involves the skull base (Figs 17–48 to 17–50).[67, 68] The tumor may extend inferiorly into the nasopharynx (Fig

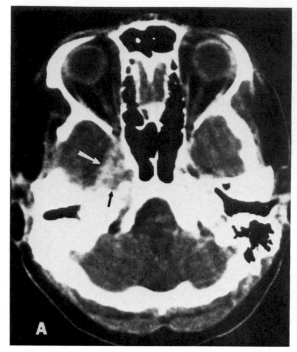 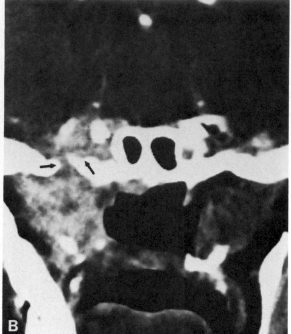

FIG 17–43.

Trigeminal schwannoma extending into the parapharyngeal soft tissues. The axial scan **(A)** demonstrates an inhomogeneously enhancing mass *(white arrow)* within the right cavernous sinus and parasphenoidal region that is producing bone erosion and destruction of the apex of the right petrous bone *(black arrow).* The patient has had a previous right temporal craniotomy for biopsy. The coronal scan **(B)** demonstrates the bone erosion and destruc-

tion at the base of the skull *(arrows),* with extension of the right parasphenoidal tumor inferiorly into the parapharyngeal soft tissues. This appearance is similar to that of the meningioma extending into the face, which is seen in Figure 17–16. (Courtesy of Drs. Modesti and Cacayorin, Upstate Medical Center, State University of New York, Syracuse.)

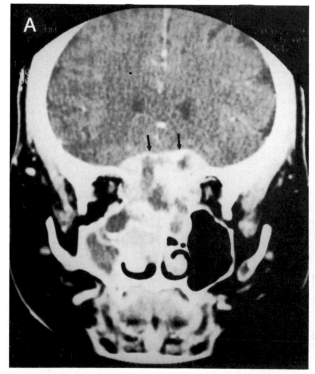 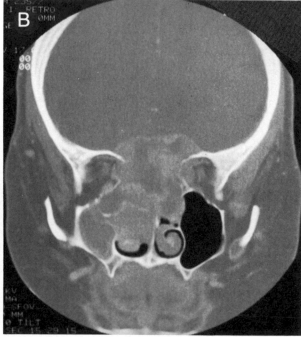

FIG 17–44.

Esthesioneuroblastoma. The enhanced coronal CT scan **(A)** demonstrates a large-mass lesion involving the ethmoid air cells, nasal cavity, and right maxillary antrum. There is destruction of the cribriform plate and floor of the anterior cranial fossae, with elevation of

the dura *(arrows).* There is nonhomogeneous enhancement of this extensive tumor. The "bone window" **(B)** nicely demonstrates the extensive destruction of the facial bones and skull base.

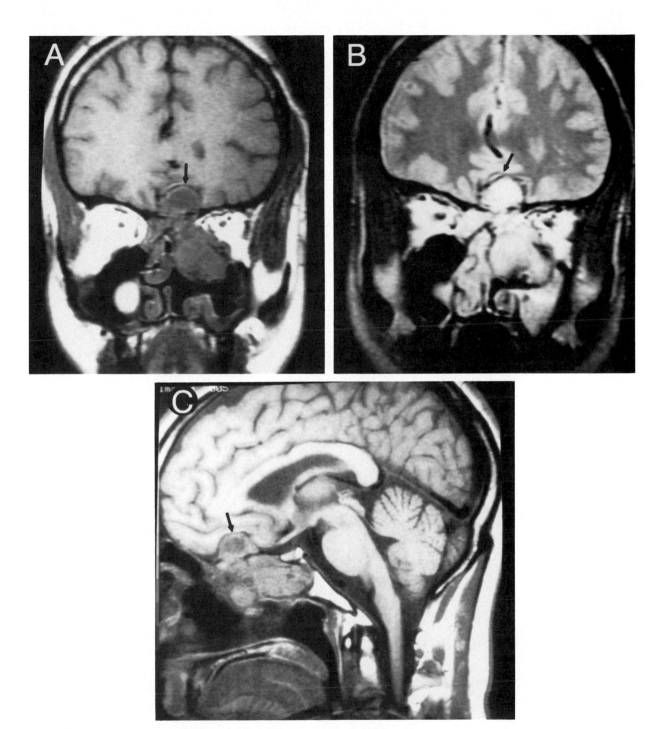

FIG 17–45.
Esthesioneuroblastoma demonstrated on MRI. The coronal short TR (**A,** TR = 600, TE – 25) and long TR/TE (**B,** TR = 2,500, TE = 75) studies and the sagittal short TR sequence (**C,** TR = 600, TE = 25) all demonstrate the extensive mass within the nasal cavity and ethmoid air cells with extension into the left orbit. There is extension superiorly to elevate the hypointense dura on all views *(ar-* *rows)* and extension posteriorly into the marrow-filled sphenoid bone **(C).** There is a sharply marginated area within the intracranial component that is of low intensity on short TR sequences **(A** and **C)** and hyperintense on the long TR study **(B);** most likely this represents a focal cyst.

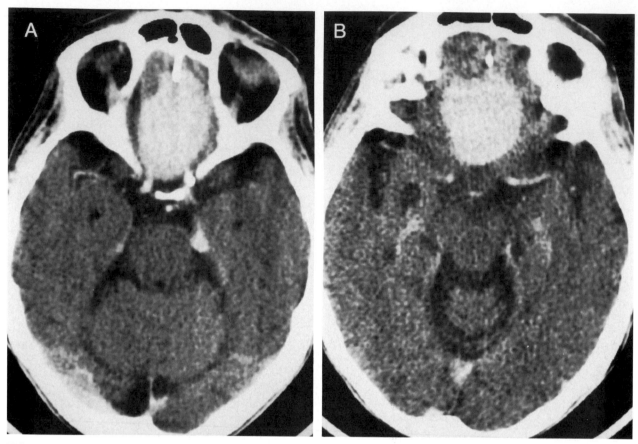

FIG 17–46.
Olfactory groove meningioma. The classic appearance on axial CT scans at the level of the crista galli **(A)** and 5 mm above that **(B)** of a sharply marginated, homogeneously enhancing meningioma.

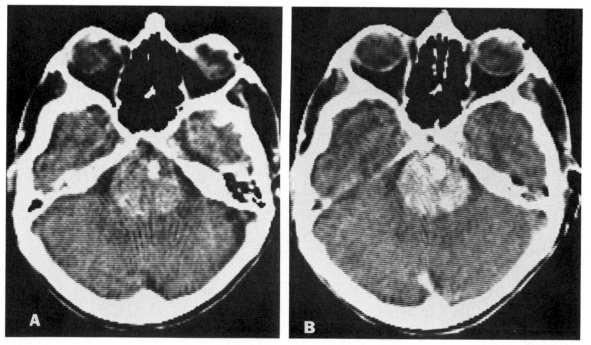

FIG 17–47.
Clival chordoma. The unenhanced scan **(A)** demonstrates a large well-circumscribed mass containing central calcification that is located in the usual region of the brain stem. The brain stem is markedly compressed and displaced posterior to this lesion. There is erosion and destruction of the clivus anterior to the mass. The enhanced scan **(B)** demonstrates a mild degree of diffuse but patchy enhancement of this slowly growing tumor.

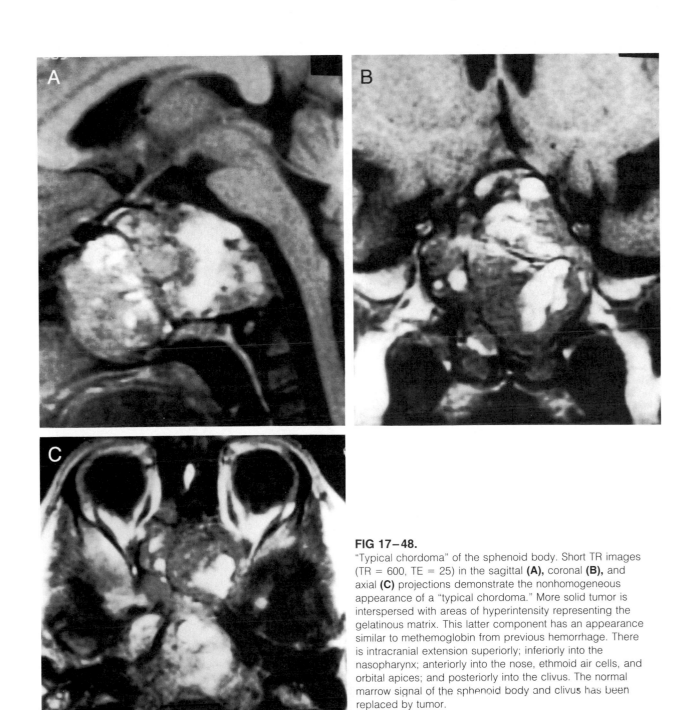

FIG 17–48.
"Typical chordoma" of the sphenoid body. Short TR images (TR = 600, TE = 25) in the sagittal **(A),** coronal **(B),** and axial **(C)** projections demonstrate the nonhomogeneous appearance of a "typical chordoma." More solid tumor is interspersed with areas of hyperintensity representing the gelatinous matrix. This latter component has an appearance similar to methemoglobin from previous hemorrhage. There is intracranial extension superiorly; inferiorly into the nasopharynx; anteriorly into the nose, ethmoid air cells, and orbital apices; and posteriorly into the clivus. The normal marrow signal of the sphenoid body and clivus has been replaced by tumor.

17–48); superiorly through the dura into the prepontine, suprasellar, and parasellar regions (Figs 17–48 and 17–50); and posteriorly into the foramen magnum (Figs 17–48 to 17–50). While the tumor generally is of a midline origin, it may occasionally present as an eccentric mass such as in a parasellar location (Fig 17–50). Rarely, it is purely intradural in origin, without bone destruction.[69]

CT scanning demonstrates increased density of this tumor on the preinfusion scan along with multiple foci of calcification and extensive destruction of the base of the skull, which are well shown with "bone windows."[67, 68] There is intense enhancement on the postinfusion scan, which demonstrates the extent of the tumor (Fig 17–47).

MRI is better for both the characterization of

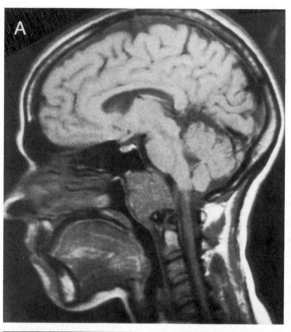

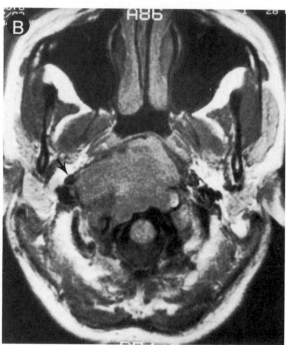

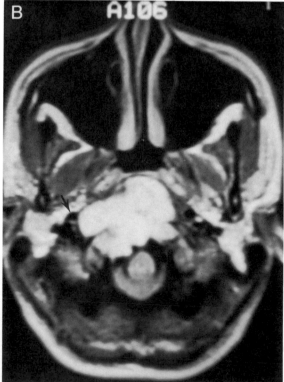

FIG 17–49.
MRI appearance of "chondroid chordoma" of the clivus. The sagittal **(A)** and axial **(B)** short TR (TR = 600, TE = 25) sequences demonstrate a homogeneous neoplasm mildly hypointense to the brain stem that is replacing the normal marrow signal of the clivus. The long TR image (**C,** TR = 2,500, TE = 25) demonstrates homogeneous hyperintensity. There is bulging into the nasopharynx and premedullary spaces, with right lateral extension in the upper portion of the neck, that is displacing the right internal carotid artery (**B** and **C,** *arrows*) laterally.

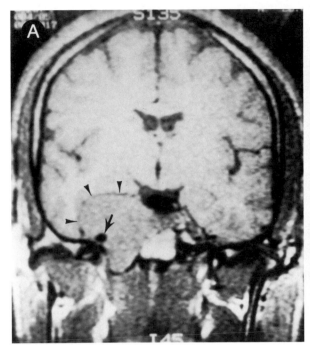
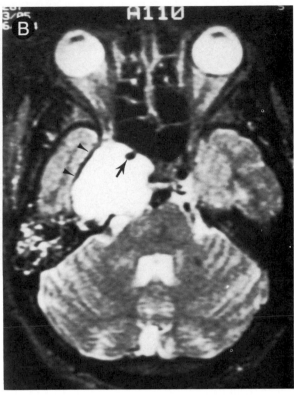

FIG 17–50.
Eccentric "chondroid chordoma." The coronal short TR image (**A,** TR = 550, TE = 25) and the long TR/TE axial sequence (**B,** TR = 2,500, TE = 75) demonstrate a right parasellar mass that is homogeneously hypointense to white matter on the short TR image **(A)** and markedly hyperintense on the long TR study **(B).** There is elevation and lateral displacement of the dura *(arrowheads)* and extension through the skull base. There is encasement of the right internal carotid artery *(arrows).* Parasellar meningioma would not be so hyperintense on the long TR study, while schwannoma would not produce the destruction of the right petrous apex as in this case, nor is it usually so homogeneous in intensity.

the tumor and definition of extension.[66, 67, 69, 70] The typical chordoma has a nonhomogeneous appearance on short TR images; the solid cords of tumor are isointense to hypointense to the brain stem, whereas the gelatinous matrix is hyperintense. Long TR images demonstrate pronounced hyperintensity (Fig 17–48).[70] On the other hand, the chondroid chordroma is isointense to hypointense to the brain stem in a homogeneous fashion on short TR images and diffusely hyperintense on long TR sequences (Figs 17–49 and 17–50).[70] Therefore, MRI characterization of tissue type is possible and may help in prognosis and patient management.[70]

MRI demonstrates the relationship of the tumor to the carotid arteries, which can be seen as flow voids (Figs 17–49 and 17–50).[67] While bone destruction is easier to see on CT,[67] short TR MRI shows the normal hyperintensity of marrow fat within the sphenoid body or clivus to be displaced by tumor of decreased signal (Figs 17–48 to 17–50). The relationship of the tumor to the dura is well demonstrated by coronal and sagittal MRI (Fig 17–50).

The differential diagnosis includes clival meningioma, chondrosarcoma, and tumors involving the sphenoid sinus. Clival meningioma has been discussed previously. Briefly, meningioma does not demonstrate the extensive bone destruction of chordoma, calcification is significantly less common, and meningioma tends to remain isointense to mildly hyperintense on long TR images. Chondrosarcoma is discussed later in this chapter. Malignant tumors involving the sphenoid sinus include sphenoid sinus carcinoma, plasmocytoma, lymphoma/leukemia, and metastases from solid tumors. Signal characteristics on MRI of any of these tumors may be identical to chondroid chordoma. Typically, these tumors do not calcify.

Occasionally, invasive benign pituitary adenoma may extend into the sphenoid and produce so much bone destruction and expansion that chordoma is simulated (Fig 17–51). The presence of a

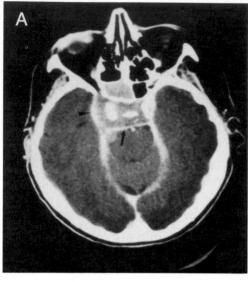

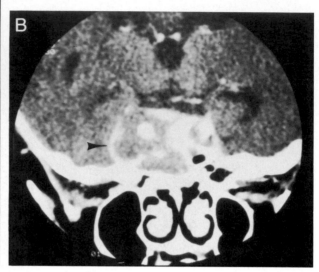

FIG 17–51.

Invasive pituitary adenoma simulating chordoma. CT scanning in the axial **(A)** and coronal **(B)** projections demonstrates a large homogeneous mildly enhancing neoplasm that expands the body of the sphenoid and invades the pituitary fossa, sphenoid sinus, and right posterior ethmoid air cells. There is posterior displacement of the dura **(A,** *arrow*) to abut the basilar artery and expansion into the right cavernous sinus and apex of the right orbit, with lateral displacement of the dura **(A** and **B,** *arrowheads*). Such a diffuse expansion by this invasive pituitary adenoma simulates chordoma.

"ballooned" sella turcica, endocrine changes, and a well-encapsulated suprasellar mass may help in differentiation. Mucocele is a nonneoplastic expansion of the sphenoid sinus due to obstruction of the ostium. Bony structures may be so expanded and thinned that chordoma is simulated. Enhanced CT does not demonstrate enhancement of the lesion unless there is secondary infection (pyomucocele). MRI demonstrates the hyperintensity of mucus, especially on long TR sequences.

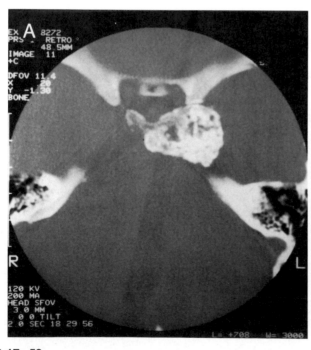

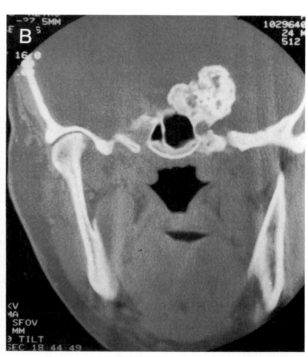

FIG 17–52.

A and **B,** sphenoid osteochondroma. There is nonhomogeneous calcification/ossification of this well-marginated osteochondroma of the left side of the dorsum sella and the body of the sphenoid. There is no bone destruction.

Chondroma, Osteochondroma, Osteoma

Chondroma, osteochondroma, and osteoma are benign lesions that commonly affect the skull base and vary in their proportions of chondroid and osteoid matrices. The osteoma is heavily ossified, osteochondroma has less homogeneous opacification/calcification than osteoma but a sharp margin of bony density, and chondroma is a sharply marginated tumor of low density/intensity that contains clumps ("popcorn") of calcification. There is no bone destruction. Figure 17–52 demonstrates the classic CT scan appearance of an osteochondroma. There is a sharply marginated inhomogeneously calcified/ossified mass extending from the left lateral and superior aspects of the sphenoid bone.[71]

Chondrosarcoma

Chondrosarcoma is a malignant tumor originating in bone that arises from cartilaginous precursors. Exuberent calcification of the cartilaginous matrix is common[72] and exhibits a "popcorn" type of calcification (Fig 17–53) similar to the benign chondroma but far exceeds the calcification of either chordoma or meningioma. Chondroma is a benign slowly growing lesion that deforms bone, whereas chondrosarcoma is malignant and destroys

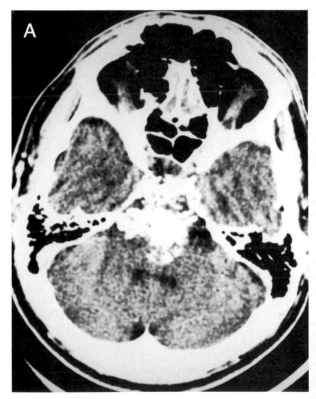

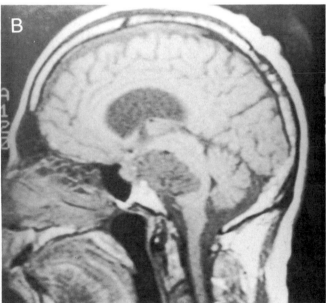

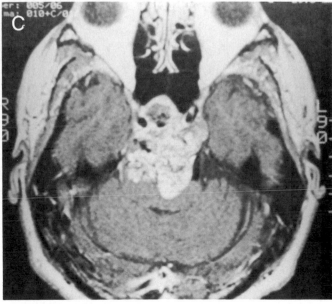

FIG 17–53.
Heavily calcified clival chondrosarcoma with enhancement on MRI. The axial enhanced CT scan **(A)** demonstrates a heavily calcified, poorly marginated, and minimally enhancing lesion of the clivus that is projecting deeply into the brain stem. The short TR sagittal unenhanced MRI study (**B,** TR = 600, TE = 20) demonstrates a lesion of the clivus that is producing an irregular margin with the clival marrow signal and projecting into the sphenoid sinus. The lesion is quite hypointense relative to the pons into which it invaginates. The calcification is not apparent because of the intermixed tumor giving signal. Imaging after the administration of gadolinium-DTPA (**C,** TR = 600, TE = 20) shows the nonhomogeneous enhancement.

bone. Chondrosarcoma may present as an isolated lesion or be part of a syndrome such as Ollier's disease (enchondomatosis) or the Maffucci syndrome (enchondromatosis and soft-tissue hemangiomas).

It may be impossible to differentiate chondrosarcoma from the chondroid form of chordoma, and in fact, chondroid chordoma may in reality be a low-grade form of chondrosarcoma.[64] Chondrosarcoma lacks the gelatinous matrix of the "typical chordoma" and therefore simulates the chondroid chordoma (see Figs 17–49 and 17–50) on MRI. It, too, is relatively isointense to mildly hypointense to cortex on the short TR sequence (Figs 17–53 to 17–55) and markedly hyperintense on long TR images (Fig 17–55). There is pronounced enhancement with gadolinium-DTPA (Figs 17–53 and 17–55). Chondrosarcoma is more commonly eccentric to the midline than is chordoma (Fig 17–55) and has more calcification, better appreciated on CT than on MRI (Fig 17–53).

The embryonal or mesenchymal form of chondrosarcoma commonly occurs in the first or second decade of life[73] and has a particular propensity to occur at the petrosphenoidal junction (Fig 17–56). It is heavily calcified like osteochondroma, grows slowly, and deforms surrounding bone. Distinction from osteochondroma can be made by the presence of focal bone destruction in addition to bone deformity and a more rapid rate of growth.

Chemodectoma

The chemodectoma (parasympathetic paraganglioma) arises from chemoreceptor tissue located in the middle ear (glomus tympanicum tumor), jugular foramen (glomus jugulare tumor), upper portion of the neck at the level of the second cervical segment (vagus body tumor), the midneck at the carotid bifurcation (carotid body tumor), or the mediastinum (aortic body tumor). Approximately 10% of patients with nonfamilial paraganglioma have at least one additional lesion, either a bilateral tumor in a similar location or a chemodectoma in another location (Fig 17–57).[74, 75] Seven percent of cases are reported to be familial,[76] with up to 35% of these patients having multiple tumors.[77, 78] All of these tumors are very vascular, with the classic angiographic findings of hypervascularity, a prolonged stain, and often, early venous opacification.

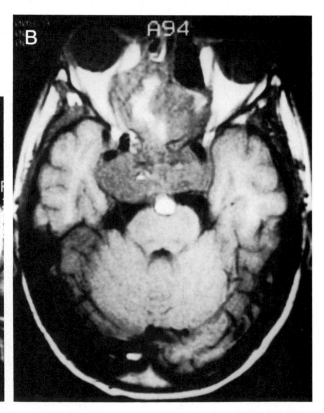

FIG 17–54.
Midline sphenoid chondrosarcoma. The short TR (TR = 800, TE = 20) sagittal **(A)** and axial **(B)** studies demonstrate a homogeneous neoplasm mildly hypointense to cerebral cortex. The appearance simulates a "chondroid chordoma" (see Figs 17–49 and 17–50). The internal carotid arteries are encapsulated by tumor **(B)** as the tumor extends anteriorly into the nose and ethmoid air cells and displaces the medial rectus muscles bilaterally **(B)**. There is a nodule of hyperintensity projecting into the pons, with focal areas of hyperintensity within the tumor, all of which may represent small areas of hemorrhage.

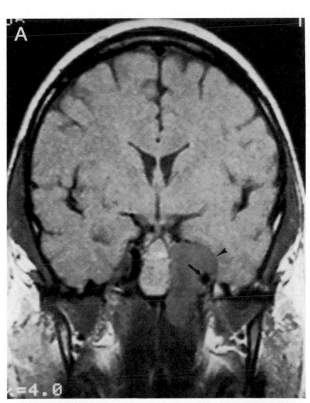

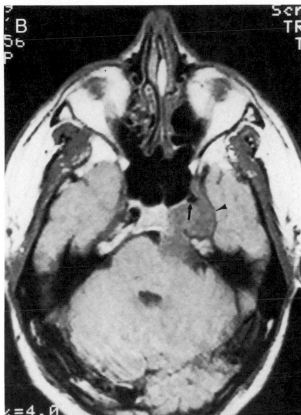

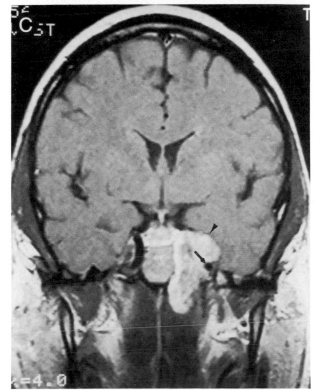

FIG 17–55.
Left parasellar chondrosarcoma. The unenhanced short TR (TR = 900, TE = 20) studies in the coronal **(A)** and axial **(B)** projections demonstrate a homogeneous tumor of low intensity to cerebral parenchyma. The mass produces bone destruction of the left lateral aspect of the marrow-filled sphenoid bone, of the left petrous apex, and of the skull base. There is a pronounced degree of nonhomogeneous enhancement **(C,** TR = 900, TE = 29, gadolinium-DTPA). There is extension of tumor into the parapharyngeal region, encasement and lateral displacement of the left internal carotid artery *(arrows)*, and lateral displacement of the hypointense dura *(arrowheads)*.

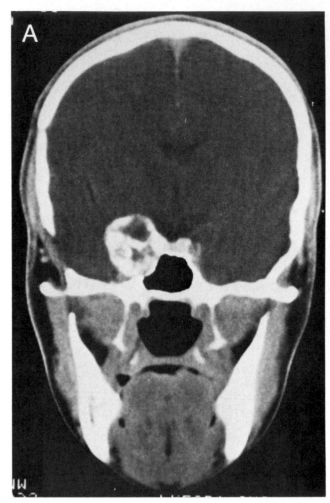

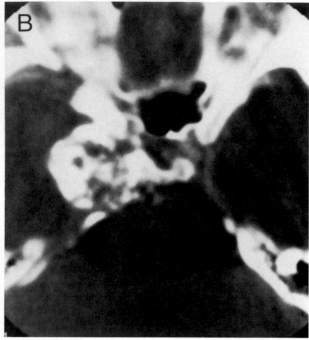

FIG 17–56.
Parasellar embryonal (mesenchymal) chondrosarcoma. The right parasellar mass is heavily calcified, but there are internal areas without calcification **(A).** While the deformity of the right lateral wall of the sphenoid sinus suggests a long-standing mass and while the mass resembles osteochondroma with its sharp margination, there are areas of bone destruction of the right petrous apex and petrosphenoidal junction **(B)** that is indicative of its more aggressive nature. The patient has had a previous right temporal craniotomy for biopsy.

The CT findings[79–82] of a glomus jugulare tumor include enlargement of a jugular foramen and focal bone erosion (Fig 17–57); enlargement alone is not a sufficient criterion for the presence of a mass because asymmetry in the size of the jugular foramina is a common and normal variant. There may be extensive infiltration and destruction of the petrous bone and skull base by this "benign" tumor (Fig 17–58). A dense mass is seen within the jugular foramen and, possibly, contiguous regions of the skull base, upper portion of the neck, and posterior fossa following contrast administration (Figs 17–57 and 17–58). Evaluation should always be made for bilateral tumors (Fig 17–57) or chemodectoma in other locations (e.g., carotid body).

Characteristically on unenhanced MRI, a glomus jugulare tumor is hyperintense relative to the surrounding jugular fossa on short TR images and is hyperintense to brain parenchyma on long TR sequences. Lesions less than 1.5 cm in size are not consistently seen on nonenhanced studies.[83] There may be flow voids either internally within the tumor or on the surface that represent enlarged vessels feeding this hypervascular mass.[83] Contrast enhancement is intense and allows visualization of tumors 5 mm or less.[83] The appearance differs from meningioma, which is usually relatively isointense on both short and long nonenhanced TR images, and from nerve sheath tumor, which is also hypointense to isointense to cerebellum on short TR images and hyperintense on long TR sequences but which may be inhomogeneous because of cyst formation. A nerve sheath tumor of cranial nerves IX, X, or X1 may produce erosion of the jugular foramen but not the extensive bone infiltration and destruction seen with some glomus tumors. Angiography may be necessary for confirmation of the diagnosis of chemodectoma, followed by preoperative embolization.

Extension may occur either inferiorly into the upper portion of the neck (Fig 17–57) or superi-

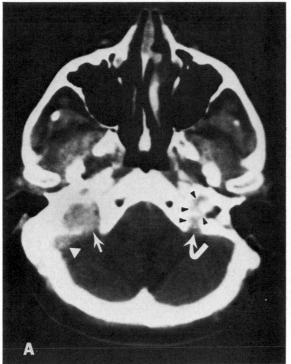

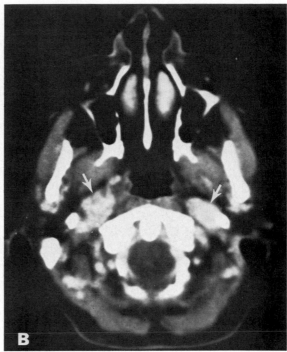

FIG 17–57.
Bilateral glomus jugulare tumors (chemodectomas). The enhanced axial scan through the jugular fossae **(A)** demonstrates enlargement of the right jugular fossa by a large soft-tissue mass *(straight arrow)*. The right sigmoid sinus is seen posterolaterally *(white arrowhead)*. On the *left,* there is irregular bone erosion and destruction *(black arrowheads)* of the jugular fossa by an enhancing soft-tissue mass *(curved arrow).* The axial scan at the level of C1 **(B)** demonstrates homogeneously enhancing, well-marginated tumors in the region of the jugular veins bilaterally *(arrows).* These represent extension of the bilateral chemodectomas into the upper portion of the neck.

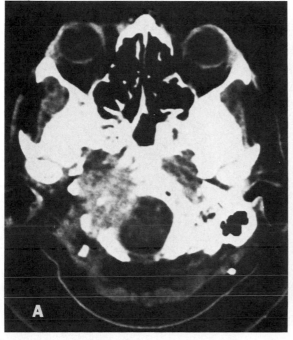

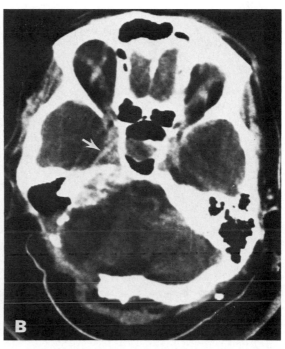

FIG 17–58.
Glomus jugulare tumor with extension into the spinal canal and middle cranial fossa. There is extensive bone destruction on the right from both the tumor itself and previous surgery in this patient with a huge recurrent glomus jugulare tumor. The lower enhanced scan **(A)** demonstrates extensive neoplasm eroding the edge of the foramen magnum and extending into the right side of the spinal canal. There is erosion of the right petrous bone **(B)** with extension of enhancing neoplasm into the right cavernous sinus to produce lateral displacement of the sinus margin *(arrow).* Right internal carotid angiography (not shown) demonstrated supply to the tumor from the petrous and cavernous portions of the artery, with encasement of that vessel.

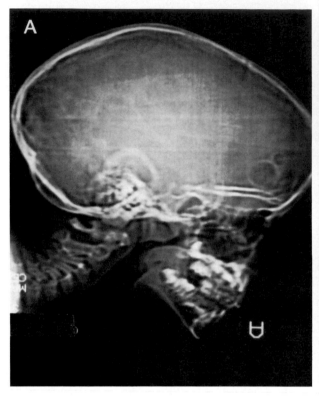

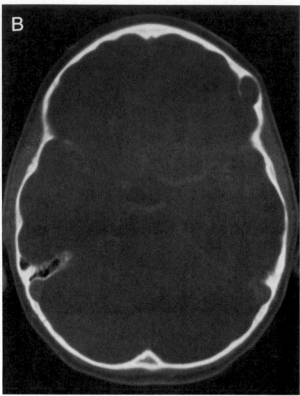

FIG 17–59.
Intradiploic dermoid. The skull film **(A)** demonstrates a sharply marginated lucency in the left frontal bone with a sclerotic rim. The CT scan with a "bone window" **(B)** demonstrates an intradiploic ex- pansion that appears homogeneous and may have broken through the inner table.

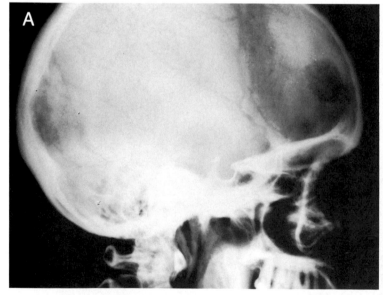

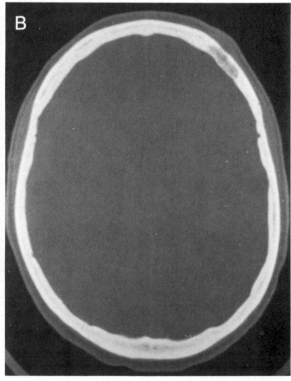

FIG 17–60.
Intradiploic hemangioma. The skull film **(A)** demonstrates a sharply marginated lucency with a reticular pattern in the left frontal bone. An axial CT scan with a "bone window" **(B)** also demonstrates a reticular pattern characteristic of hemangioma.

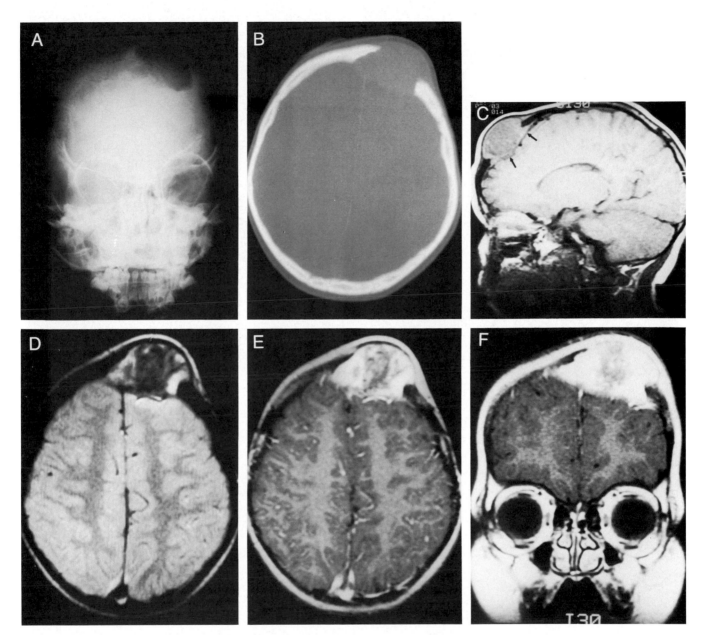

FIG 17–61.

Left frontal esosinophilic granuloma. The anteroposterior skull film demonstrates a large lytic defect in the left frontal bone with "beveled margins" characteristic of esosinophilic granuloma. The axial CT scan with a "bone window" **(B)** nicely shows the reason for the beveled margins. The lesion has produced bone erosion with oblique margins, and this accounts for the beveled contours. The bony margins are irregular, indicative of the aggressive nature of the tumor mass. Unenhanced sagittal short TR MRI **(C,** TR = 550, TE = 20) nicely demonstrates the lesion that has started within the diploic space and has extended both into the overlying scalp and into the epidural space so as to displace the dura *(arrows)* inwardly. The axial long TR study **(D,** TR = 2,600, TE = 30) demonstrates the nonhomogeneity of the lesion and crossing of the intracranial midline, indicative of its epidural location. Marked nonhomogeneous enhancement is demonstrated on the axial **(E)** and coronal **(F)** short TR enhanced studies (TR = 600, TE = 30, gadolinium-DTPA).

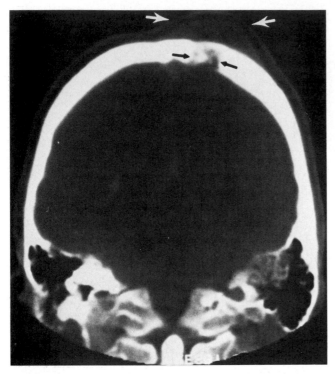

FIG 17–62.
Metastatic chondrosarcoma to the calvarium in Maffucci's syndrome (multiple enchondromatosis with soft-tissue hemangiomas). The direct enhanced coronal scan demonstrates irregular bony destruction of the high convexity of the left parietal bone near the midline *(black arrows),* with an overlying soft-tissue mass of the scalp *(white arrows).* The irregular margination of the bone destruction involves the inner and outer tables and intervening diploic space, evidence for the presence of an aggressive and destructive lesion.

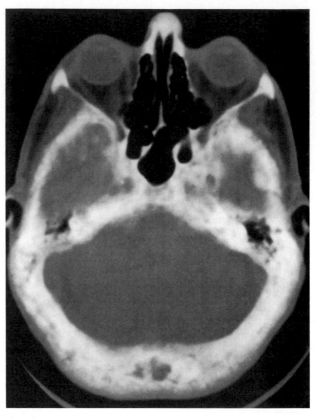

FIG 17–63.
Paget's disease. An axial CT scan with a "bone window" shows the expansion of all portions of the calvarium, with both osteolytic and osteoblastic areas. There is also involvement of the petrous bones. The appearance is characteristic of Paget's disease.

orly into the CPA (Fig 17–58).[19] While a glomus jugulare tumor is histologically benign, the tumor may produce a marked degree of bone erosion and extension into the posterior and middle cranial fossae, spinal canal, and cervical soft tissues (Fig 17–58).

TUMORS OF THE CALVARIUM

Tumors of the calvarium range from the benign dermoid and hemangioma (Figs 17–59 and 17–60), to the more aggressive eosinophilic granuloma (Fig 17–61), and finally to sarcomas and metastases (Fig 17–62). Bone erosion is best defined by using the CT "bone windows," with the degree of bony irregularity suggesting the benign or malignant nature of the lesion (Figs 17–59 to 17–62). Evaluation of the interstices of the expansion may suggest the correct diagnosis. Homogeneous intradiploic expansion is characteristic of a dermoid or epidermoid (Fig 17–59), while hemangioma appears to have linear bony septations similar to its appearance on plain skull films (Fig 17–60). However, distinguishing the various lesions on the basis of CT alone can be difficult. For example, early localized Paget's disease of the calvarium (osteoporosis circumscripta cranii) may have a similar CT appearance to metastatic disease, although in advanced cases marked thickening of the diploic space is evident, which supports the diagnosis of Paget's disease (Fig 17–63).

MRI is less efficacious than CT in evaluating small, purely bone lesions since cortical bone is more difficult to see with MRI. Visualization of the lesion depends to a large degree upon obliteration of marrow within the diploic space. However, MRI without and with contrast enhancement is superb for evaluating the tissue character of the lesion and its extension (see Fig 17–61).

An advantage of CT and/or MRI over plain skull films is the detection of a mass extending into the intracranial space (Fig 17–64). MRI is also

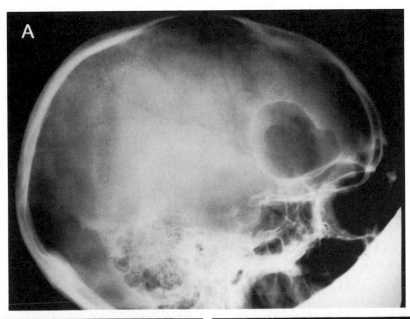

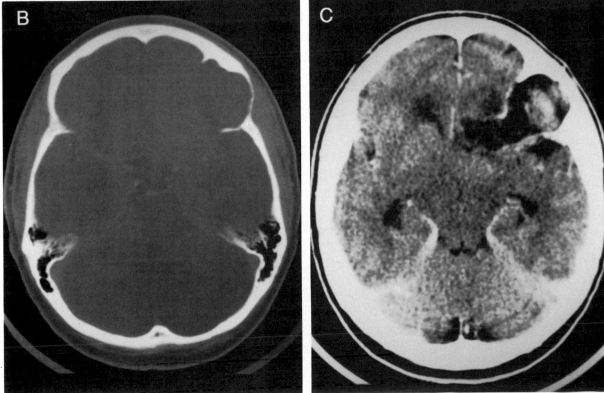

FIG 17–64.
Intradiploic dermoid with intracranial extension. The lateral skull film **(A)** demonstrates the large lytic defect in the left frontal bone with a sharp sclerotic margin. The enhanced axial CT scan with "bone" **(B)** and "soft-tissue" **(C)** windows demonstrates the intradiploic expansion, with extension of the mixed density lesion deeply into the left frontal lobe.

ideal for evaluating the dural sinuses, which may be compressed by an epidural mass.

REFERENCES

1. Wilson CB, Moossy J, Boldrey EB, et al: Pathology of intracranial tumors, in Newton TH, Potts DG (eds): *Radiology of the Skull and Brain,* vol 3. St Louis, CV Mosby Co, 1977, pp 3016–3048.
2. Quest DO: Meningiomas: An update. *Neurosurgery* 1978; 3:219.
3. Rozario R, Adedman L, Prager RJ, et al: Meningiomas of the pineal region and third ventricle. *Neurosurgery* 1979; 5:489–495.
4. Elster AD, Challa VR, Gilbert TH, et al: Meningiomas: MR and histopathologic features. *Radiology* 1989; 170:857–862.
5. Spagnoli MV, Goldberg HI, Grossman RI, et al: Intracranial meningiomas: High-field MR imaging. *Radiology* 1986; 161:369–375.
6. Zimmerman RD, Fleming CA, Saint-Louis LA, et al: Magnetic resonance imaging of meningiomas. *AJNR* 1985; 6:149–157.
7. Haughton VM, Rimm AA, Czervionke LF, et al: Sensitivity of Gd-DTPA–enhanced MR imaging of benign extraaxial tumors. *Radiology* 1988; 166:829–833.
8. Bydder GM, Kingsley DPE, Brown J, et al: MR imaging of meningiomas including studies with and without gadolinium-DTPA. *J Comput Assist Tomogr* 1985; 9:690–697.
9. Berry I, Brant-Zawadzki M, Osaki L, et al: Gd-DTPA in clinical MR of the brain; 2. Extraaxial lesions and normal structures. *AJNR* 1986; 7:789–793.
10. Watabe T, Azuma T: T1 and T2 measurements of meningiomas and neuromas before and after Gd-DTPA. *AJNR* 1989; 10:463–470.
11. New PFJ, Aronow S, Hesselink JR: National Cancer Institute study: Evaluation of computed tomography in the diagnosis of intracranial neoplasms: IV. Meningiomas. *Radiology* 1980; 136:665–675.
12. Smith HP, Cahha VR, Moody DM, et al: Biological features of meningiomas that determine the production of cerebral edema. *Neurosurgery* 1981; 8:428–433.
13. Nakagawa H, Lusino O: Biplane computed tomography of intracranial meningioma with extracranial extension. *J Comput Assist Tomogr* 1980; 4:478–483.
14. Russell EJ, George AE, Kricheff II, et al: Atypical computed tomographic features of intracranial meningioma: Radiological-pathological correlation in a series of 131 consecutive cases. *Radiology* 1980; 135:673–682.
15. George AE, Russell EJ, Kricheff II: White matter buckling: CT sign of extra-axial intracranial mass. *AJNR* 1980; 1:425–430.
16. Russell DS, Rubenstein LJ: *Pathology of Tumours of the Nervous System.* Baltimore, Williams & Wilkins, 1989, pp 500–501.
17. Alvarez F, Roda JM, Romero MP, et al: Malignant and atypical meningiomas: A reappraisal of clinical, histological, and computed tomographic features. *Neurosurgery* 1987; 20:688.
18. New PFJ, Hesselink JR, O'Carroll CP, et al: Malignant meningiomas: CT and histologic criteria, including a new CT sign. *AJNR* 1982; 3:267–276.
19. Shapir J, Coblentz C, Malanson D, et al: New CT finding in aggressive meningioma. *AJNR* 1985; 6:101–102.
20. Russell DS, Rubenstein LJ: *Pathology of Tumours of the Nervous System.* Baltimore, Williams & Wilkins, 1989, pp 479–483.
21. Russell DS, Rubenstein LJ: *Pathology of Tumours of the Nervous System.* Baltimore, Williams & Wilkins, 1989, pp 474–479.
22. Osborne DR, Dubois PR, Drayer BP, et al: Primary intracranial meningeal and spinal hemangiopericytoma: Radiographic manifestations. *AJNR* 1981; 2:69–74.
23. Russell DS, Rubenstein LJ: *Pathology of Tumours of the Nervous System.* Baltimore, Williams & Wilkins, 1989, pp 507–517.
24. Latchaw RE, Gabrielsen TO, Seeger JF: Cerebral angiography in meningeal sarcomatosis and carcinomatosis. *Neuroradiology* 1974; 8:131–139.
25. Tamura M, Kanafuchi J, Nagaya T, et al: Primary leptomeningeal melanoma with epipharyngeal invasion. *Acta Neurochir* 1981; 58:59–66.
26. Lamas E, Lobato RD, Sotelo T, et al: Neurocutaneous melanomas. *Acta Neurochir* 1977; 36:93–105.
27. Russell DS, Rubenstein LJ: *Pathology of Tumours of the Nervous System.* Baltimore, Williams & Wilkins, 1989, pp 792–797.
28. Russell DS, Rubenstein LJ: *Pathology of Tumours of the Nervous System.* Baltimore, Williams & Wilkins, 1989, pp 783.
29. Latchaw RE, Nadell J: Intra- and extracellular arachnoid cyst. *AJR* 1976; 126:629–633.
30. Starkman SP, Brown TC, Linell EA: Cerebral arachnoid cysts. *J Neuropathol Exp Neurol* 1958; 17:486–500.
31. Robinson RG: Congenital cysts of the brain: Arachnoid malformations. *Prog Neurol Surg* 1971; 4:133–174.
32. Banna M: Arachnoid cysts on computed tomography. *AJR* 1976; 127:979–982.
33. Latchaw RE, Gold LHA, Moore JS, et al: The nonspecificity of absorption coefficients in the differentiation of solid tumors and cystic lesions. *Radiology* 1977; 125:141–144.
34. Kjos BO, Brandt-Zawadzki M, Kucharczyk W, et al: Cystic intracranial lesions: Magnetic resonance imaging. *Radiology* 1985; 155:363–369.
35. Leo JS, Pinto RS, Hulvat GF, et al: Computed to-

mography of arachnoid cysts. *Radiology* 1979; 130:675–680.

36. Hayashi T, Kuratomi A, Kuramoto S: Arachnoid cyst of quadrigeminal cistern. *Surg Neurol* 1980; 14:267–273.

37. Wolpert SM, Scott RM: The value of metrizamide CT cisternography in the management of cerebral arachnoid cysts. *AJNR* 1981; 2:29–35.

38. Russell DS, Rubenstein LJ: *Pathology of Tumours of the Nervous System*. Baltimore, Williams & Wilkins, 1989, pp 533.

39. Russell DS, Rubenstein LJ: *Pathology of Tumours of the Nervous System*. Baltimore, Williams & Wilkins, 1989, pp 560–567.

40. Dolan EJ, Tacher WS, Rotenberg D, et al: Intracranial hypoglossal schwannoma as an unusual cause of facial nerve palsy. *J Neurosurg* 1982; 56:420–423.

41. Urich H: Pathology of tumors of cranial nerves, spinal nerve roots, and peripheral nerves, in Dyck PJ, Thomas PK, Lambert EH (eds): *Peripheral Neuropathy*, vol 2, ed 2. Philadelphia, WB Saunders Co, 1984, p 2253.

42. Russell DS, Rubenstein LJ: *Pathology of Tumors of the Nervous System*. Baltimore, Williams & Wilkins, 1989, p 537.

43. Davis KR, Parker SW, New PFJ, et al: Computed tomography of acoustic neuroma. *Radiology* 1977; 124:81.

44. Parker SW, Davis KR: Limitations of computed tomography in the investigation of acoustic neuromas. *Ann Otol* 1977; 86:436.

45. Dubois PJ, Drayer BP, Bank WO, et al: An evaluation of current diagnostic radiology modalities in the investigation of acoustic neurilemmomas. *Radiology* 1978; 126:173.

46. Roberson GH, Brismar J, David KR, et al: Metrizamide cisternography with hypocycloidal tomography: Preliminary results. *AJR* 1976; 127:965.

47. Rosenbaum AE, Drayer BP, Dubois PJ, et al: Visualization of small extracanalicular neurolemomas by metrizamide cisternographic enhancement. *Arch Otolaryngol* 1978; 104:239–243.

48. Kricheff II, Pinto RS, Bergeron RT, et al: Air-CT cisternography and canalography for small acoustic neuromas. *AJNR* 1980; 1:57.

49. Sortland O: Computed tomography combined with gas cisternography for the diagnosis of expanding lesions in the cerebellopontine angle. *Neuroradiology* 1979; 18:19.

50. Solti-Bohman LG, Magaram DL, Lo WWM, et al: Gas CT cisternography for detection of small acoustic nerve tumors. *Radiology* 1984; 150:403–407.

51. New PFJ, Bachow TB, Wismer GL, et al: MR imaging of the acoustic nerves and small acoustic neuromas at 0.6T: Prospective study. *AJNR* 1985; 6:165–170.

52. Enzmann DR, O'Donohue J: Optimizing MR imaging for detecting small tumors in the cerebellopontine angle and internal auditory canal. *AJNR* 1987; 8:99–106.

53. Daniels DL, Miller SJ, Meyer GA: MR detection of tumor in the internal auditory canal. *AJNR* 1987; 8:249–252.

54. Haughton VM, Rimm AA, Czervionke LF, et al: Sensitivity of Gd-DTPA enhanced MR imaging of benign extra-axial tumors. *Radiology* 1988; 166:829–833.

55. Runge VM, Sacaible TF, Goldstein HA, et al: Gd DTPA clinical efficacy. *Radiographics* 1988; 8:147–179.

56. Miller EM, Newton TH: Extra-axial posterior fossa lesions simulating intra-axial lesions on computed tomography. *Radiology* 1978; 127:675–679.

57. Goldberg R, Byrd S, Winter J, et al: Varied appearance of trigeminal neuroma on CT. *AJR* 1980; 134:57–60.

58. Zimmerman RA, Bilaniuk LT, Dolinhas C: Cranial computed tomography of epidermoid and congenital fatty tumors of maldevelopmental origin. *J Comput Tomogr* 1979; 3:40–50.

59. Chambers AA, Lubin RR, Tomsick TA: Cranial epidermoid tumors: Diagnosis by computed tomography. *Neurosurgery* 1977; 1:276–279.

60. Davis KR, Roberson GH, Taveras JM: Diagnosis of epidermoid tumors by computed tomography. *Radiology* 1976; 119:347–353.

61. Russell DS, Rubenstein LJ: *Pathology of Tumours of the Nervous System*. Baltimore, Williams & Wilkins, 1989, pp 915–920.

62. Schroth G, Gawehn J, Marquardt B, et al: MR imaging of esthesioneuroblastoma. *J Comput Assist Tomogr* 1986; 10:316–319.

63. Burke DP, Gabrielsen TO, Knake JE, et al: Radiology of olfactory neuroblastoma. *Radiology* 1980; 137:367–372.

64. Russell DS, Rubenstein LJ: *Pathology of Tumours of the Nervous System*. Baltimore, Williams & Wilkins, 1989, pp 820–821.

65. Heffelfinger MJ, Dahlin DC, MacCarty CS, et al: Chordomas and cartilaginous tumors at the skull base. *Cancer* 1973; 32:410–420.

66. Raffel C, Wright DC, Gutin PH, et al: Cranial chordomas: Clinical presentation and results of operative and radiation therapy in twenty-six patients. *Neurosurgery* 1985; 17:703.

67. Oot RF, Melville GE, Austin-Seymour M, et al: The role of MR and CT in evaluating clival chordomas and chondrosarcomas. *AJNR* 1988; 9:715–723.

68. Kendall BE, Lee BCP: Cranial chordomas. *Br J Radiol* 1977; 50:687–698.

69. Mapstone TB, Kaufman B, Ratcheson RA: Intradural chordoma without bone involvement: Nuclear magnetic resonance (NMR) appearance. *J Neurosurg* 1983; 59:535–537.

70. Sze G, Uichanco LS, Brant-Zawadzki MN, et al:

Chordomas: MR imaging. *Radiology* 1988; 166:187–191.

71. Matz SH, Israeli Y, Shalit MN, et al: Computed tomography in intracranial supratentorial osteochondroma. *J Comput Assist Tomogr* 1981; 5:109–115.

72. Grossman RI, Davis KR: Computed tomographic appearance of chondrosarcoma of the base of the skull. *Radiology* 1981; 141:403–408.

73. Russell DS, Rubenstein LJ: *Pathology of Tumours of the Nervous System.* Baltimore, Williams & Wilkins, 1989, pp 507–517.

74. Alford BR, Guilford ER: A comprehensive study of tumors of the glomus jugulare. *Laryngoscope* 1962; 72:765.

75. Spector GJ, et al: IV. Multiple glomus tumors in the head and neck. *Laryngoscopy* 1975; 85:1066.

76. Russell DS, Rubenstein LJ: *Pathology of Tumours of the Nervous System.* Baltimore, Williams & Wilkins, 1989, pp 958–962.

77. Bogdasarian RS, Lotz PR: Multiple simultaneous paragangliomas of the head and neck in association with multiple retroperitoneal pheochromocytomas. *Otolaryngol Head Neck Surg* 1979; 87:648.

78. Cook PL: Bilateral chemodectoma in the neck. *J Laryngol Otol* 1977; 91:611.

79. Marsman JWP: Tumors of the glomus jugulare complex (chemodectoma) demonstrated by cranial computed tomography. *J Comput Assist Tomogr* 1979; 3:795–799.

80. Larson TC, Reese DF, Baker HL, et al: Glomus tympanicum chemodectomas: Radiographic and clinical characteristics. *Radiology* 1987; 163:801–806.

81. Chakeres DW, LaMasters DL: Paragangliomas of the temporal bone: High-resolution and CT studies. *Radiology* 1984; 150:749–753.

82. Mafee MF, Valvassori GE, Shugar MA, et al: High resolution and dynamic sequential computed tomography. *Arch Otolaryngol Head Neck Surg* 1983; 109:691–696.

83. Vogl T, Bruning R, Schedel H, et al: Paragangliomas of the jugular bulb and carotid body: MRI imaging with short sequences and Gd-DTPA enhancement. *AJNR* 1989; 10:823–827.

18

Primary Intracranial Tumors: Tumors of Congenital, Pineal, and Vascular Origin and the Phakomatoses

Richard E. Latchaw, M.D.

David W. Johnson, M.D.

Emanuel Kanal, M.D.

Congenital tumors, pineal tumors, tumors of vascular origin, and the syndromes of the phakomatoses are all considered together in this chapter because of their multiple interrelationships. The congenital tumors include teratoma, germinoma (atypical teratoma), dermoid, epidermoid, lipoma, hamartoma, and craniopharyngioma. The teratoma is derived from all three germ cell layers (ectoderm, mesoderm, and endoderm), and therefore many different tissues may be found. Contrary to some authors, the dermoid cyst is derived from only ectoderm, not ectoderm and mesoderm.[1, 2] Both the dermoid and epidermoid are derived from ectoderm, but differ in their content of epidermal appendageal tissues and secretions.[1] A germinoma represents a form of teratoma in which a single but multipotential tissue predominates the germ cell itself. The lipoma frequently accompanies other congenital anomalies such as agenesis of the corpus callosum. It is thought to be the result of fatty differentiation of the primitive meninx. A hamartoma is a mass of normal and mature cells, but arranged in a disorganized fashion. Of particular import in this discussion is the hamartoma of the tuber cinereum that is associated with precocious

puberty. Malformations of the blood vessels, including arteriovenous malformation and capillary, venous, and cavernous angiomas, are all hamartomatous lesions involving the blood vessels. While the first three entities are discussed in earlier chapters in this book, cavernous angioma typically presents as a mass and will therefore be discussed with tumors of blood vessel origin. Finally, craniopharyngioma is thought to arise from a remnant of Rathke's pouch and is therefore of congenital origin. This entity is discussed in Chapter 23, which deals with intrasellar and suprasellar abnormalities.

One of the most common locations for the intracranial teratoma is the pineal region. The most common pineal tumor is the germinoma, although dermoid, epidermoid, and lipoma are all occasionally seen in this area. A discussion of pineal region tumors must not only include these teratomatous lesions but also the neuroepithelial tumors, including pineocytoma, pineoblastoma, and astrocytoma.

The neoplasms of blood vessel origin include hemangioblastoma, hemangioendothelioma, and angiosarcoma. (Hemangiopericytoma is considered by some to be a tumor of blood vessel origin that originates from the capillary pericyte, while others link it to the meningiomas. It is discussed with the meningiomas in Chapter 17.) Hemangioblastoma is also a component of one of the phakomatoses, the von Hippel–Lindau syndrome. The phakomatoses are those hereditary syndromes with neoplasms and/or hamartomas of the central nervous system (CNS) and skin lesions. The tuber of tuberous sclerosis is a form of hamartoma, and the angiomatous lesions of the Sturge-Weber syndrome are hamartomas of blood vessel origin. Intracranial hemangioendothelioma is a very rare lesion, as is its malignant counterpart, hemangioendotheliosarcoma (angiosarcoma). Cavernous angioma is a type of vascular malformation, i.e., a vascular hamartoma, but frequently presents as a mass lesion. It will be discussed with the tumors of blood vessel origin.

Occasionally, glioma presents in the newborn and may, therefore, be considered a "congenital" tumor. Gliomas are discussed with the other neuroepithelial tumors in Chapter 16. Ectopic gray matter may present as a focal mass and may be mistaken for a neoplasm. This topic is presented in Chapter 24, "Congenital Anomalies of the Brain."

CONGENITAL TUMORS

Teratoma

Intracranial teratoma, like any teratoma elsewhere in the body, is derived from all three germ cell layers.[3] Therefore, these tumors may contain a variety of tissue types, including ectodermal elements such as epidermis and nervous tissue; mesodermal elements such as fat, muscle, cartilage, and bone; and endodermal elements such as gastrointestinal mucosa and secretory glands. Any of these tissue types may undergo malignant degeneration.[4] Cyst formation is also typical. The most common location for these tumors is in the pineal region, with the intrasellar/suprasellar region and the posterior fossa less common sites of origin.[3, 5] Intracranial teratoma is the most common intracranial tumor in the newborn.[4, 5]

The magnetic resonance imaging (MRI) and computed tomographic (CT) appearance of these lesions depends upon the tissue(s) present.[4–6] Figure 18–1 shows the CT of a lipomyocele of the cerebellar vermis. The lesion is primarily cystic contains a great deal of fat with a large central core of muscle fibers, and has a peripheral nodule of abnormal vascularity that represents a hamartoma-

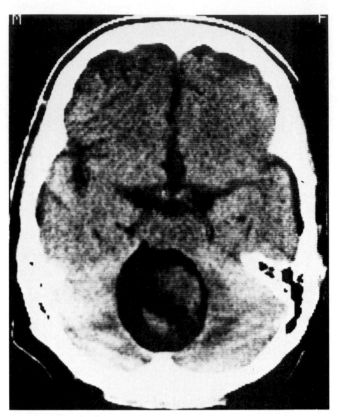

FIG 18–1.
Teratoma (lipomyocele). A nonenhanced scan demonstrates a large cystic lesion within the posterior fossa that contains a solid component centrally and low-density fat peripherally. The central solid component was primarily muscle tissue, but there were also collagenous elements and hamartomatous groups of blood vessels present, along with a minor contribution from tissues of endodermal origin.

tous collection of blood vessels. Other lesions may show the presence of cartilage, bone, glandular tissue, etc.

Dermoid

The lining of a dermoid cyst is squamous epithelium, with dermal elements present, including sebaceous and sweat glands and hair follicles.[1] All of these elements are derived from ectoderm.[1, 2] The sebaceous secretions produce very low attenuation coefficients on CT, down to −100 Houndsfield units (HU), with the hair and desquamated epithelial debris producing higher numbers, up to +16 HU (Fig 18–2). Calcification of the wall may occur (Fig 18–3), or there may be more chunklike calcifications representing either vestigial or well-formed teeth. There is no enhancement of these low-density lesions.[7] On MRI, the fatty compo-

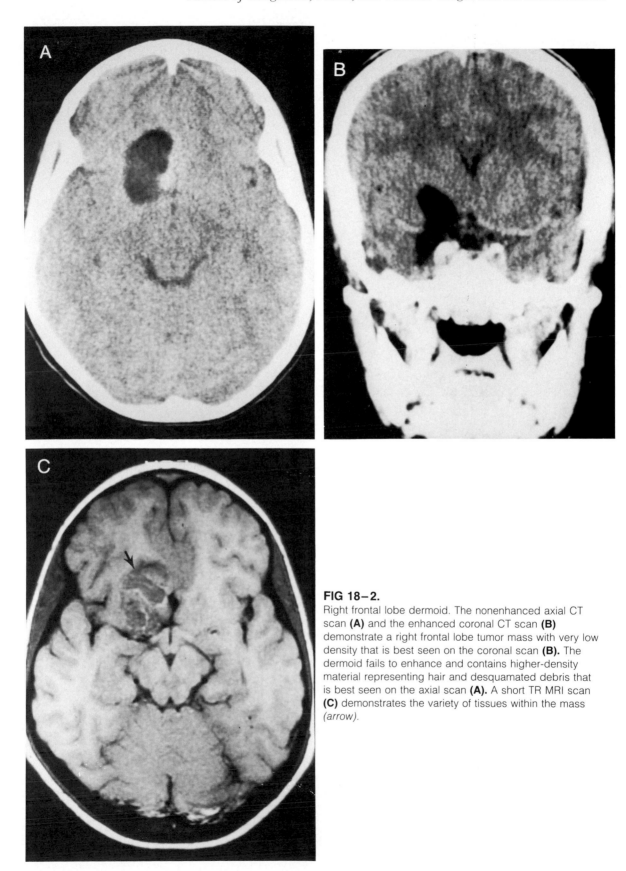

FIG 18–2.
Right frontal lobe dermoid. The nonenhanced axial CT scan **(A)** and the enhanced coronal CT scan **(B)** demonstrate a right frontal lobe tumor mass with very low density that is best seen on the coronal scan **(B).** The dermoid fails to enhance and contains higher-density material representing hair and desquamated debris that is best seen on the axial scan **(A).** A short TR MRI scan **(C)** demonstrates the variety of tissues within the mass *(arrow).*

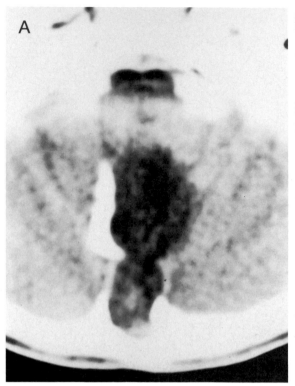
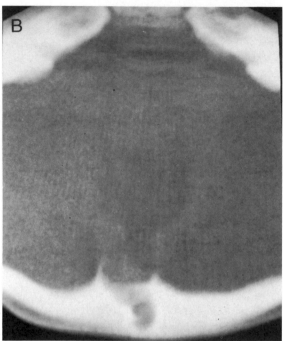

FIG 18–3.
Dermoid with a sinus tract. The nonenhanced axial CT scan with a soft-tissue window **(A)** shows a midline posterior fossa dermoid with calcification along its right lateral wall. A bone window **(B)** demonstrates the extension of the lesion through the bone to connect with a sinus tract in the scalp.

nents produce hyperintensity on short repetition time (TR) images that fades in intensity on the long TR sequences. The hair and glandular elements are closer to isointensity relative to the surrounding parenchyma.

Dermoid cysts are almost always located in or near the midline, which gives support to the theory of their development from an abnormality of the closure of the neural tube,[1] and therefore there may be associated midline abnormalities. For example, a dermoid of the posterior fossa may have an underlying dermal sinus connecting the cyst to the skin (Fig 18–3).[1] There may also be coloboma of the iris and retina[8] or other midline abnormalities.

Patients with intracranial dermoid present in a variety of fashions, including seizure disorder, hydrocephalus, or symptoms related to compression of contiguous neurologic structures.[7, 8] Rupture of a dermoid allows the sebaceous material to spread throughout the subarachnoid and/or ventricular spaces to produce a granulomatous meningitis that may be rapidly fatal.[1, 8, 9] The scan findings in such a case are those of the primary tumor along with fatty density in the subarachnoid spaces[5] or a fat–cerebrospinal fluid (CSF) level in the ventricular system (Fig 18–4).[8, 9]

Epidermoid

A congenital epidermoid is derived from ectoderm, but an acquired intraspinal epidermoid may occur following lumbar puncture that drives fragments of skin into the spinal canal. Both forms have a lining of simple stratified squamous eipthelium. There is progressive desquamation of keratinized material, which breaks down to form a thick waxy material rich in cholesterol.[1]

While these lesions may occasionally be present in the midline, such as within the fourth ventricle[10, 11] or within the suprasellar cisterns, they are generally eccentric in location, as opposed to the dermoid cyst.[1] The most common locations are the cerebellopontine angle,[12, 13] the apex of the petrous bone,[13] the middle cranial fossa, the suprasellar cisterns,[14] the diploic space of the calvarium, the fourth ventricle,[10, 11] intraspinal subarachnoid spaces, and within a lateral ventricle such as the

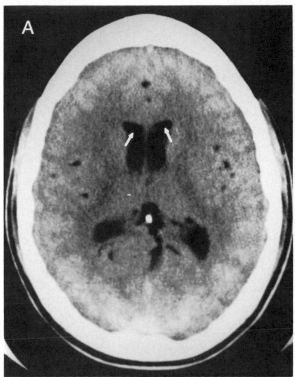 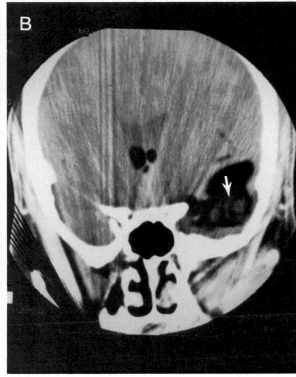

FIG 18–4.
Ruptured intracranial dermoid. Nonenhanced axial **(A)** and coronal **(B)** CT scans demonstrate the left temporal dermoid with very low density sebaceous secretions surrounding higher-density desquamated debris **(B,** *arrow*) and very low density fat within the subarachnoid spaces following rupture of the lesion. There is also in- traventricular fat, with CSF–fat fluid levels seen on the axial projection with the patient supine **(A,** *arrows*) and movement of that fat into the inferior portions of the frontal horns with the patient in the "hanging head position" for coronal scanning **(B).**

body or temporal horn.[1, 15] They grow into cisterns and crevices and may be present in two intracranial fossae such as the posterior and middle fossae. The petrous apex lesion is a congenital lesion, similar to the epidermoid of the calvarium, as opposed to the secondary cholesteotoma ("epidermoid") of the middle ear following chronic infection.[13]

The combination of desquamated epithelium and cholesterol produces CT attenuation coefficients close to that of CSF, with a range of approximately −5 to +20 HU.[7, 15, 16] The lack of fat, which produces attenuation coefficients down to −50 to −100 HU, differentiates this lesion from the dermoid or lipoma. Mural calcifications may be present as with the dermoid (Fig 18–5),[7, 15, 16] along with bony deformities reflecting the congenital nature of the lesion. When originating in the petrous apex, the lesion produces bone expansion and deformity indicative of its slow growth and bulges into the posterior and/or middle cranial fossae (Fig 18–6). The margins are commonly irregular because of both rupture of the cyst wall, thereby exposing the irregular internal architec-

ture (Fig 18–5), and the propensity to invaginate into crevices between normal tissues (Fig 18–7).

On MRI, an epidermoid is usually more intense than CSF on short TR images and very intense on the long TR sequences (Figs 18–7 and 18–8).[11, 12, 17, 18] It may be difficult to separate from surrounding CSF unless very long TR/echo time (TE) parameters are used (Figs 18–7 and 18–8). Water (and CSF) have among the longest T1 and T2 relaxation parameters in the body, and this fact may aid in the selection of scanning techniques that are optimum for defining the lesion.

Symptoms are usually related to local compression of neurologic structures, and there is no invasion of brain (Figs 18–5, 18–7, and 18–8). Because the mass is so slow growing, the epidermoid is usually large at the time of its discovery.[1] Malignant change with local invasion of brain is rare and is secondary to malignant degeneration of squamous epithelium to produce squamous cell carcinoma.[1, 19]

A major differential consideration is arachnoid cyst, which usually has more regular margins than

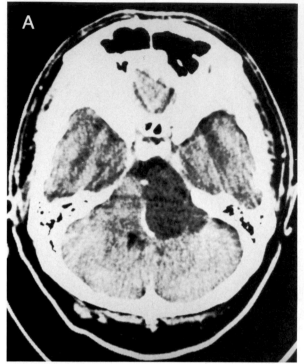

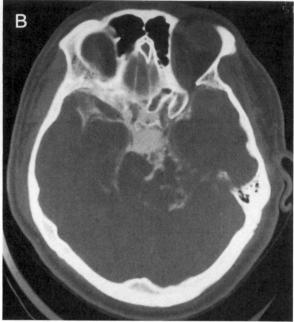

FIG 18–5.
Epidermoid with interstices demonstrated on CT cisternography. An axial CT scan through the posterior fossa demonstrates a large, low-density, well-circumscribed lesion in the left cerebellopontine angle and peripontine cistern. There is calcification in its medial wall. The density of the lesion is slightly greater than the CSF of the fourth ventricle or the prepontine cistern. There is pronounced compression and displacement of the brain stem and left cerebel-lar hemisphere. Following intrathecal injection of a water-soluble contrast agent, an axial CT scan through the mesencephalon with a "bone window" **(B)** demonstrates the irregular margin of the lesion. This irregular margination is secondary both to rupture of the capsule, which allows the contrast agent to pass into the lesion to demonstrate its "frondlike" character, and also to growth into parenchyma crevices.

FIG 18–6.
Epidermoid of the petrous apex. A long-standing expansion within the right petrous apex has totally eroded the apex and is expanding into both the posterior and middle cranial fossae. There is enhancement of the displaced dura, but the lesion has an internal density equal to CSF. These are the characteristics of a congenital petrous apex epidermoid cyst.

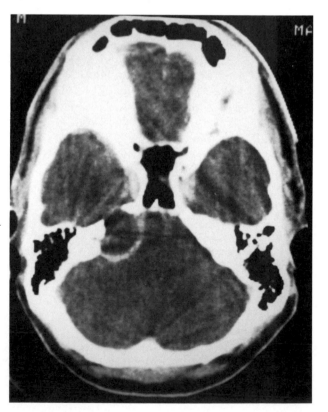

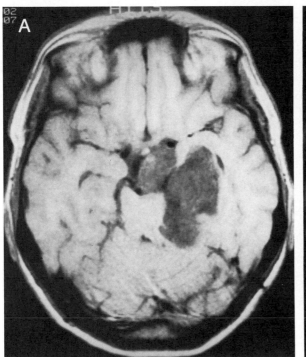 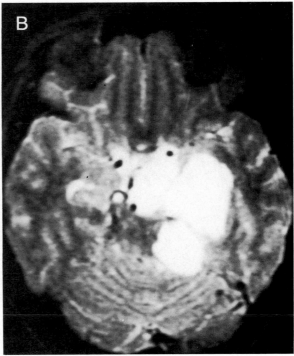

FIG 18–7.

Epidermoid invaginating into left temporal lobe, with intensity similar to CSF on a long TR/TE scan. The short TR scan (**A,** TR = 800, TE = 20) demonstrates the epidermoid, which is hypointense relative to cerebral parenchyma, within the suprasellar and perimesencephalic cisterns and invaginating deeply into the left temporal lobe. The lesion displaces cerebral parenchyma rather than invad-

ing it. On the long TR/TE sequence (**B,** TR = 2,500, TE = 100) the lesion has a similar intensity to the suprasellar CSF, which makes demarcation difficult except for the presence of hypointense arterial structures displaced by the mass. Even longer TR and TE values would be necessary to separate the suprasellar tumor from CSF.

does the epidermoid and does not have mural calcification (see Figs 17–25 to 17–31). The CT density of an arachnoid cyst is equal to CSF; the epidermoid may be slightly higher or lower. A "frondlike" appearance to the epidermoid is classically seen during pneumoencephalography because of the coating by air of the internal architecture of the cyst following capsular rupture. The same appearance may be seen with the use of positive-contrast or air cisternography and CT scanning (see Fig 18–5). On MRI, the arachnoid cyst behaves exactly like CSF, while the epidermoid has subtle intensity differences from CSF that require judicious selection of scanning parameters (Figs 18–7 and 18–8). Cholesterol granuloma of the petrous apex is hyperintense on the short TR sequence, unlike epidermoid's hypointensity. Both are hyperintense on the long TR/TE study.

Lipoma

The lipoma is probably due to abnormal differentiation of the primitive meninx[20] and is almost always located in the midline.[21] The most common locations are the genu and rostral body of the corpus callosum (Fig 18–9); the region of the pineal gland, splenium of the corpus callosum, quadrigeminal plate cistern, and velum interpositum (Fig 18–10); and the intraspinal subarachnoid spaces.[21–24] Midline dysraphism is very common with this congenital tumor, along with an absent septum pellucidum, partial or complete agenesis of the corpus callosum, agenesis of the cerebellar vermis, encephalocele, myelomeningocele, and spina bifida.[20–24] The majority of lipomas are clinically silent (Fig 18–9),[7, 21] with the patient's symptoms generally related to the associated dysraphic state.

These tumors are purely of fat density, with CT attenuation coefficients of −50 to −100 HU (Figs 18–10 and 18–11).[22–25] On MRI, hyperintensity is seen on the short TR sequence (Figs 18–9, 18–10, and 18–12) that fades on the long TR images (Fig 18–12).[26] There is no associated hair or keratinized tissue to give areas of CT density or MRI intensity different from fat, as with a dermoid cyst (see Figs 18–2 to 18–4). Calcifica-

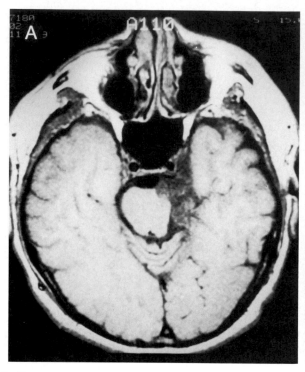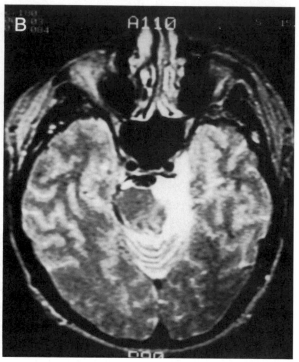

FIG 18–8.

MRI demonstration of the long T2 relaxation time of an epidermoid at the tentorial notch. The short TR scan (**A,** TR = 800, TE = 20) at the level of the tentorial notch demonstrates the epidermoid growing around the left side of the displaced brain stem as it passes through the tentorial notch, with extension of the epidermoid into Meckel's cave and the left cavernous sinus. The lesion is more in-

tense than the surrounding CSF. On the long TR/TE scan (**B,** TR = 2,500, TE = 75), the lesion cannot be separated from the surrounding CSF. Again, it is seen to extend into Meckel's cave. Separation of the lesion from CSF with its very long T2 relaxation time would require even longer TR and TE values.

FIG 18–9.

Lipoma capping the corpus callosum. A midline sagittal short TR image (TR = 600, TE = 20) demonstrates hyperintense lipomatous tissue capping the corpus callosum, which has normal thickness. Cerebral volume loss is present in this 82-year-old male being scanned for transient ischemia attacks.

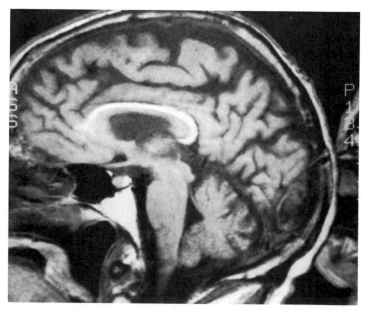

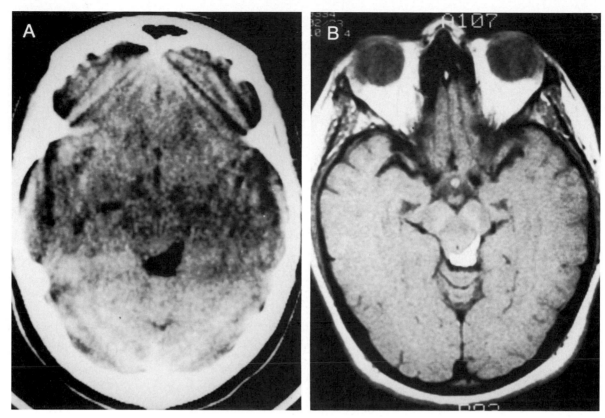

FIG 18–10.
Lipoma of the quadrigeminal plate. A nonenhanced axial CT scan **(A)** through the quadrigeminal plate demonstrates the typical density of a lipoma in the quadrigeminal plate cistern. CT density measured −90 HU. On short TR MRI (**B,** TR = 700, TE = 20), the lesion has a hyperintensity equal to orbital fat.

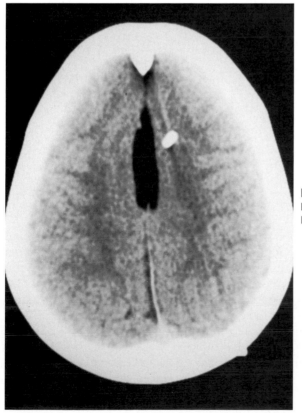

FIG 18–11.
Lipoma of the falx. A CT scan above the corpus callosum demonstrates a lipoma of the falx with a density of −85 HU.

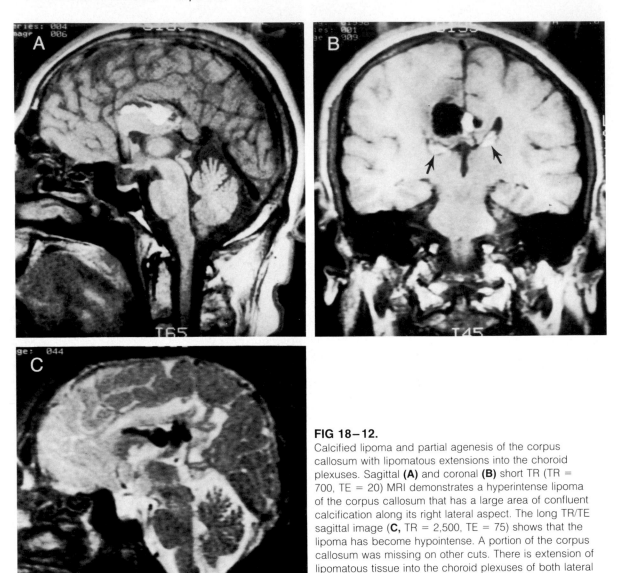

FIG 18–12.
Calcified lipoma and partial agenesis of the corpus callosum with lipomatous extensions into the choroid plexuses. Sagittal **(A)** and coronal **(B)** short TR (TR = 700, TE = 20) MRI demonstrates a hyperintense lipoma of the corpus callosum that has a large area of confluent calcification along its right lateral aspect. The long TR/TE sagittal image (**C,** TR = 2,500, TE = 75) shows that the lipoma has become hypointense. A portion of the corpus callosum was missing on other cuts. There is extension of lipomatous tissue into the choroid plexuses of both lateral ventricles (**B,** *arrows*).

tion at the periphery is a common finding, particularly with lipomas of the rostral corpus callosum (Fig 18–12).[23] The midline lipoma may also be associated with extensions of lipomas into the choroid plexus of one or both lateral ventricles (Fig 18–12).[24, 25] Change of head position may show a change of position of the choroidal lipomas as they float on the denser CSF.[24]

Theoretically, melanoma or the intracellular methemoglobin phase of hemorrhage might provide differential diagnostic difficulties on a signal pattern basis. However, the clinical history and morphology as well as the possible presence of other associated anomalies may help in differentiation. Furthermore, intracellular methemoglobin usually is part of a spectrum of signal intensities associated with the various phases of hemorrhage.

We should always be wary of the potential presence of Pantopaque, whose signal pattern may exactly follow that of a fatty-based tumor. This should not present a differential problem, however, for an intra-axial lipoma.

Hamartoma

A hamartoma is a focus of mature but disorganized or ectopic tissue. Two groups of hamartomatous lesions are of particular interest in this chapter. The first is the hamartoma that is generally attached by a thick stalk to the tuber cinereum or mammillary bodies. This lesion more commonly occurs in the male and produces precicious puberty.[27, 28] On the nonenhanced CT scan, it is isodense to brain parenchyma and is nonenhancing or minimally enhancing, which makes it difficult to define on a routine CT scan. Contrast CT cisternography is of great value in defining this mass (Fig 18–13). On MRI the mass is isointense to gray matter on short TR scans and isointense to slightly hyperintense on the long TR sequences; detection depends upon perception of the isointense mass. Enhancement would not be expected.

The second group of hamartomas of interest here are those of the phakomatoses. These will be discussed later in this chapter.

PINEAL REGION TUMORS

The term *pinealoma* refers to a group of neoplasms occurring in the pineal region, not to a single neoplasm. Included are the teratoid tumors, in-

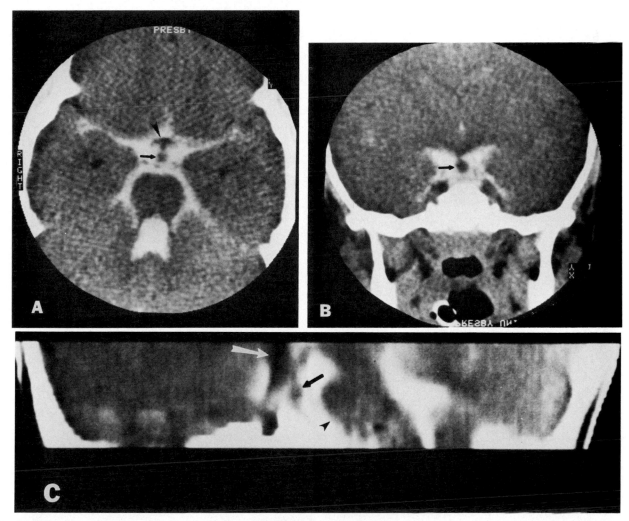

FIG 18–13.
Hamartoma of the tuber cinereum. Axial **(A)** and direct coronal **(B)** scans were performed during Amipaque cisternography. The sagittal view **(C)** is a reformatted image. There is a small mass (*black arrow,* **A–C**) that appears on the axial scan to be attached by a stalk to the posterior margin of the optic chiasm (*large arrowhead,* **A**). The sagittal image shows to good advantage the attachment of the stalk to the tissue behind the third ventricle (tuber cinereum). The third ventricle is indicated in **C** by the *white arrow,* with the *small arrowhead* denoting the pons. Multiple views with Amipaque allow for a complete evaluation of the relationships of the small mass to contiguous structures.

cluding the teratoma, germinoma ("atypical teratoma," which is the most common tumor in this region),[29, 30] epidermoid, and dermoid; embryonal cell carcinoma with its variant the endodermal sinus tumor and choriocarcinoma[31]; neuroepithelial tumors of pineal cell origin, the pineocytoma and pineoblastoma[32]; neuroepithelal tumors of glial origin, particularly astrocytoma; and lipoma. Meningioma may also extend into the region from an attachment to the falx-tentorial junction.

A number of pineal region tumors have distinctive clinical or radiologic findings. For example, the pineal region is the most common location for the intracranial teratoma,[3] which has an admixture of tissue types including fatty elements, muscle and other soft tissues, calcification, and teeth (see Fig 18–9). Lipomas occur in the pineal gland or in the region of the quadrigeminal cistern (see Fig 18–10), velum interpositum, or splenium of the corpus callosum[21] and project into the pineal area; these lesions are characterized by their uniformly low CT attenuation coefficients and the hyperintensity of fat on short TR MRI. Dermoids also have fat characteristics on CT and MRI, but have nonhomogeneous elements representing glands, follicles, and desquamated debris. Epidermoid tumors have mural calcification and are closer to CSF density and intensity characteristics than are dermoid cysts (see Fig 18–5). Germinomas account for over 50% of pineal tumors,[29, 30] while the neoplasms of pineal cell origin (pineoblastoma and pineocytoma) account for less than 20%. Teratomatous tumors, including teratoma, germinoma, and embryonal cell carcinoma, and the pineoblastoma are more common in males.[29–33]

Calcification of pineal tumors is a frequent but nonspecific finding. In one series, 75% of all pineal region tumors contained calcification, including two thirds of germinomas and 80% of pineal cell neoplasms.[34] Because the majority of pineal region tumors occur during childhood, the lower age limit for pineal calcification has been evaluated on both plain skull films and CT scans, the latter being more sensitive to the presence of small amounts of calcification than plain films are. Small specks of normal pineal calcification can be seen in children

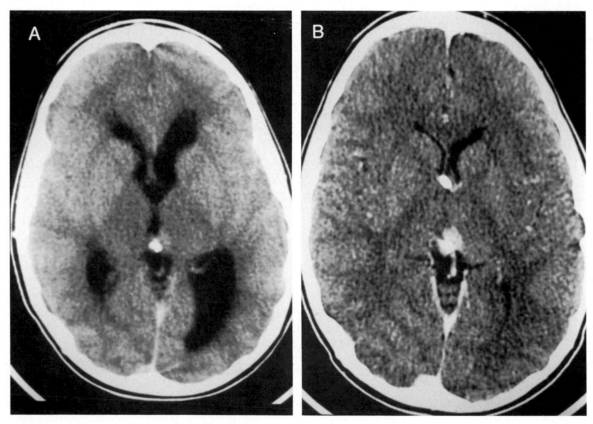

FIG 18–14.
Pineal region germinoma. An unenhanced CT scan **(A)** demonstrates an isodense soft-tissue mass surrounding pineal calcification in this 16-year-old male. The mass indents the posterior portion of the third ventricle and produces a mild degree of ventricular enlargement, the left greater than the right. Eleven months later, an enhanced CT scan **(B)** following shunting (tip of the shunt tube at the foramina of Monro) demonstrates homogeneous enhancement of the small lesion.

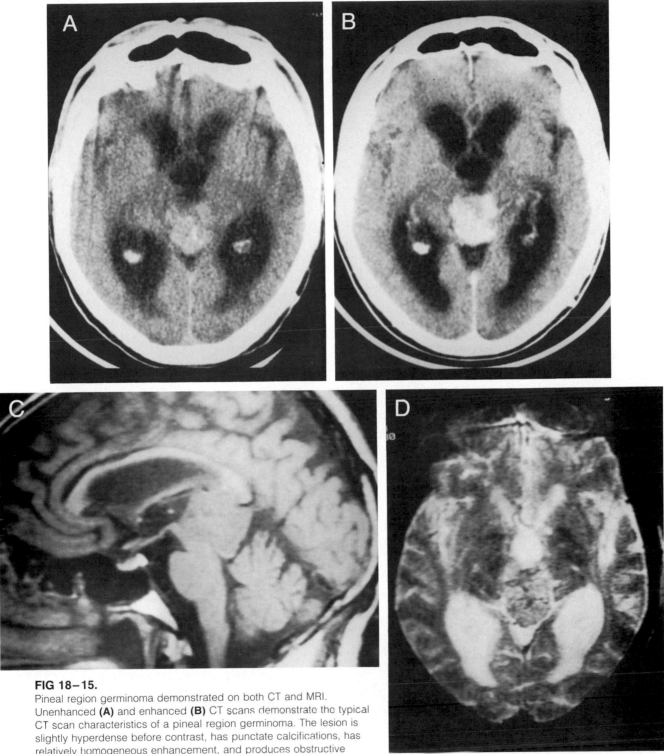

FIG 18–15.
Pineal region germinoma demonstrated on both CT and MRI.
Unenhanced **(A)** and enhanced **(B)** CT scans demonstrate the typical
CT scan characteristics of a pineal region germinoma. The lesion is
slightly hyperdense before contrast, has punctate calcifications, has
relatively homogeneous enhancement, and produces obstructive
hydrocephalus. Short TR MRI **(C,** TR = 600, TE = 20), performed 2
days later, demonstrates a lesion that is minimally hypointense relative
to gray matter. There is excellent demonstration of the relationships of
this tumor to the compressed third ventricle and aqueduct on this
midline sagittal image. The long TR/TE study **(D,** TR = 2,500, TE = 100)
shows the lesion to be relatively isointense to gray matter.

as young as 6 years, with normal pineal calcification rarely visualized as early as 2 years of age. In general, pineal calcification below the age of 6 years suggests the possibility of a pineal region tumor[35]; other authors utilize 10 years of age as the lower limit, with the upper limit of size being 1 cm.[34]

Germinomas typically have a slight increase in their density on the preinfusion CT scan and marked homogeneous enhancement (Figs 18–14 and 18–15).[33, 36] The margins may be relatively sharp, or they may be irregular, indicative of infiltration into surrounding tissues. Embryonal cell carcinoma and tumors of pineal cell origin (Fig 18–16) have a similar CT appearance to germinoma.[30] It is usually not possible to make a preoperative diagnosis of a specific histologic variety of germ cell tumor on the basis of CT characteristics alone.

Glial tumors may originate in the pineal gland or in the thalamus or mesencephalic tectum. These tumors are generally of isodensity to low density before contrast and enhance to a mild to moderate degree (Fig 18–17), generally with an inhomogeneous character so typical of low-grade glial tumors.[30] Meningioma has its typical homogeneous enhancement (Fig 18–18); sagittal or coronal reformations are helpful in defining its extrapineal origin.

The multiple planes of MRI are excellent for demonstrating the relationship of the pineal region mass to contiguous structures such as the quadrigeminal plate and aqueduct. However, calcification is not as easily detected by MRI as by CT. Since the presence of pineal calcification below the age of 6 years, even without a mass, may be the only clue to the diagnosis of neoplasm, CT remains the screening procedure of choice in the young patient, with MRI added as necessary.[37] MRI of pineal tumors demonstrates that germinoma is nearly isointense with brain parenchyma on both short and long TR sequences (see Fig 18–15). Embryonal cell carcinoma and pineoblastoma may have slightly lower intensity on short TR images and hyperintensity to brain parenchyma on long TR sequences.[37] Glioma typically shows isointensity to low intensity on short TR images and hyperintensity on long TR sequences relative to gray matter (Fig 18–17). Meningioma is isointense to gray matter on short TR studies and isointense to mildly hyperintense on long TR scans. Germinomas enhance vividly with gadolinium–diethylenetriamine pentaacetic acid (DTPA), and the other tumors usually enhance to an equal or lesser degree. Thus, early work suggests that there may be some differential signal patterns on MRI between the various tissue types.[37] However, many pineal germ cell tumors contain an admixture of tissue types, and significantly greater experience will be necessary before definitive statements regarding MRI signal characteristics of specific tissue types can be made.

A nonneoplastic cyst of the pineal gland may develop and produce a mass effect, thereby simulate a pineal neoplasm. MRI is ideal for evaluating such a cyst. The cyst contents usually have MRI characteristics similar to CSF rather than a solid neoplasm.[38] The sharp marginations of a cyst, the lack of abnormal pericystic tissue, and the lack of contrast enhancement further support a diagnosis of nonneoplastic pineal cyst.

Confusion has arisen with the term *ectopic pinealoma*, which refers to a germinoma present in the suprasellar region and is thought to represent a

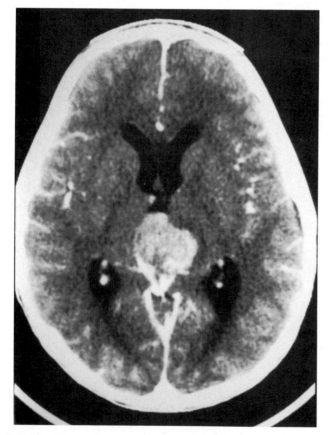

FIG 18–16.
Pineoblastoma in a 5-year-old male with Parinaud's syndrome. An enhanced axial CT scan demonstrates a homogeneously enhancing pineal region tumor that histologically was a pineoblastoma, although it has similar CT scan characteristics to germinoma.

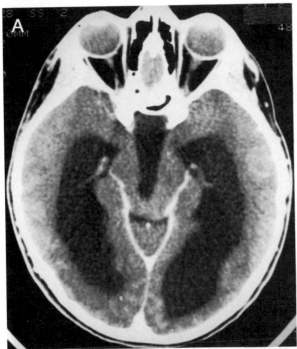

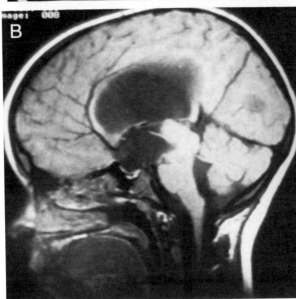

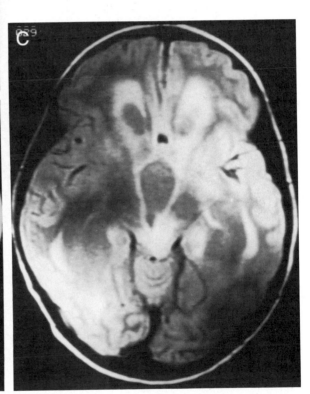

FIG 18–17.
Pineal region glioma. An enhanced axial CT scan **(A)** demonstrates an isodense mass lesion obstructing the aqueduct and producing dilatation of the third and lateral ventricles. Short TR sagittal MRI (**B,** TR = 800, TE = 25) demonstrates the mass to be slightly hyperintense relative to gray matter, pushing into the posterior portion of the third ventricle, and completely obstructing the aqueduct. The relationship of the tumor to the surrounding structures is exquisitely demonstrated. The proton-density axial MRI study (**C,** TR = 2,500, TE = 25) shows hyperintensity of the mass lesion relative to the surrounding gray matter and to the third ventricular CSF, which is relatively hypointense due to the presence of turbulence in the obstructed state. There is extensive transependymal CSF flow producing periventricular hyperintensity.

metastatic extension of a pineal region tumor. Some patients with suprasellar germinomas do indeed have pineal region tumors (Fig 18–19), and germinomas are known to seed throughout the neural axis via CSF pathways. However, a suprasellar germinoma may occur independently of a pineal region germinoma (Figs 18–20 and 18–21), and germinomas are known to occur in extracranial midline locations such as the mediastinum. With an abnormality of the closure of the neural tube, it is quite possible that germinomas and other ter-

atomatous lesions may form in either the pineal or suprasellar regions or both.[29, 30] Germinomas may also occur in a paramedian location, including the basal ganglia and thalamus.[39]

Controversy has long existed as to the role of surgery vs. radiation therapy without biopsy for the treatment of pineal region tumors. The surgical approach to this region is difficult and may produce a relatively high degree of morbidity/mortality. In addition, many of the "pinealomas" are radiosensitive, including the most common variety, the ger-

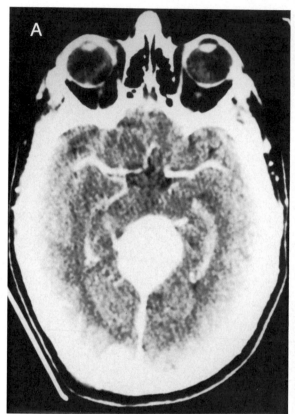

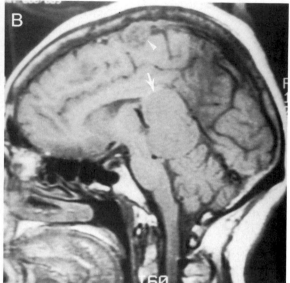

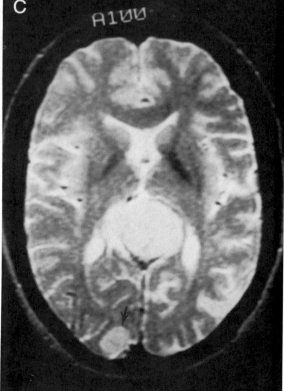

FIG 18–18.
Pineal region meningioma. This pineal region
meningioma more than likely originated from the
junction of the falx and tentorium. An enhanced CT
scan **(A)** demonstrates the typical homogeneous
intense enhancement of meningioma. Short TR,
midline sagittal MRI **(B,** TR = 600, TE = 20)
demonstrates isointensity to gray matter, typical of
meningioma *(arrow)*. The long TR study **(C,** TR =
2,750, TE = 80) shows moderate hyperintensity
relative to gray matter along with a second
meningioma *(arrow)* in the right occipital region. The
second meningioma is slightly hyperintense relative to
surrounding gray matter and was difficult to perceive
on the enhanced CT scan due to bony artifact, but is
seen in retrospect. There appears to be a third
meningioma high over the anterior parietal convexity
on the midsagittal scan **(B,** *arrowhead)*.

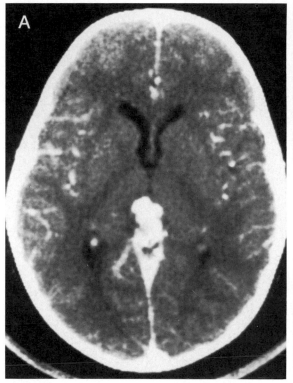

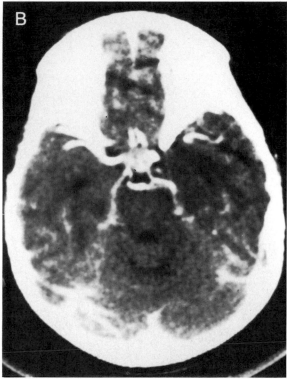

FIG 18–19.
Pineal region and suprasellar germinomas. Enhanced CT scans at the level of the pineal gland **(A)** and through the suprasellar cistern **(B)** demonstrate homogeneously enhancing germinomas in each location. Whether the suprasellar tumor represents a metastatic lesion from the pineal region tumor or whether there are two independent lesions is conjectural.

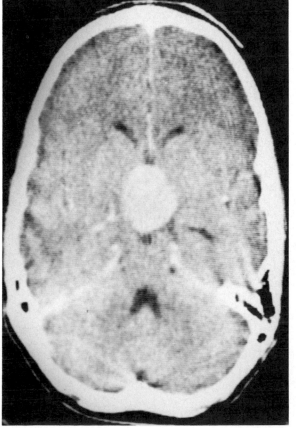

FIG 18–20.
Suprasellar germinoma. This axial enhanced CT scan demonstrates the typical appearance of a suprasellar intensely and homogeneously enhancing, well-marginated germinoma in the suprasellar cisterns that is projecting up into the third ventricle.

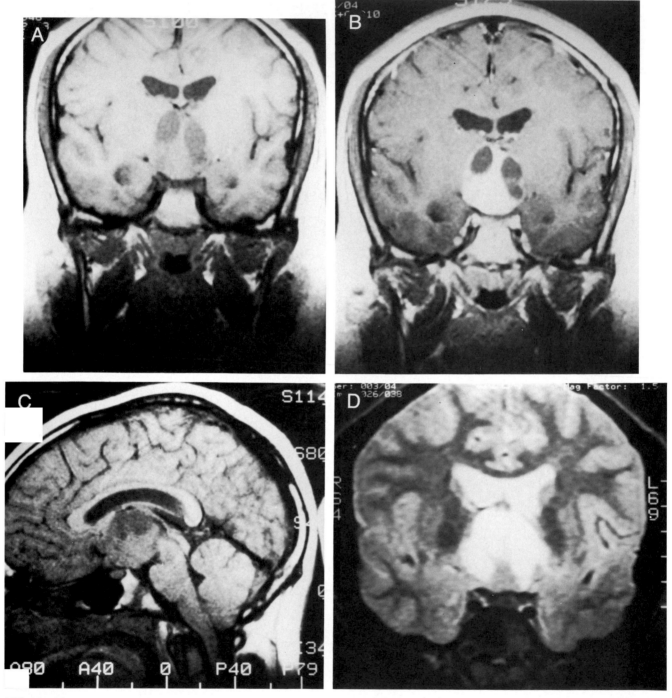

FIG 18–21.
Suprasellar germinoma demonstrated on MRI. Coronal short TR MRI (TR = 500, TE = 20) both before **(A)** and after **(B)** the administration of gadolinium-DTPA demonstrates a large mass lesion that is predominately isointense to surrounding parenchyma but contains two large cystic areas. There is intense homogeneous enhancement of the solid components but not the two cysts. Midsagittal short TR MRI (**C,** TR = 500, TE = 20) without enhancement demonstrates a mass lesion that is predominantly isointense to gray matter but contains large areas of hypointensity more superiorly. The long TR coronal study (**D,** TR = 2,875, TE = 80) demonstrates the diffuse hyperintensity of both the cystic and solid components. It would be impossible to differentiate germinoma from glioma on these MRI studies.

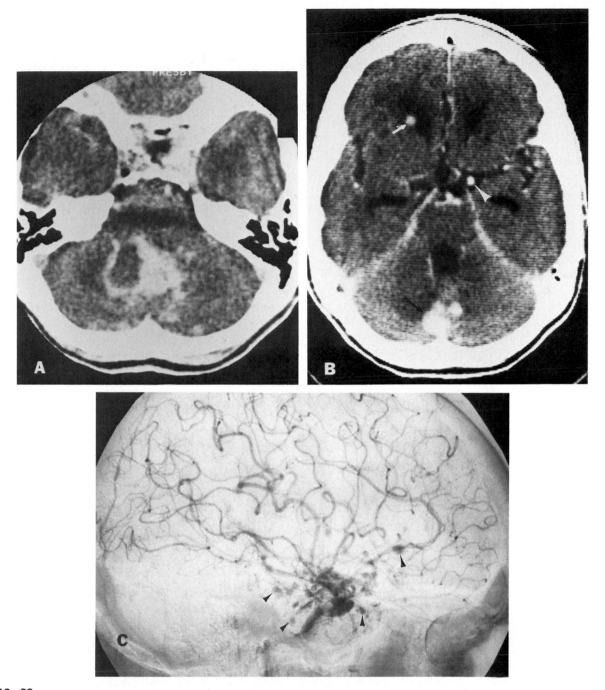

FIG 18–22.

Cerebellar hemangioblastoma with multiple supratentorial hemangioblastomas. The scan through the midportion of the cerebellum **(A)** demonstrates a large intensely enhancing mass lesion located within the cerebellar vermis and right cerebellar hemisphere. The mass is primarily solid, with an internal cyst. A higher cut **(B)** demonstrates the superior portion of the cerebellar hemangioblastoma *(black arrow)* located in the posterior portion of the cerebellar vermis. There are multiple enhancing nodules supratentorially located in the subarachnoid cisterns *(white arrowhead)* and right frontal horn *(white arrow)*. There may also be other nodules in the sylvian fissures that simulate vascular structures. A right carotid angiogram **(C)** demonstrates multiple staining nodules within the basal portions of the brain and subarachnoid cisterns, some of which are marked by *arrowheads*.

minoma, as well as pineal cell neoplasms and embryonal cell carcinoma.[30, 40] In a number of institutions, CT-guided stereotactic biopsy has given the histologic diagnosis with extremely low morbidity; this diagnostic procedure is followed by radiation therapy for a sensitive histologic type.

TUMORS OF VASCULAR ORIGIN

Hemangioblastoma

Although metastatic tumor is the most common cerebellar neoplasm in the adult, hemangioblastoma is the most common primary cerebellar neoplasm in this age group and accounts for 7% to 12% of all adult posterior fossa tumors when considering both primary and metastatic neoplasms.[41] While this tumor is associated with the von Hippel–Lindau syndrome, only approximately 20% of patients presenting with hemangioblastoma have the other manifestations of the syndrome, which include angioma of the retina (von Hippel's disease), nonneoplastic cysts of the pancreas and kidney, neoplasms of the kidney (in particular, hypernephroma) and adrenal glands (especially pheochromocytoma), and hemangioblastomas of the spinal cord.[42, 43] There may also be transitional links with the multiple endocrine neoplasia (MEN) syndrome; hence, coexistant retinal angioblastoma and paraganglioma has been reported.[42] Supratentorial hemangioblastoma has been described,[44] but the majority of such cases have probably been angioblastic meningiomas.[42] Rarely, one may see hemangioblastomas in both the infratentorial and supratentorial compartments, with this multiplicity indicative of the von Hippel–Lindau syndrome (Fig 18–22).[44, 45] Polycythemia is common in patients with hemangioblastoma, and erythopoietin has been demonstrated in the cyst fluid.[42]

Hemangioblastoma presents in three forms on the CT scan. The most common, accounting for approximately 50% of cases,[46] is that of a large cystic lesion with a mural nodule (Fig 18–23), which simulates a cystic astrocytoma of childhood. For a given size cyst, the nodule of astrocytoma is larger than that for hemangioblastoma. In addition, the thinness of the cyst wall in many cases of hemangioblastoma is helpful in differentiation from metastasis,[47] the other common adult cerebellar tumor. The nodule generally enhances homogeneously to a marked degree. The nodule may be quite small in comparison to the large cystic component[41, 47] and require multiple overlapping cuts and close scrutiny for identification. The other 50%

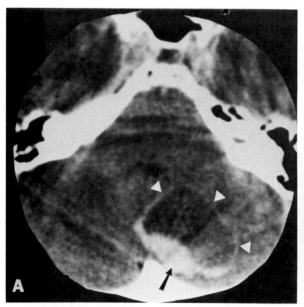
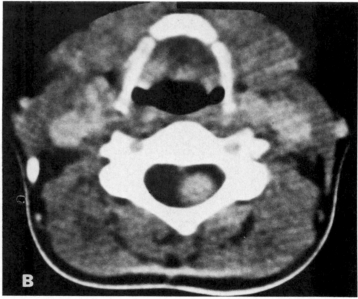

FIG 18–23.

Cerebellar and spinal cord cystic hemangioblastomas in the von Hippel–Lindau syndrome. An enhanced axial scan of the posterior fossa **(A)** demonstrates a large cystic mass *(arrowheads)* with a small mural nodule *(arrow)* that stains intensely and is located within the cerebellar vermis and left cerebellar hemisphere. A scan through the upper cervical spinal canal **(B)** following intravenous contrast enhancement demonstrates a large cystic expansion within the spinal canal and an intensely staining nodule to the left of the midline.

of tumors are split between a diffusely enhancing mass containing cystic areas (Figs 18–22 and 18–24) and a totally solid homogeneous lesion without cyst formation (Figs 18–25 and 18–26),[46] both simulating metastasis. The relative lack of edema with hemangioblastoma may help differentiate these forms of the tumor from metastasis, and the presence of feeding vessels is literally pathognomonic of hemangioblastoma (Fig 18–25).

MRI demonstrates the cystic component(s), whether the primary portion of the lesion with a mural nodule or surrounded by a peripheral solid component, to have low intensity on short TR images, usually slightly more intense than CSF due to a higher protein content, and hyperintensity on long TR sequences (Figs 18–26 and 18–27). The solid component, whether the lesion is totally solid, has central cystic areas, or is a mural nodule on the periphery of a larger cyst, is typically isointense to slightly hypointense on short TR images and become hyperintense on long TR/TE sequences (Figs 18–26 and 18–27).[48] The solid com-

ponents enhance dramatically with gadolinium (Fig 18–28). Flow void signals characteristic of rapidly flowing feeding vessels may be seen and, in conjunction with a cystic lesion containing a mural nodule, are pathognomonic of hemangioblastoma (Figs 18–26 and 18–27).[48] Hemorrhage from the hypervascular nodule may give the typical hyperintensity on both short and long TR sequences of methemoglobin or the marked hypointensity of hemosiderin.[48] Depending on its morphology, hemosiderin might be confused with flow voids of vascular structures or the hypointensity of conglomerate calcification.

The lesion is well circumscribed, and there is generally little if any surrounding cerebral edema. The mass effect, which is frequently due to the large cystic component, may produce obstructive hydrocephalus. Classically, there is intense staining of the nodular component of the tumor at angiography, and angiography is better than CT at demonstrating single or multiple small lesions.[41] Enhanced MRI with thin cuts (Fig 18–28) may be

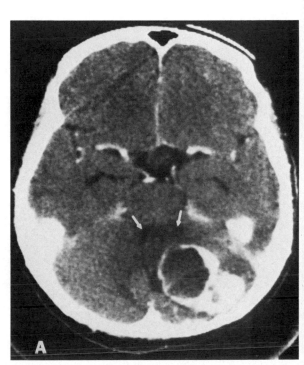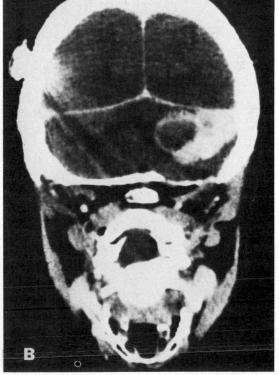

FIG 18–24.

Hemangioblastoma with an internal cyst. Rather than primarily a cyst with a mural nodule as in Figure 18–23, this hemangioblastoma is predominantly a solid tumor with an internal cyst as dem-

onstrated on both the axial **(A)** and coronal **(B)** projections. There is compression of the fourth ventricle (*arrows,* **A**) and extension of the mass to the underside of the tentorium.

FIG 18–25.
Solid hemangioblastoma. There is a solid well-circumscribed mass in the region of the fourth ventricle. The enhancement is intense and homogeneous, and there are contiguous vascular structures *(arrows).* Angiographically and histologically, this was a classic hemangioblastoma. (Courtesy of Louis Scotti, M.D., St. Francis General Hospital, Pittsburgh.)

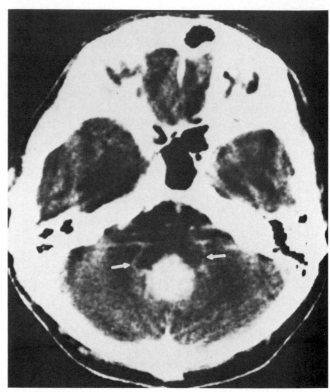

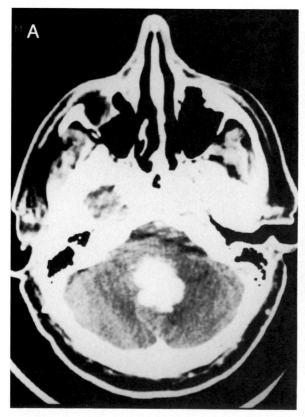

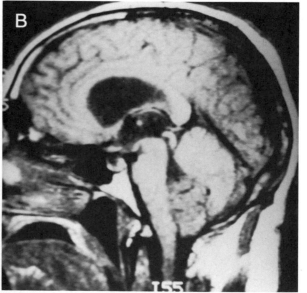

FIG 18–26.
Solid hemangioblastoma with feeding arteries detected on MRI. An axial enhanced CT scan **(A)** demonstrates the solid, intensely enhancing hemangioblastoma just below the fourth ventricle. Midsagittal, short TR MRI **(B,** TR = 700, TE = 20) shows the lesion below the fourth ventricle to be mildly hypointense to surrounding parenchyma and to have a number of linear hypointense structures representing feeding arteries coursing through the tumor.

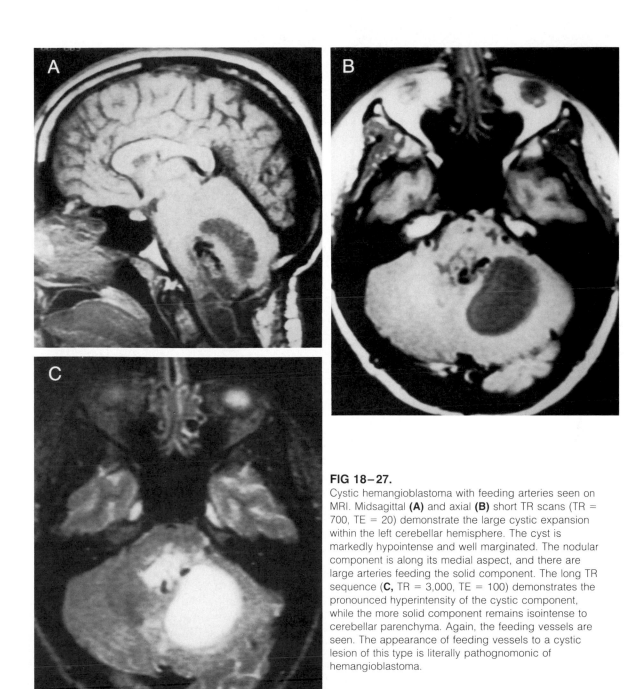

FIG 18–27.
Cystic hemangioblastoma with feeding arteries seen on MRI. Midsagittal **(A)** and axial **(B)** short TR scans (TR = 700, TE = 20) demonstrate the large cystic expansion within the left cerebellar hemisphere. The cyst is markedly hypointense and well marginated. The nodular component is along its medial aspect, and there are large arteries feeding the solid component. The long TR sequence **(C,** TR = 3,000, TE = 100) demonstrates the pronounced hyperintensity of the cystic component, while the more solid component remains isointense to cerebellar parenchyma. Again, the feeding vessels are seen. The appearance of feeding vessels to a cystic lesion of this type is literally pathognomonic of hemangioblastoma.

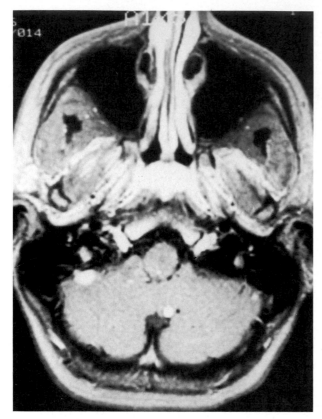

FIG 18–28.
Multiple small hemangioblastoma nodules demonstrated with enhanced MRI. This T1-weighted axial sequence (TR = 700, TE = 20) was performed following the administration of gadolinium-DTPA. A small nodule is seen near the right petrous bone, a second in the vermis, and a few tiny dots of hyperintensity in both cerebellar hemispheres and in the brain stem. Enhanced thin-section MRI may be the most sensitive technique for detecting tiny nodules.

equal in sensitivity to angiography for the detection of small nodules.

Spinal cord scans reveal similar lesions (see Fig 18–23). All patients with hemangioblastoma require excretory urography to exclude hypernephroma.

Cavernous Hemangioma

Cavernous hemangioma is a type of blood vessel hamartoma and is therefore related to arteriovenous malformation, capillary telangiectasia, and venous angioma. It is an uncommon lesion and may produce intracranial hemorrhage or present as a mass with focal neurologic deficit and/or seizures.[49] A familial form is well recognized.[50, 51]

On CT, the lesion generally is dense without the use of contrast material because of its "blood pool," although the presence of hemorrhage, fibro-

sis, and calcification may also play a role in this increased density (Fig 18–29,A). The degree of contrast enhancement varies from none to marked (Fig 18–29,B), and the amount of mass effect is generally minimal or none.[52–55] This hamartomatous lesion generally has a rounded configuration, and it may be impossible to distinguish this lesion preoperatively on the CT scan from meningioma, glioma, or simple intracerebral hemorrhage. The possibility could be suggested by a combination of an intraparenchymal location, sharply defined borders, increased density before enhancement, and an unchanged appearance on sequential CT scans.

MRI suggests that this lesion is more common than previously recognized and may be an important cause of intracerebral hemorrhage. Short TR scans demonstrate one or more well-circumscribed lesions with the hyperintensity of subacute/chronic blood (Fig 18–30). Long TR sequences show a hyperintense lesion with a low-intensity rim of hemorsiderin (Figs 18–29 and 18–30).[51] Gradient-echo sequences with low flip angles and moderate to long TEs of 20 ms or more are most sensitive at detecting such foci of hemosiderin from old hemorrhage (Figs 18–29 and 18–30). The characteristic signal patterns are therefore that of a well-circumscribed lesion with evidence of repeated hemorrhages. The lesion may grow or involute, only to grow again with another hemorrhage.[56]

PHAKOMATOSES (DYSGENETIC SYNDROMES)

The diseases herein considered are all associated with neoplasms and/or hamartomas of the CNS and have a hereditary basis. There is clinical overlap among the various phakomatoses, such as café au lait spots of the skin occurring in both neurofibromatosis and tuberous sclerosis, and less frequently in other disorders. There are a number of recorded cases with other forms of clinical and pathologic overlap indicative of the close relationship of these syndromes.[57, 58] The neoplasms and/or hamartomas of these syndromes are emphasized in this section; discussion of the hereditary patterns and extracranial manifestations of the phakomatoses is beyond the scope of this book.

The Neurofibromatoses

Two distinct forms of neurofibromatosis have long been recognized,[58] but the terms *central* and

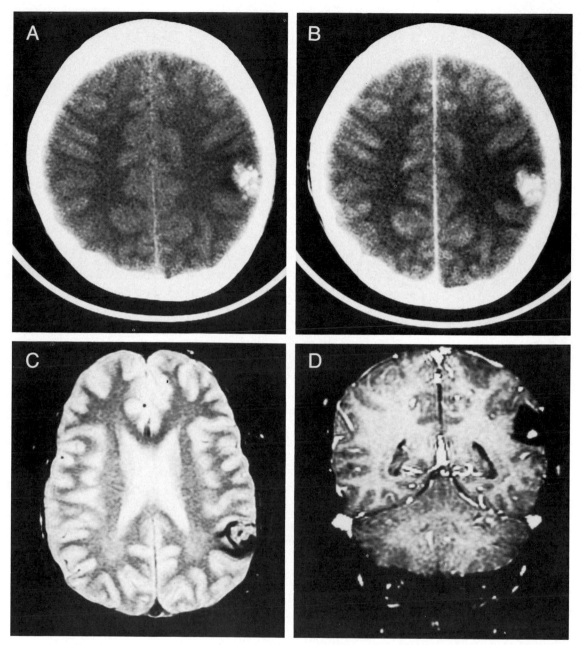

FIG 18–29.
Calcified cavernous hemangioma with an MRI demonstration of an old hemorrhage. There is a calcified mass lesion on the unenhanced CT scan **(A)** in the anterior left parietal lobe. There is only a mild degree of enhancement **(B).** Long TR MRI (**C,** TR = 2,500, TE = 75) shows pronounced hypointensity around the periphery of the lesion that is characteristic of hemosiderin from an old hemorrhage. The coronal gradient-echo study **(D)** is the most sensitive at detecting the deposits of hemosiderin and calcification.

peripheral are confusing. The National Institutes of Health Consensus Development Conference on neurofibromatosis has established neurofibromatosis, type 1 (NF-1, von Recklinghausen's disease), and neurofibromatosis, type 2 (NF-2, bilateral acoustic neurofibromatosis), as distinct disorders among several proposed categories.[59] These two disorders appear to be genetically distinct, with NF-1 having an abnormality of chromosome 17 and NF-2 having an abnormality on the long arm of chromosome 22.[58, 60]

The following are the characteristics of NF-1[60–62]: six or more café au lait spots; pigmented hamartomas of the iris (Lisch nodules); neurofibromas of peripheral and autonomic nerves; optic gliomas; astrocytomas of the cerebral and cerebellar

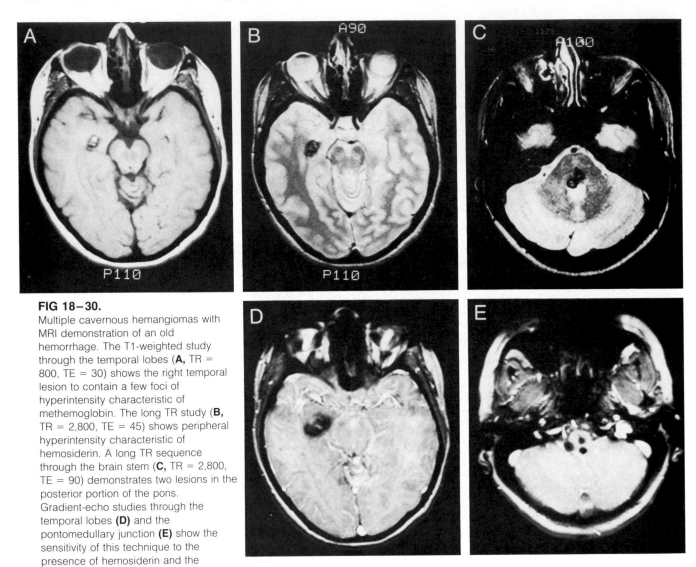

FIG 18–30.
Multiple cavernous hemangiomas with MRI demonstration of an old hemorrhage. The T1-weighted study through the temporal lobes (**A,** TR = 800, TE = 30) shows the right temporal lesion to contain a few foci of hyperintensity characteristic of methemoglobin. The long TR study (**B,** TR = 2,800, TE = 45) shows peripheral hyperintensity characteristic of hemosiderin. A long TR sequence through the brain stem (**C,** TR = 2,800, TE = 90) demonstrates two lesions in the posterior portion of the pons. Gradient-echo studies through the temporal lobes (**D**) and the pontomedullary junction (**E**) show the sensitivity of this technique to the presence of hemosiderin and the multiplicity of lesions.

hemispheres and the brain stem; "hamartomas" (foci of prolonged hyperintense signal on long TR/TE studies without significant mass effect, most notably in the cerebellar peduncles, with a lesser incidence in the brain stem, globus pallidus, thalamus, and lesser still in the cerebral white matter)[63–65]; and bony lesions with or without underlying tumors, specifically pseudoarthroses of long bones, arcuate kyphoscoliosis, and dysplasias of the sphenoid bone. The neoplasms of NF-1 therefore appear to be primarily those of astrocytes and neurons.

The pathologic findings in NF-2 are distinctly different and are as follows[60–62]: bilateral acoustic neurofibromas; multiple intracranial meningiomas; schwannomas of cranial nerves besides the 13th nerve; no parenchymal gliomas; spinal meningio-

mas and schwannomas; and occasionally peripheral nerve tumors, although much less frequently than with NF-1. In summary, NF-2 appears to be a disease primarily of the coverings of the brain and nerves, i.e., neoplasms of the meninges and Schwann cells.

As can be seen, the use of the term *central* would be confusing since NF-2 has intracranial extra-axial tumors and NF-1 has both optic glioma and parenchymal astrocytomas.[60]

The MRI and CT appearances of each of these tumors have been previously described in Chapters 16 and 17. The unusual aspects are their multiplicity and associations (Figs 18–31 and 18–32). A few additional points should be made, however. First, patients with NF-1 have a high incidence of

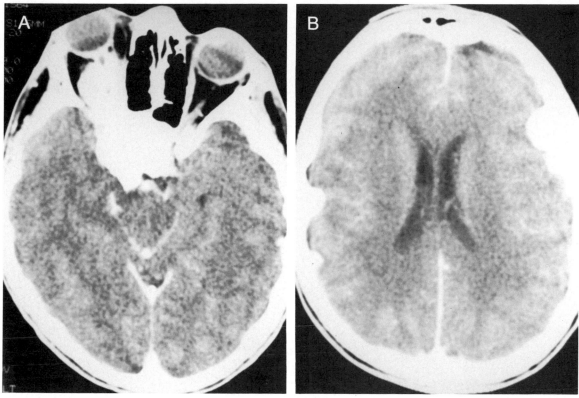

FIG 18–31.
Neurofibromatosis (NF-2) with multiple meningiomas. An enhanced CT scan at the level of the orbits **(A)** demonstrates a densely en-hancing suprasellar, parasellar, and right intra-orbital meningioma. A higher cut **(B)** shows multiple convexity meningiomas.

optic pathway gliomas, varying from 10% to 70% according to the series, but may be asymptomatic.[60] Therefore, a baseline MRI scan in any patient with known or suspected NF-1, even if asymptomatic for optic pathway disease, is strongly recommended. Second, hyperintense areas within the cerebellum, brain stem, basal ganglia, and cerebral white matter have been seen primarily on long TR studies but occasionally on short TR sequences in patients with NF-1.[64] These foci of abnormal signals appear to represent areas of heterotopia, hamartomatous tissue, or gliosis. However, they could represent subtle, low-grade gliomas, and hence serial MRI both without and with gadolinium-DTPA is recommended. Third, a patient with neurofibromatosis and macrocephaly may have head enlargement because of unilateral or bilateral megalencephaly, which is commonly associated with areas of heterotopic or hamartomatous tissue, or because of an occult periaqueductal glioma producing hydrocephalus. Enhanced MRI is therefore recommended. Fourth, the unusual location of choroidal calcification is a feature of neurofibromatosis and may be a key finding suggesting the diagnosis (Fig 18–33). Fifth, MRI may help differentiate optic nerve glioma from optic nerve sheath ectasia, which can be seen with the syndrome.

Tuberous Sclerosis (Bourneville's Disease)

Tuberous sclerosis is characterized clinically by seizures and mental retardation; cutaneous lesions including adenoma sebaceum, café au lait spots, and shagren patches; osseous lesions including cystic areas in the phalanges and flame-shaped cortical densities in periarticular locations; and the presence of tubers and patches of demyelinization in the brain. A tuber is a form of hamartoma and contains both neurons and astrocytes, with many of the latter being of giant size.[58] Tubers occur on the cortical surface and in subependymal locations. The classic appearance is the presence of raised foci of tissue below the ependymal surface of the lateral ventricles ("candle guttering"). These tubers are particularly common near the foramina of Munro, where CSF obstruction may occur.

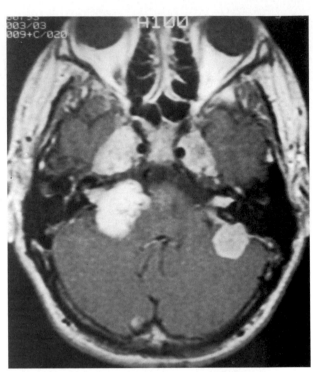

FIG 18–32.
Multiple gadolinium-enhancing acoustic schwannomas and parasellar meningiomas in a patient with NF-2. The short TR scan (TR = 600, TE = 20) performed after an injection of gadolinium-DTPA demonstrates bilateral eighth nerve tumors, a meningioma along the left petrous bone, and bilateral parasellar meningiomas.

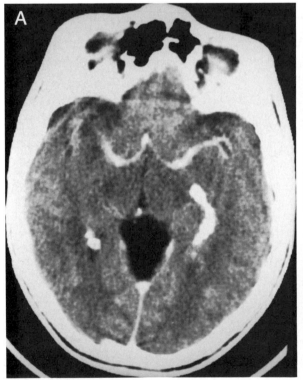

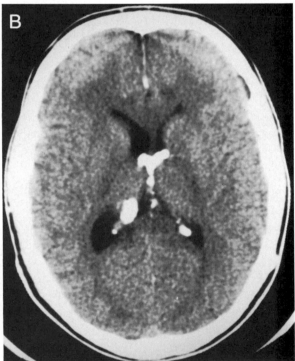

FIG 18–33.
Unusual locations of choroidal calcification in patients with neurofibromatosis. In the first patient **(A)** there is calcification along the choroid plexus within the left temporal horn. In the second patient **(B)** there is extensive calcification of choroid extending into the foramina of Monro. Both patients have neurofibromatosis.

Subependymal tubers are usually isodense to slightly hyperdense on an unenhanced CT scan and frequently calcify (Figs 18–34 and 18–35). The appearance of multiple subependymal calcifications on CT is classic for tuberous sclerosis and diagnostic even with a lack of more typical clinical features of this syndrome (up to 16% of cases have subependymal calcifications without more obvious skin lesions[66]). Multiple subependymal calcifications may also occur with one of the intrauterine inflammatory conditions such as toxoplasmosis or cytomegalic inclusion disease (see Chapter 24), but the inflammatory process generally produces other cerebral abnormalities such as hydrocephalus, microcephaly, areas of encephalomalacia, etc. Cortical tubers usually have a mixed low-density and isodensity pattern (Figs 18–34 and 18–35). Calcification of these tubers may also occur (Fig 18–34).

Tubers are usually isointense to gray matter on unenhanced short TR MRI (Fig 18–36,A). Hyperintensity is usually seen on long TR/TE sequences and may blend with ventricular CSF.[67, 68] Calcifi-

cations may be missed on MRI unless they are large and homogeneous (Fig 18–36,B).[68] MRI demonstrates the cortical tubers much better than does CT (Fig 18–36).[68] In addition, hyperintense areas on long TR/TE scans are seen in the subcortical and deep white matter (Fig 18–36,B)[67, 68]; these correspond to subtle low-density areas on CT and are thought to represent areas of hamartomatous tissue.

A tuber may undergo degeneration to a giant-cell astrocytoma,[58] and it is therefore extremely important to perform scanning both with and without contrast administration. Lesional enhancement demonstrates an abnormal blood-brain barrier and indicates that the mass is neoplastic and not a simple tuber with an intact blood-brain barrier (Figs 18–35, 18–37, and 18–38).[67]

von Hippel–Lindau Syndrome

This autosomal dominant syndrome consists of hemangioblastomas of the cerebellum, spinal cord,

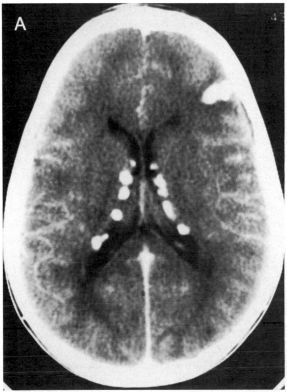
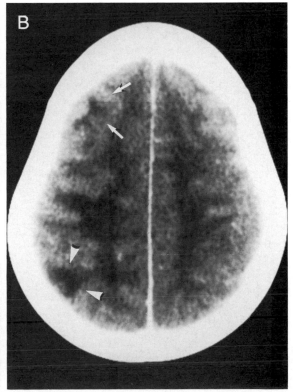

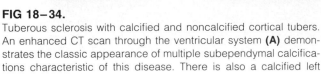

FIG 18–34.
Tuberous sclerosis with calcified and noncalcified cortical tubers. An enhanced CT scan through the ventricular system **(A)** demonstrates the classic appearance of multiple subependymal calcifications characteristic of this disease. There is also a calcified left frontal cortical tuber. A higher cut **(B)** demonstrates a mixed pattern of hypodensity and isodensity in a right frontal tuber *(arrows)* and a low-density cortical tuber in the right parietal region *(arrowheads)*.

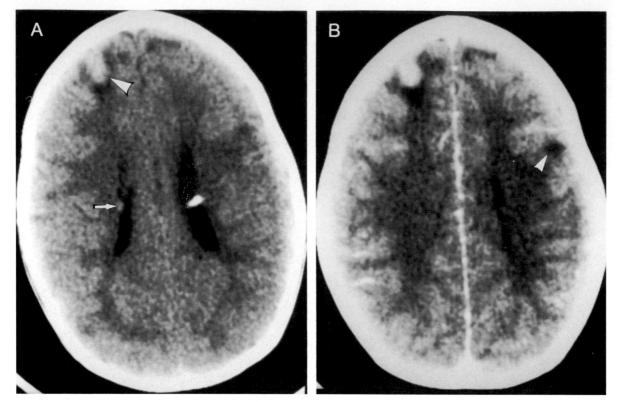

FIG 18—35.
Tuberous sclerosis with calcified and noncalcified subependymal tubers, a nonenhancing cortical tuber, and an enhancing cortical astrocytoma. The unenhanced scan **(A)** demonstrates a noncalcified isodense subependymal tuber along the body of the right lateral ventricle *(arrow)*. There is a calcified tuber along the left ventricle. A nodular density in the right frontal region is slightly hyperdense *(arrowhead)*. The enhanced scan **(B)** at a slightly higher level demonstrates homogeneous enhancement of this right frontal nodule; this represents breakdown of the blood-brain barrier, which is indicative of a giant-cell astrocytoma. There is a small low-density cortical tuber in the posterior left frontal region *(arrowhead)*.

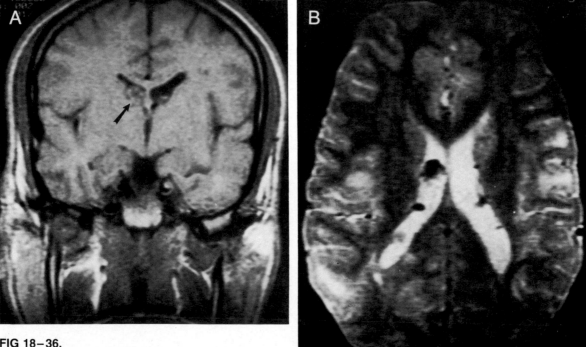

FIG 18—36.
MRI demonstration of subependymal and cortical tubers and white matter "hamartomas." The coronal T1-weighted image **(A,** TR = 700, TE = 20) shows an isodense tuber filling a portion of the right frontal horn *(arrow)*. The axial long TR image **(B,** TR = 2,500, TE = 100) demonstrates that a number of the subependymal tumors contain enough homogeneous calcification for the calcium to be visible. There are multiple hyperintense cortical tubers in both cerebral hemispheres. There is also hyperintensity in the subcortical white matter of the parietal lobes and in the deeper white matter of the right parietal lobe, which is indicative of hamartomatous tissue.

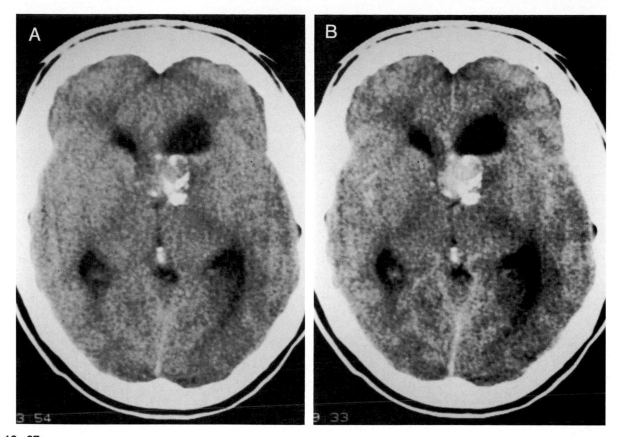

FIG 18–37.
Enhancing giant-cell astrocytoma in a patient with tuberous sclerosis. The unenhanced scan **(A)** shows calcification of a large isodense mass in the region of the foramina of Monro. There is mod-

erate enhancement on the enhanced study **(B)** in this patient with known tuberous sclerosis, and this is indicative of neoplastic degeneration.

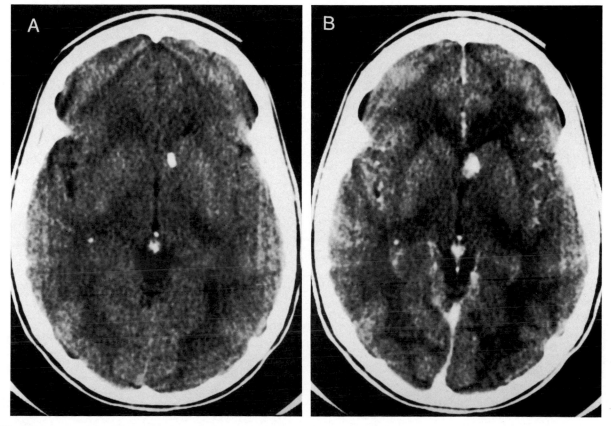

FIG 18–38.
Enhancement of a subtle subependymal mass in a patient with tuberous sclerosis. The unenhanced scan **(A)** demonstrates an area of calcification in the region of the left caudate nucleus. There is

enhancement of this lesion **(B)**. The patient has known tuberous sclerosis, and the enhancement is indicative of the degeneration of tuber into a giant-cell astrocytoma.

and rarely of the supratentorial structures (see Figs 18–12 to 18–15); retinal angiomas (von Hippel's disease); and various cysts and neoplasms of the abdominal viscera, most notably hypernephroma of the kidney and pheochromocytoma of the adrenal gland.[42, 43] Only approximately 20% of patients with hemangioblastoma are part of this diffuse syndrome. As previously discussed, hemangioblastoma presents with three appearances: a mural nodule within a cystic lesion, a solid enhancing neoplasm, and an enhancing tumor containing multiple cystic areas (see Figs 18–12 to 18–15).[41, 46–48]

Sturge-Weber Syndrome (Encephalotrigeminal Angiomatosis)

Sturge-Weber syndrome consists of blood vessel hamartoma formation involving the face and the ipsilateral cerebral hemisphere. Bilateral hemispheric involvement occurs occasionally (Fig 18–39). The cutaneous abnormality is a port-wine stain involving the cutaneous distribution of the ophthalmic division of the trigeminal nerve. Congenital buphthalmos and glaucoma may also be present.[58] The intracranial abnormality is a capil-

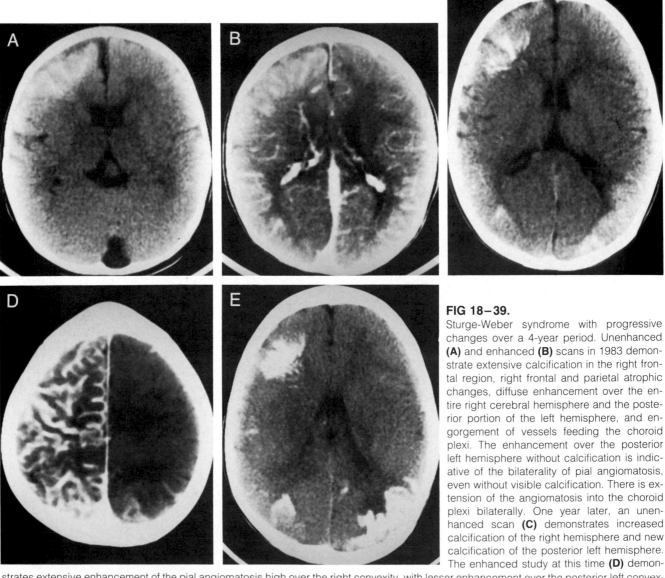

FIG 18–39.
Sturge-Weber syndrome with progressive changes over a 4-year period. Unenhanced **(A)** and enhanced **(B)** scans in 1983 demonstrate extensive calcification in the right frontal region, right frontal and parietal atrophic changes, diffuse enhancement over the entire right cerebral hemisphere and the posterior portion of the left hemisphere, and engorgement of vessels feeding the choroid plexi. The enhancement over the posterior left hemisphere without calcification is indicative of the bilaterality of pial angiomatosis, even without visible calcification. There is extension of the angiomatosis into the choroid plexi bilaterally. One year later, an unenhanced scan **(C)** demonstrates increased calcification of the right hemisphere and new calcification of the posterior left hemisphere. The enhanced study at this time **(D)** demonstrates extensive enhancement of the pial angiomatosis high over the right convexity, with lesser enhancement over the posterior left convexity. Three years later, a nonenhanced CT scan demonstrates further deposition of calcium in both cerebral hemispheres.

lary-venous malformation involving the pia and underlying cerebral cortex,[58] typically in the parieto-occipital region, although a frontal lobe distribution is occasionally seen. Calcifications in the deep layers of the cortex occur in the region of the malformation and produce parallel and wavy densities ("tramline") on skull films.

The CT scan findings are that of extensive calcification, which has the same wavy appearance as seen on the plain skull films (Figs 18–39 and 18–40), and focal or hemispheric atrophy (Fig 18–40).[69, 70] Occasionally, one may see areas of contrast enhancement representing the pial vascular malformation (Fig 18–39).[71] There may also be enlargement and increased enhancement of the choroid plexus on the side of the lesion that represent further angiomatous malformation (Figs 18–39 and 18–40).[70]

MRI does not allow visualization of the calcification as easily as does CT.[69] However, it more clearly demonstrates thickened cortex, abnormal convolutions, and abnormal white matter signals.[69, 71]

Neurocutaneous Melanosis

The predominant feature of this rare disease is the presence of an increased number of melanin-containing cells within areas of the skin and meninges.[58] Melanoma of the meninges may occur and have an appearance on CT of a homogeneously enhancing extra-axial tumor simulating meningioma.[72, 73] To our knowledge, a description of the MRI appearance of this disorder has yet to be made. However, metastatic melanoma to the CNS has a unique appearance of decreased T1 and T2 relaxation times due to the presense of melanin, hemorrhage, or both. Meningeal melanosis may have a similar appearance. If so, hyperintensity to gray matter on short TR scans and hypointensity on the long TR/TE sequence would be expected to be present. Marked enhancement with gadolinium-DTPA would parallel the CT enhancement pattern.

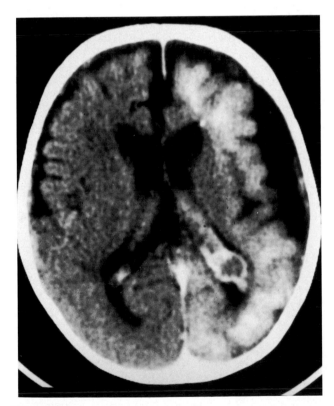

FIG 18–40.
Bilateral Sturge-Weber syndrome with pronounced atrophy and involvement of the choroid plexus. This enhanced CT scan demonstrates pronounced increased density throughout the atrophic left cerebral hemisphere, which may be a combination of both calcification and enhancement of the pial angiomatosis. There is lesser atrophy and no enhancement of the right frontal lobe, but bilateral involvement is probably present. There is enhancement of an enlarged left ventricular choroid plexus secondary to angiomatous involvement.

REFERENCES

1. Russell DS, Rubenstein LJ (eds): *Pathology of Tumours of the Nervous System.* Baltimore, Williams & Wilkins, 1989, pp 691–695.
2. Smith AS: Myth of the mesoderm (letter). *AJNR* 1989; 10:449.
3. Russell DS, Rubenstein LJ (eds): *Pathology of Tumours of the Nervous System.* Baltimore, Williams & Wilkins, 1989, pp 681–687.
4. Uken P, Sato Y, Smith W: MR findings of malignant intracranial teratoma in a neonate. *Pediatr Radiol* 1986; 16:504–505.
5. Waters DC, Venes JL, Zis K: Case report: Childhood cerebellopontine angle teratoma associated with congenital hydrocephalus. *Neurosurgery* 1986; 18:784.
6. Friedman AC, Pyatt RS, Hartman DS, et al: CT of benign cystic teratomas. *AJR* 1982; 138:659–665.
7. Zimmerman RA, Bilaniuk LT, Dolinhas C: Cranial tomography of epidermoid and congenital fatty tumors of maldevelopmental origin. *J Comput Assist Tomogr* 1979; 3:40–50.
8. Murphy JJ, Risk WX, Van Geldes JC: Intracranial dermoid cyst in Goldenhar's syndrome. *J Neurosurg* 1980; 53:408–410.
9. Healy JF, Brahme FJ, Rosenkrantz H: Dermoid

cysts and their complications as manifested by computed cranial tomography. *Comput Tomogr* 1980; 4:111–115.

10. Rosario M, Becker DH, Conley FK: Epidermoid tumors involving the fourth ventricle. *Neurosurgery* 1981; 9:9–13.

11. Yuh WTC, Barloon TJ, Jacoby CG, et al: MR of fourth-ventricular epidermoid tumors. *AJNR* 1988; 9:794–796.

12. Gentry LR, Jacoby CG, Turski PA, et al: Cerebellopontine angle—Petromastoid mass lesions: Comparative study of diagnosis with MR imaging and CT. *Radiology* 1987; 162:513–520.

13. Latack JT, Kartush JM, Kemink JL, et al: Epidermoidomas of the cerebellopontine angle and temporal bone: CT and MR aspects. *Radiology* 1985; 157:361–366.

14. Vion-Dury J, Vincentelli F, Juddane M, et al: MR imaging of epidermoid cysts. *Neuroradiology* 1987; 29:333–338.

15. Chambers AA, Lybin RR, Tomsick TA: Cranial epidermoid tumors: Diagnosis by computed tomography. *Neurosurgery* 1977; 1:276–279.

16. Davis KR, Roberson GH, Taveras JM: Diagnosis of epidermoid tumors by computed tomography. *Radiology* 1976; 119:347–353.

17. Olson JJ, Beck DW, Crawford SC, et al: Comparative evaluation of intracranial epidermoid tumors with computed tomography and magnetic resonance imaging. *Neurosurgery* 1987; 21:357.

18. Tampieri D, Melanson D, Ethier R: MR imaging of epidermoid cysts. *AJNR* 1989; 10:351–356.

19. Dubois PJ, Sage M, Luther JS, et al: Malignant change in an intracranial epidermoid cyst. *J Comput Assist Tomogr* 1981; 5:443–445.

20. Budka H: Intracranial lipomatous hamartomas (intracranial "lipomas"). *Acta Neuropathol (Berl)* 1974; 28:205–222.

21. Russell DS, Rubenstein LJ (eds): *Pathology of Tumours of the Nervous System.* Baltimore, Williams & Wilkins, 1989, pp 706–708.

22. Faerber EN, Wolpert SM: The value of computed tomography in the diagnosis of intracranial lipomata. *J Comput Assist Tomogr* 1978; 2:297–299.

23. Zee C-S, McComb JG, et al: Lipoma of the corpus callosum associated with frontal dysraphism. *J Comput Assist Tomogr* 1981; 5:201–205.

24. Yock DH: Choroid plexus lipomas associated with lipoma of the corpus callosum. *J Comput Assist Tomogr* 1980; 4:678–682.

25. Buxi TBS, Mathur RK, Doda SS: Computed tomography of lipoma of corpus callosum and choroid plexus lipoma: Report of two cases. *J Comput Tomogr* 1987; 11:57–60.

26. Kean DM, Smith MA, Douglas HB, et al: Two examples of CNS lipomas demonstrated by computed tomography and low field (0.08T) MR imaging. *J Comput Assist Tomogr* 1985; 9:494–496.

27. Russell DS, Rubenstein LJ (eds): *Pathology of Tumours of the Nervous System.* Baltimore, Williams & Wilkins, 1989, pp 710–714.

28. Diebler C, Ponsot G: Hamartomas of the tuber cinereum. *Neuroradiology* 1983; 25:93–101.

29. Russell DS, Rubenstein LJ (eds): *Pathology of Tumours of the Nervous System.* Baltimore, Williams & Wilkins, 1989, pp 665–676.

30. Zimmerman RA, Bilaniuk LT, Wood JH, et al: Computed tomography of pineal, parapineal, and histologically related tumors. *Radiology* 1980; 137:669–677.

31. Russell DS, Rubenstein LJ (eds): *Pathology of Tumours of the Nervous System.* Baltimore, Williams & Wilkins, 1989, pp 677–681.

32. Russell DS, Rubenstein LJ (eds): *Pathology of Tumours of the Nervous System.* Baltimore, Williams & Wilkins, 1989, pp 380–394.

33. Chang T, Teng MMH, Guo W-Y, et al: CT of pineal tumors and intracranial germ-cell tumors. *AJNR* 1989; 10:1039–1044.

34. Lin SR, Crane MD, Lin ZS, et al: Characteristics of calcification of tumors of the pineal gland. *Radiology* 1980; 126:721–726.

35. Zimmerman RA, Bilaniuk LT: Age-related incidence of pineal calcification detected by computed tomography. *Radiology* 1982; 142:659–662.

36. Futrell NN, Osborn AG, Cleson BD: Pineal region tumors: Computed tomographic–pathologic spectrum. *AJNR* 1981; 2:415–420.

37. Kilgore DP, Strother CM, Starshak RJ, et al: Pineal germinoma: MR imaging. *Radiology* 1986; 158:435–438.

38. Lee DH, Norman D, Newton TH: MR imaging of pineal cysts. *J Comput Assist Tomogr* 1987; 11:586–590.

39. Kobayashi T, Kageyama N, Kida Y, et al: Unilateral germinomas involving the basal ganglia and thalamus. *J Neurosurg* 1981; 55:55–62.

40. Inoue Y, Takeuchi T, Tamaki M, et al: Sequential CT observations of irradiated intracranial germinomas. *AJR* 1979; 132:361–365.

41. Seeger JF, Burke DP, Knake JE, et al: Computed tomographic and angiographic evaluation of hemangioblastomas. *Radiology* 1981; 138:65–73.

42. Russell DS, Rubenstein LJ: Tumours of vascular origin, in *Pathology of Tumours of the Nervous System.* Baltimore, Williams & Wilkins, 1989, pp 639–651.

43. Russell DS, Rubenstein LJ: Von Hippel–Lindau disease, in *Pathology of Tumours of the Nervous System.* Baltimore, Williams & Wilkins, 1989, pp 784–787.

44. Tomasello F, Albanese V, Iannotti F, et al: Supratentorial hemangioblastoma in the child: Case report. *J Neurosurg* 1980; 52:578–583.

45. Diehl PR, Simon L: Supratentorial intraventricular

hemangioblastoma: Case report and review of the literature. *Surg Neurol* 1981; 15:435–443.

46. Naidich TP, Lin JP, Leeds NE, et al: Primary tumors and other masses of the cerebellum and fourth ventricle: Differential diagnosis by computed tomography. *Neuroradiology* 1977; 14:153–174.

47. Ganti SR, Silver AJ, Hilal SK, et al: Computed tomography of cerebellar hemangioblastomas. *J Comput Assist Tomogr* 1982; 6:912–919.

48. Lee SR, Sanches J, Mark AS, et al: Posterior fossa hemangioblastomas: MR imaging. *Radiology* 1989; 171:463–468.

49. Russell DS, Rubenstein LJ (eds): *Pathology of Tumours of the Nervous System.* Baltimore, Williams & Wilkins, 1989, pp 730–735.

50. Bicknell JM, Carlow TJ, Kornfeld M, et al: Familial cavernous angiomas. *Arch Neurol* 1978; 35:746–749.

51. Rigamonti D, Drayer BP, Johnson PC, et al: The MRI appearance of cavernous malformations (angiomas). *J Neurosurg* 1987; 67:518–524.

52. Ishikawa M, Handa H, Moritake D, et al: Computed tomography of cerebral cavernous hemangiomas. *J Comput Assist Tomogr* 1980; 4:587–591.

53. Pozzati E, Padorani R, Morrone B, et al: Cerebral cavernous angiomas in children. *J Neurosurg* 1980; 53:826–836.

54. Bartlett JE, Kishore PRS: Intracranial cavernous angioma. *AJR* 1977; 128:653–656.

55. Ahmadi J, Miller CA, Segall HD, et al: CT patterns in histologically complex cavernous hemangiomas. *AJNR* 1985; 6:389–393.

56. Pozzati E, Giuliani G, Poppi M: Growth of cerebral cavernous angiomas. *Neurosurgery* 1989; 25:92–97.

57. Bouge M, Pasquini V, Salvalini U: CT findings of atypical forms of phakomatosis. *Neuroradiology* 1980; 20:99–101.

58. Russell DS, Rubenstein LJ (eds): *Pathology of Tumours of the Nervous System.* Baltimore, Williams & Wilkins, 1989, pp 766–808.

59. National Institutes of Health Consensus Development. Neurofibromatosis. *Arch Neurol* 1988; 45:575–578.

60. Aoki S, Barkovich AJ, Nishimura K, et al: Neurofibromatosis types 1 and 2: Cranial MR findings. *Radiology* 1989; 172:527–534.

61. Riccardi VM: Neurofibromatosis. *Neurol Clin* 1987; 5:337–349.

62. Huson SM: The different forms of neurofibromatosis. *Br Med J* 1987; 294:1113–1114.

63. Bognanno JR, Edwards MK, Lee TA, et al: Cranial MR imaging in neurofibromatosis. *AJNR* 1988; 9:461–468.

64. Mirowitz SA, Sartor K, Gado M: High-intensity basal ganglia lesions on T1-weighted MR images in neurofibromatosis. *AJNR* 1989; 10:1159–1163.

65. Hurst RW, Newman SA, Cail WS: Multifocal intracranial MR abnormalities in neurofibromatosis. *AJNR* 1988; 9:293–296.

66. Kingsley DPE, Kendall BE, Fitz CR: Tuberous sclerosis: A clinicoradiological evaluation of 110 cases with particular reference to atypical presentation. *Neuroradiology* 1986; 28:38–46.

67. Altman NR, Purser RK, Post MJD: Tuberous sclerosis: Characteristics at CT and MR imaging. *Radiology* 1988; 167:527–532.

68. Nixon JR, Houser OW, Gomez MR, et al: Cerebral tuberous sclerosis: MR imaging. *Radiology* 1989; 170:869–873.

69. Chamberlain MC, Press GA, Hesselink JR: MR imaging and CT in three cases of Sturge-Weber syndrome: Prospective comparison. *AJNR* 1989; 10:491–496.

70. Stimac GK, Solomon MA, Newton TH: CT and MR of angiomatous malformations of the choroid plexus in patients with Struge-Weber disease. *AJNR* 1986; 7:623–627.

71. Jacoby CG, Yuh WTC, Afifi AK, et al: Accelerated myelination in early Sturge-Weber syndrome demonstrated by MR imaging. *J Comput Assist Tomogr* 1987; 11:226–231.

72. Tamura M, Kanafuchi J, Nagaya T, et al: Primary leptomeningeal melanoma with epipharyngeal invasion. *Acta Neurochir* 1981; 58:59–66.

73. Lamas E, Lobato RD, Sotelo T, et al: Neurocutaneous melanomas. *Acta Neurochir* 1977; 36:93–105.

19

Metastases

Richard E. Latchaw, M.D.

David W. Johnson, M.D.

Emanuel Kanal, M.D.

Metastatic involvement of the brain takes many forms, ranging from hematogenous metastases to the brain and meninges, direct spread to the brain and meninges from primary tumors of the skull base and face, or intracranial dissemination of primary and secondary brain tumors via cerebrospinal fluid (CSF) pathways. Likewise, metastases may primarily involve the bones of the calvarium or skull base.

This chapter will be divided into four sections, beginning with hematogenous metastases to the brain and meninges. The involvement of the brain and meninges by systemic lymphoma and leukemia warrants a separate section because there is a characteristic pattern of initial meningeal involvement followed by infiltration into the contiguous parenchyma. Bony involvement is divided into metastatic lesions involving the calvarium and metastases to the base of the skull. Finally, dissemination of primary and secondary tumors to other portions of the brain via the CSF will be discussed.

HEMATOGENOUS METASTASES TO THE BRAIN AND MENINGES

The most common primary tumors producing intracranial metastases are carcinoma of the lung and breast, malignant melanoma, lymphoma, and leukemia; less common are carcinoma of the kidney, paranasal sinuses, stomach, prostate, and thyroid, and the various sarcomas.[1, 2] Hematogenous metastases are frequently to the gray matter/white matter junction (Figs 19–1 and 19–2), probably because they impact in small arterioles.[1] Metastatic involvement of the deeper parenchymal structures is also frequent, probably for the same reason (Fig 19–2). Metastases to the brain stem (Fig 19–3) and choroid plexus are significantly less common.[3, 4]

The findings on the unenhanced computed tomographic (CT) scan are extremely variable. Areas of low density have been seen, particularly with metastases from carcinomas of the lung, breast, and kidney.[2, 5] In many cases, the decreased density on unenhanced CT that is seen with metastatic lesions is probably a reflection of the amount of surrounding cerebral edema. Metastases with increased attenuation coefficients have been seen with carcinomas of the lung, kidney (Fig 19–4), and colon; melanoma (Fig 19–5); choriocarcinoma; and various sarcomas (Fig 19–6), particularly osteogenic sarcoma. All of these latter lesions are known to be frequently hemorrhagic or contain calcium or mucoid degeneration, which may account for their increased density (see Fig 19–3).[2, 6, 7] However, hemorrhage, calcification, or mucoid degeneration has not always been found pathologically in metastases of increased density,[5, 7, 8] with the increased density probably resulting from a compact cellular architecture (Fig 19–7).[7]

Many metastatic tumors are isodense on the unenhanced CT scan, without much surrounding edema (Figs 19–8 and 19–9). These lesions may be extremely difficult to detect without the use of

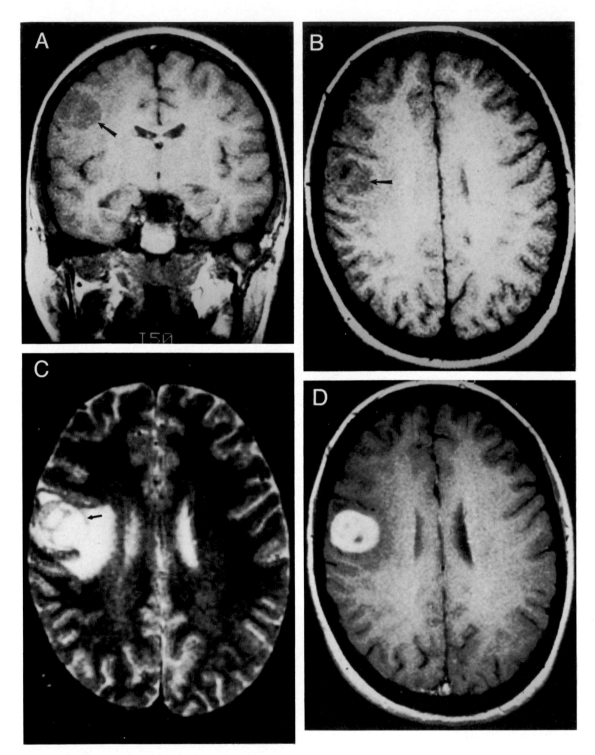

FIG 19–1.
Metastatic melanoma to the gray/white junction. The short repetition time (TR) (TR = 400, echo time [TE] = 20) axial **(A)** and coronal **(B)** unenhanced magnetic resonance imaging (MRI) scans demonstrate a hypointense metastasis to the gray/white junction at the right frontoparietal junction *(arrows)*. There is a rim of cortex overlying the lesion that is indicative of its intra-axial location. The long TR/TE study **(C,** TR = 2,400, TE = 80) shows the lesion to be predominantly hyperintense and separated from the surrounding hyperintense edema by a thin line isointense to cortex *(arrow)*, which may represent compressed normal parenchyma. There is relative homogeneous enhancement of the metastasis on the enhanced short TR image **(D,** TR = 700, TE = 28, gadolinium–diethylenetriamine pentaacetic acid (DTPA).

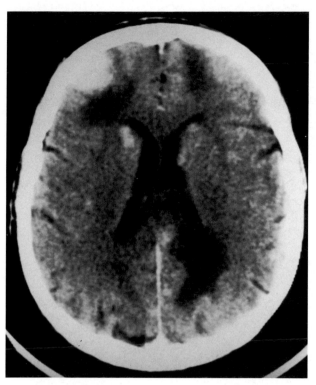

FIG 19–2.
Metastases to both corticomedullary junctions and deep gray matter. This enhanced CT scan demonstrates a large right frontal metastasis to the corticomedullary junction. The densely enhancing tumor appears to be contiguous to the inner table of the skull; the relative density of the two structures does not allow visualization of the compressed intervening cortex. There are multiple metastases to the caudate nuclei and other deep structures. Extensive edema surrounds some metastatic deposits but not others.

contrast material. Multiple bilateral lesions may be present and "balance" each other so that there is no detectable assymetrical mass effect. A contrast-enhanced CT scan is therefore imperative when evaluating by CT the possibility of metastatic tumor, not only to better visualize a lesion with obvious mass effect but also to look for occult lesions not detectable on the unenhanced scan. Multiple lesions tend to confirm the diagnosis of metastatic tumor (Fig 19–10). While most hematogenous metastases enhance to a moderate or marked degree, occasionally some metastases are difficult to define with a single dose of contrast material. Some authors have advocated performing a high-dose delayed contrast-enhanced CT scan with the administration of over 80 g of iodine and scanning 1 to 2 hours after infusion whenever there is a question of metastatic disease. In such cases, lesions difficult to define may become evident, and multiple lesions not otherwise detected with a single dose of contrast material may be seen.[9, 10] In one series,

44% of patients undergoing this delayed high-dose technique had additional lesions seen with more information provided by this technique than on the conventional enhanced CT scan in two thirds of the cases; 11.5% of the cases were false-negative until the delayed high-dose technique was utilized.[10]

Unenhanced short TR MRI studies of nonhemorrhagic metastases demonstrate low intensity to isointensity of the lesion relative to normal brain and pronounced hyperintensity on long TR/TE sequences (see Fig 19–1) (melanocytic melanoma and hemorrhagic metastases are exceptions). Much of the low intensity on the short TR scans and the hyperintensity on long TR/TE scans represents vasogenic edema surrounding a sharply demarcated nodule of tumor. That nodule may be slightly more intense than the edema on the short TR study and allow separation (see Fig 19–1,A and B). On the long TR sequences, there may be a line isointense to gray matter separating the hyperintense nodule from the hyperintense edema (see Fig 19–1,C). The line represents compressed nonneoplastic parenchyma or viable tumor between necrotic tumor and edema if necrosis is present. If the line of separation is of even lower intensity on the long TR scan, hemosiderin from previous hemorrhage (Fig 19–11) or collections of ionic iron known to accompany both primary and secondary tumors may be responsible. Cystic or necrotic metastases appear on short TR studies as areas of intensity between that of CSF and gray matter/white matter (Fig 19–12,A); while quite hyperintense on long TR/TE studies (Fig 19–12,B), the intensity fades relative to CSF if very long TR and TE values are used. A rim of viable tumor may separate the necrotic core from surrounding edema (Fig 19–12,B).

Contrast-enhanced short TR MRI demonstrates a hyperintense enhancing nodule surrounded by low or isointense edema (see Figs 19–1, 19–3, and 19–11). Because MRI is more sensitive than CT for the detection of soft-tissue differences and because enhanced MRI defines the enhancement better than enhanced CT with minimal disruption of the blood-brain barrier,[11–14] we do not use the double-dose enhancement technique with CT any longer but prefer to evaluate for metastatic disease by MRI using a combination of a long TR/TE sequence and an enhanced short TR study (Fig 19–13).

Melanoma metastases present an unusual appearance on MRI. While most tumors have longer T1 and T2 relaxation values than normal brain pa-

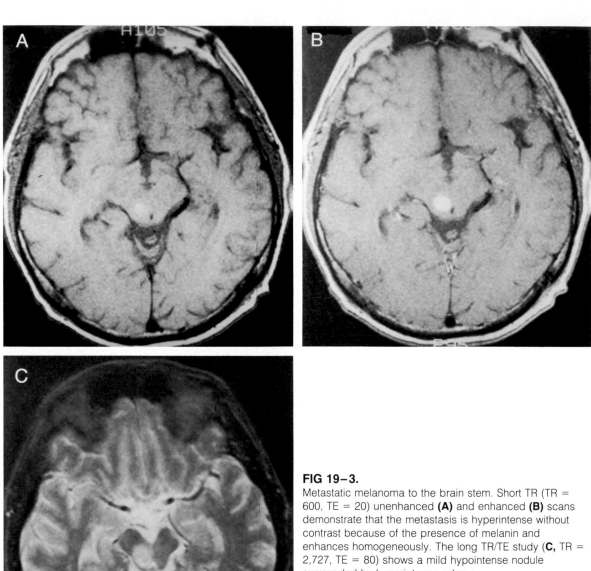

FIG 19–3.
Metastatic melanoma to the brain stem. Short TR (TR =
600, TE = 20) unenhanced **(A)** and enhanced **(B)** scans
demonstrate that the metastasis is hyperintense without
contrast because of the presence of melanin and
enhances homogeneously. The long TR/TE study **(C,** TR =
2,727, TE = 80) shows a mild hypointense nodule
surrounded by hyperintense edema.

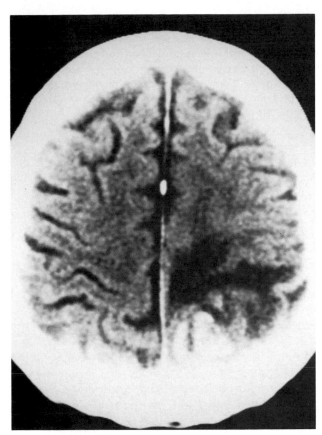

FIG 19–4.
Metastatic hypernephroma, dense on CT scan without contrast enhancement. This nonenhanced scan demonstrates a hyperdense metastatic deposit without the use of contrast enhancement. The etiology of this hyperdensity is unknown.

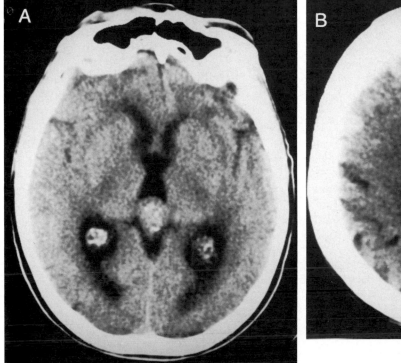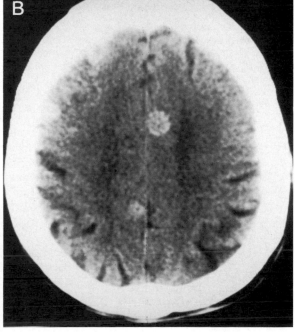

FIG 19–5.
Hyperdense deposits of metastatic melanoma on unenhanced CT. Unenhanced scans through the region of the pineal **(A)** and supraventricular **(B)** regions demonstrate multiple hyperintense nodules within the pineal **(A)** and at corticomedullary junctions of numerous regions within the parietal and right frontal lobes. There is no significant edema surrounding any of the deposits.

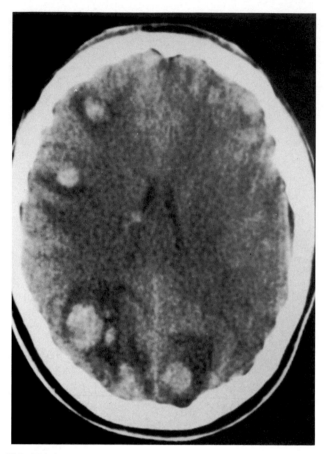

FIG 19–6.
Metastatic epithelioid sarcoma with hyperdense deposits on unenhanced CT. scan. This single nonenhanced CT scan demonstrates multiple hyperdense metastases in both cerebral hemispheres. The metastases are relatively "balanced," so there is no shift of the compressed ventricular system. Moderate edema surrounds the metastatic deposits. The reason for their hyperdensity is unknown.

renchyma does, melanocytic melanoma usually has short T1 and T2 relaxation rates (see Fig 19–3). This results in hyperintensity on short TR scans and hypointensity on long TR/TE sequences. This may be the result of the melanin alone, hemorrhage into the tumor, or both.[15, 16]

While many metastatic lesions have a round, homogeneously enhancing appearance on the enhanced scan (see Figs 19–1 to 19–3), the "ring sign" is also a frequent finding (Figs 19–12 and 19–14). The appearance of rim enhancement is nonspecific and may occur with either primary or secondary tumors, abscesses, resolving hematomas, and occasionally infarcts. The CT-lucent or MRI-hyperintense (on a long TR/TE scan) area within the metastatic tumor represents necrosis as the tumor outgrows its blood supply. Extracellular fluid or blood accumulation within the cavity may

produce a fluid level; contrast material may also leak into the cavity to produce a fluid-fluid level on the enhanced scan.[17] Metastases may be truly cystic (Fig 19–15), and there may be both a solid and a cystic component, with the solid portion appearing like a mural nodule and suggesting cystic astrocytoma or hemangioblastoma.[18] A metastasis may also have multiple cysts (see Fig 19–10). CT absorption coefficients do not separate a true cyst from necrosis; a true cyst is differentiated from necrosis on CT when the margins of the lucency within the ring of enhancement are sharp (Fig 19–15). MRI may be more helpful in this differentiation. A true cyst tends to be more uniformly hypointense on short TR scans than necrosis is, although the protein content of the tumoral cyst generally makes it more intense than CSF. The diagnosis of a cystic component can be surgically important because drainage of the cyst without complete tumor removal may give temporary palliation of the mass effect.

The amount of edema surrounding a metastatic lesion is variable, but generally moderate to marked (see Figs 19–1, 19–2, 19–6, 19–10 to 19–12, and 19–14).[2] However, only minimal or no edema may be present (see Figs 19–3, 19–5, 19–8 to 19–10, and 19–13), and when associated with an isodense mass on a precontrast CT scan, the metastasis may be difficult or impossible to detect without the use of contrast material (see Figs 19–8, 19–9, and 19–13). Because MRI demonstrates the presence of edema far better than does CT, subtle lesions are more easily detected by MRI, which makes it the preferred screening examination when compared with CT. Long TR MRI scans demonstrate that edema. However, contrast-enhanced short TR MRI scans not uncommonly detect metastatic disease not identified even in retrospect on long TR/TE images (see Fig 19–13). Therefore, a combination of a long TR/TE MRI sequence and an enhanced short TR study is the screening procedure of choice for metastatic disease to the brain.

Certain metastatic tumors have a high propensity to bleed, and acute intracranial hemorrhage or a strokelike clinical picture may be the initial neurologic presentation.[19] The most common metastases presenting with hemorrhage are metastatic choriocarcinoma and melanoma, with lung and kidney cancers being less common.[19–21] The appearance of hemorrhage into the tumor itself or into the surrounding parenchyma is the same as for nontumorous hemorrhage: acutely, hyperdense on

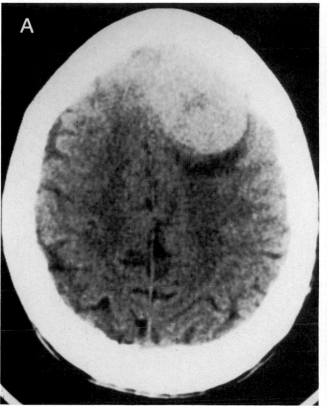

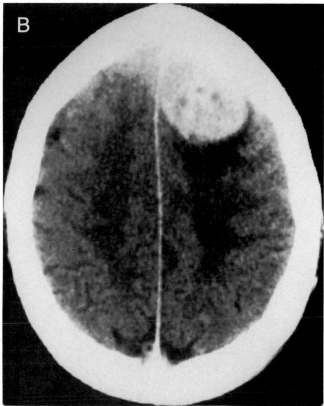

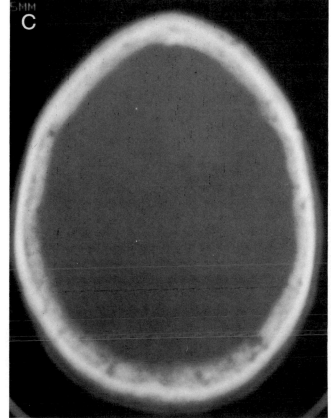

FIG 19–7.
Metastatic myeloma simulating meningioma. An unenhanced CT scan **(A)** demonstrates a large neoplasm that is hyperdense without contrast material and is apparently based along the inner table of the left frontal bone. There is homogeneous enhancement of this lesion **(B)**. The appearance is "typical" of meningioma, except for the few hypodense areas within the tumor and the involvement of the right frontal region, which are indicative of an epidural location. A "bone window" of the calvarium **(C)** demonstrates multiple diploic lucencies in this patient with known multiple myeloma. The density without contrast enhancement is secondary to the dense cellularity of the neoplasm.

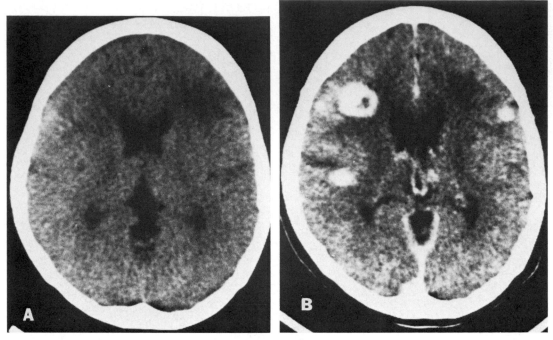

FIG 19–8.
Enhancement of multiple isodense metastases. This 38-year-old woman with metastatic melanoma has an unenhanced CT scan **(A)** with left frontal lobe edema and some patchy edema in the left temporal and right frontal regions. The enhanced scan **(B),** however, demonstrates intense enhancement of multiple metastatic nodules that is not seen on the unenhanced scan.

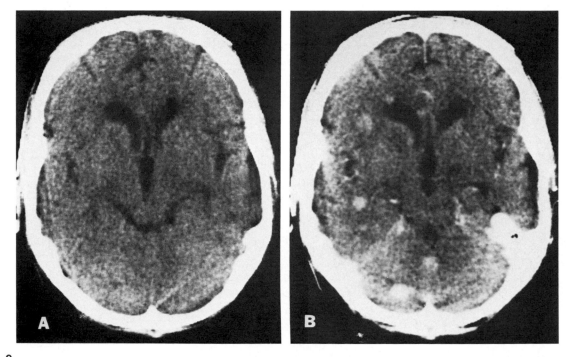

FIG 19–9.
Enhancement of multiple occult metastases. The unenhanced scan **(A)** is unremarkable in this patient with known metastatic oat cell carcinoma. The enhanced scan **(B)** at a very slightly different angle demonstrates multiple enhancing cerebral and cerebellar nodules. None of these nodules could be identified on the preinfusion study, nor was there evidence of edema or mass effect to suggest multiple tumor deposits.

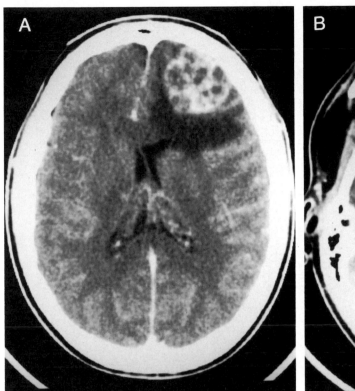 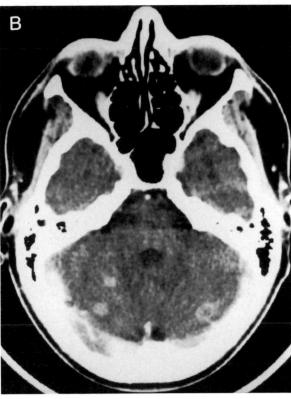

FIG 19–10.

Large multicystic left frontal metastasis with occult posterior fossa metastases. An enhanced CT scan through the level of the ventricular system **(A)** demonstrates a large multicystic neoplasm in the left frontal lobe with abundant surrounding edema. The lesion could be either primary or metastatic. A scan through the posterior fossa, however, reveals multiple metastases to both cerebellar hemispheres without edema **(B)**.

unenhanced CT (see Fig 21–5), isointense on short TR studies, and hypointense on long TR/TE scans; and in the subacute to chronic stage, hypodense on CT but hyperintense on both short TR and long TR/TE scans, possibly accompanied by hemosiderin deposition (Figs 19–16 and 19–17).[22] The important differential diagnostic features from simple hemorrhage include an atypical location of the hemorrhage relative to that expected from aneurysm, arteriovenous malformation, or hypertension; contrast enhancement in the area of hemorrhage, particularly during the acute phase when delayed enhancement around a resolving hematoma would not be expected; and the multiplicity of lesions (see Fig 19–5).[20] Occult vascular malformation deep in the parenchyma and hemorrhagic metastasis may have a similar appearance.[22] The presence of multiple lesions (although cavernous angiomas may be multiple) and abundant edema favors metastases. In cases where MRI differentiation is difficult, CT may be helpful since cryptic malformations are frequently isodense to

mildly hyperdense on unenhanced CT, as opposed to the very dense appearance of the acutely hemorrhagic metastasis, and commonly calcify (see Fig 18–29).[22]

Certain metastases may be CT dense because of calcification/ossification, such as metastases from osteogenic sarcoma or mucinous carcinoma of the colon (Figs 19–6 and 19–18).[7] These lesions have a variable intensity pattern on MRI, depending upon the concentration of specific components.

Unless specific constituents such as hemorrhage, calcification, or paramagnetic compounds such as melanin are present that might help in defining a particular subgroup of metastatic lesions, it is usually impossible to differentiate one source of metastatic tumor from another by either CT or MRI. Likewise, it may be difficult to distinguish a solitary metastasis from a primary brain tumor. In one series, only 40% of single melanoma metastases seen on CT had the characteristics most commonly associated with hematogenously disseminated tumor, including a round enhancing

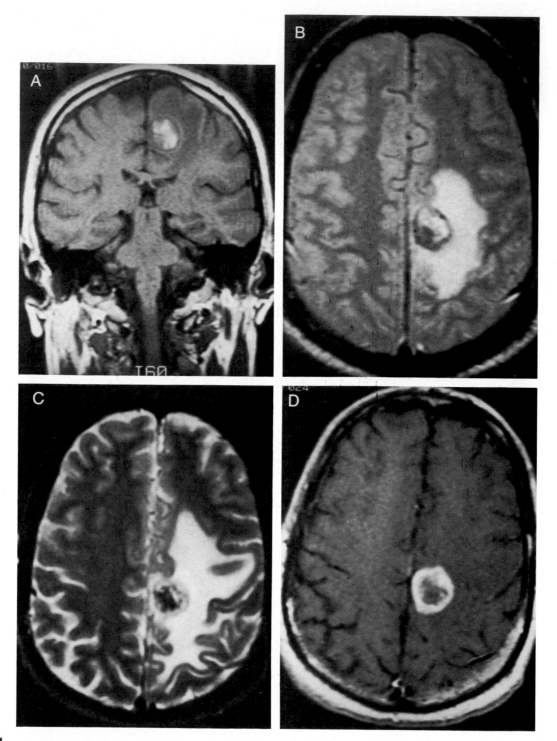

FIG 19–11.
Hemorrhagic metastasis with evolution over 7 months. The coronal short TR MRI study (**A,** TR = 600, TE = 20) demonstrates a left parietal metastasis that is hyperintense—indicative of the presence of methemogloblin. A long TR axial image (**B,** TR = 2,875, TE = 30) shows both methemoglobin and hemosiderin within the lesion and a rim of hemosiderin on the periphery. There is abundant surrounding edema. Seven months later there is less methemoglobin and more hemosiderin within the lesion (**C,** TR = 2,400, TE = 80). The rim of viable tumor enhances brightly (**D,** TR = 600, TE = 20, gadolinium-DTPA), while the old hemorrhagic core does not enhance.

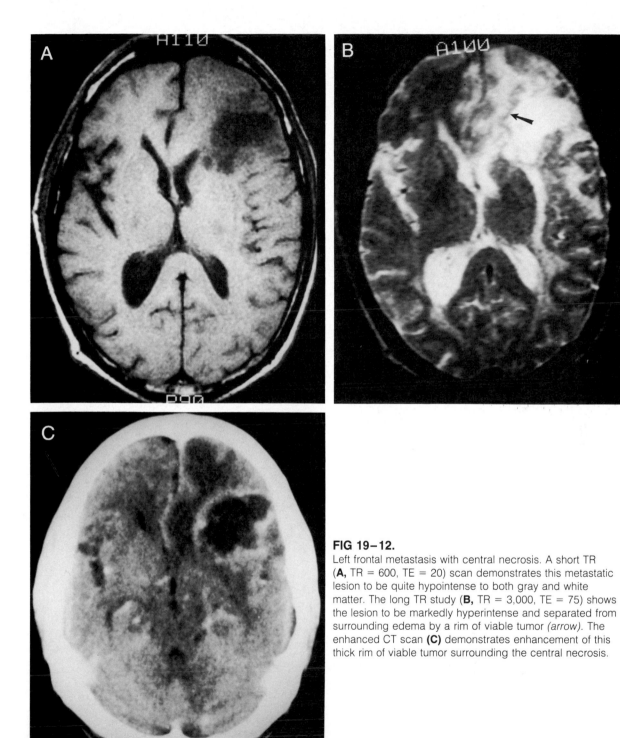

FIG 19–12.
Left frontal metastasis with central necrosis. A short TR
(**A,** TR = 600, TE = 20) scan demonstrates this metastatic
lesion to be quite hypointense to both gray and white
matter. The long TR study (**B,** TR = 3,000, TE = 75) shows
the lesion to be markedly hyperintense and separated from
surrounding edema by a rim of viable tumor *(arrow).* The
enhanced CT scan **(C)** demonstrates enhancement of this
thick rim of viable tumor surrounding the central necrosis.

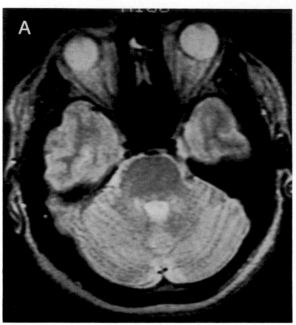

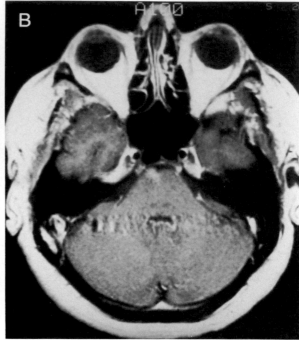

FIG 19–13.

Subtle melanoma metastasis to the brain stem, shown only on enhanced MRI. The long TR/TE image through the pons (**A,** TR = 2,500, TE = 75) does not demonstrate a metastasis in the pons. However, the enhanced short TR study (**B,** TR = 600, TE = 20, gadolinium-DTPA) defines the metastasis to the anterior portion of the right side of the pons. While MRI is extremely sensitive to edema, some metastasis have minimal edema and are better shown with an enhanced study. The combination of a long TR/TE sequence and enhanced MRI is the screening procedure of choice for intracranial metastases.

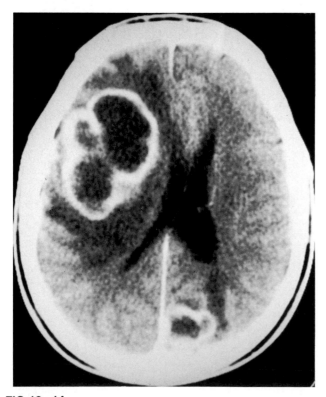

FIG 19–14.

Multiple thick-rimmed metastases from carcinoma of the lung. This enhanced CT scan demonstrates multiple large thick-rimmed, centrally necrotic/cystic metastases.

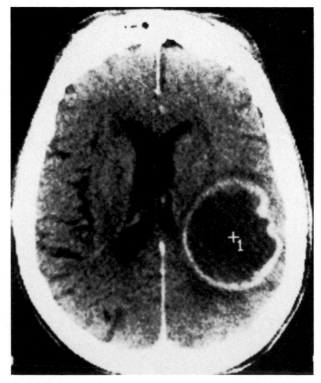

FIG 19–15.

Thin-rimmed cystic left parietal metastasis. This enhanced CT scan demonstrates a thin-rimmed cystic metastasis. The presence of a true cyst is denoted by the sharp demarcation between the enhanced rim and the internal hypodensity.

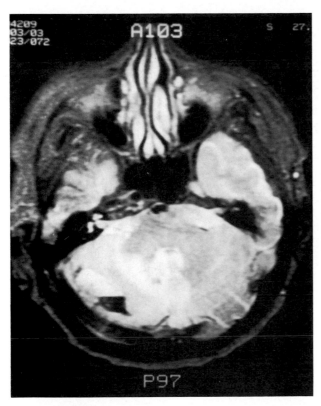

FIG 19–16.
Hemorrhagic right cerebellar metastasis. This long TR/TE (TR = 2,500, TR = 75) scan through the posterior fossa demonstrates a metastatic lesion in the right cerebellar hemisphere with old hemorrhage. The hyperintensity represents methemoglobin, and the pronounced hypointensity is hemosiderin. Interestingly, there appears to be a fluid-fluid level between the two components.

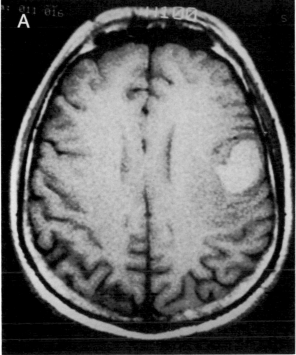

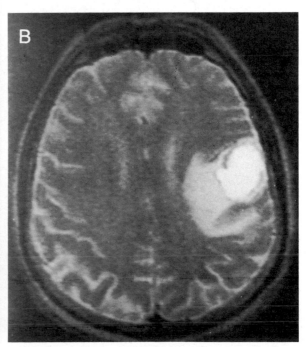

FIG 19–17.
Probable hemorrhagic metastasis, left parietal lobe. This metastasis from adenocarcinoma of the lung to the anterior left parietal lobe is hyperintense on an unenhanced short TR/TE image (**A,** TR = 600, TE = 20). The hyperintensity suggests the presence of methemoglobin. The long TR/TE study (**B,** TR = 2,650, TE = 100) demonstrates not only an increase in this hyperintensity but also a peripheral hypointense line, probably hemosiderin, separating the tumor nodule from surrounding edema.

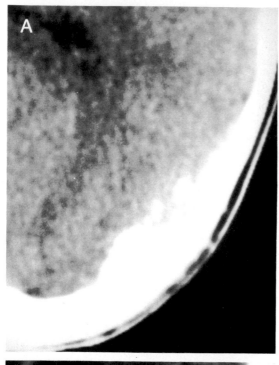

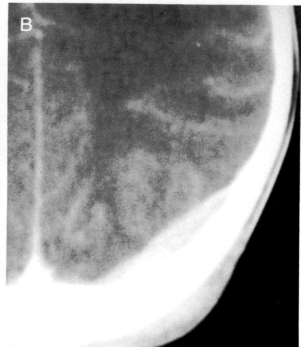

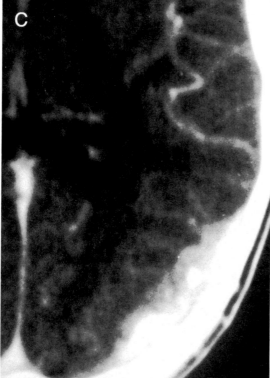

FIG 19–18.
Metastatic osteogenic sarcoma to the skull, with invasion through the dura. A blowup of the left parieto-occipital region of a nonenhanced CT scan **(A)** demonstrates a dense collection of calcium beneath the inner table of the skull. The enhanced scan slightly higher **(B)** demonstrates tumor deposits in the scalp and epidural region from osteogenic sarcoma metastatic to the calvarium. A cut just below this **(C)** shows the calcium seen on the unenhanced scan and a wavy line of enhancement, different from the straight margin representing dura on the higher cut **(B).** This wavy line probably represents extension of tumor through the dura into the underlying meninges and brain.

mass and moderate-to-marked edema. Many of the lesions had an appearance more typically associated with primary brain tumor, including less enhancement and edema than typically seen with metastatic tumor.[23] MRI is far more sensitive than CT at detecting multiple lesions, so the discovery of a solitary metastatic lesion by MRI is less common than with CT, thus making the question of primary vs. secondary tumor less difficult.

It may be difficult to distinguish a solitary metastasis from a meningioma on CT, particularly if the metastatic tumor is based along the falx or if axial cuts through the high convexity appear to show the mass to be based along the inner table of the skull (Figs 19–7, 19–19, and 19–20). Coronal or sagittal projections in such a case may be of more value. The multiple MRI projections usually allow differentiation of an extra-axial from an intra-axial mass more easily than does CT (Fig 19–20). A rim of cortex surrounding the metastasis may be difficult to see with CT but more easily detected with MRI (see Fig 19–1).

Finally, differentiation of a solitary metastasis with a ring of enhancement from other lesions such as primary brain tumor, abscess, or a resolving hematoma may be impossible by CT. For example, while it has been said that abscesses typically have a thin wall while tumors have a thicker, more irregular wall, metastatic tumors may have either a thick rim of enhancement (see Figs 19–12 and 19–14) or a thin rim (see Fig 19–15) mimicking abscess. On MRI, primary brain tumor, solitary metastasis, and abscess may all look identical. A resolving hematoma has the typical MRI appear-

ance of subacute and chronic hemorrhage (see Chapter 9), which is distinctly different from non-hemorrhagic tumor or abscess; however, it may be difficult or impossible to exclude a hemorrhagic metastasis.

Metastatic tumors generally respect dural boundaries as they grow, similar to primary central nervous system (CNS) parenchymal tumors. While a tumor may invade a dural structure, actual growth through that structure into contiguous parenchyma is rare. For example, the spread of metastatic tumor from one hemisphere to another does not usually occur through the falx but requires passage through a connecting structure such as the corpus callosum. Rarely, a very aggressive metastatic neoplasm may grow through the dura or falx (Figs 19–18, 19–21, and 19–22). Periventricular spread of metastatic tumor may also occur (Fig 19–23), as with primary CNS tumors.[24]

Certain primary tumors have a propensity to metastasize to the meninges to produce meningeal carcinomatosis. Of particular note are the adenocarcinomas of the lung, breast (Fig 19–23), stomach, and colon (Fig 19–24) and lymphoma and leu-

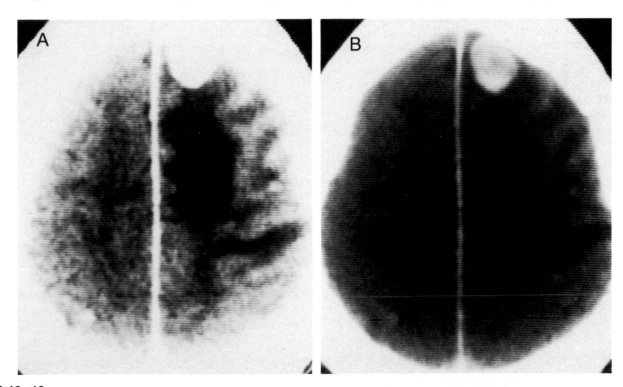

FIG 19–19.
Metastatic carcinoma of the breast that is simulating meningioma. An enhanced CT scan in the supraventricular region **(A)** demonstrates a dense nodule of metastatic carcinoma of the breast that lies below the inner table of the skull. The density of this homogeneous enhancement and its contiguity to the inner table of the skull makes it difficult to differentiate an intraparenchymal neoplasm such as metastasis from an extraparenchymal tumor such as meningioma. Using a wider window **(B)** helps to separate a tumor nodule from bone, with the acute margins of the nodule suggesting its intraparenchymal location.

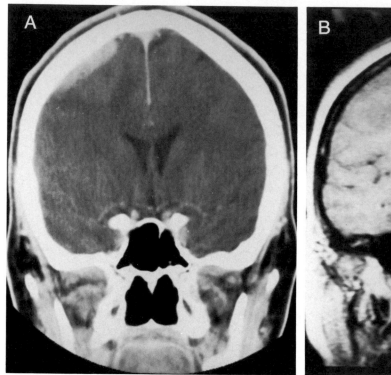
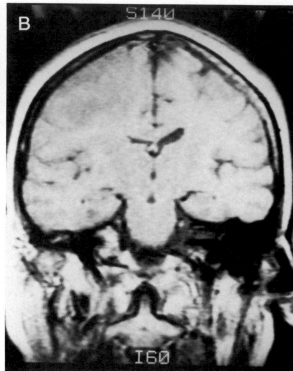

FIG 19–20.

Metastatic carcinoma of the breast to the calvarium that is simulating *en plaque* meningioma. The coronal enhanced CT scan **(A)** in this patient with known carcinoma of the breast demonstrates a linear deposit of tumor along the inner table of the skull. Although the patient has known carcinoma of the breast, this could represent *en plaque* meningioma, not metastasis. An unenhanced short TR MRI scan (**B,** TR = 600, TE = 25) demonstrates a hypointense region below the inner table of the skull, with a larger less hypointense region deep to the tumor representing edema. The key in this case is the hypointensity of the calvarium, which represents replacement of marrow fat by tumor and therefore allows the diagnosis of calvarial metastasis with epidural extension.

kemia.[1, 25] Visualization of meningeal deposits without evidence of parenchymal metastases is inconstant by enhanced CT.[26, 27] In one series, 44% of patients with proven meningeal carcinomatosis had pathologic enhancement of the meninges, 100% of patients with metastatic melanoma had visualization, but there was visualization in only 3% of patients with proven meningeal involvement by leukemia and lymphoma.[26] One problem in visualization by CT is that enhancement of the dura normally occurs with iodinated contrast material. Metastases must demonstrate greater-than-normal enhancement to be identified. A second problem is the overlying bone with its density and artifact production that makes difficult the perception of subtle meningeal abnormalities. Third, meningeal infiltration may be at a microscopic level, too subtle for detection by any imaging system. Visualization of meningeal carcinomatosis is also difficult with nonenhanced MRI.[28] A tumor that is isointense relative to cortex is difficult to perceive when it is contiguous to that cortex. Likewise, low-intensity tumor is difficult to perceive because of its contiguity to low-intensity CSF. Enhanced MRI fares much better (see Figs 19–23 and 19–24).[29] The dura normally enhances only to a mild degree with gadolinium-DTPA, and there is no overlying cortical bone signal to hinder visualization. Enhanced MRI is therefore much more sensitive to neoplastic involvement than is CT. In a recent report, 66% of patients with proven meningeal carcinomatosis had visualization of their meningeal deposits on enhanced MRI.[30] Still, there was a significant percentage of patients who did not show an imaging abnormality. When there is a high degree of clinical suspicion for meningeal carcinomatosis, the best test is probably still lumbar puncture with cytologic evaluation of the CSF.

LYMPHOMA/LEUKEMIA

Lymphoma

Cerebral involvement by systemic lymphoma typically begins in the leptomeninges rather than the parenchyma (Fig 19–25), while primary malig-

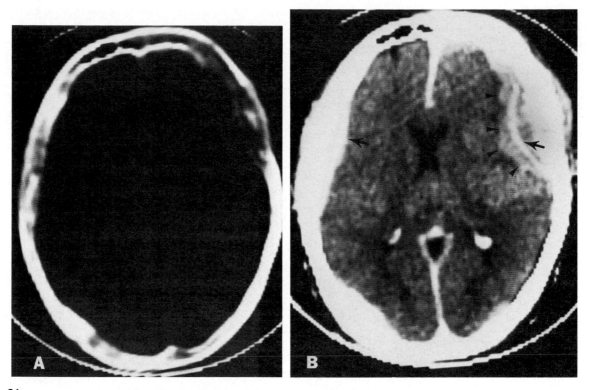

FIG 19–21.

Metastatic carcinoma of the prostate to the calvarium with dural penetration. An axial scan with a wide window (bone window) **(A)** demonstrates multiple areas of bone destruction involving the calvarium, most prominent in the frontal regions bilaterally. An enhanced scan of the head with windowing for the cerebral paren- chyma **(B)** shows elevation of the dura *(arrows)* in the regions of the bone destruction that is indicative of epidural extension of tu- mor. This aggressive neoplasm has penetrated the dura on the left, with spread into the contiguous cerebral parenchyma *(arrow-heads)*.

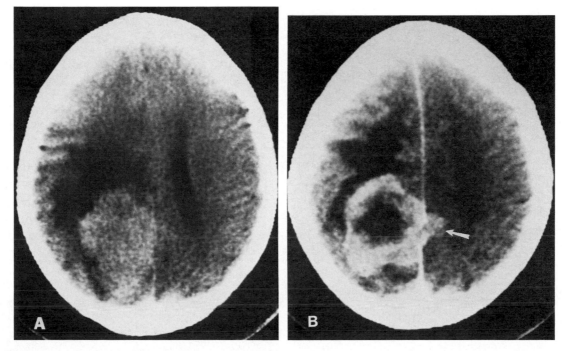

FIG 19–22.

Metastatic oat cell carcinoma penetrating the falx. An unenhanced scan **(A)** demonstrates a relatively dense large metastasis of oat cell carcinoma with abundant surrounding cerebral edema. The enhanced study **(B)** demonstrates intense enhancement with cen- tral necrosis. The aggressive nature of the lesion is demonstrated by the growth of tumor through the falx into the opposite cerebral hemisphere *(arrow,* **B**) in this 35-year-old woman with rapid deteri- oration.

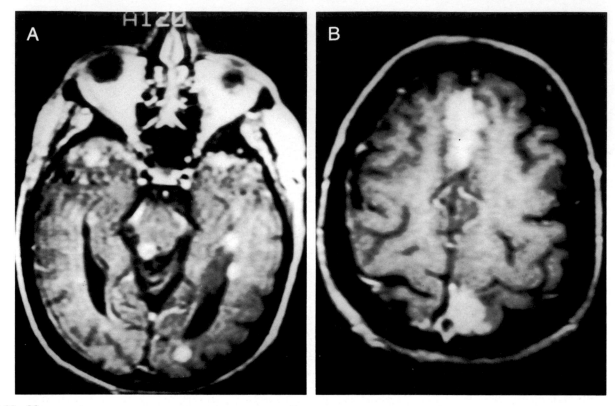

FIG 19–23.
Metastatic carcinoma of the breast with periventricular nodules and meningeal carcinomatosis. Enhanced short TR images (TR = 800, TE = 30, gadolinium-DTPA) at the levels of the mesencephalon **(A)** and the high convexities **(B)** demonstrate multiple metastatic nodules, a number of which are subependymal in location. There is extensive enhancement along the surfaces of the temporal tips **(A)** and in the interhemispheric fissure **(B)** that represents meningeal deposits of tumor.

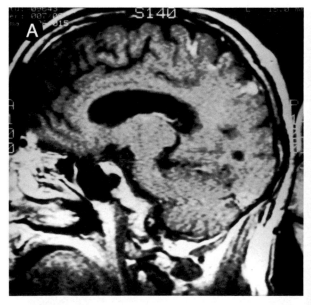

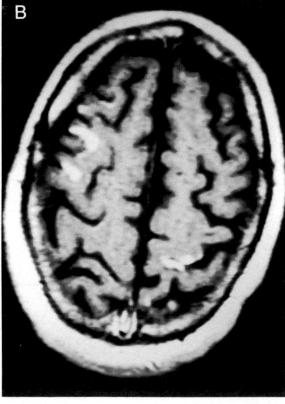

FIG 19–24.
Meningeal carcinomatosis from adenocarcinoma of the colon. Enhanced short TR MRI (TR = 600, TE = 20, gadolinium-DTPA) in the sagittal **(A)** and axial **(B)** projections demonstrates multiple areas of meningeal enhancement that are consistent with meningeal metastases.

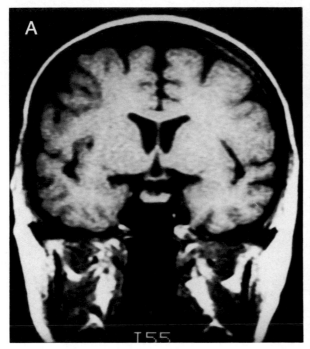

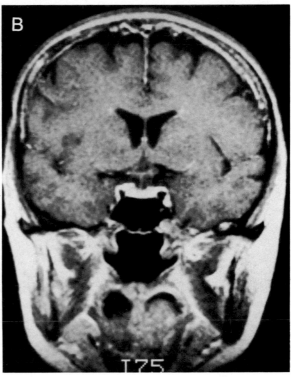

FIG 19–25.
Enhanced MRI demonstration of leptomeningeal involvement by systemic lymphoma. The coronal unenhanced short TR MRI scan (**A,** TR = 600, TE = 20) is unremarkable. The enhanced study (**B,** TR = 450, TE = 30, gadolinium-DTPA) demonstrates bright enhancement of the meninges over the frontal convexities, left greater than right.

nant lymphoma of the brain (also called reticulum cell sarcoma or histiocytic lymphoma) is a parenchymal tumor, as discussed in Chapter 16.[31, 32] Metastatic lymphoma spreads along the leptomeninges and dips into the Virchow-Robin spaces along with the pial vasculature. Occasionally, tumor may spread into the contiguous gray matter to form a parenchymal mass (Fig 19–26).[31, 33, 34] Circulation of tumor cells via the CSF into the ventricular system will result in subependymal growth and periventricular spread.[35]

Identification by CT of lymphomatous involvement of only the meninges, without parenchymal tumor, is unusual.[26, 33, 34] This is true even if a double dose of contrast material is utilized.[33] This is so because the tumor deposits may be quite thin, the meninges normally enhance on CT, and the density of the overlying calvarium makes visualization difficult. When seen, there is thickening of the normal meningeal enhancement. The only clue to the presence of leptomeningeal disease on a CT scan may be a mild communicating hydrocephalus due to impaired CSF circulation.[27] Leptomeningeal lymphoma is not easily detected on un-

enhanced MRI (Fig 19–25,A).[28] Only large deposits can be seen and are generally seen as isointense to gray matter on short TR scans and hyperintense on long TR/TE sequences, the same as the contiguous CSF. Enhanced MRI provides significantly better visualization than with either unenhanced MRI or enhanced CT.[29, 30] The dura normally enhances only mildly, and there are no bony densities to obscure detection. This allows detection of the brightly enhancing deposits of a size smaller than that seen on CT (Fig 19–25,B).[29, 30]

Parenchymal extensions of tumor, which may be multiple, are generally moderately hyperdense or less commonly isodense relative to the surrounding brain on the precontrast CT scan (Fig 19–26) and usually enhance homogeneously but have irregular margins (Figs 19–26 to 19–28).[33–35] This is the same appearance as primary malignant lymphoma of the brain (but not that seen with acquired immunodeficiency syndrome [AIDS]).[32, 36–40] The parenchymal mass(es) usually have surrounding edema of minimal to mild degree (Figs 19–26 to 19–28). This appearance of minimal edema and margins that are less sharp than he-

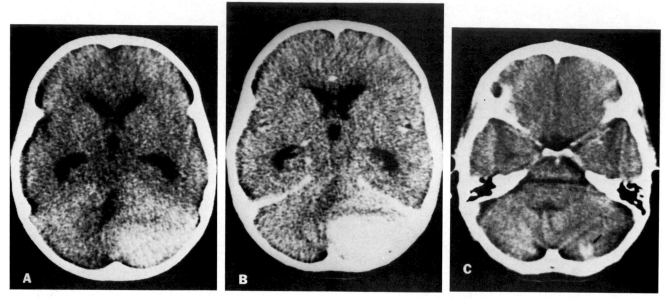

FIG 19–26.
Non-Hodgkin's lymphoma of the cerebellar hemisphere. The unenhanced scan **(A)** demonstrates a highly dense mass within the left cerebellar hemisphere that is contiguous to the inner table of the left occipital bone and producing compression of the fourth ventricle and obstructive hydrocephalus. There is intense enhancement of the postinfusion study **(B).** Although of a high density on the unenhanced scan, the appearance is not typical of hemorrhage because the mass was not as highly dense as the typical hematoma, nor were the margins as sharp, and enhancement occurred, which is characteristic of neoplasm. This child had a history of diffuse systemic involvement with lymphoma, and the intracranial mass undoubtedly began in the meninges with spread into the contiguous cerebellum. Following radiation therapy, there has been a rapid diminution in the size of the cerebellar mass in only 10 days **(C),** with only a small tumor nodule remaining *(arrow)*.

FIG 19–27.
Superficial and periventricular deposits of lymphoma. This enhanced CT scan demonstrates a superficial deposit of intensely enhancing lymphoma within the anterior right frontal lobe. Note the irregular margins, representing infiltration into the surrounding parenchyma, and the lack of edema. The tumor probably invaded from leptomeningeal disease. Spread via the CSF pathways has led to penetration of the ependyma and enhancing periventricular deposits.

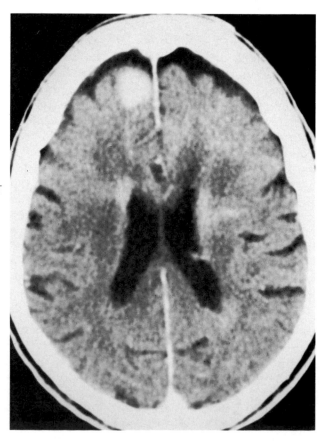

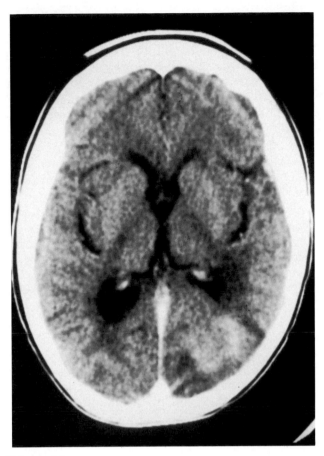

FIG 19–28.
Irregularly marginated lymphomatous deposit in the left parieto-occipital region. This enhanced scan demonstrates an irregularly marginated, mildly enhancing deposit of lymphoma. Note the minimal edema. There is some increased density below the inner table of the skull in the right parieto-occipital region, but it is difficult to be sure whether there is leptomeningeal or cortical lymphomatous deposition because of the artifact from bone.

matogenous metastases (Figs 19–26 and 19–28) is different on CT from that usually seen with hematogenous metastatic tumor and may suggest the appropriate diagnosis. Spread via the CSF may result in periventricular (Fig 19–27) and deep gray and white matter deposits.

Up to two thirds of the parenchymal lymphomatous deposits in patients with AIDS have a cystic or necrotic center.[36, 37] This is a distinctly different appearance on CT from the typical homogeneity of non–AIDS-related primary lymphoma[36–40] and of secondary parenchymal involvement by systemic non-AIDS lymphoma.[33–35]

Parenchymal non-AIDS lymphamatous deposits usually appear isointense or mildly hypointense to gray matter on unenhanced short TR scans, with isointensity to slight hyperintensity relative to gray matter on unenhanced long TR/TE sequences.[41]

Enhanced short TR scans demonstrate homogeneous enhancement like contrast-enhanced CT scans. This appearance is different from most metastatic lesions, which are more hyperintense on the long TR sequences. Irregular margination of the enhancing portion, indicative of parenchymal infiltration, with proportionately less cerebral edema than found with comparably sized hematogenous metastases may also suggest the appropriate diagnosis. AIDS-related lymphoma is commonly cystic or necrotic.[36, 37]

Leukemia

Leukemic involvement of the CNS, like lymphoma, generally starts by involving the leptomeninges (Fig 19–29), with spread along the Virchow-Robin spaces.[31] There may be enough penetration into contiguous brain to form a focal leukemic mass ("chloroma") (Fig 19–28).[42–45] With spread via CSF pathways into the ventricular system, a chloroma may be present within the deep periventricular parenchyma (Fig 19–30).

Leptomeningeal leukemia, like lymphoma, is rarely visualized on CT (Fig 19–29). The only clue on the CT scan to the presence of the disease may be slight ventricular enlargement due to a slowing of CSF circulation over the convexities by the leptomeningeal tumor.[27, 45] Again, like with lymphoma, enhanced MRI is better than enhanced CT for detection.

Parenchymal leukemic deposits are generally isodense or of slight increased density on the nonenhanced CT scan (Fig 19–30) and enhance homogeneously (Figs 19–29 and 19–30).[33, 42–45] The borders of the enhancing mass may be relatively sharp,[42] but infiltration into surrounding parenchyma with irregular margination is common (Figs 19–29 and 19–30). Such irregular margination may allow differentiation of a solitary focus of leukemia (Fig 19–30) from a solitary hematogenous metastasis (see Fig 19–1) when there is inadequate history of the type of systemic tumor.

MRI descriptions of parenchymal leukemic deposits are uncommon. One case report showed deposits of myelogenous leukemia to be isointense to white matter on both unenhanced short TR and long TR sequences and referenced two other similar cases.[44] This is an unusual appearance and has been described in some meningiomas.[44] Contrast enhancement was not performed. Figure 19–30 shows a different appearance in that there is pronounced hyperintensity on the long TR/TE se-

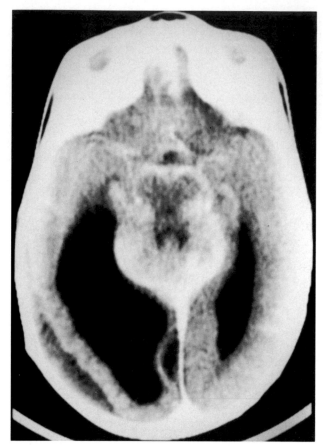

FIG 19–29.
CT demonstration of leptomeningeal leukemia with infiltration into the mesencephalon. This enhanced CT scan demonstrates dense enhancement of the meninges at the tentorial notch, with tumor infiltrating into the mesencephalon. There is also leptomeningeal tumor in the anterior portion of the interhemispheric fissure. Communicating hydrocephalus is present.

quence. The frequency of the different appearances is unknown.

Differential Diagnosis

The CT appearance of parenchymal involvement by non-AIDS systemic lymphoma and leukemia is important to recognize relative to other pathologic conditions that occur in patients with these diseases, particularly cerebritis/abscess, hemorrhage, and infarction. Infarction is generally of low density on the precontrast CT scan, while the enhanced study shows peripheral enhancement, involvement of both gray and white matter, and a wedge-shaped configuration in a vascular distribution. Acute hemorrhage is dense without the use of contrast material, cerebritis is generally patchy in its enhancement pattern, and abscess usually is seen as a ring of enhancement. All of these CT appearances are different from the appearance of parenchymal involvement by either leukemia or non-AIDS lymphoma, and in most cases, parenchymal involvement by tumor should be readily distinguished from these other complications. AIDS-related lymphoma may have a ring pattern, and biopsy may be necessary for differentiation from abscess.

MRI often helps distinguish parenchymal involvement by lymphoma or leukemia from other acute complications. Infarction is hypointense on an unenhanced short TR study and quite hyperintense on long TR sequences. Tumorous deposits are usually isointense to slightly hypointense, depending upon the amount of contiguous edema, on short TR studies and isointense to only slightly hyperintense on most long TR sequences (Fig 19–30, with its hyperintensity on the long TR/TE sequence, may be an exception). Peripheral infarction is in a vascular distribution. Since lymphomatous and leukemic deposits are commonly deep in the basal ganglia or periventricular tissues, differentiation is with infarction from lenticulostriate disease, which should not be difficult. Contrast enhancement is usually peripheral with infarction, if present, as opposed to the homogeneous enhancement of the tumor. Acute hemorrhage is hypointense on long TR/TE sequences as opposed to the isointensity to slight hyperintensity of neoplasm. Subacute blood is quite hyperintense on long TR/TE sequences and short TR scans as opposed to the relative isointensity of tumor. Finally, cerebritis usually is significantly brighter on long TR sequences than are lymphomatous to leukemic deposits (again, Fig 19–30 may be an exception) and has a patchy enhancement pattern. Abscess has a ring of enhancement, as opposed to the homogeneous enhancement of non-AIDS lymphoma and leukemic deposits. Differentiation between abscess and AIDS-related lymphoma with its common ring of enhancement may require aspiration biopsy.

METASTASES TO THE CALVARIUM AND SKULL BASE

Metastases to the calvarium in the adult age group may occur from a wide variety of tumors, with metastases from carcinoma of the breast (see Fig 19–20), the prostate (see Fig 19–21), and mul-

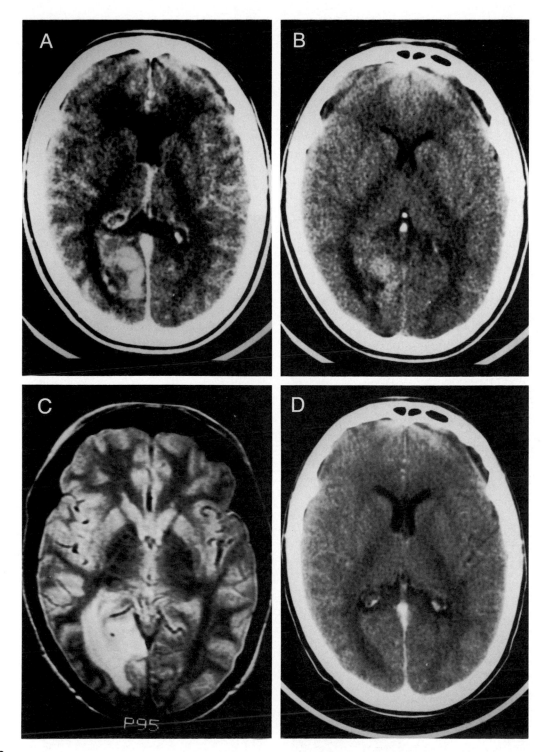

FIG 19–30.

Periventricular and parenchymal leukemic deposits demonstrated by CT and MRI. A 48-year-old female with acute myelogenous leukemia has an unenhanced CT scan **(A)** where a leukemic deposit in the medial right parieto-occipital region is seen to be mildly hyperdense. There is intense enhancement on the enhanced scan **(B),** with tumor along the medial margin of the right occipital horn. Dissemination from leptomeningeal disease via CSF pathways and pooling in the right occipital horn has resulted in the growth of tumor through the ependymal surface into the adjoining parenchyma. A long TR, short TE MRI scan **(C,** TR = 3,000, TE = 30) demonstrates pronounced hyperintensity throughout the entire region of involvement that has produced a blending in intensity of the tumor, the CSF within the ventricle, and any peritumoral edema. Following chemotherapy, enhanced CT scanning was repeated 25 days after the first study. The scan **(D)** now shows normal anatomy.

tiple myeloma (see Fig 19–27) being particularly common offenders.[46] The dural boundary is almost always respected by metastatic lesions, even when there is extensive bony involvement (Fig 19–31). Rarely, aggressive metastases may break through the dura to invade the brain (see Figs 19–18 and 19–21). Carcinoma of the prostate frequently involves the calvarium and produces either a mixed lytic and blastic appearance (see Fig 19–21) or possibly an osteoblastic response that mimics the hyperostosis of meningioma.

Calvarial involvement in the pediatric age group is generally from neuroblastoma (Fig 19–32), lymphoma, leukemia, or any of the sarcomas (Figs 19–18 and 19–33).[46–48] Deposits of neuroblastoma may spread along the epidural

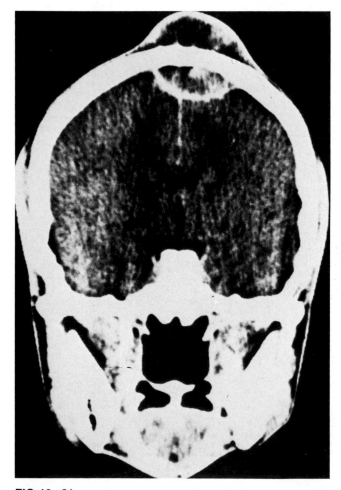

FIG 19–31.
Ewing's sarcoma metastasis to the calvarium with epidural deposit. This enhanced scan in the coronal projection demonstrates a mass in the left frontal bone that is producing elevation of the scalp. There is extension of neoplasm into the epidural space with inferior displacement of the enhancing dura. The epidural location is denoted by intracranial tumor crossing the midline.

spaces to the cranial sutures and produce sutural erosion that simulates the split sutures of increased intracranial pressure (Fig 19–32).[47, 48]

Certain tumors of the face have a propensity to extend in retrograde fashion along nerves through the neural foramina to produce intracranial deposits. This perineural extension is particularly common with adenocystic carcinoma of the paranasal sinuses (Fig 19–33). Other tumors may extend directly through the base of the skull, such as squamous cell carcinoma of the nasopharynx or facial structures in the adult. Metastases from more distant sources to the skull base may come from a variety of primary tumors in the adult and produce epidural deposits of tumor displacing neural structures. In the child, skull base involvement is most common with extracranial rhabdomyosarcoma (Fig 19–34),[49] neuroblastoma (Figs 19–32 and 19–35),[47] lymphoma, and histiocytosis X.

A patient presenting with a tumor in the parapharyngeal region or face requires intracranial imaging in order to evaluate the possibility of parameningeal involvement (Fig 19–33). Such involvement will alter the therapeutic regimen, with the addition of radiation therapy to the cranial cavity or intrathecal chemotherapy. Thin-section (3 mm or less) CT scanning with a bone algorithm is excellent for demonstrating bone destruction (Fig 19–36). While enhanced CT with a soft-tissue algorithm is very good for demonstrating a mass lesion, subtle meningeal involvement may be missed. Enhanced MRI demonstrates this meningeal involvement much better than CT does.[29, 30] Enhanced tumor deposits are easier to see because of the lack of contiguous signal and artifact from cortical bone that plague CT at the skull base. Bone destruction, on the other hand, is more difficult to see with MRI. Typical findings on MRI include blurring of the sharp low-intensity margins of cortical bone (see Fig 19–33) and a change in the marrow signal on short TR sequences (see Fig 19–20).

By and large, the scan findings are nonspecific, and the primary tumor of origin cannot be distinguished on the scan alone. However, there are a few tumors that have distinctive metastases. In the adult, metastasis from adenocystic carcinoma frequently presents as a cavernous sinus mass, and the presence of a paranasal sinus mass should suggest the correct diagnosis. In children, neuroblastoma commonly metastasizes early to the periorbital bony structures (see Figs 19–32 and 19–35). A young patient presenting with sphenoid bone

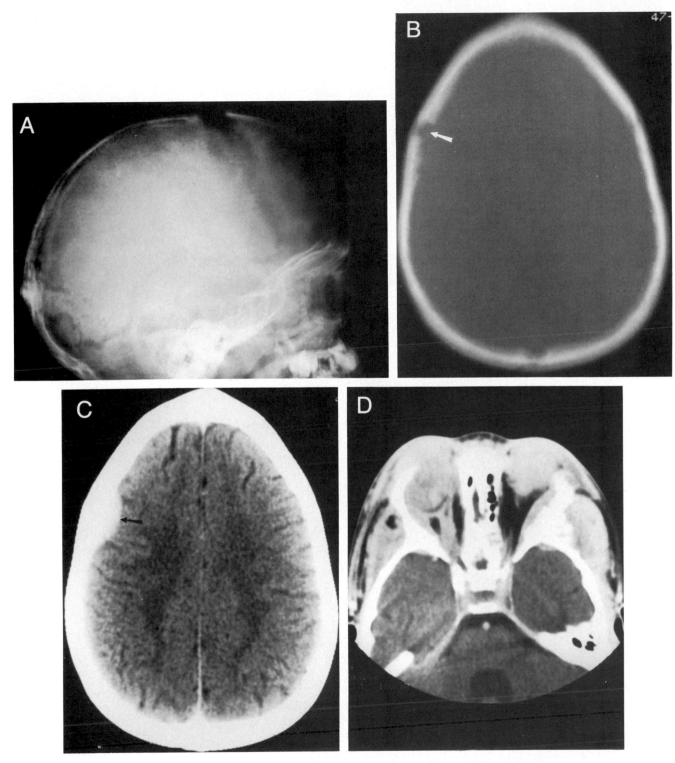

FIG 19–32.
Metastatic neuroblastoma to the calvarium, with epidural spread producing sutural erosion and metastases to the orbits. A lateral skull film **(A)** demonstrates widening of the coronal sutures. Rather than being from increased intracranial pressure, there are metastases to the calvarium, as defined by the "bone window" of the CT scan **(B,** *arrow*), and spread of tumor in the epidural space **(C,** *arrow*) producing sutural erosion that simulates the widened sutures found with increased intracranial pressure. There are also metastases to the periorbital bony structures bilaterally that are displacing the lateral rectus muscles inward, extending into the periorbital soft tissues bilaterally, and extending along the right optic sheath **(D).**

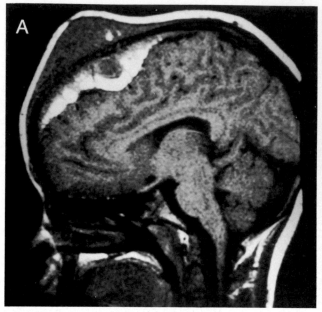

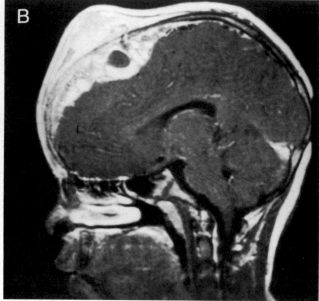

FIG 19–33.

Metastatic rhabdomyosarcoma to the calvarium. An unenhanced sagittal short TR image (**A,** TR = 500, TE = 20) demonstrates a large mass in the scalp, erosion of the calvarium with decreased sharpness of the cortical bone of both the outer and inner tables, a nodule that is isointense to gray matter, and pronounced hyperintensity that is probably in a subdural location. This hyperintensity is most likely subacute extracerebral hemorrhage. The enhanced study (**B,** TR = 500, TE = 20, gadolinium-DTPA) demonstrates extensive enhancement of tumor within the scalp and bone and tumor extending into the region of the subacute hemorrhage. The nodule does not enhance, and its histology is unknown.

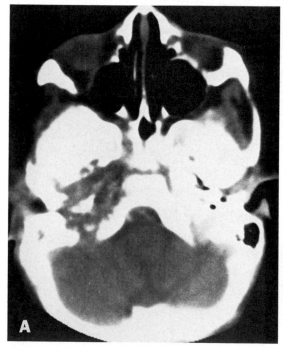

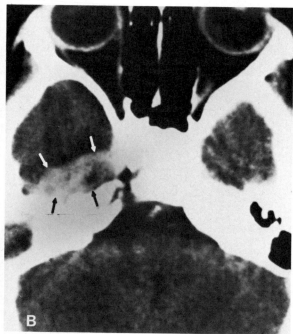

FIG 19–34.

Rhabdomyoscarcoma of the nasopharynx with extension into the middle and posterior cranial fossae. This 3-year-old child with previous treatment for rhabdomyosarcoma of the nasopharynx presented with palsies of the right 5th through 12th cranial nerves. A scan at the base of the skull **(A)** demonstrates extensive bone destruction involving the base of the skull on the right, right petrous and temporal bones, and the right side of the body of the sphenoid bone. An enhanced intracranial scan **(B)** demonstrates a large focal tumor within the inferior and posterior portion of the right temporal fossa *(arrows)*. There was undoubtedly parameningeal extension of tumor as well for lower cranial nerve palsies to be produced.

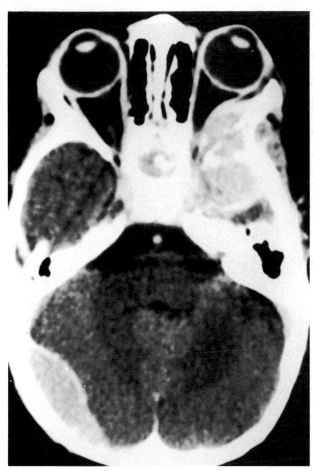

FIG 19–35.
Metastatic neuroblastoma to left greater wing of the sphenoid and skull base and to the right occipital bone. This enhanced CT scan demonstrates a large mass lesion destroying the left greater wing of the sphenoid, extending inferiorly into the skull base, and producing large epidural soft-tissue masses that bulge into the left middle cranial fossa and into the left orbit and displacing the lateral rectus inward. There is another area of metastasis involving the right occipital bone, with a large epidural collection of tumor. The dura enhances densely at both sites.

destruction should suggest neuroblastoma as a strong possibility; calcifications in an abdominal mass ensures the diagnosis. Bone destruction and enhancing soft-tissue masses in the orbital, sellar, and/or petrous regions suggest histiocytosis X.

Benign tumors may bulge intracranially if they erode the skull base. For example, angiofibroma of the nasopharynx frequently extends laterally into the subtemporal fossa or into the sphenoid sinus. Erosion of the lateral walls of the sphenoid sinus or of the bony margins of the temporal fossa will allow tumor to extend intracranially.

SPREAD OF NEOPLASM THROUGH CSF PATHWAYS

Many primary and secondary tumors involving the cerebral parenchyma may be seeded to other portions of the brain via CSF pathways. While any tumor that extends to a cortical or ventricular surface will have access to the CSF with the potential for seeding of tumor cells, malignant tumors originating around the ventricular system have a greater propensity to produce such internal metastases. Of the primary CNS tumors, medulloblastoma, ependymoma, and glioblastoma frequently produce meningeal seeding as denoted by meningeal or ependymal enhancement on the contrast-enhanced scan (see Figs 16–23 and 16–49 to 16–51). There may be extension of this leptomeningeal tumor through the cortical surface to produce a focal parenchymal mass. Multiple foci of glioblastoma may result from seeding of this type (see Fig 16–5), although multiple focal masses can result from the spread of fingers of glial tumor through the parenchyma (see Fig 16–9). Occasionally, primary multifocal glioblastoma occurs. The distinction of this entity from spread of a single tumor requires pathologic confirmation of separate lesions not connected by fingers of tumor and the location of the second tumor away from the cortical surface, where spread via CSF pathways would have placed the lesion.[50]

Metastatic tumors may also spread via CSF pathways. Most commonly, tumor spreads directly to the meninges to produce meningeal carcinomatosis (see Figs 19–23 and 19–24). Occasionally, however, parenchymal metastases may gain access to a cortical or ventricular surface to spread via the CSF.

Periventricular spread of tumor occurs with many malignant primary and metastatic tumors (see Figs 16–23, 19–23, 19–26, and 19–29). Tumor may invade the brain to reach the subependymal tissues, with spread of tumor along the ventricular margins,[24] or tumor spreads into the ventricular system via CSF movement and grows through the parenchyma. Unenhanced CT scanning demonstrates periventricular low density, while MRI shows low intensity on short TR scans and hyperintensity on long TR/TE sequences. This appearance is nonspecific and compatible with radiation injury, ventriculitis, or shunt malfunction.[28] An enhanced MRI or CT scan demonstrates a dense rim of enhancement around the ventricles (see Figs 19–26 and 19–29)[24] and may also dem-

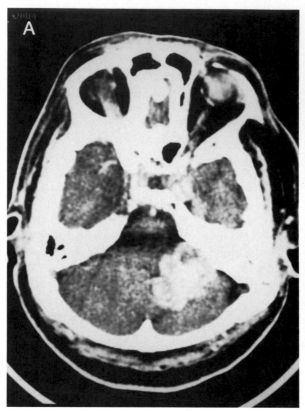
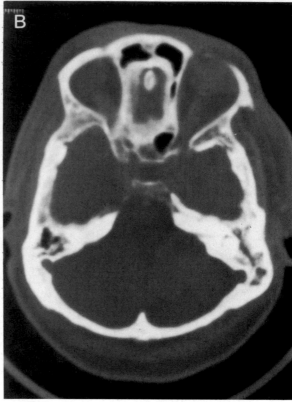

FIG 19–36.
Metastatic thyroid carcinoma to the posterior fossa and left cavernous sinus, with bone destruction demonstrated on a CT "bone window." The enhanced CT scan **(A)** demonstrates a large mass lesion in the left cerebellar region and a second mass in the region
of the left cavernous sinus. The wide window **(B)** demonstrates destruction of the left lesser and medial margin of the greater wings
of the sphenoid bone and erosion of the medial side of the left petrous bone.

onstrate the focal mass or masses of the primary or
metastatic tumor. The major differential consideration on the enhanced scan is ventriculitis, with an
easy clinical distinction between these two entities
in most cases. Periventricular spread of tumor is
generally an ominous sign, even when the patient
appears to be unchanged neurologically.[24] Whenever CSF seeding of a neoplasm is in the differential diagnosis, enhanced CT or MRI scanning is indicated.

REFERENCES

1. Russell DS, Rubenstein LJ (eds): *Pathology of Tumours of the Nervous System.* Baltimore, Williams
   & Wilkins, 1989, pp 825–841.
2. Potts DG, Albott GF, von Sneidern JV: National
   Cancer Institute study: Evaluation of computed tomography in the diagnosis of intracranial neoplasms: III. Metastatic tumors. *Radiology* 1980;
   136:657–664.
3. Weiss HD, Richardson EP: Solitary brainstem metastasis. *Neurology* 1978; 28:562–566.
4. Healy JF, Rosenkrantz H: Intraventricular metastases demonstrated by cranial computed tomography. *Radiology* 1980; 136:124.
5. Deck MDF, Messina AV, Sackett JF: Computed
   tomography in metastatic disease of the brain. *Radiology* 1976; 119:115–120.
6. Danzinger J, Wallace S, Handel SF, et al: Metastatic osteogenic sarcoma to the brain. *Cancer* 1979;
   43:707–710.
7. Ruelle A, Macchia G, Gambini C, et al: Unusual
   appearance of brain metastasis from adenocarcinoma of colon. *Neuroradiology* 1986; 28:375.
8. Gouliamos AD, Jimenez JP, Goree GA: Computed
   tomography and skull radiology in the diagnosis of
   calcified brain tumor. *AJR* 1978; 130:761–764.
9. Hayman LA, Evans RA, Hinch VC: Delayed high
   iodine dose contrast computed tomography: Cranial
   neoplasms. *Radiology* 1980; 136:677–684.
10. Shalen PR, Hayman LA, Wallace S, et al: Protocol
    for delayed contrast enhancement in computed to-
    mography of cerebral neoplasia. *Radiology* 1981;
    139:397–402.

11. Claussen C, Laniado M, Schorner W, et al: Gadolinium-DTPA in MR imaging of glioblastomas and intracranial metastases. *AJNR* 1985; 6:669–674.

12. Felix R, Schorner W, Laniado M, et al: Brain tumors: MR imaging with gadolinium-DTPA. *Radiology* 1985; 156:681–688.

13. Healy ME, Hesselink JR, Press GA, et al: Increased detection of intracranial metastases with intravenous Gd-DTPA. *Radiology* 1987; 165:619–624.

14. Russell EJ, Geremia GK, Johnson CE, et al: Multiple cerebral metastases: Detectability with Gd-DTPA–enhanced MR imaging. *Radiology* 1987; 167:609–617.

15. Atlas SW, Grossman RI, Gomori JM: Hemorrhagic intracranial malignant neoplasms: Spin-echo MR imaging. *Radiology* 1987; 164:71–77.

16. Woodruff WW, Djang WT, McLendon RE, et al: Intracerebral malignant melanoma: High–field-strength MR imaging. *Radiology* 1987; 165:209–213.

17. Dublin AB, Norman D: Fluid-fluid level in cystic cerebral metastatic melanoma. *J Comput Assist Tomogr* 1979; 3:650–652.

18. Whelan MA, Ascheri GF, Schlesinger EB: Cerebellar metastases from ovarian carcinoma. *J Comput Assist Tomogr* 1981; 5:583–585.

19. Mandybur TI: Intracranial hemorrhage caused by metastatic tumors. *Neurology* 1977; 27:650–655.

20. Gildersleeve N Jr, Koo AH, McDonald CJ: Metastatic tumor presenting as intracerebral hemorrhage. *Radiology* 1977; 124:109–112.

21. Ginoldi A, Wallace S, Shalen P, et al: Cranial computed tomography of malignant melanoma. *AJNR* 1980; 1:531–535.

22. Sze G, Krol G, Olsen WL, et al: Hemorrhagic neoplasms: MR mimics of occult vascular malformations. *AJNR* 1987; 8:795–802.

23. Enzmann DR, Kramer R, Norman D, et al: Malignant melanoma metastatic to the central nervous system. *Radiology* 1978; 127:177–180.

24. McGeachie RE, Gold LHA, Latchaw RE: Periventricular spread of tumor demonstrated by computed tomography. *Radiology* 1977; 125:407–411.

25. Latchaw RE, Gabrielsen TO, Seeger JF: Cerebral angiography in meningeal sarcomatosis and carcinomatosis. *Neuroradiology* 1974; 8:131–139.

26. Enzmann DR, Krikorian J, Yoke C, et al: Computed tomography in leptomeningeal spread of tumor. *J Comput Assist Tomogr* 1978; 2:448–455.

27. Lee YY, Glass JP, Geoffray A, et al: Cranial computed tomographic abnormalities in leptomeningeal metastasis. *AJNR* 1984; 5:559–563.

28. Davis PC, Friedman NC, Fry SM, et al: Leptomeningeal metastasis: MR imaging. *Radiology* 1987; 163:449–454.

29. Lee YY, Tien RD, Bruner JM, et al: Loculated intracranial leptomeningeal metastases: CT and MR characteristics. *AJNR* 1990; 10:1171–1179.

30. Sze G, Soletsky S, Bronen R, et al: MR imaging of the cranial meninges with emphasis on contrast enhancement and meningeal carcinomatosis. *AJNR* 1989; 10:965–975.

31. Russell DS, Rubenstein LJ (eds): *Pathology of Tumours of the Nervous System.* Baltimore, Williams & Wilkins, 1989, pp 590–638.

32. Enzmann DR, Krikorian J, Norman D, et al: Computed tomography in primary reticulum cell sarcoma of brain. *Radiology* 1979; 130:165–170.

33. Pagani JJ, Libshitz HI, Wallace S, et al: Central nervous system leukemia and lymphoma: Computed tomographic manifestations. *AJNR* 1981; 2:397–403.

34. Brandt-Zawadski M, Enzmann DR: Computed tomographic brain scanning in patients with lymphoma. *Radiology* 1978; 129:67–71.

35. Dubois PJ, Martinez AJ, Myerowitz RE, et al: Subependymal and leptomeningeal spread of systemic malignant lymphoma demonstrated by cranial computed tomography. *J Comput Assist Tomogr* 1978; 2:217–221.

36. Lee Y-Y, Bruner JM, Van Tassel P, et al: Primary central nervous system lymphoma: CT and pathologic correlation. *AJNR* 1986; 7:599–604.

37. Smirniotopoulos JG, Murphy FM: Radiology of CNS lymphoma. Presented at the 27th annual meeting of the American Society of Neuroradiology, Orlando, Fl, March 1989.

38. Holtas S, Nyman U, Cronqvist S: Computed tomography of malignant lymphoma of the brain. *Neuroradiology* 1984; 26:33–38.

39. Jack CR Jr, O'Neill BP, Banks PM, et al: Central nervous system lymphomas: Histologic types and CT appearance. *Radiology* 1988; 167:211–215.

40. Kasner E, Wilshe J, Steinhoff H, et al: Computer assisted tomography in primary malignant lymphomas of the brain. *J Comput Assist Tomogr* 1978; 2:125–134.

41. Schwaighofer BW, Hesselink JR, Press GA, et al: Primary intracranial CNS lymphoma: MR manifestations. *AJNR* 1989; 10:725–729.

42. Wendling LR, Cromwell LD, Latchaw RE: Computed tomography of intracranial leukemic masses. *AJR* 1979; 132:217–220.

43. Sowers JJ, Moody DM, Naidich TP, et al: Radiographic features of granulocytic sarcoma (chloroma). *J Comput Assist Tomogr* 1979; 3:226–233.

44. Leonard KJ, Mamourian AC: MR appearance of intracranial chloromas. *AJNR* 1989; 10(suppl):67–68.

45. Pederson H, Clausen N: The development of cerebral CT changes during treatment of acute lymphocytic leukemia in childhood. *Neuroradiology* 1981; 22:79–84.

46. Healy JF, Marshall WH, Brahme PJ, et al: CT of intracranial metastases with skull and scalp involvement. *AJNR* 1981; 2:335–338.

47. Latchaw RE, L'Heureux PR, Young G, et al: Neuro-

blastoma presenting as central nervous system disease. *AJNR* 1982; 3:623–630.

48. Chirathivat S, Post MJD: CT demonstration of dural metastases in neuroblastoma. *J Comput Assist Tomogr* 1980; 4:316–319.

49. Scotti G, Harwood-Nash DC: Computed tomography in rhabdomyosarcoma of the skull base in children. *J Comput Assist Tomogr* 1982; 6:33–39.

50. Kieffer SA, Salibi NA, Kim RE, et al: Multifocal glioblastoma. Diagnostic implications. *Radiology* 1982; 143:709–710.

20

Differential Diagnosis of Intracranial Tumors

Richard E. Latchaw, M.D.

David W. Johnson, M.D.

Emanuel Kanal, M.D.

Two aspects of the differential diagnosis of cerebral neoplasms utilizing computed tomography (CT) and magnetic resonance (MR) scan characteristics are emphasized in this chapter: first, those characteristics that help in distinguishing one type of tumor from another; second, those characteristics that are of value in distinguishing a neoplasm from a non-neoplastic process. No one scan characteristic can be utilized in differentiating one type of tumor from another, or in separating neoplastic from non-neoplastic processes. However, a combination of findings will generally improve the probability of the diagnosis of a particular neoplasm. While biopsy will always be necessary to ensure the correct histologic finding, the diagnosis of neoplasm can be made preoperatively in most cases, and many times the specific tumor type itself can be accurately predicted.

COMPUTED TOMOGRAPHY AND MAGNETIC RESONANCE SCAN CHARACTERISTICS FOR DIFFERENTIATING TUMOR TYPES

The five most common tumor types have been selected for analysis and evaluation according to their CT and MR scan characteristics. They are (1) benign astrocytoma, (2) malignant astrocytoma and glioblastoma multiforme, (3) meningioma, (4) hematogenous metastasis, and (5) lymphoma (both primary and secondary) and leukemia. While lymphoma has not been a common tumor until recently, the advent of the acquired immunodeficiency syndrome (AIDS) and the increase in the number of patients undergoing immunosuppression mean that this tumor, which is related to the change in immunologic state, will become increasingly more common.

The CT and MR scan characteristics include the density and intensity before contrast enhancement, the degree and homogeneity of enhancement, the speed of the enhancement and the sharpness of the tumor margins following enhancement, and the degree of peritumoral edema and mass effect (Table 20–1). The characteristics for a given tumor are obviously generalizations, and exceptions will always be found. In addition, each generalization concerns the usual supratentorial tumor in an adult, which may differ for a different location or age group. For example, a low-grade pilocytic astrocytoma of the cerebellum in a child usually enhances to a rather marked and homogeneous degree, whereas most low-grade supratentorial astrocytomas in the adult demonstrate a patchy pattern of low-level enhancement. In addition, there is a subset of astrocytomas that are of a purely decreased density or intensity without evidence of enhancement, but are varied in degree of histologic malignancy. These tumors are also exceptions to the generalizations in this chapter.

Of all the neuroepithelial tumors, only the be-

TABLE 20–1.
Differential Diagnostic Features of Cerebral Neoplasms

Characteristic	Supratentorial Astrocytoma	Malignant Astrocytoma/Glioblastoma	Meningioma	Hematogenous Metastasis	Lymphoma (Primary and Secondary)/Leukemia
CT density without contrast	Decreased to isodense, mixed	Variable: decreased to increased, mixed	*Isodense to increased, homogeneous	Variable: decreased to increased	Isodense to hyperdense
MR intensity without contrast Short TR	Hypo- to isointense	Hypo- to isointense rim; hypointense center	Isointense	Hypo- to hyperintense (melanoma, bleed) nodule, hypointense periphery (edema)	Lymphoma: slightly hypointense to gray matter Leukemia: isointense to white matter
Long TR/TE	Hyperintense	Hyperintense	*Isointense to mildly hyperintense	Hyperintense	*Lymphoma: isointense to slightly hyperintense to gray matter Leukemia: isointense to white matter
Calcification	Common	Uncommon, unless malignant degeneration of benign astrocytoma	Frequent	Uncommon	Unknown
Hemorrhage	Rare	Common	Rare	Common in certain metastases	Rare
Degree of enhancement	*None to moderate	Moderate to marked, occasionally minimal	Marked	Moderate to marked	Moderate to marked
Homogeneity of enhancement	Unusually patchy	Ring, solid	Homogeneous	Homogeneous or ring	Homogeneous
Enhancement over time	*Slow	Moderate to rapid; ring may fill in	Rapid	Moderate to rapid; ring may fill in	Moderate
Tumor margins after contrast	Irregular, poorly defined	Mixed: sharp, irregular	Sharp	Sharp	Irregular
Edema	Minimal	Abundant	Minimal to mild	Abundant	Minimal
Mass effect	Variable: none to moderate	Moderate to marked	Variable: slight to moderate	Frequently marked	Slight

*Denotes significant differential characteristics.

nign and malignant astrocytomas are considered in this evaluation. Other neuroepithelial tumors such as oligodendroglioma, ependymoma, and primitive neuroectodermal tumors (PNET) (including medulloblastoma) have scan characteristics that are sufficiently different from the generalizations given that they cannot be included in this discussion. The specific appearances of these latter tumors are described more fully in Chapter 16. The congenital tumors and associated neoplasms discussed in Chapter 18 are sufficiently uncommon, with specific radiographic or clinical findings (patient age, anatomic position, clinical syndromes, presence of fat, etc.), that they usually do not enter into the differential diagnosis of the five major classes of neoplasms to be compared and contrasted in this chapter.

In summary, this evaluation of the features of differential diagnosis emphasizes the five most common types of neoplasms seen in the adult, and their most typical appearances on MR and CT scans. The generalization for each scan characteristic is listed in Table 20–1; only brief additional comments are presented on the following pages.

CT Density Before Contrast Enhancement

The measured CT density of a cerebral neoplasm depends upon whether evaluation is made of the tumor itself or the peritumoral edema. For a meningioma, hematogenous metastasis, and lymphoma and leukemia, a nodular mass of tumor tissue is well demarcated from low density that may be properly called edema since the tumor is relatively circumscribed and creates an area of surrounding vasogenic edema without fingers of tumor infiltrating the parenchyma. For astrocytoma and glioblastoma, on the other hand, tumor infiltrates into the contiguous parenchyma creating an admixture of vasogenic edema, tumor, and normal glia. When describing the CT scan characteristics of a lesion, it is helpful to make the distinction, if possible, between a relatively well-circumscribed mass, which itself may be either homogeneous or patchy in its hyper-, iso-, or hypodensity, and the surrounding low-density edema.

The precontrast CT scan may be helpful in the differential diagnosis. As seen in Table 20–1, benign (see Figs 16–1 to 16–3) and malignant astrocytoma[1] and hematogenous metastasis[2–6] are variable in density on the precontrast scan, whereas meningioma (see Fig 17–1) and lymphoma and leukemia (see Figs 16–63, 16–64,A, 19–26, and

19–30)[7–10] tend to be homogeneously isodense to moderately hyperdense. If there is a large amount of edema surrounding the meningioma or the deposit of lymphoma or leukemia, the appearance may be similar to a hematogenous metastasis, which may also have a relatively homogeneous tumor nodule on the preinfusion scan and a large amount of surrounding edema. The presence of diffuse low density tends to exclude the diagnosis of meningioma.

MR Intensity Before Contrast Enhancement

The preenhancement MR intensity patterns are divided between those seen on the short TR scans and those on the long TR/TE sequences. On the short TR scans, the low-grade astrocytoma tends to be a patchy admixture of hypo- and isointensity with poorly defined borders (see Fig 16–6). Glioblastoma with a ring of viable neoplastic tissue surrounding a necrotic center has hypo- to isointensity of its rim and hypointensity of the central necrosis.[11–14] Meningioma is typically isointense to mildly hypointense with respect to gray matter (see Fig 17–5).[15–17] Hematogenous metastasis usually has a hypointense (see Fig 19–1) to hyperintense nodule (especially if hemorrhagic, or melanoma) surrounded by hypointense edema. Lymphomatous deposits are slightly hypointense to gray matter,[18] and leukemic deposits are isointense to white matter.[19]

On the long TR/TE sequences, benign astrocytoma (see Figs 16–3, 16–6, and 16–7) is hyperintense as is glioblastoma (see Fig 16–4). The rim of more viable tissue surrounding a necrotic center usually is less hyperintense than the center. Meningioma generally maintains the same intensity relative to gray matter on the long TR/TE scan as was present on the short TR sequence, or becomes mildly hyperintense (see Figs 17–5 through 17–8),[17–19] which is a distinguishing feature among all the tumors considered. The hematogenous metastasis generally becomes hyperintense, although the central nodule may be less hyperintense than the peritumoral edema (see Fig 19–1). Lymphomatous deposits maintain isointensity to gray matter or slight hyperintensity. This, too, is a distinguishing feature for intraaxial masses, since gliomas and hematogenous metastases tend to become more hyperintense on the long TR sequences.[18] Leukemia may stay isointense to white matter, or become hyperintense (see Fig 19–30).[19] It should again be stressed, however, that there can be considerable variation in these patterns. For example, as discussed and illustrated in Chapter 17, meningioma can occasionally become quite hyperintense relative to gray matter on long TR/ TE studies.

Calcification

Calcification is a rather nonspecific finding and may be seen with many neuroepithelial tumors,[20] even the more malignant varieties such as the benign astrocytoma that has undergone malignant degeneration (see Fig 16–18). Calcification is uncommon in most metastases, although certain metastatic tumors such as osteogenic sarcoma (see Fig 19–18) and adenocarcinoma of the gastrointestinal tract may have well-defined foci of calcification. In addition, the increased density on nonenhanced CT scans of some metastatic tumors is on the basis of hemorrhage (see Fig 19–5) or mucoid degeneration. Others, however, are dense because of their high cellularity (see Fig 19–7). Calcification is common in meningioma (see Figs 17–3 and 17–4). To our knowledge, it has not been reported in lymphoma (primary or secondary) or leukemia.

Hemorrhage

Hemorrhage is distinctly rare in meningioma, lymphoma (primary and secondary) and leukemia, and benign astrocytoma, but is relatively common in malignant neoplasms as they rapidly outgrow their blood supply (see Figs 16–17, 19–5, 19–11, and 19–16).[21–23] The presence of hemorrhage tends to exclude a diagnosis of benign astrocytoma, lymphoma or leukemia, and meningioma.

Degree of Enhancement

Malignant astrocytoma and glioblastoma (see Fig 16–8),[24–26] meningioma (see Fig 17–1),[26–28] and many metastatic tumors (see Fig 19–1)[2, 3, 29, 30] enhance to a marked degree. Lymphomatous and leukemic deposits usually have moderate-to-marked enhancement (see Figs 16–63, 16–64, 19–26, 19–27, and 19–30).[7–10] On the other hand, benign astrocytoma tends to have a relatively intact blood-brain barrier (BBB), and therefore there is a degree of enhancement that varies from minimal to none in a large number of cases (see Figs 16–1 and 16–2),[25,31,32] to moderate in a few of the cases. Again, one must realize that many low-grade astrocytomas, particularly those in children, may have a moderate-to-marked degree of enhancement (see Figs 16–19 and 16–29). There is also a subset of glial tumors, from benign to malignant, that are hypodense on CT and have little or no enhancement.[33]

Homogeneity of Enhancement

The texture of enhancement is frequently helpful in distinguishing the five types of tumors. Benign astrocytoma tends to be patchy in its enhancement pattern (see Figs 16–1 and 16–2),[25,31,32] whereas malignant astrocytoma and glioblastoma vary from a relatively well-circumscribed although irregular appearance (see Fig 16–8) to a ring of enhancement. The ring appearance is common with glioblastoma (see Fig 16–11), with irregular margins of the ring being characteristic.[24,31] Meningioma is usually homogeneous in its enhancement pattern (see Fig 17–5),[15–17, 27–29] although up to 15% of meningiomas may have unusual appearances such as hemorrhage, cyst formation, or irregular margins.[34] Hematogenous metastasis usually has either a homogeneous (see Fig 19–1) or a ring type of enhancement (see Fig 19–12). Deposits of lymphoma or leukemia are usually homogeneous in enhancement (see Figs 16–63, 16–64, 19–27, and 19–30).[7–10]

It should also be stressed that the homogeneity of enhancement may be in part time-dependent. A ring lesion may partially fill in over time, and this has been seen with both primary gliomas and metastatic lesions.[2–4]

In summary, the heterogeneity of enhancement usually excludes meningioma; the presence of a ring of enhancement tends to exclude benign astrocytoma; and patchy enhancement usually excludes most hematogenous metastases, although some metastases may have this pattern.

Time-Dependent CT and MR Enhancement Characteristics

The CT scan characteristic depends upon the serial observations of the neoplasm over time, with an evaluation of the changing attenuation coefficients. Early studies by Hatam and co-workers[35] and by Lewander[36] suggested that tumor diagnosis may be facilitated by such serial observation. Graphic representation of the enhancement pattern of various tumors demonstrated that relatively vascular meningiomas and metastases enhance quickly, while the benign glioma tends to enhance over a slower period of time. Unfortunately, these early studies relied upon relatively slow scanners. Follow-up studies to this early work have been uncommon.[26, 37-39]

Gadolinium diethylenetriamine pentaacetic acid (DTPA) enhancement characteristics for magnetic resonance imaging (MRI) are similar, both anatomically and temporally, to iodinated contrast enhancement for CT. However, the sensitivity to such enhancement appears to be greater for MRI than for CT.

In general, benign astrocytoma tends to enhance relatively slower over time than its more malignant counterpart. The enhancement of a metastatic lesion depends upon the degree of alteration of the BBB, which is variable with different metastatic tumors. Enhancement of lymphomatous and leukemic deposits parallels that of metastatic lesions. The rings of both malignant astrocytomas and hematogenous metastases may fill in over time as previously indicated. Extraaxial tumors such as meningioma, nerve sheath tumor, and pituitary tumor all lack a BBB, and all enhance rapidly with the movement of contrast material across the blood-tissue interface. Meningiomas tend to have a relatively rapid clearance of that enhancement, while the clearance may be slower in schwannomas.[38]

Tumor Margins

Most hematogenous metastases tend to be sharply demarcated on the enhanced scan, with a sharp margin separating the actual tumor nodule from the peritumoral edema (see Figs 19-1 and 19-10). Some metastases, however, have irregular margins indicating infiltration into surrounding tissue. Lymphomatous and leukemic deposits have such margins (see Figs 16-64 and 19-28). Sharp margination is characteristic of meningiomas (see Fig 17-1). Malignant astrocytoma and glioblastoma may have either an irregular enhancing margin or a relatively sharp margin (see Fig 16-8). When a ring of enhancement is present, it is typically thick and irregular in contour (see Figs 16-11, 16-12). Finally, benign astrocytoma generally has poorly defined, irregular margins, as the tumor blends imperceptibly into the surrounding parenchyma (see Figs 16-1 and 16-2).[11-14, 33]

Edema

It must be stressed that the low density surrounding an astrocytoma or glioblastoma usually represents a combination of edema and poorly enhancing fingers of tumor. In general, however, most benign astrocytomas have minimal surrounding edema because of the relatively intact BBB, whereas there is usually abundant edema surrounding a malignant glial tumor (see Fig 16-17). Likewise, the edema surrounding metastatic tumors is generally abundant (see Fig 19-2). Edema around lymphomatous and leukemic deposits is usually minimal to mild in degree (see Figs 16-63, 16-64, 19-27, and 19-30),[7-10, 18] a feature that helps distinguish this class of tumors from other intraaxial neoplasms. Peritumoral edema surrounding meningioma is quite variable. The stated classic appearance is that of minimal edema (see Fig 17-11), whereas up to 47% of meningiomas may have a moderate or occasionally even a marked degree of peritumoral edema (see Fig 17-1).[40]

Mass Effect

The amount of mass effect from the malignant tumors, whether of primary glial or metastatic origin, tends to be moderate to marked, secondary to the amount of peritumoral edema that is present (see Figs 16-11 and 19-10). Lymphomatous and leukemic deposits differ, in that edema is minimal to mild in degree (see Figs 16-63 and 19-27). Benign astrocytoma may have a mass effect that varies from none to moderate, depending upon the amount of associated edema and the size of the lesion. With minimal mass effect and only patchy enhancement (see Figs 16-1 and 16-2), infiltrating low-grade astrocytoma frequently resembles cerebritis, infarction, and demyelinating disease. Meningioma grows very slowly, frequently indenting the brain[41] and causing little diffuse mass effect even when very large (see Fig 17-7). Peritumoral edema may be moderate to marked, however, with that edema occurring very quickly in some cases (see Fig 17-1). The reason for this rapid accumulation of edema fluid with meningioma is unknown, but may produce a marked degree of mass effect and rapid neurologic change.[42]

Summary

It can be seen from Table 20-1 and the generalizations described that no one feature of the MR and CT scan appearances of these five major classes of intracranial tumors is sufficient for distinguishing the tumor type. Rather, it is generally a combination of features that points to the correct diagnosis. The salient features for each tumor type can be listed as follows:

1. *Benign astrocytoma:* Hypodense-to-isodense lesion with inhomogeneous and patchy texture on CT before enhancement; hypointense to isointense on short TR unenhanced MR scans and hyperintense on long TR/TE sequence; may be calcified, but no evidence of hemorrhage; slight-to-moderate enhancement occurs slowly and gives a nonhomogeneous texture with poor visualization of the margins; there is slight or no edema and mild mass effect.

2. *Malignant astrocytoma and glioblastoma:* Inhomogeneous low-to-isodense lesion without calcification but possibly hemorrhage on the unenhanced CT scan; hypo- to isointense rim with a hypointense central area on short TR MR scans, and hyperintensity on long TR/TE sequences; moderate-to-marked enhancement occurs rapidly, producing either an inhomogeneous texture, a relatively homogeneous appearance, or a ring of enhancement; margins are frequently sharply defined, particularly when a ring is present, although margins are thick and ragged in contour; there is moderate-to-marked surrounding edema and mass effect.

3. *Meningioma:* Extraaxial homogeneous isodense to moderately hyperdense lesion on the nonenhanced CT scan, frequently containing calcifications, but no hemorrhage; isointense lesion on short TR MR sequence that maintains the same or mildly increases the intensity on long TR/TE MR scans; rapid, marked, and homogeneous enhancement; sharp margination with minimal-to-mild surrounding edema and mass effect.

4. *Hematogenous metastasis:* Variable density on noncontrast CT scan; may have hemorrhage; calcification is specific to certain histologic types; hypo- to hyperintense nodule (melanoma, hemorrhagic) with a hypointense periphery on short TR MR scans and hyperintensity on long TR/TE sequences; enhancement in a moderately rapid period of time, and to a moderate or marked degree; texture is usually either homogeneous or a ring, with sharp margination and abundant surrounding edema; the nodule and edema may be separable on long TR/TE MR scans and on postcontrast studies.

5. *Lymphoma (primary or secondary) and leukemia:* Isodense to hyperdense on precontrast CT; hemorrhage is rare and calcification unknown; lymphoma is slightly hypointense to gray matter on the short TR MR study that becomes slightly hyperintense on the long TR/TE sequence; leukemia is either isointense to white matter on both short TR and long TR/TE studies, or changes from mild hypointensity (short TR) to hyperintense (long TR/TE); there is moderate-to-marked homogeneous enhancement in a moderate time period; tumor margins are irregular; there is minimal edema with only slight mass effect.

MAGNETIC RESONANCE AND COMPUTED TOMOGRAPHY SCAN CHARACTERISTICS DIFFERENTIATING NEOPLASTIC FROM NON-NEOPLASTIC LESIONS

The major disease categories to be differentiated from cerebral neoplasm are infarction; infection producing cerebritis and abscess; noninfectious granulomatous disease such as sarcoidosis, demyelinating disease, aneurysm, and arteriovenous malformation (AVM); radiation necrosis; and non-neoplastic mass such as arachnoid cyst. The specific CT scan features of infarction, inflammatory lesions, and aneurysms and AVM are presented elsewhere in this book. Radiation necrosis is discussed in this chapter and in Chapter 21, while arachnoid cyst has been extensively discussed in Chapter 17.

Infarction

Neoplasms are included in the differential diagnosis of lesions producing acute cerebrovascular symptoms. While the rapid onset of symptoms in a particular vascular distribution generally suggests thrombosis, embolism, or hemorrhage, a mass lesion such as neoplasm or subdural hematoma may occasionally produce a sudden change in neurologic status and, therefore, mimic a vascular lesion.[43] In such a case, the appearance of the lesion on the MR or CT scan will generally distinguish neoplasm from infarction.

Leptomeningeal arterial occlusion leads to infarction that involves the gray matter in almost all cases, and a combination of gray and white matter in two thirds of cases.[44] It occurs in the vascular distribution specific for that vessel, and frequently has a wedge-shaped configuration, the apex of which

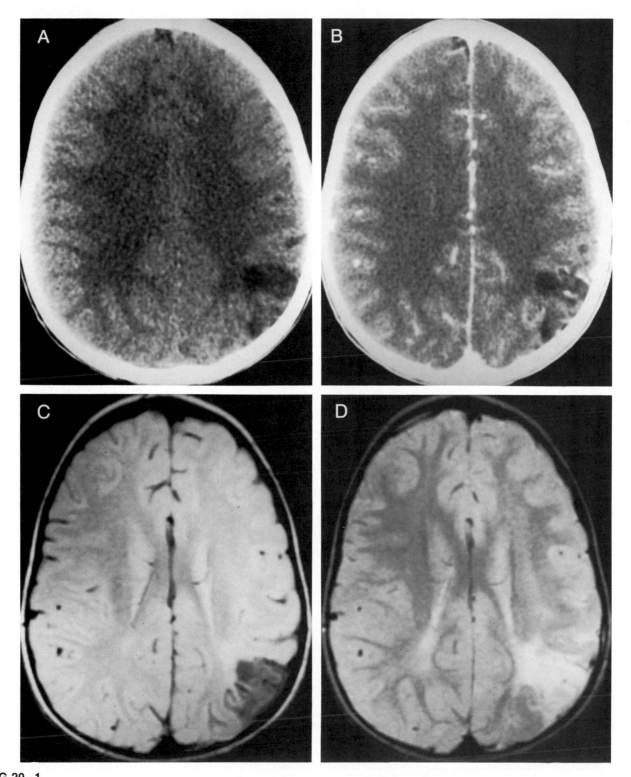

FIG 20—1.
Left parietal infarct. **A,** the unenhanced CT scan demonstrates a low-density abnormality involving both cortex and subcortical white matter in the left parietal lobe. There is mixed isodensity within the area of low density, representing an area that is not infarcted. **B,** the enhanced scan shows peripheral enhancement characteristic of infarction. **C,** the long TR, short TE MR examination (TR 2,000, TE 20) demonstrates an area of pronounced hypointensity which is quite homogeneous in contradistinction to the mixed isodense and hyperdense appearance on CT (**A** and **B**). **D,** the long TR/TE study (TR 2,000, TE 80) demonstrates the classic appearance of an infarct with its pronounced hyperintensity involving both cortical and subcortical white matter, extending to the edge of the ventricle. The extension is greater than appreciated on the CT scan.

points toward the ventricular system (Fig 20–1). Deep white matter infarction occurs in the watershed between branches of the leptomeningeal arteries and the lenticulostriate vessels. Glial tumors involve gray or white matter or both but not in a discrete vascular distribution. Hematogenous metastases involve the gray-white interface, or the deep gray or white matter structures but have a discrete nodule with surrounding edema. Meningioma indents the cortex, but does not destroy superficial gray matter,[41] and its appearance is distinctly different from that of infarction.

Infarcts have peripheral nonhomogeneous or gyriform enhancement beginning no earlier than 24 hours after ictus on CT and 4 to 6 hours on MRI, maximizing at 7 to 14 days and lasting up to 8 weeks.[45] This enhancement is at the margin of viable tissue where there is still a BBB, albeit damaged, whereas the central portion of the infarct is devascularized and undergoes necrosis (see Fig 20–1). An intense gyriform enhancement pattern on MRI, especially in the subacute phase, may be quite impressive in degree and extent (much

greater than suggested on the unenhanced short or long TR studies), strongly suggesting the correct diagnosis. It is rare for glial tumors to demonstrate this cortical ribbon of enhancement.[46] Both primary and secondary neoplasms may have a rim of enhancement (see Figs 16–11, 19–15), and at times the peripheral enhancement of an infarct may simulate the ring enhancement of a neoplasm. However, the peripheral enhancement of an infarct is generally an incomplete ring, and this finding in combination with the position of the lesion in a vascular distribution and the clinical history will differentiate infarction from neoplasm in the overwhelming majority of cases.

Infectious Lesions

When discussing infection, a distinction must be made between cerebritis and abscess. Cerebritis is a diffuse encephalitic process with poor margins and irregular enhancement (Fig 20–2) that may go on to frank abscess formation with relatively sharp margins and the appearance of a ring

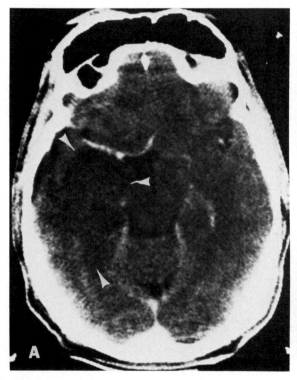
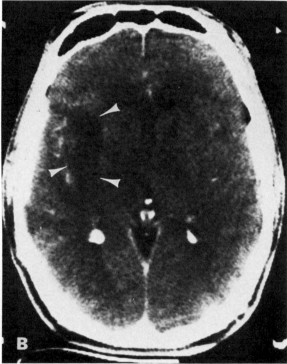

FIG 20–2.
Herpes encephalitis of the right temporal lobe. **A,** the lower enhanced axial scan demonstrates a poorly marginated area of moderate decreased density and no enhancement *(white arrowheads)* involving the inferior portion of the right temporal lobe. There is some anterior displacement of the middle cerebral artery. **B,** a higher cut demonstrates a more sharply circumscribed area of low density *(arrowheads)* within the superior right temporal lobe. Intracellular inclusion bodies typical of herpes simplex encephalitis were found by stereotactic biopsy (scans performed in stereotactic frame).

lesion (Fig 20–3). It may be extremely difficult to distinguish cerebritis from a diffuse infiltrating neoplasm on MRI or CT alone. In both, irregular borders and heterogeneous density and intensity may be present on CT and MR scans, respectively, with and without contrast enhancement. The distinction between cerebritis and infarction also may be extremely difficult. Infarction has a vascular distribution, involving both cortex and white matter in most cases, whereas cerebritis may involve primarily deep structures outside of a classic vascular distribution (see Fig 20–2). The correct distinction between infiltrating neoplasm, cerebritis, and infarction may depend upon the patient's history, the clinical findings, and the progression of the lesion. Biopsy may be necessary in early stages for appropriate diagnosis.

Likewise, it may be impossible to distinguish abscess with its ring formation from either primary malignant glioma or metastatic tumor. Abscess commonly has a sharp inner margin to the ring of enhancement, while the inner margin of a necrotic tumor is usually shaggy (see Fig 19–14). However, the "ring sign" is nonspecific. Abscess may be seen to have a relatively shaggy margin (Fig 20–3), while both primary and secondary neoplasms may have sharply marginated rings (see Figs 16–11 and 19–15). The appearance of the ring of an abscess is time-dependent, with a more shaggy margination occurring in the early stages of abscess formation. A sharp inner margin of the ring of a neoplasm is indicative of its cystic nature. In any given case, the distinction between abscess and tumor may be impossible. The clinical history, including the rapidity of progression and the presence of extracranial infection, may be necessary for the appropriate diagnosis. Biopsy and drainage under CT or ultrasonic guidance may be both diagnostic and therapeutic.

Tuberculous involvement of the cerebral parenchyma varies from the ring enhancement of an abscess to the solid nodule of a tuberculoma. In addition, there may be a diffuse meningitis, particularly at the base of the brain, characterized by meningeal enhancement. It is said that a tuberculous abscess frequently has thick irregular walls and is multilocular, whereas bacterial abscesses classically have thinner walls[47]; given that appearance, distinguishing tuberculous abscess from primary or metastatic tumor would probably be impossible on the scan alone. Tuberculoma may be isodense on CT before contrast enhancement, with either a homogeneous or a ring appearance pro-

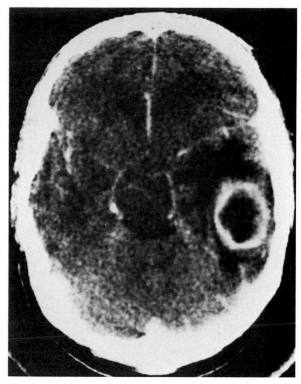

FIG 20–3.
Left temporal lobe abscess. The enhanced axial scan demonstrates the classic ring of enhancement within this left temporal lobe abscess. There is abundant surrounding edema and a moderately irregular and shaggy rim.

duced on the postinfusion CT scan.[48] Calcification may or may not be present to help in distinguishing such a nodule from metastatic tumor.

Sarcoid

Up to 14% of patients with systemic sarcoidosis will have meningeal or parenchymal deposits of sarcoid. Meningeal involvement is more common, with parenchymal involvement usually being peripheral as a result of spread of the lesion through the meninges. The lesion(s) occasionally may be isolated to periventricular or deep white matter.[49–53] The MR or CT scan appearance will vary from only meningeal enhancement, similar to meningitis or meningeal carcinomatosis of any form, to a parenchymal mass lesion that enhances homogeneously and mimics neoplasm[49–53] to multiple deposits (Fig 20–4) simulating diffuse metastatic disease.[51] The combination of meningeal and peripheral parenchymal involvement of a homogeneous nature is also found in lymphoma and leukemia (see Figs 19–25 through 19–30), and distinction from sarcoid proba-

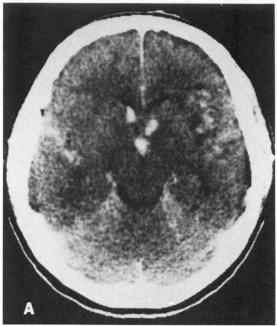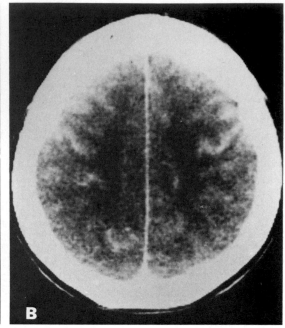

FIG 20–4.

Meningeal and parenchymal sarcoid. **A,** the lower cut demonstrates multiple nodular deposits of sarcoid in the region of the left hypothalamus, right caudate nucleus, and third ventricle. There is a propensity for sarcoid involvement of the hypothalamus, pituitary, and basal ganglia. There are also further deposits of sarcoid in the temporal lobes bilaterally. **B,** a higher scan demonstrates multiple areas of gyral enhancement, similar to the appearance of leptomeningeal neoplasm or pyogenic meningitis.

bly cannot be made without a history of the particular systemic disease, or biopsy.

Demyelinating Disease

The most common demyelinating disease is multiple sclerosis (MS), which is characterized by a history of waxing and waning of neurologic symptoms, including blurred vision, ataxia, incoordination, and slurred speech. Multiple periventricular lucencies on the CT scan, and multiple hypointense foci on the short TR scan which become hyperintense on long TR sequences are classic findings. Involvement of the brain stem and cerebellum is common, with a lower incidence of spinal cord involvement. Some of these plaques may enhance with contrast material during an acute exacerbation, representing a transient breakdown of the BBB (see Figs 13–15 and 13–16). Usually only a few of the plaques enhance at any given time. Occasionally, enhancement of multiple nodules may suggest a diagnosis of metastases in a case without the typical clinical history. However, MS is suggested by the location of the nodular enhancement in a periventricular distribution rather than at the corticomedullary junctions so typical of metastases, by the lack of perinodular edema typical of most metastases, and by the enhancement of only a few of the hyperintense lesions seen on the long TR study.

Rarely, a previously normal patient will present with a solitary enhancing lesion on the CT scan accompanying the acute onset of neurologic symptoms as the earliest manifestation of MS. That lesion may have heterogeneous enhancement with irregular borders simulating a primary neoplasm (see Fig 13–17). The correct diagnosis may be impossible by CT alone. High gamma globulin levels (IgG) in the cerebrospinal fluid (CSF) or subtle historical points such as transient visual blurring may give a hint to the correct diagnosis. MR scanning will usually show multiple lesions in MS even when the CT only shows one, differentiating primary tumor and MS.

Other forms of demyelinating disease may present with acute symptomatology and lesions that simulate neoplasm on imaging studies (see Fig 13–18). Bilateral frontal lobe demyelinating lesions of adrenoleukodystrophy with involvement of the corpus callosum may simulate a "butterfly glioma."[54] In such cases, the diagnosis of demyelinating disease will require biopsy and/or evaluation of other organ systems.

Aneurysm and Arteriovenous Malformation

A giant aneurysm presents as a mass, with a well-circumscribed homogeneously enhancing density on CT scan when the aneurysm is patent (see Fig 11–5). The presence of the lesion in the distribution of one of the major cerebral blood vessels may arouse suspicion for the presence of an aneurysm. Laminated clot may fill the aneurysm so that there is only peripheral enhancement, representing relative vascularity of the wall. A central nodule of enhancement may also be seen, representing that portion of the lumen remaining patent, surrounded by laminated clot (see Fig 11–6). Calcification of the wall is common. A parasellar aneurysm that is dense before the administration of contrast material because of the presence of the "blood pool," which does not have calcification in the wall and which enhances homogeneously, will simulate a meningioma or trigeminal schwannoma on the CT scan (see Fig 23–44).

MRI is the method of choice for distinguishing aneurysm from neoplasm. Rapidly flowing blood in a totally patent aneurysm has a characteristic marked hypointensity on both short and long TR sequences (see Fig 11–5). Partially or totally thrombosed aneurysms have components characteristic of subacute and chronic hemorrhage, thrombosis, and fibrosis (see Figs 11–7 and 11–8). These appearances allow easy differentiation from neoplasm.

The classic racemose AVM has large serpentine structures representing feeding arteries and draining veins. The typical MR and CT appearances are unlike any typical neoplasm, allowing the distinction between AVM and neoplasm to be made (see Figs 11–11 to 11–13). Unfortunately, some cases of AVM present primarily as irregular nonhomogeneous but relatively confluent densities on the enhanced CT scan, thereby simulating neoplasm. The presence of increased density on the preinfusion CT scan may suggest an increased blood pool. Hemorrhage in the vicinity may strongly suggest a vascular lesion such as AVM, although hemorrhage into a tumor is not uncommon.[21–23] The distinction may be possible with MRI. The hypointensity of flowing blood, the hyperintensity of subacute blood, and the pro-

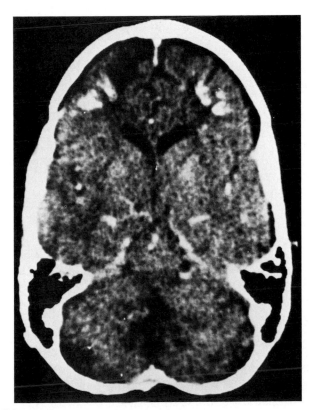

FIG 20–5.
Frontal lobe calcifications following methotrexate and cranial irradiation for medulloblastoma. This single enhanced axial view demonstrates midline oncephalomalacia within the posterior fossa following previous resection, chemotherapy, and irradiation for medulloblastoma. There are areas of frontal lobe encephalomalacia bilaterally, associated with multiple nodular calcifications in both frontal lobes.

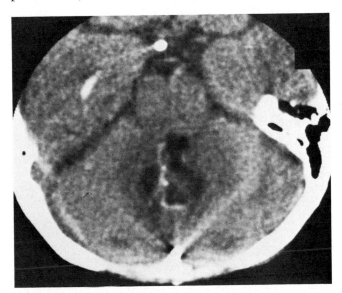

FIG 20–6.
Radiation necrosis of the cerebellar vermis. This axial enhanced scan through the posterior fossa demonstrates that a previous midline posterior fossa craniotomy has been performed for ependymoma in this adolescent girl. There is curvilinear enhancement just to the right of the midline. The patient had symptoms of progressive ataxia and midline cerebellar dysfunction, prompting surgical exploration for possible recurrent ependymoma. Surgery and pathologic examination revealed only radiation necrosis.

nounced hypointensity of hemosiderin on long TR/TE scans and gradient echo sequences are characteristic of AVM. An occult or "cryptic" AVM may have these MR findings[55] without enlarged hypointense feeding or draining vessels. Old hemorrhage into tumor may look similar, although there is usually solid tumor evident on the enhanced MR scan.

Venous angioma has a classic appearance on high-resolution CT or MR scans, with radiating venules converging into a nidus, from which exits a large transparenchymal vein (see Fig 11–17).[56] The classic appearance should not be confused with neoplasm.

Finally, mass effect with a ring of enhancement on CT scan may be present with a resolving hematoma. If no history of previous hemorrhage is available, this ring may be thought to represent abscess, primary glioma, or metastatic neoplasm. The ring represents a vascular capsule and the abnormality of the BBB surrounding the resolving hematoma, with the more central low CT density being the liquefying portion of the clot. MRI easily

detects the subacute-to-chronic clot with intensities unlike nonhemorrhagic neoplasm. Old hemorrhage into a tumor may obscure the diagnosis of underlying neoplasm.[54] Enhancement of the solid neoplastic component or sequential MR or CT scans demonstrating progression or resolution usually resolve the dilemma. Occasionally, tumors such as metastatic melanocytic melanoma with hemorrhage might provide differential diagnostic difficulty on MRI, mimicking the multiple sites of non-neoplastic hemorrhage from a coagulopathy.

Radiation Necrosis

Irradiation of the head has been reported to produce numerous findings, including osteoradionecrosis of the calvarium[57]; radiation-induced sarcoma, such as fibrosarcoma in the parasellar region following pituitary irradiation[58–60]; parenchymal calcification with areas of white matter hypodensity and atrophy (Fig 20–5) following the combined use of radiation and chemotherapy for intracranial leukemia, lymphoma, and other neoplasms[61, 62]; CT hy-

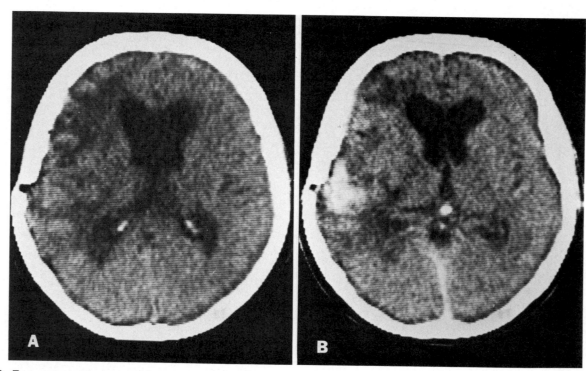

FIG 20–7.
Right frontotemporal radiation necrosis. The patient had multiple previous craniotomies for attempted removal of a right sphenoid wing meningioma. Radiation therapy was administered in an attempt to prevent recurrence. **A,** the unenhanced scan demonstrates multiple patchy high- and low-density areas within the right frontal and temporal lobes. **B,** the enhanced scan shows a confluent and homogeneously enhancing focus in the right parietotemporal region. The enhancing focus simulates neoplasm. Surgery revealed radiation necrosis only. (Courtesy of Lawrence Gold, M.D., University of Minnesota, Minneapolis.)

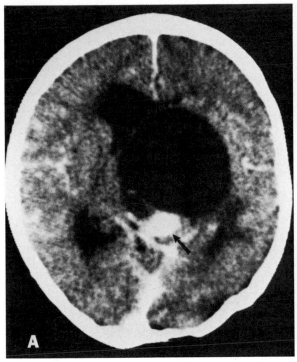 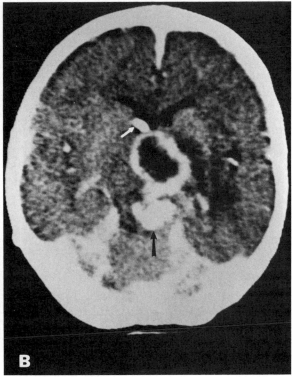

FIG 20–8.
Radiation necrosis following interstitial irradiation. **A,** enhanced CT scan demonstrates a large recurrent thalamic glioma with both a cystic component anteriorly and a solid component posteriorly *(arrow).* The patient went to Stockholm for the placement of yttrium into the cyst cavity in an attempt to decrease the mass effect and the rate of recurrence. **B,** follow-up scanning 6 months later shows a nodular component *(black arrow)* more posteriorly, a shunt within the right lateral ventricle *(white arrow)* decompressing the ventricular system, but an area of ring enhancement in the midline. Fearing further tumor recurrence, surgery was performed, which revealed extensive radiation necrosis without evidence of tumor, thereby accounting for the ring of enhancement.

podensity or MR hyperintensity (long TR/TE scans) of white matter; and patchy or well-circumscribed contrast enhancement with or without mass effect, representing radiation necrosis (see Chapter 21).[62–71] Acute radiation edema occurs during treatment and apparently subsides spontaneously. Radiation necrosis of the brain has a latent period of 6 months to 14 years after treatment and occurs with doses of 6,000 rad or greater.[63] The occurrence of a mass long after treatment may therefore represent recurrent primary tumor, radiation-induced neoplasm, or radiation necrosis alone.

An area of radiation necrosis may appear on the enhanced CT scan as an irregular region of enhancement without mass effect (Fig 20–6),[63] a solid area of enhancement with or without mass effect (Fig 20–7),[65] or a ring lesion simulating malignant primary brain tumor, metastatic tumor, recurrent or persistent tumor, or abscess (Fig 20–8).[63–65] On MRI, the appearance is equally confusing, with mixed hypo- and isodensity on short TR

scans, hyperintensity on long TR/TE sequences, and the same type of enhancement patterns as on CT.[67–71]

MRI has not been successful at differentiating recurrent tumor from radiation necrosis. It has been suggested that radiation dose curves can be compared to the zones of CT or MR scan abnormality, with areas of enhancement corresponding to regions receiving less than 5,500 rad of radiation probably representing recurrent tumor and not radiation necrosis.[72] However, in the majority of cases it is virtually impossible to definitely distinguish areas of radiation necrosis from recurrent tumor on CT or MRI (Figs 20–8 and 20–9), and biopsy is necessary for diagnosis.[66] Positron emission tomography (PET) scanning with deoxyglucose appears to be helpful in distinguishing the etiology of a large mass. Glucose metabolism is increased in neoplasm and decreased with necrosis and infarction.[73] However, less homogeneous areas of necrosis could also contain viable neo-

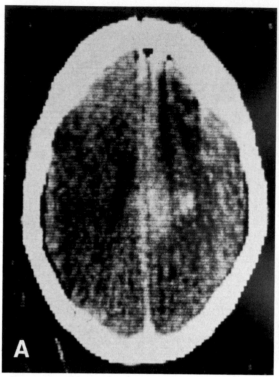
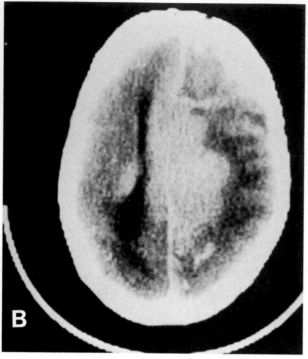

FIG 20–9.
Radiation necrosis simulating recurrent neoplasm. **A,** the initial enhanced scan demonstrates an enhancing mass in the region of the posterior portion of the corpus callosum. Unfortunately, the scan is marred by artifact. Biopsy revealed malignant astrocytoma, and the patient underwent radiation therapy. Four months later, the patient became markedly somnolent, and CT scanning revealed a massive area of enhancement involving the medial portions of both cerebral hemispheres **(B).** Autopsy revealed that the majority of the enhancing mass represented radiation necrosis, with only a small amount of tumor present. (Courtesy of Robert Selker, M.D., Montefiore Hospital, Pittsburgh.)

plasm and metabolic studies would be inconclusive.

Non-neoplastic Cysts

Non-neoplastic cysts include arachnoid cyst, and neurepithelial cyst and its subtype, colloid cyst. As discussed in Chapter 17, arachnoid cyst is an extraaxial mass characterized by sharp regular margins, lack of contrast enhancement, and MR relaxation parameters equal to CSF.[74] Differentiation from a low-density, low-intensity neoplasm such as epidermoid or oligodendroglioma, or old infarction, is by the combination of the marginal characteristics and relaxation parameters. Any deviation suggests tumor or infarct.

Neurepithelial cyst, discussed in Chapter 16, is an intraaxial nonenhancing mass with sharp margins (see Fig 16–32).[75] Because the protein concentration in the cyst fluid may be slightly higher than in CSF, MR relaxation parameters may not exactly parallel CSF and differentiation from a low density, low-intensity neoplasm (see Fig 16–27) may be difficult, requiring aspiration biopsy. Colloid cyst has a characteristic location. It is usually hyperdense on CT, but occasionally is isodense to gray matter (see Fig 16–59). Its MR intensity pattern on short and long TR sequences has been shown to be quite variable. However, these patterns still generally allow differentiation from the rare septal or periventricular glioma (see Chapter 16).

REFERENCES

1. Tchang S, Scotti G, Terbrugge K, et al: Computerized tomography as a possible aid to histological grading of supratentorial gliomas. *J Neurosurg* 1977; 46:735–739.
2. Potts DG, Albott GF, von Sneidern JV: National Cancer Institute study: Evaluation of computed tomography in the diagnosis of intracranial neoplasms: III. Metastatic tumors. *Radiology* 1980; 136:657–664.

3. Deck MDF, Messina AV, Sackett JF: Computed tomography in metastatic disease of the brain. *Radiology* 1976; 119:115–120.

4. Danzinger J, Wallace S, Handel SF, et al: Metastatic osteogenic sarcoma to the brain. *Cancer* 1979; 43:707–710.

5. Ruelle A, Macchia G, Gambini C, et al: Unusual appearance of brain metastasis from adenocarcinoma of colon. *Neuroradiology* 1986; 28:375.

6. Gouliamos AD, Jimenez JP, Goree GA: Computed tomography and skull radiology in the diagnosis of calcified brain tumor. *AJR* 1978; 130:761–764.

7. Enzmann DR, Kirkorian J, Norman D, et al: Computed tomography in primary reticulum cell sarcoma of brain. *Radiology* 1979; 130:165–170.

8. Holtas S, Nyman U, Cronqvist S: Computed tomography of malignant lymphoma of the brain. *Neuroradiology* 1984; 26:33–38.

9. Pederson H, Clausen N: The development of cerebral CT changes during treatment of acute lymphocytic leukemia in childhood. *Neuroradiology* 1981; 22:79–84.

10. Kasner E, Wilshe J, Steinhoff H, et al: Computer assisted tomography in primary malignant lymphomas of the brain. *J Comput Assist Tomogr* 1978; 2:125–134.

11. Lunsford LD, Martinez AJ, Latchaw RE: Magnetic resonance imaging does not define tumor boundaries. *Acta Radiol* [Suppl] *(Stockh)* 1986; 369:370–373.

12. Kelly PJ, Daumas-Duport C, Kispert DB, et al: Imaging-based stereotactic biopsies in untreated intracranial glial neoplasms. *J Neurosurg* 1987; 66:865–874.

13. Earnest F, Kelly PJ, Scheithauer BW, et al: Cerebral astrocytomas: Histopathologic correlation of MR and CT contrast enhancement with stereotactic biopsy. *Radiology* 1988; 166:823–827.

14. Johnson PC, Hunt SJ, Drayer BP: Human cerebral gliomas: Correlation of postmortem MR findings and neuropathologic findings. *Radiology* 1989; 170:211–217.

15. Elster AD, Challa VR, Gilbert TH, et al: Meningiomas: MR and histopathologic features. *Radiology* 1989; 170:857–862.

16. Spagnoli MV, Goldberg HI, Grossman RE, et al: Intracranial meningiomas: High-field MR imaging. *Radiology* 1986; 161:369–375.

17. Zimmerman RD, Fleming CA, Saint-Lois LA, et al: Magnetic resonance imaging of meningiomas. *AJNR* 1985; 6:149–157.

18. Schwaighofer BW, Hesselink JR, Press GA, et al: Primary intracranial CNS lymphoma: MR manifestations. *AJNR* 1989; 10:725–729.

19. Leonard KJ, Mamourian AC: MR appearance of intracranial chloromas. *AJNR* 1989; 10:S67–S68.

20. Atlas SW, Grossman RI, Gomon JM, et al: Calcified intracranial lesions: Detection with gradient-echo-acquisition rapid MR imaging. *AJNR* 1988; 9:253–259.

21. Atlas SW, Grossman RI, Gomori JM: Hemorrhagic intracranial malignant neoplasms: Spin-echo MR imaging. *Radiology* 1987; 164:71–77.

22. Zimmerman RA, Bilaniuk LT: Computed tomography of acute intratumoral hemorrhage. *Radiology* 1980; 135:355–359.

23. Destian S, Sze G, Krol G, et al: MR imaging of hemorrhagic intracranial neoplasms. *AJNR* 1988; 9:1115–1122.

24. Steinhoff H, Lanksch W, Kazner E, et al: Computed tomography in the diagnosis and differential diagnosis of glioblastomas: A qualitative study of 295 cases. *Neuroradiology* 1977; 14:193–200.

25. Silverman C, Marks JE: Prognostic significance of contrast enhancement in low-grade astrocytomas of the adult cerebrum. *Radiology* 1981; 139:211–213.

26. Latchaw RE, Payne JT, Gold LHA: Effective atomic number and electron density as measured with a computed tomography scanner: Computation and correlation with brain tumor histology. *J Comput Assist Tomogr* 1978; 2:199–208.

27. Haughton VM, Rimm AA, Czervionke LF, et al: Sensitivity of Gd-DTPA-enhanced MR imaging of benign extraaxial tumors. *Radiology* 1988; 166:829–833.

28. Berry I, Brant-Zawadzki M, Osaki L, et al: Gd-DTPA in clinical MR of the brain: 2. Extraaxial lesions and normal structures. *AJNR* 1986; 7:789–793.

29. Healy ME, Hesselink JR, Press GA, et al: Increased detection of intracranial metastases with intravenous Gd-DTPA. *Radiology* 1987; 165:619–624.

30. Russell EJ, Geremia GK, Johnson CE, et al: Multiple cerebral metastases: Detectability with Gd-DTPA-enhanced MR imaging. *Radiology* 1987; 167:609–617.

31. Butler AR, Horii SC, Kricheff II, et al: Computed tomography in astrocytomas. A statistical analysis of the parameters of malignancy and the positive contrast-enhanced CT scan. *Radiology* 1978; 129:433–439.

32. Joyce P, Bentson J, Takehasin M, et al: The accuracy of predicting histologic grades of supratentorial astrocytomas on the basis of computerized tomography and cerebral angiography. *Neuroradiology* 1978; 16:346–348.

33. Latchaw RE, Gold LHA, Moore JS, et al: The nonspecificity of absorption coefficients in the differentiation of solid tumors and cystic lesions. *Radiology* 1977; 125:141–144.

34. Russell EJ, George AE, Kricheff II, et al: Atypical computed tomographic features of intracranial meningioma: Radiological-pathological correlation in a series of 131 consecutive cases. *Radiology* 1980; 135:673–682.

35. Hatam A, Bupvall U, Lewander R, et al: Contrast medium enhancement with time in computer to-

mography: Differential diagnosis of intracranial lesions. *Acta Radiol [Suppl] (Stockh)* 1975; 346:63–81.

36. Lewander R: Contrast enhancement with time in gliomas. Stereotactic computer tomography following contrast medium infusion. *Acta Radiol [Diagn] (Stockh)* 20:689, 1979.

37. Latchaw RE, Payne JT, Loewenson RB: Predicting brain tumor histology: Change of effective atomic number with contrast enhancement. *AJNR* 1980; 1:289–294.

38. Takeda N, Ranaka R, Nakai I, et al: Dynamics of contrast enhancement in delayed computed tomography of brain tumors: Tissue-blood ratio and differential diagnosis. *Radiology* 1982; 142:663–668.

39. Schorner W, Laniado M, Niendorf HP, et al: Time-dependent changes in image contrast in brain tumors after gadolinium-DTPA. *AJNR* 1986; 7:1013–1020.

40. New PFJ, Aronow S, Hellelink JR: National Cancer Institute study: Evaluation of computed tomography in diagnosis of intracranial neoplasms: IV. Meningiomas. *Radiology* 1980; 136:665–675.

41. George AE, Russell EJ, Kricheff II: White matter buckling: CT sign of extra-axial intracranial mass. *AJNR* 1980; 1:425–430.

42. Smith HP, Cahha VP, Moody DM, et al: Biological features of meningiomas that determine the production of cerebral edema. *Neurosurgery* 1981; 8:428–433.

43. Weisberg LA, Nice CM: Intracranial tumors simulating the presentation of cerebrovascular syndromes: Early detection with cerebral computed tomography (CCT). *Am J Med* 1977; 63:517–524.

44. Monajati A, Heggeness L: Patterns of edema in tumors vs. infarcts: Visualization of white matter pathways. *AJNR* 1982; 3:251–255.

45. Inoue Y, Takemoto K, Miyamoto T, et al: Sequential computed tomography scans in acute cerebral infarction. *Radiology* 1980; 135:655–662.

46. Masdeu JC: Infarct versus neoplasm on CT: Four helpful signs. *AJNR* 1983; 4:522–524.

47. Reichenthal E, Cohen ML, Schujman E, et al: Tuberculum brain abscess and its appearance on computerized tomography. *J Neurosurg* 1982; 56:597–600.

48. Price HI, Danzinger A: Computed tomography in cranial tuberculosis. *AJR* 1978; 130:769–771.

49. Kendall BE, Tatler GLV: Radiological findings in neurosarcoidosis. *Br J Radiol* 1978; 51:81–92.

50. Cahill DW, Salamon M: Neurosarcoidosis: A review of the rarer manifestations. *Surg Neurol* 1981; 15:204–211.

51. Kempe DA, Ras CVGK, Garcia JH, et al: Intracranial neurosarcoidosis. *J Comput Assist Tomogr* 1979; 3:324–330.

52. Brooks J, Steckland MC, Williams JP, et al: Computed tomography changes in neurosarcoidosis, clearing with steroid treatment. *J Comput Assist Tomogr* 1979; 3:398–399.

53. Smith AS, Meisler DM, Weinstein MA, et al: High-signal periventricular lesions in patients with sarcoidosis: Neurosarcoidosis or multiple sclerosis? *AJNR* 1989; 10:485–490.

54. Reith KG, DiChiro G, Cromwell LD, et al: Primary demyelinating disease simulating glioma of the corpus callosum. *J Neurosurg* 1981; 55:620–624.

55. Sze G, Drol G, Olsen WL, et al: Hemorrhagic neoplasms: MR mimics of occult vascular malformations. *AJNR* 1987; 8:795–802.

56. Hacker DA, Latchaw RE, Chou SN, et al: Bilateral cerebellar venous angioma. *J Comput Assist Tomogr* 1981; 5:424–426.

57. Latchaw RE, Gabrielsen TO: Osteoradionecrosis of the skull. *Univ Mich Med Center J* 1973; 39:166–169.

58. Kingsley DPE, Kendall BE: CT of the adverse effects of therapeutic radiation of the central nervous system. *AJNR* 1981; 2:453–460.

59. Robinson RG: A second brain tumor and irradiation. *J Neurol Neurosurg Psychiatry* 1978; 41:1005–1012.

60. Martin WH, Cail WS, Morris JL, et al: Fibrosarcoma after high energy radiation therapy for pituitary adenoma. *AJNR* 1980; 1:469–472.

61. Peylan-Ramu N, Poplack DG, Pizzo PA, et al: Abnormal CT scans of the brain in asymptomatic children with acute lymphatic leukemia after prophylactic treatment of the central nervous system with radiation and intrathecal chemotherapy. *N Engl J Med* 1978; 298:815–823.

62. Shalen PR, Ostrow PT, Glass PJ: Enhancement of the white matter following prophylactic therapy of the central nervous system for leukemia: Radiation effects and methotrexate leukoencephalopathy. *Radiology* 1981; 140:409–412.

63. Mikhael MA: Radiation necrosis of the brain: Correlation between patterns on computed tomography and dose of radiation. *J Comput Assist Tomogr* 1979; 3:241–249.

64. Baron SH: Brain radiation necrosis following treatment of an esthesioneuroblastoma olfactory neurocytoma. *Laryngoscope* 1979; 89:214–223.

65. Sundersen N, Galicich JH, Deck MDF, et al: Radiation necrosis after treatment of solitary intracranial metastases. *Neurosurgery* 1981; 8:329–333.

66. Deck MDF: Imaging techniques in the diagnosis of radiation damage to the central nervous system, in Gilbert HA, Kagan AR (eds): *Radiation Damage to the Nervous System.* New York, Raven Press, 1980.

67. Atlas SW, Grossman RI, Packer RJ, et al: Magnetic resonance imaging diagnosis of disseminated necrotizing leukoencephalopathy. *CT* 1987; 11:39–43.

68. Tsuruda JS, Kortman KE, Bradley WG, et al: Radiation effects on cerebral white matter: MR evaluation. *AJR* 1987; 149:165–171.

69. Curnes JT, Laster DW, Ball MR, et al: Magnetic

resonance imaging of radiation injury to the brain. *AJNR* 1986; 7:389–394.

70. Dooms GC, Hecht S, Brant-Zawadski M, et al: Brain radiation lesions: MR imaging. *Radiology* 1986; 158:149–155.

71. Grossman RI, Hecht-Leavitt CM, Evans SM, et al: Experimental radiation injury: Combined MR imaging and spectroscopy. *Radiology* 1988; 169:305–309.

72. Mikhael MA: Radiation necrosis of the brain: Correlation between computed tomography, pathology, and dose distribution. *J Comput Assist Tomogr* 1978; 2:71–80.

73. Lilja A, Lundqvist H, Olsson Y, et al: Positron emission tomography and computed tomography in differential diagnosis between recurrent or residual glioma and treatment-induced brain lesions. *Acta Radiol [Diagn]* 1989; 30:121–128.

74. Kjos BO, Brant-Zawadzki M, Kucharcyzk W, et al: Cystic intracranial lesions: Magnetic resonance imaging. *Radiology* 1985; 155:363–369.

75. Numaguchi Y, Connolly ES, Kumra AK, et al: Computed tomography and MR imaging of thalamic neuroepithelial cysts. *J Comput Assist Tomogr* 1987; 11:583–585.

21

Imaging of the Brain Following Surgery, Radiation Therapy, and Chemotherapy

David W. Johnson, M.D.

Richard E. Latchaw, M.D.

Over the last two decades increasingly aggressive therapeutic modalities have been used in the treatment of brain tumors. The frequent combination of surgery, radiation therapy, and chemotherapy lead to nonneoplastic parenchymal changes that can themselves be confused with tumor recurrence. Improved survival times have allowed primary tumors to recur in distant sites and new tumors, possibly radiation induced, to appear. The intent of this chapter is to give the radiologist an introduction to the issues important to this subject. Unfortunately, in many cases imaging alone may not distinguish between post-therapeutic change and tumor recurrence, but it is hoped that a knowledge of the pathophysiology of the treatment modalities will provide a better understanding of the differential diagnostic possibilities.

POSTOPERATIVE IMAGING

The bane of the radiologist is the evaluation of the postoperative patient. Computed tomography (CT) or magnetic resonance imaging (MRI) is often used because it is adequate to evaluate ventricular size, the presence or absence of mass effect, and edema. Nonenhanced scanning becomes necessary if there is a need to rule out hemorrhage. In this respect, in the acute phase (less than 2 to 3 days) CT is better than MRI because acute blood is relatively isointense to normal brain tissue on MRI whereas it is unmistakably dense on CT. But once acute blood (hemoglobin) has begun to change to methemoglobin, MRI becomes very useful and is more sensitive than CT in the detection of minute amounts of hemorrhage. A "stain" of methemoglobin can persist at the margin of a surgical defect for many weeks but means little in the management of the patient (Fig 21–1). This represents only petechial, not frank hemorrhage.

Gelfoam, Surgicel, and gauze packing have a variable appearance depending upon their admixture with blood, cerebrospinal fluid (CSF), or even air.[1] Proper interpretation of their presence may require consultation with the neurosurgeon (Figs 21–2 and 21–3).

Enhanced scanning is required when there is a need to evaluate the possibility of recurrent or residual tumor or abscess formation. Enhancement of operative contusion and/or infarction may mimic residual tumor or abscess formation depending upon the time interval following surgery. Early investigators have described ringlike enhancement on CT at the margin of a lobectomy.[2, 3] Similar ringlike enhancements are produced by resolving hematomas and infarcts.[4–7] Their appearance and disappearance have been found to be time dependent, with enhancement seen from 1 to 10 weeks. Vascular proliferation from operative injury can be seen as early as 4 days.[8] Jeffries et al., using a dog model, reported marginal enhancement at the surgical site from 1 week to 4 weeks.[9] Enhancement was minimal in the first and fourth weeks, with the greatest enhancement during the second to third weeks. Enhancement correlated closely with the development and maturation of reactive vascular-

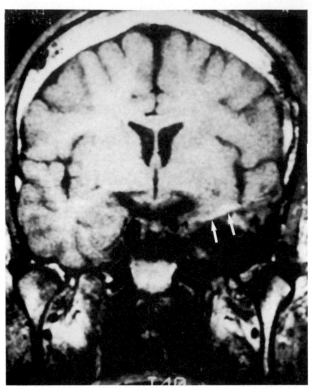

FIG 21–1.
A 37-year-old male with temporal lobe epilepsy. Preoperative scan results were normal. A left temporal lobectomy was done 5 weeks earlier. MRI (TR/TE, 500/20) shows increased signal representing methemoglobin at the surgical margin *(arrows)*. The surgeon left a clean resection margin, and no excessive bleeding was encountered.

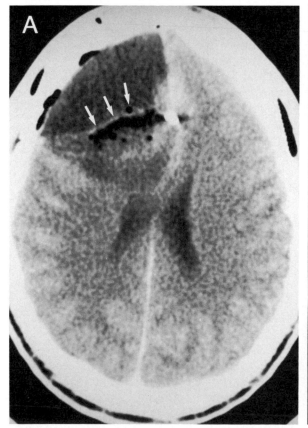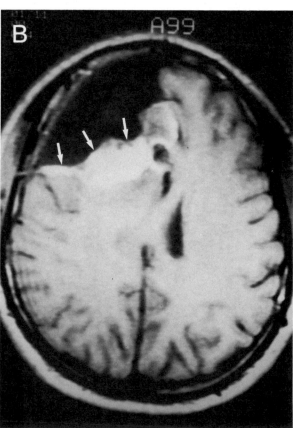

FIG 21–2.
A 26-year-old male with a history of a right frontal lobe anaplastic astrocytoma treated with surgical resection. Vigorous bleeding was encountered during surgery, but hemostasis was obtained. Avitene wrapped in Surgicel was placed in the tumor bed. **A,** contrast-enhanced CT shows the Avitene/Surgicel dressing in the tumor bed mixed with some air *(arrows)*. A surgical clip is seen with metal artifact in the midline, frontally. **B,** 4 days later, MRI (TR/TE, 700/20) shows high signal in the Avitene/Surgicel dressing that is compatible with methemoglobin *(arrows)*.

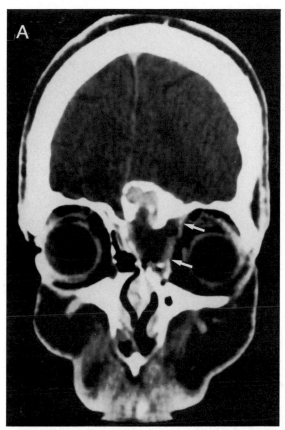

FIG 21–3.
A 38-year-old male with osteogenic sarcoma of the anterior cranial fossa. **A,** coronal contrast-enhanced CT shows a partially calcified tumor of the floor of the anterior cranial fossa and opacification of the ethmoid sinus due to tumor and/or postoperative changes *(arrows).* Postoperative scans with soft-tissue **(B)** and bone **(C)** windows show mixed low density in the tumor bed due to air in the gauze packing placed at the time of surgery.

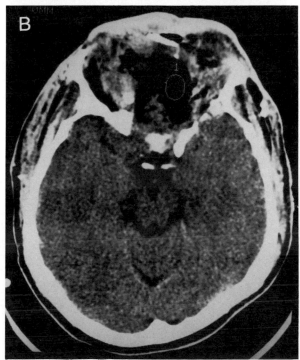

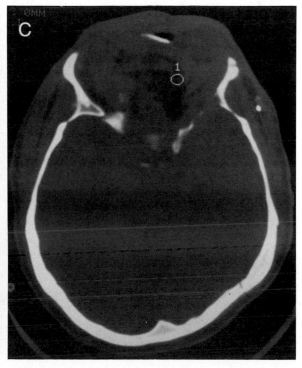

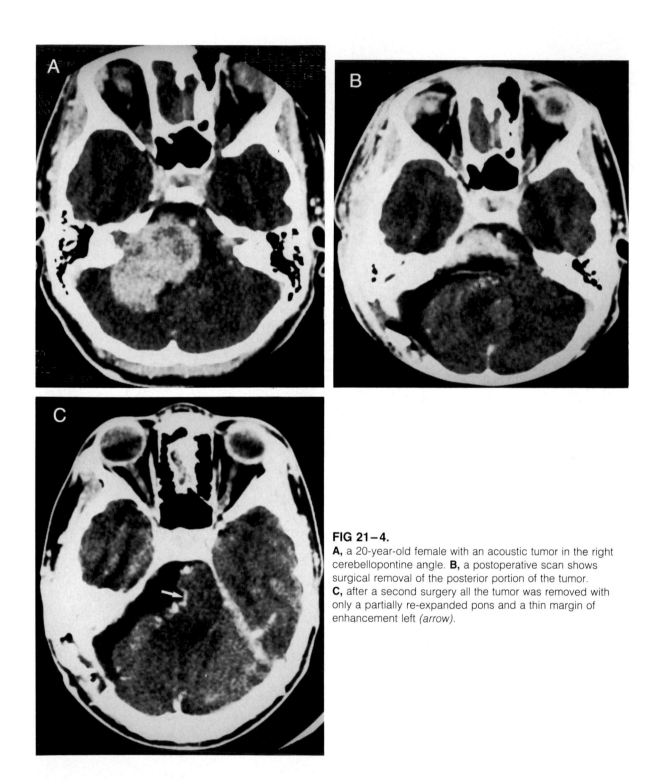

FIG 21–4.
A, a 20-year-old female with an acoustic tumor in the right cerebellopontine angle. **B,** a postoperative scan shows surgical removal of the posterior portion of the tumor. **C,** after a second surgery all the tumor was removed with only a partially re-expanded pons and a thin margin of enhancement left *(arrow).*

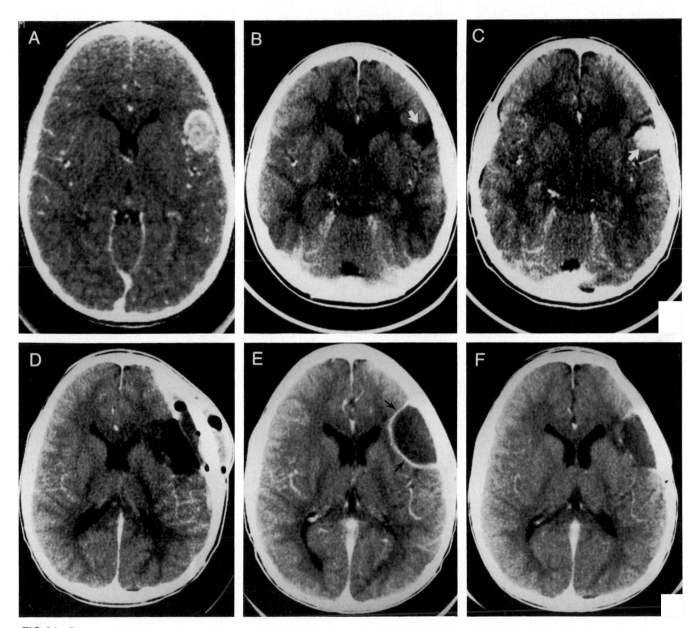

FIG 21–5.
A 9-year old male with a history of anaplastic mixed glioma. **A,** the initial scan shows tumor in the left frontal lobe. **B,** the next scan shows the operative defect 3 months after surgery *(arrow).* **C,** the tumor recurs 8 months later along the posterior margin *(arrow).* **D,** a scan done 3 days after the second surgery shows no contrast enhancement in the tumor bed. **E,** 10 weeks later a thin rim of enhancement outlines the surgical bed *(arrows).* **F,** 3 months later the marginal enhancement has almost completely resolved.

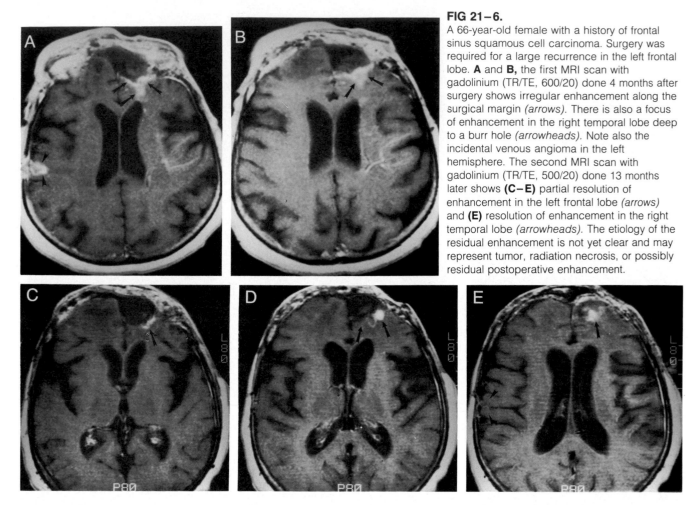

FIG 21–6.
A 66-year-old female with a history of frontal sinus squamous cell carcinoma. Surgery was required for a large recurrence in the left frontal lobe. **A** and **B,** the first MRI scan with gadolinium (TR/TE, 600/20) done 4 months after surgery shows irregular enhancement along the surgical margin *(arrows).* There is also a focus of enhancement in the right temporal lobe deep to a burr hole *(arrowheads).* Note also the incidental venous angioma in the left hemisphere. The second MRI scan with gadolinium (TR/TE, 500/20) done 13 months later shows **(C–E)** partial resolution of enhancement in the left frontal lobe *(arrows)* and **(E)** resolution of enhancement in the right temporal lobe *(arrowheads).* The etiology of the residual enhancement is not yet clear and may represent tumor, radiation necrosis, or possibly residual postoperative enhancement.

ity in the brain tissue at the margin of the surgical defect. Dural enhancement was also observed locally by the second week and was due to the formation of granulation tissue. One would conclude from the data of Jeffries and associates that in order to rule out residual tumor in the postoperative patient a scan must be obtained within the first week and optimally in the first 3 postoperative days before any vascular proliferation is known to occur. Similarly, in order to rule out recurrent tumor another study at 6 to 8 weeks may be necessary after normal postoperative enhancement has faded (Figs 21–4 to 21–6). We have found, however, that occasionally postoperative enhancement can persist to 3 months. A similar study has not yet been done with MRI and gadolinium, but because of the greater sensitivity of MRI for enhancement with gadolinium, marginal and dural enhancement may be appreciated sooner and for a longer period of time than with contrast-enhanced CT. Normal postoperative enhancement is usually thin rimmed and without mass effect, whereas recurrent tumor will usually show thickened, irregular enhancement and may be nodular and/or have mass effect.

Lanzieri et al. studied the meningogaleal complex (MGC) with CT in postcraniectomy patients and found that the smooth thickening often indicated postoperative infection, nodular thickening indicated recurrent extra-axial tumor, whereas recurrent intra-axial tumor did not change the MGC itself.[10]

IMAGING FOLLOWING RADIATION THERAPY

Mechanisms of Injury

Most investigators feel that the basic mechanism of injury from radiation therapy is damage to the capillary endothelial cell.[11–14] Still capable of replication, these cells are most sensitive to radiation. Radiosensitivity is greatest in the mitotic (m) phase and early DNA synthesis (s) phase.[15] When DNA strand damage outpaces repair, replication is halted, and cell death occurs.[16, 17] Such damage to the capillary endothelium inevitably leads to breakdown of the blood-brain barrier (BBB). Glial elements are also radiosensitive, particularly in the young patient,[18, 19] and white matter is more radiosensitive than is gray matter.[20]

Types of Radiation Therapy

Most patients are treated with x-ray (photon) external-beam therapy from a variety of sources such as cobalt-60, linear accelerators, and betatrons capable of producing electron beams from 4 to 45 million electron volts (meV). Beam columnation is achieved with lead shaped to include the tumor with an acceptable margin and to exclude normal tissue, particularly tissue that is very radiosensitive. Normal tissue interposed between the tumor or directly behind the tumor but in line with the source of radiation cannot be protected in this manner. Dose distribution can be influenced, however, by increasing beam energy and the use of multiple ports. Unavoidable exposure of normal tissue may lead to adverse changes to be discussed later.

Brachytherapy with radioisotope seed implantation is one attempt to limit exposure of surrounding tissue while boosting the dose to the tumor. This requires stereotactic localization of the tumor and placement of seeds containing a measured amount of a radioactive isotope into the tumor or around the margin. Tumor cysts may be punctured stereotactically for the injection of radioactive phosphorus. Recently the development of gamma-knife radiotherapy using 201 cobalt-60 sources has been developed to increase target dose and limit exposure to surrounding normal tissue.

All of these techniques deliver lower doses to surrounding normal tissue and therefore leave fewer radiation changes on follow-up scans. The following discussion is drawn from the literature using conventional external-beam radiation. Any attempt to extrapolate these data to other forms of radiotherapy is hazardous.

Acute Reactions

This form of radiation injury syndrome occurs during therapy. Signs and symptoms are mild and may resolve with corticosteroid therapy. The incidence is related to fraction size, frequency of irradiation, and total dose.[21–23] A smaller fraction size will allow greater frequency and total dose. Similarly, a larger fraction size will limit frequency and

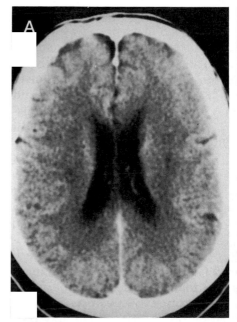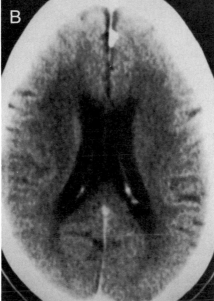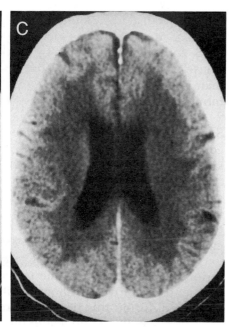

FIG 21–7.
A 56-year-old female with small-cell carcinoma of the lung metastatic to the cerebellum. Two years ago she received 3,000-rad whole-brain irradiation and 1,000-rad boost to the cerebellar vermis in 16 treatments over a period of 23 days. She also received cyclophosphamide, doxorubicin (Adriamycin), vincristine, cisplatinum, and VP-16. **A,** 8 days after completion of radiation therapy the first scan is normal. **B,** 8 months later lucencies are developing in the white matter. **C,** 18 months after completion of radiation therapy the lucencies are more widespread.

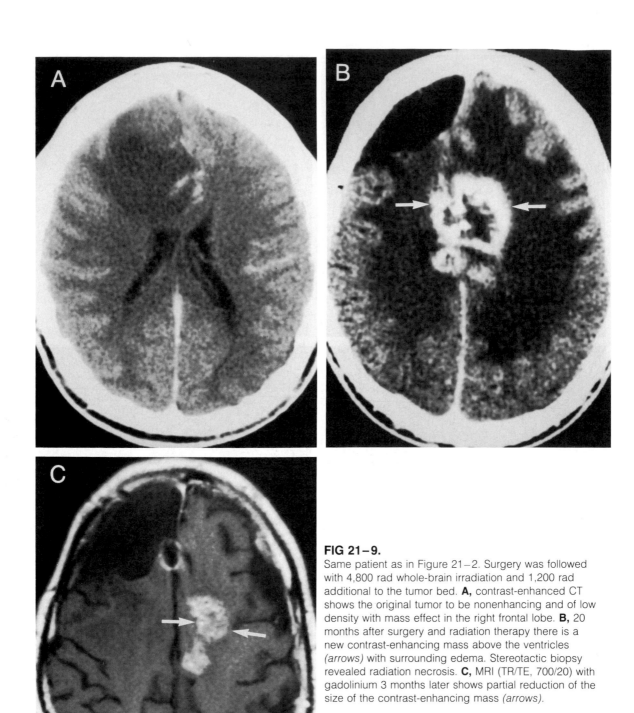

FIG 21–9.
Same patient as in Figure 21–2. Surgery was followed
with 4,800 rad whole-brain irradiation and 1,200 rad
additional to the tumor bed. **A,** contrast-enhanced CT
shows the original tumor to be nonenhancing and of low
density with mass effect in the right frontal lobe. **B,** 20
months after surgery and radiation therapy there is a
new contrast-enhancing mass above the ventricles
(arrows) with surrounding edema. Stereotactic biopsy
revealed radiation necrosis. **C,** MRI (TR/TE, 700/20) with
gadolinium 3 months later shows partial reduction of the
size of the contrast-enhancing mass *(arrows).*

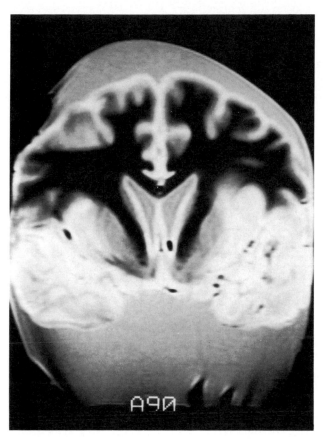

FIG 21–10.
A 43-year-old male with a history of a pituitary adenoma. The patient received 5,600 rad in 28 fractions over 44 days via the left and right lateral pituitary fields. Fourteen months later CT showed bilateral contrast-enhancing masses in the temporal lobes at the level of the sella. The patient died 2 months later. Postautopsy coronal MRI (TR/TE, 2,500/25) of the formalin-fixed brain shows increased signal in both temporal lobes. Neuropathology revealed radiation necrosis in both temporal lobes.

dolinium, chemical shift imaging and phosphorus spectroscopy showed no changes.[39]

The one imaging modality that appears to differentiate recurrent tumor from radiation necrosis is positron-emission tomography (PET) with[18]F-deoxyglucose (FDG). Hypometabolism is seen in the area of radiation necrosis, whereas recurrent tumor will demonstrate hypermetabolism.[40] However, infiltrative tumor cells can be intermixed with radiation necrosis, and it remains to be seen whether this technique can detect small amounts of tumor mixed with radiation necrosis.

Despite its irreversible and progressive nature, radiation necrosis is treatable if focal. Edwards and Wilson concluded that resection of focal necrosis can improve symptoms.[41] The importance to the radiologist here is to keep radiation necrosis in the differential diagnosis of tumor recurrence. Recurrent malignant tumor may be a relative contraindication to surgery, but surgery may be curative in the patient with radiation necrosis.

Tumor Induction

A very late complication of CNS irradiation is tumor induction. Tumors known to occur following irradiation include meningioma, sarcoma, glioma, and nerve sheath tumors.[42–47] The latent interval is on the order of years, and there is a strong dose-response relation.[42] These tumors are usually solitary but can be multiple.[48, 49] There are three criteria that must be satisfied in order to establish the likely diagnosis of a radiation-induced tumor: (1) it must appear in the field of irradiation, (2) it must appear after a latent interval of several years, and (3) it must be histologically different from the first tumor.[50] Imaging characteristics will be identical to their spontaneously occurring counterparts (Figs 21–11 and 21–12).

Large-Vessel Occlusive Vasculopathy

Rarely, large-vessel occlusive disease can develop following irradiation of the brain. The latent period can be years.[51] These lesions may appear identical to atherosclerotic narrowing at angiography. There are three patterns: (1) large-vessel stenoses, (2) moyamoya collateral formation in addition to large-vessel stenoses, and (3) diffuse cerebral arteritis.[52] Pathologically, there are subintimal collections of foam cells.[53] There is a wide variation in the range of radiation necessary to produce these lesions, which indicates there is considerable differences in individual susceptibility. A review of the literature in children by Wright and Bresnan reports a range of 1,000 to 8,500 rad.[51]

Other Irreversible Changes Due to Radiation Therapy

Depending upon the study, one third to one half of individuals receiving cranial radiation therapy will develop atrophy.[54–57] Children seem to be more susceptible than adults, and the combination with chemotherapy leads to atrophy at a lower dose of radiation exposure. Calcification has been found in 28% of children, most frequently in the subcortical white matter.[56] Sites of calcification

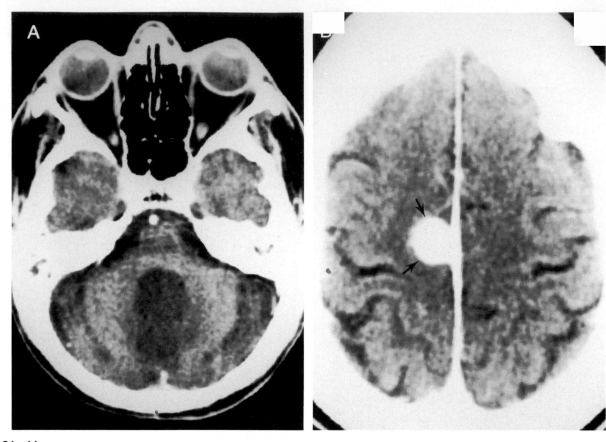

FIG 21–11.

A 39-year-old female with medulloblastoma treated with surgery and radiation therapy (dose unknown) 29 years ago. Two years ago the patient had a seizure and struck her head. **A,** contrast-enhanced CT reveals the postsurgery/postradiation therapy changes in the posterior fossa. **B,** a higher level from the same scan revealed a falx meningioma *(arrows)* that was subsequently followed, found to enlarge, and finally removed.

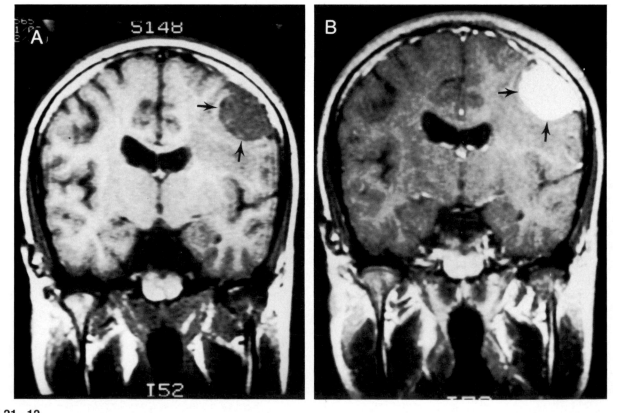

FIG 21–12.

A 16-year-old male had a posterior fossa ependymoma diagnosed and treated at 2 years of age with surgery and radiation therapy. He did well until 1 month prior to this scan when he had a right-sided seizure. MRI (TR/TE, 400/20) **(A)** without and **(B)** with gadolinium–diethylenetriamine pentaacetic acid (DTPA) revealed an extra-axial tumor of the convexity *(arrows)* on the left that had a low-signal precontrast that enhanced following contrast. Pathology revealed a mixed mesenchymal benign pseudosarcoma.

correlated with pathologic findings of mineralizing microangiography and demyelination.

IMAGING FOLLOWING CHEMOTHERAPY

The use of prophylactic irradiation and systemic or intrathecal methotrexate for the prevention of cerebral spread of ALL have resulted in increased survival times.[58, 59] This has also led to the occurrence of a progressive leukoencephalopathy.[60, 61] The individual contribution of radiation or chemotherapy to these CNS side effects is difficult to assess, but similar findings have been reported in patients receiving high doses of only methotrexate[61, 62] or high doses of only cranial irradiation.[63]

Methotrexate, a folic acid antagonist, does not cross the BBB well. Cranial irradiation disrupts the BBB and allows increased brain penetration of methotrexate,[64] which is probably the reason why combination chemotherapy and radiation therapy lead to these changes with lower doses of each modality than when these modalities are used alone.

Methotrexate is the best-known chemotherapeutic agent responsible for white matter changes. However, other agents are also known to do the same. Furthermore, in an attempt to limit systemic toxicities and at the same time increase delivery to the tumor, intrathecal and intra-arterial administration of drugs has become more commonplace. Therefore, lower doses of these focally administered drugs are capable of causing the same white matter changes.

Disseminated necrotizing leukoencephalopathy (DNL) is a particularly severe form of demyelination seen in patients receiving intrathecal methotrexate; shortly thereafter they develop severe encephalopathic symptoms including somnolence, confusion, ataxia, and seizures, which can culminate in coma and death. Investigators have found multifocal coagulative necrosis of the white matter with demyelination and axonal swelling.[65] The characteristic change by CT is the appearance of white matter lucencies, with or without mass effect and rarely contrast enhancement.[66, 67] MRI is more sensitive than CT in detecting these changes.[68]

Other findings include ventricular and sulcal dilatation and parenchymal calcification. Calcification most commonly occurs in the basal ganglia, brain stem, and subcortical white matter.[69] Calcification and demyelination were felt by some in the past to be pathologic hallmarks of methotrexate

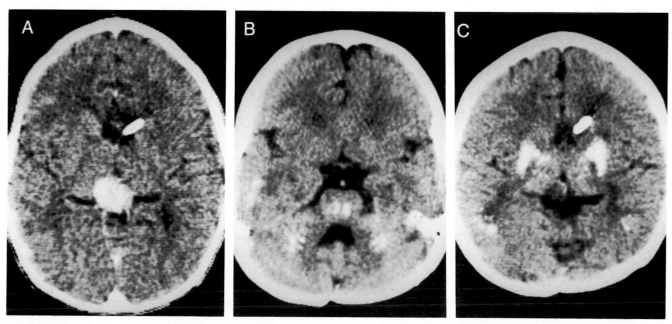

FIG 21–13.
A 6-year-old female presented at the age of 3 years with pineoblastoma and had subtotal resection of the tumor. She received 3,960 rad whole-brain irradiation in 22 fractions and an additional 1,400 rad to the pineal region in 20 fractions as well as five courses of cisplatin. **A,** the original scan shows the pineal tumor and no calcification. **B** and **C,** a follow-up scan 3 years later reveals sulcal enlargement and calcification in the basal ganglia, thalamus, parietal subcortical white matter, brain stem, and cerebellum. (Courtesy of Samuel M. Wolpert, M.D., Tufts New England Medical Center.)

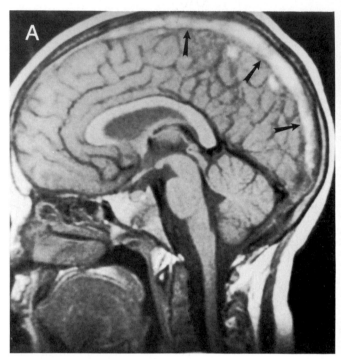

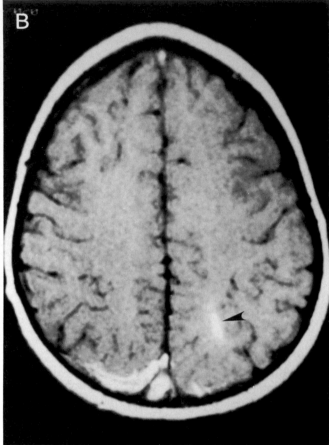

FIG 21–14.
A 6-year-old male with ALL treated with L-asparaginase subsequently developed **(A)** superior sagittal sinus thrombosis *(arrows)* and **(B)** intracerebral hemorrhage *(arrowhead).*

leukoencephalopathy[65, 70] but can occur with other chemotherapeutic agents (Fig 21–13).

Another effect of chemotherapy is cerebral hemorrhage, infarct, or venous thrombosis due to hemostatic abnormalities caused by the agent L-asparaginase, probably by the inhibition of the synthesis of various clotting proteins.[71]

Patterns of Recurrence and Results of Aggressive Treatment

The most illustrative example of the results of aggressive treatment for cancer is the rise in CNS recurrence of ALL prior to the establishment of CNS prophylaxis. The success of systemic chemotherapy that could not cross the BBB well increased the life span of these children but allowed tumor to recur in the CNS. More aggressive treatment with relatively toxic combinations of chemotherapy and radiotherapy have resulted in control of CNS dissemination but not without parenchymal alterations (Fig 21–14).

Patterns of recurrence of primary CNS tumors

is another prime example. Because more than 90% of glioblastoma recur within a 2-cm margin of the original tumor,[72] survival times have improved with aggressive local control including surgery and brachytherapy. Indeed, local control does result in reduction of tumor size and occasionally complete disappearance of tumor.[73, 74] Systemic chemotherapy and more recently intra-arterial chemotherapy have been employed with some reports of success, but also with complications.[75–82] Better local control of tumor recurrence has been observed only to give way to tumor extension or growth outside of the vascular bed being perfused (Figs 21–15 and 21–16).[74] Spinal "drop metastasis" and systemic occurrence of glioblastoma have been observed at the time of recurrence, uncommon before such therapies.[83] The optimistic view of malignant glioma and glioblastoma is that of a local disease process that can be controlled if surgery and enough radiation therapy and chemotherapy can be locally applied. Imaging often suggests a localized tumor with surrounding normal brain. Contrast enhancement can have very sharp margins,

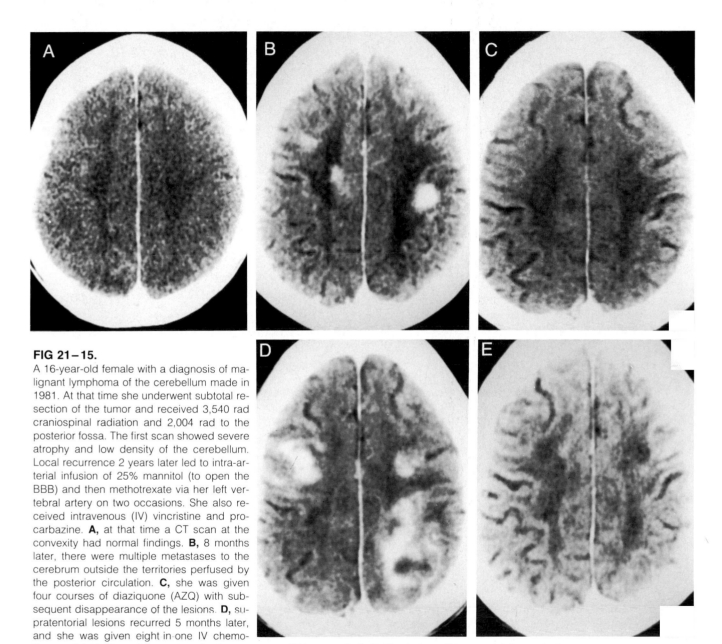

FIG 21–15.
A 16-year-old female with a diagnosis of malignant lymphoma of the cerebellum made in 1981. At that time she underwent subtotal resection of the tumor and received 3,540 rad craniospinal radiation and 2,004 rad to the posterior fossa. The first scan showed severe atrophy and low density of the cerebellum. Local recurrence 2 years later led to intra-arterial infusion of 25% mannitol (to open the BBB) and then methotrexate via her left vertebral artery on two occasions. She also received intravenous (IV) vincristine and procarbazine. **A,** at that time a CT scan at the convexity had normal findings. **B,** 8 months later, there were multiple metastases to the cerebrum outside the territories perfused by the posterior circulation. **C,** she was given four courses of diaziquone (AZQ) with subsequent disappearance of the lesions. **D,** supratentorial lesions recurred 5 months later, and she was given eight in-one IV chemotherapy (eight chemotherapy agents given over one 24-hour period). **E,** The lesions disappeared 2 months later and left white matter lucencies. Note the steady progression of atrophy and white matter lucencies.

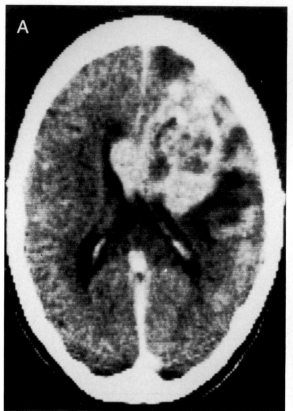

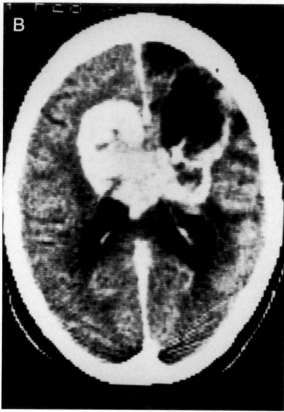

FIG 21–16.

A 27-year-old female with a right frontal lobe grade II astrocytoma resected 5 years prior to the first scan. She was treated with external-beam radiation therapy and had documented recurrence of the tumor leading to the infusion of three courses of 1,3-bis-(2-chloroethyl)-1-nitrosourea (BCNU) into the left internal carotid artery. **A,** the first scan shows tumor mostly in the left frontal lobe. **B,** 5½ months after the first scan there is a large area of necrosis in the tumor in the left frontal lobe, but it has enlarged greatly in the opposite hemisphere outside of the vascular territory perfused with BCNU. (From Johnson DW, Parkinson D, Wolpert SM: *Neurosurgery* 1987; 20:577–583. Used by permission.)

and a tumor may appear to have very well defined boundaries. Pathologic studies and comparison with CT and MRI have shown that tumor does occur beyond the margins of enhancement and neither CT nor MRI can differentiate nonenhancing tumor from surrounding edema.[84, 85] Even normal-appearing structures by CT or MRI do not rule out the presence of tumor without edema or BBB breakdown.

In summary, the issues of post-therapy changes are complex. In order for CT and MRI to differentiate postsurgical changes from recurrent or residual tumor, timing of the scans becomes important. Postradiation and chemotherapy changes have been carefully described in the literature, but in the individual case radiation necrosis may also be confused with tumor. PET may make the differentiation but is not always available, and tissue biopsy may ultimately be necessary. As therapies become more directed to the tumor in an effort both

to control local disease and to more effectively exclude surrounding normal tissue, fewer adverse effects of therapy will be seen in surrounding tissues. However, more unusual patterns and locations of recurrence of the primary tumor will be seen, and the radiologist will be further challenged by new and unusual diagnostic dilemmas.

REFERENCES

1. Dubin LM, Quencer RM, Green BA: A mimicker of a postoperative spinal mass: Gelfoam in a laminectomy site. *AJNR* 1988; 9:217–218.
2. Krishna Rao CVG, Kishore PRS, Bartlett J, et al: Computed tomography in the post-operative patient. *Neuroradiology* 1980; 19:257–263.
3. Grand W, Kinkel WR, Glasauer FE, et al: Ring formation on computerized tomography in the post-operative patient. *Neurosurgery* 1978; 2:107–109.
4. Zimmerman RD, Leeds NE, Naidich TP: Ring

blush associated with intracerebral hematoma. *Radiology* 1977; 122:707–711.

5. Yock DH Jr, Marshall WH Jr: Recent ischemic brain infarcts at computed tomography: Appearance pre- and post-contrast infusion. *Radiology* 1975; 117:599–608.

6. Messina AV: Computed tomography: Contrast enhancement in resolving intracerebral hemorrhage. *AJR* 1976; 127:1050–1052.

7. Laster DW, Moody DM, Ball MR: Resolving intracerebral hematoma: Alteration of the "ring sign" with steroids. *AJR* 1978; 130:935–939.

8. Enzmann DR, Britt RH, Yeager AS: Experimental brain abscess evolution: Computed tomographic and neuropathologic correlation. *Radiology* 1979; 133:113–122.

9. Jeffries BF, Kishore PRS, Singh KS, et al: Contrast enhancement in the postoperative brain. *Neuroradiology* 1981; 139:409–413.

10. Lanzieri CF, Som PM, Sacher M, et al: The postcraniectomy site: CT appearance. *Radiology* 1986; 159:165–170.

11. Clemente CD, Holst EA: Pathological changes in neurons, neuroglia and blood-brain barrier included by x-irradiation of heads of monkeys. *Arch Neurol Psychiatry* 1954; 71:66–79.

12. McDonald LW, Hayes TL: The role of capillaries in the pathogenesis of delayed radionecrosis of brain. *Am J Pathol* 1967; 50:745–764.

13. Reinhold HS, Busiman GH: Radiosensitivity of capillary endothelium. *Br J Radiol* 1973; 46:54–57.

14. Reinhold HS, Busiman GH: Repair of radiation damage to capillary endothelium. *Br J Radiol* 1975; 48:727.

15. Denekamp J, Fowler JF: Cell proliferation kinetics and radiation therapy, in Becker FE (ed): *Cancer—A Comprehensive Treatise.* New York, Plenum Publishing Corp, 1977, pp 101–137.

16. Bonura T, Town CD, Smith KC, et al: The influence of oxygen on the yield of DNA double strand breaks in x-irradiated *Escherichia coli* K12. *Radiat Res* 1975; 63:567.

17. Lohman PHM: Induction and rejoining of breaks in the deoxyribonucleic acid of human cells irradiated at various phases of the cell cycle. *Mutat Res* 1968; 6:449.

18. Korr H, Schultze B, Maurer W: Autoradiographic investigations of glial proliferation in the brain of adult mice. I. The DNA synthesis phase of neuroglia and endothelial cells. *J Comp Neurol* 1973; 150:169–176.

19. Korr H, Schultze B, Maurer W: Autoradiographic investigations of glial proliferation of the brain of adult mice. II. Cycle time and mode of proliferation of neuroglia and endothelial cells. *J Comp Neurol* 1975; 160:477–490.

20. Kingsley DPE, Kendall BE: CT of the adverse effects of therapeutic radiation of the central nervous system. *AJNR* 1981; 2:453–460.

21. Salazar OM, Rubin P, McDonald JV, et al: High dose radiation therapy in treatment of glioblastoma multiforme: A preliminary report. *Int J Radiat Oncol Biol Phys* 1976; 1:717–727.

22. Young DF, Posner JB, Chu F, et al: Rapid-course radiation therapy of cerebral metastases: Results and complications. *Cancer* 1974; 34:1069–1076.

23. Zeman W, Shidnia H: Post-therapeutic radiation injuries of the nervous system. Reflections on their prevention. *J Neurol* 1976; 212:107–115.

24. Almquist S, Dahlgren S, Notter G, et al: Brain necrosis after irradiation of the hypophysis in Cushing's disease. *Acta Radiol* 1964; 2:179–188.

25. Wendling LR, Bleyer WA, DiChiro G, et al: Transient, severe periventricular hypodensity after leukemic prophylaxis with cranial irradiation and intrathecal methotrexate. *J Comput Assist Tomogr* 1978; 2:502–505.

26. Rider WD: Radiation damage to the brain—a new syndrome. *J Can Assoc Radiol* 1963; 14:67–69.

27. Druckman A: Schlafsucht als Folge der Rontgenbestrahlung. Beitrag zur Strahlenempfindlichkeit des Gehirns. *Strahlentherapie* 1929; 33:382–384.

28. Freeman JE, Johnston PGB, Voke JM: Somnolence after prophylactic cranial irradiation in children with acute lymphoblastic leukaemia. *Br Med J* 1973; 4:523–525.

29. Boden G: Radiation myelitis of the cervical spinal cord. *Br J Radiol* 1948; 21:464–469.

30. Jones A: Transient radiation myelopathy (with reference to Lhermitte's sign of electrical paresthesia). *Br J Radiol* 1964; 37:727–744.

31. Hoffman WF, Levin VA, Wilson CB: Evaluation of malignant glioma patients during the postirradiation period. *J Neurosurg* 1979; 50:624–628.

32. Curnes JT, Laster DW, Ball MR, et al: Magnetic resonance imaging of radiation injury to the brain. *AJNR* 1986; 7:389–394.

33. Kramer S: The hazards of therapeutic irradiation of the central nervous system. *Clin Neurosurg* 1968; 15:301–318.

34. Burger PC, Mahaley MS Jr, Dudka L, et al: The morphologic effects of radiation administered therapeutically for intracranial gliomas. A postmortem study of 25 cases. *Cancer* 1979; 44:1256–1272.

35. Pratt RA, DiChiro G, Weed JC Jr: Cerebral necrosis following irradiation and chemotherapy for metastatic choriocarcinoma. *Surg Neurol* 1977; 7:117–120.

36. Dooms GC, Hecht ST, Brant-Zawadzki M, et al: Brain radiation lesions: MR imaging. *Radiology* 1986; 158:149–155.

37. Hecht-Leavitt C, Grossman RI, Curran WJ, et al: MR of brain radiation injury: Experimental studies on cats. *AJNR* 1987; 8:427–430.

38. Mikhael MA: Radiation necrosis of the brain: Corre-

lation between computed tomography, pathology, and dose distribution. *J Comput Assist Tomogr* 1978; 2:71–80

39. Grossman RI, Hecht-Leavitt CM, Evans SM, et al: Experimental radiation injury: Combined MR imaging and spectroscopy. *Radiology* 1988; 169:305–309.

40. DiChiro G, Oldfield E, Wright DC, et al: Cerebral necrosis after radiotherapy and/or intra-arterial chemotherapy for brain tumors. *AJNR* 1987; 8:1083–1091.

41. Edwards MS, Wilson CB: Treatment of radiation necrosis, in Gilbert HA, Kagan AR (eds): *Radiation Damage to the Nervous System.* New York, Raven Press, 1980, pp 129–143.

42. Ron E, Modan B, Boice JD, et al: Tumors of the brain and nervous system after radiotherapy in childhood. *N Engl J Med* 1989; 319:1033–1039.

43. Bogdanowicz WM, Sachs E: The possible role of radiation in oncogenesis of meningioma. *Surg Neurol* 1974; 2:379–383.

44. Modan B, Baidatz D, Mart H, et al: Radiation induced head and neck tumors. *Lancet* 1974; 1:2267–2274.

45. Norwood CW, Kelly DL, Davis CH, et al: Irradiation induced mesodermal tumors of the central nervous system: Report of two meningiomas following x-ray treatment for gliomas. *Surg Neurol* 1974; 2:161–164.

46. Waga S, Handa H: Radiation induced meningioma with review of the literature. *Surg Neurol* 1976; 5:215–219.

47. Watts C: Meningioma following irradiation. *Cancer* 1976; 38:1939–1940.

48. Patronas NJ, Brown F, Duda EE: Multiple meningiomas in the spinal canal. *Surg Neurol* 1980; 45:2051–2055.

49. Rubinstein AB, Shalit MN, Cohen ML, et al: Radiation-induced cerebral meningioma: A recognizable entity. *J Neurosurg* 1984; 61:966–971.

50. Cliffon MD, Amromin GD, Perry MC, et al: Spinal cord glioma following irradiation for Hodgkin's disease. *Cancer* 1980; 45:2051–2055.

51. Wright TL, Bresnan MJ: Radiation-induced cerebrovascular disease in children. *Neurology* 1976; 26:540–543.

52. Brant-Zawadski M, Anderson M, DeArmond SJ, et al: Radiation-induced large intracranial vessel occlusive vasculopathy. *AJR* 1980; 134:51–55.

53. Fajardo LF, Barthong M: Radiation injury in surgical pathology, part I. *Am J Surg Pathol* 1978; 2:159–199.

54. Pay NT, Carella RJ, Lin JP, et al: The usefulness of computed tomography during and after radiation therapy in patients with brain tumors. *Radiology* 1976; 121:79–83.

55. Kingsley DPE, Kendall BE: Cranial computed to-

mography in leukemia. *Neuroradiology* 1978; 16:543–546.

56. Davis PC, Hoffman JC, Pearl GS, et al: CT evaluation of effects of cranial radiation therapy in children. *AJNR* 1986; 7:639–644.

57. Wang AM, Skias DD, Rumbaugh CL, et al: Central nervous system changes after radiation therapy and/or chemotherapy: Correlation of CT and autopsy findings. *AJNR* 1983; 4:466–471.

58. Liu HM, Maurer HS, Vongsvivut S, et al: Methotrexate encephalopathy. A neuropathologic study. *Hum Pathol* 1978; 9:635–648.

59. Ch'ien LT, Aur RJA, Stagner S, et al: Long-term neurological implications of somnolence syndrome in children with acute lymphocytic leukemia. *Ann Neurol* 1980; 8:273–277.

60. Peylan-Ramu N, Poplack DG, Pizzo PA, et al: Abnormal CT scans on the brain in asymptomatic children with acute lymphocytic leukemia after prophylactic treatment of the central nervous system with radiation and intrathecal chemotherapy. *N Engl J Med* 1978; 298:815–818.

61. Skullerud K, Halvorsen K: Encephalomyelopathy following intrathecal methotrexate treatment in a child with acute leukemia. *Cancer* 1978; 42:1211–1215.

62. Allen JC, Thaler HT, Deck MDF, et al: Leukoencephalopathy following high-dose intravenous methotrexate chemotherapy: Quantitative assessment of white matter attenuation using computed tomography. *Neuroradiology* 1978; 16:44–47.

63. Di Lorenzo N, Nolletti A, Palma L: Late cerebral radionecrosis. *Surg Neurol* 1978; 10:281–290.

64. Rottenberg DA, Chernik NL, Deck MDF, et al: Cerebral necrosis following radiotherapy of extracranial neoplasms. *Ann Neurol* 1977; 1:339–357.

65. Rubenstein LJ, Herman MM, Long TF, et al: Disseminated necrotizing leukoencephalopathy: A complication of treated central nervous system leukemia and lymphoma. *Cancer* 1975; 35:291–305.

66. Bjorgen JE, Gold LHA: Computed tomographic appearance of methotrexate-induced necrotizing leukoencephalopathy. *Radiology* 1977; 122:377–378.

67. Shalen PR, Ostrow PT, Glass PJ: Enhancement of the white matter following prophylactic therapy of the central nervous system for leukemia. *Radiology* 1981; 140:409–412.

68. Atlas SW, Grossman RI, Packer RJ, et al: Magnetic resonance imaging diagnosis of disseminated necrotizing leukoencephalopathy. *CT* 1987; 11:39–43.

69. Mueller S, Bell W, Seibert J: Cerebral calcifications associated with intrathecal methotrexate therapy in acute lymphocytic leukemia. *J Pediatr* 1976; 88:650–653.

70. Smith B: Brain damage after intrathecal methotrexate. *J Neurol Neurosurg Psychiatry* 1975; 38:810–815.

71. Priest JR, Ramsey NKC, Latchaw RE, et al: Throm-

botic and hemorrhagic strokes complicating early therapy for childhood acute lymphoblastic leukemia. *Cancer* 1980; 46:1548–1554.

72. Alvord EC: Why do gliomas not metastasize? *Arch Neurol* 1976; 33:75.

73. Marks JE, Gado M: Serial computed tomography of primary brain tumors following surgery, irradiation and chemotherapy. *Radiology* 1977; 125:119–125.

74. Johnson DW, Parkinson D, Wolpert SM, et al: Intracarotid chemotherapy with 1, 3-bis(2-chloroethyl)-1-nitrosourea (BCNU) in D$_5$W in the treatment of malignant glioma. *Neurosurgery* 1987; 20:577–583.

75. Walker MD, Alexander E, Hunt WE, et al: Evaluation of BCNU and/or radiotherapy in the treatment of anaplastic gliomas. *J Neurosurg* 1978; 49:333–343.

76. Hochberg FH, Pruitt AA, Beck DO, et al: The rationale and methodology for intra-arterial chemotherapy with BCNU as treatment for glioblastoma. *J Neurosurg* 1985; 63:876–880.

77. Grimson BS, Mahaley MS, Dubey HD, et al: Ophthalmic and central nervous system complications following intracarotid BCNU (carmustine). *J Clin Neuro Ophthalmol* 1981; 1:261–264.

78. Omojola MF, Fox AJ, Auer RN, et al: Hemorrhagic encephalitis produced by selective non-occlusive intracarotid BCNU injection in dogs. *J Neurosurg* 1982; 57:791–796.

79. Stewart DJ, Grahovic Z, Benoit B, et al: Intracarotid chemotherapy with a combination of 1,3-bis (2-chloroethyl)-1-nitrosourea (BCNU), cis-diaminedichloroplatinum (cisplatin), and 4′0-demethyl-1-0-(4,6-0-2-thenylidene-β-D-glucopyranosyl)epipodo-phyllotoxin (VM-26) in the treatment of primary and metastatic brain tumors. *Neurosurgery* 1984; 15:828–833.

80. Theron J, Villemure JG, Worthington C, et al: Superselective intracerebral chemotherapy of malignant tumors with BCNU. *Neuroradiology* 1986; 28:118–125.

81. Bonstelle CT, Kori SH, Rekate H: Intracarotid chemotherapy of glioblastoma after induced blood-brain barrier disruption. *AJNR* 1983; 4:810–812.

82. Kapp J, Vance R, Parker JL, et al: Limitations of high dose intra-arterial 1,3-bis(2-chloroethyl)-1-nitrosourea (BCNU) chemotherapy for malignant gliomas. *Neurosurgery* 1982; 10:715–719.

83. Heros DO, Renkens K, Kasdon DL, et al: Patterns of recurrence in glioma patients after interstitial irradiation and chemotherapy: Report of three cases. *Neurosurgery* 1988; 22:474–477.

84. Burger PC, Dubois PJ, Schold SC, et al: Computerized tomographic and pathologic studies of the untreated, quiescent, and recurrent glioblastoma multiforme. *J Neurosurg* 1983; 58:159–169.

85. Johnson PC, Hunt SJ, Drayer BP: Human cerebral gliomas: Correlation of postmortem MR imaging and neuropathological findings. *Radiology* 1989; 170:211–217.

Index

ATLAS OF
AFRICAN-AMERICAN
HISTORY

James Ciment

Facts On File, Inc.

....

Atlas of African-American History

Copyright © 2001 by Media Projects Inc.

Media Projects, Inc. Staff
Executive Editor: C. Carter Smith Jr.
Project Editor: Carter Smith III
Principal Writer: James Ciment
Associate Editor: Karen Covington
Production Editors: Anthony Galante, Aaron Murray
Indexer: Marilyn Flaig

Checkmark Books
An imprint of Facts On File, Inc.
11 Penn Plaza
New York NY 10001

Library of Congress Cataloging-in-Publication Data
Ciment, James.
  Atlas of African-American history / James Ciment.
    p. cm.
  Includes bibliographic references and index.
  ISBN 0-8160-3700-0 (hardcover: acid-free paper)—ISBN 0-8160-4127-X (pbk.)
    1. Afro-Americans—History. 2. Afro-Americans—History—Maps. I. Facts On File, Inc.
II. Title

E185.C55 2001
973'.0496073—dc21

                                                                    00-049047

Cover design by Nora Wertz
Text design by Paul Agresti
Layout by Anthony Galante and Aaron Murray
Maps by Anthony Galante, Aaron Murray, and David Lindroth

Printed in Hong Kong

CREATIVE USA FOF 10 9 8 7 6 5 4 3 2 1
         (pbk) 10 9 8 7 6 5 4 3 2 1

This book is printed on acid-free paper.

CONTENTS

Note on Photos

Some of the illustrations and photographs used in this book are old, historical images. The quality of the prints is not always up to modern standards, as in many cases the originals are from old negatives or the originals are damaged. The content of the illustrations, however, made their inclusion important despite problems in reproduction.

INTRODUCTION

"We hold these truths to be self-evident... That all men are created equal." So wrote Thomas Jefferson in the Declaration of Independence, in 1776. This founding principle outlined what was at the time a quite radical idea, but that idea has remained one of the cornerstones upon which the United States has been built.

Of course, when the U.S. Constitution was ratified thirteen years later, the exceptions to that principle were made clear. Voting rights, one of the preeminent badges of individual equality, were denied to women outright. What is more, while the Declaration of Independence pronounced the equality of "all men," only landowning white men were deemed fit to vote by the drafters of the Constitution. Enslaved Africans, in fact, were not even acknowledged as fully human. In deciding how to allot state-by-state representation in the U.S. Congress, each slave was declared equal to three-fifths of a man.

This conflict between the lofty promise of Jefferson's Declaration of Independence and the U.S. Constitution's limitations on that promise are at the heart of what may well be the central dilemma of U.S. history. Jefferson himself was a slaveowner, who unlike other founding fathers never freed the majority of his slaves, even upon his death.

In many ways, this book depicts the struggle that the United States has undergone to live up to the promise spelled out by the Declaration of Independence. While it is expressly concerned with the African-American experience, the history of African Americans cannot be separated from the story of all Americans, any more than the story of the nation's presidents or military conflicts can.

In addition to the national struggle to fulfill the promise of "life, liberty and the pursuit of happiness" for all Americans, readers will find other themes running throughout this story.

One such theme has been the conflict between the goal of integration into the larger American community on the one hand and separation from that community on the other. Whether the figures or organizations involved are the African Colonization Society in the early 19th century, Marcus Garvey's United Negro Improvement Association in the early 20th century, or Louis Farrakhan's Nation of Islam in the present-day, the impulse toward separatism has been a consistent response to the scourge of racism.

By the same token, those calling for an equitable integration have held their position with an equal fervor, and that struggle is well documented in these pages, from the quiet nobility of Benjamin Banneker, who lobbied Jefferson to recognize that achievement was less a matter of race than of opportunity, to the commanding stature of former general Colin Powell, who proved through his actions and character that he was fit for any office in the land, if he chose to pursue it.

The struggle for African-American equality, then, should not be defined by a series of government laws passed over time granting increased rights to black citizens. Instead, it is the story of African Americans and their allies forcing these changes through concerted action. It is the story of well-known heroes such as Harriet Tubman and Frederick Douglass, of Booker T. Washington and W. E. B. DuBois, and of Martin Luther King Jr. and Malcolm X. However, it is equally the story of those unknown, everyday heroes who face the enormous obstacles of personalized and institutionalized racism, have not only maintained their dignity and strength but have moved mountains in the process.

In many ways, movement itself is yet another crucial theme of this book. In one sense, the struggle for civil rights is referred to as a movement. On a more basic level, the migration of people from place to place is another form of movement. This form of movement, as much as any other theme stated above, is at the heart of the African-American experience. Beginning with the epoch of the African enslavement and diaspora, movement has defined African-American history. As enslaved Africans from diverse regions of Africa arrived in first in the Caribbean and Latin America, and then in the North American colonies, they carried old traditions—and formed new ones—that reshaped their new world. With emancipation came new eras of movement, as freedpersons traded shackles for life in the North, in the West, and elsewhere, once again transforming their new homes. It is for this reason that the form of this book—an atlas—is especially appropriate. It is our hope that the maps included in these pages will help give concrete life to the story of how geographic as well as cultural and political borders have been crossed over the centuries. Likewise, we hope readers come away with an understanding of the consequences of these crossings, and the barriers that remain in the road to fulfilling the promise of Thomas Jefferson's revolutionary vision of equality for all.

ACKNOWLEDGMENTS

The author and editors wish to thank the many people who have contributed greatly to this project. It was first conceived by Facts On File's Eleanora von Dehsen. Although the road to this book's completion has had its stops and starts, and bumps and turns, Eleanora and her noble team of successors Nicole Bowen, Terence Maikels and Gene Springs have together exhibited, not only an unerring editorial sense of what the project demands, but also perseverance, patience, and expertise. It was a pleasure working with them all.

The maps too were a collaborative effort. Most were prepared by David Lindroth, a very skilled independent illustrative cartographer. Anthony Galante and Aaron Murray of Media Projects Incorporated contributed maps also, as well as handling production and layout work.

On the editorial side, an enormous amount of research went into this project, and we are grateful for all the hard work on that front performed by Melissa Hale, Karen Covington, Kenneth West, and Kimberly Horstman.

THE AFRICAN HERITAGE
A Short History of a Continent

Mother Africa, the land has been called, for it is in East Africa's Rift valley that scientists believe that humans first evolved. These human ancestors, current archaeological findings indicate, emerged as a distinctive genus, or grouping of species, within the primate order (apes, monkeys, lemurs, etc.) of mammals approximately 5 million years ago. There is little resemblance, of course, between these ancient hominids, roughly defined as primates who walked on two legs, and people today. It would take millions of years of evolution to transform these small-statured and -brained primates into modern human beings. Nonetheless, archeologists say that fossil evidence confirms that humanity first emerged in East Africa.

According to scientific evidence, the roots of humankind reach deep into African soil. Indeed, all humans—when traced back far enough—come from the world's second-largest continent. The African heritage, then, is the the heritage of humankind.

THE BIRTHPLACE OF HUMANKIND

Evidence of the very first hominids is scant: an arm bone at Kanapoi, part of a jaw at Lothagam, a molar at Lukeino—all archaeological digs in the modern-day nation of Kenya. The earliest substantial fossil find was made at a place called Laetoli, in neighboring Ethiopia, in 1974. It was so complete a skeleton that the archaeologists who discovered it gave it a name—Lucy. About 3.5 million years old, Lucy was an *Australopithecine*, part of a genus of the hominid family about four to five feet tall and with a brain about one-third the size of the modern human brain. More precisely, she was labeled an *Australopithecus afarensis*. (Archaologists are always careful to note that the precise line of descent from Lucy to modern humans is not always direct. This fact should be kept in mind in the following discussion. Some of the different species listed below lived side by side, and some died out rather than evolving into more modern human form.)

For the next 1.5 million years—or about 75,000 generations—*A. afarensis* evolved through a series of *Australopithecus* species, including *A. africanus* and *A. robustus*, each somewhat larger and bigger-brained than its predecessors. Then, about 2 million years ago, humanity's first direct ancestors arrived on the scene, the genus *Homos*.

It was the great archaeologist Richard Leakey who discovered the first of the *Homo* species, *habilis*, at Olduvai Gorge in Kenya in the early 1960s. The name *Homo habilis* means "handy man," and it comes from the fact that *H. habilis* is the first human ancestor whose remains have been found accompanied by evidence of tool-making. About half a million years later came *H. ergaster*, "upright man," which lived beside *A. robustus*.

Homo sapiens, or "thinking man," appears in the East African fossil record about 500,000 years ago. Here was a human ancestor with our physical size, a brain almost equal to our own, and the ability to make tools and harness fire. *H. sapiens*, like some of the earlier *Homo* species, made its way out to southern Africa and out of the continent to Asia and Europe.

Finally, about 100,000 years ago, however, *Homo sapiens sapiens* or "wise thinking man"—a being biologically identical to ourselves—appeared in East Africa. *H. sapiens sapien*s would migrate even farther than earlier *Australopithecus* and *Homo* species, settling not just in Asia and Europe, but in Australia (about 40,000 years ago) and the Americas (about 15,000 years ago) as well. And wherever it went it displaced—through competition or mating—more primitive forms of human beings. Halfway between the emergence of *H. sapiens sapiens* and today comes evidence of multipiece weapons, tools, and even jewelry. And, again, it shows up in eastern and southern Africa first.

For the next 40,000 years or so—until the end of the last ice age 10,000 years ago—human beings in Africa and elsewhere largely lived as bands of hunters and gatherers. Groups remained small—probably no more than 150 or so persons—and ranged widely, requiring up to 300 square miles to support each group. The entire continent of Africa supported perhaps a million

The Origins of Human Beings

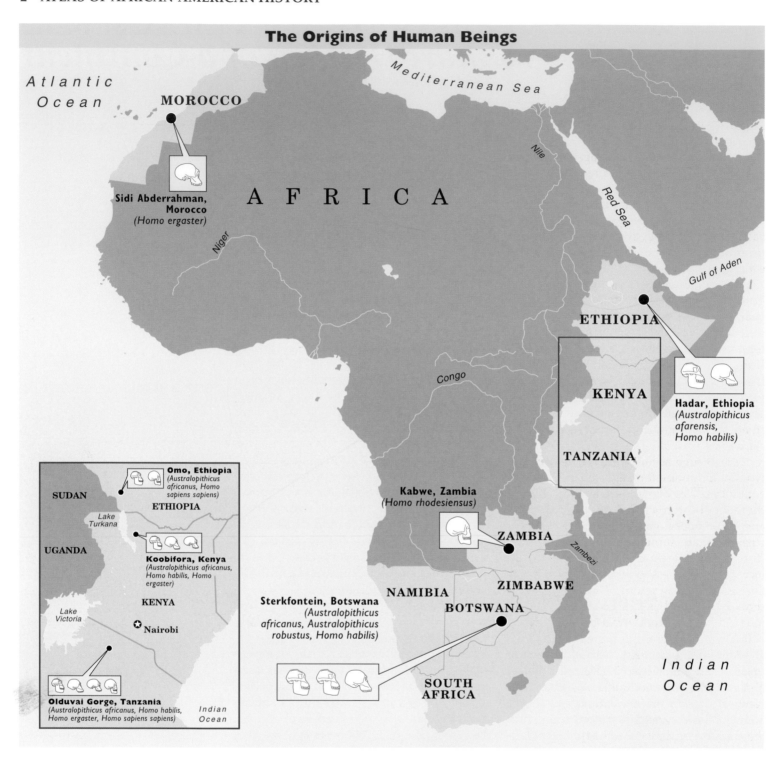

people. Many of them, surprisingly, lived in what is now the Sahara Desert, which was much wetter and greener then. There they hunted big game with spears and bows and arrows, gathered edible plants and insects, and recorded what they saw on the sides of rocks and caves.

A MASTERY OF NATURE

Drawings on rocks and cave walls reveal a fascinating story. Etchings from 12,000 years ago depict the wild beasts—giraffes, elephants, and rhinoceroses—hunted by these Paleolithic, or Old Stone Age, people. In art from approximately 7,000 years ago, both the subject and the style begin to change. Etchings are replaced by paintings made from oxidized minerals and clay, mixed perhaps with blood, animal fat, or urine to make the colors bind to the rock. Along with pictures of wild animals, these paintings also depict people hunting and herding. Archaeologists theorize that this new emphasis on human beings in control of the animal world reflects a new mastery of nature, as the people of Africa had begun to domesticate animals such as cattle, sheep, and goats.

But even during the wetter and greener eras of long ago, the Saharan climate—punctuated by long periods of drought—made life difficult and uncertain for its inhabitants. As historian John Reader has written, "the Sahara acted as a pump, drawing people from surrounding regions into its watered environments during the good times, and driving them out again as conditions deteriorated (though not necessarily returning them to their point of origin)." Among the places of refuge in dry times was a green and narrow valley near the eastern end of the desert, watered by a meandering river that would come to be called the Nile.

Modern human beings probably lived in the Nile valley for tens of thousands of years, but the best picture of what their life was like comes from 19,000-year-old remains at an archaeological dig at Wadi Kubbaniya, in modern-day Egypt. Hunting, while still practiced, was rarer in the valley than in the surrounding territories. There were just too many people in too small an area. Fishing, however, was critical, as was the gathering of seeds, fruit, and root crops such as nut-grass tubers. And, as would be the case for thousands of years to come, the lives of the people followed the rhythms of the river. Indeed, the vegetable and fish stocks gathered after the river crested in late summer and early fall were stored away against the lean times. The incredible richness of the valley and the need to protect agricultural surpluses led to settlement in villages of up to 500 persons or more by about 7000 B.C., 4,000 years before the first pyramids were built.

The development of agriculture marked the great leap between the Paleolithic times, or Old Stone Age, and the Neolithic times, or New Stone Age. Most archaeologists agree that it first occurred in the Fertile Crescent of the Middle East, a particularly fertile region stretching from modern-day Iraq to Israel. But the legumes and grains first domesticated there soon found a home in the Nile valley, along with a locally domesticated grain from North Africa called sorghum. The seeds of a future civilization, both literally and figuratively, had now been planted.

ANCIENT CIVILIZATIONS

The Nile valley of Egypt—along with Mesopotamia, China, the Indus Valley, and Meso-America—is often referred to as one of the "cradles of civilization." While the term civilization can be and has been defined in numerous ways, it is meant here in its conventional sense. The civilization that arose along the lower reaches of the Nile—between the cataracts at Aswan in the south to the Mediterranean Sea in the north—was a unified state with a common culture. It was ruled by a king, or pharaoh, and administered by an army of literate bureaucrats. It developed an indigenous form of writing, art, and religion and built massive monuments and engineering projects, many of which have weathered the millennia and are visited today by millions of tourists.

ANCIENT EGYPT

It is no accident that civilization first arose in the Nile valley. Archaeologists and historians have long noted that most of the early civilizations on Earth arose in river valleys.

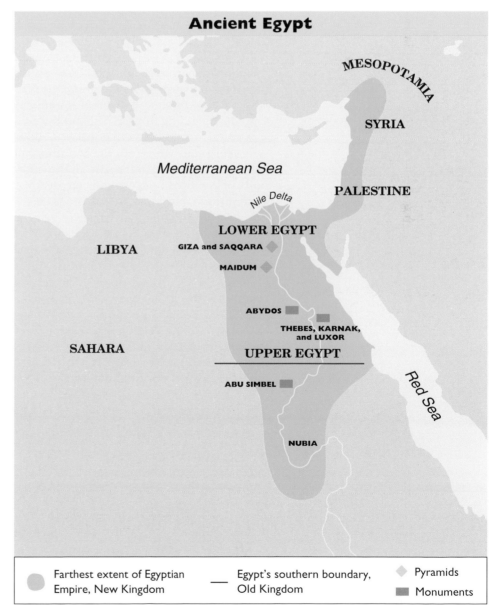

Ancient Egypt

MESOPOTAMIA

SYRIA

Mediterranean Sea

PALESTINE

Nile Delta

LOWER EGYPT

LIBYA

GIZA and SAQQARA

MAIDUM

ABYDOS

THEBES, KARNAK, and LUXOR

SAHARA

UPPER EGYPT

Red Sea

ABU SIMBEL

NUBIA

Farthest extent of Egyptian Empire, New Kingdom

Egypt's southern boundary, Old Kingdom

Pyramids

Monuments

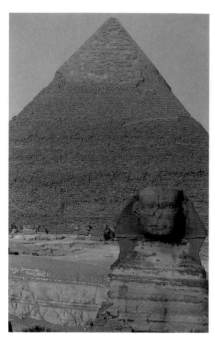

The Great Pyramids and the Sphinx in a late-19th-century photograph (Library of Congress)

There is no great mystery to this phenomenon. River valleys, such as the Nile, have rich soils and access to stable supplies of water. Thus, they can support larger numbers of people and agricultural surpluses. These surpluses relieve some members of society from raising food, leaving them free to devote themselves to art, crafts, engineering, writing, religion, war-making, and governing. River valleys also create connectedness, unity, and ease of transportation, allowing for the spread of ideas, inventions, culture, and law. The process eventually becomes self-sustaining. Surpluses support greater numbers of officials and soldiers who can command greater numbers of people to produce greater surpluses. Large numbers of laborers could be conscripted to work on—or taxed to pay for—large irrigation and other engineering projects. These, in turn, would create greater surpluses, which would result in larger populations and larger bases for taxation and labor, and so on.

But while all of this explains why and how civilization arose in ancient Egypt, it doesn't explain why that civilization took the form that it did. Two other features of the Nile are necessary for that. First, unlike the rivers of nearby Mesopotamia, the Nile is stable, flooding in predictable amounts at a predictable time of year. This produced a remarkable continuity in Egyptian civilization over time. Moreover, the continuity of the river helped instill the idea of the continuity of life. Egyptians saw life and death as a continuum and built great monuments—the massive pyramids at Giza are just the most famous examples—to ensure that their pharaohs would live on forever to protect Egypt and ensure the continuity of the Nile and its life-giving floods. The second unique feature of the Nile valley is its location. Surrounded by great deserts to the east and west, it was relatively isolated. Over the course of its first 2,500 years, Ancient Egypt was conquered only once by foreign invaders. This security added to the sense of continuity inherent in Egyptian history and culture.

EGYPT'S AFRICAN ROOTS

There is another feature of Egypt's location that is important. As a quick glance at a map shows, the Nile valley is located in the northeastern corner of Africa but connected to the Middle East and the Mediterranean world as well. Although Egypt is on the African continent, scholars continue to debate the degree to which Ancient Egypt was of Africa. In other words, how African was Egyptian culture and how Egyptian is African culture? The first of these questions is the easier one to answer. As noted above, Egypt was largely settled by peoples from all over Africa, even though a significant minority did come from what is now the Middle East and the Mediterranean parts of Europe. In that sense, Egypt is most certainly African.

Regarding the question of Egypt's influence on the rest of the African continent, there can be little doubt that Egyptian culture heavily influenced the Nubian civilizations that bordered it immediately to the south, a region the ancient Egyptians referred to as Punt. As early as 2450 B.C., the pharaoh Sahure sent an expedition to the region, in what is today the nation of Sudan. Its mission was not a friendly one. Upon their arrival in Punt, the invading Egyptian military plundered or demanded in tribute a king's ransom of timber, precious metals, and incense. Later expeditions from Egypt would bring back grain, ivory, cattle, slaves, even an "exotic" Mbuti (or pygmy, as they have been commonly called). The enormous value that Egyptians placed on African commodities—as well as the resistance put up by the Nubians—can be measured by the extremes the Egyptian pharaohs went to acquire such treasures. In 1472 B.C., for example, Egyptian Queen Hatshepsut had an armada of ships carried across the desert from the Red Sea to the upper reaches of the Nile. Gradually, Egypt established control over the region, turning Nubia, or Kush, as the Egyptians referred to it, into a vassal state, or virtual colony.

THE KINGDOM OF KUSH

The Egyptians, however, offered as much as they took. The merchants of Kush soon grew rich on trade and adopted Egyptian art, culture, and religion. Indeed, Kush grew so rich and powerful that it was able to conquer and rule Egypt itself for about a 60-year period in the 8th and 7th centuries B.C. By the time the Romans conquered Egypt in the last century before Christ, Meroë, the capital of Kush, was among the wealthiest cities in the world, where the kings and queens erected massive monuments—in Egyptian style—to assure their eternal life. But what made Kush and Meroë great also unmade them. Unlike Egypt—where softer bronze tools and weapons predominated—Kush was built on iron. More heavily wooded than its neighbor to the north, it had the timber resources necessary to fuel its forges. Gradually, however, these forests were depleted, leading to heavy erosion and a collapse of the critical agricultural base. By the 2nd century A.D., Meroë had fallen.

For a long time, historians believed that the people of Meroë fled their dying civilization for the heartland of the continent, bringing their iron-making technology with them to West and Central Africa. Indeed, there is some evidence that both Meröe and Egypt had a linguistic influence across the breadth of the continent. For example, there are numerous words in the language spoken by the Wolof people of modern-day Senegal, at Africa's most-western extreme, that bear a strong resemblance to Egyptian. Where the Wolof say *gimmi* for "eyes," the Egyptian used *gmk* for "look"; Wolofs say *seety* for "prove" where Egyptians used *sity* for "proof." More recently, however, historians have become skeptical of this earlier theory, since no material evidence of such a technology transfer exists.

While some scholars—pointing to distinct kinds of iron-smelting furnaces found in different parts of the continent—argue that iron-making technologies were entirely indigenous to Africa, most historians and archaeologists believe that iron-making emerged from the Middle East, where iron was first forged 4,500 years ago in Anatolia, a region in modern-day Turkey. From there, they say, it spread throughout the Middle East, was brought to North Africa by the seafaring Phoenicians, and then traded across the Sahara by Berbers, the indigenous people of North Africa. Early forges, dating back to about 600 B.C.—as old as those in Meroë—have been found in what is now Nigeria.

The importance of iron cannot be overestimated. It is stronger and more versatile than copper or bronze—the earliest metals to be forged—and its ores are far more widespread, though making it requires furnaces that can reach much higher temperatures. A culture that possesses iron-making technology has a distinct advantage over one that does not. And while there is evidence of the effects of this technological edge in many parts of the world, nowhere is it more obvious than in sub-Saharan Africa. It is not a coincidence, say historians, that the earliest sub-Saharan cultures to adopt iron-making—that is, those in modern-day Nigeria and Cameroon, the so-called Bantu-speaking people—were the ones that came to dominate the entire continent below the Sahara Desert.

The iron-making technologies also served as an engine that propelled social and economic change in sub-Saharan

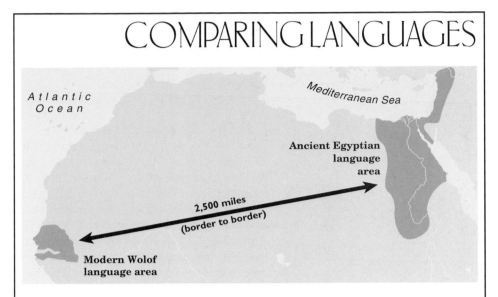

COMPARING LANGUAGES

Atlantic Ocean

Mediterranean Sea

Ancient Egyptian language area

2,500 miles (border to border)

Modern Wolof language area

Egyptian word	Meaning	Wolof word	Meaning
nb	basket	ndab	calabash
ro	mouth	roh	to swallow
tpn	example	top	to follow
gmk	look	gimmi	eyes
sity	proof	seety	to prove
kite	ring	khet	ring
r db	in exchange	dab	to shake hands
ta tenem	first land made by the gods	ten	clay God used to make the first humans
aar	paradise	aar	divine protection
tefnut	the god that created the sun by spitting it out	tefnit	to spit
geb	dirt	gab	to dig
kau	above	kaou	heaven
auset	Isis, wife of Osiris	set	wife
tiou	five	diou-rom	five
etbo	floating sun at the beginning of time	temb	to float

Africa. Large-scale iron-making required specialized craftspeople who ate the agricultural surpluses of farmers who, in turn, became more productive through the iron tools they used. Regions where iron was forged became food importers, creating a network of trade and exchange that can still be traced in many parts of the continent. At the same time, the use of iron had its consequences. High-temperature iron furnaces (2,200°F/1,200°C) have an insatiable appetite for wood charcoal. Some archaeologists theorize that the ecological deterioration caused by deforestation delayed the rise of large centralized states in some parts of sub-Saharan Africa, although by A.D. 1000 empires and federations of trading cities stretched across Africa from modern-day Ethiopia in the east to Senegal in the west.

THE BANTU MIGRATION

The sheer scale of the Bantu conquest and its impact on the natural and human environment of Africa makes it one of the most important developments in human history, and one of the most remarkable. Beginning about 2,000 years ago, many Bantu-speaking peoples begin migrating to central Africa. By at least 1,000 years ago, they had reached east to modern Tanzania, south to Mozambique and southwest to Angola. In West Africa, they mixed with Sudanic peoples from modern Chad and Sudan.

Again, the reasons for the success of this massive migration over the centuries

can be found in the unique properties of iron and the special requirements of iron-making. First, the strength of the metal makes it ideal for weapons. According to archeologists and historians who have found few weapons in sites dating back to the migration epoch of 2,000 to 2,500 years ago, the Bantu-speaking peoples—unlike many other great conquerors of history—achieved most of their success wielding the hoe and not the sword. Iron hoes allowed the Bantu-speakers to produce more food on more land, allowing for greater population growth and spread. Local hunters and gatherers, such as the Mbuti (often referred to as pygmies) of central Africa and the Khoisan (sometimes called bushmen) of southern Africa were pushed into marginal lands, such as the deep rain forests of the Congo River basin and the Kalahari Desert of southern Africa. Indeed, there is no geographically larger region of the world with such a wide array of closely related languages as in sub-Saharan Africa, with the Bantu family spoken today in countries as far afield as South Africa, Senegal in West Africa, and Kenya in East Africa. Even American English has been affected. Such common everyday American words as banjo, jiffy, and bozo have their roots in the Bantu language.

AFRICAN KINGDOMS

The Bantu peoples enter recorded, or written, history—as opposed to the history recreated through archaeological finds and oral traditions—around 1,000 years ago. During the early centuries of the past millennium, there arose in West Africa a series of kingdoms and empires. Based on trade, they mixed elements of the indigenous cultures of the region with the Islamic civilization of North Africa and the Middle East, a culture to be discussed at greater length in the next section of this chapter.

The wealth of these kingdoms—and most especially of Mali—is revealed in the spending of their rulers. In the 13th century A.D., one ruler named Kankan Mansa Musa led a caravan of 25,000 camels to Mecca, as part of the pilgrimage all good Muslims are expected to take at least once in their lifetime. Indeed, Mansa Musa ordered the construction of a new mosque—or Islamic temple—every Friday, to honor the weekly Muslim sabbath. Moreover, the caravan contained so much gold that it brought down the price of the precious metal wherever it went.

The Bantu Migration

Mediterranean Sea

AFRICA

Red Sea

MODERN NIGERIA

Original Bantu area

LIMIT OF BANTU MIGRATION (ca. A.D. 1000)

WESTERN BANTU

EASTERN BANTU

LIMIT OF BANTU MIGRATION (ca. A.D. 1000)

Atlantic Ocean

Retreat of Khoisan (bush) people

Indian Ocean

→ Route of Bantu migration ▪▪▪▪ Border between Bantu-speaking regions

▪ Geographical limit of Bantu migration

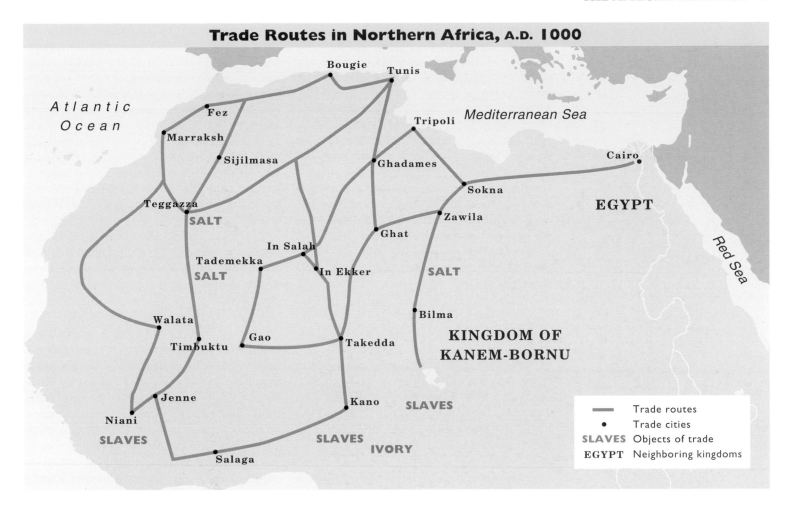

Trade Routes in Northern Africa, A.D. 1000

As with much of African history, the origins of Mali lie in a complex interplay of indigenous developments and outside influences. Around 1000 B.C., the Mande-speaking people of what is now western Sudan and Chad shifted their economy from hunting and gathering to agriculture, domesticating native plants like sorghum and millet. Farming, of course, can support far greater numbers of people than hunting. Among the Mande it produced a population explosion that led them to settle across a vast territory stretching to the Atlantic Ocean by A.D. 400. As population densities increased, federations of villages under a single king spread across the Sahel, the semi-dry grassland region south of the Sahara. But what turned these small federations into great empires—of which Mali was just one—was only partly the doing of the Mande. In fact, the foundations of Mali and the other great Sahelian empires rested on the back of the camel.

TRADE ROUTES
OF NORTH AFRICA

While camels are difficult to handle, they are ideally suited for desert travel and desert commerce—able to carry 500 pounds 25 miles a day and do so without a sip of water for a week at a time. Not surprisingly, the camel—originally from Asia—spread rapidly through North Africa after its introduction around 200 A.D. It opened up an immensely lucrative trans-Saharan trade network between the Mediterranean and sub-Saharan Africa, a network that put the Mande in the middle. Great cities arose at the southern edge of the Sahara, where the main caravan routes emerged from the desert: Walata (in present-day Mauritania); Tekedda and Agades (Niger); and, most famously, Gao and Timbuktu (Mali). There, Arab, Berber, and Mande merchants—all Muslim peoples from North and West Africa—exchanged silk cloth, cotton cloth, mirrors, dates, and salt (essential to the diets of people in tropical climates) for ivory, gum, kola nut (a stimulant), and gold. By the 11th century, the mines of West Africa had become the Western world's greatest source of gold, turning out nine tons of the precious metal annually.

Also making its way across the Sahara—not on the backs of camels but in the minds of the merchants who drove them—was a new faith. Islam was born in the Arabian cities of Mecca and Medina in the early 7th century. A crusading religion that preached the power of Allah and the equality of all men, Islam—under the Prophet Muhammed and his successors—quickly spread throughout the Middle East and North Africa. By A.D. 1100, the Maghreb—Arabic for "land of the setting sun," that is, modern-day Morocco, Algeria, and Tunisia—boasted major Berber and Arabic Islamic empires. South of the Sahara, a major kingdom—built on the wealth of the trans-Saharan trade—was emerging in what is now Mauritania and Mali. While its subjects—a Mande-speaking people known as the Soninke—called it Aoukar, outsiders referred to it as Ghana, after the title taken by its warrior-kings, and the name stuck.

GHANA, MALI, AND SONGHAI

By any name, Ghana was a remarkable place, so well-administered that scholars throughout the Western world praised it as a model for other kingdoms. To assure the royal lineage, for example, the kingdom was inherited not by the king's son—in an age before genetic testing, paternity could never be determined with one hundred percent accuracy—but by his nephew, that is, his sister's son. And while the king and his people retained their ancestral religion—

commissioning exquisite altars and statues to worship ancestors and guardian saint-like spirits—much of the merchant class and the government bureaucracy were Arabic-speaking Muslims. It was a potent combination of ideas, wealth, and military strength. By the end of the first millennium, Ghana had conquered almost all of the trading cities of the western Sahel, covering a territory roughly the size of Texas, where it exacted tribute, or taxes, from trans-Saharan merchants, subordinate kings, and local chiefs.

Despite its good governance, Ghana collapsed around 1100 and divided into small kingdoms, which warred on each other for more than a century until a new dynasty of warrior-kings, founded by the great Sundiata, united the region from their capital at Niani (present-day Mali). Even more extensive than Ghana, the kingdom of Mali and its successor—the Songhai Empire—dominated much of West Africa from the 13th to 16th centuries. Even more than Ghana, these were thoroughly Islamic empires, where many of the rulers, such as Mansa Musa, were driven as much by faith as power. And as medieval Islam valued literacy and learning above all other earthly pursuits, the kingdoms of Mali and the Songhai were renowned for their scholarship. By the late 15th century, Timbuktu

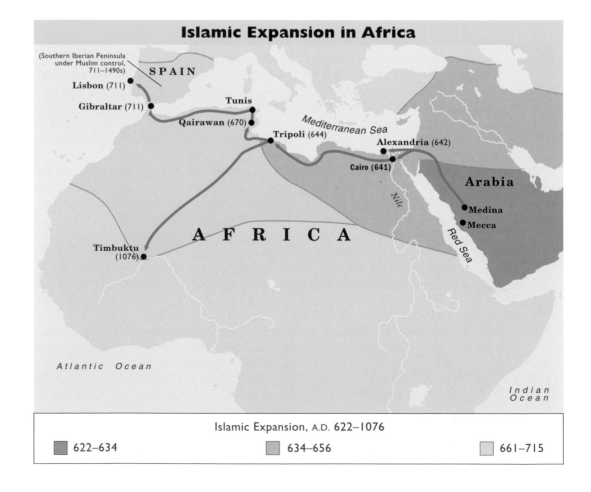

Kingdoms of Africa

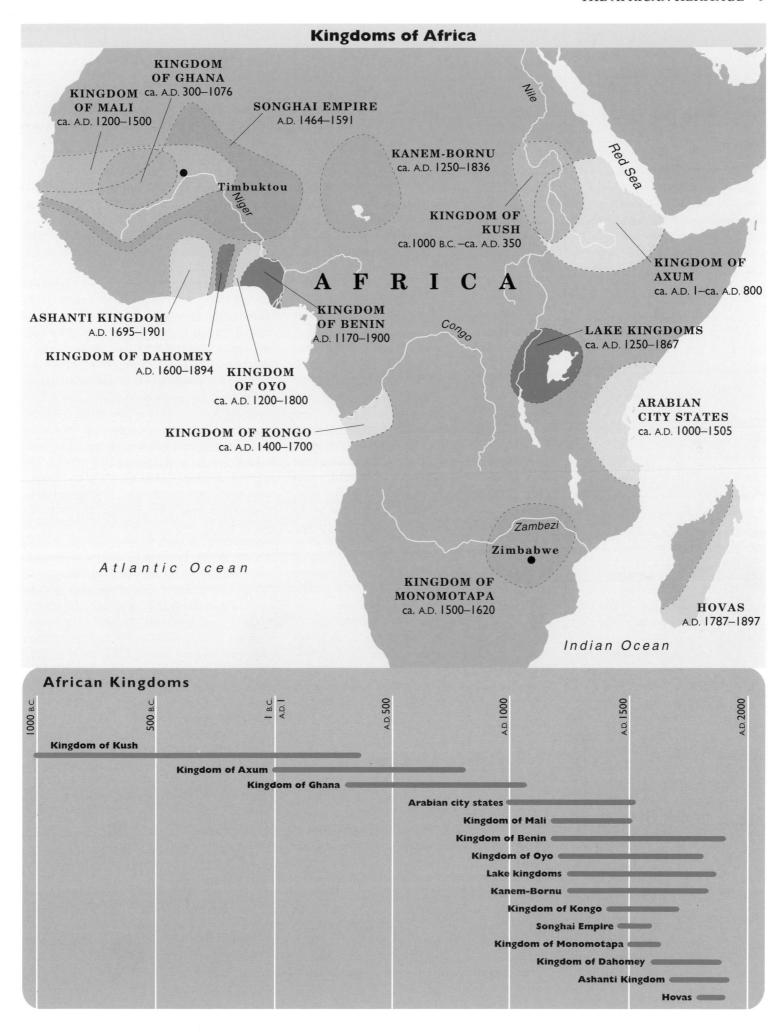

KINGDOM OF GHANA ca. A.D. 300–1076

KINGDOM OF MALI ca. A.D. 1200–1500

SONGHAI EMPIRE A.D. 1464–1591

Nile

Red Sea

KANEM-BORNU ca. A.D. 1250–1836

Timbuktou

Niger

KINGDOM OF KUSH ca.1000 B.C. –ca. A.D. 350

KINGDOM OF AXUM ca. A.D. 1–ca. A.D. 800

A F R I C A

ASHANTI KINGDOM A.D. 1695–1901

KINGDOM OF BENIN A.D. 1170–1900

Congo

LAKE KINGDOMS ca. A.D. 1250–1867

KINGDOM OF DAHOMEY A.D. 1600–1894

KINGDOM OF OYO ca. A.D. 1200–1800

ARABIAN CITY STATES ca. A.D. 1000–1505

KINGDOM OF KONGO ca. A.D. 1400–1700

Atlantic Ocean

Zambezi

Zimbabwe

KINGDOM OF MONOMOTAPA ca. A.D. 1500–1620

HOVAS A.D. 1787–1897

Indian Ocean

African Kingdoms

1000 B.C. | 500 B.C. | 1 B.C. | A.D. 1 | A.D. 500 | A.D. 1000 | A.D. 1500 | A.D. 2000

Kingdom of Kush

Kingdom of Axum

Kingdom of Ghana

Arabian city states

Kingdom of Mali

Kingdom of Benin

Kingdom of Oyo

Lake kingdoms

Kanem-Bornu

Kingdom of Kongo

Songhai Empire

Kingdom of Monomotapa

Kingdom of Dahomey

Ashanti Kingdom

Hovas

MAJOR THEMES IN AFRICAN ART

Traditionally, African art exhibits several features: 1. It always serves a purpose or conveys a message; 2. It is usually produced to be used by the community of the artist who made it; 3. It often has a spiritual element to it. The art below, though created by 20th century artists, maintains these traditions.

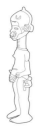

Fertility/Fortune
This piece was produced by an artist of the Bena Lulua ethnic group of contemporary Congo. The stomach and navel symbolize female fertility. Note the baby clinging to the mother's side.

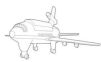

Death
This coffin from modern-day Ghana is an example of how African art adjusts to changes in the cultural environment. The coffin shown here was built for an airplane pilot by a member of a community of woodcarvers working outside of the Ghanian capital of Accra.

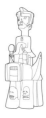

Protection of the Living
This *ejiri*, or altar, was created by an artist from the Ijo ethnic group of Nigeria. It depicts a man riding a trunkless elephant. The man is the head of a family, two members of which are represented by faces on elephant's legs. Together, man and elephant represent a spirit of family protection. The altar is meant to be kept in the home.

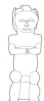

Ancestor Adoration
This piece is a *bieri*, produced by a member of the Fang ethnic group of Gabon. It was meant to be fitted into a container and carried in spiritual processions.

was home to the largest university in Africa, outside of Egypt, funded by the wealth derived from trans-Saharan trade.

But while that wealth went to build mosques, universities, and great cities, it came at an immense cost. Along with the gold, salt, and cloth transported by trans-Saharan caravans, there was human cargo—slaves.

While never reaching the scale of the transatlantic slave trade of the 16th through 19th centuries, the trans-Saharan trade was still immense. It is estimated that up to 10,000 slaves were annually carried northward across the Sahara (along with a small trickle southward) at the height of the trade in the 10th and 11th centuries. In all, historians estimate over 4 million men, women, and children were transported from West Africa to the Islamic realms of the Mediterranean and Middle East between the years 650 and 1500. As in the Americas, the black slaves of the Arab world were largely put to work as laborers—in mines, plantations, workshops, and households.

Still, there were significant differences between Islamic and transatlantic slavery. For one thing, many of the Islamic slaves became soldiers, where they could often earn their freedom through military valor. And because race and color had little to do with status—the Arab world also imported slaves from Europe and western Asia—there was far more social intermingling of free people and slaves, including extensive intermarriage. Indeed, it was in this multicultural Mediterranean setting that African slaves first came to the attention of European Christians, including the Spanish and Portuguese. And when these Europeans looked for people to work the plantations of their transatlantic empires after 1500, they increasingly turned to Africa.

THE SLAVE TRADE

"Sir," began the letter that the king of Kongo, Nzinga Mbemba, wrote in 1526 to King João III of Portugal. "Your Highness should know how our Kingdom is being lost in so many ways . . . by the excessive freedom given by your agents and officials to the men and merchants who are allowed to come to this Kingdom to set up shops with goods and many things which have been prohibited by us, and which they spread throughout our Kingdoms and Domains in such abundance that many of our vassals [subjects], whom we had in obedience, do not comply because they have the things in

greater abundance than we ourselves; and it was with these things that we had them content and subjected under our vassalage and jurisdiction. . . ."

Mbemba, the son of the first central African king to encounter Europeans, was probably not the first African ruler, and certainly not the last, to learn that the trade goods that Europeans brought with them in their ships came with a steep price tag. In 1506, Mbemba had invited Portuguese merchants, administrators, and government officials to live in his central African kingdom and introduce European ideas, faith, and commodities to his subjects. But as the 1526 letter between Mbemba and King João III makes clear, the European presence proved to be destructive. Portugal's representatives freely sold Mbemba's subjects alcohol, firearms, and other goods, thereby undermining the Kongo government. And, of course, the goods were only part of the trade. In exchange, the Portuguese demanded the kingdom's most valuable asset. "We cannot reckon on how great the damage is," Mbemba's letter goes on to say, "since the mentioned merchants are taking every day our natives . . . and get them to be sold; and so great, Sir, is the corruption of licentiousness [sin] that our country is being completely depopulated." The king of Portugal's response to the African leader was less than encouraging; Kongo, he argued, had nothing else of value to Europeans. If Mbemba wanted to continue to receive the European goods that his kingdom now depended on, he would have to let Portuguese slave traders conduct their business without interference from his government. Although Mbemba's successors would attempt to prevent Portugal from dominating the kingdom's affairs by fostering trade with the Dutch as well, by the late 17th century, Kongo had splintered apart. Two centuries later, French and Belgian colonies, known as French Congo and Congo Free State (later renamed Belgian Congo) would complete Kongo's transformation from independence to colonial subjegation.

SLAVERY IN PRE-COLONIAL AFRICA

As in many regions of Earth in ancient times—including Asia, Europe, and the Americas—slaves and slavery were part of everyday life in Africa. As the biblical book of Exodus recounts, the Egyptians enslaved thousands of Hebrews—and Nubians—putting them to work constructing some of the greatest monuments of the ancient world. The Phoenician trading empire of Carthage—in modern-day Tunisia—exported African slaves throughout the Mediterranean world several centuries before Christ. And, as in everything they did, the Romans took the trade to another level, enslaving tens of thousands of Africans (including a small number of black Africans), slaves, and others to work the plantations and crew the sea-going galleys of the empire. The fall of Rome in the 5th century did not end slavery, although it did temporarily curb the trafficking in human beings in the Western world. Still, the barbarian successors to Rome in North Africa maintained slavery, and the coming of the Arab armies in the 7th and 8th centuries expanded the trade, although the religion they brought with them established some of the first moral codes on the treatment of slaves.

As noted earlier, human beings were among the most common and valuable commodities of the trans-Saharan trade, with Arab merchants working hand in hand with local officials and traders to secure the cargo. While evidence of slavery in all great medieval kingdoms of Africa is relatively scarce, a pattern seems to emerge: the more trade-oriented the kingdom, the more common was slavery. Thus, in the relatively self-contained and long-lived Christian kingdom of Axum—which existed in what is now modern-day Ethiopia from the 3rd to 11th centuries—slavery appears to have been somewhat rare. But in the great West Africa trading empires of Mali and Songhai, forced labor played a much greater role in economic life, with slaves doing much of the back-breaking labor in salt mines and on plantations, as well as serving as a lucrative export.

Evidence of a significant trade in human beings—as well as the widespread use of slaves for agriculture and mining—exists for the early kingdoms of Oyo and Benin (in the modern-day countries of Benin and Nigeria) from the 15th century onward and in the kingdom of Great Zimbabwe in southern Africa from 1200 to 1500. The slave trade was also an essential component of the economies of the Islamic city-states established by Arab merchants along the Indian coast of Africa from modern-day Eritrea to Mozambique. Finally, many smaller African societies kept slaves, although the institution there was very different from what it was in the great empires and trading states of West Africa and the East African coast.

Amongst the villages and tribal confederations of sub-Saharan Africa, slavery was a more intimate affair. In terms of numbers, it was much smaller in scale and slaves lived with, worked among, and often married into the families who owned them. Before the arrival of European slavers and outside the orbit of the great Islamic and African empires, slaves were not simply commodities in a vast trading system. While slaves in such societies were not always treated benignly—wherever one person holds power over another there is the potential for abuse—they were still treated as human beings. A person became a slave because of misfortune—losing a war and becoming a prisoner or losing a crop and being a debtor—or because of individual misdeeds, as in the case of criminals. Thus, slavery was rarely an inherited status and slaves were not necessarily viewed as an inferior form of humanity.

THE TRANSATLANTIC SLAVE TRADE

While the transatlantic slave trade organized first by the Portuguese and later by other Europeans is more properly the subject of chapter 2, a few comments about its impact on Africa are appropriate here. First, the Europeans expanded the slave trade beyond any scale ever dreamt of by the most ambitious trans-Saharan merchant. The development of New World plantation agriculture and the decimation of Native American populations by disease and war after 1500 led to an insatiable demand for labor, and the African slave trade was expanded exponentially to meet that demand. Over the course of the 16th century, the trade gained momentum slowly, with the Portuguese dominating. By 1600, the transatlantic trade drew, even with the trans-Saharan network, about 5,000 slaves being transported every year along each of these routes. With the arrival of the more efficient Dutch, British, and French traders in the 17th and 18th centuries, the transatlantic trade easily outdistanced the trans-Saharan trade. By 1800, nearly 80,000 Africans were being forcibly transported to the New World. During the course of the 19th century, the numbers leveled off and then declined, as first Great Britain, then the United States, and finally other European countries banned first the trade in slaves and then the practice of slavery itself.

All of these numbers represent controversial estimates. But one fact should always be kept in mind: the numbers of slaves actually taken to the New World represents only a fraction—probably less

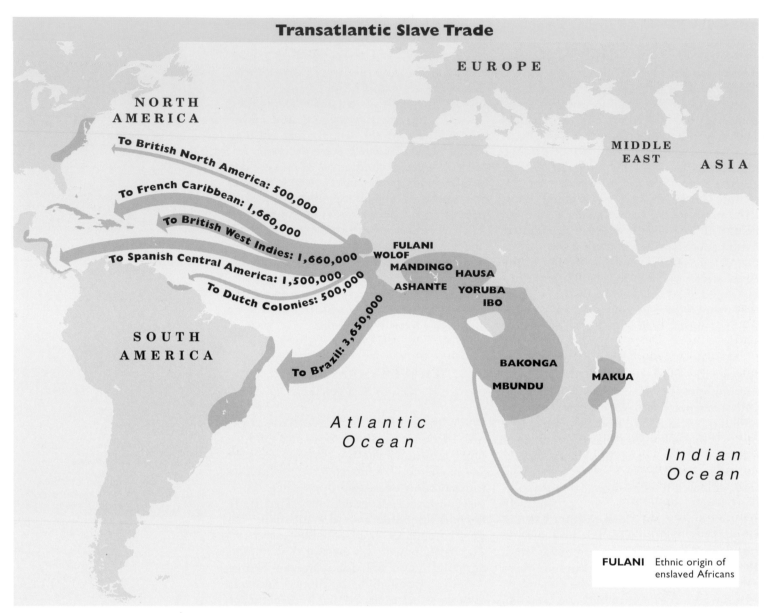

Transatlantic Slave Trade

EUROPE

NORTH
AMERICA

MIDDLE
EAST   ASIA

To British North America: 500,000

To French Caribbean: 1,660,000

To British West Indies: 1,660,000

To Spanish Central America: 1,500,000

To Dutch Colonies: 500,000

FULANI
WOLOF
MANDINGO   HAUSA
ASHANTE   YORUBA
            IBO

SOUTH
AMERICA

To Brazil: 3,650,000

BAKONGA

MBUNDU   MAKUA

Atlantic
Ocean

Indian
Ocean

FULANI Ethnic origin of
enslaved Africans

Between 1505 and 1870, over 9 million Africans were forcefully transported to the Americas as slaves. It is estimated that approximately one in six enslaved Africans died en route to their destinations. All told, 3.6 million Africans were sent to Brazil, with most of the rest heading for European colonies in the Caribbean. The map above outlines the main points of origination and destination in the transatlantic slave trade and the number of Africans involved.

than half—of the total numbers of Africans enslaved. For example, historian Patrick Manning has estimated that approximately 9 million persons were brought to the Caribbean, Brazil, and the United States as slaves at the height of the trade between 1700 and 1850. But, he adds, some 12 million died within a year of their capture and another 7 million were enslaved for domestic use within Africa. Altogether, for the length of the transatlantic slave trade—from about 1500 to the late 1800s—it is estimated that as many as 18 million persons were forcibly taken from tropical Africa: 11 million from West Africa across the Atlantic; 5 million more from the Sahel across the Sahara and Red Sea; and yet another 2 million from central and southern Africa

to the Middle East and the sugar islands of the Indian Ocean. The demographic effect of this trade was even greater than these numbers indicate. Scholars estimate the population of sub-Saharan Africa at about 50 million in 1850; absent the slave trade, however, it would have been closer to 100 million.

SLAVERY'S IMPACT ON AFRICA

While the cultural impact of the slave trade on those transported to the New World was profound beyond measure, the political and economic impact of the business on the lands they were taken from is more difficult to gauge. Indeed, there are two mutually exclusive schools of thought on the subject. One argues that slavery—horrendous as it was—had little impact because it was spread so thinly over so vast a territory. As one historian points out, an African's chance of being enslaved at the height of the trade was no worse than that of a modern American being killed in a car crash. It is also pointed out that new food crops brought eastward across the Atlantic from the Americas—like cassava and corn—made African agriculture significantly more productive, counterbalancing the demographic impact of the westward trade in slaves.

Other historians disagree and use a number of convincing arguments to bolster their cases. First, they point to the dramatic demographic impact that the population drain caused by the slave system produced. Despite the fact that most of the territory south of the Sahara is adequately watered and fertile enough for agriculture, the African continent remains significantly underpopulated, despite the population explosion of the late 20th century. While China and India together have only 60 percent of the amount of territory of Africa, they contain roughly three times as many people. This underpopulation, say scholars, has hampered the development of agriculture, trade, manufacturing, and nation-building. Furthermore, slave traders preyed upon the youngest, healthiest, and most productive members of African society.

Slave trading also created great insecurity and fear wherever it existed. Most slaves were captured in raids, either conducted on a major scale by armies or on a smaller scale by professional kidnappers. Precious resources in societies living on the very edge of subsistence had to be devoted to defense, and fear of capture kept villagers close to home, limting their ability to trade or farm far afield. Olaudah Equiano—who wrote his autobiography years after being captured as a slave in what is now Nigeria—explained the anxieties engendered by the slave trade. "Generally, when the grown people in the neighborhood were gone far in the fields to labour, the children assembled together . . . to play; and commonly some of us used to get up a tree to look out for any assailant, or kidnapper, that might come upon us; for they sometimes took these opportunities of our parents' absence to attack and carry off as many as they could seize." Indeed, Equiano and his sister were taken from their own frontyard.

Politically, the slave trade encouraged the growth of predator states. The Dahomey and Oyo kingdoms of modern-day Benin and Nigeria grew rich and powerful in a vicious cycle of trading slaves for firearms, with the latter being used to capture more slaves. But as these kingdoms drained whole territories of people, they too collapsed as the European traders moved elsewhere in their search for cheap and plentiful human beings. The trade in slaves also stunted local industry, as Africans traded slaves for cheap European cloth and metal goods, thereby undermining local producers, as was the case in Mbemba's Kongo of the 16th century. At the same time, alcohol became more plentiful, while the problems associated with it spread throughout slave-trading territories.

Perhaps worst of all, the transatlantic and Indian Ocean slave trades expanded the use of slaves within Africa itself, spreading violence, destroying legitimate trade, disrupting the social order, and undermining the freedom of millions who never even had to see the inside of a slave ship before becoming enslaved. Historian Joseph Miller likens the effect of slave-trading in Africa to a tidal wave. "It tossed people caught in its turbulence about in its wildly swirling currents of political and economic change. Like an ocean swell crashing on a beach, it dragged some of its victims out to sea in the undertow of slave exports that flowed from it, but it set most of the people over whom it washed down again in Africa, human flotsam and jetsam exposed to slavers combing the sands of the African mercantile realms left by the receding waters." Ultimately, the slave trade would render Africa far more vulnerable to European colonization and would place the African people in a politically and economically subservient role —a role from which they have yet to fully emerge.

EUROPEAN COLONIZATION

If, by some magic, all European settlers had disappeared from sub-Saharan Africa in 1800, they would have left behind scant evidence of their presence: some British, and French slave forts along the coasts of western and southwestern Africa, a few Portuguese trading posts along the southern and east African coast and, most

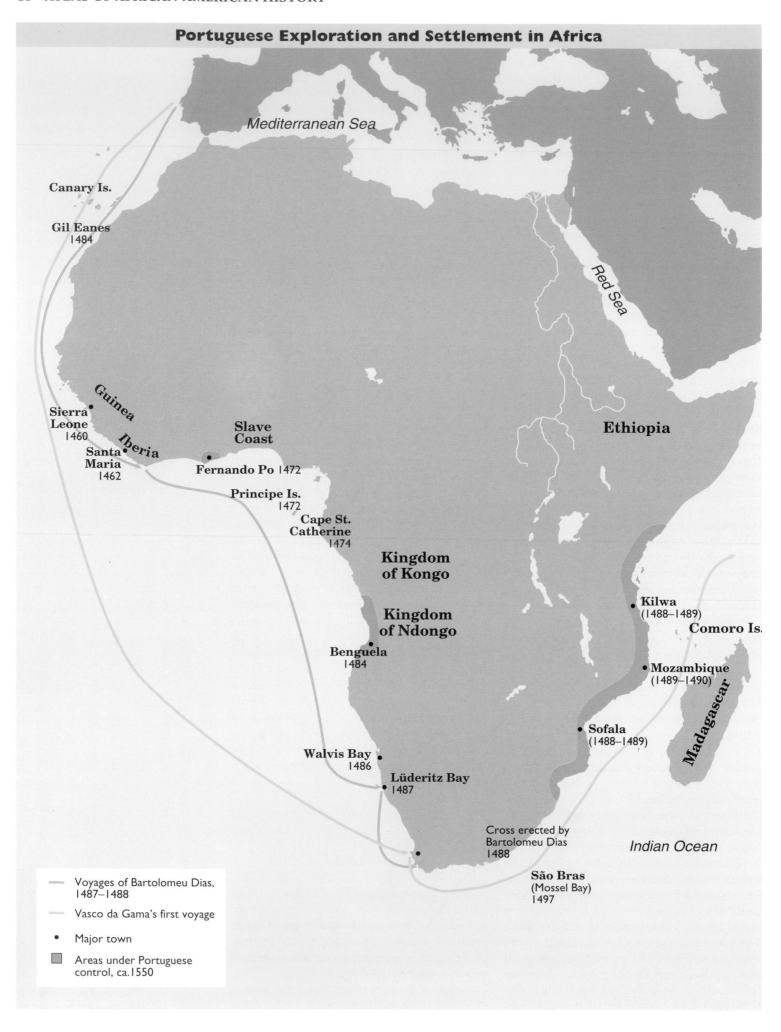

Portuguese Exploration and Settlement in Africa

Mediterranean Sea

Canary Is.

Gil Eanes
1484

Red Sea

Guinea

Sierra
Leone
1460

Slave
Coast

Iberia

Santa
Maria
1462

Fernando Po 1472

Principe Is.
1472

Cape St.
Catherine
1474

Ethiopia

**Kingdom
of Kongo**

Kilwa
(1488–1489)

Comoro Is.

**Kingdom
of Ndongo**

Benguela
1484

Mozambique
(1489–1490)

Walvis Bay
1486

Lüderitz Bay
1487

Sofala
(1488–1489)

Madagascar

Cross erected by
Bartolomeu Dias
1488

Indian Ocean

São Bras
(Mossel Bay)
1497

Voyages of Bartolomeu Dias,
1487–1488

Vasco da Gama's first voyage

• Major town

Areas under Portuguese
control, ca.1550

notably, a scattering of Dutch towns and farms at the Cape of Good Hope (modern South Africa), where the Mediterranean climate was more conducive to European settlement. Until the 19th century, European settlers and colonists kept their distance from Africa, and for good reasons. First, the tropical parts of the continent were full of diseases deadly to outsiders, with malaria in particular felling most of those who tried to settle there. Even the freed slaves from North America who settled in Liberia—all distant descendants of the African motherland—often succumbed to disease. Not for nothing had tropical Africa earned the terrifying name "white man's grave."

Topography also played a role in keeping the Europeans at bay. Much of interior Africa is made up of high plateaus, which drop off steeply near the coast. Turbulent rapids and falls mark the lower reaches of most of the great African rivers, making them all but impassable to navigation. Finally, there was the human factor. For European governments and merchants of the 17th and 18th centuries, there was no need and little chance to penetrate more than a few miles from the coast. Africa's most valuable and coveted export—slaves—was largely controlled by powerful, militaristic African states. Until the advent of more sophisticated and deadly weaponry in the late 19th century—such as the Maxim gun—no European force could effectively challenge the African middlemen of the slave trade, armed as they were by those same Europeans.

EUROPEAN SETTLEMENTS

As with exploration and the slave trade, the Portuguese were the first to settle in sub-Saharan Africa. For much of the 15th century, the Portuguese monarchs—most notably Prince Henry the Navigator—sent ships southward, looking for an all-sea route to the Indies. Two years after Christopher Columbus's 1492 "discovery" of America, Pope Alexander VI helped arrange the Treaty of Tordesillas, dividing the non-European world into Spanish and Portuguese spheres: most of the Americas and the Pacific for Spain; Asia, Brazil, and Africa for Portugal. In 1497, Portuguese explorer Vasco da Gama finally rounded the Cape of Good Hope at the southern tip of Africa, sailed on to India, and returned to Portugal. Although his expedition was less than successful

financially—his European trinkets were of little interest to local African merchants—it did prove three things: the voyage was possible; the Portuguese had bigger guns than the locals (and could force them to sell); and the spice price differential between India and Europe (the source of profits) was enormous.

Over the next several decades, the Portuguese would establish trading posts and factories at Elmina (modern-day Ghana) and Luanda (Angola), while forcibly taking the Arab trading cities of Sofala, Moçambique, Pemba, Zanzibar, and Mombasa on the Indian Ocean coast. In 1652, the Dutch East India Company established a colony of farmers and traders in the region around the modern-day city of Capetown, to serve as a provisioning station for ships bound to and from the East Indies. At the same time, and on through the 18th century, British, Dutch, French, Spanish, and even Danish merchants built slave factories, or fortified trans-shipment centers, along the West African coast from Senegal to Nigeria, many of which thrived well into the 19th century.

But while the early years of the 19th century saw the peaking of the transatlantic slave trade, subsequent decades would see its decline, outlawing, and disappearance. In 1807, the British—then the most powerful maritime power in the world—banned the trade in slaves, followed by the Americans a year later. Naval patrols scoured the Atlantic in an effort to prevent the illegal trade. But the struggle was a long and frustrating one. As the quantity of slaves diminished, prices went up, encouraging even more ruthless and greedy traffickers in human flesh. Eventually, as first the British (1833), then the French (1848), the Americans (1865), and the Spanish and Portuguese (1880s) outlawed slavery in territories under their control, the transatlantic slave trade died out. (The trans-Saharan trade continued well into the 20th century; while internal African slavery survives in pockets—such as Sudan—today.)

THE SCRAMBLE FOR AFRICA

Yet even as they halted their slave trading, Europeans were expanding their holdings on the African continent. During the first 75 years of the 19th century, the French invaded Algeria and pushed into Senegal, the British established a protectorate over the

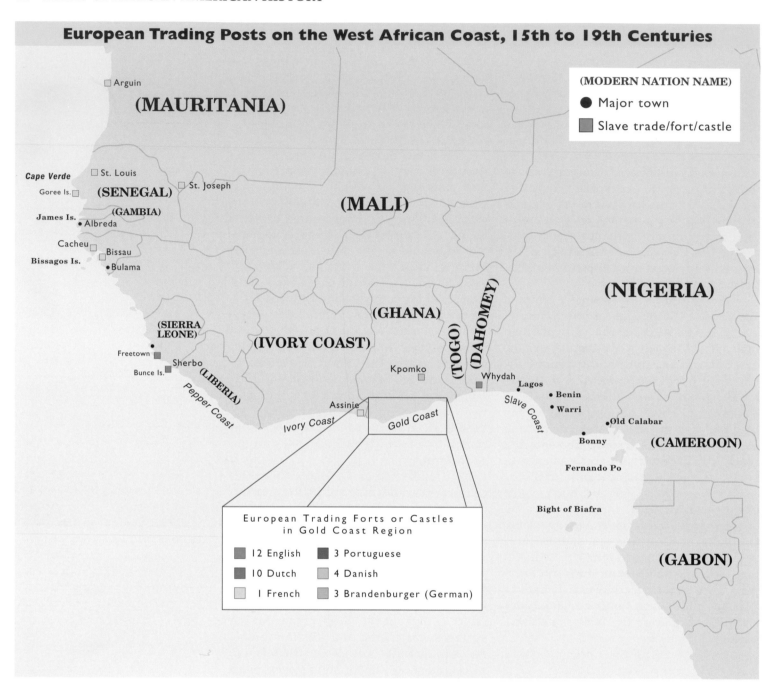

European Trading Posts on the West African Coast, 15th to 19th Centuries

(MODERN NATION NAME)
● Major town
■ Slave trade/fort/castle

□ Arguin

(MAURITANIA)

Cape Verde   □ St. Louis
Goree Is.□   (SENEGAL)   □ St. Joseph

(MALI)

(GAMBIA)
James Is.□
● Albreda

Cacheu □
□ Bissau
Bissagos Is.
● Bulama

(SIERRA
LEONE)

(IVORY COAST)   (GHANA)   (TOGO) (DAHOMEY)   (NIGERIA)

Freetown ■
Sherbo   Kpomko
Bunce Is.■   Whydah ■   ● Lagos
(LIBERIA)   ● Benin
Pepper Coast   Assinie□   ● Warri
Ivory Coast   Gold Coast   Slave Coast   ● Old Calabar
Bonny   (CAMEROON)

Fernando Po

Bight of Biafra

(GABON)

European Trading Forts or Castles
in Gold Coast Region

■ 12 English   ■ 3 Portuguese
■ 10 Dutch   ■ 4 Danish
■ 1 French   ■ 3 Brandenburger (German)

Gold Coast (modern-day Ghana) and took possession of the Cape Colony from the Dutch, forcing the latter to trek northward into the interior, and the Portuguese expanded their settlements into the Zambezi River valley of Mozambique. The goals were generally the same in each; establish direct control over a small but growing trade in gold, palm oil, dyewoods, and other tropical products. Still, as late as 1875—decades after the colonization of India and centuries after the conquest of the Americas—the vast interior of Africa remained under the control of indigenous African empires, kingdoms, and chiefdoms. Several related events, however, would bring this era to an abrupt close and usher in, in less than a quarter of a century, the direct colonization of African territories nearly six

times the collective size of the colonizing countries themselves—Belgium, Britain, France, Germany, Italy, Portugal, and Spain.

First came the explorers. As late as 1800, much of the African interior was unknown to outsiders and unmapped. Over the next 75 years, however, numerous European expeditions had crossed Africa from north to south and east to west, discovering interior highlands conducive to European settlement in the Eastern and Southern Africa and two vast, navigable river networks—the Congo and its tributaries and the Niger—in the center and west of the continent respectively. Next came the miners. In the 1870s and 1880s, the world's richest deposits of gold and diamonds were discovered in South Africa, spurring a rush of miners that would bring much of southern

EUROPEAN COLONIZATION OF AFRICA

1415	The Portuguese capture the North African city of Ceuta.
1441	Antonio Gonsalvez of Portugal, at the request of Prince Henry the Navigator, travels down the west coast of Africa and kidnaps 12 Africans, taking them back to Lisbon.
1453	The Ottoman Turks capture Constantinople, blocking Europe's overland routes to East Asia.
1469–1475	Portuguese navigator Gernao Gomes explores the African coast from Sierra Leone to Gabon.
1487–1488	The Portuguese explorer Bartolomeu Dias rounds the Cape of Good Hope.
1494	Pope Alexander VI divides the world into Spanish and Portuguese spheres; Africa is given to the latter.
early 1500s	The Portuguese destroy Islamic forts along the east coast of Africa.
1505	The first African slaves are transported to the Western Hemisphere; by 1870 an estimated 12 million Africans are forcefully removed to the Americas.
1517–1574	The Ottoman Turks conquer Egypt and North Africa.
1571	The Portuguese establish the colony of Angola.
1600s	British, Dutch, and French displace Portuguese from West Africa and establish their own slaving forts.
1652	The Dutch East India Company founds a settlement at Cape of Good Hope when Jan van Riebeeck and a small group drop anchor in Table Bay.
1698	Fort Jesus, a Portuguese fortification in Mombassa, in East Africa, falls to the Imam of Oman, signaling the waning power of Portugal's African empire.
1717	The Dutch East India Company announces that the use of African slave labor would be favored over the use of free labor in the Cape of Good Hope settlement.
1787	The British establish the colony of Sierra Leone for freed slaves from the Americas.
1806	The British take Cape Colony from Holland. The Dutch settlers, or Boers, decide to escape northward. In doing so they will come into increasing conflict with the Zulu.
1807	The British ban the international slave trade and establish patrols in the Atlantic.
1816	Shaka, king of the Zulus, begins to turn his army into the most powerful, well-trained military force in black Africa.
1822	Freed slaves from the United States found Liberian settlements.
1830	France invades Algeria.
1833	The British outlaw slavery in their empire.
1835	The Boers begin what is known as "The Great Trek," in which 12,000 men, women, and children head northward from their former Cape Colony. Despite fierce resistance from the Zulu people, the Boers found new republics, which they call Natal and the Orange Free State.
1847	Liberia declares itself the first independent black republic in Africa.
1848	The French outlaw slavery in their empire.
1854–1856	Scotsman David Livingstone explores central Africa from east to west and promotes the commercialization of Africa by Europeans.
1856	Britain takes control of Zanzibar.
1860	The French expand into West Africa from Senegal.
1866	Diamonds are discovered in southern Africa.
1869	The Suez Canal opens in Egypt.
1874	The British attack the Ashanti in West Africa.
1879	The Zulu Nation routs the British at Islandhlwana only to later be destroyed by a heavily armed British force.
1881–1885	Sir Charles George Gordon, military governor of the Anglo-Egyptian territory of Sudan, angers Muslim leaders by waging a campaign against slavery. Muslim rebels besiege Gordon and an Egyptian garrison for ten months. Despite a British rescue mission, Gordon is killed.
1882	The British take control of Egypt.
1884	Germany takes control of the West African territories of Togoland and Cameroon.
1884–1885	At the Berlin Conference, Africa is divided between English, French, German, Spanish, and Portuguese colonizers.
1885	Leopold II of Belgium sets up the colony of the Belgian Congo, not in the name of his country but in the name of a private company, which he heads.
1886	Gold is discovered in South Africa. Industrialist Cecil Rhodes begins to envision British rule extending from Egypt to the Cape Colony.
1890	Cecil Rhodes becomes prime minister of Cape Colony. That same year, he takes control of mines in Rhodesia (named after him in 1895 and since renamed Zimbabwe).
1896	The forces of King Menelik I of Ethiopia defeat the Italian army when it attempts to conquer that nation.
1899–1902	Dutch Boers fight British troops in South Africa's Boer War.
1904–1907	Germany pushes Herero men, women, and children into the Omaheke Desert of present-day Namibia. After poisoning water holes, the Germans surround the desert and bayonet all who try to crawl out. Survivors are sent to forced labor camps. By 1911, over 80 percent of the Herero are dead.
1911	Italy conquers Libya.
1914–1915	During World War I, the British and French seize German colonies.
1935	Italy invades Ethiopia.
1942	The Allies defeat Nazi armies at El Alamein, Egypt, beginning the drive of Germans from North Africa.
1948	The apartheid system is established in South Africa.
1952	The Mau Mau rebellion begins in Kenya.
1954–1962	Algerians wage a war of independence.
1957	Ghana becomes the first European colony in sub-Saharan Africa to win its independence.
1960	The Year of African Independence. Dozens of countries earn freedom from European colonizers.
1965	Whites of Rhodesia declare independence from Britain.
1975	Angola, Mozambique, and other Portuguese colonies gain their freedom.
1975–1994	Civil wars, with rebels armed by both the United States and South Africa, occur in Angola and Mozambique.
1989–1990	Namibia gains independence from South Africa.
1994	Nelson Mandela becomes the first majority-elected president of South Africa.

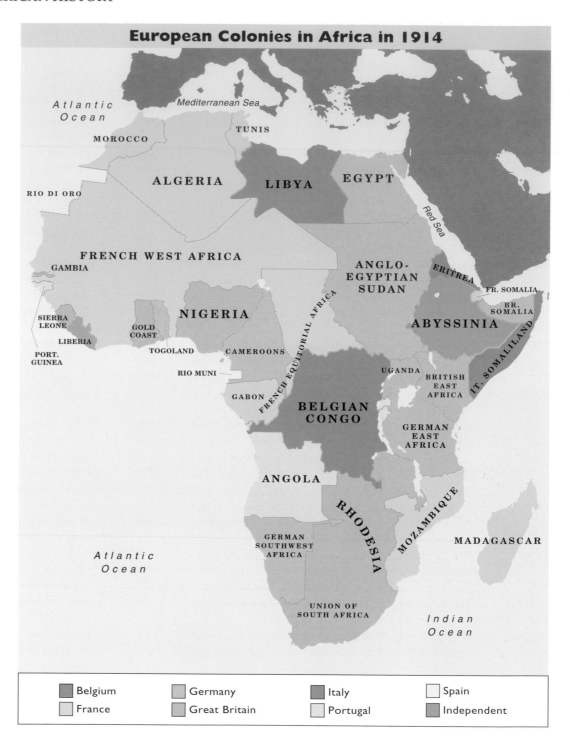

European Colonies in Africa in 1914

Atlantic Ocean

Mediterranean Sea

TUNIS

MOROCCO

ALGERIA

LIBYA

EGYPT

RIO DI ORO

Red Sea

FRENCH WEST AFRICA

GAMBIA

ANGLO-EGYPTIAN SUDAN

ERITREA

FR. SOMALIA

BR. SOMALIA

SIERRA LEONE

NIGERIA

GOLD COAST

ABYSSINIA

LIBERIA

PORT. GUINEA

TOGOLAND

CAMEROONS

RIO MUNI

GABON

UGANDA

BRITISH EAST AFRICA

IT. SOMALILAND

FRENCH EQUITORIAL AFRICA

BELGIAN CONGO

GERMAN EAST AFRICA

ANGOLA

RHODESIA

MOZAMBIQUE

MADAGASCAR

Atlantic Ocean

GERMAN SOUTHWEST AFRICA

UNION OF SOUTH AFRICA

Indian Ocean

	Belgium		Germany		Italy		Spain
	France		Great Britain		Portugal		Independent

Africa under the sway of the British Empire. Finally came the imperialist governments in a grab for territories that would see the entire continent—except for Ethiopia and Liberia—divided among seven European powers in little more than 20 years.

If one man could be said to be responsible for the "great scramble," it was the king of Belgium, Leopold II. Frustrated by his relative weakness as titular ruler of one of Europe's smallest countries, Leopold had great ambitions to carve out a personal empire in the heart of Africa by using his vast fortune. Beginning in the late 1870s, the Belgian monarch laid a personal claim to the vast Congo River basin of Central

Africa, establishing a colony called the Congo Free State that he ruled not in the name of Belgium, but as a personal kingdom, with the primary aim of extracting as much of the Congo's natural resources—particularly rubber—as possible, regardless of the human cost to Congo's population, who were treated as his personal slave labor force. Leopold's actions set off alarm bells in other European capitals, though not for any moral reasons. Leopold's European competitors were concerned that if they did not act quickly, the opportunity to exploit Africa's resources would be lost to them. Soon Britain, France, and Germany were scrambling for control over territories from one end of the continent to the other, while Portugal attempted to maintain its hold on Angola and Mozambique.

THE IMPACT OF COLONIALISM

To prevent a conflict that might spill over to Europe itself, the great powers met in the winter of 1884–1885 to resolve their conflicting territorial claims in Africa. At the Berlin conference, the politicians and diplomats considered a host of items: African resources, colonial borders, existing European settlements—everything but the African people themselves, none of whom were invited to attend. By the time they were through, the governments of Europe had created a web of internal boundaries that paid little heed to existing African patterns of ethnicity, language, or trade. In some places, ethnic groups were divided by the new borders; in others, antagonistic peoples were lumped together in the same colony.

But the European colonizers had just begun the process of stamping their will on the African continent. First came the struggle for colonial political control, as expeditionary forces—officered by Europeans, soldiered by African mercenaries, and armed with the latest rapid-fire guns—broke the power of African kingdoms throughout the continent. In Southwest Africa (now Namibia), German colonizers launched the 20th century's first genocide, virtually exterminating the region's Herero people after they rose up against European land grabs and forced labor demands. Colonial administrators were then sent in to collect taxes and forcibly recruit laborers. In Leopold's misnamed Congo Free State (which he ruled as his own personal colony), tens of thousands of Africans were slaughtered as Leopold's representatives sought to exploit the rich rubber resources of the territory, setting off the first international human rights crusade, which eventually forced Leopold to turn his personal colony over to the Belgian government.

"UNDERDEVELOPING" AFRICA

The Europeans masked their greed with righteousness. The French called their African campaigns a *mission civilatrice*, a civilizing mission, bringing legitimate (non-slave) commerce, European technology and ideas, and religion to the "dark continent." But much of this so-called development offered little for the Africans themselves.

Indeed, much of the infrastructure developed by the colonizers was designed to better exploit the colonized. Mines and plantations—using cheap African labor and exploiting African lands and resources—generated enormous profits for foreign investors, while railroads and highways linked the mines and plantations to ports, leaving Africa with a disconnected transportation system that largely served the interests of the European colonizers. Even to this day, it is far easier to fly or make a telephone call from Abidjan (Ivory Coast) to Paris (capital of the former colonizing power)—a distance of 3,000 miles—than it is to Accra (in neighboring Ghana), less than one-tenth the distance. It was for these reasons that famed African historian Walter Rodney titled his best-known book *How Europe Underdeveloped Africa*.

Even as Europeans were exploiting the wealth of Africa, they were trying to establish control over the minds of Africans. Christianity took hold wherever missionaries were present. While many of the missionaries spent their time railing against what they called "African superstition," some—like France's Albert Schweitzer—offered more practical help, establishing clinics, schools, and hospitals, as well as churches. But even the most beneficent facilities were often established for ulterior motives. Essentially, the schools and missions served three purposes: to instill obedience to European rule, to inculcate a belief in the superiority of European civilization and, during the latter years of the colonial enterprise, to train cadres of civil servants to run local affairs. Ironically, it would be these same schools and missions that bred the nationalist leadership that would overthrow colonialism in the mid-20th century.

The process by which a pro-European curriculum turned into an African nationalism is a fascinating one. While the colonizers tried to keep schools focused on technical training and loyalty to empire, bigger and more dangerous ideas tended to creep in. French teachers, for example, in recounting their nation's history, could hardly avoid the great revolutionary ideas that shaped it: "liberty, equality, and brotherhood." African students could not help but notice how little their colonial masters practiced the ideals they preached. The European missions and schools, by bringing together different ethnic groups from around each colony, also helped undo some of the destructive divisiveness European governments had fostered.

To step back a moment, most European colonizers practiced a simple method of

Independence in Africa

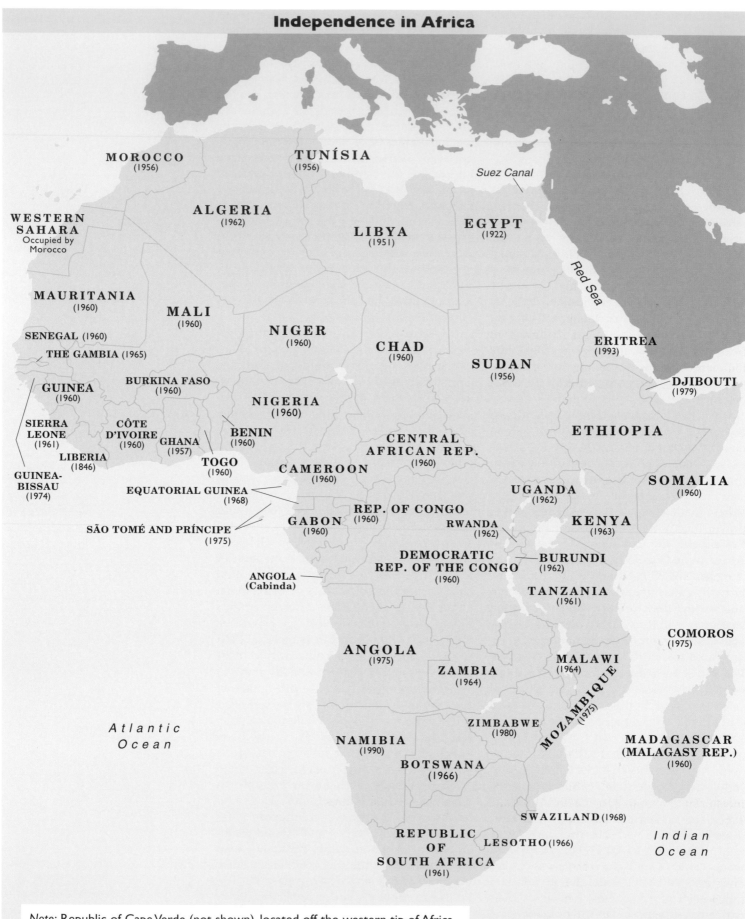

MOROCCO
(1956)

TUNÍSIA
(1956)

Suez Canal

WESTERN
SAHARA
Occupied by
Morocco

ALGERIA
(1962)

LIBYA
(1951)

EGYPT
(1922)

Red Sea

MAURITANIA
(1960)

MALI
(1960)

NIGER
(1960)

CHAD
(1960)

SUDAN
(1956)

ERITREA
(1993)

SENEGAL (1960)

THE GAMBIA (1965)

DJIBOUTI
(1979)

GUINEA
(1960)

BURKINA FASO
(1960)

NIGERIA
(1960)

ETHIOPIA

SIERRA
LEONE
(1961)

CÔTE
D'IVOIRE
(1960)

GHANA
(1957)

BENIN
(1960)

CENTRAL
AFRICAN REP.
(1960)

LIBERIA
(1846)

TOGO
(1960)

CAMEROON
(1960)

SOMALIA
(1960)

GUINEA-
BISSAU
(1974)

EQUATORIAL GUINEA
(1968)

UGANDA
(1962)

SÃO TOMÉ AND PRÍNCIPE
(1975)

GABON
(1960)

REP. OF CONGO
(1960)

RWANDA
(1962)

KENYA
(1963)

ANGOLA
(Cabinda)

DEMOCRATIC
REP. OF THE CONGO
(1960)

BURUNDI
(1962)

TANZANIA
(1961)

COMOROS
(1975)

ANGOLA
(1975)

ZAMBIA
(1964)

MALAWI
(1964)

MOZAMBIQUE
(1975)

Atlantic
Ocean

ZIMBABWE
(1980)

MADAGASCAR
(MALAGASY REP.)
(1960)

NAMIBIA
(1990)

BOTSWANA
(1966)

SWAZILAND (1968)

Indian
Ocean

REPUBLIC
OF
SOUTH AFRICA
(1961)

LESOTHO (1966)

Note: Republic of Cape Verde (not shown), located off the western tip of Africa,
gained independence from Portugal in 1975. The Republic of Seychelles, made
up of 90 widely scattered islands located roughly 1,000 miles east of Kenya and
Tanzania in the Indian Ocean, gained independence from Great Britain in 1976.

control—"divide and rule"—which pitted one African ethnic group against another. The tiny central African nations of Rwanda and Burundi provide examples with the most horrific consequences. For centuries, the Tutsis—just 10 percent of the population—and the majority Hutus had together created feudal kingdoms in which elite Tutsis ruled over Hutu farmers and non-elite Tutsi cattle-herders. Hutus and poor Tutsis paid tribute to their rulers and, in turn, were protected by them. Although tensions occasionally broke into violence, the two ethnic groups lived amongst each other and frequently intermarried.

Like other European colonialists, the Germans and Belgians (the latter taking over the colonies from the former during and immediately after World War I) created misconceived racial myths about the peoples they conquered in Africa. In the case of Burundi and Rwanda, they imagined the taller and less Negro-looking Tutsis to be a superior, more intelligent ruling race (some even said, ridiculously, that they were actually distant relations of the Europeans) and the Hutus a race of subservient, less intelligent farmers. Tutsis were given special rights, education, and police powers over the Hutus. This bred contempt among the Tutsis and resentment among the Hutus. When the Belgians left in 1962, they turned power over to the Tutsis in both countries. In Rwanda, the Hutu majority quickly overthrew the Tutsis; in Burundi, the Tutsis clung to power. Both countries would then be plunged into decades of bloodshed, with Tutsi killing Hutu in Burundi and Hutu killing Tutsi in Rwanda, a trend that culminated, in the latter country, in the genocide of 1994, in which 800,000 Tutsis and their Hutu sympathizers were slaughtered in a few months.

INDEPENDENCE

Indeed, independence—which came to most of sub-Saharan Africa in the 1950s and 1960s—began with great hopes that were quickly disappointed. The problems inherited by the first national leaders of Africa were many. The European colonialists had done very little to prepare their colonies for independence. In most new African nations, there were a handful of trained civil servants and but a few university-educated people. The economies—geared to meet the needs of the European colonizers—were oriented toward the export of raw materials. During the boom years of international capitalism in the 1960s, some African nations prospered. But with the oil crisis and worldwide recession of the 1970s and 1980s, prices for natural resources—except oil, for a time—collapsed. Declining revenues and rising foreign debt produced internal tensions that resulted in coup after coup across Africa. Making things worse were the ethnic rivalries fostered by Europeans and the internal ethnic divisions created by European-imposed borders. In 1967, Nigeria—the most populous nation in Africa—was plunged into a brutal, ethnic civil war. By the 1980s and 1990s, such conflicts had spread to Algeria, Angola, Congo, Ethiopia, Liberia, Mozambique, Sierra Leone, and a host of other countries—in some cases fueled by cold war tensions between the United States and the Soviet Union.

APARTHEID

While hardly spared the conflict that engulfed much of the rest of the continent, southern Africa experienced a different kind of struggle, a result of its special geography and history. Like Rhodesia (today's Zimbabwe)—its smaller neighbor to the north—South Africa possesses a mild climate conducive to white settlement. That climate and the fabulous mineral wealth of the region created a different kind of African colony—a settler colony of minority whites ruling over a majority African population. Over the course of much of the 20th century, the white farmers, businessmen and skilled workers of South Africa and Rhodesia enjoyed great economic and political privileges, while blacks were forced to farm marginal lands or work the mines, often separated from their families for months on end. In South Africa especially, a system of apartheid, or racial separation by law, was instituted. Virtually everything that was fine and good in the country—the best schools, jobs, lands, restaurants, hotels, parks, and beaches— were reserved for whites only.

The black majority hardly took this injustice lying down. In 1960, they protested in the black township of Sharpeville and were gunned down. In the early 1970s, guerrilla movements rose up to challenge white rule in Rhodesia, eventually forcing the minority to cede power to the majority in 1980 elections. Meanwhile, new protests erupted in Soweto and other black townships around Johannesburg in the mid-1970s, leading to a nationwide struggle that lasted through the 1980s. For a time, the white government cracked down on the protesters with unprecedented brutality. By the decade's end, however, some of those in power recognized that the apartheid system was doomed. Adding to its troubles was a growing international movement to end investment and trade with the minority-ruled regime. In 1990, President F. W. de Klerk freed Nelson Mandela, the leader of the anti-apartheid African National Congress (ANC), after Mandela had spent more than a quarter of a century in prison, and legalized his organiza-tion. Four years later—in what many considered a political miracle—Mandela was elected the first president of majority-ruled South Africa and the ANC became the country's dominant political party. While serious problems like crime, health issues and black economic underdevelopment inherited from the apartheid regime continue to plague the country, South Africa, by far the wealthiest nation on the continent, has the potential to lead Africa into a more prosperous and peaceful 21st century.

SLAVERY IN EARLY AMERICA

In 1441, a Portuguese sea captain named Antam Gonçalvez led nine of his crewmen ashore in a place they called Rio d'Ouro, or River of Gold. It lay along the northwest African coast, in what is now the territory of Western Sahara. Known locally as Baldaya, Rio d'Ouro had been renamed five years earlier by the first Portuguese explorers to encounter it. At first, those earlier adventurers thought it was a waterway that led deep into the legendary gold fields of West Africa. But a quick reconnaissance of the area revealed otherwise. Rio d'Ouro had no river and no gold, being merely a bay, on a parched stretch of coastline where the Sahara Desert met the sea.

Gonçalvez knew that. But he was after another prize. As darkness fell along the African coast, Gonçalvez and his crew—augmented by men from another Portuguese ship—descended on some tiny villages. The ship's chronicler related what happened next: "And when our men had come nigh to them [the African villagers], they attacked them very lustily, shouting at the top of their voices . . . the fright of which so abashed [surprised] the enemy, that it threw them all into disorder. And so, all in confusion, they began to fly without any order or carefulness."

No Portuguese were hurt in the encounter, but four Africans were killed. More significantly, ten were taken prisoner and brought back to Portugal. And Gonçalvez—knighted for his efforts by the Portuguese king—found a place in the history books as the first European since ancient times to enslave Africans.

Not that Africans were unknown in Europe before 1441. Indeed, blacks were so highly prized in the palaces of Renaissance Europe that they fetched many times the price of white servants. Like women, they were considered tokens of wealth. At the same time, Africans were widely sought after as actors, musicians, and dancers. But as Portuguese ships sailing the West African coast brought an increasing number of Africans, a new and more ominous role for blacks in Europe emerged—as slaves. In 1444, the first sizable shipment arrived in Lisbon.

By the late 1400s, thriving slave markets emerged in the ports of Portugal, Spain, France, and Italy, with a thousand Africans arriving annually in the Portuguese capital of Lisbon alone. A century later, black Africans represented roughly 10 percent of Lisbon's population. Even distant Great Britain had a population of some 15,000 Africans by 1600, around the time William Shakespeare created one of the most memorable African characters in English literature, Othello.

Ultimately, black slavery did not take root in Europe for a variety of reasons—religious, political, economic, even climatic. Traditionally, slavery was justified in medieval and Renaissance Europe on religious grounds. Enslaving Muslims and "heathens" was not only acceptable, it was considered a righteous crusade, according to a papal bull of 1452. The problem was what happened to a slave's status if he or she converted to Christianity, as many slaves did as it often allowed one one's freedom. Nor did slavery make economic sense in Europe. Slavery worked best on plantations in tropical lands where the workforce labored throughout the year. Most of Europe had neither the open space nor the warm climate for such a plantation regime.

In the end, however, slavery was doomed in Europe because it ran against political and historical events and trends. By the 1400s, slavery and similar forms of labor—such as serfdom—were fast disappearing across the face of western Europe. Peasants were gaining their freedom and a new economic and political system was emerging on the ruins of the old feudal order of lord and serf. An attempt to revive an archaic form of labor like slavery was economically counterproductive and politically explosive. And so it was never seriously tried.

Even as slavery was dying out in Europe, it was gaining a new and far more vigorous lease on life in those parts of the world coming under European hegemony—first the Atlantic Islands, and then the Americas. Madeira, an island 600 miles southwest of Portugal, and the Canary islands, 300 miles south of that, were "discovered" by Portugal and Spain respectively in the 14th century, although both had probably been known to the Romans more than a millenium before. Their settlement in

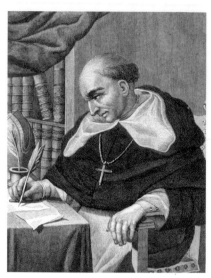

Bartolomé de Las Casas
(Library of Congress)

the following century would set a pattern that would hold true for the conquest of the Americas as well. The Atlantic islands would prove an ideal laboratory in which to establish what would become the trans-Atlantic slave trade.

SLAVERY IN THE SPANISH COLONIES

With rich soil and subtropical climates, Madeira and the Canary Islands were well suited for the growing of sugarcane, a crop originally from Southeast Asia and introduced to Europeans by the Arabs in the Middle Ages. By the early 1500s, the Spaniards had wiped out the indigenous people of the Canaries, the Guanche. (The name Canaries comes not from birds but from the archipelago's many large dogs, *canes* in Latin.) They imported thousands of slaves from West Africa to work the sugarcane plantations. The Portuguese did the same in Madeira, except there were no indigenous people to exterminate. Both Madeira and the Canary Islands also served as important provisioning stops for exploratory voyages down the African coast and, after 1492, to the Americas. But significant as the islands were as a template for conquest and plantation agriculture, their output of sugar—and their plantations' needs for African slaves—soon paled beside that of the Caribbean islands and tropical Latin America.

Christopher Columbus's 1492 voyage to America introduced Europeans to a whole "new world" across the Atlantic, even if Columbus himself went to his grave believing he had reached Asia. In the century after Columbus, much of the Americas—including the Caribbean, Mexico, Central America, and large parts of South America—was utterly transformed by Europeans.

Between 1492 and the late 1700s, European explorers—who often traveled with multiethnic crews that included Africans—visited and charted every major landmass in the world, with the exception of Antarctica. Within the first 100 or so years after Columbus's voyage, Spanish and Portuguese explorers led expeditions to virtually all of the islands of the Caribbean, as well as the Central, South, and North American mainlands. Exploration of the Caribbean and the American mainland was followed by conquest and, for the original inhabitants of the Caribbean, death. Within 50 years after Columbus's first major landfall, the native Taino and Carib population on the island of Hispaniola (modern Dominican Republic and Haiti) had fallen to 200, from a precontact level of between 250,000 and 500,000—near total annihilation. In the rest of the Caribbean, the story was much the same. Some native peoples were killed by Spanish swords, muskets, and dogs; the vast majority, however, were felled by hidden marauders: diseases such as smallpox and measles. On the American mainland, the numbers were even more appalling, with millions dying. Again, most succumbed to disease, though a significant minority were worked to death in mines or starved when their lands were taken from them to raise Spanish cattle. Horrified by the enormous carnage he was witnessing, Spanish priest Bartolomé de Las Casas pleaded for mercy for his Indian charges. "For God's sake and man's faith in Him, is this the way to impose the yoke of Christ on Christian men?" he asked King Charles I. "They are our brothers."

Ultimately, the king agreed with Las Casas. But if not American Indians, then colonizers would need others to work the mines that fed the Spanish treasury and the ranches and farms that fed the miners. Las Casas suggested Africans, though he would later regret the idea and condemn African slavery as well. There was both precedence and practicality behind his suggestion. By the early 1500s, there were thousands of African slaves living in Spain and the Canary Islands. Moreover, Africans—living in roughly the same disease environment as Europeans—did not succumb as easily to pathogens carried by the Spaniards. Africans could and did convert to Christianity, especially after they arrived in the Americas. But the Europeans—desperate for slave labor—changed the rules, eliminating baptism or conversion as a justification for emancipation.

Azores, Madeira, and the Canary Islands

PORTUGAL

Azores

SPAIN

Madeira

Atlantic Ocean

Canary Islands

AFRICA

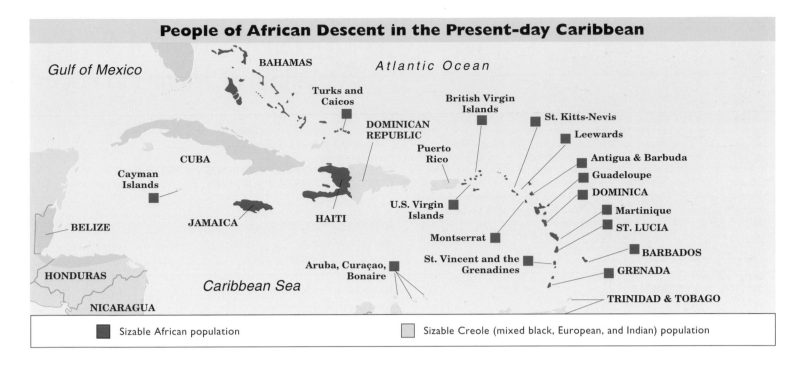

People of African Descent in the Present-day Caribbean

Gulf of Mexico

Atlantic Ocean

BAHAMAS

Turks and Caicos

British Virgin Islands

St. Kitts-Nevis

Leewards

DOMINICAN REPUBLIC

Puerto Rico

Antigua & Barbuda

Guadeloupe

CUBA

DOMINICA

Cayman Islands

Martinique

ST. LUCIA

U.S. Virgin Islands

BELIZE

JAMAICA

HAITI

BARBADOS

Montserrat

St. Vincent and the Grenadines

GRENADA

HONDURAS

Aruba, Curaçao, Bonaire

Caribbean Sea

NICARAGUA

TRINIDAD & TOBAGO

⬛ Sizable African population   ⬜ Sizable Creole (mixed black, European, and Indian) population

SLAVERY IN THE CARIBBEAN

Still, African slavery would only take root on the periphery of the Spanish empire in the Americas. Despite the decimation of Native Americans, millions survived in Central and South America. (Because Spanish settlement in North America did not begin until the very end of the 16th century—and remained relatively sparse even as late as the the early 18th century—the scope of the threat from Spanish settlement was not as great for Native Americans in North America as it was for their counterparts in other parts of New Spain.) And while formal Indian slavery was banned after 1542, other forms of coerced labor—such as the *encomienda* system—assured a steady supply of Indian muscle for Spanish mines and ranches during the 16th and 17th centuries. Equally important, the Spanish—more interested in plundering American gold and silver than settling there—were slow to make the kinds of investments that would assure new sources of wealth, like plantation agriculture. It would take the more enterprising and emigration-oriented countries of northern Europe to realize that wealth and economic development could be realized through new products, new markets, and new sources of labor. During the 1500s and 1600s, the Dutch, the English, and the French would come to supplant the Spanish in much of the Caribbean and the southern part of the North American mainland, turning these tropical islands and subtropical lands into vast areas of plantations worked largely by African slaves growing crops for a mass European market.

The records show that the profits from plantation economy could be quite substantial, as the ledger of one Jamaican sugar grower makes clear. Investing some £41,480 in land, buildings, and stock—including 250 African slaves at an average £70 each—Bryan Edwards was able to realize an annual net profit of £2,990, (or roughly $750,000 in current U.S. dollars) for a profit percentage of more than 7 percent. While some planters complained that profit margins such as these were far too low, some sources suggest that many planters did far better than Edwards—often netting as much as a 21 percent profit. Moreover, unlike Spanish wealth in gold and silver, plantation profits were self-sustaining, although subject to fluctuations in the world price for sugar and other commodities. In addition, slavery offered profits in two ways—the trade in products realized by slave labor and the profits realized in the slave trade itself.

THE TRIANGLE AND RECTANGLE TRADES

The transatlantic triangle slave trade began with the Portuguese and Spanish in the 1400s, and was greatly expanded by Dutch, English, and French slavers in the 1600s and 1700s. North American—and, after 1776, U.S.—slavers were also active, particularly toward the end of the 18th century. In the early 19th century, first England, then the United States, France, and other powers outlawed the trade. But with slavery legal in the British Empire (until 1833), French

THE BUSINESS OF SLAVERY: A Caribbean Planter's Ledger

Caribbean planters often complained about what they considered the high costs and thin profit margins of the slave economy. In 1793, Bryan Edwards, an English planter on Jamaica, published this ledger sheet, showing a profit of 7 percent on an initial investment of over 41 thousand pounds in English currency. Whether that rate of return gave Edwards cause for complaint is a subjective question. However, it should be noted that other sources have put typical profits at a rate three times that level. According to one source, Jamaican planters reaped a 21 percent annual profit between 1687 and 1787. At any rate, the human cost of this equation was left out entirely. Note the manner in which "250 Negroes" were listed no differently than mules or steers.

Ledger Sheet
INITIAL INVESTMENT

Lands	£ 14,100
Buildings	£ 7,000
Stock	
250 Negroes @ £70 ea	£ 17,500
80 steers @ £15	£ 1,200
60 mules @ £28	£ 1,680
Total in Stock	£ 20,380
TOTAL INITIAL INVESTMENT	£ 41,480 (Jamaican currency)

INCOME FROM CROPS

200 Hogshead of sugar, @ £15 sterling £ 3,000 sterling per hogshead	
130 Puncheons of rum @ £10 sterling £ 1,300 sterling	
GROSS RETURN FROM CROPS	£ 4,300 (sterling)
GROSS RETURN FROM CROPS	£ 6,020 (Jamaican currency)

PLANTATION EXPENSES

ANNUAL SUPPLIES (Imported from Great Britain and Ireland)
(Estimates not available for each item)
Negro Clothing
1,500 yards of Osnaburgh cloth or German linen
650 yards of blue bays, or pennistones, for a warm frock for each negro
350 yards of striped linseys for the women
250 yards of coarse check for shirts for the boilers, tradesmen, domestics, and the children
3 dozen coarse blankets for lying-in women and sick negroes
18 dozen coarse hats

Tools
For the carpenters and coopers, to the amount of £ 25 sterling, including 2 or three dozen falling axes.
Miscellaneous

COST OF IMPORTED SUPPLIES	£ 850 (sterling)
COST OF IMPORTED SUPPLIES	£ 1,190 (Jamaican currency)

ANNUAL EXPENSES (Not imported)
(Jamaican currency)

Overseer's or manager's salary	£ 200
Distiller's salary	£ 70
Two other white servants, £60 each	£ 120
A white carpenter's wages	£ 100
Maintenance of 5 white servants, £40 each exclusive of their allowance of salted provisions	£ 200
Medical care of the negroes (at 6 s per annum for each negro and extra cases, paid for separately)	£ 100
Millright's, coppersmith's, plumber's, and smith's bills, annually	£ 250
Colonial taxes, public and parochial	£ 200
Annual supply of mules and steers	£ 300
Wharfage and storeage of goods land and shipped	£ 100
American staves and heading, for hogsheads and puncheons	£ 150
A supply of small occasional supplies of different kinds, supposed	£ 50
COST OF NON-IMPORTED SUPPLIES (Jamaican currency)	£ 1,840
GRAND TOTAL OF ANNUAL EXPENSES (Jamaican currency)	£ 3,030

GROSS RETURN FROM CROPS (Jamaican currency)	£ 6,020
GRAND TOTAL OF ANNUAL EXPENSES (Jamaican currency)	£ 3,030

PROFIT (Jamaican currency)	£ 2,990
PROFIT PERCENTAGE	7.2 %

Source: History, Civil and Commercial of the British Colonies in the West Indies

overseas holdings (until 1848), the United States (until 1865), Brazil (until 1888), and the Spanish Caribbean islands (Cuba and Puerto Rico, until the 1880s), the smuggling of Africans remained big business through much of the 19th century.

A great debate has emerged about the number of Africans transported across the Atlantic as slaves. Most scholars estimate the figure at roughly 9 to 12 million, with about 50,000 coming in the 15th century, 300,000 in the 16th, 1.5 million in the 17th, 5.8 million in the 18th, and 2.4 million in the 19th, many of the latter being smuggled despite international sanctions against the slave trade. About 40 percent during the entire period came from the coasts of West Central Africa (modern-day Angola, Congo, Gabon), another 35 percent from the Bights of Benin and Biafra (Cameroon and Nigeria), 10 percent from the Gold Coast (Ghana), 5 percent from the Windward Coast (Ivory Coast, Liberia, Sierra Leone), 5 percent from Senegambia (Gambia, Guinea, Senegal) and 5 percent from southeastern Africa (Mozambique, Tanzania).

Over the centuries, the source of slaves changed. During the early years of the trade—through 1600—90 percent came from the West Central African coast. That declined to 55 percent in the 1600s and 37 percent in the 1700s, only to climb back to 48 percent in the 19th century. Meanwhile, the percentage coming from the Bights of

THE TRAVELS OF ESTÉBAN DORANTES

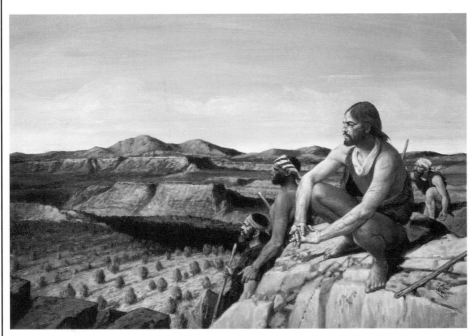

Estéban Dorantes, second from left in this modern depiction of the journey of Cabeza de Vaca, who is seen in the foreground, to the right of Estéban. (National Park Service)

Among the most remarkable stories of early European exploration took place in what is now the American Southwest. It was led by a Spanish-speaking African slave named Estéban Dorantes. Born in Morocco, Estéban Dorantes had first come to the Americas in 1527 as a member of an expedition led by Pánfilo de Narváez, the newly commissioned Spanish governor of Florida. Landing near what is now Sarasota, Florida, the 500-man expedition wandered through what is now the southeastern United States and northern Mexico. Poorly managed and struck down by disease, the crew was eventually reduced to four men, who survived by convincing local people that they were healers and shamans. According to Álvar Núñez Cabeza de Vaca, the surviving leader, Estéban "was our go-between; he informed himself about the ways we wished to take, what towns there were, and the matters we desired to know." Eight years after setting out, Estéban and his three companions reached a Spanish outpost in Mexico.

Three years later, Estéban became the logical choice for guide of an expedition to the American Southwest launched in search of Cibola, or El Dorado, the legendary "seven cities of gold." To mark his progress, Estéban was told to send back crosses to the Mexican governor. For a time, they arrived, each larger than the last, along with stories of hundreds of Indian followers showering Estéban in jewels and gold. Then the crosses stopped coming; Estéban had disappeared, fate unknown. Some say Estéban lived on, shedding his slave status for that of American Indian shaman. But a legend among the Zuni— a people living in the region Estéban explored—say the "black Mexican" was killed by one of their own in about 1539.

Benin and Biafra stayed at roughly 35 percent from 1600 to 1800, dropping off in the 19th century to just about 25 percent. Meanwhile, southeast Africa saw its proportion rise from 1 percent in the 1600s to roughly 15 percent by the 1800s, although many of the slaves taken from this region ended up on the French sugar islands of the Indian Ocean rather than in the Americas.

Africans were settled across the length and breadth of North, Central and South America and the Caribbean. Overall, about 40 percent (or 4 million) of all enslaved Africans were sent to the Portuguese colony of Brazil. The next most common destination were the British holdings in the Caribbean, with about 20 percent of all slaves (or 2 million). Spanish American colonies on the mainland and in the Caribbean took about 17.5 percent (or 1,750,000), French holdings in the Caribbean (mostly, Saint-Domingue, modern Haiti) took in 13.5 percent (or 1,350,000), and the tiny Dutch and Danish Caribbean islands received about 2.5 percent (or 250,000). Finally, British North America and, after independence the United States, took in 650,000 slaves, or 6.5 percent of the total.

SLAVERY IN SOUTH AMERICA

As with the source of slaves, the destinations changed over time, depending on economic and political developments in the Americas. For example, in the early years of the slave trade, fully 75 percent of all enslaved Africans ended up in the Spanish colonies, a figure that declined to 35 percent in the 1600s, and 20 percent in the 1700s, only to climb to 30 percent with the growth of the sugar industry in Cuba and Puerto Rico in the 19th century. Maintaining its slave system well into the late 1800s meant that Brazil's percentage of slave arrivals reached some 65 percent of the total in that century. As for the British mainland colonies and the United States, they never reached 10 percent of the total in any century, peaking at some 9 percent in the 1700s.

THE MIDDLE PASSAGE

The slave trade was enormously profitable. In the context of the transatlantic trading system, the shipment of slaves from Africa to the Americas represented what was known as the Middle Passage, one leg of a

Peoples of African Descent in South America

The map above, illustrating which present-day South American nations have the highest concentrations of peoples of African descent, documents the ethnographic impact of the African slave trade on South America.

triangular trade that saw European manufactures transported to Africa, where they were exchanged for slaves, and American plantation crops carried to Europe. (In reality, the system was far more complex, with ships traveling to and from many different ports in many different lands and with all kinds of goods.) At the height of the trade in the 1700s, an adult male slave could be purchased at a slave-trading post on the African coast such as Goree Island off French Senegal; Bonny, off British Nigeria; or Benguela, off Portuguese Angola, where hundreds or even thousands of captured Africans were kept in holding pens called barracoons. While a slave ship merchant might pay about 12 ounces in gold for a slave in Africa, Africans sold for several times that amount in an American port. Therefore, with ships carrying anywhere from a few dozen to more than 100 slaves, the human cargo on a larger ship could equal more than a million dollars in today's money.

Slave ships ranged in size from small sloops to ships weighing several hundred tons, the latter with extensive crews that included doctors, carpenters, and other skilled workers, as well as sailors. Upon arriving on the African coast, ship captains would have to pay a variety of fees to local rulers, merchants, and pilots, the latter to guide them over the numerous sandbars. While some crewmen gathered provisions, the captain and his guards went ashore to purchase slaves, kept in densely crowded cells in coastal barracoons. Because the supply of slaves and the arrival of ships were irregular, many Africans were forced to live in the crowded barracoons, for weeks or months. Added to the miserable conditions was terror. Rumors circulated through the cells that a captured slave's destiny was not the other side of the Atlantic but the dinner plates of the strange men with white faces and heavy beards that seemed to have the run of the forts.

Indeed, by the time the enslaved Africans reached the coast, they were so terrorized and exhausted that they were ready to believe the worst, for the process of enslavement was both capricious and brutal. Some were captured in raids by neighboring tribes; others were kidnapped by slave-hunting bandits; some were sold into slavery by their own chiefs. Captured, they were roped or shackled together and marched to the coast, sometimes across hundreds of miles of scorching tropical grassland and dank and muddy rain forest. Poorly fed and barely clothed, many grew weak and sick. But the pace remained relentless, as the raiders were eager to deliver their human cargo to the Europeans on the coast. If a prisoner faltered, he or she was beaten and forced to move on. If captives proved physically unable to continue, they were left by the side of the trail to die.

Once at the ocean-side slave fort, the misery continued. In the hot and humid climate of the West African coast—a climate

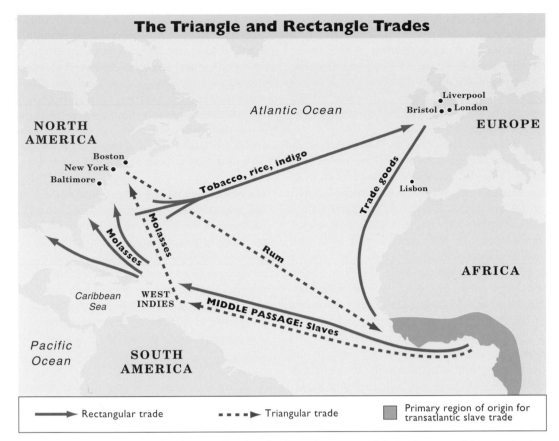

The Triangle and Rectangle Trades

Rectangular trade | ▪▪▪▪► Triangular trade | Primary region of origin for transatlantic slave trade

The term triangle trade *has often been used to describe the trade routes used during the years of the tranatlantic slave trade. For example, African slaves would be traded in the Caribbean for molasses, which would then be sent to North America, where it would be used to produce rum, which in turn would then be traded in Africa for more slaves. In recent years, historians have also begun referring to the* rectangle trade, *in which North American agricultural products such as tobacco, rice, and indigo were sent to Great Britain, which in turn would send trade goods to Africa in exchange for slaves, thus adding another leg to the trade cycle.*

unfamiliar and uncomfortable to the many Africans coming from the drier interior— the slaves remained in their barracoons even after they were purchased. For the slaves ships that would take them across the Atlantic often lay at anchor for weeks and months waiting for a full cargo.

Conditions aboard ranged from the awful to the horrendous, depending on the attitude of the captain, the company he worked for, the quality of the ship, and the length of the voyage. Some slavers believed in tight-packing, cramming as many slaves into the hot and unsanitary holds as possible, while others were loose packers. The former, of course, meant more cargo, but also more loss of lives and potential profits. Death rates for slaves in the Middle Passage

Captured Africans in the hold of a slave ship (Library of Congress)

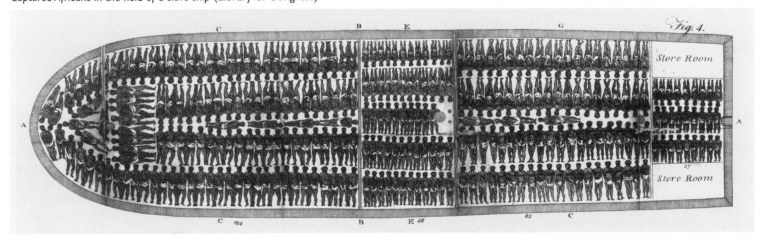

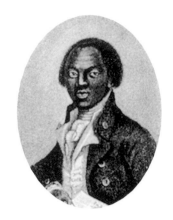

Olaudah Equiano (Library of Congress)

therefore ranged greatly between voyages, but they averaged about 15 to 20 percent in the first couple of centuries of the trade, dropping off to about 5 to 10 percent in the latter years. (Nor was the crew much better off, suffering similar mortality rates on the voyage from diseases picked up on shore or from the slaves themselves.)

But while these numbers explain deadliness of the business, it requires the words of participants to convey the true horrors of the middle passage. "I was soon put down under the decks, and there I received such a salutation in my nostrils as I had never experienced in my life: so that with the loathsomeness of the stench and crying together, I became so sick and low that I was not able to eat," wrote Olaudah Equiano, an African enslaved near the Bight of Benin in the 1750s. He continued, "I now wished for death to relieve me." Not surprisingly, during this loading period—as during the transatlantic trip itself—the crew had to remain ever vigilant. Escapes, rebellions, and suicides were common occurrences throughout the process, but particularly so in the first few weeks. Indeed, crews let the slaves out of the holds for only a few brief moments while the ship was still in sight of land, and sometimes confined them to the hold for the entire voyage.

To keep their human cargo alive on the voyage, the crews sometimes forced food on them. The provisions—usually little more than a mealy porridge and perhaps some fish heads for protein—was unfamiliar to the Africans. Moreover, in the tropical climate, it often became rotten and bug-infested, leading to stomach illness, diarrhea, and vomiting, which further polluted the crowded holds in which they were kept. Alexander Falconbridge, a doctor who served aboard British slave ships in the 1770s and 1780s, described conditions thus:

Upon the Negroes refusing to take sustenance, I have seen coals of fire, glowing hot, put [on] a shovel, and placed so near their lips, as to scorch and burn them. Exercise being deemed necessary . . . they are sometimes obliged to dance. . . . If they go about it reluctantly, or do not move with agility, they are flogged. . . . The poor wretches are frequently compelled to sing also; but when they do so, their songs are generally, as may naturally be expected, melancholy lamentations of their exile from their native country.

After a voyage that could take several weeks or many months, the vessel arrived in port, usually on one of the Caribbean islands or in Brazil. Slaves were then prepared for sale by being given plentiful fresh water and local produce and meats, so as to make them appear healthier and hence more valuable. Depending on the facilities available, the slaves would either be herded ashore or local slave traders would come on board to examine the merchandise. The first to go were the youngest and strongest, with

Slave traders inspect captured Africans (Library of Congress)

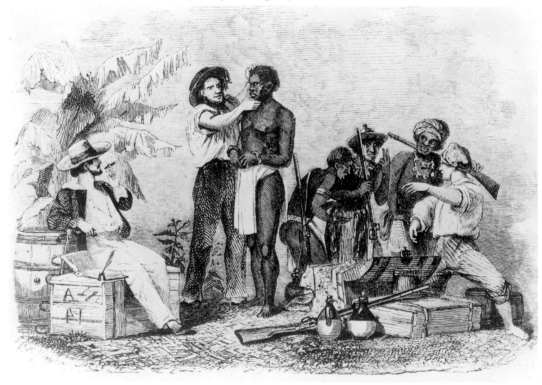

the sick and the old being sold to the poorest colonists. It was, recounts Equiano, yet another terrifying episode in a saga of fear and suffering. "Without scruple," he later wrote, "are relations and friends separated, most of them never to see each other again."

THE CARIBBEAN PLANTATION SYSTEM

Africans came to be the labor of choice for the grueling work on the sugar plantations of the Caribbean, particularly after the Dutch, English, and French secured Hispaniola (Saint-Domingue, later Haiti), Jamaica, and most of the Lesser Antilles in the 1600s. (The Spanish-speaking islands of the Caribbean took a different course. Cuba and Puerto Rico—which remained in Spanish hands until the Spanish-American War of 1898—would not see large-scale plantation agriculture and importation of slaves until the 19th century. The Dominican Republic on the eastern two-thirds of Hispaniola was politically and economically linked to Saint-Domingue or Haiti almost continuously through 1844.)

Barbados, the first Caribbean island extensively settled by the British, offered a model for African life and labor in much of the English-speaking Caribbean. Conquered by the Spanish—who killed or drove away the entire native population of Carib in the 16th century—Barbados was first encountered by the English in 1625. Two years later, a ship carrying 80 British colonists and 10 African slaves arrived. Laboring on small tobacco and cotton farms, much of the population consisted of white indentured servants until the 1640s, when sugar cultivation was introduced from Brazil by Dutch traders. Involving grueling work and large-scale capital investment for refining equipment, sugar cultivation soon displaced cotton and tobacco, even as plantations took over farms and African slave labor replaced independent white farmers and servants. In 1645, Barbados counted just under 6,000 slaves; by 1685, there were ten times that number; and by the end of the century, some 135,000. In the process, the vast majority of whites—some 30,000—fled to other Caribbean islands, England, or the British colonies in North America, particularly South Carolina. Thus, like much of the Caribbean but unlike mainland North American colonies, Barbados became predominantly black. More than 90 percent of its population was of African descent by the end of the 1700s.

SOCIAL CONDITIONS IN THE CARIBBEAN

Another factor differentiated Barbados and other Caribbean islands from the mainland of North America—a constant influx of new African slaves, until the outlawing of the slave trade in the early 1800s. While it might seem pointless to discuss the relative merits of slavery in one place or another—slavery was brutal business wherever it took hold—it was less fatal on the North American mainland than it was in the Caribbean, mostly due to two inter-related reasons. First, North American slaves ate better. For example, while mainland slaves enjoyed diets with ample vitamins and minerals, it is estimated that Caribbean slaves received only 90 percent of their vitamin A needs, less than 50 percent of their calcium needs, and only a third of the vitamin C they required. Second, the more poorly fed Caribbean slaves were more likely to succumb to disease. A look at mortality statistics bears this out. Nearly 40 percent of Jamaican slaves were listed as dying from fevers, compared to just 11 percent of Virginia slaves. At the same time, twice as many slaves in Virginia—albeit a still miniscule 7.3 percent—died of old age.

This difference was due more to economic calculation than the relative kindness of the mainland master class. On tiny Caribbean islands, most of the land was devoted to sugar, forcing planters to resort to costly imported foodstuffs, which they rationed out parsimoniously. Plentiful land in North America allowed planters and farmers to raise both commercial and food crops. Moreover, mainland planters soon came to the realization that healthy slaves worked harder, had more babies, and did not need to be replaced. Thus, by the early 1700s, the North American slave population had reached a point where it could sustain growth without further imports while the English-speaking Caribbean islands required slave imports right up until abolition in 1833 to sustain their populations. (It should be noted that sugar cultivation in a tropical climate is far more grueling than tobacco or cotton farming in a temperate climate.)

Quality of life issues go beyond nutrition, disease, and work. Because of the high proportion of Africans in the population and the constant influx of new Africans, Caribbean blacks were able to retain more of their culture, especially in terms of language, religion, and social customs. Even today, Caribbean blacks are more likely

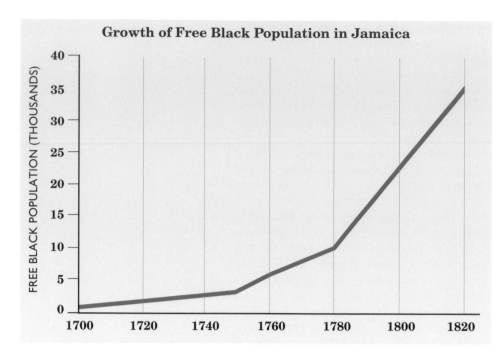

Growth of Free Black Population in Jamaica

overwork, and murder within a few decades. First settled in 1506, Jamaica developed slowly under the Spanish, with only about 1,000 white and black inhabitants in 1655 when it was conquered by the British, who quickly took advantage of its tropical climate and, for the Caribbean, abundant land. Soon, more than 100,000 African slaves—along with 10,000 European masters, overseers, and skilled workers—were working in gangs producing the largest sugar crop in the English Caribbean.

THE MAROONS

While Jamaica's abundant land produced abundant sugar, it also offered opportunity for runaway and rebellious slaves. From the late 1600s onward, Jamaican runaway slaves established numerous independent settlements in the mountainous interior, where they effectively fought off British soldiers and Mosquito Indian troops, recruited by the English from Central America. Known as maroons (from the Spanish *cimarrones*, or runaway cattle), they numbered nearly 40,000 by the time slavery was prohibited in 1833.

The first maroons, known as *libertos* (Spanish for liberated ones), emerged in 1655 when their Spanish masters freed them as the English captured the island. British forces tried to recapture them but the maroons' growing familiarity with the nearly impenetrable interior frustrated

than their North American counterparts to practice a faith that blends Christianity with traditional African religions, and their English is laced with more Africanisms. Moreover, their demographic dominance also gave birth to a fuller history of rebellion and resistance, especially on the largest of the English-speaking Caribbean islands, Jamaica.

Encountered by Columbus on his second voyage to the Americas in 1494, Jamaica saw virtually its entire indigenous population of Taino wiped out by infection,

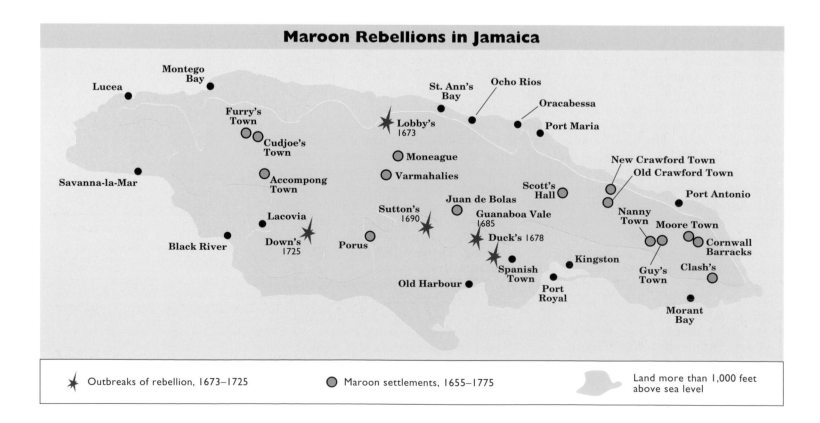

Maroon Rebellions in Jamaica

★ Outbreaks of rebellion, 1673–1725   ⬤ Maroon settlements, 1655–1775   Land more than 1,000 feet above sea level

their efforts. In the 1680s, a guerrilla war broke out between the maroons and the British. Led by such legendary fighters as Accompong, Quao, and Nanny, the maroons held out for some 50 years.

In 1739, however, maroon leaders signed a controversial treaty with the British. While granted their freedom, the maroons agreed to stop raiding European plantations, stop protecting runaways, and assist the British in quelling slave insurrections. The treaty preserved the maroon communities, but at the cost of dividing them from the much larger slave population. Still, after the 1833 declaration of emancipation in the British Empire, many former slaves migrated to the maroon communities, rather than work as wage laborers on the European-owned sugar plantations of the lowlands.

THE HAITIAN REBELLION

Still, impressive as the Jamaican maroon experience was, it did not end European rule or the plantation system. As is discussed later in this chapter, the United States would become the first nation in the Americas to free itself from European colonialism when it won independence from Britain in the Revolutionary War of 1775–1783. That victory, however, did not end the plantation system. That would not be achieved anywhere in the Americas until the start of the 19th century—not in the United States, but on a Caribbean island 120 miles to Jamaica's east.

Unlike Jamaica, Hispaniola was heavily settled by the Spanish, who established their first city in the Americas at Santo Domingo. Indeed, through Santo Domingo came the first African slaves to the New World. With virtually the entire native population wiped out in the first 50 years of Spanish conquest, Hispaniola supported a population of 6,000 Europeans and 30,000 Africans by the 1540s. The vast majority lived on the eastern two-thirds of the island (modern-day Dominican Republic), leaving the western third (Haiti) largely uninhabited. In 1697, France began settling in Haiti. Over the next century, France turned Saint-Domingue, as they called it, into the "pearl

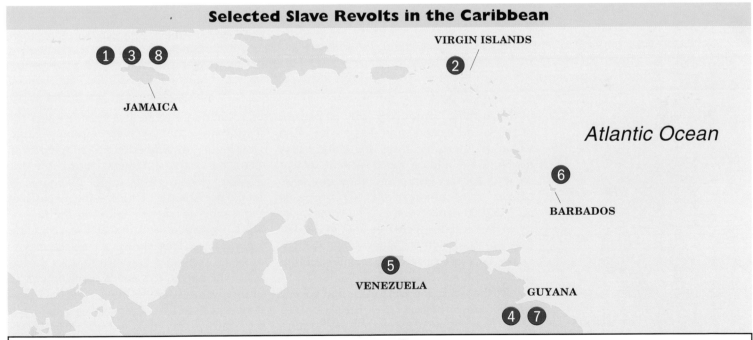

Selected Slave Revolts in the Caribbean

1 1663 The first serious slave revolt in Jamaica takes place. It involves 400 slaves.

2 1733 At least 150 slaves are implicated in a slave revolt on St. John in the Danish West Indies.

3 1760 On Jamaica, an uprising known as Tacky's rebellion involves about 1,000 slaves.

4 ca. 1763 Two thousand slaves revolt in Berbice, Guyana, and kill 200 of the settlement's 350 whites.

5 1795 Three hundred slaves rise up at Coro, Venezeuela.

6 1816 On Easter Sunday, slaves on approximately 60 plantations rise up on Barbados.

7 1823 Between 10,000 and 20,000 slaves on 50 plantations revolt in Demerara, Guyana.

8 1831 The Christmas Uprising of 1831, a revolt by 20,000 slaves, takes place in Jamaica. The revolt leads to the end of slavery in the British Caribbean.

The Haitian Rebellion

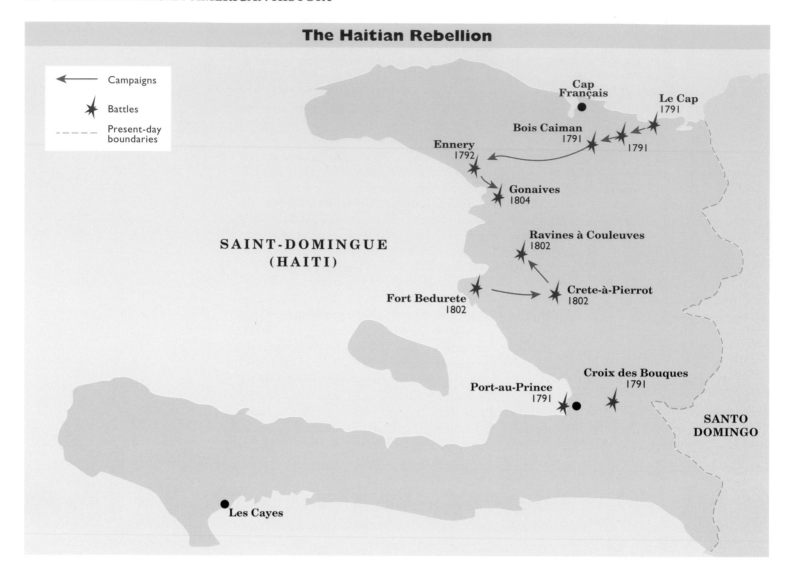

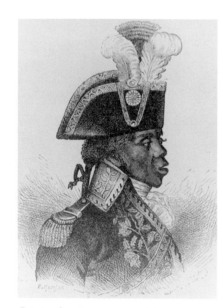

François Dominique Toussaint Louverture
(Library of Congress)

of the Antilles," producing fully 60 percent of the world's coffee and 40 percent of its sugar. At the same time, the colony also developed a unique racial system, where some 25,000 mixed-race mulattos, or *gens de couleur*, lived amongst 30,000 Europeans and 450,000 African slaves. The vast majority of the mulattos were free and, to the dismay of local whites, a growing number were becoming wealthy, slave-holding planters themselves.

By the 1780s, the Europeans had passed a series of laws banning these free people of color from possessing firearms and holding political office. In 1789, the growing resentment at these restrictions by the free people of color was fanned by the startling news from Paris: revolution had overthrown the *ancien régime*. Calls for freedom and citizenship by the free people of color were soon taken up by the African majority, leading to a slave insurrection in the north of the country in August 1791. Under the leadership of an ex-slave named François Dominique Toussaint Louverture, an army of freedpersons (ex-slaves) and free people

of color had driven the French—and the institution of slavery—from Saint-Domingue, now called Haiti (adapted from *Ayti*, the native Arawak word for the island). French efforts under Napoleon to retake the island—including the dispatch of thousands of troops—failed in the face of black resistance and tropical disease. Under Jean-Jacques Dessalines, an ex-slave who replaced Toussaint Louverture, after the latter's surrender to and imprisonment in France, Haiti became the second independent nation in the Americas, after the United States, and the world's first black republic.

As will be seen in chapter 3, the black revolution in Haiti spread fear through the corridors of power in Washington and Paris. In 1793, Congress passed the first fugitive slave law, allowing owners to reclaim escaped slaves who had crossed state lines. A decade later, a humbled Napoleon decided to sell France's largest American possession—popularly called the Louisiana Purchase—to the United States. For Haiti itself, the revolution proved a mixed blessing. Dessalines was assassinated just two years after independence and was replaced by Henry Christophe, a paranoid dictator who nearly bankrupted the country by building huge forts and castles for protection against French forces that never came. The tensions between the free people of color and pure Africans intensified over the years, leading to numerous coups, U.S. military invasions, political repression, and economic stagnation, which have continued to this day.

Far to Haiti's south was Brazil, a country now home to the largest black population in the world outside of Africa. Claimed and settled by the Portuguese in the 1500s, Brazil became a major sugar producer and, as noted earlier, the largest recipient of slaves from 1600 through the end of the transatlantic trade in the late 1800s, 3.75 million Africans in all. Unlike its Spanish colonial neighbors, Brazil achieved independence peacefully, in 1821. At the same time, slavery lingered on far longer in Brazil than anywhere else in South America, and was finally prohibited in 1888.

Many scholars have compared Brazilian to North American slavery favorably, pointing out the tradition of social intermingling and even intermarriage between slaves and masters and the protections offered slaves by the powerful Catholic Church, which sanctified slave marriages, making it illegal for masters to separate husband and wife. Moreover, the continuous arrival of large numbers of Africans assured a cultural continuity to the old country that can be seen in Brazilian music, religion, and such traditions as *capoeira*, a martial art and dance with African roots. (Originally, capoeira was a form of self-defense and combat that employed swift and subtle physical movement to compensate for the slaveowners' edge in weaponry.) Still, the reason so many Africans were imported into Brazil was that so many died from overwork, poor diet, and disease. Slaves in the North American colonies (and later, the United States) experienced fertility rates—a good measure of overall health—twice those of slaves in Brazil. And as for the claim that Brazil's milder forms of slavery led to a more racially tolerant country, the record is mixed. Brazilian blacks never suffered from the kinds of degrading segregation that North American blacks had to endure. At the same time, by virtually every measure of health, wealth, and education, Brazilians of African descent still lag significantly behind whites, who continue to control both the country's economy and government.

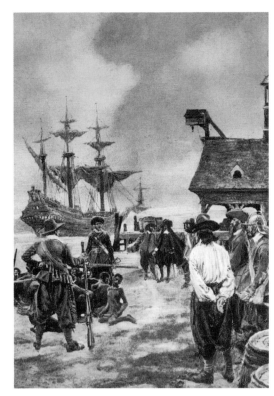

The first Africans in North America, at Jamestown, in 1619 (Library of Congress)

SLAVERY COMES TO NORTH AMERICA

In 1619, slaves—if not slavery itself—came to Jamestown, Virginia, Britain's first permanent colony on the North American mainland. As would become the pattern in British North America, the 20 or so slaves aboard the Dutch ship probably came from the Caribbean, and not directly from Africa. While they were quickly sold off to local tobacco farmers, it is not clear if these transactions were in property or persons. In other words, Virginia's first Africans might have been slaves or servants. Nor is it clear that they inherited a status that condemned them and their offspring to perpetual servitude.

Jamestown was founded in 1607 by the Virginia Company, a business enterprise chartered by Britain's King James I to settle the region around the Chesapeake Bay, "propagate the Christian religion" among the "savages," and reap profits for the company's investors. The plan sounded good on paper, but it proved disastrous in execution. Expecting to find large Indian populations eager to be "civilized" and work for the English—or, at least, trade with them—the early settlers were entirely unprepared to do the hard work of carving farms out of forests. But the Indians had little gold or wealth to exchange, and absolutely no intention of serving these invading white

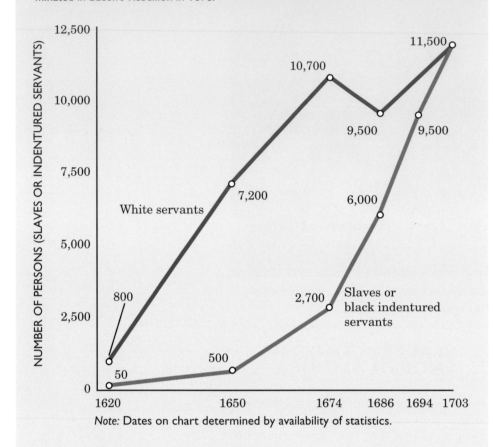

Slave Region of the Atlantic Coast

The number of African slaves in the Virginia colony during the 17th century rose rapidly, while the number of indentured servants declined before rising again at a slower rate, particularly after armed white servants and small farmers began a series of revolts, which culminated in Bacon's Rebellion in 1676.

Note: Dates on chart determined by availability of statistics.

Source: American Slavery, American Freedom: The Ordeal of Colonial Virginia

first turned to their homeland, importing thousands of indentured servants who agreed to seven years' labor in exchange for their passage, some land, and the supplies needed to set up on their own once their indentureship was up. It was in this context that the first Africans arrived in a colony that had yet to draw up slave codes.

For the first 50 or so years, however, the African population in Virginia remained small. By 1670, they represented just 5 percent of the estimated 40,000 settlers in the colony. Slavery also came equally slowly to the colony, even though slave laws began to appear on the books by the 1640s. A simple calculation explains the reluctance. With most people dying within a few years of their arrival—often in their first year, the so-called seasoning period—it made no sense to pay the higher initial cost of a slave. Two things, however, altered the calculation. First, as the colony became more firmly established, more settlers survived the "seasoning" and became independent farmers, or yeomen. Second, these yeomen—both white and black—were becoming increasingly discontented with their lot. Because the best land along the tidewater was already owned by planters, yeomen were forced to work for planters or stake out tobacco farms on the frontier, where they fought incessantly with Indians outraged at the Englishmen's greed for their land. Meanwhile, the colony's government—the House of Burgesses—was largely a tool of the planters and had little sympathy for the yeomen's demands of fairer taxes and more protection.

men. When the malaria-ridden and starving English tried to raid Indian food stores, the latter fought back or moved away. Of the first 120 settlers who arrived, less than a third survived.

Still, the colony limped on, saved by a local Indian ruler named Powhatan who saw in the English a useful ally against his native enemies. The great breakthrough, however, occurred in 1612 when Jamestown leader John Rolfe imported tobacco seeds from the West Indies. Smoked for centuries among the local tribes—and increasingly popular in England and Europe—tobacco grew extremely well in Virginia. By the end of the decade, plantations were being established up and down the rivers and estuaries around the Chesapeake, sparking conflicts with the Indians that culminated in major wars in 1622 and 1644. Because the Indians refused to be part of the British scheme, the planters needed to look elsewhere for labor. They

THE CODIFICATION OF SLAVERY

In 1676, the yeomen's anger boiled over. In an uprising known as Bacon's Rebellion after its ringleader, Nathaniel Bacon, a former aristocrat who sided with the poor farmers, the yeomen turned on the Indians first. But when the natives proved elusive, the rebels turned on the planters and would have driven the latter into the sea but for the fortuitous arrival of an English warship and the death of Bacon himself. Among the last to surrender was a mixed regiment of black and white yeomen. Victorious, the planters and burgesses were also wiser for the near-death experience. Indentured servants became yeomen and yeomen insisted on their rights as Englishmen, even if some of them were African. Slaves could make no such claims. But—for both cultural and legal reasons—it was not possible to enslave Englishmen. Borrowing a page from the English colony of Barbados, the Virginia planters turned to Africans. But instead of going to Africa for their laborers, the tobacco farmers went to the Caribbean, importing slaves who had already been "seasoned" to plantation agriculture. By 1700, the population of Africans in Virginia—the vast majority enslaved—had multiplied tenfold to 20,000. Over the course of the next 50 years, no less than 100,000 slaves would be imported into the Chesapeake region.

Changes in labor reflected—and drove—changes in the law. In the 1660s and 1670s, a series of new statutes discriminated on the basis of race and turned informal slavery into an institution. For example, white servants who ran away were punished with added years tacked onto their indentureship, while black runaways received a life sentence. In the wake of Bacon's Rebellion, whites were placed in jail; blacks received corporal punishment—the thinking being that only physical pain would teach them a lesson. Most crucial were a series of laws passed between 1667 and 1671 that said baptism and Christianity did not qualify African servants for eventual freedom. In 1692, marriage and sexual relations between whites and blacks were outlawed. Finally, in 1705, the burgesses ended all half measures by passing a law that read: "All servants imported or brought into this country by sea or land who were not Christians in their native

country shall be accounted and be slaves."

There was both economic and racial reasoning behind these decisions. Not only did the laws assure a secure and docile labor force—and one that could be easily identified by skin color—it also made race, rather than class, the dividing line of Virginia politics. Even the poorest and most disenfranchised whites now had a stake in the existing order of things. They owned property—their white skin—and this fact would help ally them to their social and financial betters among the ruling planter class, even if their economic interests differed. The pattern set in Virginia would soon be adopted in, then adapted to, all of

---

SLAVERY IN EARLY VIRGINIA

1607	Jamestown is founded.
1617	Tobacco is planted for the first time.
1619	First shipment of Africans arrives in the colony.
1623	William Tucker, born in Jamestown, becomes the first black child born in the English colonies.
1639	The Virginia legislature enacts a law that provides arms and ammunition to all colonists except blacks.
1642	Virginia passes a fugitive slave law to penalize those who help slaves escape.
1649	The Virginia colony's black population reaches 300.
1657	A Virginia law establishes a colonial militia to track down runaway servants.
1658	To encourage slave trade, Virginia lowers import duties for merchants who carry slaves into the colony.
1661	The Virginia legislature legally recognizes slavery.

THE LEGAL FOUNDATIONS OF SLAVERY

While slavery did not officially begin in the Chesapeake Valley until the latter half of the 17th century, the region's courts distinguished between white and black indentured servants from the beginning. This chart of court cases illustrates the different punishments held for whites and blacks.

YEAR	CRIME COMMITTED	OFFENDER	PUNISHMENT
1630	Sleeping with a black maidservant	White servant	Whipped for "defiling his body by lying with a Negro"
1640	Conspiracy to escape	Four white servants and one black servant	White servants are sentenced to extra service; black servant is whipped, branded, and required to wear shackles for a year
1641	Running away	Two white servants, and John Punch, a black servant	An extra year of service for the whites, lifetime servitude for Punch
1661	Running away in the company of slaves	White servant	2 years of extra service
1660s	Maidservant becomes pregnant	White servant	2 years of extra service
1660s	Stealing a hog	White servant	1,000 pounds of tobacco or a year's extra service
1660s	22 days absent	White servant	3 months of extra service and the loss of one year's crop
1669	Disobeying the master	Black slave	Toes cut off
1707	Killing a slave	White master	No penalty

the English colonies of North America. And with it, "black" and "African" became synonymous with slave and inferior in the eyes of white America for generations to come.

SLAVERY IN GEORGIA AND THE CAROLINAS

Aside from the Chesapeake region—which included parts of both Virginia and Maryland, a colony established in the 1630s for persecuted English Catholics—slavery's deepest roots developed in British North America along a stretch of coastline several hundred miles to the south in what is now the Carolinas and Georgia. Of these the colony of Carolina (which was located mostly in modern-day South Carolina) was the earliest to be founded and the most important. It was supposed to be different than the Chesapeake, based not on narrow commercial gain but political and social

The Slave Economy of the 17th and 18th Centuries

Pennsylvania

New Jersey

Maryland

Delaware

Virginia

North Carolina

South Carolina

Georgia

Tobacco

Rice and indigo

idealism—its first constitution was written by philosopher John Locke—where small land-holding farmers would govern themselves, enjoy a host of freedoms, and trade harmoniously with the Indians. To that end, land-hungry white settlers—already "seasoned" to life in the colonies—would be recruited from the British West Indies. At first, the plan seemed to work. Small farmers—generally older than settlers in the Chesapeake and with families in tow—poured in, mostly from Barbados. Lacking a commercial crop, most lived on small farms near the coast, growing food for their own consumption.

Soon, however, things began to change. The younger sons of wealthy West Indian planters—short on land, but rich in slaves—settled the Carolina low-country, taking control of millions of the best acres. They raised cattle and engaged in trade with the Indians (including enslaving Indians and selling them to the Caribbean), both only nominally profitable businesses. To escape the worst effects of the subtropical climate and diseases, many of the wealthier landowners settled in Charleston, which became the largest seaport south of the Chesapeake. Combined with the fact that cattle-raising on lands that were unfenced required slaves to roam far and wide, this urban-rural split produced a very different pattern of slave-master relations in Carolina, with slaves living and working separately from their owners and enjoying an unusual degree of cultural autonomy. This would become even more the case once Carolina discovered a lucrative commercial crop.

Rice is not an easy crop to grow or process, even under ideal conditions like those in the wet and fertile lowlands of Carolina. Hydraulic systems had to be created to periodically flood the fields; large numbers of workers were necessary to separate the tough outer husk from the edible grain within. Englishmen knew nothing of rice farming because the plant cannot be grown in such a northern clime. And the first efforts made by white settlers to grow rice in Carolina failed dismally. But West Africans—particularly those from the Windward Coast (modern-day Sierra Leone and Liberia), where a bag of rice remains an alternate unit of currency—were accomplished rice farmers. They brought the rice-growing skills and technology to the Carolina coast, which led to enormous wealth for the planter class that exploited their knowledge and labor. Beginning in the 1680s, rice exports rose from almost none to 17 million pounds in 1730 and 75 million pounds by the American Revolution, not including millions more that were consumed locally.

The slave population of the colony grew in stride from a few thousand at the beginning of the 18th century to nearly 40,000 seventy years later. Moreover, by the eve of the American Revolution, there were two blacks for every white in South Carolina. And because whites dreaded the malarial rice-growing districts and avoided it much of the year, the African population was left pretty much to its own devices. Slaves—under sporadic white supervision—were organized into teams who were required to produce a certain quantity of the grain each year. As with earlier cattle herding—but on a far vaster scale—rice planting produced a more autonomous black culture than that in the Chesapeake. This development was most notable for the rise of the Gullah community and its language, a hybrid of English and various African dialects unique to the region. (Although still spoken in isolated areas, the Gullah language is fast disappearing as the Carolina coast and Sea Islands have shifted to an economy based on the tourism and retirement industries.) The work environment and the climate and weather put enormous strain on the African slaves. The hot and humid climate was often brutal in the growing season. Malaria and other diseases were rampant in the swamps. Slaves saw little of the wealth that their labor generated, and enjoyed even fewer material comforts than their counterparts in the Chesapeake.

Moreover, the fact that South Carolina remained a majority black and slave colony (and later, state) made whites particularly edgy. The opinions of its citizens and leaders, and the laws they enacted, reflected a most virulent kind of racism, as a 1712 slave code attests:

Whereas, the plantations and estates of this province cannot be well and sufficiently managed and brought into use, without the labor and service of negroes and other slaves; and forasmuch as the said negroes and other slaves brought into the people of this Province for that purpose, are of barbarous, wild, savage natures, and such as renders them wholly unqualified to be governed by the laws, customs, and practices of this Province; but that it is absolutely necessary, that such other constitutions, laws, and orders, should in this Province be made and enacted, for the good regulating and ordering of them, as may restrain the disorders, rapines and inhumanity, to which they are naturally prone and inclined, and may also tend to the safety and security of the people of this Province and their estates; to which purpose, be

it therefore enacted . . . that all negroes, mulattoes, mestizoes [mixed white and Indian], or Indians, which at any time heretofore have been sold, or now are held or taken to be, or hereafter shall be bought and sold for slaves, are hereby declared slaves; and they, and their children, are hereby made and declared slaves, to all intents and purposes. . . .

The citizens of South Carolina—and their Georgian neighbors to the south—had good reason to worry about the docility of the slave population. Situated near the edge of British North America, they represented the first line of defense against a hostile Spanish regime in Florida that offered freedom and land to any black who fled the colony. In 1738, that defense was tested when some 69 slaves made their way to St. Augustine, leading to rumors of an even bigger "Conspiracy . . . formed by Negroes in Carolina to rise and make their way out of the province." When war broke out between England and Spain the following year, rumor became reality as some 75 slaves killed several whites, seized weapons, and headed for Florida "with Colours displayed and two Drums beating." Most of the Stono rebels—named after the river where they plotted their uprising—were quickly hunted down and killed before they could make it to Florida or spark a general uprising. Still, the Stono Rebellion put enough fear into the hearts of southern planters that imports of African slaves declined for a time, for fear that the slave to citizen ratio was becoming dangerously high.

SLAVE COMMUNITY AND CULTURE

In addition to outright rebellion, enslaved Africans asserted themselves in the face of their condition in other ways. While the slave system actively worked to destroy any tangible links to the African past, enslaved Africans in the New World retained critical elements of their culture, particularly in those areas—like the South Carolina and Georgia Sea Islands—where slaves represented the vast majority of the population. Not surprisingly, it was those cultural elements most easily transported that survived: music, dance, names, and faith. African rhythms and instruments—like the banjo and drums—remained popular throughout the Americas. Traditional faiths—often fused with the Christianity of the European enslavers—lived on. Even in areas like the inland American South—where Africans represented a minority—

cultural traits persisted. Historian Herbert Gutman notes that North American slaves continued to follow West African customs when naming their children, who often refused to answer to the names given to them by their masters.

By 1750, a distinctive slave system—and, within it, a unique African-American culture—had emerged in the British North American colonies from the Chesapeake south—a system that would remain relatively unchanged until its destruction in the Civil War more than a century later. It was a system based on harsh laws, rigorous policing, and unspeakable brutality, made more horrifying by its very ordinariness. Thomas Jefferson—one of history's most eloquent spokespeople for freedom and a large slave-holder himself—spoke of generations of whites "nursed, educated, and daily exercised in tyranny." The relationship between slave and master, he wrote, "is a perpetual exercise of the most unremitting despotism on the one part, and degrading submission

THE PRESERVATION OF CULTURE:
Griots, Talking Drums, and Call and Response Singing

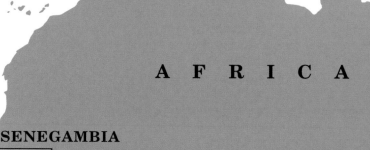

Although slavery did much to disconnect slaves from their African heritage, many African traditions not only survived but adapted and shaped American culture as well. Music is one such tradition. As Africans were taken from Senegambia, from the Slave Coast stretching from Sierra Leone to Cameroon, and finally from Congo-Angola, the musical traditions of each of these regions traveled with them.

THE GRIOTS: In Senegambia, singers and musicians belong to a social class known as griots. Griots often sing songs of praise about the rich and powerful in return for payment. Because those songs turn to insults if the griots are not paid, griots are both respected and feared. Griots also serve as musical historians by singing songs that tell the stories of their people. Some griots play in groups to provide accompaniment to farmers and other workers. Griots have often been compared to the songsters and blues musicians who traveled the Mississippi Delta in the first decades of the 20th century.

THE BANJO: Partly because there are few forests from which large drums can be made, Senegambian music emphasizes stringed instruments. Music historians trace the roots of the modern banjo to this region.

THE TALKING DRUM: The complex music of the Slave Coast region relies heavily on drums, rattles, bells, and other percussion instruments. Western jazz drumming has much in common with this sound. Among the most famous drums of West Africa is the "talking drum" used by Nigeria's Yoruba people. The talking drum has strings that when squeezed vary the tension on the drumhead, thus altering the sound the drum produces. Drummers also use a curved drumstick and, by changing pitch and rhythm, can make the instrument "talk" in "language" based on spoken language.

The people of the Congo-Angola river basin are best known for complex singing, often containing whoops, shouts, and hollers. Some music historians have compared this style to that of Western artists such as James Brown.

CALL AND RESPONSE: Music has always been at the center of West African life. Religious rites, farming, building houses, and other activities all have their own songs, often performed by entire villages in a musical pattern known as "call and response." A lead vocalist sings a line, then everyone else sings a response. Call and response singing has influenced American popular music, from gospel to rhythm and blues to hip-hop.

VOCAL MASKING: In village rituals, celebrants often wear masks to represent various gods or other figures. These masked figures would also "mask" their singing voices by drastically changing the pitch and tone of songs, using growls, shrieks, and other unusual effects. Some masks have layers of material in their mouthpieces, which change the singer's voice even more. In America, vocal masking can be heard in many African-American church sermons, as well as in a wide range of popular music.

on the other. Our children see this and learn to imitate it." With cruelty came want. The material poverty of the slaves' lives was acute, especially when set against the lavish lifestyle of many of their owners. A European traveler visiting the slave quarters on a mid-18th century plantation described them as

> *... more miserable than the most miserable of the cottages of our peasants. The husband and wife sleep on a mean pallet, the children on the ground; a very bad fireplace, some utensils for cooking.... They work all week, not having a single day for themselves except for holidays.... The condition of our peasants is infinitely happier.*

Yet despite the squalid living conditions, the exhausting work regimen, and the brutality of the master class, the African-American population of the southern colonies thrived, at least demographically. While less than 250,000 slaves were imported into British North America between 1619 and the beginning of the Civil War, the African-American population in the colonies stood at more than 500,000 in 1770. Indeed, the share of the population of the southern colonies—and, after 1776, the southern states—that was of African descent remained consistently between one-third and two-fifths during the 1700s. With free white immigration into the region roughly balancing slave imports, this meant that the reproductive rates of black slaves equaled those of free whites, a rather remarkable fact when compared to the Caribbean and Brazil, where only through the massive import of new slaves was the black population sustained. The fact that the slave population in North America reproduced in such significant numbers would have profound effects on African-American culture.

A population that grows through natural reproduction is going to be quite different than one that grows through importation. While slave-traders preferred males, they could not control the male-female balance in natural birth rates. For this reason, the enslaved African population in North America was far more balanced between males and females, and also featured more offspring being born than was the case in the Caribbean. The higher birth rate in North American slave communities was also partly due to the fact that North American slaves were generally better fed and clothed than their Caribbean and Brazilian counterparts. In short, family life took hold more firmly among Africans in the British North American mainland. Of course,

because slaves were merely property under English (and pre–Civil War American) law, slaveowners had the right to do with them as they wished, including breaking up married couples and families for sale. This was a relatively regular occurrence in colonial times when slaveowners—like everyone else—died young and their estates were split up among heirs or sold off to pay debts. This was the fate of Jefferson's Monticello plantation, for instance.

Still, in the face of such obstacles, African Americans began to create families, kinship networks, and communities as their numbers increased. Indeed, one half of African Americans in the 18th century lived on plantations with at least 20 slaves. And even those who lived on smaller farms experienced a sense of community in more densely settled areas. Recalling West African custom, African Americans created elaborate kinship networks of aunts, uncles, and cousins—both biological and fictive—which were reinforced by traditional naming patterns. These patterns and networks assured that each child belonged to a family and would have a guardian in the event of sale or death of a parent.

Slave families and community also allowed for development of a distinct African-American culture—some of it inherited from the old country, some of it borrowed from the European-American community, much of it a hybrid of the two. The development of this culture—thwarted by the fact that slaves came from so many different societies in Africa and spoke so many different languages—came into full flowering once the majority of slaves had been born and raised in America. It was a culture created out of a life of pain and poverty. It included art forms—like music, dance, and oral storytelling—that required little in the way of material wealth, though wood carvings, daily utensils, and even housing fashioned by slaves bore a remarkable resemblance to African forms and styles. Increasingly anchored in a deep and ecstatic Christianity that promised release from suffering and an ultimate judgement against the sin of slaveholding, the culture of African-American slaves in the southern colonies extolled resistance and rebellion as the spiritual duty of believers.

AFRICAN AMERICANS IN THE NORTHERN COLONIES

Not all 18th-century African Americans were slaves and not all lived in the southern colonies. Small communities of free blacks

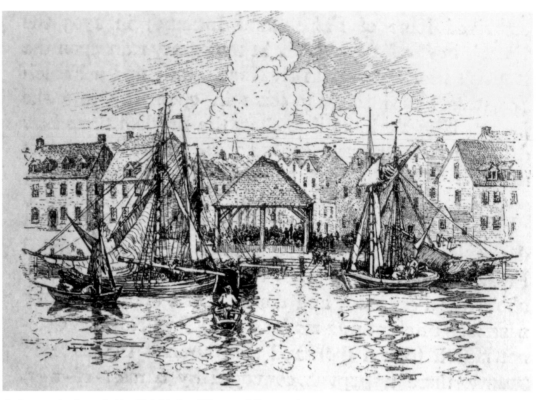

A slave auction house in New York Harbor (Library of Congress)

survived, in southern ports like Charleston, in older rural regions like the Chesapeake, and in the growing cities of the northern colonies. Although commonly associated with the South—where it survived much longer—slavery was also both legal and practiced in all of the British North American colonies, including New England. Particularly in the middle colonies—and especially New York—slavery thrived, though in a very different and far more truncated form than the South. According to the first national census in 1790, 7.6 percent, or 25,875 persons, of the population of New York State was African American; in Pennsylvania, the figure was 2.4 percent, or 10,238 persons, and in Massachusetts just 1.4 percent, or 5,369.

In rural areas of the North, African Americans—either slave or free—were indeed rare. Slavery did not take hold in the northern colonies for one simple reason: climate. Colder weather and a shorter growing season made it impossible to farm labor-intensive crops like tobacco, sugar, and rice, which required nearly year-round maintenance. Those commercial crops that did thrive in the North—largely grains— had highly seasonal labor demands. Lots of hands were only needed at planting and harvest time. Thus, it made little economic sense to buy and maintain slaves who only worked part of the year. It was better to hire labor as it was needed. But while African

Americans were rare in rural areas of the North, they were common in the tiny colonial cities. Approximately 10 percent of Boston and fully 20 percent of New York— both with total populations under 20,000— were black. Whether slave, indentured, or free, African Americans were often among the most impoverished urban residents, consigned to the poorest-paying professions like day laborers, cartmen, or merchant seamen.

The harsh conditions bred discontent and, on some occasions, rebellion. Not surprisingly, given the multicultural nature of the city, African Americans often found allies among other the members of oppressed groups. In 1712, about 25 Indian and black slaves set fire to an outhouse, then lay in ambush, killing nine men and wounding seven others who came to put the fire out. The punishment meted out was even more horrific than the crime. More than 20 slaves—including a pregnant woman—were hanged; another three were burned to death; one was broken on the wheel. Moreover, slave codes were toughened—slaves found meeting in groups larger than three were subject to a punishment of 40 lashes—and arson was made punishable by death for anyone in the colony.

Harsh codes, however, did little to assuage the fear of wealthy white New Yorkers living in a city increasingly dominated by the poor and nonwhite. A series of suspicious fires in 1741—just two years after the Stono Rebellion in South Carolina—led to rumors of a slave and indentured servant insurrection. Although no conclusive evidence of a conspiracy could be found, authorities rounded up poor African Americans and whites. Some of them were tortured; others were offered a reward for turning in other slaves and servants. In all 30 blacks and four whites were executed for their supposed roles in the alleged conspiracy. This episode illustrates that although not as dependent on slaves for their wealth as southern planters, northern merchants nevertheless feared those whom they had enslaved—the black people who served them daily and helped keep the city running.

THE AMERICAN REVOLUTION

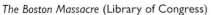

The American Revolution represented the first great colonial rebellion in modern times, and it also contributed ideas of freedom and citizenship that served as an inspiration to revolutionaries in France and Latin America in the late 1700s and early 1800s, and later to peoples all around the world. Indeed, many anticolonial leaders in Africa of the 20th century found in those revolutionary ideals inspiration for their own struggles against British, French, and Portuguese imperialists. At the same time, the Revolution was a deeply flawed affair that left African Americans—fully 20 percent of the population of the country in 1776—mired in bondage or forced to live on the margins of freedom.

By the mid-18th century, Britain had established a string of 13 colonies stretching from New Hampshire in the north to Georgia in the south, with a population of about 2 million, including almost half a million people of African descent. Under the principle of mercantilism, the colonies were supposed to serve imperial interests, providing raw materials for the home country as well as a market for finished goods from Britain. Moreover, all trade was supposed to be kept within the empire and under Britain's control. The slave-based economies of the southern colonies largely fulfilled that role, producing tobacco, rice, and cotton for the home market. But the northern colonies, with their growing manufacturing base and

The Boston Massacre (Library of Congress)

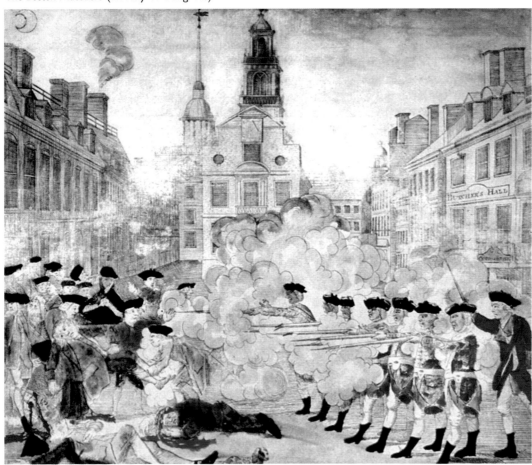

merchant fleets, increasingly competed with British economic interests. In response, Britain instituted a series of laws designed to enforce the mercantilist system. But with the colonies continuing to enrich Britain, these were enforced lackadaisically.

All that changed after 1763 when Britain emerged triumphant, although financially strained, from a seven-year war with France. To help pay its wartime debt, the British government issued a series of especially unpopular taxes, duties, and mercantilist laws. Parliament's thinking was simple: the colonists benefited from the war and the elimination of the French enemy in North America. Therefore, they should pay their fair share. Moreover, as Parliament represented all the peoples of the empire—what political thinkers of the time called "virtual" representation—it was perfectly within its rights to impose such taxes, even if there were no colonial representatives. But the Americans had other ideas. For over a century, they had been largely left to their own devices, permitted to govern themselves and their affairs as they saw fit. During that period, the colonists had developed a very different idea of governance—local representation. By their thinking, taxation imposed by this distant parliament was "taxation without representation."

BLACK PATRIOTS

In 1765 Parliament imposed the Stamp Act—placing a tax on dozens of items of everyday use. Colonists up and down the Atlantic seaboard refused to pay, forcing London to back down. Parliament was determined to prevail and followed with the Townshend duties on imported goods two years later. The colonists responded with a boycott of British products, as urban crowds attacked customs officers and their houses. On March 5, 1770, a crowd confronted British redcoats in Boston, provoking a fusillade that felled five of the protesters. One of the leaders of the demonstrators—and the first to die in America's struggle with Britain—was a half-Indian, half-black dockworker named Crispus Attucks. A freed slave, Attucks had grown up in a highly stratified colonial society where lowly workmen—white or black—deferred to their social superiors on political matters. Participation in acts of rebellion—and, later, the American Revolution—would change all that.

In short, colonial elites who wanted to free themselves from British rule needed the support of the masses of poor and working colonists to win independence. But while men like John Adams and even George Washington would have preferred to keep the struggle confined to home-rule, ordinary colonists insisted the revolution also be about who should rule at home. On January 13—less than six months since the Declaration of Independence was proclaimed in Philadelphia—a petition was presented to the legislature. Signed by dozens of enslaved blacks in Massachusetts, it read:

[We] have in common with all other men a natural and inalienable right to that freedom which the Great Parent of the heavens has bestowed equally on all mankind and which [we] have never forfeited by any compact or agreement whatever.... Every principle from which America has acted in the course of their unhappy difficulties with Great Britain pleads stronger than a thousand arguments in favor of your petitioners ... [that] they may be restored to the enjoyments of that which is the natural right of all men—and their children who were born in this land of liberty—not to be held as slaves.

When war between the colonists and Britain finally began in April 1775, African Americans—at least, the small proportion not enslaved—were faced with a dilemma: fight alongside their fellow colonists who denied them full membership in society or side with the British. In fact, black colonists had a long tradition of military service by 1775, having served as militia men in various colonial wars fought between Britain and its European rivals, France, Holland, and Spain, as well as in numberless skirmishes with Native Americans. Even slaves fought, occasionally winning their freedom in the bargain. At the same time, free blacks and runaway slaves signed up for naval duty, usually aboard independent privateers. Unlike the militia—where they were generally relegated to support positions—the privateers offered black sailors near equality of pay, while the camaraderie of close-quarter shipboard life eliminated segregation and undermined white racist attitudes.

The tradition of black military service, then, continued with the Revolution, with African-American militia men fighting alongside whites at the battles of Lexington and Concord and Bunker Hill in 1775 and at numerous other major engagements throughout the war. Still, racial prejudice remained deeply entrenched. George Washington, commander of the Continental Army, did not open the ranks to free blacks until 1777, and only then because he was

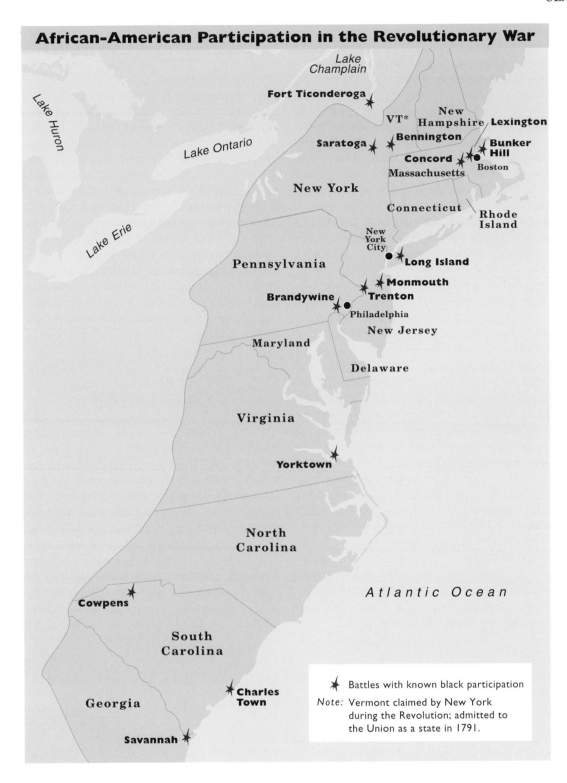

African-American Participation in the Revolutionary War

Lake Champlain

Lake Huron

Fort Ticonderoga

Lake Ontario

VT*

New Hampshire

Lexington

Bennington

Saratoga

Bunker Hill

Concord

Boston

Massachusetts

New York

Connecticut

Rhode Island

Lake Erie

New York City

Long Island

Pennsylvania

Monmouth

Brandywine

Trenton

Philadelphia

Maryland

New Jersey

Delaware

Virginia

Yorktown

North Carolina

Atlantic Ocean

Cowpens

South Carolina

Charles Town

Georgia

Savannah

★ Battles with known black participation

Note: Vermont claimed by New York during the Revolution; admitted to the Union as a state in 1791.

suffering manpower shortages. Soon thereafter, colonies in the North and upper South—where slavery was becoming less important to the agricultural economy—passed laws permitting the manumission (or freeing) of any slaves who joined up to fight against the British. Ultimately, about 5,000 African Americans—both slave and free—joined the Continental Army between 1777 and the end of the war in 1781. Others joined the various colonial militias—including an all-black Massachusetts company nicknamed the "Bucks"—as well as the Continental navy.

BLACK SOLDIERS ON THE BRITISH SIDE

As with white colonists, North American blacks were divided in their loyalties, especially after the British began to promise emancipation in exchange for military service. In late 1775, for example, more than a thousand blacks answered the plea of Lord Dunmore ("Liberty to slaves!"), royal governor of Virginia, to form the all-black Ethiopian Regiment. In the end, however, it was not so much black soldiers—who remained small in number on both sides— but African-American slaves that nearly changed the outcome of the war.

The decision by France and Spain's to back the colonists, along with Patriot victories in the North, forced the British to launch a new attack plan in 1778: an invasion of the southern colonies. The decision made sense both strategically and tactically. First, the British valued the commercial agricultural colonies of the South far more than they did those of the North, where a growing manufacturing base competed with British imports. Second, British commanders understood that the slavery system burdened southern colonists with an extra handicap. Planters did not dare to arm their slaves—who outnumbered whites in many areas and who were also critical to the economy of the region—nor did they risk leaving the plantations themselves to enlist in the American cause, which would have left their slaves free to escape. But escape they did. As British forces marched from victory to victory through Georgia and the Carolinas, tens of thousands of escaping slaves flocked to their ranks. In exchange for their freedom, they were put to work carting supplies, constructing earthworks, and doing all the other hard labor required of an army in the field. Indeed, Britain's "southern strategy" almost worked, right up to Yorktown, the decisive October 1781 defeat in southeastern Virginia that forced the main British armies in North America—surrounded by Washington's troops on land and the French fleet at sea—to surrender.

AFRICAN AMERICANS IN THE FEDERAL PERIOD

The American Revolution offered an ambivalent legacy for African Americans. For black Loyalists—free blacks who joined the British cause—defeat brought exile. Like their white counterparts, they were forced to flee. Most were first transported by the British to Nova Scotia. But the cold climate, poor lands, and lingering prejudice caused many to emigrate once again, this time to Sierra Leone, a British colony for freed slaves established on the coast of West Africa. As for slaves, the British largely honored their promise of freedom—shipping thousands to the Bahamas and elsewhere— though some runaways were returned to their masters.

SLAVERY AND THE CONSTITUTION

On the American side, emancipation became—for a brief moment—the order of the day, particularly in the states of the upper South and North. The impetus came from both idealism and economics. For many whites, the contradictions of the independence struggle were too much to bear. "It always appeared a most iniquitous Scheme to me," Abigail Adams wrote to her husband, patriot leader John Adams, "to fight ourselves for what we are daily robbing and plundering from those who have as good a right to freedom as we have." By

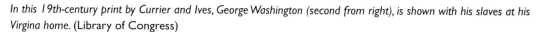

In this 19th-century print by Currier and Ives, George Washington (second from right), is shown with his slaves at his Virgina home. (Library of Congress)

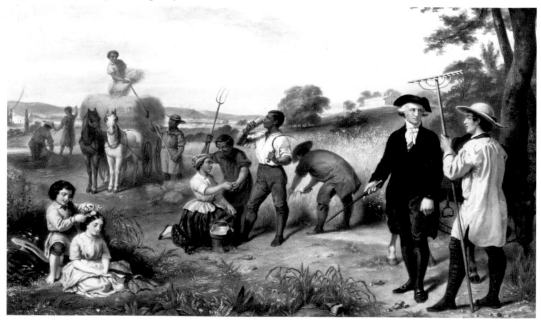

1784, four northern states—including Adams's Massachusetts—had abolished slavery. Within the next 15 years, every state north of Delaware would do the same, though some did so far more gradually than others. A 1799 law in New York, for example, offered emancipation to the children of slaves only, and then only when they reached 25 years of age. Thus, as late as 1810, nearly one-fourth of the black population in the North remained in bondage.

In the upper South, slavery was retained, but laws were passed making manumission easier. Within a decade, Virginia's planters had freed upward of 10,000 slaves. Indeed, many of the great Virginian leaders of the Revolution had decidedly mixed feelings about free blacks. Washington, Jefferson, and Constitution author James Madison all expressed support for abolition, but only Washington was willing to free his slaves in his will, though only upon the death of his wife, Martha, and only then, say critics, because he had no other heirs to will them to. In fact, the motives of many emancipation-minded Virginia planters were not always purely idealistic. As the colony's economy shifted from one based on a labor-intensive tobacco plantation system to one based on grain-based farming, large slave forces were less economically critical.

To Virginia's south, however, two factors led to a hardening, rather than easing, of slavery. First, the labor-intensive plantation agriculture in the region—notably, rice, indigo, and long-staple cotton crops—required an inexpensive labor force that

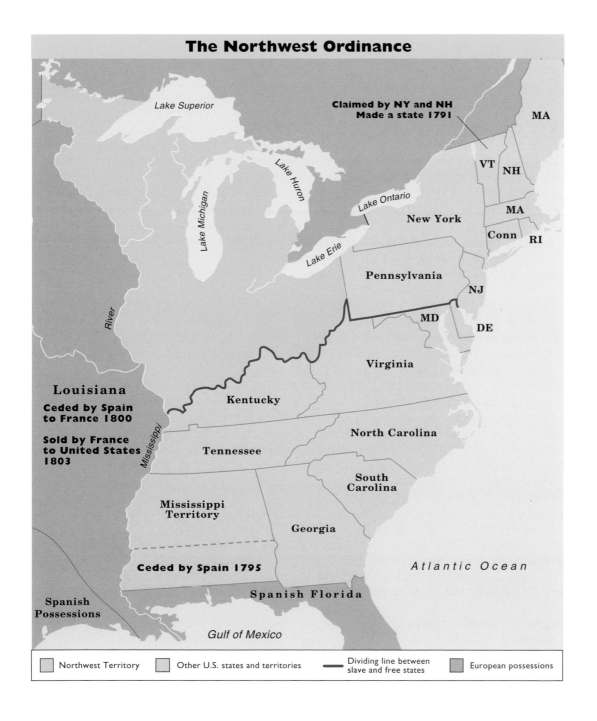

The Northwest Ordinance

Lake Superior

**Claimed by NY and NH
Made a state 1791**

MA

Lake Huron

VT   NH

Lake Ontario

MA

New York

Conn   RI

Lake Erie

Lake Michigan

Pennsylvania

NJ

River

MD

DE

Virginia

Louisiana

**Ceded by Spain
to France 1800**

Kentucky

**Sold by France
to United States
1803**

Mississippi

Tennessee

North Carolina

South
Carolina

**Mississippi
Territory**

Georgia

Ceded by Spain 1795

Atlantic Ocean

**Spanish
Possessions**

Spanish Florida

Gulf of Mexico

| | Northwest Territory | | Other U.S. states and territories | Dividing line between slave and free states | | European possessions |

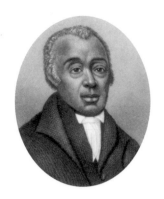

Richard Allen, founder of the African Methodist Episcopal Church (Library of Congress)

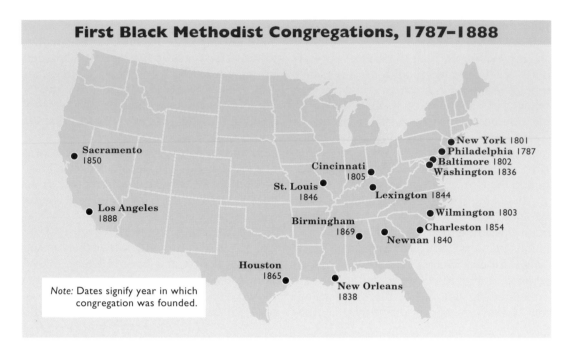

First Black Methodist Congregations, 1787–1888

New York 1801
Philadelphia 1787
Baltimore 1802
Washington 1836
Cincinnati 1805
St. Louis 1846
Lexington 1844
Sacramento 1850
Los Angeles 1888
Wilmington 1803
Charleston 1854
Birmingham 1869
Newnan 1840
Houston 1865
New Orleans 1838

Note: Dates signify year in which congregation was founded.

could be forced to work in disease-ridden swamps. Only slaves would suit the purpose. Second, the maintenance of a large slave population led to fears of uprising among planters and other whites. And those fears bred harsher slave codes and policing. The Revolution's powerful rhetoric of freedom was clearly meant, as far as the Deep South was concerned, for white ears only.

When it came time to forge a new system of government for the fledgling country, southerners were determined to ensure that nothing threatened their "peculiar institution." Concerned about the passage of the Northwest Ordinance in 1787—which outlawed slavery in the territories between the Ohio River and the Great Lakes—southern delegates to the 1787 Constitutional Convention in Philadelphia wrung a compromise from northerners on the slavery question. For the purposes of apportioning representation, slaves—though the word never actually appears in the Constitution—would be counted as three-fifths of a person, giving southern states controlling power in the Congress and the ability to squash any abolitionist legislation. The southerners were also able to win a postponement in the abolition of the international slave trade for 20 years.

THE AFRICAN METHODIST EPISCOPAL CHURCH

Still, for many African Americans, the effects of the American Revolution were both powerful and lasting. For one thing, there were more free blacks. From a few

thousand strong in 1776, the free black population of the North and upper South grew to 200,000 in less than 50 years. For the first time, there was the critical mass necessary to create independent black communities and institutions, including voluntary mutual aid associations like the African Union Society of Rhode Island and the Free African Society of Philadelphia. Perhaps the most important development, however, was the rise of free black congregations. Among these, the African Methodist Episcopal (AME) Church was the most significant.

Richard Allen, its founder, was arguably the most influential black American of his day. Born a slave in 1760, Allen experienced a religious awakening in his late teens, purchased his freedom at 20, and became an itinerant preacher in his early twenties. In 1786, the Methodists of Philadelphia asked him to preach to free blacks in the congregation. Although liberal for its time on racial issues, the white Methodists of Philadelphia were too controlling for Allen's taste and, in 1816, he founded the AME Church, the first independent black religious organization in the United States. To win their independence from the existing white Methodist church, Allen and his congregation successfully sued in the Pennsylvania Supreme Court.

While the AME retained the baptism and communion practices of the Methodist church, it made them distinctly African American. The hymn-singing that predominated in both the white and black churches became more spontaneous in the AME church and services were marked by shouting and praying out loud. It was also more

BENJAMIN BANNEKER

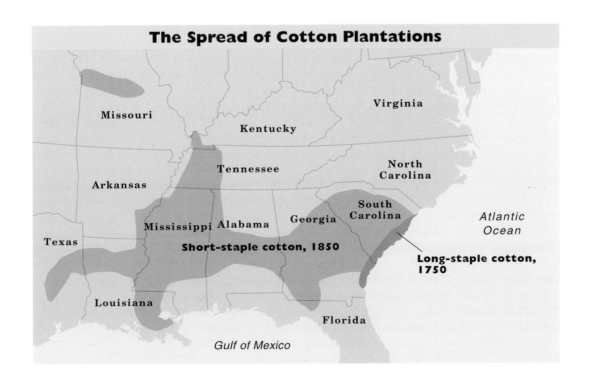

BANNEKER's ALMANACK, AND EPHEMERIS
FOR THE
YEAR OF OUR LORD 1793;

E *Nt*

BEING

THE FIRST AFTER BISSEXTILE OR LEAP-YEAR:

CONTAINING

THE MOTIONS OF THE SUN AND MOON;
THE TRUE PLACES AND ASPECTS OF THE PLANETS;
THE RISING AND SETTING OF THE SUN;
RISING, SETTING, AND SOUTHING OF THE MOON;
THE LUNATIONS, CONJUNCTIONS, AND ECLIPSES;
AND
THE RISING, SETTING, AND SOUTHING OF THE PLANETS AND NOTED FIXED STARS,

PHILADELPHIA:
PRINTED AND SOLD BY JOSEPH CRUKSHANK, NO. 87, HIGH-STREET.

Banneker and his almanac (Library of Congress)

Along with the expanded numbers, the growth of free African-American communities, and the development of independent black institutions came a newfound confidence. No individual better personified the new free black identity of the early American republic better than Benjamin Banneker. Born to free black parents in 1731, Banneker grew up and lived on the Maryland tobacco farm he inherited from his father. From an early age, Banneker showed an aptitude for science and mathematics, building one of the first mechanical clocks in the colonies at age 21. In the late 1780s, he developed an interest in astronomy and, borrowing books and instruments from a neighboring white planter, Banneker published his first astronomical almanac in 1791. After reading Jefferson's *Notes on the State of Virginia*—and taking exception to the author's remarks about black mental inferiority—Banneker sent the Declaration of Independence author a copy. The two began an exchange of letters on the subject of African-American intelligence and ability. While recognizing Banneker's extraordinary achievement—Jefferson helped get him appointed surveyor for the new capital city of Washington—the Virginia planter nevertheless ignored the astronomer's arguments against slavery and privately remained skeptical that Banneker had produced the almanac on his own.

openly political, engaging in social activism and promoting the idea of black nationalism, or a separate culture for African Americans within the United States. Evangelical like the white Methodist church, the AME targeted black communities in the American South, the Caribbean, and Africa for religious outreach. Today, the AME has branches in 20 countries on three continents. In the 20th century, the church provided much needed social services and a religious community for the millions of rural blacks migrating to northern cities. And, from the very beginning, the AME church played a very active role in the civil rights movement, including the filing of lawsuits against segregation in public education.

THE COTTON GIN

For all of the strides made by African Americans in the wake of the Revolution, the gains were dwarfed by the obstacles that remained. Slavery was still entrenched in half the nation; 90 percent of blacks remained in bondage; and, even in the so-called free states, legal restrictions and racial prejudice made a mockery of the democratic ideals so recently fought for by Americans of all colors. Moreover, a dark shadow loomed over the future of African Americans and the union itself. In 1793, Eli Whitney—a New England teacher working as a tutor on a Georgia plantation—came up with a solution to the age-old problem of

The Spread of Cotton Plantations

Missouri

Virginia

Kentucky

Tennessee

North Carolina

Arkansas

South Carolina

Mississippi Alabama Georgia

Short-staple cotton, 1850

Atlantic Ocean

Texas

Long-staple cotton, 1750

Louisiana

Florida

Gulf of Mexico

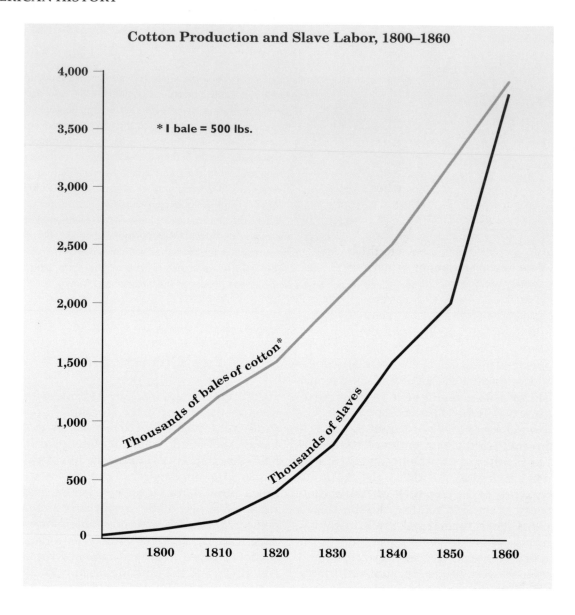

Cotton Production and Slave Labor, 1800–1860

* I bale = 500 lbs.

*Thousands of bales of cotton**

Thousands of slaves

cotton processing. For years, American planters were confined to growing only long-staple cotton, a seedless variety that can only be grown in a subtropical environment, such as the Sea Islands of Georgia and South Carolina. With its numerous seeds that had to be picked from the boll by hand, the far hardier short-staple cotton remained economically impractical. Whitney's gin—which did the work of 50 persons—changed all that.

The implications were enormous. Overnight, much of the southern United States—including a vast area in the southwestern territories—was rendered ideal and economically viable cotton growing land. Fueled by the growing demand of textile mills in Great Britain and, later, the northern states, cotton farming spread rapidly and, with it, the institution of slavery. Thus, a slave population of roughly 200,000 in 1790 had grown to nearly 4 million by 1860. By the end of that period, the

southern states were producing two-thirds of the world's cotton. The white stuff had become far and away America's number one export, drawing in foreign capital that helped finance canal, railroad, and factory construction. Northern merchants and bankers—as well as southern planters—grew rich off the trade. It was a rare politician that dared to challenge the institution.

In 1790, many people in both the North and South were convinced that slavery was on the road to gradual and peaceful extinction. Fifty years later—with slavery and cotton fields spread across the South from Virginia to East Texas and the "slave power" entrenched in the capital at Washington—few subscribed to that view. As the fiery abolitionist John Brown—on trial for launching a failed slave uprising in 1859—presciently told the nation: "I . . . am quite certain that the crimes of this guilty land . . . will never be purged away; but with Blood."

"Cruel, unjust, exploitative, oppressive, slavery bound two peoples together in bitter antagonism while creating . . . [a] relationship so complex and ambivalent that neither could express the simplest human feelings without reference to the other." So wrote the historian of American slavery Eugene Genovese.

Indeed, American slavery was complex. On the one hand, masters and slaves were part of a modern and dynamic economic system that yoked together one of civilization's oldest forms of labor—slavery—with modern, global free markets. Planters were businessmen (and occasionally women), willing to use any means necessary to realize the maximum return from their investments in human flesh. And their slaves were hyper-exploited workers who saw virtually all of their surplus labor value—that is, the value of what they produced minus the cost of keeping them alive—taken from them, literally by force.

At the same time, slavery was more than just a labor relationship. Slavery—as encoded in the laws and customs of the 19th century South—gave to one class of people absolute control over the lives of another. Slave masters had the power over every aspect of slaves' lives—where they lived, what kind of work they did, and whom they associated with. For slaves, marriage, family, friendship, home, labor, leisure—all depended upon the whims of the master.

Thus, slaves were more than workers and masters were more than employers. The two shaped each others lives and identities in ways that went far beyond a simple economic relationship. Together, the descendants of Africa and the descendents of Europe created a unique southern American culture and civilization that, despite the destruction of slavery, exists to this day.

THE EXPANSION OF SLAVERY

As noted in the previous chapter, slavery appeared to be on the road to gradual extinction in the years immediately following the American Revolution. Revolutionary ideals about "all men [being] created equal" prompted some planters to manu-mit, or legally free, their slaves. More important, grain farming was on the rise in the North and the upper South. Grains—like wheat and corn—required heavy labor at sowing and harvest times only. It made more economic sense to hire labor when it was needed than to make a heavy investment in slaves who would only be used part of the year. Thus, in 1790, the institution of slavery thrived largely along a narrow, coastal corridor of rice and long-staple cotton plantations in South Carolina and Georgia. While hugely profitable, the agricultural economy of this region was not replicable in the territories of the West for climatic reasons. Eli Whitney's simple invention of the cotton gin changed all that. By making short-staple cotton—which could be grown across much of the lower South—profitable, the gin revived slavery as an institution. And by creating an insatiable demand for the commodity, the Industrial Revolution—which began in England and soon spread to New England—made short-staple cotton farming hugely profitable.

A slave at work (Library of Congress)

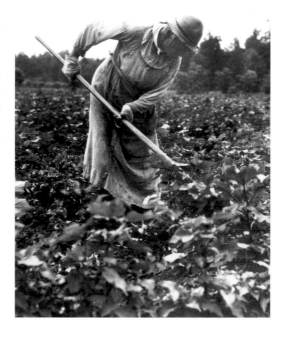

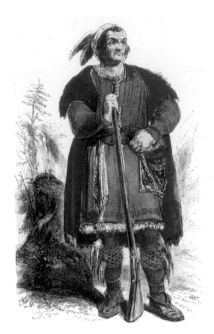

Tecumseh (Library of Congress)

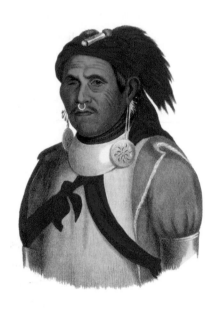

Tenskwatawa, the Shawnee Prophet
(Library of Congress)

Between 1800 and 1860, cotton production doubled every 10 years. By the latter year, the American South was producing two-thirds of the world's supply. At the same time, cotton exports were worth double the amount of all other goods and crops exported by the United States. Although of paramount importance, cotton was not the only commercial crop grown in the slave South. Rivaling the spectacular growth of cotton—although on a much smaller geographic scale—was sugar. Primarily grown in Louisiana, sugar production multiplied by a factor of five between 1800 and 1860. Meanwhile tobacco remained important, with exports doubling between 1790 and 1860, even though its percentage within the total exports of the country fell from 15 to 6 percent. In short, slavery—and the agricultural commodities it produced—was a very big business in antebellum America.

Production of the commercial crops—sugar, tobacco, rice, and above all cotton—of the South required three critical ingredients: land, capital, and labor. Land, of course, was the foundation. In 1790, the farms and plantations of the South—from Maryland in the north to Georgia in the south—were largely confined to a strip of land between the Atlantic coast and the Appalachian Mountains, although pioneers had begun to settle the future states of Tennessee and Kentucky. Divided into low-lying tidewater and upland piedmont areas (areas by the base of the mountain), the settled territories of the eastern seaboard ranged between 50 and 200 miles in width.

RESETTLEMENT OF NATIVE AMERICANS

West of the Appalachian crest was Indian country, primarily occupied by the so-called Five Civilized Tribes: the Cherokee and Creek of the western Carolinas and eastern Alabama and Tennessee; the Choctaw and Chickasaw of western Alabama and Mississippi; and the Seminole of Florida. These Indian nations were designated "civilized" for a simple reason: their societies most resembled that of whites. They were settled and agrarian. Some even produced commercial crops for sale and owned black slaves, although on a smaller scale and with a far more relaxed attitude about interracial mixing.

Yet despite their "civilized" ways, the Native Americans of the trans-Appalachian South saw virtually all of their lands seized by whites between 1800 and 1840. At first, these seizures occurred on a case by case

basis, as the federal and various state governments insisted that traditional communal lands be divided into individual property holdings, a form of land tenure unfamiliar to most Indians. Lent money by local merchants, many Native American landholders saw their lands seized when they could not pay the interest on their debts, the concept of interest also being completely alien to them. This led to clashes between whites and Native Americans, including an uprising of a confederacy of Indian groups organized by two Shawnee brothers—Tecumseh and Tenskwatawa—between 1809 and 1814. Their defeat at the Battle of Horseshoe Bend in Alabama ended much of the armed resistance.

By the time the federal government decided to remove all of the remaining Native Americans east of the Mississippi River to Oklahoma in the 1830s, it encountered little armed resistance, although the forced midwinter marches—known as the Trail of Tears, for the thousands who died from malnutrition, cold, and disease—remains one of the most brutal episodes in American history. At the same time, the settlement of these new lands in the Old Southwest (Alabama, Arkansas, Mississippi, Lousiana, Tennessee, and the western parts of Georgia and North Carolina) was accelerated by developments in transportation technology, most notably the steamboat. This linked the South and West into an integrated economic region based on the Mississippi River and its tributaries, until the development of the railroad network re-oriented trade along an east-west pattern in the 1840s and 1850s. This early economic integration had important political repercussions, creating a South-West alliance in Congress dedicated to the protection of slavery, at least in the South and Old Southwest. (The Old Northwest Territory was declared free under the Northwest Ordinance of 1787, with most new states there banning both slavery and the in-migration of free blacks.)

FINANCING THE SLAVE SYSTEM

Meanwhile, former tribal lands in the Old South began to fill up with white farmers and planters determined to expand the cotton empire. And to the hundreds of thousands of square miles of ideal short-staple cotton-growing land now available, the planters and farmers of the antebellum South now added the two other crucial ingredients mentioned in a previously—

capital and labor. The former came largely from Britain and the northern states. Like all commercial farmers, the cotton growers of the Old South were perpetually in debt, borrowing to meet this year's living and operation expenses against next year's crop. To meet this economic contingency, there arose a financing system stretching as far as New York City and London and linking northern and British money and textile interests with southern farmers and planters. Much of the business was handled by commission merchants or "factors"— some independent and some working directly for northern and English financial interests—who lived in the South and offered a variety of services to planters, including loans, warehousing, and ship-

ping. In addition, these factors helped finance western settlement, providing large loans to cover the first four or five costly years of plantation development. But these services came at a high price. Factors typically skimmed off a fifth to a quarter of the crop in payment. By the 1850s, more than $100 million in cotton profits was annually siphoned off to northern banks, giving major financial centers in the North a direct stake in preserving the slave-based cotton system of the South.

This outside financing was also heavily responsible for supplying the final ingredient in the spread of slavery to the territories of the Old Southwest: labor. New plantations needed new labor forces, and factors helped finance the huge growth in the

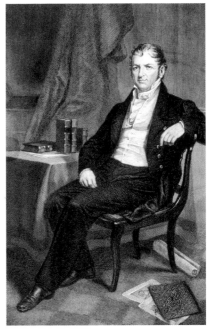

Eli Whitney (Library of Congress)

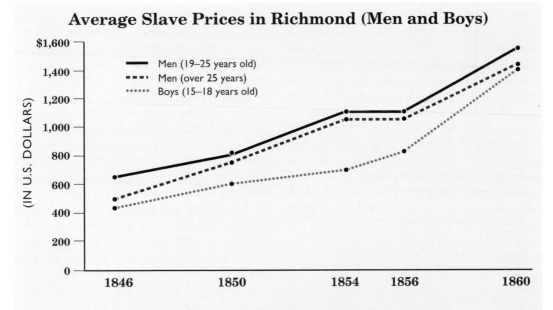

Average Slave Prices in Richmond (Men and Boys)

Legend:
— Men (19–25 years old)
- - - Men (over 25 years)
····· Boys (15–18 years old)

Y-axis: (IN U.S. DOLLARS), $1,600 / 1,400 / 1,200 / 1,000 / 800 / 600 / 400 / 200 / 0

X-axis: 1846 1850 1854 1856 1860

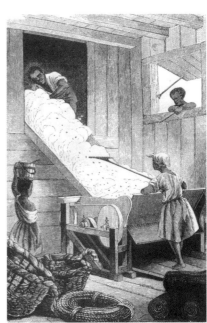

The cotton gin (Library of Congress)

Average Slave Prices in Richmond (Women and Girls)

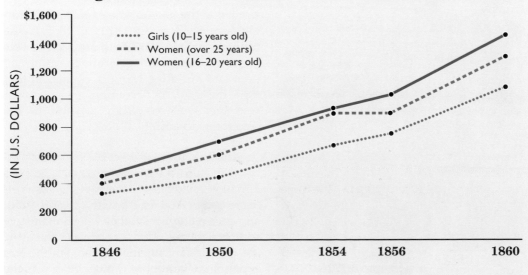

Legend:
····· Girls (10–15 years old)
- - - Women (over 25 years)
— Women (16–20 years old)

Y-axis: (IN U.S. DOLLARS), $1,600 / 1,400 / 1,200 / 1,000 / 800 / 600 / 400 / 200 / 0

X-axis: 1846 1850 1854 1856 1860

Percentage of Sales Involving the Breakup of Marriages and/or Families, 1850			
Children Sold Without Either Parent as Percentage of All Trades		**Married Adults Sold Without Spouse**	
AGE IN YEARS	PERCENT	GENDER/AGE	PERCENT
0–7	2	Women (15–19)	12
8–11	8	Women (20 and over)	7
12–14	15	Men (20–24)	11
		Men (25 and over)	8

domestic slave trade between 1820 and 1860. Like many aspects of slavery, the domestic trade and price of slaves was a market-driven phenomenon. With the growth of slavery increasing demand and the abolition of the international slave trade in 1807–1808 reducing supply, the price of slaves began to climb. Indeed, areas of early slave population concentrations along the eastern seaboard began to see rising profits from the sale of slaves, even as their depleted land (both cotton and tobacco drain nutriments from the earth) resulted in decreased productivity. By the 1850s, slaveowners were shipping more than 25,000 slaves from east to west, in the process breaking up African-American families and communities. (Westward expansion was not the only cause for the breakup of slave families and communities, as planters often divided their estates—including their labor force—among various heirs.)

Slave sales represented some of the most cruel and frightening moments in an African American's life. Often purchased by slave traders—notorious even among whites for their vicious barbarity—slaves would be shackled and forcibly marched up to hundreds of miles to auction houses, where they were kept in barracks and pens for days, weeks, and months on end. Paraded in front of potential buyers—who poked and prodded them like cattle, often peering into their mouths to check their teeth—slaves were auctioned off to the highest bidder, often with little regard to family and marriage ties. (Some planters—both as buyers and sellers—made a point of keeping families together for fear that breaking them up would produce an unhappy and, hence, unproductive or recalcitrant slave force.)

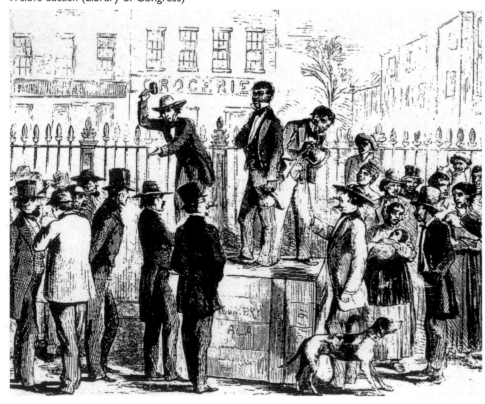

A slave auction (Library of Congress)

LIFE ON THE PLANTATION

The slave-owning population increased alongside the geographic expansion of cotton farming. Between 1820 and 1860, it rose from just under 200,000 to around 400,000, many of them coming from the ranks of poor and middling farmers. Indeed, at that time the goal of becoming a slaveowner was the southern white version of the American dream.

SLAVE OWNERS

Slave ownership was, however, confined to an increasingly smaller percentage of southern whites. This was because the overall population of the white South was expanding even more rapidly than was the number of slave owners. Between 1830 and

1860, the percentage of southern whites who owned slaves fell from 36 to 26, a drop of more than 25 percent. Still, despite the diminishing rate of slave ownership, the institution itself was strongly defended by virtually the entire white population of the South, which would partly explain why massive numbers of poor whites volunteered to fight for the Confederacy in the Civil War.

Nonslaveholding whites stood by the system for two reasons. As noted above, poor and property-less whites were elevated in their social standing by the existence of a class—and race—of people whose very skin color assigned them the lowest rung on the societal ladder. As Frederick Douglass, an abolitionist born into slavery, argued, the poorest white could always lord it over any black he/she encountered, thereby enhancing his or her own self-esteem and allying him/her politically with planters. In addition, poor southern whites—like all Americans—believed strongly in social mobility, the opportunity to rise out of their social station through native ability and hard work. In the South, that meant buying and working slaves, most likely on western lands. Indeed, the very system of slavery relied on the cooperation of poor whites. More numerous than planters, they could be called upon to act as a police force, questioning, detaining, and returning any slave found off the plantation.

There were also great economic disparities within the slaveholding class. Most owned just a few slaves and perhaps $3,000 in land, making them economically far better off than nonslaveholders but poor in comparison with the middling and large planters, who might own from 10 to 50 slaves in the former case and from 50 to several hundred in the latter. Indeed, most small slave owners—as well as poorer nonslaveholders who might rent their slaves at critical periods in the growing season—were highly dependent on the large planters, turning to them to help process, store, and market their crops. This created a system in which a small number of planters controlled the governments of the South, with poorer white elements deferring to them on political matters. The skewed distribution of slaves also created a demographic paradox. Simply put, the vast majority of slave owners owned few slaves, but well over 50 percent of southern African Americans lived on plantations with 20 or more slaves. These numbers—combined with the fact that most plantations lay in so-called black belts (named for the richness of the soil and not the color of the laborers'

skin)—meant that the majority of slaves lived in places where African-American communities could develop. This fact would have enormous consequences for the development of a distinct black culture in the antebellum South.

WHITE PATERNALISM

Most male slave owners—and the vast majority were men—fancied themselves aristocrats and modeled their lives after English country squires. They tried to cultivate an aristocratic way of life, which placed an emphasis on culture, elegance, refined manners, and leisure, as opposed to the hectic pace and moneyed pursuits among their northern counterparts in finance and manufacturing. Most lived on isolated plantations where, like the lords of the manor celebrated in the novels of Walter Scott, the Old South's favorite writer, they controlled all aspects of the lives of their subordinates. Out of this mentality grew a self-styled system of control known as paternalism. That is to say, planters imagined themselves as father figures—strict but essentially caring—of a vast family of slaves, an ideal they clung to in the face of northern criticism. According to the planters, theirs was a system superior to that of the North, where laborers were hired and fired as needed, with little concern for their well-being and livelihood.

The whole notion of paternalism was deeply flawed, though, for several reasons. First, it was based on an extremely racist conception of African-American capabilities. A slave, wrote Virginia planter George Fitzhugh, "is but a grown-up child, and must be governed as a child [while] the master occupies toward him the place of parent or guardian." Over the years, slave masters elaborated an ideology in defense of slavery that slipped from an argument of "necessary evil" to "positive good." That is to say, in the early years of the 19th century, the planters of the South and their intellectual defenders in the press and academia argued that because blacks and whites were inherently different, the two could not live on an equal social and economic footing. Forced to survive amidst a superior white population, the argument went, blacks would sink into poverty, crime, and violence. Slavery, then, was necessary to keep southern society and the economy that underpinned it functioning.

Gradually, the "necessary evil" argument metamorphosed into one that insisted slavery was a "positive good." As James

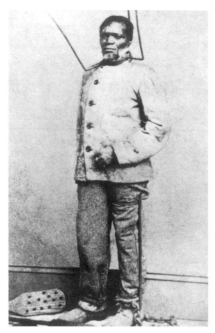

A slave wearing shackles around his neck
(Library of Congress)

Hammond, a South Carolina planter and senator, put it, every society had to have a "mud-sill class" of people who did the hard and dirty work of heavy labor and domestic servitude. In societies where these tasks were performed by free laborers, such as the North, dangerous rifts in the social and political order could result. But the South, he said, had found a perfect solution to this dilemma in assigning those tasks to an "inferior" race perfectly suited and willing to performing them, albeit under close white supervision. Later, the absurdity of this racist proposition would be put to the test in the immediate post–Civil War era. While planters expected either violent retribution from blacks—based on the racist notion that blacks were savages and prone to violence—or incapacity that would lead to a new dependence on whites—based on the paternalistic idea of blacks as "grown-up children"—former slaves proved neither particularly vengeful nor helpless.

A second flaw in white paternalism was its tendency to gloss over the essential brutality of the slave system, in which the threat or practice of corporal punishment—often times slipping over the line into outright torture—was ever-present. In the antebellum South—as in every society—practice varied from individual to individual. Some masters could be quite harsh in their treatment of slaves; others more benevolent. However, the system and the

racist ideology it perpetuated rested on inherent brutality for two reasons. First, slaves were legally considered as chattel, that is, living property, not unlike livestock. For both social and psychological reasons, reducing someone to less than human status—that is, making someone the property of another—invites cruelty and abuse, as abolitionists were wont to argue when the slave masters offered up their system as one inherently more benevolent than the northern wage labor system.

Second, slaves were not just property but workers who had virtually all of the wealth produced by their labor taken from them by force. Without the positive incentives of wages, few slaves were willing to perform the back-breaking labor of plantation agriculture without the threat or application of force. To get labor out of their slaves, then, planters employed a host of punishments that included beating, branding, shackling, and the selling off of recalcitrant slaves or their loved ones. (Some planters also offered a few meager incentives like an extra day or two off at Christmas, a larger tobacco ration, or the right for their slaves to earn a few dollars raising crops on their own plots or from selling their labor.)

Next to physical punishment, the most important method for labor control was maintaining ignorance. Masters—and southern state law—prohibited teaching slaves reading and writing. This had immediate and practical reasons, as well as more subtle, longterm ones. When masters sent slaves off the plantation on errands, they supplied them with written passes to explain their presence. A slave who could write was also a slave who could counterfeit a pass. But more profoundly, masters did not want their slaves learning of the outside world. They did not want them to know that there was any world other than that of the plantation and any authority other than that of the planter. Thus, planter regimes in the South made it a point to ban all abolitionist literature, for fear it might fall into the hands of the few free blacks or slaves who could read and would pass the ideas on to the majority who could not.

Ultimately, however, the idea of the plantation as family was undermined by the contradiction inherent in a system where slavery and capitalism were intimately linked. That is to say, planters had to make a profit, or they would fail. In a competitive world market, where planters and farmers had little control over the prices their crops fetched—that meant lowering the costs of production. This could be done

A Louisiana sugar plantation

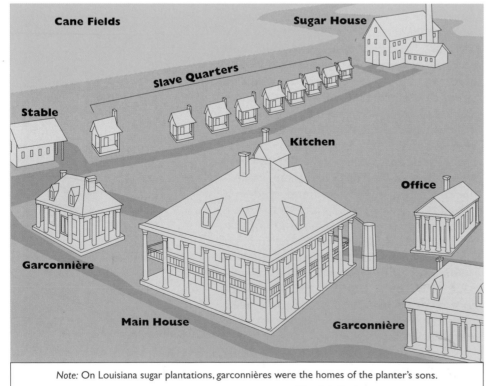

Note: On Louisiana sugar plantations, garconnières were the homes of the planter's sons.

by finding more and better land—hence the move westward—or by lowering labor costs. Since slaves were not paid a wage, lowering labor costs meant scrimping on necessities, driving the labor force harder, or both when prices for crops dropped. These imperatives usually overrode any paternalistic pretensions toward benevolence. Planters who truly tried to live up to some fictional aristocratic ideal were likely to find themselves in financial trouble, forced to sell off their human property—a slave's greatest fear as it meant separation from family and friends—to meet debt payments. Thomas Jefferson, for example, who had a reputation for lenience, lived on the edge of bankruptcy most of his life.

Thus, slaves worked far harder and with far less return, if any, than even the most exploited farm laborer or factory worker in the North. While a few of the wealthier planters tried to make showcases of their plantations, most slaves were housed in windowless, dirt-floored cabins. Furnishing usually amounted to little more than a roughhewn table and chairs, a few utensils, and itchy straw-tick mattresses. Clothing was skimpy and of the cheapest grades of cloth, often reduced to rags because they were rarely replaced. And while food was often plentiful, it was usually of the poorest and most basic quality. A weekly ration typically included a few pounds of salt pork and a quarter-bushel, or 16 pounds, of cornmeal—a diet lacking in essential vitamins and minerals. (To supplement this unhealthful and monotonous diet, many slaves fished, trapped, or worked small vegetable gardens of their own, though this meant laboring on their one day of rest a week.)

SLAVES

Because southern plantations were often self-contained economic units—with all but the luxuries gracing the planters' lives grown or manufactured on the premises—African Americans found themselves asked to perform a host of tasks. Thus, some slaves were skilled workers—blacksmiths, carpenters, coopers (barrel-makers), as well as other craftspersons. A few slaves were promoted to overseer status—although this position was often reserved for poor whites—which put them in the delicate position of having to drive or discipline their fellow slaves. But the most significant division in the labor force—and one with the most profound ramifications for the African-American slave community—was

that between house slaves and field slaves. The former were usually lighter-skinned and sometimes, as in the case of the Jefferson household, were offspring of the planter. Although under the close supervision of whites who could call on them day and night, house slaves often had an easier workload and a higher standard of living. This could produce tensions in the slave community as the house slaves sometimes saw themselves as superior, while field slaves saw the house slaves as allies of the planters.

The vast majority of slaves worked in the fields. But even here the types of labor varied depending on the crop produced. As discussed previously, there were essentially two kinds of field labor. Most typical was gang labor, the kind usually employed on cotton plantations. Here, slaves worked in gangs under the close supervision of overseers, with the pace of planting or picking set by the fastest-working slave. The other form of labor was called the task-system and was usually employed on rice or tobacco plantations, which required more skilled and delicate work than cotton farming. Here, groups of slaves were given specific tasks for the day, week, or season. Involving greater autonomy, the task system allowed slaves less white supervision and even time off for themselves once the task was completed. Finally, many slaves were rented out by their masters to work for others. Often, the hirers of slaves had little incentive to properly care for them since the slaves' long-term health was of little concern to them.

In any case—gang, task, or rental—the slave system allowed for little gender difference. While 19th-century white America believed in a strict differentiation of women's work from men's—or, in the case of upper class families, exempted women from labor altogether—slave owners demanded that all hands—female or male—work in the fields. Children, too, were put to work as soon as they could, while infants and toddlers were left in the care of slaves too old to work.

FAMILY LIFE

Meanwhile, amidst the grueling work, grinding poverty, and abject cruelty of the plantation—and constantly haunted by the specter of sale and separation—African Americans in bondage forged a uniquely powerful and sustaining social order, based primarily on family and religion. The preservation of a coherent and nurturing

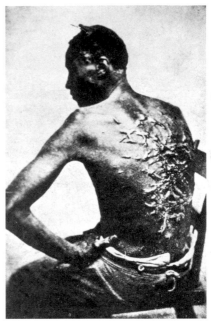

A whipping victim (Library of Congress)

family life in spite of the cruelty of the slave regime of the antebellum South is one of the most remarkable achievements of African-American history.

The obstacles against maintaining such a structure were significant. One obstacle was the law. Unlike Catholic slave countries of Latin America, slave marriages—even those performed by a black preacher—did not have legal standing. The North Carolina Supreme Court offered a typical interpreta-tion of the matter in an 1853 ruling: "Our law requires no solemnity or form in regard to the marriage of slaves, and whether they 'take up' with each other by express per-mission of their owners, or from a mere impulse of nature, in obedience to the [bib-lical] command 'multiply and replenish the earth' cannot, in the contemplation of the law, make any sort of difference."

Another obstacle was the auction block. While some slaves might live out their lives

SLAVERY'S IMPACT ON AFRICAN-AMERICAN CUISINE

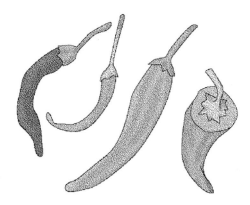

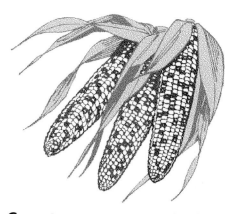

Peppers: According to an old Yoruba proverb, "The man who eats no pepper is weak, for pepper is the staff of life." Hot and sweet ground red pepper and red pep-per oil were commonly used to season meals in Africa. In slave cooks' efforts to enliven their food, they used generous amounts of red pepper, which they brought with them, or green peppercorns and cayenne pepper. A typical dish using pepper was okra soup infused with fresh mashed green peppers, which became a plantation staple in antebellum days.

Corn: Corn was a common staple food for enslaved Africans. Weekly rations typically included about a peck (16 pounds) of cornmeal, which when mixed with salt and water made cornbread, or as it was also variously called pone, johnny cake, corn dodger, or hoecake. On some large plantations, owners used a ritual called the shucking party to squeeze extra work out of slaves. Husking parties occurred at night, with the slaves singing as they worked. When work was done, the slaves took the corn directly into the plantation kitchen where they received a special meal—commonly thick soup and small amounts of whiskey—in return. The meal was often followed by a dance.

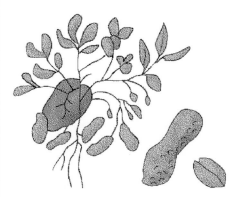

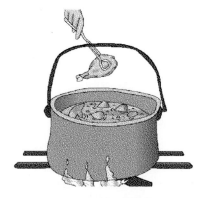

Peanuts: Africans used peanuts in their cuisine in dif-ferent ways. For example, they often served fresh peanuts as a vegetable or ground them up as a soup base. This tradition continued especially in the South, and many typical southern dishes used peanuts in versa-tile ways. Peanuts were often prepared in a cream sauce, or for more exotic tastes, were mashed with yams and eggs, sprinkled with crumbs and seasoning, and formed into cakes and fried.

Deep Frying: African cooks used animal fat or palm oil to deep-fry their foods. Using big pots of oil, they fried a variety of foods, such as yams, okra, plan-tains, and bananas. Slaves continued this cooking style on the plantations, using the lard available from their pork rations. Fish such as catfish, butterfish, haddock, and trout were often prepared this way.

on a single plantation, most would be transferred to another owner at least once in their lives, even if it was just to the plantation of their first owner's heir. Similarly, while most slaves were sold locally, leaving the possibility of visiting spouses and children on Sundays, many were not, especially as the long-distance domestic slave trade between the eastern seaboard and the Old Southwest increased after 1820. Despite their profession of deep Christian faith, slave owners routinely ignored one of the bedrocks of the faith—marriage and family—as far as slaves were concerned. Again, racist ideas offered a rationalization that overrode reality. African Americans, it was argued, could not understand the meaning of holy matrimony and, being childlike, did not share the emotional sophistication necessary for romantic love—this, despite the common scenes of heartbreaking grief, repeated endlessly across the antebellum

THE PRESERVATION OF CULTURE: Slave Crafts

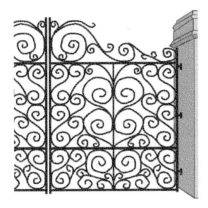

Blacksmithing: Many enslaved Africans possessed sophisticated metal working skills closely rooted in traditional African techniques. These slaves often helped build the lavish antebellum plantations of the American South, forging practical and ornamental objects such as wrought-iron balconies, grilles, doors, tools, and kitchenware. The wrought-iron gates shown here illustrate the high-quality detail present in African artisans' work.

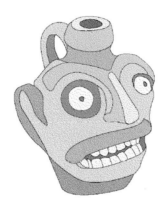

Pottery: A number of pottery "face vessels" have been attributed to 19th-century slaves. Ranging in height from one inch to one foot, they are typically glazed in dark colors such as green, brown, or black. Certain characteristics, such as large inlaid eyes and wide mouths, displaying prominent teeth, also appear in ancient sculptures found in what is now the Democratic Republic of Congo. Although the function of these vessels is debated, they appear to have been of personal value, as many of them were found near Underground Railroad homes.

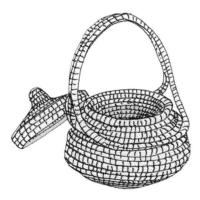

Basket Weaving: Basket weaving has a long African heritage, and the tradition was preserved by African slave communities in the antebellum South. Sweetgrass baskets, still commonly found in South Carolina, are similar to those found in West Africa. These baskets have distinct geometric patterns. Craftspeople weave tan-colored sweetgrass with darker strips of pine needles, binding them together with palmetto leaves. They still prefer to use traditional tools, such as nails, the flat ends of teaspoons, and even sharpened oyster shells.

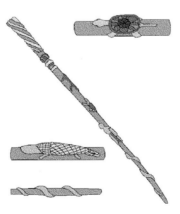

Wood Carving: Many slaves of the American South were also familiar with West African wood carving techniques. The tradition of carving wooden canes and walking sticks with reptilian imagery (symbolic of spiritual strength) continued in bondage. The cane shown here is attributed to Henry Gudgell, who lived and worked on a 19th-century Missouri plantation. The motifs—the lizard, the tortoise, and the serpent wrapped around the base—are all of African derivation.

VOODOO

During the first half of the 19th century, New Orleans, Lousiana, was an important center for free blacks. Many had come to New Orleans from Haiti during that country's revolution. They brought with them many of the spiritual traditions of the Yoruba religion to their new home. These rites were known as voudun, or voodoo, meaning "spirit" or "deity" in the West African Ewe language. Adherants of voodoo believe that life can be improved or destroyed by any of the over 400 spirit forces, or *loas*, in the voodoo pantheon. Worshippers pray for good fortune and protection from evil using amulets, dolls, spells, and rituals. Voodoo thrived in New Orleans's black community despite laws dating back to 1724 requiring all Africans to be baptized into the Roman Catholic Church. Voodoo thus coexisted and even mingled with Catholicism, creating a system of syncretic imagery and belief that exists to this day. During the 19th century, Marie Laveau (1796–1879) reigned as Queen of Voodoo in New Orleans. Born a free Catholic, her reputation as a voodoo priestess solidified soon after she became a member of the religion in 1826. In her house near Congo Square, she practiced her religious magic, making and selling charms, or *gris-gris*. Mesmerized by her beauty and spiritual powers, both Africans and whites consulted her on matters such as love, wealth, death, and happiness. Laveau sometimes invited whites suspicious of voodoo to rituals, thus helping dispel mistaken beliefs that these events were barbaric and rife with human sacrifice. To this day, voodoo worshippers pay homage to Laveau, visiting her grave and making offerings.

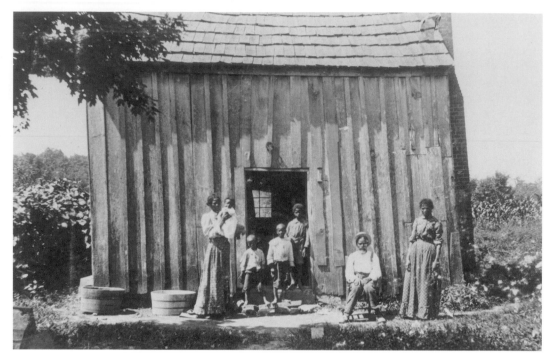

A slave family (Library of Congress)

South, of spouses and parents suddenly separated on the auction block from thier loved ones.

But if racism offered a justification for ignoring Christian tradition, the bedrock reason for ignoring slave marriage was economic. Slaves were property pure and simple. If a master needed to break up a slave marriage or family for economic necessity, then the state—controlled by that same master class—was not going to get in the way with laws in defense of slave marriages. In registering newly freed slaves after the Civil War, Union army officials in Mississippi found that fully one quarter of all male slaves had been torn from their wives at least once by sales.

Highlighted in much of the antislavery literature of the day, though couched in delicate language, was yet another—and deeply shameful—obstacle placed in the path of African-American family life on the plantation. As anyone familiar with the plantation system understood, it was not uncommon for slave owners, their sons, and the white overseers they hired to take mistresses from among the slave quarters. Some did it by coercion—even rape—others used incentives to gain the company of slave women. Whatever the method, the taking of mistresses by white masters cast a dark shadow over the security and sanctity of families and marriages within the slave quarters.

Yet despite all of these obstacles the African-American family survived, largely by retaining African customs and adapting

theem to the painful and disruptive daily life under the slave regime. Despite the fact that slave marriages carried no legal weight, African Americans married outside the law in ceremonies—such as jumping over the broom to symbolize domestic wedlock—that resonated with African tradition. Unless broken up by sale, these marriages often lasted a lifetime and were the core of strong nuclear families. Beyond that, African Americans retained the extended family networks familiar back in the homeland. To establish heritage in a world where families could be broken up at any moment at the will of the master or the market, children were named in ways that created links with the past—such as being named after the day of the week on which they were born, a customary practice in West Africa. Or they might be named after an aunt, grandparent, or cousin who had been sold off or died, in order to establish family lineage.

Extended families might also include fictive kin, or close friends who were not actually related by blood or by marriage but who nonetheless considered themselves part of an extended family through a form of unofficial adoption. Like extended families, this was a practice that hailed back to the West African homeland and adapted to slave society in the America. By these methods of naming and adoption, enslaved African-American parents could be fairly certain that their children would be taken care of should they themselves die or be sold off.

RELIGION

Religion was the other mainstay of African-American life on the plantation. In certain isolated areas like the Louisiana Delta or the Sea Islands off South Carolina and Georgia—where blacks vastly outnumbered whites and imports from Africa and the Caribbean continued right up to the international slave trade ban in 1807–1808—this religion might include strong African elements, as was the case with voodoo practices in New Orleans. But for the most part, slave religion was Christian, usually Baptist or Methodist, but occasionally Episcopalian. Despite the European roots of these religions, African Americans adapted them to their own needs.

Planters could hardly deny religion to their slaves. One of the pillars of the slaveholder ideology was that slavery was a halfway house on the path from savagery to civilization. Civilization in 19th-century America was synonymous with Christianity. Thus, masters often encouraged religious practice on their plantations as they hoped it might inculcate the values they wanted in their slaves—loyalty, obedience, submission to a God-given order where blacks were subservient to whites, and the reward of everlasting freedom in the afterlife. But slave congregations were taught and absorbed a very different Christian message. In secret meetings, self-taught slave or itinerant free black preachers emphasized liberation in this world and not just the next, with an emphasis on the Book of Exodus and its story of Moses leading the Hebrews out of their Egyptian bondage.

As all faith is intended to do, the Christian religion of the slaves attempted to fuse daily practice with a larger meaning and purpose to life. Slavery, black preachers sermonized, was a wicked and sinful institution created and maintained by the devil. As good Christians, slaves were bound by their faith to fight sin and wickedness—hence, to fight slavery. Every act of resistance, every attempt to subvert the will of the master, then, was infused with a higher purpose, fulfilling God's will.

RESISTANCE AND ESCAPE

Indeed, the record of African-American resistance to slavery is a long and proud one. Some of it—particularly the Underground Railroad and the great slave rebellions, like the one led by Nat Turner in 1831—are well chronicled in most history books and are discussed in a later section of this chapter. But most went on quietly, in everyday life. For example, slaves stole from their masters. George Washington once complained that his slaves were drinking more of his wine than he was. To many whites, thievery by slaves only confirmed the racist belief that it was in the very nature of the black man to steal.

At the most basic level, the main cause of stealing by slaves was that they were all too often underfed. But, to slaves, stealing also had a moral element—for to them, stealing was really an act of taking back what properly belonged to them, the fruits of their labor confiscated by their masters.

SUBVERSION AND RESISTANCE

Taking a master's property was only one form of everyday subversion. Slaves also found effective ways to withhold their labor power as well. Slaves sometimes feigned illness to get out of work. Many African-American communities had developed a whole host of herbal concoctions that were not just used to cure the sick but to make someone appear to be so. Slaves also sabotaged equipment. By breaking a hoe, a slave in the fields would have to make the long walk back to the toolshed to get a replacement or have their broken one fixed. This provided both a much-needed break from their back-breaking labor and the satisfaction of knowing they had put one over on the master. Indeed, out of this tradition of quietly subverting the will of the master came an oral literary tradition some of which was eventually written down after the Civil War as the tales of Br'er (short for Brother) Rabbit and Br'er Fox. Based on the West African figure of the trickster, Br'er Rabbit—though physically weak and helpless—was always outsmarting Br'er Fox and getting him to do what he wanted him to.

Ultimately, these small acts of rebellion by slaves were intended—consciously or unconsciously—to maintain a sense of power and control over one's life in a world where slaves had little or none. But they also signified that deep down slaves occupied a critical place in the southern order of things. Planters were after profits; profits came from crops; crops were raised by slaves. If a slave could deny his or her labor, he or she could exert power. Of course, this had to be done very carefully, since planters had a host of punishment available to them all the way up to exile (that is, sale) and

THE ORAL TRADITION

The African-American oral tradition was, in many ways, a direct response to the powerlessness that enslaved blacks felt. Numerous stories were passed from generation to generation in a subtle expression of subversion. The most famous of these stories were the Br'er (Brother) Rabbit tales, featuring a cunning protaganist based on West African trickster figures. Below are a few other examples, collected by the early 20th century writers Langston Hughes and Arna Bontemps in their seminal 1958 work, *The Book of Negro Folklore*, followed by explanations:

Story:
They say that in the beginning, God was getting the races together and He told the people, He say, "now, yawl git to the right." But He couldn't hear so good, so he make them all "white." Then He say, "yawl standin' aroun', stand aroun', git aroun!" They all got brown.

Explanation:
Many black folktales tried to make sense of the race question. In this story, the reasons for racial differences are made to look silly—that God simply made a mistake.

Story:
Dese two old black slaves and their massa were waiting in line at St. Peter's gate to be let into hebbin [heaven]. Ol' St. Peter, he say, to the two blacks, you two go on over there to those little cabins by the creek. Then he say to their massa, you there, you got that big white house on the hill. The first slave, he say, dis ain't fair. That bad ol' master gettin' the fine house in hebbin and we gettin' the same ol' cabins like back on de earth. How come? And ol' St. Peter, he say, you two dumb as wood. We got plenty o' black men up here, but dat one be the first white man we ever got.

Explanation:
In most slave stories, the white man is usually punished in the afterlife. But in this one, he is rewarded. The twist of the story, of course, is that white men generally are made to look bad.

even execution (masters were never prosecuted for killing slaves, though few did so since it meant loss of a major investment).

Unlike free laborers, of course, slaves could not go on strike, at least not overtly. And yet, there was a way to strike out against the master, and that way was to escape. Slaves escaped frequently or, at least, temporarily absented themselves from the plantation. Most slaves who ran away did so locally, to the nearby woods, and for short periods of time, not permanently (the odds against long-distance escape were enormous and will be looked at below in the discussion on the Underground Railroad). The reasons were many: to visit a loved one on another plantation, to supplement a meager diet by hunting or fishing, or to escape punishment. This could be a form of negotiation, particularly at critical points in the growing season when all hands were needed to bring in the

crop. Desperate to recover the lost slave, a master might send another slave to talk the runaway into coming back (often, other slaves secretly brought food to a runaway and knew his or her whereabouts). All of this did not mean that planters and slaves negotiated as equals on questions of punishment and other matters, but simply that slaves did exert some power in their own way. They were not the completely helpless victims of the master's will.

THE UNDERGROUND RAILROAD

While most slaves made their escapes temporary, thousands of African Americans did manage to break free of slavery altogether and escape the South, usually by escaping to the North and Canada. A few in the Deep South made it to the swamps of Florida, where they joined the Seminole Nation or stowed away on boats bound for the Caribbean, while some Texan slaves made their escape to Mexico, which had banned slavery upon independence from Spain in 1821. But the odds against escaping the South were long. The distances were enormous. White patrols, supplemented with bloodhounds, constantly patrolled the roads. Any black person off the plantation was presumed to be a runaway—and if stopped by a white, who was usually armed—would be forced to produce a pass. Thus, the odds were best for those who lived near the free states. Still, it is estimated that approximately 1,000 slaves annually made it to freedom during the 1840s and 1850s. Many, if not most, were aided in their escape by a network of black and white abolitionists—that is, those who opposed slavery on moral grounds—that came to be called the Underground Railroad.

Because of the intense secrecy that shrouded its operations, much about the Underground Railroad has been lost to history. As slaves were property, freeing them was a form of theft under state and federal law. Penalties for those who participated were severe, especially for blacks. While whites risked arrest, prison, and fines, black "conductors" and "station masters"—as guides and owners of safe houses (places where runaway slaves could hide) were respectively called—risked being sent back into slavery. Even free blacks in the North could be re-enslaved if caught aiding runaways. For instance, abolitionist Frederick Douglass, born a slave on the Eastern Shore of Maryland, made his way north by borrowing the papers of a free black sailor. Had

The Underground Railroad

Douglass been caught, it is highly likely that the sailor would have been punished by enslavement.

While some slaves, like Douglass, made their way north by boat, most traveled by land routes. In general, a slave's best chance of escape came if he or she was escorted northward by a "conductor," a free black or former slave living in the North who traveled South to serve as a guide. The most famous of these was Harriet Tubman. Like Douglass, Tubman was born a slave on Maryland's Eastern Shore, not far from the free state of Pennsylvania. As a teen, she was severely injured when her owner threw a two-pound weight at a runaway slave Tubman was shielding. The weight hit Tubman in the head, leaving a deep scar and a propensity for headaches and dizzy spells the rest of her life. After marrying a free black in 1844, Tubman searched for ways to escape bondage. She first tried the law and, when that failed, she escaped to the North in 1849. (Her husband refused to go along so she went alone.)

Working as a maid and cook in Philadelphia, Tubman saved her earnings and plotted a trip to Baltimore to free her sister and her sister's two children in 1850. Between that year and the outbreak of the Civil War, Tubman—despite a bounty on her head, dead or alive—made more than 15 trips into the South, liberating some 200 slaves, including her entire family. Unlike in the early years of the Railroad—when most runaways were settled in the free black communities of the North—Tubman was forced to deal with the Fugitive Slave Act, which required northern authorities return all runaways or face federal criminal prosecution. To cope, she connected up with a network of safe houses and guides who could lead escaped slaves to Canada.

As noted above, for those slaves living in the Deep South, escape to Mexico and Florida were alternatives to the North. Before the Civil War, hundreds of black Texas slaves made their way to freedom in Mexico. In the mid-1850s, noted landscape architect Fredrick Law Olmstead reported meeting an escaped slave in Mexico:

He very civilly informed me ... that he was born in Virginia, and had been brought South by a trader and sold to a gentleman who had brought him to Texas, from whom he had run away four or five years ago. He would like ... to see old Virginia again, that he would—if he could be free. He was a mechanic, and could earn a dollar very easily, by his trade, every day. He could speak Spanish fluently, and had traveled extensively in Mexico, sometimes on his own business, and sometimes as a servant or muleteer.... He

had joined the Catholic Church, he said, and he was very well satisfied with the country. Runaways were constantly arriving here; two had got over, as I had previously been informed, the night before. He could not guess how many came in a year, but he could count forty, that he had known of, in the last three months....

THE SEMINOLE WARS

Far more runaways found their way to Florida, a then sparsely settled territory of marshes, subtropiocal forests, and scrubland. Ensconced in these wilds were runaway blacks and a nation of Indians, known as the Seminole, who continued to resist southern planters and even the U.S. Army right up to the verge of the Civil War. The Seminole—named from a Creek version of the Spanish word for "runaway" or "wild"—had been one of the "Five Civilized Tribes" of the Southeast, displaced by white settlers and the government in the late 1700s and early 1800s. Rather than being moved to Oklahoma, however, most of the Seminole escaped to Florida—a land of dense forests and extensive swamps that, as a Spanish colony, lay outside the jurisdiction of the United States.

There, the two communities—Native American and African American—developed a symbiotic relationship whereby the latter did much of the agricultural work while the former offered land and protection against invading whites. Technically, the blacks were slaves of the Native Americans but that was largely for legal cover. In fact, the two lived largely as equals, with blacks assuming many positions of leadership within the tribe. For blacks, the existence of an independent mixed race society on slavery's southern border was a ready inducement for escape. For British and later American planters, the existence of this independent black and Indian community was a major irritant. During colonial times, the Spanish—who owned Florida—encouraged these runaways, going so far as to arm them as a defense against British incursions. In the early years of the American republic, planters and militiamen from Georgia would launch periodic raids to recapture runaways.

Beginning in 1816, U.S. Army troops got into the fight. In that year, General Andrew Jackson—who, later, as president set the Trail of Tears into motion—led a major expedition against the Seminole and their stronghold on Apalachicola Bay, a place known as Fort Negro. Surrounded by cannon fire from land and sea, 300 Seminole

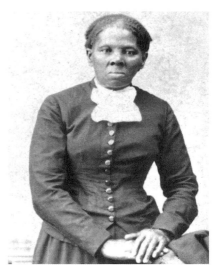

Harriet Tubman (Library of Congress)

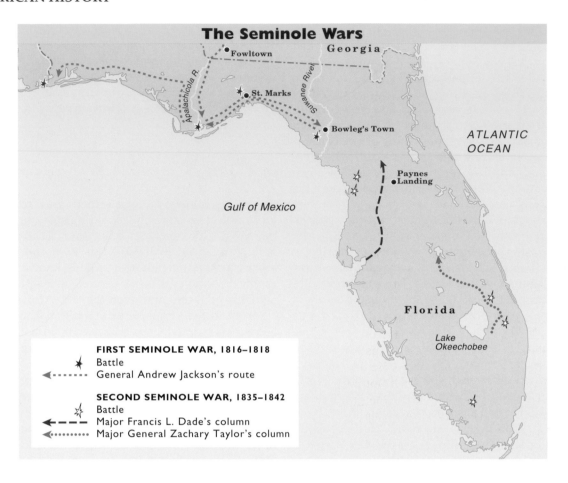

The Seminole Wars

FIRST SEMINOLE WAR, 1816–1818
✱ Battle
◄┄┄┄┄ General Andrew Jackson's route

SECOND SEMINOLE WAR, 1835–1842
✩ Battle
◄━ ━ ━ Major Francis L. Dade's column
◄┄┄┄┄ Major General Zachary Taylor's column

men, women, and children held out until a well-placed shot from a U.S. warship struck the fort's ammunition dump, causing an explosion that killed most of the defenders. Hundreds of other Seminole living in the Pensacola region continued to resist. By 1818, the year before Florida itself was purchased from the Spanish and incorporated as a U.S. territory, most Seminole had been pushed farther south. With this U.S. victory, what is known as the First Seminole War had ended, although scattered skirmishes continued over the next several years.

Then U.S. policy was to make promises of land to the Native Americans, in exchange for the return of runaway slaves. While Seminole leaders generally refused to turn over runaway slaves, fear of such a deal caused many black Seminole to set up separate communities within the wilds of Florida, although many blacks continued to live among and marry Native Americans. In the 1830s, the U.S. government again began pressuring Seminole to join the other "civilized tribes" in emigrating to Oklahoma and other lands west of the Mississippi River. In 1835, some of the Seminole chiefs were tricked into signing a misleading treaty that appeared to promise them the right to remain in Florida but actually called for their removal. When the truth about the treaty was revealed, an army of

black and Native American Seminole launched attacks on white plantations and U.S. Army outposts, sparking the Second Seminole War.

For several years, the U.S. Army and the Seminole fought skirmishes and battles throughout northern and central Florida. Under the leadership of chiefs Osceola, King Philip, and Wild Cat, Seminole warriors pursued a guerrilla strategy of hitting the U.S. Army when they least expected it, and then disappearing into the swamps they had come to know so well. With Seminole facing extradition to Oklahoma and blacks re-enslavement, the fighting became bitter. General Thomas Sidney Jesup, commander of U.S. forces in the Second Seminole War, recognized the importance of the black Seminoles in the resistance. "This, you may be assured," he told his superiors in Washington, "is a negro and not an Indian war. . . . Throughout my operations I found the negroes the most active and determined warriors; and during my conferences with the Indian chief [Osceola] I ascertained that they exercised an almost controlling interest over [him]."

However, using trickery and overwhelming force, Jesup and the U.S. Army were eventually able to capture Osceola and wear down much of the Seminole's resistance. By 1842, most of the Seminole had surrendered, with hundreds sent west to Arkansas and Oklahoma and many blacks forced back into slavery. A reporter for *Harper's Weekly* noted in that year, "The negro slaves are, in fact, the masters of their own red owners. . . . The negroes were the master spirits, as well as the immediate occasion, of the Florida wars. They openly refused to follow their masters if they removed to Arkansas; it was not until they capitulated that the Seminoles ever thought of emigrating."

Still, a small band of African Americans and Seminole continued to hold out in the Everglade swamps of southern Florida. A series of sporadic skirmishes, sometimes called the Third Seminole War, continued until 1858. These last survivors won a major concession from the federal government, which allowed them to stay on in southern Florida, where they live to this day. Today's mixed-race Florida Seminole are proud to say that they fought the longest war in American history against the U.S. government and that they never signed a treaty ending the war.

Slave Rebellions

The mixed-race Seminole represent the most long-lived armed resistance to the slave regime in American history and the best example of a runaway slave community surviving within U.S. territory. But armed resistance to the slave regime of the South was hardly confined to Florida and the Seminole. The first major slave uprising in American history occurred in South Carolina on September 9, 1739, when hundreds of slaves gathered along the Stono River and then marched from plantation to plantation killing masters and freeing slaves. The rebellion, which lasted but a single day, resulted in the deaths of some 60 people including 35 slaves and was put down by colonial militias. The Stono Rebellion resulted in a series of harsh edicts that restricted freedom of movement and assembly and banned the right of slaves to earn money or learn to read. In addition, the colonial assembly outlawed the "speaking drum," an African instrument that was

SLAVE UPRISINGS IN NORTH AMERICA, 1663–1831

1 **1663** African slaves join white indentured servants in Gloucester County, Virginia, to plan a revolt. When the plan is discovered, the black leaders are beheaded and their heads publically displayed in the village square.

2 **1712** Twenty-one slaves are executed in New York City for their part in an uprising.

3 **1739** Fifty to 100 slaves at Stono, South Carolina, flee the South with stolen arms, killing all whites who attempt to stop them. They are later captured.

4 **1741** Although the evidence is scant, 31 slaves are charged with burning down several properties in New York and exectuted.

5 **1741** In Boston, slaves are caught trying to escape to Florida in a stolen boat.

6 **1800** Gabriel Prosser, a Virginia slave, plans an attack on Richmond, Virginia. Most of the 40,000 slaves living in the region were thought to know the plan. Before the revolt is set to take place, the plan is discovered and Richmond placed under martial law. Then torrential rains on the evening that the uprising is set to begin disrupt the plan completely. Prosser is captured and hanged a month later.

7 **1822** Denmark Vesey, a free black carpenter, plans a revolt to conquer Charleston, South Carolina. When his plan is discovered, he and 47 others are executed.

8 **1831** Nat Turner, a slave whose father had escaped to freedom, leads a group of slaves through Southampton County, Virginia, after swearing to kill all whites in surrounding plantations. Just over 24 hours later, he and his men have killed more than 60 white men, women, and children. In retalliation, whites throughout the South kill more than 100 blacks, regardless of their involvement in the revolt.

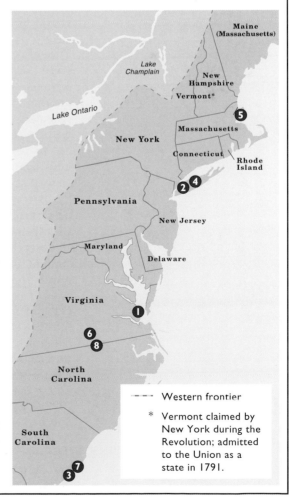

- - - Western frontier

* Vermont claimed by New York during the Revolution; admitted to the Union as a state in 1791.

used at Stono to call slaves to rebellion. While numerous acts of violent resistance continued throughout the colonial period, most were small-scale and many have been lost to history. It would take more than 60 years for African Americans of the South to attempt another major uprising against the slave regime, this time in the Virginia area.

The 1790s and 1800s were a tense time in the upper South; the wave of manumissions following the Revolution had largely come to an end. As discussed in the previous chapter, however, planters in the United States had closely followed the violence in Haiti that began in 1791 and ended with the overthrow of the white regime in 1804. Two years after the Haitian rebellion started, the U.S. Congress passed the first fugitive slave law, allowing owners to reclaim escaped slaves who had crossed state lines. In 1800, a self-educated blacksmith in the Richmond area named Gabriel Prosser organized a rebellion that may have involved up to 600 slaves. Angry at the fact that his master kept most of his earnings as an itinerant craftsman—and believing that the nation was facing an imminent political crisis during an election year that saw Democrats take over the government from Federalists—Prosser selected the night of August 30 for the uprising. But a major thunderstorm forced him to postpone the rebellion for 24 hours, during which time several slaves betrayed the plot to whites. Though hundreds of African Americans were arrested, Prosser escaped on a schooner to Norfolk. Unfortunately for him, another slave—enticed by a $300 reward—revealed his whereabouts. Prosser, along with 26 other slaves, were tried and executed. In response, Virginia strengthened its laws against slave assemblies and literacy, as well as bolstering its militia.

Betrayal also doomed the new republic's second major rebellion, this one in Charleston, South Carolina, in 1822. Fear of slave uprisings was particularly acute in the state as the population of blacks had outnumbered that of whites for nearly a century. Moreover, Charleston was one of the few cities of the Deep South with a significant number of free blacks. Among these was Denmark Vesey, a former slave who had purchased his freedom after winning a state lottery in 1799. A successful carpenter, Vesey had amassed $8,000 in savings by 1822, a fortune for a free black man of the South in those years. Yet, despite his personal prosperity, Vesey dedicated his life to destroying the institution of slavery, speaking at gatherings in black churches and workshops. By 1822, he had gathered a small cadre of like-minded blacks—both enslaved and free—willing to launch an uprising against the white population. Planned for late July, the conspiracy was betrayed by several slaves in May. Cash awards were offered to those who turned in conspirators and, on July 2, Vesey was arrested. Refusing to confess, Vesey and 34 other African Americans were executed. Once again, harsh laws were passed following the discovery of the conspiracy, including a law that required all free black sailors be jailed while their ships were in port.

Despite such measures, rebellions large and small continued across the South, reaching a culmination in the bloodiest slave uprising in American history: the Nat Turner revolt of 1831. Turner was born a slave in Virginia's Southampton County on October 2, 1800, just five days before the execution of Gabriel Prosser. His father had run away when Turner was a boy, where it is believed he lived out his life as a runaway slave in the Great Dismal Swamp along the North Carolina border. Turner's mother was just seven years removed from Africa when she gave birth to Nat and constantly told her son that he was destined for great things. Deeply spiritual and a self-educated biblical scholar, Turner claimed to receive visions all of his life. In 1821, his master, Benjamin Turner, hired a particularly violent overseer and Nat escaped for a month, during which time he claimed God told him to lead a slave rebellion. Over the next decade, Turner became an itinerant preacher, traveling from plantation to plantation giving sermons on the necessity of violent liberation. An eclipse of the sun in February 1831 was, in Turner's mind, a signal that the time for revolt was ripe. He soon began recruiting a small cadre of followers with the symbolic date of July 4 as their day to launch the rebellion. When Turner got sick, the date was pushed back six weeks.

On August 22, Turner and his band of followers began their attack, striking first on the plantation of Joseph Travis, where Turner then lived. The strategy was simple and brutal; they would move from plantation to plantation slaughtering masters and their families until they had intimidated the local white community and raised an army of rebel slaves. At that point, the killing would cease and the slave army would head for Jerusalem, Virginia, Southampton's county seat and the site of a major arsenal. Armed, they would make their way to the Great Dismal Swamp where they would establish an armed free black community impervious to white counterattack. Over the next couple of days, the rebels—

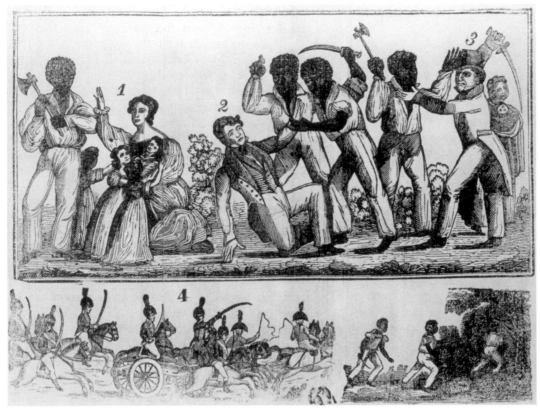

The broadside above depicts Nat Turner's Rebellion as follows: 1. A woman pleads for the life of her children; 2. Mr. Travis is murdered by his own slaves; 3. Mr. Barrow defends himself so his wife can escape; 4. Mounted dragoons in persuit of slaves. (Library of Congress)

now some 60 or 70 in all—murdered 57 whites, though it is believed that Turner himself killed no one. But as the element of surprise faded, local white militias counterattacked, killing some 100 blacks in the process and ending the uprising. Turner, however, escaped and was not apprehended until October 30. Following a brief trial, he was executed on November 11, 1831, after offering a detailed confession and biography to a court-appointed attorney.

Like the Prosser and Vesey rebellions before it, the Nat Turner uprising led to harsh new disciplinary edicts and practices. Beyond that, the Turner rebellion marked a pivotal moment in the history of American slavery and in the development of the antislavery movement. The uprising ended any lingering thoughts that slavery might fade away peacefully in the upper South while, at the same time, dispelling the belief that slaves were largely contented with their lot. Coming in the same year that William Lloyd Garrison launched his fiercely abolitionist newspaper—*The Liberator*—Turner's rebellion sharpened the conflict between antislavery and proslavery forces in the North and South. It also strengthened the idea—particularly in the upper South, where slavery was increasingly seen as no longer economically viable—that the only way to effectively deal with the presence of blacks in America was to eliminate it, banishing blacks to Africa.

ANTISLAVERY MOVEMENT

The idea of sending African Americans back to their African homeland was not a new one in the 1830s. Indeed, many of the founding fathers, including Thomas Jefferson, believed that the African and Caucasian races—given the history of black subjugation and the supposedly different abilities of the two races—could not live in peace in the same land. As a Virginia legislator, Jefferson had advocated sending freed blacks to "a far away place selected as the circumstances of the time should render most proper." As hopes that the American Revolution might lead to a more equal society for African Americans faded in the late 18th century and early 19th century, the idea of "colonization"—as the return to Africa proposal was called—caught on among leading whites and a few free blacks.

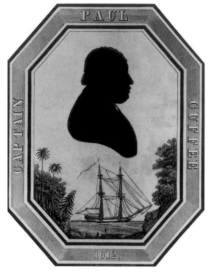

Paul Cuffe (Library of Congress)

AFRICAN COLONIZATION

Among the free blacks who supported re-Africanization was Paul Cuffe, a wealthy black shipowner from New Bedford, Massachusetts. Cuffe believed he had a duty to help his fellow Africans, both in America and Africa. Sending blacks back to Africa offered a way to do both. For African Americans, it would mean an opportunity to escape white racism and build a community of their own, proving to the world that blacks were capable of self-government. At the same time, these settlers would bring civilization and Christianity to their long-lost brothers in Africa. In 1811, Cuffe visited Sierra Leone, a British colony established as a haven for former slaves from Britain, North America and the Caribbean. Four years later, he sent the first shipload of settlers to Sierra Leone at his own expense. But his death two years later ended the project.

Meanwhile, a group of influential whites—including Kentucky senator Henry Clay, future president Andrew Jackson, "Star Spangled Banner" author Francis Scott Key, and Bushrod Washington, nephew of George—established the American Colonization Society (ACS) in Washington in 1816. The goals of the society were decidedly mixed ones. "Can there be a nobler cause," Clay, a wealthy planter and slaveowner, asked his fellow colonizationists, "than that which, while it proposes to rid our own country of a useless and pernicious, if not dangerous, portion of the population, contemplates the spreading of the arts of civilized life, and the possible redemption from ignorance of a benighted portion of the globe?" Indeed, from the beginning, colonization was tainted by its association with slaveholders and denounced by free blacks and, later, abolitionists as a way to force free African Americans—many of whom traced their ancestry in America back for generations—out of the country, while preserving slave status for the vast majority of blacks. "We have no wish to separate from our present homes for any purpose whatsoever," declared a statement issued by 3,000 African Americans meeting at Philadelphia's Bethel Church in 1817, adding "we only want the use of those opportunities . . . which the Constitution and the laws allow to us all."

Still, the ACS achieved some success. In 1820, it sponsored its first shipment of 86 blacks to the British colony of Sierra Leone. After a sojourn ridden with disease, colonists moved southward to found the colony of Liberia. Over the next four decades, more than 10,000 African Americans settled in Liberia. In 1847, the colonists—a mix of free blacks from the North, freed slaves from the South, and Africans recaptured from slavers on the high seas—declared their independence from the ACS, making Liberia Africa's first republic. Indeed, aside from Ethiopia, it would remain the only part of Africa to escape European colonialism in the 19th and 20th centuries. For roughly 150 years, Liberia was ruled by the descendents of African Americans—the so-called Americo-Liberians—until their regime was overthrown in a 1980 coup.

ABOLITIONISM

Although somewhat successful, the colonization idea was displaced in the 1830s by a new and more radical movement—abolitionism. While colonizationists spoke of a gradual end to slavery through emigration—an impossible proposal given the millions of blacks already living in America—abolitionists called for the institution's immediate demise. They dismissed the colonizationists as co-conspirators of planters, seeking to rid the country of its unwanted free black population.

Meanwhile, throughout the North, free black communities in the 1820s were endorsing ever more radical measures to end slavery, even if they involved violence.

Freetown, the present-day capital of Sierra Leone, was founded in 1787 by the British Sierra Leone Company as a haven for former slaves from Great Britain, North America, and the Caribbean. In 1820, the American Colonization Society (ACS) sent the first group of freedpersons from the United States to Sierra Leone. Two years later, that group moved south to present-day Liberia, where they founded the city that would later become Monrovia. Liberia became the first independent republic in 1847.

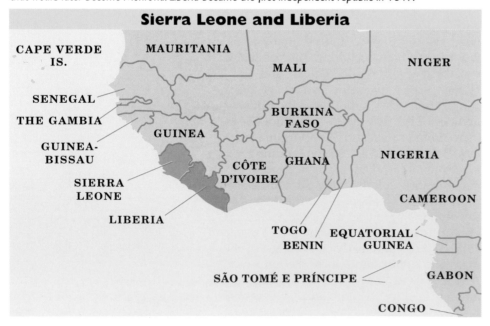

Sierra Leone and Liberia

CAPE VERDE IS.
MAURITANIA
MALI
NIGER
SENEGAL
THE GAMBIA
GUINEA-BISSAU
GUINEA
BURKINA FASO
SIERRA LEONE
CÔTE D'IVOIRE
GHANA
NIGERIA
LIBERIA
CAMEROON
TOGO
BENIN
EQUATORIAL GUINEA
SÃO TOMÉ E PRÍNCIPE
GABON
CONGO

In 1829 came the most incendiary statement yet. The pamphlet *An Appeal . . . to the Colored Citizens of the World* declared to whites: "We must and shall be free . . . in spite of you. . . . And woe, woe, will be it to you if we have to obtain our freedom by fighting." Written by David Walker, a used clothing salesman and pamphleteer living in Boston, and commonly known as Walker's Appeal, the tract also violently refuted white claims to racial superiority. "I do declare that one good black man can put to death six white men," wrote Walker, who soon gained an enthusiastic black audience. The pamphlet went through three printings and even showed up among free black communities in the South.

Meanwhile, sentiment was shifting among white opponents of slavery as well. The wave of evangelical Christianity that swept much of the upper Midwest, upstate New York, and New England in the 1820s inspired a new condemnation of slavery. The religious message of the Great Awakening—as the movement was called—emphasized the individual moral agency of all human beings. Being a good Christian meant choosing to follow God's plan. By keeping African Americans in bondage, slave owners were keeping them in darkness, unable to make the moral choice God had given all human beings. The implications of this argument were clear: slavery was a sin and slaveholders were contravening God's will. To many evangelicals, there could be no compromise with slavery, no gradualist approach to its extinction. Nat Turner's 1831 uprising seemed like a sign to many that God's patience with America and its compromise with the forces of evil—that is, with slavery—was running thin.

That same year, William Lloyd Garrison, a Boston-based printer and evangelical Christian, launched a weekly abolitionist newspaper, *The Liberator*. In its first issue, the editor made his intentions clear: "I will be harsh as truth and as uncompromising as justice. . . . I am in earnest—I will not equivocate—I will not excuse—I will not retreat a single inch—AND I WILL BE HEARD." In later issues, Garrison would go on to denounce the American Constitution—with its unwritten acceptance of slavery—as "a covenant with death, an agreement with Hell." Garrison's fiery language and uncompromising convictions attracted other like-minded opponents of slavery. In 1833, Garrison joined with Theodore Weld—an upstate New York preacher—and Arthur and Lewis Tappan—wealthy merchant brothers from New York City—to form the American Anti-Slavery Society.

The society's members took two approaches to their crusade. The first was aimed at the public. Borrowing techniques from the revivalist churches, they held public meetings where eloquent and passionate speakers offered the equivalent of sermons on the theme of abolitionism. Many evangelical women became caught up in the crusade, going so far as to speak to mixed sex audiences on the subject, unprecedented events that shocked the gender sensibilities of the day. (Indeed, the antislavery movement proved to be one of the seedbeds of the women's movement, which grew to fruition in the same abolitionist strongholds and culminated in the first women's rights convention in American history, held at Seneca Falls, New York, in 1848.)

And, of course, the abolitionist movement drew on black speakers as well. In 1841, a white abolitionist in New Bedford, Massachusetts invited a young, escaped slave named Frederick Douglass to speak at a meeting on Nantucket Island. The power and conviction of Douglass's testimony

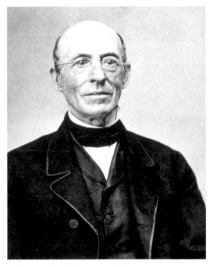

William Lloyd Garrison (Library of Congress)

William Lloyd Garrison's The Liberator (Library of Congress)

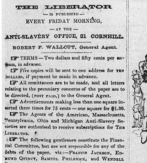
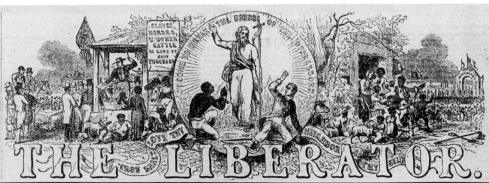

THE LIFE OF FREDERICK DOUGLASS

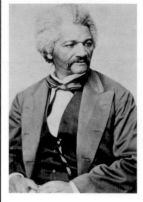

". . . If there is no struggle there is no progress. Those who profess to favor freedom and depreciate agitation are men who want crops without plowing up the ground, they want rain without thunder and lightning, they want the ocean without the awful roar of its mighty waters."

—Frederick Douglass

Of figures from the 19th century, Frederick Douglass is among the most revered. Following his escape from slavery in 1838 at the age of 21, he became an international figure, speaking out against the "peculiar institution" of slavery throughout the North and in England. Although the abolition of slavery was his primary concern, he increasingly spoke out on a wide range of human rights causes, from prison reform and public education to international peace. His speeches often pointed out the hypocrisy of the fact that the same patriotic Americans who fought for liberty and freedom could enslave an entire people. His ties were particularly strong with the women's suffrage movement until he broke with movement leaders in 1866 over whether black men should be granted voting rights before women. Through his alliances with other abolitionists such as William Lloyd Garrison, the publisher of *The Liberator*, he was able to further the cause of emancipation for the enslaved.

1817 or 1818	Frederick Augustus Washington Bailey is born in Tuckahoe, Maryland.
1826	At age nine, he is sent to Baltimore, Maryland, to work as a houseboy. While there, his master's wife teaches Bailey to read and write, although educating slaves was forbidden by law.
1833	He is returned to his plantation home as a field hand.
1836	He attempts an escape but fails; soon thereafter, he is sent back to Baltimore to work as an apprentice to a ship's caulker. Soon after arriving there, he meets Anna Murray, a free black woman and his future wife.
1838	After Anna Murray gives him money for an escape attempt, Bailey borrows a sailor suit and some official looking papers and escapes by sea. He makes his way to New York City, where he is joined by Anna Murray. The two then move to the Quaker fishing center (an abolitionist stronghold) of New Bedford, Massachusetts, where the newlyweds adopt the last name Douglass.
1841	Without the benefit of written notes, Douglass gives an impassioned address to the Massachusetts Anti-Slavery Society in Nantucket and is immediately employed as one of their agents. For the next four years, he travels on speaking engagements throughout the North.
1843	On speaking tours of New England and the Midwest, Douglass is joined on the podium by a former slave named Isabella Baumfree, who states that she has been called by God to rename herself Sojourner Truth. Although she is illiterate, she matches Douglass in her powerful oratory skill.
1845	Douglass publishes his autobiography *Narrative of the Life of Frederick Douglass, An American Slave* in order to refute those who claim that because of his powerful speaking ability he could not actually have been a slave. Following the publication of the book, he moves to England to avoid recapture. While there, he continues to speak out publicly against slavery. He also broadens the scope of his efforts

won him a role as abolitionism's most famous and effective spokesperson. In addition, abolitionists published hundreds of thousands of pamphlets, flooding the North and the South with antislavery propaganda. The purpose of this approach, known as "moral suasion," was to create a moral climate in which slave owners would recognize the error of their ways and move to end slavery. While the campaign did little to change the moral stance of most slave owners, it did increase the public pressure on them. In response, southern officials began routinely raiding post offices to seize and destroy the literature.

The abolitionists also published—and sometimes ghost-authored—slave narratives. Usually written in the melodramatic style of 19th century literature, these narratives told of the unspeakable barbarities of the slave regime—beatings, torture, rape, and the anguished cries of mothers torn from their children at slave auctions. To modern readers, the most powerful narratives were those written in the clear and unadorned prose of the former slaves themselves. Among the most famous of these tracts are Frederick Douglass's *Narrative of the Life of Frederick Douglass, an American Slave*, Solomon Northrup's *Twelve Years a Slave*, and Harriet Jacobs's *Incidents in the Life of a Slave Girl*.

A second strategy of the abolitionists was aimed at politicians. In order to convince Congress of the depth of antislavery sentiment in the North, the Anti-Slavery Society encouraged local chapters to inundate Congress with petitions calling for laws that were in its purview to pass, including the abolition of slavery in Washington, D.C.; a ban on the interstate slave trade; the removal of the "three-fifths compromise" in the Constitution, which enhanced southern legislative representation; and a ban on the admission of new slave states. (As slaves were considered legal property, slavery was protected by the Constitution; banning slavery required a

	by speaking in favor of Irish home rule, on behalf of landless European peasantry, and on such issues as prison reform, free public education, and women's suffrage.
1847	As Douglass prepares to return from England, a group of British female abolitionists pay $711.96 to buy him his freedom. They also supply him with a printing press. Rejoining his family, Douglass moves to Rochester, New York, and begins to publish his antislavery newspaper *The North Star*. Douglass is also elected president of the New England Anti-Slavery Society.
1848	Douglass becomes president of the Colored Convention Movement, which advocates racial solidarity and economic improvement. He is a featured speaker at the Seneca Falls, New York convention at the Wesleyan church chapel, organized by Elizabeth Cady Stanton and Lucretia Mott, that launches the women's suffrage movement.
1849	The Women's Association of Philadelphia forms to help Douglass raise money for *The North Star*. By this time, the Douglass's household has become an Underground Railroad "station." Although Frederick Douglass is often away from home, Anna Murray Douglass sees that runaways are always welcome.
1851	Douglass publicly splits with William Lloyd Garrison over the issue of moral pressure versus political participation as a means towards abolition of slavery. Douglass joins the abolitionist Liberty Party and is named its candidate for vice president.
1855	He publishes a revision of his autobiography entitled *My Bondage and My Freedom (Part I: Life as a Slave, Part II: Life as a Freeman)*. The Liberty Party nominates him for the post of New York secretary of state, making him the first African American nominated for statewide office.
1859	Douglass is invited by John Brown to participate in his raid on Harpers Ferry, Virginia. Douglass denounces the plan as

	suicide. Nonetheless, following the attack, he is accused of supporting it and is forced to flee to Canada and then London.
1860	Douglass returns from England after learning of the death of Annie, his youngest child, at age 11. He campaigns for the repeal of a New York law that requires black men to own $250 in order to vote.
1861	Douglass campaigns for blacks to be allowed to serve in the Union army.
1863	Douglass helps recruit African Americans in Massachusetts, New York, and Pennsylvania to serve in the all-black Fifty-fourth Massachusetts Regiment and visits President Abraham Lincoln to protest discrimination against black troops.
1864	Douglass appeals for black male suffrage.
1866	Douglass attends an Equal Rights Association convention and breaks with women's rights leaders over whether African-American men should receive the vote before the same right is given to all women as well.
1872	After the Douglass home in Rochester is destroyed by fire, the family moves to Washington, D.C.
1874	Douglass becomes president of the financially troubled Freedmen's Bank. To encourage investment, Douglass deposits his own money and appeals to the U.S. Senate for aid. Nonetheless, confidence in the bank continues to fall, and the bank collapses.
1877–1881	Douglass serves as marshal of the District of Columbia.
1881–1884	Douglass serves as recorder of deeds for the District of Columbia.
1889–1891	Douglass serves as minister to Haiti.
1895	Douglass dies in Anacostia Heights, D.C. Congressman George Washington Murray (R-SC) attempts to have his body lie in state in the Capitol rotunda, but House Speaker Charles Crisp (D-GA) refuses to permit it.

constitutional amendment.) So many petitions flooded Washington that, in 1836, southern Congressmen and their northern sympathizers pushed through the "gag rule," whereby all petitions against slavery were automatically tabled so that they could not become the subject of debate. The law—a clear denial of the 1st amendment—would remain in effect for eight years.

Eventually, the efforts of the political wing of the abolitionist movement led to the establishment of the Liberty Party in 1840, the first political party in American history expressly devoted to ending slavery. Although winning less than 3 percent of the northern vote in the 1844 presidential elections, the Liberty Party eventually gave way to the Free Soil Party in the late 1840s, a much larger party with a more popular—although, less radical—mandate of preventing the spread of slavery to the West. The Free Soil Party—with expresident Martin Van Buren as its nominee—won more than 10 percent of the vote in 1848 and paved the

way for the antislavery Republican Party of the 1850s.

Despite this success, the political strategy helped split the abolitionist movement. Radical white abolitionists—led by Garrison—believed that working with politicians compromised the idea of abolitionism as a moral crusade against evil. At the same time, more moderate white abolitionists and the majority of black abolitionists—coalescing around Douglass—took a more pragmatic approach, hoping that political and legislative action would gradually put slavery on the road to extinction. Ultimately—with proslavery power increasing in the 1850s—Douglass and anti-Garrisonian radicals like John Brown would come to the conclusion that neither the political nor the moral suasion route offered a solution to the slavery problem. Instead, direct action was necessary, though when Brown and a number of radical white abolitionists suggested an invasion of the South in 1859, Douglass dismissed the idea as folly.

The abolitionists' place in history—and their role in ending slavery—is a complicated one. On the one hand, most of their efforts—either radical or pragmatic—failed. Few slave owners were ever convinced of the errors of their ways and Congress failed to pass any of the legislation desired by the abolitionists, at least until the Civil War. Indeed, the rhetoric and action of the abolitionists stirred up a hornet's nest of protest in the North, where many whites feared a flood of unwanted black migrants should slavery be ended in the South. Abolitionist speakers like Douglass and Garrison were often attacked verbally and even physically by antiabolitionists. In 1837, the movement got its first martyr in Elijah Lovejoy, an abolitionist editor murdered by a white mob in Alton, Illinois.

And yet through this very controversy, abolitionists achieved success of a kind. Until the crisis decade of the 1850s, most Americans accepted slavery as a fact of national life. For southerners, it was a way of life; for northerners, it was a distant and abstract issue. For almost all Americans, it didn't seem worth fighting over. And politicians did their best to keep things that way. Slavery was a no-win issue; support it too strongly and one offended northerners; oppose it, and one alienated the South. It was best to just ignore it. But abolitionists, with their speeches, pamphlets, and petitions, made it increasingly hard to ignore slavery as a political and moral issue. Moreover, as proslavery politicians and white mobs attacked abolitionists, they turned them into martyrs, not so much to the cause of black freedom but to the causes of freedom of speech, assembly, and press. Most northerners were both racist and against slavery. They wanted to keep blacks—enslaved or free—out of the North and West. As southern politicians and their northern allies passed proslavery legislation, northerners felt that their political will was being ignored or actively subverted. Abolitionists, then, were critical in raising the national political temperature to a degree high enough to spark the Civil War, which ultimately destroyed slavery.

THE MARCH TOWARD WAR

Slavery as a political issue went back all the way back to the Constitution. In creating a document that would appeal to southerners, northern statesmen—who wanted a constitution that created a strong, pro-trade central government—agreed to a compromise whereby slaves would count as three-fifths persons for the purposes of apportioning representation. As the South was then the largest region of country, it was expected that it would have the largest population and the most representatives. In short, northerners got the kind of government they wanted but at the price of allowing southerners to run it. This compromise rested, however, on a premise that ultimately proved to be false. Because of the presence of a slave labor force, few immigrant laborers moved to the South and the North soon surpassed it in population.

MISSOURI COMPROMISE

In 1819, a challenge to the three-fifths compromise emerged. After accepting the admission of several slave states in the 1810s, northern politicians finally put their foot down when Missouri asked to join the Union as yet another. For two years, Congress divided bitterly over the issue, until a compromise was hammered together by House Speaker Henry Clay of Kentucky. Under the Missouri Compromise, that state would join the Union alongside the free state of Maine. Thus was inaugurated a new sectional balancing act, whereby states would enter in pairs—one free state for every slave state. And so while the House of Representatives—which was based on population—came to be dominated by northerners, the Senate—which guaranteed each state two members—would maintain a balance of power between the two regions. Moreover, to satisfy lingering northern suspicions of slavery dominating the West, a line was drawn from Missouri's southern border—at 36° 30' latitude—to the Pacific Ocean, even though most of this territory belonged to the newly independent country of Mexico. To many Americans—including an aging Thomas Jefferson—the Missouri Compromise portended dangerous divisions within the republic. "This momentous question, like a firebell in the night," wrote the retired president, "awakened and filled me with terror."

THE MEXICAN WAR AND THE COMPROMISE OF 1850

Jefferson's fears were not idle ones. In the mid-1830s, Texas won its independence from Mexico—partly to escape the latter's edicts against slavery—and sought to enter the American Union as a slave state, a move

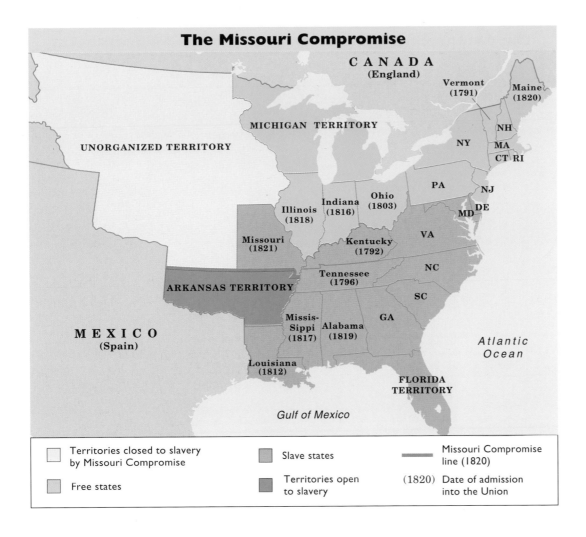

The Missouri Compromise

| | Territories closed to slavery by Missouri Compromise | | Slave states | | Missouri Compromise line (1820) |
| | Free states | | Territories open to slavery | (1820) | Date of admission into the Union |

blocked by antislavery forces in the North. Angry southerners then began pressuring the national government to acquire western lands open to slavery below the Missouri Compromise line, a plan that was bound to lead to hostilities with Mexico. In 1845, southerners won the admission of Texas into the Union as a slave state. A year later, President James Polk, a slave owner from Tennessee and a determined expansionist, provoked a war with Mexico by sending American troops into disputed territory along the Rio Grande. When Mexican soldiers fired on the Americans, Polk and southerners in Congress declared war. David Wilmot, a Free Soil congressman from Pennsylvania, tried to undermine the southerners' plans by introducing a proviso making all territories acquired from Mexico free, but his efforts were brushed aside by proslavery forces in Congress.

From the beginning, the war was an unequal one. Mexico proved to be no match for the United States and, after two years of hostilities, was forced to cede the northern third of its territory to the United States for a nominal payment of $15 million. Suddenly, southerners had what they wanted—vast new American territories for the expansion of slavery. Although somewhat

mollified by the acquisition of the Oregon territory from Britain in 1846, northerners cried foul, arguing that the war was part of a southern conspiracy to spread slavery and dominate the Union. The sense of crisis was stoked by the discovery of gold in newly acquired California in 1848. With hundreds of thousands of settlers—largely from the North—pouring in, the Pacific Coast territory asked to join the Union as a free state in 1850.

But with no equivalent slave territory ready to enter the Union, California's request provoked the most serious sectional crisis since Missouri. Over the course of the year—and after some of the bitterest debate in congressional history—an elaborate new compromise was reached. Although involving a series of delicately balanced elements, the Compromise of 1850 boiled down to two controversial provisions. First, California would be admitted into the Union as a free state, giving the North a 16 to 15 state advantage in the Senate. Second, as a concession to southerners, Congress passed the infamous Fugitive Slave Act. For the first time, the federal government became a seriously active participant in enforcing the law against runaway slaves. Under the act, fugitive slaves and even free blacks anywhere

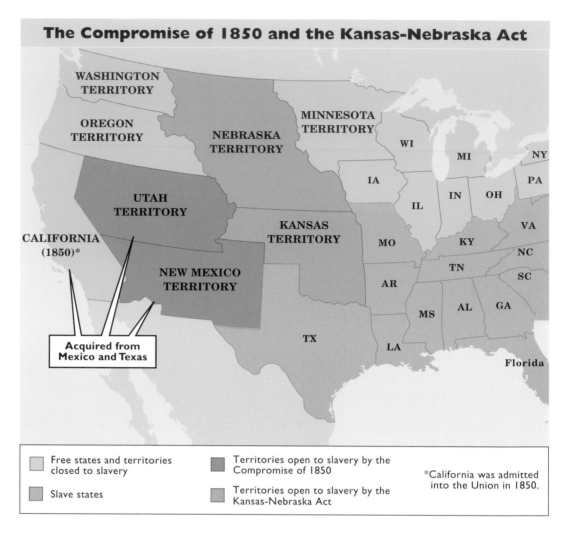

The Compromise of 1850 and the Kansas-Nebraska Act

☐ Free states and territories closed to slavery	■ Territories open to slavery by the Compromise of 1850
■ Slave states	■ Territories open to slavery by the Kansas-Nebraska Act

*California was admitted into the Union in 1850.

in the Union were subject to potential enslavement or re-enslavement. Moreover, the Fugitive Slave Act made it a crime for any northerner to interfere in the apprehension of an alleged escapee. Northerners were outraged, and not just because law-abiding blacks were subject to arrest. Suddenly, it seemed to them as if the entire federal government had been hijacked by what was coming to be called the "slave power conspiracy."

"POPULAR SOVEREIGNTY" AND THE DRED SCOTT DECISION

The events of the 1850s only seemed to confirm those fears, even as southerners believed they were offered evidence of a widespread abolitionist plot to destroy the institution of slavery altogether. With pioneers beginning to settle the lands to the immediate west and northwest of Missouri, a proposal was floated by the powerful Illinois senator Stephen Douglas to establish two organized territories—Kansas and Nebraska. To gain southern support for the measure, Douglas insisted that the settlers decide their status as slave or free. Because

the territories lay north of the Missouri Compromise line, antislavery northerners cried foul, arguing that the lands were supposed to be free. Despite their protestations, the "popular sovereignty" elements of the Kansas-Nebraska bill passed, providing yet more evidence to suspicious northerners that the "slave power conspiracy" was determined to enforce its will on the entire country.

In fact, as some contemporaries pointed out, the debate was misguided. The cold, dry plains of Kansas and Nebraska—as well as the deserts of the southwestern territories taken from Mexico—were hardly places to support cotton and other slave-based plantation crops. But in the heated political climate of the 1850s, few people were able to think in such terms. For both southerners and northerners, the West represented the future, a land of opportunity for poor but aspiring white settlers. Yet northerners feared the competition of slave labor in the West, while southerners worried that the presence of antislavery northerners in the territories would make the institution of slavery untenable there.

Meanwhile crisis followed crisis as the decade unfolded. In 1856, violence erupted

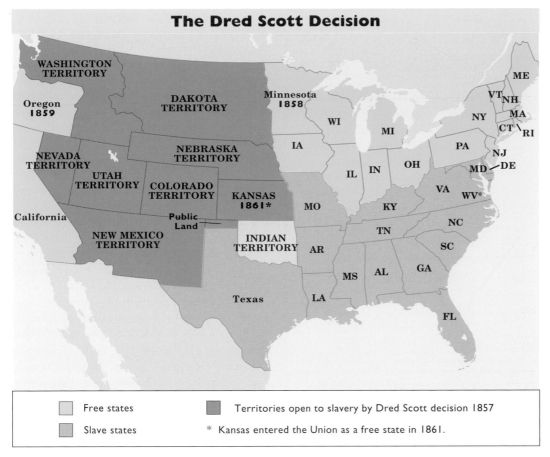

The Dred Scott Decision

WASHINGTON TERRITORY
Oregon 1859
Minnesota 1858
DAKOTA TERRITORY
ME
VT
NH
MA
NY
CT
RI
WI
MI
IA
NEVADA TERRITORY
UTAH TERRITORY
NEBRASKA TERRITORY
COLORADO TERRITORY
KANSAS 1861*
PA
NJ
DE
OH
IN
IL
MD
VA
WV*
KY
California
New Mexico Territory
Public Land
MO
INDIAN TERRITORY
AR
TN
NC
SC
MS
AL
GA
LA
Texas
FL

☐ Free states   ■ Territories open to slavery by Dred Scott decision 1857
☐ Slave states   * Kansas entered the Union as a free state in 1861.

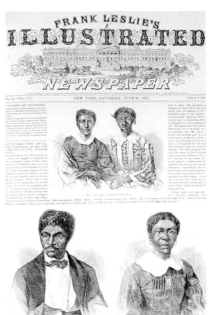

Dred Scott and his wife (Library of Congress)

in Kansas as pro- and antislavery forces clashed, leading to murders, skirmishes, and massacres. In the summer, more than 700 proslavery men attacked the free town of Lawrence, burning it to the ground. In response, abolitionist John Brown and a small gang of followers descended on a settlement at Pottawatomie Creek, where they murdered five proslavery settlers in their homes. The violence over the slavery issue even penetrated Capitol Hill. Following a fiery speech on the floor of Congress—in which he denounced South Carolina senator Andrew Butler for taking up with "the harlot slavery"—Massachusetts senator Charles Sumner was beaten unconscious by Butler's nephew, Representative Preston Brooks.

With Kansas in flames and Congress bitterly divided, the Supreme Court moved into the breach, seeking to resolve the issue through a broad judicial ruling. The case that came to them involved a slave named Dred Scott who, with the help of abolitionist lawyers, was suing for his freedom. Scott's master, an army surgeon, had taken his slave with him when assigned to serve in the free state of Illinois and the free territory of Wisconsin. When his master died, Scott—citing his habitation on free soil—claimed his freedom. His late master's heirs insisted he belonged to them. In a highly controversial decision, the Supreme Court ruled against Scott in March 1857, saying that he was a slave no matter where he lived. To northerners, the implications were dire. Legally, a slaveowner could now bring his slaves with impunity to any northern state, rendering the entire Union slave territory. Once again, it seemed to many in the North that the "slave power conspiracy" was winning the day.

JOHN BROWN'S RAID AND THE ELECTION OF 1860

Southerners, meanwhile, had their own fears. Outnumbered and outpaced by a rapidly growing and industrializing North, they felt hemmed in on all sides. Britain had outlawed slavery in its empire in 1833, followed by France in 1848. The bestselling novel of the day—popularized in countless theatrical productions across the North—was Harriet Beecher Stowe's *Uncle Tom's Cabin*, a powerful melodrama on the evils of slavery. A new and popular antislavery party—the Republicans—was fast becoming the majority in the northern states. Then, in 1859, came the final blow. In October, John Brown—the abolitionist fighter from Kansas—led an armed gang on a raid of the federal armory at Harper's Ferry, Virginia

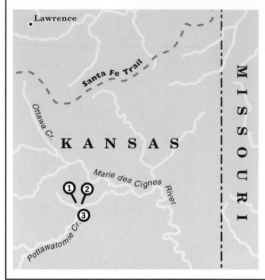

THE POTTAWATOMIE CREEK MASSACRES, MAY 24, 1856

① John Brown and his gang drag James Doyle and his sons, William and Drury, from their home and hack them to death with swords. They spare the lives of Mrs. Doyle, a daughter, and 14-year-old John.

② Brown and his men move to the home of Allen Wilkinson and take him prisoner. They also steal two saddles and a rifle.

③ The group moves on to the home of James Harris, where Harris, his wife, young child, and three other men, including William Sherman, are sleeping. Sherman is executed. Brown makes off with more weapons, a saddle, and a horse.

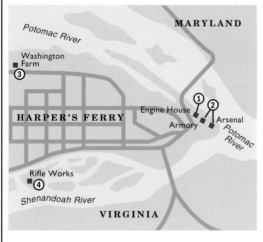

RAID ON HARPER'S FERRY, OCTOBER 16, 1859

① **The Engine House:** Brown and his men use the engine house as a base of operations.

② **The Federal Armory and Arsenal:** After capturing these installations, Brown distributes weapons to all his troops and then steals enough weapons to arm a force of 1,500.

③ **Washington Farm:** Brown and his men kidnap Colonel L. W. Washington and a number of his slaves. At the height of Brown's assault, he and his men hold 40 captives in the engine house.

④ **Rifle Works:** Brown's men also hold the rifle works until they are killed or captured by local townspeople.

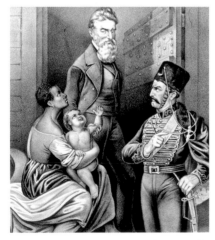

The capture of John Brown, by Currier and Ives (Library of Congress)

(now West Virginia), hoping to launch and arm a general slave insurrection in the process. Brown's plan was as crazy as it was audacious. There were few African Americans in the mountainous region around Harper's Ferry and Brown's small force was quickly killed or dispersed by a Virginia militia company headed by Robert E. Lee, future commander of Confederate forces in the Civil War. Brown himself was captured alive.

At first, northerners and southerners were largely in agreement on Brown; he was seen as a dangerous and misguided fanatic who threatened the peace and wel-

fare of the country. But during his trial, Brown spoke with such great eloquence on the evils of the slavery system and on the necessity of destroying it that he won over the majority of public opinion in the North. Following his conviction and subsequent death by hanging, Brown's body was shipped northward to a burial site in New York's Adirondack Mountains, where he had lived much of his life. In Philadelphia, his body was taken from its original coffin—which had been built by slaves—and placed in one made by free blacks. Along the train's route, large crowds came out to pay their respects to the man they now viewed as a national hero. To proslavery southerners, this was further proof that all northerners were secret abolitionists. This was a mistaken assumption, of course. Most northerners did not want to ban slavery in the South, but instead just prevent it from spreading to the West. But, in politics, opinion often counts for more than fact, a rule that would be proven—with disastrous results—in the presidential election year of 1860.

By the end of the 1850s, many of the institutions that had previously bound the nation together had divided into mutually hostile northern and southern wings. Fraternal organizations, churches, and the Whig Party had all broken over the question of slavery. During the election campaign of 1860, the only remaining national party—the Democrats—would come apart as well. At their national convention in Charleston, South Carolina, southern and northern delegates debated the question of popular sovereignty and the expansion of slavery in the western territories. When the northerners—who only weakly supported both—won out, the southerners walked out on the convention. Ultimately, the Democratic Party ran two candidates for president—Stephen Douglas and Kentucky senator John Breckinridge. Along with a third party candidate, former Tennessee senator John Bell, who ran under the banner of the Constitutional Union Party, the Democrats split the southern and border states of Delaware, Kentucky, Maryland, and Missouri between them. Meanwhile the Republicans, united behind Lincoln, swept the northern states and took the election with a plurality of just 40 percent of the national popular vote.

As far as southerners were concerned, the election results were the final straw. In their opinion, Lincoln was a closet abolitionist, despite his protestations that he did not intend to ban slavery where it already existed. Lincoln had also made clear his

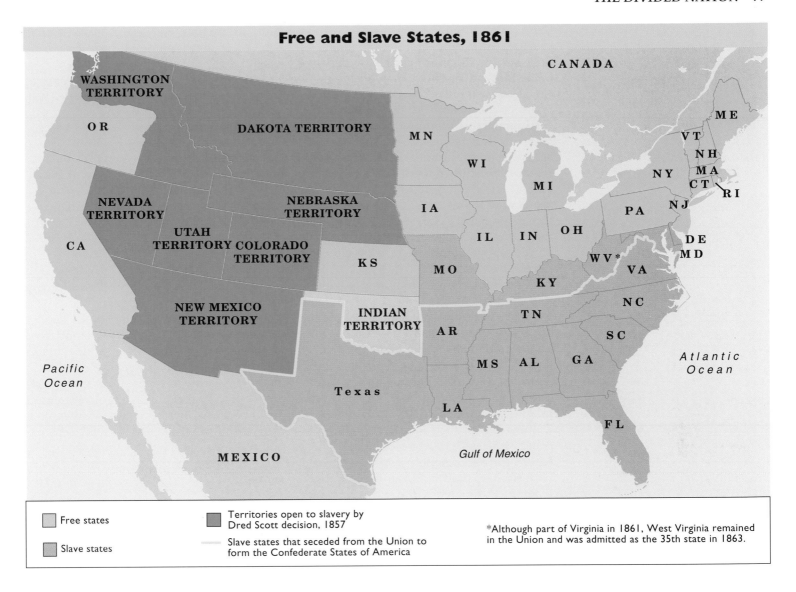

Free and Slave States, 1861

Free states

Slave states

Territories open to slavery by Dred Scott decision, 1857

Slave states that seceded from the Union to form the Confederate States of America

*Although part of Virginia in 1861, West Virginia remained in the Union and was admitted as the 35th state in 1863.

belief that the Union would "become all one thing, or all the other."

CIVIL WAR

On December 20, 1860, a convention to consider secession from the Union was held in Charleston. The meeting was dominated by so-called fire-eaters, who argued several points. First, they insisted the Union was a voluntary compact of states, making secession legitimate, even though the Constitution offered no clear language on the subject. They also argued that the original Constitutional Compromise—in which the North got the strong central government it wanted as long as the South dominated it—had been violated by the election of an anti-southern president. Finally, pointing out that Lincoln had received almost no votes south of the Mason-Dixon Line, southerners argued they no longer had a government to represent them. Thus, like the Patriots of 1776, the secessionists of

1860–1861 believed they had a perfect right—in the words of the Declaration of Independence—"to throw off such Government, and to provide new guards for their future security."

SECESSION AND FORT SUMTER

In the end, the fire-eaters won the day. Over the next six weeks, six more states—Alabama, Florida, Georgia, Louisiana, Mississippi, and Texas—joined South Carolina. In February, commissioners from the seven seceded states met in Montgomery, Alabama to form a new nation, the Confederate States of America. Meanwhile, in Washington, Kentucky senator John Crittenden offered a compromise—renewing the Missouri Compromise line and adding a Constitutional amendment defending slavery forever. But President-elect Lincoln and congressional Republicans rejected the compromise.

More worrisome for the Union were military developments. Throughout the

South, pro-secession forces had seized federal forts, all except Fort Sumter, situated on an island in Charleston harbor; that was being blockaded. Thus, upon his inauguration, President Lincoln was facing the worst crisis in the history of the Republic. His inaugural speech offered familiar concessions to the South—no punishment for secession and assurance that slavery would remain undisturbed there—and tough measures if the seceding states did not return to the Union. It was a difficult balancing act, threatening the Deep South with punishment while easing fears in the critical states of the upper South, most especially Virginia.

Fort Sumter presented Lincoln with his first immediate decision. To abandon it would be to destroy the Union's credibility. To break the blockade by armed force risked making the North the aggressor and thereby causing the states of the upper South to join their Deep South sisters in secession. Ultimately, Lincoln chose the middle ground. With the fort's defenders running out of food and fresh water, Lincoln dispatched a relief expedition. With the new supplies, southern leaders realized, Fort Sumter could hold out for months. A federal fort situated in the symbolic capital of the South was intolerable to Confederate leaders, who began an artillery barrage against the fort on April 14. Ironically, given the enormous bloodshed of the Civil War that began there, no one died in the two-day bombardment of Fort Sumter. And, though lost to the South, the fort represented a symbolic victory for Lincoln: he had forced the other side to fire first. Within days, his call for 75,000 new federal soldiers had been easily met, though the call to arms was enough to push Arkansas, North Carolina, Tennessee, and Virginia to secede. The Civil War had begun in earnest.

only to punish the secessionist planters who most northerners felt had started the war.

Meanwhile, as Union armies pushed into the South, a new problem arose: runaway slaves. When three showed up at a Union army encampment on the Virginia coast in 1861, commanding officer General Benjamin Butler refused to return them to their masters, declaring them "contraband" of war, that is, property of the enemy. It was, in short, a legal cover for emancipation. With white southerners off at war, those three Virginia slaves were soon joined by thousands of African Americans.

In Washington, changing opinion and the problem of runaway slaves was forging an ever more radical antislavery coalition between Lincoln and congressional Republicans. In April 1862, slavery was outlawed in the District of Columbia; in June, it was outlawed in the territories. Neither act freed many slaves, but it showed a growing commitment to immediate abolition, a commitment bolstered by the Second Confiscation Act passed in July. Under this bill, all "contraband" was declared "forever free." The way was being paved for the most radical measure of all. On September 22, 1862, Lincoln issued the historic Emancipation Proclamation, declaring all slaves in rebel-held territories free as of January 1, 1863. Technically speaking, the proclamation did not free a single slave. Slaves in Union-held territory would remain in bondage (to maintain the support of border state leaders); and slaves held in rebel territory were out of reach of the act. But, the reality was that the proclamation forever changed the meaning of the war. From then on it was about abolishing slavery and, with every mile of territory captured by Union armies, African Americans would be emancipated by an act of the federal government.

EMANCIPATION

From the beginning, both northerners and the Republican Party were divided over the war's meaning. To Democrats, moderate Republicans, and Lincoln himself, the main aim of the conflict was to preserve the Union. But to abolitionists, free blacks, and the so-called Radical Republicans, the war was about saving the Union and destroying slavery. At first, the former group—with its talk of gradually abolishing slavery over many years—predominated. But as casualties mounted in the first year of fighting, public and congressional opinion began to shift toward more immediate abolition, if

AFRICAN-AMERICAN SOLDIERS

Moreover, just as African Americans had helped force emancipation by their decision to leave the plantations, so black leaders helped push into effect the recruitment of black soldiers into the Union army. At the beginning of the war, few people outside the abolitionist and free black communities believed in recruiting blacks. There was just too much prejudice. In the racist thinking of the day, blacks were considered too cowardly and undisciplined for soldiering. And the notion of giving guns to blacks in order to kill whites—even if those whites were traitors to the Union—was anathema to the vast majority of northerners. But as the war ground on—and casualties mounted—the unthinkable became possible then desirable.

On the other hand, from the moment southern guns opened up on Fort Sumter in April 1861, African Americans clamored to serve in the military. Unlike whites, blacks understood from the beginning that the war would ultimately decide the fate of American slavery. This, they believed, was their struggle. And, as Frederick Douglass understood, "once let the black man get upon his person the brass letters, 'U.S.,' let him get an eagle on his buttons and a musket on his shoulder and bullets in his pockets, and there is no power on earth which can deny that he has earned the right to citizenship in the United States." Indeed, in 19th-century America, citizenship was often defined by one's willingness to serve one's country in the military. Still, the politicians hesitated, fearing northern public opinion and potential racial conflict in the ranks of soldiers.

But public opinion in the North was changing and changing fast. As the idea that the war was about abolition—as opposed to simply preserving the Union—began to sink in, more and more whites came to accept the idea that if blacks were going to benefit by the war, they ought to share in the fighting and the dying. New technologies—including the grooved bore rifle that allowed for greater accuracy over long distances—led to unprecedented carnage on the battlefield, as commanders were slow to adjust their tactics from older patterns of massed troop firing. Adding to the bloodshed was the recognition that the Civil War as a war of attrition. In other words, northern commanders were increasingly coming to the realization that the only way to win the war was to grind down both southern armies and the South's ability to make war. Such a strategy required the North to sacrifice enormous numbers of soldiers and material, knowing that the region's greater population and resources would outlast those of the South.

Another factor in changing northern public opinion—and U.S. government policy—on recruiting African Americans was the field performance of black regiments. In January 1863, Thomas Wentworth Higginson, an abolitionist-turned-commander,

Recruitment of African Americans	
STATE/DISTRICT	NUMBER OF ARMY RECRUITS
Kentucky	23,703
Missouri	8,766
Maryland	8,718
Pennsylvania	8,612
Ohio	5,092
New York	4,125
District of Columbia	3,269
Massachusetts	2,966
Rhode Island	1,837
Illinois	1,811
Other*	110,076
Union Total	**178,975**

*From the Confederacy and other northern states

Fifty-fourth Massachusetts Regiment storming Fort Wagner, South Carolina (Library of Congress)

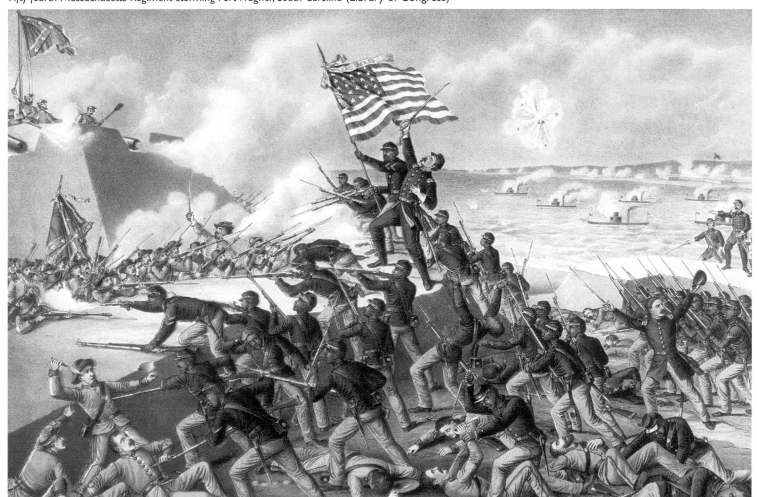

wrote a well-read newspaper account, praising the African-American First South Carolina Volunteers. "No [white] officer in this regiment," Higginson noted, "now doubts that the key to the successful prosecution of the war lies in the unlimited employment of black troops." Shortly thereafter, the War Department authorized the enlistment of troops from the free black community of the North and from among runaway slaves in the South.

At the same time, the abolitionist and free black communities of Boston organized the Fifty-fourth Massachusetts Regiment, an all-black regiment commanded by white abolitionist Robert Gould Shaw. At first, the Fifty-fourth was either kept in camp or ordered to perform routine noncombat duties. They were not even issued guns or ammunition. But protests by Shaw and his men—as well as drops in white recruitment—pushed higher-ups in the military to authorize combat duty for the regiment. In July 1863, during a heroic, but ultimately doomed, assault on South Carolina's Fort Wagner, black soldiers had finally proved to whites that they were able to fight and were willing to die in the cause of freedom. Nor could the pride and satisfaction in their new duties be disguised. One black soldier, seeing his former master among the prisoners he was guarding, greeted him with: "hello massa, bottom rail on top dis time."

Still, even as military commanders recognized the valor and discipline of black troops, racist attitudes prevailed. Black troops were kept in segregated camps and usually assigned to menial labor or guard duty. And, until mass protests by black troops in June 1864, they received little more than half the pay of white soldiers: $7 versus $13 a month. Even as black troops experienced discrimination within the Union army, they faced a threat on the battlefield that whites did not. That is to say, as the number of black troops rose, the Confederate government issued a dire warning: any blacks captured in war would either be executed or returned to slavery. When word came back that black prisoners of war were being routinely executed by southern military authorities, Lincoln cut off all prisoner exchanges, although he did not carry through on his own threat to begin executing southern POWs in retaliation.

Yet despite discrimination on the northern side and the executions on the southern side, blacks continued to flock to the military. By the end of the war, approximately 200,000 African Americans were serving in the Union army and navy, about 10 percent of the total fighting force. (Due to the close quarters of shipboard life, segregation was impossible in the navy and blacks and whites served together.) Their critical role in the war effort was recognized by Lincoln in an 1864 campaign speech, when he said that without black soldiers, "we would be compelled to abandon the war in three weeks." Yet despite black willingness to serve the Union cause, prejudice in the North remained high. Many parts of the Midwest, largely inhabited by migrants from the South, were bastions of pro-southern sympathizers. These so-called copperheads—named after a particularly venomous snake of the region—turned increasingly against the Union war effort as it became associated with abolitionism.

NEW YORK CITY DRAFT RIOTS

Ironically, however, the most violent demonstrations against the war effort, abolitionism, and blacks was in a place far from the South—both geographically and demographically: New York City. When the war began, New Yorkers—like the majority of northerners—supported the Union cause enthusiastically. The largely working-class and immigrant communities of the city had little sympathy for white planters, even if the city's economy was closely bound up with that of the South. Moreover, most New Yorkers—like most northerners—believed the war would be short, glorious, and relatively bloodless. When that proved to be far from the case, sentiment began to change and, by 1863, recruitments began to dry up. To maintain, effective troop numbers, Lincoln and his War Department authorized two measures: one, mentioned above, was the recruitment of black soldiers; the other was the Enrollment Act of 1863, the nation's first military draft. Among the provisions of the act was a commutation fee. Any draftee who could come up with $300—more than half a year's income for the average worker—could buy his way out of the war.

By the summer of 1863, when the draft was set to commence, tensions in working-class neighborhoods of the city were high. There was resentment. The largely Democratic population was not particularly fond of Lincoln and the Republicans, whom they saw as agents of the city's business leaders. There was also anger over high prices and war profiteering by the same merchants and factory owners who could pay the commutation fee. And there was fear. Immigrant and working-class New Yorkers believed that abolition would lead to a flood of southern black workers into the city who would drive wages down as they competed for the same unskilled positions.

Thus, when draftee names were announced in early July, the city exploded, particularly its Irish neighborhoods. The draft office was the first to receive the rioters' torch, then the mobs attacked buildings associated with the Republican Party and business elites. While the undermanned metropolitan police force was able to keep the rioters out of the wealthier residential neighborhoods, they lost control over most of the city. Ultimately, the mobs turned their wrath against the city's free black community, lynching dozens of African Americans and burning the Colored Orphans Asylum to the ground, forcing hundreds of terrified children to flee the city in the middle of the night. It took several days for Lincoln and the federal government to react, but, when they did, they came down hard. Federal troops were rushed back from their battlefield victory over the Confederacy at Gettysburg to put down the rioting. Dozens of rioters were shot and thousands were arrested. In the end, more than 100 people died in the New York City draft riots of 1863, making them the worst civil disturbance in American history.

THE NORTH VICTORIOUS

Yet for all the bitter divisions within northern society—as exemplified by the riots—the ultimate outcome of the war was hardly in doubt after Gettysburg. By the end of 1863, the South was split in two down the Mississippi and effectively blockaded at sea. During the course of 1864 and early 1865, Union armies under generals William Tecumseh Sherman and Philip Sheridan destroyed some of the most productive regions of the South, including much of Georgia and Virginia. Meanwhile, the main Union army, led by Ulysses S. Grant, was conducting a bloody war of attrition against the Army of Northern Virginia, under the command of Robert E. Lee. By early spring, Lee recognized that the struggle was lost. On April 9, at the courthouse in Appomattox, Virginia, he surrendered to Grant, ending the four-year-long war that had cost the lives of more than 600,000 Americans, far and away the bloodiest in the nation's history.

Historians have debated why and how the North won the war ever since. Most point to its vastly greater population and manufacturing capacity. Indeed, these were critical to winning the "first modern war"

THE NEW YORK DRAFT RIOTS

July 13

1. No-Draft demonstration and arson at 9th District draft office, 9–10am
2. Riot, noon
3. 8th District marshal's office burned, 5pm
4. Lexington Avenue, wealthy homes burned
5. 18th Ward arsenal raided for weapons, evening
6. Colored Orphans' Asylum burned, evening

July 14

7. Rioting spreads to 6th Ward
8. Union Steam Works (East 21st Street)—crowds and troops clash, afternoon

July 15

9. Crowds and militia clash on First Avenue, afternoon

✖ Blacks murdered

in world history, where the total destruction of the other side's capacity to make war was the ultimate object.

When the South went to war in 1861, it was largely to preserve slavery. For all the talk of state's rights, southerners would have not have gone to war unless they felt that slavery and white supremacy were threatened by the North. Ironically, by the end of the war, the South was fighting to

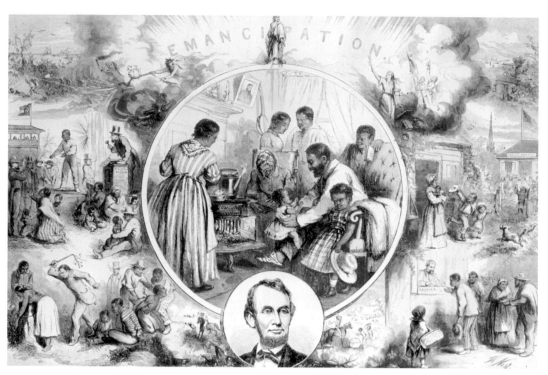

The Emancipation Proclamation is celebrated. (Library of Congress)

preserve its existence, even if that jeopardized slavery. One of the last acts the Confederate Congress passed was a bill—never implemented, because the war ended first—to offer freedom to any slave that took up arms in defense of the Confederacy.

As with the South, the war started out as one thing for the North and ended up as another. In the beginning, it was fought to preserve the Union or, as Lincoln put it at Gettysburg, to ensure that "government of the people, by the people, for the people, shall not perish from the earth." But by the end, the North was fighting for an entirely different reason: ending slavery and bringing the long-postponed promise of freedom to the nation's African-American population. Sadly, the man most responsible for that transformation—President Abraham Lincoln—did not live to see it through to completion; he was assassinated just five days after the surrender at Appomattox. For the civil war he presided over was just half a revolution. It destroyed the slavery regime forever. But the struggle over the other half—that is, what would be constructed or, rather, reconstructed in its place—had just begun.

UP FROM SLAVERY
African Americans in the Late 19th Century

4

B etween 1865 and 1877, the United States of America embarked on one of the greatest experiments in social transformation ever attempted in human history. The period—known as Reconstruction—has often been called the "second American Revolution," for its far-reaching efforts to fulfill the political and social promise of the first. Beginning during the Civil War and reaching its culmination in the decade that followed, Reconstruction saw the near total—albeit temporary—transformation of southern politics, economy, and society. Reconstruction involved several elements: reintegration of southern states into the Union, the punishment and rehabilitation of southern whites who had fought against their country in the Civil War, and a battle between Congress and the White House for political supremacy. But, above all, Reconstruction was the story of African Americans and their struggle for integration into the mainstream of southern and American society.

RECONSTRUCTION

The pace of change during this period was breakneck. In 1861, 4 million African Americans in the South lived in bondage, the chattel property of their masters. Several hundred thousand other blacks—in both the South and North—lived in a twilight zone between freedom and servitude with, in the words of Chief Justice Roger Taney, "no rights which the white man was bound to respect." Less than a decade later, not only had 4 million slaves been removed from bondage, but all African-American males (black women—like their white counterparts—were still denied basic civil rights) had achieved political and legal

African-American troops arrive home after the Civil War (Library of Congress)

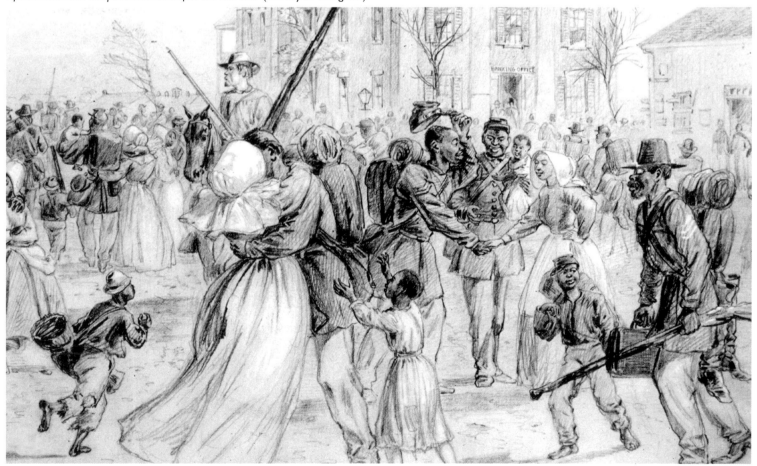

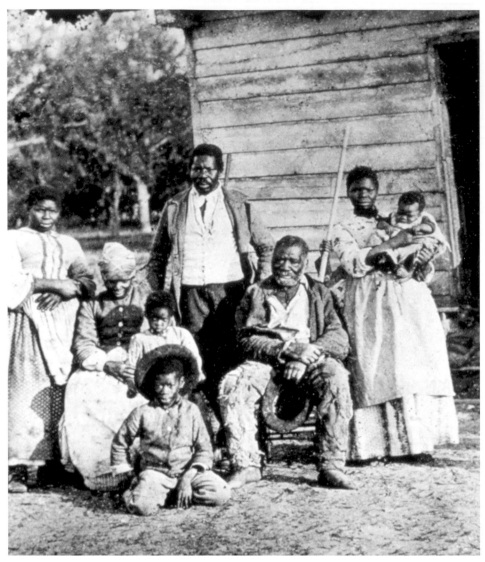

A family of freedpersons (Library of Congress)

although that event has been used as the starting point for Reconstruction by the eminent historian Eric Foner. In most regions of the South, freedom was either seized by the slaves themselves or offered by advancing Union armies. Emancipation came whenever slaves sensed that the authority of the master no longer held sway. Emancipation, then, was not just a legal act, but a psychological and existential event in the lives of every African American emerging from bondage.

Among the first places to experience emancipation—more than a year before the Emancipation Proclamation went into effect—were the Sea Islands off the coast of South Carolina and Georgia. Occupied by the Union army as part of the North's wartime strategy of blockading the Confederacy by sea, the islands saw the white planter class flee at the first sign of trouble. When planters tried to force their slaves to follow them to the mainland, most of the latter refused. With northern armies coming, slaves understood that the disciplinary structure of the slave regime—and the authority of the slaveowners themselves—had crumbled. They were, in short, emancipated at that moment.

Emancipation meant many things to former bondsmen and bondswomen. On the Sea Islands, it meant liberation from the grinding gang labor of the cotton plantation. Indeed, one of the first things that the freedpersons did was destroy the cotton gins and other property of the former masters. As emancipation advanced across the South, so the freedpersons took advantage of their newfound freedom. Some shed their slave surnames and took on ones appropriate to the times, like Freeman. Others sought out local black preachers and Union army chaplains to legitimize the informal marriage arrangements of slavery times. Many took to the road—some for the purposes of finding loved ones separated on the auction block; others to experience the sheer joy of freedom of movement.

There were changes on the land as well. On most plantations, slave cabins were situated around the planter's house, so that the activities of the slaves could be easily monitored. With emancipation, many freedpersons moved their cabins to the far reaches of the plantations, to get away from white oversight. Former slaves also shifted their labor from cotton and other commercial crops to the raising of food for personal and family consumption. While planters and other apologists of the slave regime had long argued that African Americans would never work unless coerced, freedpersons

equality with whites, including the right to vote. While it is true that this era of equality was short-lived—largely dying with the end of Reconstruction in 1877—it established the constitutional basis for the civil rights movement of the mid-20th century.

EMANCIPATION AND WARTIME RECONSTRUCTION

Reconstruction would have been impossible without the Civil War. And, of all the cataclysmic changes wrought by the Civil War on southern society, none was more important than the emancipation of African Americans from centuries of bondage and servitude. To understand the significance of emancipation, it is useful to examine what it was not. Emancipation was not a single event, but millions of individual events involving millions of individuals. Nor was emancipation primarily set in motion by Lincoln's Emancipation Proclamation,

proved them wrong. If hard work was necessary for survival or if it brought returns like a better diet or some cash in hand, then former slaves proved themselves more than willing to work hard. At the same time, absorbing the belief system of 19th-century America, the freedperson community also made it clear that they did not want their women to work in the fields. Thus, nearly half the labor force once available for commercial agriculture in the plantation South was lost.

Emancipation also meant the little things that might seem to trivial to anybody who had never been forced to do without them. In many towns and cities, African Americans took to promenading on streets and in neighborhoods where they had previously been banned. Freedpersons also began wearing more fashionable clothing, which was denied to them under slavery. And, most disturbingly to white southerners, blacks refused to pay their former masters the deference those masters had come to expect. "It is impossible to describe the condition of the city," one South Carolina planter said, describing postwar Charleston. "It is so unlike anything we could imagine—Negroes shoving white persons off the walk—Negro women drest in the most outré style, all with veils and parasols, for which they have an especial fancy."

The Sea Islands were not only where emancipation happened first; they were also where the first efforts at Reconstruction began. As one historian described them, wartime events in the Sea Islands represented a "rehearsal for Reconstruction." And, as would be the case in other parts of the South, the course of Reconstruction was determined by victorious white northerners as much as it was by liberated black southerners. Two groups of the former descended on the Sea Islands within months of their liberation. One included abolitionists who wanted to prove that black people were "reasonable beings" who had a "capacity for self-government." Alongside former slaves, the abolitionists established schools and churches, in order to prepare the freedpersons for eventual citizenship. Their dream—a goal that was shared by the former slaves—was to create a community of small land-owning farmers, harking back to the Jeffersonian ideal—still widely held in much of America and shared by Lincoln himself—wherein political freedom was achieved through economic independence. Some modest steps in this direction were taken when several groups of blacks pooled their resources and bought several thousand acres of plantation land auctioned off by the federal government.

Other northerners had different ideas about the direction the Sea Island "rehearsal for Reconstruction" should take. Beginning in 1863—as the federal government began auctioning off lands that

A Reconstruction school (Library of Congress)

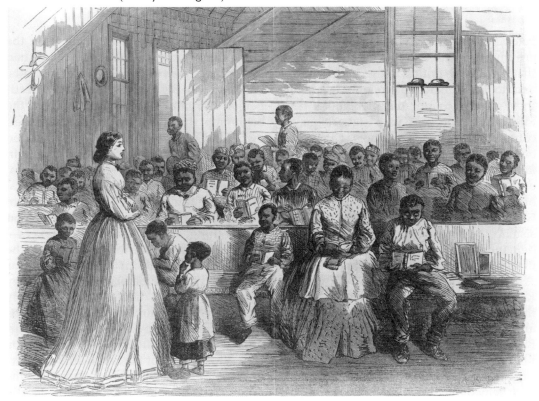

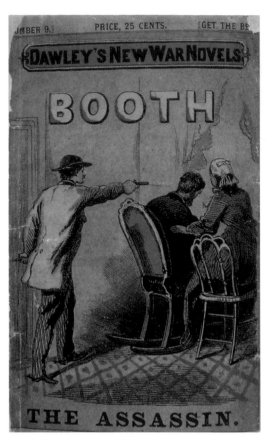

Lincoln's assassination (Library of Congress)

rehabilitation and limited black freedom, Congress established the Bureau of Refugees, Freedmen, and Abandoned Lands in March 1865. Popularly known as the Freedmen's Bureau, the agency took on the task of feeding and clothing black and white refugees, renting out confiscated planter land to "loyal" whites and freedpersons, and writing up and enforcing labor contracts between freedpersons and planters. In addition, the bureau worked with northern volunteer associations to establish schools and to send teachers throughout the South. By the end of the war, the Freedmen's Bureau had settled about 10,000 black and white families on lands seized from planters in Georgia and South Carolina. While it was not its intention, the bureau often encouraged blacks—in the hopes of gaining land of their own—to hold out against signing labor contracts with their former masters. As one freedperson told South Carolina planter Thomas Pinckney, "we ain't going nowhere. We are going to work right here on the land where we were born and what belongs to us."

Land and labor were not the only wartime Reconstruction issues on the table. There were also the matters of political power and civil rights, questions that first came to the fore in Louisiana. With their base in New Orleans, the largest free black community in the South—allied with many antiplanter, pro-Union whites among the city's working class population—began to demand civil rights, including the vote, even before the war ended. At first, Lincoln made it clear that he hoped that the state government could be turned over to moderate white planters. In December 1863, the president announced his "10 percent plan." Under the proposal, any confederate state where 10 percent of the voters took a loyalty oath to the Union would be readmitted to the Union. But as black protests continued, Lincoln shifted his opinion, requesting that the state's 1864 constitutional convention grant the voting rights to "intelligent blacks" and black soldiers. Still, he did not make black voting rights a requisite for readmission to the Union. Whether he would have shifted further in favor of black civil rights—as some historians claim—is impossible to ascertain.

On April 14, just five days after General Robert E. Lee surrendered to Ulysses S. Grant in Virginia, effectively ending the Civil War, Lincoln and his wife Mary Todd decided to relax by attending an English theatrical comedy at Washington's Ford Theatre. During the performance, a southern assassin named John Wilkes Booth put a bullet in Lincoln's head, killing the president within hours. The assassination was part of a larger conspiracy to avenge the Confederacy's defeat. Other targets included the Lincoln cabinet—Secretary of War William Seward was also stabbed—and Vice President Andrew Johnson, who escaped attack. In fact, Johnson, a southern loyalist whom Lincoln had selected as his running mate in 1864 in hopes of reconciling a postwar South—proved to be the best friend the planter class could possibly have had in Washington in the early years of Reconstruction.

ANDREW JOHNSON AND PRESIDENTIAL RECONSTRUCTION

While racism permeated 19th-century America, Andrew Johnson—a former Democratic senator and military governor of Tennessee—was in a class by himself. In one address to Congress, Johnson insisted African Americans had less "capacity for government than any other race of people . . . [W]herever they have been left to their own devices they have shown a constant tendency to relapse into barbarism." Still, many Radical Republicans held out hope for a pro–civil rights, antiplanter policy in the early days of the Johnson administration, as the new president—a self-made man from the hill country of eastern Tennessee—was also known to hold deep suspicions and even animosity toward the planter class of the South. But when faced with a decision to back freedperson versus planter aspirations, Johnson sided with his fellow whites.

Like his predecessor in the White House, Johnson believed that the secession states had never legally left the Union and, therefore, their readmission did not require acts of Congress. Assuming Executive Branch control over the process, Johnson merely requested that southern states ratify the 13th Amendment—banning slavery—and revoke their acts of secession. Once southerners took an oath of allegiance to the Union, they would get back all of their civil rights and all their property, minus the slaves. Exempted persons—including high-ranking Confederate officials and officers and persons with taxable property exceeding $20,000—could personally petition Johnson, who turned virtually no one away. Southerners immediately moved to take back property seized by the Union army during and immediately after the war. In October, Johnson ordered Freedmen's Bureau head General Oliver Howard to tell Sea Island blacks that they had no legal title to the land they were working. When Howard reluctantly agreed, he was met with a barrage of protests. "Why do you take away our lands?" a petition from a group of dispossessed farmers begged to know. "You take them from us who have always been true, always true to the Government. You give them to our all-time enemies!" When blacks resisted, Union soldiers forced them off or ordered them to work for their former masters.

Despite interference from the federal government, the struggle over the two critical ingredients to the southern economy—land and labor—continued. Planters, of course, had lost much economically by the war—namely $3 billion in human property. Most had also seen their savings wiped out, as Confederate currency became worthless after surrender. Still, if they could regain control of their land and their labor, they felt they could return to economic health and political power. But they continued to meet black resistance. Many of the latter voted with their feet, moving to towns and cities where they could find better-paying jobs. Others retreated to subsistence farming, raising crops for their own consumption on small plots of land. And, as noted

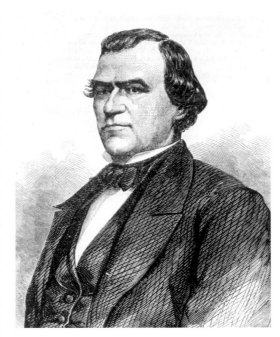

President Andrew Johnson (Library of Congress)

above, even where the labor force remained on the plantation, many black families insisted on pulling their women from the fields, thereby cutting the labor force significantly.

To counter these moves, the new postwar southern state governments—largely run by planters and their sympathizers—passed a series of strict new laws governing the freedperson population. The so-called black codes were essentially designed to return the social and economic order of the South to a facsimile of antebellum times. Indeed, in writing the new laws, postwar southern legislatures often turned to the old slave codes, merely replacing the word *slave* with *negro* or *freedman*. Many of the laws concerning vagrancy were so loosely worded that they made it possible to arrest any black person who was not actually working at the moment when confronted by a law enforcement official. Faced with fines that they could not pay, the "guilty" parties were then hired out to employers, often the former masters. In some states, codes were passed setting long hours of work and onerous duties for freedpersons. Anybody who refused to abide by the laws was deemed a vagrant. To keep blacks on the plantations, some states passed laws requiring licenses to take "irregular work," that is, jobs off the plantation. Legislation was also passed making it illegal for blacks to leave the plantation without a pass signed by their employer.

Harsh as the black codes were, they proved difficult to enforce. Supported by Freedmen's Bureau officials and Union

THE BLACK CODES

In the aftermath of the Civil War, southern state governments passed a series of strict new laws governing the freedperson population. The so-called black codes were intended to return the social and economic order of the South to the way it had been lived under slavery. Listed below are a number of black codes passed in Mississippi in 1865.

Apprentice Law

• All freedmen under 18 years who are orphans or financially unprovided for by their parents, shall be forcibly apprenticed.

• If apprentice escapes and is caught, master may reclaim him. Apprentice faces imprisonment if he or she refuses to comply.

• Employer is legally allowed to punish freedman in any way a parent or guardian might their own child or ward.

• Apprentice shall be indentured until 21 years of age if male and 18 years if female.

Vagrancy Law

• All freedmen over the age of 18 who do not have written proof of employment at the beginning of each year are vagrants.

• All vagrants shall be fined up to $50 and jailed up to 10 days.

• If freedman cannot pay the fine, he shall be hired out to any white man who will pay it for him, with the amount deducted from his wages.

• Freedmen between 18 and 60 years of age will pay a tax up to $1 per year toward the Freedman's Pauper Fund.

• If a freedman cannot pay a tax, he is a vagrant and will be hired out to any white man who will pay it for him.

Civil Rights of Freedmen

• Freedmen are forbidden to marry any white person upon penalty of life imprisonment.

• Reward offered to any person who catches a freedman who quits their employer's service prior to official termination.

• Penalty of up to $200 for any white man who employs or aids a runaway freedman.

Penal Code

• Illegal for freedmen to carry firearms.

• Illegal for freedmen to sell liquor, participate in riots, use insulting language or gestures, or preach the Gospel without a license.

• Freedmen are liable for fines for the above, and if a freedman refuses to pay, he will be hired out to any white man who will pay for him.

---

army officers, many blacks refused to abide by them. Making things more difficult for planters was the overall postwar labor shortage. While laws might be passed making it illegal for one planter to entice another's labor force away, desperate planters often ignored the law. Still, the general tendency in the southern states in the first year after the Civil War, was a return—sanctioned by President Johnson—to the social, economic, and political order of the slavery regime, less the legal status of slavery itself.

But if the black codes were less than fully effective in maintaining tight control over the African-American labor force of the South, they had a more lasting and dramatic effect in Washington and the North generally. Seeing former Confederates back in power in the South and passing laws aimed at overturning the objectives of the Civil War, many northerners—most of whom had had immediate family members killed or wounded in the fighting—were upset. In Washington, Radical and many moderate Republicans were outraged, especially as there was little any of them could do. Until the passage of the 20th Amendment in 1933, Congress was largely in recess during its

second year. In the year after the Civil War, that meant Congress was not in session until December 1865. As the months rolled by, and the South was reconstructed under prosouthern rules set by President Johnson, frustration among congressmen grew and, with it, a consensus that Congress should take control of the Reconstruction process.

This feeling was nothing new. In July 1864, Radical and moderate Republicans in Congress had offered an alternative to what they saw as Lincoln's overly lenient Reconstruction policies. The Wade-Davis Bill set up a strict set of guidelines for a southern state's readmission to the union. Like Lincoln's plan, the states had to ratify the 13th Amendment. But rather than 10 percent signing oaths of allegiance, a majority of white adult males would have to do so. Furthermore, so-called ironclad oaths—whereby delegates to the conventions held to write new state constitutions had to swear they had never taken up arms against the Union—were required. This, of course, excluded the vast majority of southern whites. Finally, the Confederacy's military and civilian leaders were permanently disenfranchised. Lincoln—loath to turn over

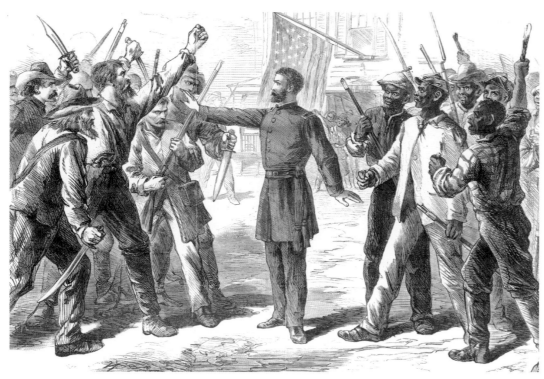

U.S. Army officer protects freedmen (Library of Congress)

Reconstruction authority to Congress—found the requirements too onerous and pocket-vetoed, or refused to sign, Wade-Davis, thereby postponing Congress's role in Reconstruction until well after the war.

CONGRESSIONAL RECONSTRUCTION

By December 1865, then, Republicans were itching for a showdown with Johnson over Reconstruction policy. And while the Republican delegation was divided between minority Radicals—led by Pennsylvania congressman Thaddeus Stevens and Massachusetts senator Charles Sumner—and majority moderates—under senators William Fessenden of Maine and Lyman Trumbull of Illinois—it did agree on one thing: outrage at the arrival of former Confederate officials—including Confederate vice president Alexander Stephens, as the new Senator from Georgia—in Congress. As the Constitution mandates, "each House [of Congress] shall be the Judge of the Election, Returns, and Qualifications of its own Members." Congressional Republicans exercised that right by refusing to recognize the representatives sent to Washington by the southern states.

Next, Congress acted on the controversial issue of confiscated lands. While moderate Republicans voted down a measure by Thaddeus Stevens to turn over the "forfeited estates of the enemy" to freedper-

sons, they did move to countermand Johnson's orders to the Freedmen's Bureau evicting blacks from lands in the Sea Islands. And, in early 1866, Congress passed the Southern Homestead Act, opening up 45 million acres in the region to anyone—black or white—who cultivated 80-acre plots for five years. The legislation typified northern attitudes toward the freedpersons and Reconstruction. Where

Thaddeus Stevens (Library of Congress)

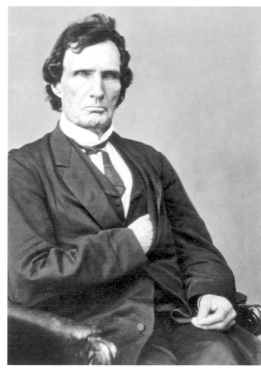

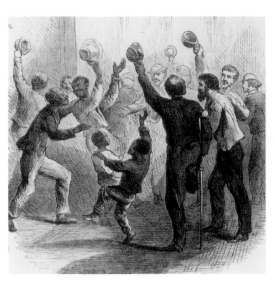

Celebrating passage of the Civil Rights Act of 1866
(Library of Congress)

Radicals wanted active measures to guarantee black rights—including gifts of former planter estates—moderates believed in equality of opportunity, whereby both blacks and whites would be given a chance to earn their land. This fit in with both northern policy—as exemplified in the similar Homestead Act of 1862 that opened up lands in the West—and averted Radicals' precedent-setting measures. After all, the reasoning of many moderate Republicans went, if southern property could be confiscated and given to the poor, so could northern factories and businesses, though this was hardly the intention of Stevens, himself the owner of an ironworks in Pennsylvania.

In February, Congress's showdown with Johnson intensified, when the president—citing the unconstitutionality of a "system for the support of indigent persons"—vetoed legislation extending the life of the Freedmen's Bureau. Unable to bring northern Democrats and conservative Republicans on board, the Radicals failed to override Johnson's veto. But then, adding fuel to the fire, an allegedly inebriated Johnson celebrated with prosouthern sympathizers in Washington, denouncing Radical Republicans as traitors in an impromptu speech. Both the veto and the ill-advised speech pushed many moderates into the arms of the Radicals. In March, Congress passed the Civil Rights bill. For the first time in its history, the federal government had passed legislation defining citizenship rights, including the right to own or rent property, the right to make contracts, and the right for access to the courts. In addition, the historic act authorized federal officials to sue on behalf of persons whose rights had been violated and guaranteed

that civil rights suits would be heard in federal court.

Although advised by his cabinet that many of his moderate and conservative Republican allies were turning against him, Johnson vetoed the bill. To many, the justification he offered—that the bill offering immediate citizenship to former slaves violated the rights of white immigrants who had to wait five years—was far-fetched. And so this time, moderate Republicans—still stinging from Johnson's ill-advised remarks on the treasonous behavior of their fellow party members—overrode the president's veto. Now fully convinced that Congress had to take control of Reconstruction away from an increasingly reactionary and irresponsible president, moderate Republicans passed a watered-down extension of the Freedmen's Bureau extension—requiring Sea Island blacks to buy, rather than be given, confiscated lands—and then overrode a second Johnson veto in July.

Meanwhile, the Joint Committee on Reconstruction—established by both houses of Congress to recommend further measures—was drawing up a plan to place the question of black civil rights and federal guarantees of citizenship beyond the law, that is, by anchoring them in the Constitution itself. In April, the committee submitted to the Congress the 14th Amendment. Although failing to offer guarantees of black suffrage—a key demand of Radical Republicans—the 14th Amendment represented perhaps the most far-reaching extension of federal powers in the history of the republic. Until its passage, the civil rights of all Americans were largely guaranteed by the states. The 14th Amendment put the federal government on record as the guarantor of the citizenship rights of "all persons born or naturalized in the United States." Moreover, the amendment made it unconstitutional for any state to abridge "the privileges or immunities of citizens of the United States" or deprive "any person of life, liberty, or property, without due process of law." Finally, the 14th Amendment penalized states that denied suffrage to any male by decreasing that state's representation in Congress proportional to the numbers of adult males denied the vote. (Much to the chagrin of women's rights supporters, this was the first time that gender-specified rights entered the Constitution.) Prompted by increasing violence against blacks in the South, including rioting that left 48 persons dead—all but two black—in Memphis, Tennessee, Congress submitted the amendment for state ratification in June.

Johnson, needless to say, was outraged by what he considered to be a barely disguised black civil rights amendment to the Constitution. Under his urging, border states and former Confederate states refused to go along, denying amendment supporters the three-quarter state majority required for ratification under the Constitution. The president also attempted to create a political consensus against congressional control of Reconstruction by forming a new national party of Democrats and conservative Republicans. With violence rising in the South—in New Orleans, a white, largely Democratic mob attacked a black suffrage convention in July, leaving 37 African Americans dead—Republicans refused to join Democrats, and Johnson's National Union Convention failed. Still, the president remained determined. In late summer, he sought to win support through a railroad tour of the nation, even though personal campaigning by a sitting president was considered undignified at the time. Nor did Johnson help his case by drinking heavily and engaging in verbal shouting matches with hecklers, once again asserting his claim that the real root of treachery lay not in the South but in Congress.

Republicans responded in kind, initiating a political strategy that would prove successful through much of the late 19th century. Known as "waving the bloody shirt," the strategy involved charging Democrats as the party of treason. It worked marvelously, especially in the congressional elections of 1866, when the party won a three-to-one majority in both the House and the Senate, as well as gaining control of the governorships and legislatures in every northern and most border states. Indeed, Republicans continued to "wave the bloody shirt" until the end of the 19th century, and the tactic proved successful up to and including the pivotal election year of 1896, when Republicans established a political hegemony over the national government that would continue nearly unbroken until the rise of Franklin Roosevelt and the New Deal Democratic coalition in the 1930s.

With overwhelming control of Congress and state governments, the Republican majority gave its radical wing the lead in setting Reconstruction policy. First, in March 1867, came the Reconstruction Act, which divided the South into five military districts, each headed by Union army generals. Before a southern state could return to

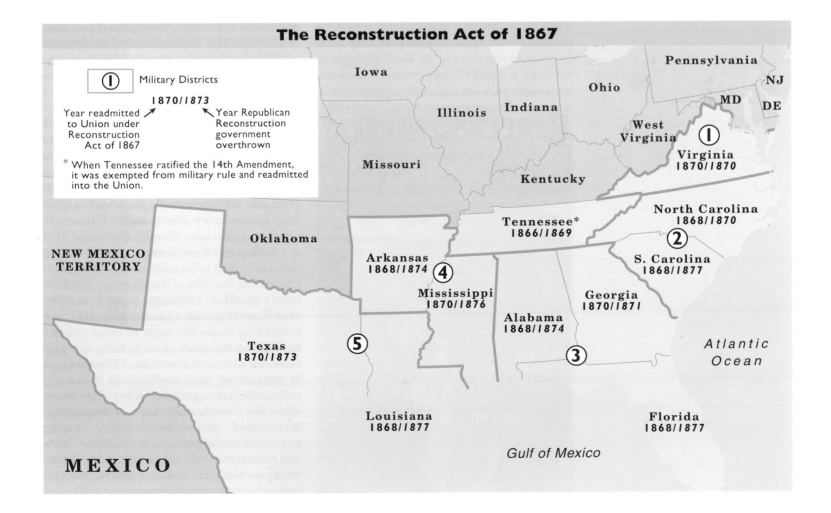

The Reconstruction Act of 1867

① Military Districts

1870/1873

Year readmitted ↗ to Union under Reconstruction Act of 1867   ↖ Year Republican Reconstruction government overthrown

* When Tennessee ratified the 14th Amendment, it was exempted from military rule and readmitted into the Union.

Iowa · Pennsylvania · NJ · Ohio · MD · DE · Illinois · Indiana · West Virginia · ① Virginia *1870/1870* · Missouri · Kentucky · North Carolina *1868/1870* · Tennessee* *1866/1869* · ② S. Carolina *1868/1877* · NEW MEXICO TERRITORY · Oklahoma · Arkansas *1868/1874* ④ · Mississippi *1870/1876* · Georgia *1870/1871* · Alabama *1868/1874* · ⑤ · ③ · Texas *1870/1873* · Louisiana *1868/1877* · Florida *1868/1877* · Atlantic Ocean · Gulf of Mexico · MEXICO

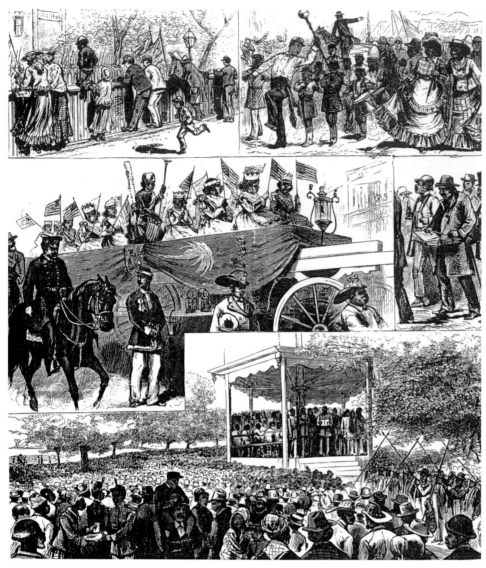

Scenes from a Union League parade in South Carolina, celebrating the anniversary of Emancipation Day (Library of Congress)

most northern states—was introduced, including state hospitals, asylums for orphans and the insane, and more modern and humane prisons. Some southern states outpaced their northern counterparts, introducing social welfare programs that would not be seen in much of the country until the 1960s. For example, the Reconstruction regimes of South Carolina and Alabama respectively offered free medical care and legal counsel for the poor. (For the most part, the schools and other institutions created by the Reconstruction-era governments of the South remained strictly segregated along racial lines, prefiguring developments in the post-Reconstruction era.)

To pay for this vast expansion of government services, new taxes were passed. Not surprisingly, this served to create more opposition than almost anything else attempted by the Reconstruction governments. For years, the South had lagged behind the North in taxation. With their governments run by planters, land and personal property taxes were kept to a minimum. State budgets were balanced by offering almost no government services. But with their ambitious agendas, Reconstruction governments passed a series of property taxes. As with all progressive taxation schemes, those with more paid more. And, in the South, that meant the planters. The Reconstruction governments had a threefold agenda in imposing taxes on this group: to make them pay their fair share in rebuilding a backward and war-torn South; to diminish their economic power; and to force them to sell their land, making more land available to poor blacks and whites. Intensifying the hostility of the planters were the methods employed to assess and collect the taxes. Because counties with significant numbers of plantations usually had majority black populations, many of the new assessors and collectors were African Americans. Indeed, it was not unusual for a planter to find that the person forcing him to pay taxes—with the power of the state government behind him—was a former slave.

Nor was tax assessing unique in this regard. Just as some African Americans—largely freeborn elites—were gaining power during Reconstruction at the state and even federal level, many former slaves were winning office and gaining power at the local level. In fact, the freedpersons recognized early on that achieving social and economic gains depended upon who had power on the land. Thus, even as Reconstruction regimes were taking control of

Reconstruction South rewrote their constitutions, extending the vote and making more offices elective. Laws were updated to northern standards. For example, in some southern states, statutes allowing for the imprisonment of debtors were still on the books in 1865. By the end of the Reconstruction period, those had disappeared. Women were aided by the new governments as well. Laws that turned over a married woman's property to her husband were done away with and divorce—virtually illegal in most southern states—was made fairer and easier to obtain.

The Radical Reconstruction governments also attempted to rebuild, diversify, and expand the southern economy. The railroad network of the region was repaired and expanded and new manufacturing enterprises were promoted and subsidized. New roads were built into rural areas and city streets were paved. In addition, a host of new institutions—already familiar in

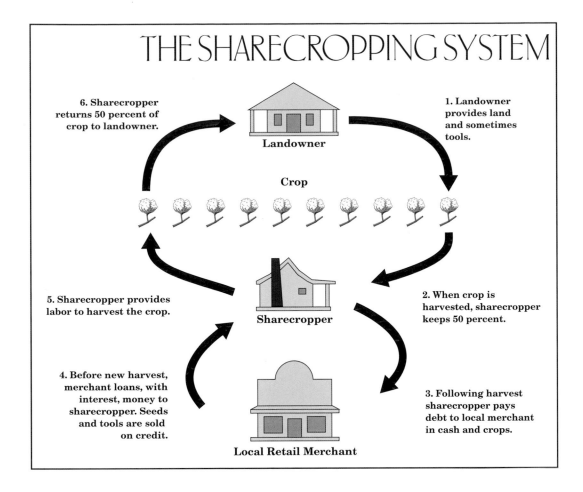

THE SHARECROPPING SYSTEM

6. Sharecropper returns 50 percent of crop to landowner.

1. Landowner provides land and sometimes tools.

Landowner

Crop

5. Sharecropper provides labor to harvest the crop.

Sharecropper

2. When crop is harvested, sharecropper keeps 50 percent.

4. Before new harvest, merchant loans, with interest, money to sharecropper. Seeds and tools are sold on credit.

3. Following harvest sharecropper pays debt to local merchant in cash and crops.

Local Retail Merchant

state governments, the Union (or Loyal) League was asserting power in localities throughout the South. Begun during the war as a northern organization to support the Union cause, the league quickly spread to the South when black and white organizers—often following in the wake of the Union army—founded chapters, largely in areas with significant African-American populations. These chapters soon became more than patriotic clubs. Many became self-help centers, helping to finance and construct local schools and churches. Most also had a political agenda, offering a civics education to newly freed slaves as well as promoting the candidacies of Radical Republican politicians at the local, state, and national levels. Finally, many Union League chapters—often filled with former Union army veterans, who retained their military rifles—formed militia companies to defend themselves against white violence and to protect those engaging in strikes against their landlords.

League chapters, militias, and local officials sympathetic to the plight of the freedperson were critical to the economic well-being of African Americans throughout the South. While some freedpersons migrated to southern towns and cities in search of work, the vast majority of the population remained on the land. In some cases, they became agricultural laborers and were paid a wage for working a planter's land. As with northern factory work, there was a constant struggle during the Reconstruction period over wages and working conditions in the cotton fields, with strikes breaking out in various parts of the region. The existence of Union League chapters and militia companies meant that black—and poor white—strikers would not be met with violence or, at least, could defend themselves against it.

Still, while some freedpersons became agricultural laborers in the Reconstruction era, most turned to sharecropping. As its name implies, sharecropping was a system of sharing, whereby planters provided the land, while "croppers" added the labor. When the crop was harvested, the two shared the proceeds—usually on a fifty-fifty basis. "Cropping," as it was popularly called, provided a reasonable solution to the many problems facing southern agriculture in the immediate post-war years. For cash-poor planters, it offered a guaranteed labor force without the need for wages. (In fact, it often increased the labor force as croppers, eager to maximize their own returns, reintroduced women into the fields at critical periods in the crop cycle.) For the former freedpersons, it meant relative independence. Croppers worked the land at

Acres per Worker on White and Black Family Cotton Farms, 1880

The amount of land acreage available to African-American farmers was consistantly less than that available to whites.

Form of Tenure	White Farms	Black Farms
Owner-operated farms	12.5 acres	6.6 acres
Rented farms	14.5 acres	7.3 acres
Sharecropped farms	11.7 acres	8.0 acres
All farms	**12.4 acres**	**7.5 acres**

their own pace and without direct white supervision, two benefits of supreme importance to people who had known the lash and the auction block all of their lives.

At first, "cropping" effectively served all parties. Cotton prices remained high during the first years after the Civil War and so returns to both planters and croppers were good. At the same time, as long as there were local black militias and officials, the cropper could be assured of a fair deal. Since the system inherently favored the planter—who controlled the weighing of the crop and offered credit for seeds, tools, and food against next year's crop—it was critical that croppers could turn to the law to protect their interests. Under Republican Reconstruction regimes, black or procropper sheriffs, judges, and other local officials made sure that croppers could turn to the courts and find justice in the law if they felt their landlord planters were trying to cheat them. Planters—so recently used to having absolute command over their labor force—found the new arrangements difficult to adjust to. Sharecropping, said one, "is the wrong policy. It makes the laborer too independent; he becomes a partner, and has a right to be consulted." Thus, from the very beginning of the post–Civil War era, the planter class of the South was determined to reassert its economic control over the region. But, as long as blacks, northerners, and their white progressive southern allies held the balance of political power, the planters were held in check. Not surprisingly,, destroying that political power became the number one priority of the southern planter class during the Reconstruction era.

REACTION AND "REDEMPTION"

Aside from the Civil War itself, the Reconstruction era is unquestionably the most violent period in American history, as planters and their allies among the white population of the region employed systematic terror to destroy black political power and the Republican Party in the South. The backlash began just one year after war's end. In 1866, a group of planters and other whites met in Pulaski, Tennessee to form a secret organization dedicated to white power and white supremacy in the South. Led by Nathan Bedford Forrest, a vicious Confederate army leader who had massacred northern black troops after they surrendered in the 1864 Battle of Fort Pillow, the group called itself the Ku Klux Klan. Allied closely with the Democratic Party in the South, the Klan—the name derived from a Greek word for "circle of men"—quickly spread across the region and, by decade's end, was operating in every southern state. It was particularly active in rural areas and in those parts of the South where the population of whites and blacks was relatively evenly balanced.

And while most of the Klan's membership was drawn from the ranks of poor southern whites, its leadership was largely composed of planters, merchants, and other elites of the region, including large numbers of Democratic Party officials. As a white minister traveling in Alabama noted, the Klan was organized by "the leading men of the state. They had lost their property, and worst of all, their slaves were made their equals and perhaps their superiors to rule over them." While a bit of an exaggeration—with little land of their own, freedpersons were hardly in a position to rule over

African-American Land Ownership in Rural Georgia, 1876

During the 1870s, African Americans made up just under half of the population of Georgia. Not surprisingly, however, they owned almost none of the land and held very few other assets.

Type of Asset	Percentage Owned by African Americans
Land	1.0%
City/town property	2.7%
Money/liquid assets	0.4%
Furniture	5.2%
Livestock	1.1%
Tools	4.9%
All other property	13.1%
Total taxable wealth	**2.5%**

CHRONOLOGY OF THE KU KLUX KLAN

April 1865	Confederacy surrenders; President Abraham Lincoln assassinated by southerner; Vice President Andrew Johnson, a southerner, becomes president.	May 1867	Klan becomes national organization and elects former Confederate general Nathan Bedford Forrest its first Grand Wizard in Nashville, Tennessee.
December 1865	Congress passes 13th Amendment banning slavery.	Winter–Spring 1868	Klan quickly spreads across the South, from Virginia to Texas.
March 1866	First Civil Rights Act passed by Congress.	May 1868	U.S. House of Representative impeaches President Andrew Johnson. The Senate vote to remove him from office fails by one vote.
June 1866	First Klan chapter organized in Pulaski Tennessee; Congress passes 14th Amendment, guaranteeing equal civil rights to blacks.	November 1868	Republican Ulysses S. Grant, the former commander of the Union army, is elected president.
July 1866	Tennessee becomes first Confederate state officially readmitted into the Union.	February 1869	Congress passes 15th Amendment, giving black males the vote.
November 1866	Republicans sweep Congress.	April 1871	Congress passes Ku Klux Klan Act, making violent anti–civil rights actions federal crimes.
March 1867	Congress passes Military Reconstruction Act, putting most of the South under martial law.		

the planters—the minister's remarks captured the resentment permeating white society in the Reconstruction era.

At first, the organization was largely a social fraternity, focusing on ritualistic ceremonies that celebrated white southern heritage. The events of the mid-1860s—including the rise of the Republican Party in the South, as well as black economic and political gains—soon turned the Klan into a vigilante organization that used violence and terror to achieve its ends, which included the return to power of the white planter class; the re-establishment of white social, economic, and political supremacy; and the resurrection of the Democratic Party in the

South. By early 1868, with chapters throughout the South, the Klan had turned to physical intimidation and violence. While white Republicans and other pro-black sympathizers were attacked by the Klan, the group's primary targets were the black population of the South and freedmen organizations, such as Union League chapters and local branches of the Republican Party. Indeed, Klan violence was rarely random. Singled out were black Union army veterans—most of whom were armed and many of whom were leaders in their local communities—as well as freedpersons who appeared to be succeeding economically, especially those who had been able to buy land of their own and thus escape the control of local planters.

Testimony gathered by federal investigators at the time provides a vivid depiction of Klan methods. "They took me to the woods and whipped me three hours or more and left me for dead," explained Abram Colby, a black member of the Georgia legislature, in 1869. "They said to me, 'Do you think you will ever vote for another damned radical ticket?' . . . I said, 'If there

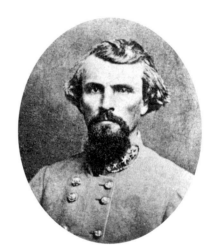

Nathan Bedford Forrest
(Library of Congress)

Early members of the Ku Klux Klan
(Library of Congress)

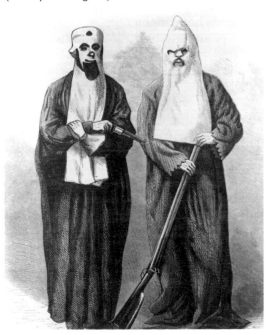

Other Racist Organizations During Reconstruction

Constitutional Union Guard (North Carolina)
Knights of the Rising Sun (Texas)
Knights of the White Camelia (Louisiana)
Knights of the White Carnation (Alabama)
Knights of the White Cross (Mississippi)
White Brotherhood (North Carolina)
Young Men's Democratic Clubs (Tennessee)

Republican hands and the House in Democratic hands, the balance of power lay with southern Democrats, and Hayes and other Republican leaders began to woo them in secret negotiations. Historians are not sure exactly who agreed to what—if anything—during these talks. But the outcome—the so-called compromise of 1877—led to the final dismantling of the Reconstruction governments of the South. Not only were Florida, Louisiana, and South Carolina turned over to Democratic rule, but the new president agreed to confine all federal troops in the South to their barracks.

Reconstruction—which had been undergoing a slow death since the late 1860s—was not killed off by the "compromise" but it was hastened to its end. Southern blacks would continue to vote and elect their own to local, state, and federal office through the end of the century. Segregation and the full imposition of the misnamed "separate but equal" doctrine were still a decade or more in the future. Still, the "compromise of 1877" did mark the end of the federal government's commitment to one of the most remarkable efforts at social reconstruction in the nation's history. And nowhere was the loss of that commitment more sharply felt than on the plantations of the South and in the economic relations between sharecroppers and their landlords.

As noted earlier, the presence of local politicians, judges, and law enforcement officials sympathetic to the plight of the freedperson was critical in assuring that fairness prevailed in the economic relations of sharecropping. It is not surprising, then, that the planter-led Ku Klux Klan specifically targeted African Americans, Republicans, and the candidates they voted for through intimidation, violence, and even murder. By destroying black political power in the South, the planters hoped to return the black population to economic subservience and assure that the bulk of the profits generated from sharecropping would accrue to those who owned the land. This goal became increasingly critical to cash-strapped planters as the price of cotton began to decline from the highs that prevailed in the immediate post–Civil War shortage years. Thus, even as the price of cotton and other commercial crops in the South declined, planters moved to take a bigger share of the profits that remained.

They did so through a system that came to be known as "debt peonage" or, as African Americans pointedly came to call it, "debt slavery." Croppers were usually forced to borrow from the planter to meet the farming and living expenses they accrued during the growing season. Sometimes this lending took the form of cash, but usually it was in goods such as seed, tools, foodstuffs, and cloth. The interest and/or prices charged by the planter were often exorbitant. A sharecropper might find that at the end of the season—when the crop was weighed and the profits divided—he or she owed more to the planter than the cropper's half of the crop was worth. Moreover, operating the scales and keeping the books—many croppers remained illiterate, especially after white "redemption" governments cut the budgets for public education—offered the planters many opportunities to cheat their tenants. If a tenant complained or threatened to find a better deal on another plantation, the planter could use law enforcement and the courts to keep the cropper in line. Laws were also passed at the state level to make it a crime to try and induce croppers away from a planter, and local industrialists and railroads were warned not to recruit black workers, except for the lowliest, poorest-paying positions. Gradually, croppers—and this included both blacks and poor whites—found themselves so deeply in debt to their landlords that they could never leave. And if they tried, they could be arrested and rented out by the state to work on their former master's land.

THE LATE 19TH CENTURY

Given the conditions that freedmen in the South had to live under, it is not surprising that many African Americans who were able to leave the South in the years immediately following the collapse of Reconstruction did so. And, like many Americans, some African Americans looked to the West for salvation. The so-called Exoduster movement of the late 1870s and early 1880s saw thousands of sharecroppers flee the South for the open farmlands of Kansas, Nebraska, and Oklahoma, where homesteading laws made it possible to stake out free claims on government land. Of course, the Exodusters were not the first blacks to head West. Although few in number, African Americans were critical to the history of the American West. Thus, before turning to the Exodusters, it is useful to examine the long, illustrious, and often overlooked history of blacks in the American West.

The first non–Native Americans to explore what would become the American West were the Spanish conquistadores of the 16th and 17th centuries. As discussed in chapter 2, one of the most famous of these

"Spanish" explorers was Estéban Dorantes, a Moorish slave whose search for the mythical Seven Cities of Gold ended in his mysterious disappearance in the deserts of the Southwest. But the tradition of black exploration of the West did not die with Estéban Dorantes. Indeed, the African-American experience in the West followed the general outlines of the region's history—first exploration and surveying; then exploitation of natural resources and the military conquest of the Native-American peoples; and finally the wholesale settlement of ranches and farms by westward migrating Americans.

AFRICAN AMERICANS
IN THE WEST

Among the first black explorers in North America was Jean-Baptiste Pointe du Sable. Born in Haiti to a French sailor and African-American slave woman in 1745, du Sable was sent by his father to Paris for an education, eventually working as a seaman on one of his father's ships. Shipwrecked near New Orleans in 1765 and fearful of being enslaved, he fled the region for what was then the Old Northwest, working as a fur trapper. Like most in his profession, du Sable took an Indi-

an woman for his wife. By 1779, he had built a cabin on the southern shores of Lake Michigan, at a site local Indians called *Eschikagou*, or "land of wild onions." Eventually, du Sable would buy land, on which he would establish a thriving farm and mill there, earning himself a historical claim as the founder of the nation's third largest city which, adapting the Indian name, would come to be known as Chicago.

Estéban and du Sable represented the black presence among Europeans in the American Midwest and West. But with the Louisiana Purchase of 1803, all of the land east of the Rocky Mountains came under American control. To learn what was there and to chart possible routes to the Pacific Ocean, President Thomas Jefferson recruited his personal secretary Meriwether Lewis and an army officer named William Clark to lead an expedition to the Pacific Northwest. Among the party was Clark's slave. Known to history by his Christian name only, York proved a critical member of the expedition. His great size, athletic prowess, and African features fascinated local Indians along the route, a phenomenon that greatly aided the progress of the largely white expedition as his presence often smoothed over relations with curious Native Americans.

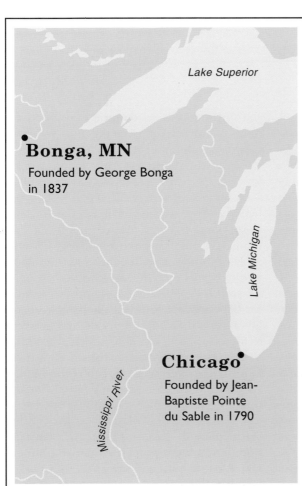

Bonga, MN
Founded by George Bonga
in 1837

Lake Superior

Lake Michigan

Chicago
Founded by Jean-
Baptiste Pointe
du Sable in 1790

Mississippi River

JEAN-BAPTISTE POINTE DU SABLE
AND THE BONGA FAMILY

Jean-Baptiste Pointe du Sable was born in 1745 in Saint-Domingue. In 1773, he purchased a home and land in Old Peoria Fort, Illinois. Five years later, he founded a trading post at the mouth of the Chicago River. From that post, he established himself as a successful fur trapper and trader as well as a miller and cooper. In 1790, he built the first permanent settlement in what is now Chicago, Illinois. After selling his holdings in Chicago, du Sable retired in 1800 to a stone mansion in St. Charles, Missouri. He died in 1818.

Among the most important families in Minnesota history, Jean Bonga, his son Pierre, and his grandsons George and Stephen, were instrumental in opening the Northwest Territories to settlement.

Jean Bonga, a former slave, opened the first inn on Mackinaw Island sometime after 1787.

His son, Pierre, was a reknowned explorer and translator who joined the North West Company in 1803. Married to a Chippewa (Ojibway) Indian, he served as the chief guide during the British exploration of the Red River Valley.

Grandson Stephen was a skillful negotiator who helped convince Chippewa Chief Hole-in-the-Day to negotiate with the American government.

Of all the Bongas, grandson George had the most illustrious career. He too was a trader, negotiator, translator, and guide. In 1820, he helped lead the Cass expedition in search of the source of the Mississippi River. Standing 6'6" tall and weighing well over 200 pounds, George was a commanding presence, whose half-black, half-Indian heritage won him the respect of Native American leaders.

In 1837, George founded a town in Cass County County, Minnesota, that bears his family name. His death in 1885 was noted in the U.S. Congress was well as in newspapers in New York, Chicago, and elsewhere.

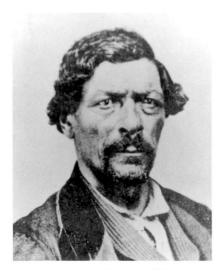

James Beckwourth (Library of Congress)

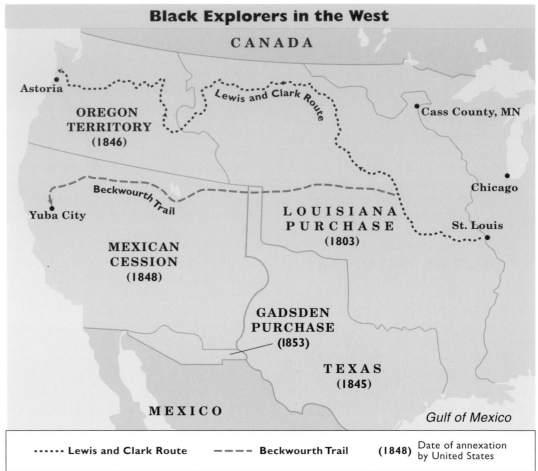

York, an enslaved African serving William Clark, played a crucial role during the Lewis and Clark expedition. The American explorers were guided by a Frenchman named Jean-Baptiste Charbonneau and his Native American wife Sacagawea. Because York spoke a little French as well as English, he served as company translator, not only within the company, but with Native Americans encountered along the way. The red line on the map above shows the westward route of the expedition. The Beckwourth Trail, forged by famed African-American mountain man James Beckwourth several decades later, is shown in green.

While the Lewis and Clark expedition focused on exploring and mapping, those who soon followed were more interested in exploiting the resources of the region, even as they explored and mapped much of this territory. The trailblazers in this endeavor were the fur trappers, men who ranged far and wide across the plains and mountains of the West in search of beaver and other pelts. Generally working alone or in small parties, they often traded with, lived among, and even married Native Americans. Among the most famous of these trapper/explorers was James Beckwourth. Born in 1798 and, like du Sable, of mixed heritage, Beckwourth began his trapping days at age 19, working for the Rocky Mountain Fur Company. By the time of the California gold rush of the late 1840s, he was ranging as far west as the Sierra Nevada. In April 1850, he discovered one of the key passes through those intimidating mountains—a pass that still bears his name—and set up a farm and trading post at its western end,

just in time to take advantage of the many miners and settlers pouring into northern California after gold was discovered in 1848.

Indeed, among the forty-niners were a few African Americans, largely brought as slaves by southern gold seekers. But the freewheeling atmosphere of the mining camps and the instant metropolis of San Francisco made escape easy. Most slaves quickly broke free of their masters and worked on claims of their own, or as wage laborers for other miners—some white miners believed blacks were good luck—or in businesses that offered goods and services to miners. Some, like land speculator Biddy Mason, became entrepreneurs of their own. Others, like Mifflin Gibbs, who founded the state's first black newspaper, took on the role of civil rights activists. Nor were American blacks the first Africans in the Golden State. Many members of the state's Mexican population were of mixed Spanish, Indian, and African heritage, including Pío Pico, a wealthy rancher and the first governor of

California following its annexation after the U.S.-Mexican War.

The coming of the Civil War interrupted black migration to the West, just as it did for the population in general. But in the wake of the conflict a new surge of settlement began, particularly in the territories of the Great Plains and Mountain West. The intrusion of these settlers on their ancestral lands angered the Native Americans of the region and set off a series of wars between the U.S. Army and various Indian nations that would last until 1890 and the Wounded Knee Massacre in what is now South Dakota. Taking part in this bloody and oftentimes unjust struggle were several regiments of black soldiers—many of them veterans of the Civil War—that Native Americans came to call Buffalo Soldiers, after their curly black hair, which the Indians believed looked like buffalo fur.

Divided into four regiments—two infantry and two cavalry, the latter making up 20 percent of all U.S. cavalry in the late 19th century—the Buffalo Soldiers patrolled the region between the Mississippi River and the Rocky Mountains. It was, of course, a physically and morally challenging task for many of the soldiers. For $13 per month, they divided their time between stays in rough-hewn forts and long, hard rides across the western landscape. They chased down outlaws and cattle rustlers and kept the peace in territories where sheep and cattle ranchers settled their differences with gunfire. Later, many of the black cavalrymen would see service in the Spanish-American War where they fought alongside Teddy Roosevelt's "Rough Riders" in the Battle of San Juan Hill. Black troops of the Ninth and 10th Cavalry overwhelmed a Spanish fort and cut though barbed wire, thus providing an opening for the Rough Riders to attack. In response, Roosevelt remarked, "Well, the Ninth and 10th men are alright. They can drink out of our canteens." The Buffalo Soldiers continued their service in the Philippines, helping to put down a revolt against American occupation in the early years of the 20th century, and Mexico, where they fought revolutionaries and bandits in 1916 after the latter conducted raids across the U.S. border.

But, mostly, the Buffalo Soldiers attacked Indians. Former slaves, they were given the task of forcing another oppressed people off the land to make way for a white population that had little respect for either group. Indeed, local whites often failed to pay the Buffalo Soldiers the respect that was given to other cavalrymen. In 1878, a

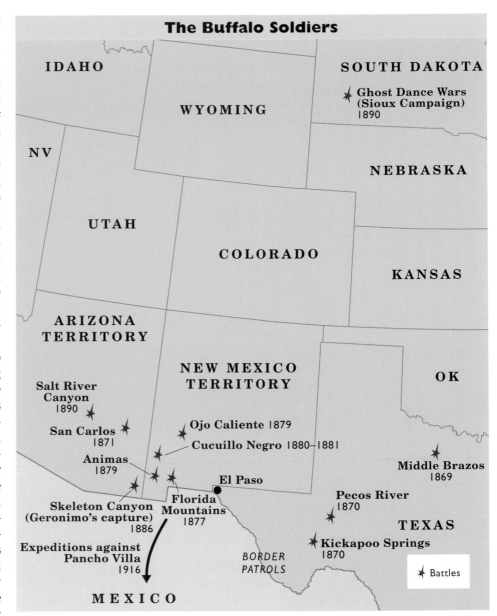

The Buffalo Soldiers

IDAHO

WYOMING

SOUTH DAKOTA

✴ **Ghost Dance Wars (Sioux Campaign)** 1890

NV

NEBRASKA

UTAH

COLORADO

KANSAS

ARIZONA TERRITORY

NEW MEXICO TERRITORY

OK

Salt River Canyon 1890 ✴

San Carlos ✴ 1871

Animas 1879

✴ **Ojo Caliente** 1879

— **Cucuillo Negro** 1880–1881

Middle Brazos 1869

El Paso

Pecos River 1870

Skeleton Canyon (Geronimo's capture) 1886

Florida Mountains 1877

Expeditions against Pancho Villa 1916

BORDER PATROLS

TEXAS

✴ **Kickapoo Springs** 1870

✴ Battles

MEXICO

major gunfight between white cowboys and black cavalry broke out in San Angelo, Texas, after the barroom murder of a Buffalo Soldier by a white cowhand who boasted that he committed the crime for "sport." Sometimes, they faced hostility from the army bureaucracy itself. Benjamin O. Flipper, West Point's first black graduate, was assigned to the 10th Cavalry, and was drummed out of the service after being caught riding with a white woman. As historian William Loren Katz noted, "it is ironic that these brave black soldiers served so well in the final and successful effort to crush American Indians, the first victims of white racism in this continent. But serve they did." In fact, they served with distinction, earning 23 Medals of Honor for their bravery in the Indian wars and the Spanish-American War.

Blacks in the West, however, were not always on the side of the law. A number of

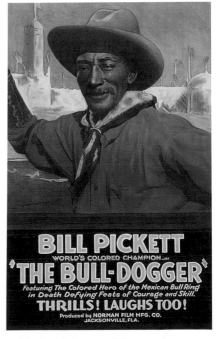

Bill Pickett (Library of Congress)

African-American Participation in the Spanish-American War's Cuban Campaign

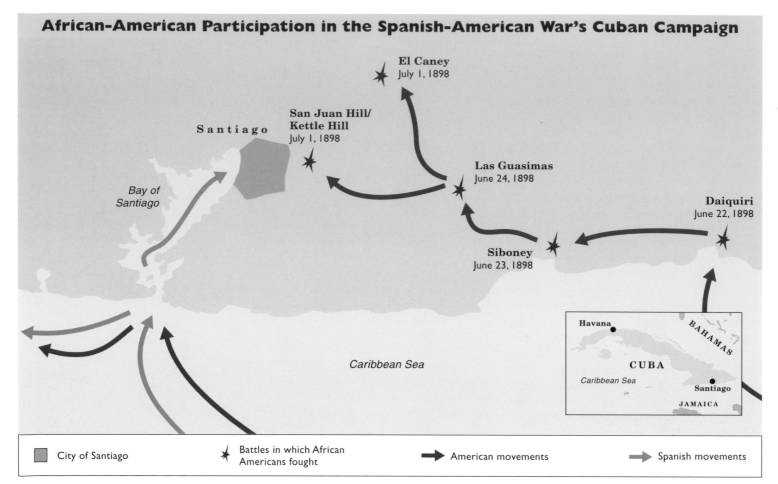

African-American troops played a significant role in the Spanish-American War, including at the famous Battle of San Juan Hill. The map shown here illustrates battles during the campaign for Cuba in which African-American troops played a part.

the more notorious outlaws of the old West were African American, including cattle rustler Isom Dart, gunfighter Cherokee Bill, and con man Ben Hodges, who once swindled the president of the Dodge City National Bank out of thousands of dollars.

Most black cowboys were honest, hardworking men. Making up an estimated 25 percent of all Texas cowhands in the late 19th century, black cowboys were such a part of the western scene that several became western legends. Bill Pickett is widely credited as the inventor of bulldogging, the popular rodeo sport of chasing down a steer on horseback, jumping off, and wrestling the animal to the ground. Pickett later went on to a lucrative career as a star of rodeo and the early movie screen. Nat Love—known as "Deadwood Dick"— was perhaps the most famous of the black cowboys, largely because of his autobiography which, in the tradition of western truth-stretching, painted Love as a man who could out-rope, out-shoot, and out-drink any man alive.

Still, the days of the open range—for both blacks and whites in the West—were numbered. Eventually, farming followed ranching. As with whites, many African Americans saw an opportunity to improve their lot by homesteading western lands. It also offered—or so many blacks thought— an escape from racism in the South. Rising white violence and the collapse of pro-black Reconstruction regimes in 1877 left many freedpersons in despair and terror. Then, as in a religious revival, promoters like Benjamin "Pap" Singleton spread the word

Blacks in the Spanish-American War

Federal
Ninth Cavalry
10th Cavalry
24th Cavalry
25th Cavalry

State
Ninth Ohio
Third Alabama
Third North Carolina
Sixth Virginia
23rd Kansas
Eighth Illinois

Two Indiana infantry companies
Company L of the Sixth Massachusetts

Congressional Medal of Honor Winners
Pvt. Dennis Bell, 10th Cavalry, born in
    Washington, D.C.
Pvt. Fitz Lee, 10th Cavalry, born in Virginia
Pvt. William Thompkins, 10th Cavalry,
    born in New Jersey
Pvt. George Wanton, 10th Cavalry,
    born in Wyoming

Black Towns in Oklahoma and Kansas, ca. 1900

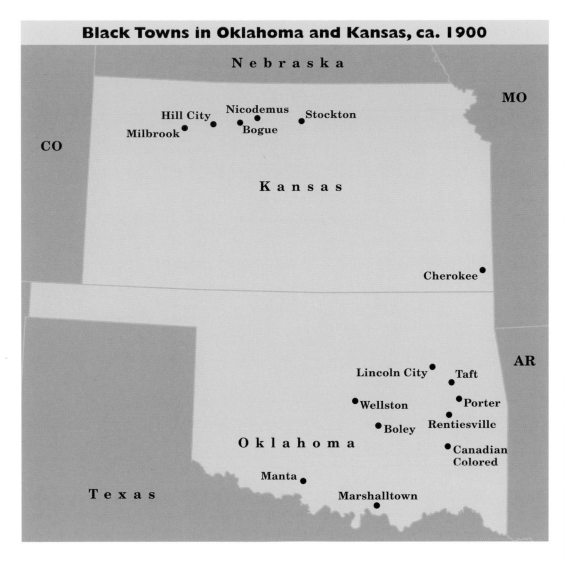

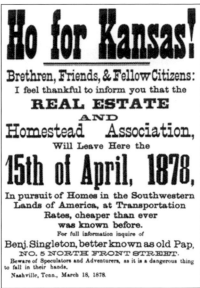

A recruitment sign for Singleton's
Homestead Association
(Library of Congress)

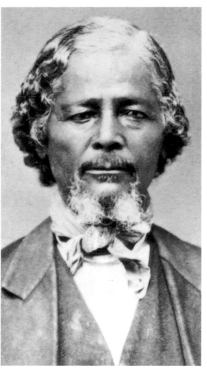

"Pap" Singleton (Library of Congress)

through freedperson communities of the South that there was free land and freedom from white racism in the West. During the spring of 1879, thousands heeded his call. By May, more than 6,000 Exodusters were camped out along the St. Louis riverfront, awaiting riverboats that would take them upriver to Kansas and Nebraska. Many were impoverished, with no money for fares and little more than the clothes on their backs. Still, by 1880, the U.S. Census reported more than 40,000 black people in the state of Kansas, making it the second-largest black population in the West, after Texas. Twenty years later, a second exodus brought the black population of Oklahoma to more than 130,000, including several thousand who lived in "planned," all-black towns like Boley and Langston City. As in other such real estate ventures, streets were carefully laid out on grids and lots set aside for parks, schools, and other public buildings. Sadly, both efforts at homesteading would be largely defeated in the late 19th and early 20th centuries, broken by drought, low crop prices, and racist institutions, including milling operations and rail-roads that discriminated against black farmers.

THE RISE OF JIM CROW

While the end of Reconstruction came in 1877—with President Hayes's order to end active federal army supervision of the South—the impact of the nation's first great experiment in racial equality lingered on for at least another generation. Segregation—while widespread—was not absolute and had yet to be enshrined in law in the late 1870s and 1880s. In many regions of the South, for example, blacks continued to vote and elect other African Americans to local and state office through the end of the 19th century. In Mississippi and South Carolina, the two southern states with proportionally the largest black populations, voters sent African Americans to Congress through the end of the century. Still, there were critical differences between the Reconstruction era and the "redemption" period of renewed white rule that succeeded it.

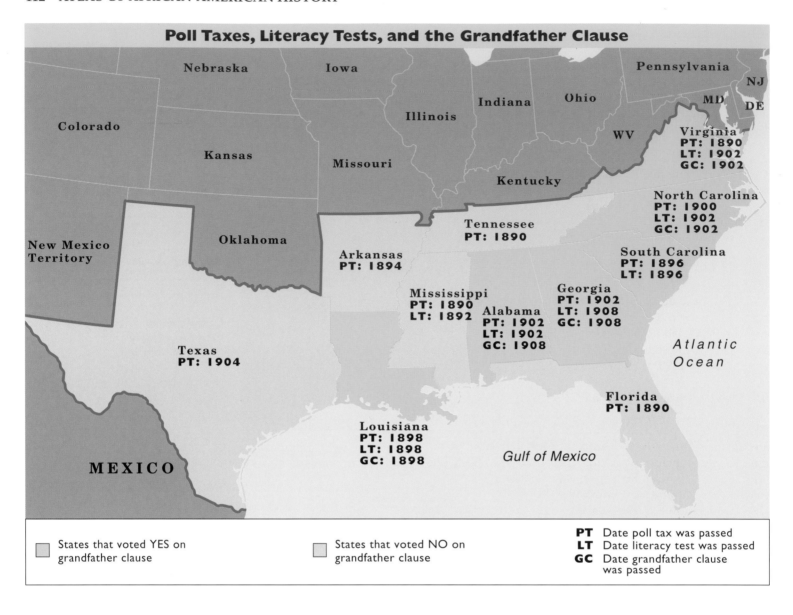

Poll Taxes, Literacy Tests, and the Grandfather Clause

Nebraska
Iowa
Pennsylvania
NJ

Colorado
Indiana
Ohio
MD
DE

Kansas
Illinois
WV
Virginia
PT: 1890
LT: 1902
GC: 1902

Missouri
Kentucky

North Carolina
PT: 1900
LT: 1902
GC: 1902

New Mexico
Territory
Oklahoma
Tennessee
PT: 1890

Arkansas
PT: 1894

South Carolina
PT: 1896
LT: 1896

Mississippi
PT: 1890
LT: 1892
Alabama
PT: 1902
LT: 1902
GC: 1908
Georgia
PT: 1902
LT: 1908
GC: 1908

Texas
PT: 1904

Atlantic
Ocean

Florida
PT: 1890

Louisiana
PT: 1898
LT: 1898
GC: 1898
Gulf of Mexico

MEXICO

States that voted YES on grandfather clause

States that voted NO on grandfather clause

PT Date poll tax was passed
LT Date literacy test was passed
GC Date grandfather clause was passed

During the former, blacks and white Republicans had political power somewhat commensurate to their numbers in the population, often vying with white Democrats for local and state government control. In the latter period, blacks and Republicans voted and won office as a distinctly minority force. Blacks continued to vote in large numbers in the late 1870s and 1880s but their vote was tightly controlled. Moreover, there was no institutional challenge to the rule of planters and other elites, as the Republican party—castigated as the party of northern carpetbaggers—virtually disappeared as a political force in the white South, not to be revived for another century. The South had become a one-party region and that party—the Democrats—had clearly become the voice of white supremacy and planter power.

Yet, despite the hegemony of the Democratic Party, there were deep divisions within southern society, and not just between blacks and whites. Resentment of planter wealth and political power ran deep even before the Civil War among many poor southern whites, particularly those who had been relegated to marginal hill-country lands. The huge losses suffered by white farmers in the war—a popular slogan of the day was that the conflict had been "a rich man's war but a poor man's fight"—added to the anger. But it was economic concerns that turned this resentment into political revolt, with enormous consequences for the black population of the South.

Following a short-lived, postwar boost in the value of cotton and other commercial crops, prices began to fall in the 1880s. Many poor southern farmers fell into debt to local merchants who fronted them food and supplies for the growing season. With prices for their crops falling, many farmers found themselves unable to pay their debts and were forced to sell their lands. The result was a burgeoning population of white sharecroppers across the South. As the economic distress grew, poor white farmers and sharecroppers formed the Southern Alliance, a populist-style movement aimed at addressing low crop prices and burdensome debt. Blacks followed suit with the Colored Farmers' Alliance. The organizations grew rapidly. By the late 1880s, the two organizations boasted a membership of 3 million between them.

Nor were the Southern Alliance and many poor white farmers generally slow to realize the obvious racial implications of their struggle. That is, poor white farmers and the Southern Alliance had far more in common with black croppers and the Colored Farmers' Alliance than they did with planters and the Democratic Party. As populist leader Tom Watson of Georgia remarked, "the accident of color can make no difference in the interest of farmers, croppers, and laborers. You are kept apart that you may be separately fleeced of your earnings." By 1890, both alliances were rallying behind the single largest challenge to the two-party system in the late 19th century—the Peoples' Party, also known as the Populists. A movement designed to alleviate agricultural poverty through government action—including nationalization of the railroads, government purchase of crops, and inflationary monetary policy (inflation, by lowering the value of money and raising the price of crops, makes it easier for farmers to pay back their debts)—the Populists demonstrated enormous political appeal in both the South and Midwest.

Sadly, particularly for its black supporters, the Populist movement was broken in the South by the Democratic Party and its appeals to white supremacy. With money, power, and influence on their side, white elites and Democratic Party politicians appealed to the lowest instincts of poor white southerners. Arguing that economic and political cooperation with blacks would lead to social equality—and even sexual intermixing—southern political leaders were able to browbeat many poor whites into voting Democratic. Indeed, Democratic rallies often featured bevies of white women appealing to their menfolk to protect them from the black man. When visceral appeals to racial intolerance failed, white elites employed fraud, running up huge pro-Democratic tallies in the largely African-American counties that they controlled. As Frank Burkitt, a Mississippi populist, complained, "a class of corrupt office-seekers . . . hypocritically raised the howl of white supremacy while they debauched the ballot boxes . . . disregarded the rights of the blacks . . . and actually dominated the will of the white people through the instrumentality of the stolen negro vote." Sometimes, as in the case of the secret White Man's Union of Grimes County, Texas, the old, anti-Reconstruction methods of violence and intimidation were used to keep blacks from the polls in the late 1890s.

Yet, despite the shared economic concerns of blacks and poor whites, fraud and the appeals to white racism worked. Nationally, the Populist Party—torn by divisions over its national alliance with Democratic presidential candidate William Jennings Bryan—virtually disappeared as a political force after 1896. Regionally, future Populist threats to Democratic Party rule were met by reinforcing white supremacy and disenfranchising black

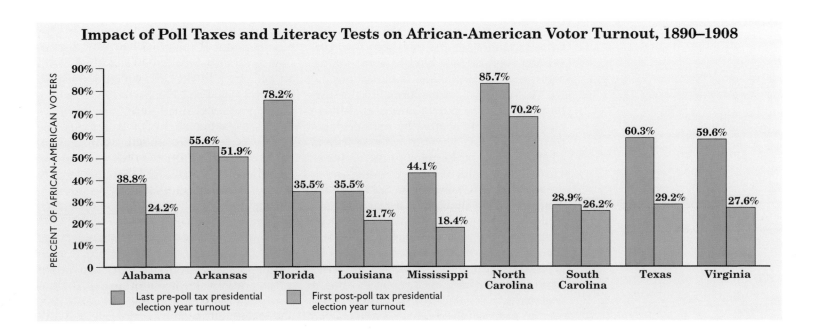

Impact of Poll Taxes and Literacy Tests on African-American Voter Turnout, 1890–1908

PERCENT OF AFRICAN-AMERICAN VOTERS

Alabama: 38.8% / 24.2%
Arkansas: 55.6% / 51.9%
Florida: 78.2% / 35.5%
Louisiana: 35.5% / 21.7%
Mississippi: 44.1% / 18.4%
North Carolina: 85.7% / 70.2%
South Carolina: 28.9% / 26.2%
Texas: 60.3% / 29.2%
Virginia: 59.6% / 27.6%

■ Last pre-poll tax presidential election year turnout   ■ First post-poll tax presidential election year turnout

SELECTED SEGREGATION LAWS

Separation in Railroad Cars by State	Year Law Passed
Georgia	1891
South Carolina	1900
North Carolina, Virginia	1901

State	Year Law Passed
Louisiana	1902
Arkansas, Tennessee	1903
Mississippi, Maryland	1904

Examples of Segregation Laws by State	Law	Year Law Passed
Alabama	Separate school system	1868*
Georgia	Separate parks	1905
Alabama	Separate street cars	1906
Baltimore, Maryland	Separate neighborhoods	1910
Louisiana	Separate entrances and seating at circuses	1914
South Carolina	Separate entrances, working facilities, pay windows, water glasses, etc. in factories	1915
Oklahoma	Separate telephone booths	1915
Mississippi	Separate taxicabs	1922
Atlanta, Georgia	African-American barbers forbidden from cutting the hair of white women	1926
Atlanta, Georgia	White and black baseball teams banned from playing within two blocks of each other	1932
Texas	Whites and blacks forbidden from wrestling together	1933
Oklahoma	Whites and blacks forbidden from fishing or boating together	1935
Arkansas	Segregated race tracks	1937
Virginia	Segregated waiting rooms at airports	1944

* By 1885, all states in the South required separate schools for white and black children.

voters. Segregation. or "Jim Crow" as it was called, once enforced by custom, became enshrined in law. All public places and conveyances were either strictly divided by race or restricted to whites only. At the same time, state after state in the South passed poll taxes and literacy tests to prevent blacks from voting. Sometimes, these also had the potential to disenfranchise poor whites, but the rules were rarely enforced in white counties.

An even more effective method of disenfranchising blacks was the "grandfather clause," which denied the vote to anyone whose grandfather had not been free, preventing almost all blacks from voting, regardless of their finances or educations.

As with the retreat from Reconstruction, the white South's efforts to reverse black gains were abetted by northern apathy and acquiescence. During the 1880s and 1890s, a series of Supreme Court decisions virtually undid all of the civil rights laws of the Reconstruction era. In an 1883 case, the court virtually eliminated the "equal protection" clause of the 14th Amendment by exempting the actions of private citizens. That is to say, the court declared that the U.S. Constitution only applied in cases where the state itself discriminated. Thus, it was perfectly legal for a restaurant or a railroad to practice discrimination in its hiring or its offering of services to black citizens. The most infamous case reversing the gains of the Reconstruction era, however, was the 1896 *Plessy v. Ferguson* opinion in which the Court decided that governments—local, state, and even federal—could practice segregation, as long as they provided "separate but equal" facilities and services to both races. *Plessy v. Ferguson* resulted in the "separate" but not the "equal."

The 1890s and the early 20th century mark, perhaps, the nadir of post–Civil War racial tolerance. In the South, lynching—the arbitrary torture, execution, and even dismemberment of those suspected of disobedience or rule-breaking—flourished, with an average of 100 blacks killed every year between 1890 and 1910. In the North, where blacks remained small in number until the Great Migration of World War I and the 1920s, racism was equally widespread, based on the "scientific" principles of social Darwinism that deemed blacks genetically inferior to whites. Still, despite oppression, intimidation, and violence, individual blacks and black organizations continued to challenge the ideas and practices of late 19th- and early 20th-century racism. But the means to best accomplish that—separation or integration—created a rift in the African-American community that, arguably, has not healed to this day.

THE "NEW NEGRO"
African Americans in the Early 20th Century

The two decades following the collapse of the Reconstruction era in 1877 witnessed a rolling back of civil rights gains for African Americans both in the South and in the North. The black presence in local, state, and federal politics gradually eroded as various methods of disenfranchisement were employed in the southern states. These included literacy tests, poll and property taxes, grandfather clauses (denying the vote to those whose grandfathers could not vote in 1866, before the 15th Amendment gave blacks the right to vote), and whites-only primaries (a considerable restriction given the de facto one-party system in the South). At the same time, laws were passed to formalize and extend the daily racial segregation of southern life, with separate places on streetcars, railroads, and other forms of transportation set aside for whites and blacks. In other public facilities, blacks were banned altogether—as in restaurants and hotels—or made to use back entrances.

explain the evolution of species—scientists and philosophers applied a version of the ideas the ideas of the English naturalist to the social sciences. This school of thought—known as social Darwinism—argued among other things that certain races and ethnicities were inherently superior or inferior to others, as could be proved by their ranking in the social order. As African Americans were considered at the bottom of this order, they were thought of as biologically inferior to whites. The widespread acceptance of this pseudoscience among educated people both in the North and the South goes a long way in helping explain why one of the few presidents in American history with a doctoral degree—history professor and Princeton University president Woodrow Wilson (1913–1921)—was among the most racist men to occupy the office, going so far as to segregate all government facilities in Washington and restrict blacks to the most menial jobs within the federal government.

THE EARLY CIVIL RIGHTS MOVEMENT

Even as southern states passed discriminatory laws, these laws were being upheld by the U.S. Supreme Court. A series of cases over a 25-year period eroded the legal and constitutional protections for freedpersons that were created during the Reconstruction period. The 1896 *Plessy v. Ferguson* decision represented the culmination of this process when it declared that "separate but equal" facilities did not violate the "equal protection" clause of the 14th Amendment. In practice, of course, facilities were hardly equal, if they existed at all for black citizens. Writing for the seven-to-one majority, Justice Henry Brown claimed that "legislation is powerless to eradicate racial instincts or to abolish distinctions."

The decision was both a surrender to—and confirmation of—the racial prejudice of the day. Indeed, the late 19th and early 20th centuries represented the culmination of racially deterministic thinking in America. Building on the work of Charles Darwin—whose "survival of the fittest" theory helped

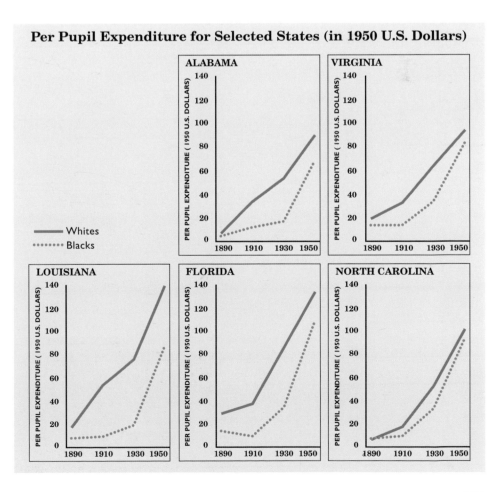

Per Pupil Expenditure for Selected States (in 1950 U.S. Dollars)

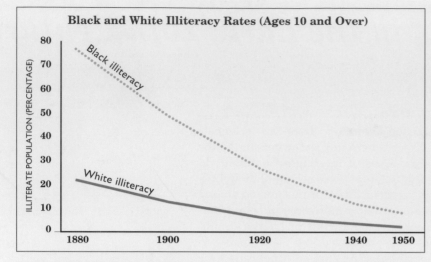

Black and White Illiteracy Rates (Ages 10 and Over)

Black illiteracy

White illiteracy

ILLITERATE POPULATION (PERCENTAGE)

80 70 60 50 40 30 20 10 0

1880   1900   1920   1940   1950

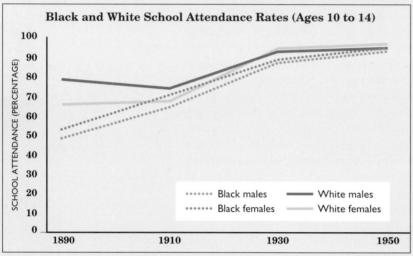

Black and White School Attendance Rates (Ages 10 to 14)

SCHOOL ATTENDANCE (PERCENTAGE)

100 90 80 70 60 50 40 30 20 10 0

1890   1910   1930   1950

········· Black males   ——— White males
········· Black females ——— White females

Meanwhile, in the South, violence against blacks—sometimes approaching the widespread murder of the late Reconstruction–Ku Klux Klan period—remained endemic, with the lynching of blacks in the 1890s for reasons as trivial as looking at a white woman or accumulating too much property. In that ten-year period, more than 1,100 blacks—mostly young men—were beaten, hanged, or burned to death, oftentimes in festival-like surroundings.

When not confronting the direct violence of the lynch mob, most African Americans in the South—and the small minority who lived in the North—faced the day-to-day economic assault of poverty. For example, in Georgia, where blacks represented about one-third of the population in 1880, they owned but 1.6 percent of all farm acreage and represented just 7.3 percent of all skilled laborers. And while the *Plessy* decision was based on the idea of "separate but equal" facilities for both races, in the realm of education it was far from the case. Illiteracy among blacks over 20 years old in the Deep South stood at more than 75 percent, compared to just 17 percent of whites of the same age. Legal slavery was no more, but a system of debt peonage—in which black sharecroppers remained unable to pay off the loans fronted to them by their landlords—kept them tied to the cotton plantation as in antebellum times.

A mother teaches her children at home (Library of Congress)

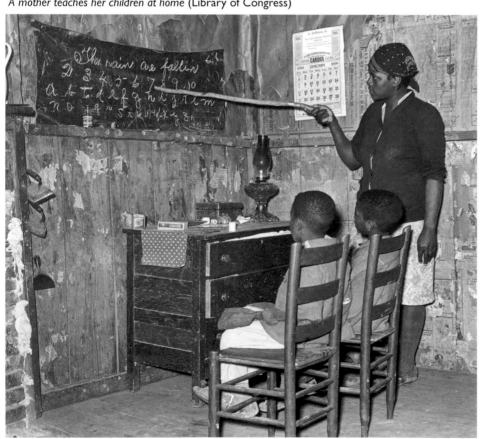

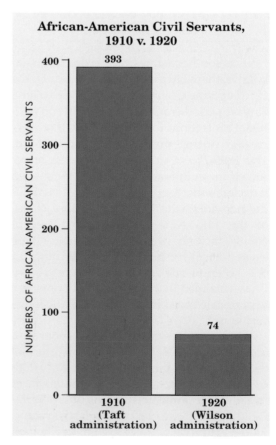

African-American Civil Servants, 1910 v. 1920

NUMBERS OF AFRICAN-AMERICAN CIVIL SERVANTS

400   393

300

200

100   74

0

1910
(Taft administration)

1920
(Wilson administration)

Booker T. Washington and the Tuskegee Institute

Widespread segregation and extreme discrimination was the context in which the civil rights leaders of the era tried to advance the interests of African Americans. Among these was a former slave named Booker T. Washington, the most widely recognized black spokesperson since Frederick Douglass and easily the most influential African-American leader of the late 19th century. Born to a black mother and an unknown white father in rural Virginia, Washington was liberated by Union troops near the end of the Civil War. At 16, he left home for Virginia's Hampton Institute, one of the few higher educational facilities set up for blacks in the Reconstruction era. Under the guidance of Hampton's principal—a white former Union general named Samuel Chapman Armstrong—Washington imbibed a self-help philosophy as he received an education in both the liberal and manual arts. Armstrong also helped Washington financially, finding him a white benefactor who paid for his living and educational expenses. Both to Washington's later admirers and critics, this experience of white beneficence goes a long way in explaining the man's philosophy and his willingness not to challenge in any radical way the racial prejudices of his day.

In 1881, the state of Alabama asked Armstrong to recommend a principal for a new school for blacks to be opened at Tuskegee. Although Alabama asked for a white principal, Armstrong suggested Washington, and the state agreed. Apportioned just $2000 for teachers' salaries—but nothing for land and buildings—Tuskegee quickly came to reflect the ideas for black education Washington picked up at Hampton. The emphasis was on manual skills, with boys learning carpentry, shoemaking, and other skills and girls being taught cooking and sewing. Students were also put to work raising money and helping construct buildings, aided by the donations of white philanthropists. Within a decade, Tuskegee was training 500 African Americans a year in the manual arts and agricultural sciences.

But while Tuskegee earned Washington a modest reputation among wealthy white benefactors interested in black self-improvement, real prominence—and status as a national black spokesperson acceptable to the white community—came with his widely quoted speech at Atlanta's Cotton States and International Exposition in 1895, the year of Frederick Douglass's death. Speaking to a largely white audience,

GEORGE WASHINGTON CARVER

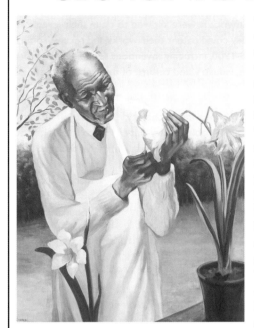

George Washington Carver
(Library of Congress)

George Washington Carver was born a slave during the Civil War, and died 80 years later an internationally renowned agricultural scientist. Carver was the most famous teacher at Booker T. Washington's Tuskegee Institute and is remembered for urging southern farmers to end their reliance on cotton, which left the soil depleted and worthless, and to start planting nutrient-rich, soil-renewing crops, such as peanuts and sweet potatoes. To further encourage the switch to peanuts and sweet potatoes, Carver created hundreds of money-making by-products, including coffee substitutes, flour, shaving cream, ink, dyes, plastics, vinegar, and more, giving small farmers hope for self-sufficiency. Throughout his career, Carver experimented with improved methods of cultivation. In his later years, he became a symbol of black achievement and was widely celebrated in the United States and throughout the world.

Washington advised his fellow African Americans to "cast down your bucket where you are." By this he meant that they should remain in the South, on the farm, and to accept the society as it was. "In all things that are purely social," he said of the

Booker T. Washington (center) with President William Howard Taft (left) and industrialist Andrew Carnegie (right) outside the White House (Library of Congress)

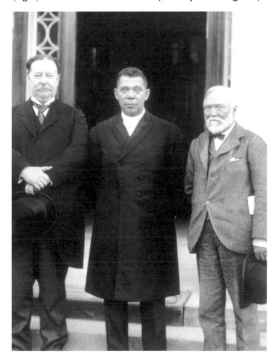

Annual Lynchings of African-Americans, 1882–1925

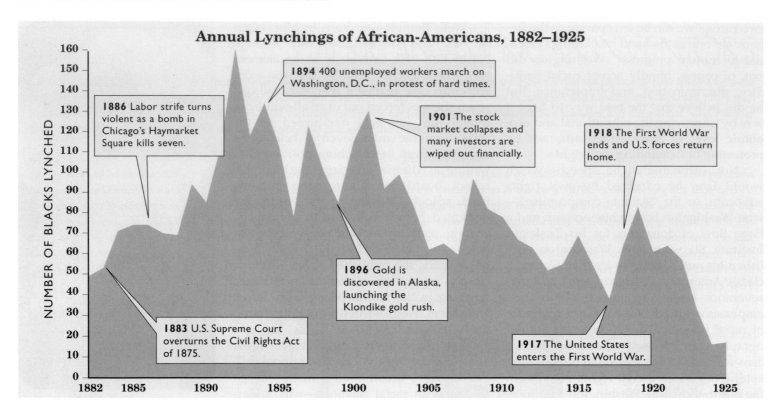

1886 Labor strife turns violent as a bomb in Chicago's Haymarket Square kills seven.

1894 400 unemployed workers march on Washington, D.C., in protest of hard times.

1901 The stock market collapses and many investors are wiped out financially.

1918 The First World War ends and U.S. forces return home.

1883 U.S. Supreme Court overturns the Civil Rights Act of 1875.

1896 Gold is discovered in Alaska, launching the Klondike gold rush.

1917 The United States enters the First World War.

W. E. B. DuBois (National Portrait Gallery)

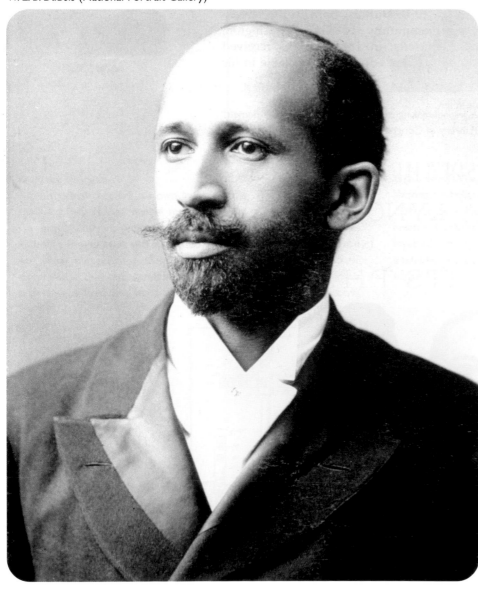

day to a man of any color. First attending Fisk University, he then received his bachelor's degree from Harvard, attended the University of Berlin for two years, and went on to earn his Ph.D. in sociology from Harvard, studying under the guidance of some of the leading intellectuals of the time, including philosophers George Santayana, William James, and Josiah Royce.

Despite this exceptional academic background, DuBois still faced the prejudice of his day and was forced to accept a low paying teaching position at Wilberforce College. Having moved on to Atlanta University, DuBois published *The Souls of Black Folks* in 1903, widely considered to be among the most important books ever published on African-American culture and American racial relations. The book passionately yet analytically examines the tortured role and place of black people in American history and society. He also used the book to criticize Booker T. Washington's philosophy of accomodation. "[When he] apologizes for injustice, does not rightly value the privilege and duty of voting, belittles the emasculating effects of caste distinctions, and opposes the higher training and ambition of our brighter minds," DuBois wrote, "we must unceasingly and firmly oppose [him]."

DuBois was as much a political activist as he was an intellectual. In 1905, he joined William Monroe Trotter, editor of the *Boston Guardian*, a radical African-American newspaper, in founding the Niagara Movement, named after the upstate New York town where it was begun. In a speech inaugurating the movement, DuBois laid out a series of demands, each of which was considered quite radical for their the time: "First . . . we want full manhood suffrage . . . Second. We want discrimination in public accommodation to cease . . . Third. We claim the right of freemen to walk, talk, and be with them that wish to be with us. Fourth. We want the laws enforced . . . against white as well as black. Fifth. We want our children . . . trained as intelligent human beings should be."

While the Niagara Movement was short-lived, it laid the foundation for DuBois's most lasting contribution to the institutionalization of the struggle for African-American civil rights in the United States—the National Association for the Advancement of Colored People (NAACP). Unlike the Niagara Movement, the NAACP—which was founded in 1909—included members of all races. Indeed, much of its early leadership was white. In 1910, DuBois moved from Atlanta to New York City to take an assignment as the editor of the organization's magazine, *Crisis*. For the next 25 years, DuBois would use the publication as a forum for his views on civil rights. Despite these notable accomplishments, DuBois was not above criticism. Many civil rights leaders charged him with elitism for his belief that the educated and "talented tenth" of African Americans were best suited to promote the interests of the race. In his later years, DuBois would increasingly come to embrace the cause of international communism. His controversial criticism of what he called American imperialism and his praise for the Soviet Union—which he saw as a society free of racial prejudice and class distinctions—landed him in frequent trouble with the U.S. federal government during the height of the cold war years of the 1950s. Invited by the socialist government of Ghana to live in that country— the first black African nation to break free of European colonial domination—DuBois died in Africa in 1963, having lived for nearly a century. By the time of his death, DuBois had long since given up hope that racial equality would ever be acheived in the United States. In an interesting twist of historical fate, the very same day he died, a young African-American minister from Atlanta, Georgia, Dr. Martin Luther King Jr., would deliver his famous "I Have a Dream" speech to a large multiracial crowd from steps of the Lincoln Memorial in Washington, D.C.

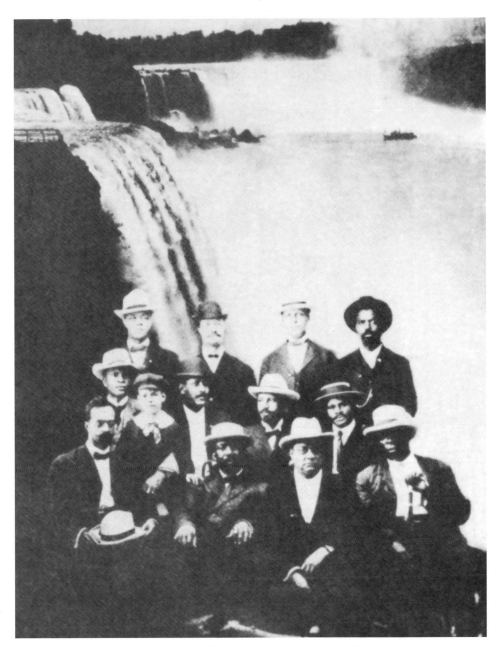

Participants at the the first meeting of the Niagara Movement (Library of Congress)

WORLD WAR I AND THE GREAT MIGRATION

In *The Souls of Black Folks*, W. E. B. DuBois wrote with foresight that, "[t]he problem of the twentieth century is the problem of the color-line," thereby identifying racial relations as the most critical issue of the then-new 20th century. Indeed, as the history of the century proved, DuBois was right, not just for the United States but for the world generally. While the first great conflagration of the new century—the Great War as contemporaries called it, or World War I as it is better known today—was not directly about race per se, it had an enormous effect on relations between white and nonwhite peoples in the United States and around the world.

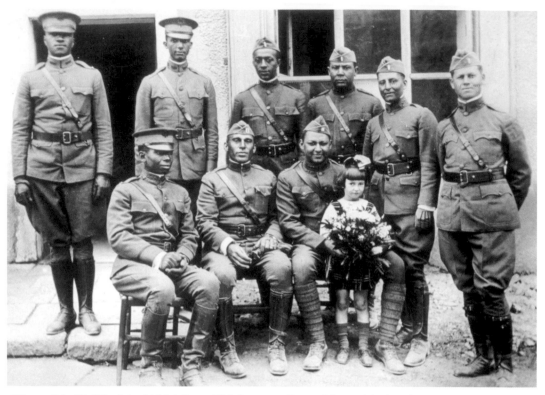

Officers of the "Buffalos," the 367th Infantry, 77th Division, in France (National Archives)

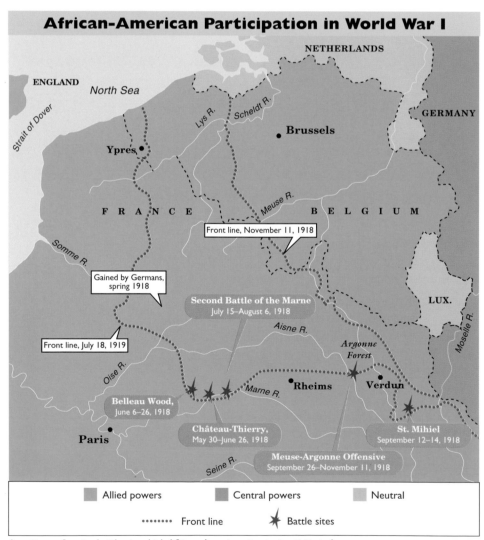

African-American Participation in World War I

NETHERLANDS

ENGLAND

North Sea

GERMANY

Strait of Dover

Lys R.

Scheldt R.

Brussels

Ypres

F R A N C E

Meuse R.

B E L G I U M

Front line, November 11, 1918

Somme R.

Gained by Germans, spring 1918

LUX.

Second Battle of the Marne
July 15–August 6, 1918

Aisne R.

Moselle R.

Front line, July 18, 1919

Argonne Forest

Oise R.

Rheims

Verdun

Marne R.

Belleau Wood,
June 6–26, 1918

Château-Thierry,
May 30–June 26, 1918

St. Mihiel
September 12–14, 1918

Paris

Seine R.

Meuse-Argonne Offensive
September 26–November 11, 1918

▨ Allied powers	▨ Central powers	▨ Neutral
•••••• Front line	★ Battle sites	

Locations of major battles in which African-American troops participated

WORLD WAR I

Among the many causes of the war was the imperialist scramble for African colonies in the last two decades of the 19th century. At various points in that period, England, France, and Germany nearly came to blows over African territory, creating tensions that would play themselves out in European politics of the early 20th century. Moreover, the war itself would greatly debilitate the European imperialist powers. Not only was the loser—Germany—forced to cede its African colonial holdings, but even the winners found themselves substantially weakened vis-à-vis the nonwestern world. The idea that a superior European civilization was destined to rule the world was forever destroyed in the barbaric carnage of World War I trench warfare. Indeed, many of the great independence leaders of the post–World War II era cite the beginning of the end of colonialism in the catastrophe of First World War.

For the United States, of course, World War I represented something altogether different. Rather than its world status being undermined by the war, the country found itself in a position of unrivaled power and prosperity in the wake of World War I, even if it failed to exploit that dominance and assert world leadership, as it would after World War II. Part of the reason the United States did not suffer as much from the war

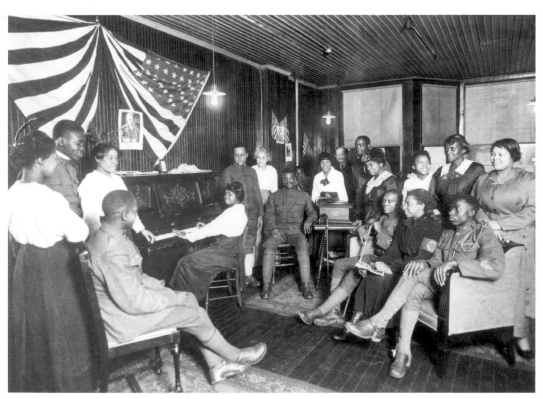

African-American soldiers at women's club before leaving for Europe (National Archives)

was its late entry. For nearly three years—beginning in August 1914—the United States watched the bloody struggle at a distance. Finally, after suffering enormous losses of ships to German submarines in the Atlantic—America continued to trade with Britain and France during the conflict—the country was drawn in to the war in April 1917.

As was the case in the Civil War and, as would later be the case in World War II, African Americans soldiers hoped that their patriotic service in the war effort would help win them recognition, acceptance, and equality in American society. Even the critical and skeptical DuBois urged blacks to fight for their country. But resistance was great, particularly in the South, where whites feared that a uniform and a military record would make blacks unwilling to accept their inferior status in society. But the persistence of black leaders and the great need to fill the military ranks overcame these reservations and, by war's end, more than 365,000 blacks were drafted, virtually all of them into the army. (The U.S. Navy had few black sailors; the Marine Corps was white-only; and the air force did not yet exist.) At the same time, blacks were kept in the lowest ranks, with only 639 trained as officers at the Colored Officers' Training Camp, located at Fort Dodge, Iowa.

Prejudice also persisted against black soldiers off-base, particularly in the South. Protests and threats of violence against blacks training at nearby army facilities in Spartanburg, South Carolina, caused the military to send the unit—the soon-to-be highly decorated 369th U.S. Infantry—to France. Violence, however, was not avoided in Houston where black troops—incensed by the abusive treatment they received from local whites—rioted, leaving 16 whites and four blacks dead. Ultimately, the military executed 19 black soldiers and sentenced dozens more to long prison sentences for their participation in the rioting.

By war's end, some 200,000 black American soldiers served in Europe. Although most were consigned to Service of Supplies units and labor battalions, several combat regiments were organized. Ironically, it was the prejudice of the American Expeditionary Force commander, John J. Pershing, that gave black soldiers their greatest opportunity to display valor and heroism. When France—desperate for soldiers to fill their depleted ranks—asked the Americans for more troops, General Pershing turned the 369th over to them. Spending more time on the front lines than any other American unit that served in the war, the men of the 369th earned an unprecedented 171 croix de guerre, or Legions of Merit, France's highest military medals.

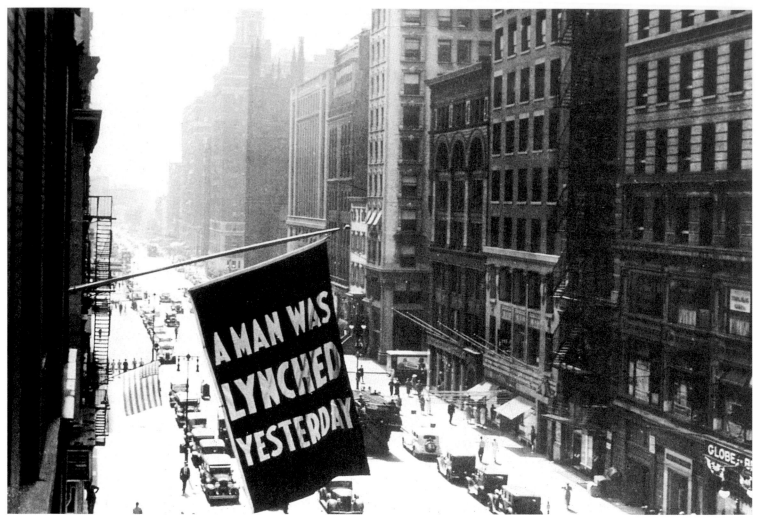

To bring attention to escalating violence against African Americans after World War I, the NAACP flew this flag outside of its headquarters office in New York (National Archives)

An NAACP march against lynching during the "Red Summer" of 1919 (Library of Congress)

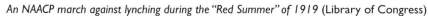

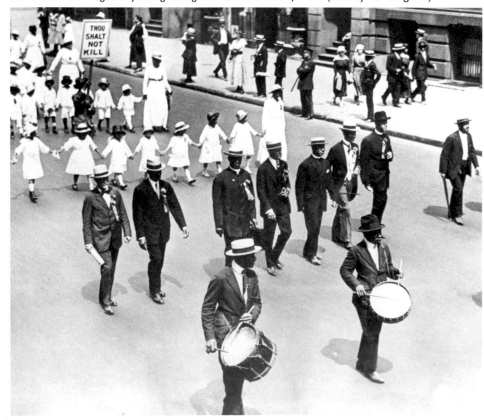

(No U.S. Medals of Honor were awarded to black troops at the time, although one was bestowed posthumously in 1991.)

Despite their military service—and disappointing their hopes for equal treatment—African-American soldiers were met with disdain and even lynchings by whites upon their return to the United States from Europe after the war. As one New Orleans city official in told black veterans, "you are going to be treated exactly like you were before the war; this is a white man's country, and we expect to rule it." Nor was the harsh welcome confined to the South. During the "Red Summer"—named after the fear of reds, or communist-sympathizing radicals, sweeping the country during the time—major civil disturbances broke out in two dozen cities nationwide, including one particularly violent one in Chicago that left 23 blacks and 15 whites dead, and another 520 persons injured. While the return of black soldiers was occasionally the spark that set off a riot, there also were much deeper social causes for the escalating postwar violence.

fraud in 1922 sank the Black Star Line and permanently crippled the UNIA. A petition drive by Garvey's wife helped win the former UNIA leader a release from prison after three years, but he was immediately deported to Jamaica, where he tried to resuscitate the organization. In 1935, Garvey moved to London, and died there of a stroke in 1940. While the UNIA barely remains alive as an organization today—with a just few small chapters here and there—its ideological legacy remains strong

and Garvey is still a figure of great respect in many African-American homes. His emphasis on the pursuit of black economic independence and self-determination—as opposed to an emphasis on civil rights and integration—profoundly influenced the thinking and work of the Nation of Islam, Malcolm X, and the Black Panthers, among others.

HARLEM RENAISSANCE

Along with black politics, the Great Migration had an enormous impact on the arts and culture of African Americans in the post–World War I era. Rural blacks from the Mississippi Delta region brought blues music—a hybrid of West African rhythms, slave field hollers, and gospel hymns that emerged at the turn of the century—to cities like St. Louis and Chicago, while musicians from New Orleans carried north a blues-influnced style of music known as jazz. While the basic blues structure is characterized by the use of a three-line stanza in which the words of the second line repeat the first, in a call and response pattern similar to tose found in West Africa, jazz used the blues form merely as a starting point, emphasizing the improvised interplay of weaving and contrasting elements. By 1920, Chicago had overtaken New Orleans as the center of jazz music in America. But the real center of black culture in the 1920s was neither the Crescent City nor the Windy City, it was New York.

Even before World War I—but certainly by the beginning of the 1920s—the Harlem district of New York City—roughly that part of Manhattan stretching north a mile or so from Central Park—had become the unofficial "Negro capital of the world." As Reverend Adam Clayton Powell Sr., pastor of Harlem's influential Abyssinian Baptist Church, put it, Harlem represented "the symbol of liberty and the Promised Land to Negroes everywhere." Here for the first time in American history was a large, confident, and vibrant urban black community, based in the cultural hub of the country. Its artistic flowering—popularly known as the Harlem Renaissance—was felt in music, dance, the visual arts, theatre, and literature. And just as the Lost Generation of white writers of the 1920s represents, perhaps, the greatest literary decade of the 20th century, so the Harlem Renaissance—or the New Negro movement—stands, arguably, as the greatest artistic flowering in African-American history. And like the largely apolitical Lost Generation, the artists of the

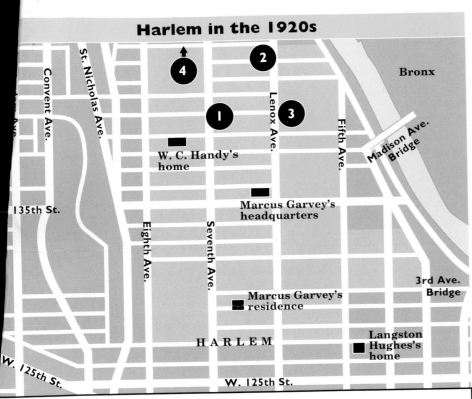

Harlem in the 1920s

Bronx

W. C. Handy's home

Marcus Garvey's headquarters

3rd Ave. Bridge

Marcus Garvey's residence

HARLEM

Langston Hughes's home

W. 125th St.

1. Founded in 1809 as the Free Baptist Church of New York City, the **Abyssinian Baptist Church** became a center of civil rights activism when a young preacher named Adam Clayton Powell Sr. took over the pulpit a century later. The church building, dedicated in 1923, was a cavernous Gothic structure, featuring an Italian marble pulpit and imported stained glass windows. The congregation numbered more than 7,000.

2. Opened in 1922, the **Cotton Club** became the premier showcase in America for black musicians. The elegant interior, featuring primitivist decor, helped to inspire the "jungle sound" of Duke Ellington, who opened there in 1927. Other jazz greats who played there included Cab Calloway, Louis Armstong, and singer Lena Horne. Sadly, during the 1920s, black audiences could not listen to these musicians since the club was for whites only.

3. **The Harlem YWCA**, completed in 1919, offered some of the finest athletic facilities in New York City at the time. It also sponsored a host of conferences on subjects like women's suffrage, antilynching legislation, and civil rights activism. Among the figures who spoke there were Ida Wells, Mary McLeod Bethune, and Booker T. Washington.

4. **The Dunbar Apartments**, located at W. 149th and 150th Streets between Seventh and Eighth Avenues and financed by John D. Rockefeller Jr., were the first large cooperative built for African Americans. Among the prominent African Americans who lived at the Dunbar Apartments were W. E. B. DuBois, actor and singer Paul Robeson, labor leader A. Philip Randolph, and Arctic explorer Matthew A. Henson.

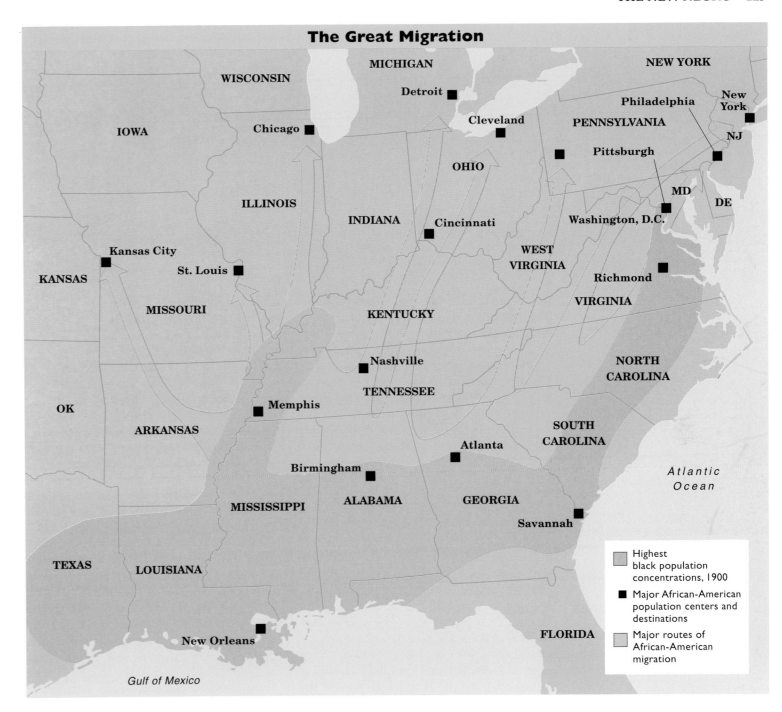

The Great Migration

Highest black population concentrations, 1900

Major African-American population centers and destinations

Major routes of African-American migration

THE GREAT MIGRATION

In 1910, roughly 90 percent of all African Americans lived in the South, and nearly 80 percent of those worked in agriculture, figures not much changed from Civil War days. The next decade, however, would set in motion a dramatic demographic and geographic transformation that would see millions of blacks moving to northern cities by the 1960s. It has since been referred to as the Great Migration and, like other vast movements of humanity over the course of world history, it was triggered by both push and pull factors. Depressed cotton prices and infestations by the boll weevil—an insect pest that destroys the cotton plant—pushed

many black (and white) tenant farmers and sharecroppers off the land in the second decade of the 20th century.

At the same time, there was a great demand for labor in northern and western factories. European immigration—the source of so much cheap labor in American history—had been cut off, first by the war and then by restrictive legislation. Adding to the shortage was America's entry into World War I. That is, just as the demand on industry was peaking to meet defense needs, millions of young men were drafted into the military. With wages rising correspondingly, word soon spread across the black South of unprecedented economic opportunities up North and out West. Moreover, while northerners held their own

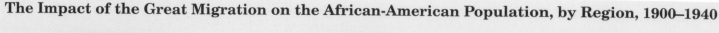

The Impact of the Great Migration on the African-American Population, by Region, 1900–1940

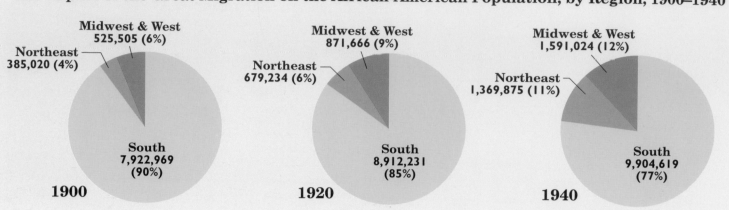

1900

Midwest & West
525,505 (6%)

Northeast
385,020 (4%)

South
7,922,969
(90%)

1920

Midwest & West
871,666 (9%)

Northeast
679,234 (6%)

South
8,912,231
(85%)

1940

Midwest & West
1,591,024 (12%)

Northeast
1,369,875 (11%)

South
9,904,619
(77%)

racial prejudices, discrimination was far less institutionalized there. Blacks in the North could vote; their children had a better chance of attending school; and there was far less violence directed against them. Many northern cities saw their black populations more than double in the 1910s. Where Chicago had roughly 35,000 African Americans in 1910, it claimed 90,000 ten years later. Southern planters and the newly revived Ku Klux Klan tried to stop the flow through violence, the banning of northern black newspapers—which promoted migration—and even the jailing of potential migrants.

But the draw was too strong and it only intensified in the decade following the war. With agriculture in a slump nationwide and relative prosperity buoying the urban economy, migration from the rural black South to the urban North and West accelerated. Nearly one million African Americans made the trek on the "chicken bone express"—named after the imagined trail of refuse left from the lunches packed for the migrants—in the 1920s. The demographic effects on northern and western cities was nothing less than transformative. Where Detroit's black population, for example, was a miniscule 6,000 before World War I, it stood at 120,000 by the time of the Great Crash in 1929. In New York, the numbers were 100,000 and 330,000 respectively.

The dramatic growth of the urban black population set off predictable fear and hostility among whites. During the war, there was intense competition for limited housing in growing industrial areas, one of the sources of white rioting in East St. Louis, Illinois, in 1917. Real estate interests and politicians responded with discriminatory housing practices, attempting to confine blacks to the worst parts of town. But housing was only one source of the friction. Many blacks were refused membership in

unions and were thereby forced to work as "scabs" or strikebreakers, a trend exacerbated by industrialists who used racial differences to divide the labor force and forestall union solidarity. When the war ended, a wave of strikes spread across the country and further antagonized relations between non-union black workers and unionized white ones. The recession of the early 1920s intensified the competition, although the subsequent boom of the latter half of the decade eased it somewhat. Still, for all the prejudice, hostility, and even violence blacks faced in the North, the Great Migration created something that had never existed before in American history—large, black urban communities. For the first time, great numbers of African Americans lived free of rural ignorance and oppression. The result of this liberation was a remarkable and unprecedented flowering of black political and artistic expression. It was, to use a term coined by African-American writer Alain Locke, the birth of a "new Negro," who proudly defied the old white stereotypes imposed on African Americans in favor of a new racial conciousness that celebrated black achievement on its own terms. This new conciousness not only reflected cultural and artistic achievement but also inspired a growing political spirit that demanded equality in all spheres of life.

AFRICAN AMERICANS IN THE 1920s

Several trends came together to galvanize African-American politics in the 1920s. As in the case of the Civil War 60 years earlier and the Second World War a generation to come, World War I raised black expectations. Both service to country and the ideals for which the war was supposedly fought—

"to make the world safe for democracy," in President Woodrow Wilson's high-minded words—led many African Americans to believe that a new dispensation of justice and equality was around the corner. However, unlike those two other wars, World War I resulted in little white acceptance for African Americans. That disappointment—combined with the confidence that came from their new demographic strength in the urban North—produced a political activism among African Americans unseen since Reconstruction days. Yet, it was a very different kind of politics, bent less on integrating into the majority white–controlled establishment and the Republican Party than on creating an independent and self-sufficient economic and political order within the black community itself. Something else in this period differed from the Reconstruction Era as well—leadership. Unlike black politics in the post–Civil War era, the activism of the post–World War I years was largely influenced by one man, Marcus Mosiah Garvey.

MARCUS GARVEY AND THE UNIVERSAL NEGRO IMPROVEMENT ASSOCIATION

Born in rural Jamaica in 1887, Garvey moved to the island's administrative capital—Kingston—at age 16 and soon became involved in the anti-imperialist, black nationalist politics of the British colony. After traveling through Central America and Europe, Garvey settled briefly in England, where he worked on a pan-African journal, before returning to Jamaica on the eve of World War I. Initially influenced by Booker T. Washington's self-help philosophy, he founded the Universal Negro Improvement Association (UNIA) and attempted to build a Tuskegee -like institute in Jamaica. Disappointed in his failedefforts, Garvey then went on a speaking tour of North America, before ending up in Harlem in 1917 where, influenced by the excitement of the burgeoning center of black life in America, he restarted the UNIA. Garvey combined principles—economic self-reliance, political self-determination, and independence for black Africa—with panache. In the ritualistic style of the day, he held parades and created elaborate uniforms and insignias for organization members. A charismatic leader, Garvey soon founded chapters of the UNIA throughout the United States, Canada, the West Indies, Africa, Latin America, and Great Britain.

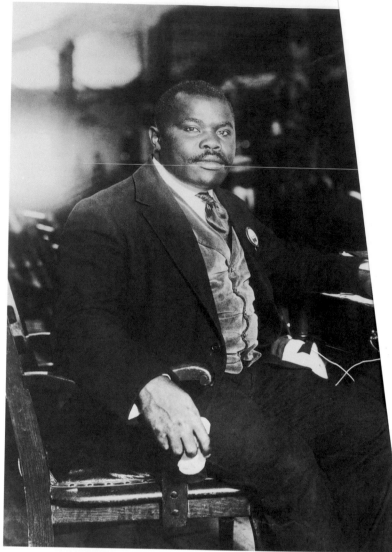

Marcus Garvey (Library of Congress)

Garvey's most ambitious project, however, involved the establishment of the Black Star Steamship Line. The company aimed to fulfill two goals: first, to create an independent transportation network for black trade, and second, to provide passage to African Americans who wanted to return to the African homeland. A symbol of pride, the Black Star Line drew thousands more into the UNIA. In August 1920, the organization held a convention in New York's Madison Square Garden that drew 25,000 people. Delegates drew up A Declaration of Rights of the Negro Peoples of the World, voted on an anthem—the "Universal Ethiopian Anthem"—and elected Garvey president-general of the organization. Plans were also laid to develop a UNIA colony in Liberia, black Africa's only independent republic.

Heavy debt, poor management, constant criticism from DuBois and his integrationist allies in the NAACP, and—most critically—Garvey's indictment for mail

Harlem Renaissance—disappointed by the backlash against blacks in the wake of World War I—focused on artistry rather than politics in their writing and theater.

Several trends came together to produce the Harlem Renaissance. First was the vast expansion of Harlem itself, from a tiny black community of several thousand at century's turn to a city-unto-itself of a quarter of a million African Americans by the end of the 1920s. The dynamism of Harlem could be seen everywhere, in the spread of street corner speakers, religious cults, and health fads. The excitement of the neighborhood's nightlife also drew white patrons eager to break free of the confining and straitlaced life of Prohibition America. Ironically, many of the hottest spots—like the premier showcase for black musical talent, the Cotton Club—were restricted to white patrons only who flocked uptown to hear the so-called jungle sound of Duke Ellington, as well as other jazz greats like Cab Calloway and Louis Armstrong.

Along with music, the greatest legacy of the Harlem Renaissance was in the field of literature. Two magazines—and the organizations that sponsored them—were primarily responsible for popularizing the literature of the period's black writers. The first was the NAACP's *Crisis*, edited by DuBois. DuBois both published the work of others and, in his own editorials, emphasized the need for a literature that emphasized black themes and an independent and assertive black voice. Even more critical to the movement was the National Urban League's journal, *Opportunity*. The National Urban League (NUL) was founded in 1911 to promote scientific social work in the black community. Under the editorship of the University of Chicago Ph.D. Charles Johnson, its journal not only published the works of young Harlem Renaissance writers but attempted to create a sense of community and purpose for the fledgling movement. In 1924, it hosted a gathering of white and black intellectuals and writers that, in the following year, turned into the movement's most important honors ceremony, the "Opportunity Awards." In 1926, literary critic Alain Locke—a contributor to *Opportunity*—edited *The New Negro*, an anthology that exposed Harlem Renaissance writers to a national audience.

Those whom DuBois, Johnson, and Locke sought to nurture and honor included a variety of poets, novelists, playwrights, and visual artists. Most prominent among the writers were Claude McKay, Jean Toomer, Countee Cullen, and Zora Neale Hurston.

Born in Jamaica in 1889, McKay moved to the United States in 1912 and attended Tuskegee Institute and Kansas State University before moving to Harlem for seven years, where he wrote poetry while working on railroad dining cars. After a short stint in Europe, McKay returned to Harlem in 1921 and produced such memorable novels as *Home to Harlem* (1928) and *Banjo* (1929), where he explored issues of race,

The Crisis (Library of Congress)

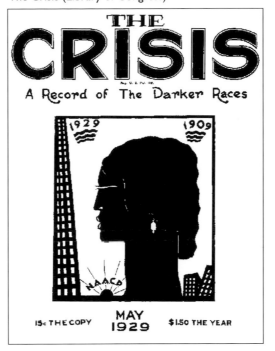

Zora Neale Hurston (Library of Congress)

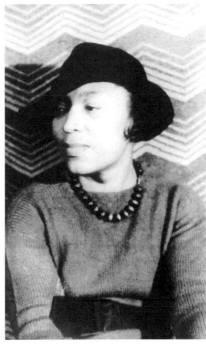

Below, left: *Duke Elington* (Library of Congress); below, right: *Jazz orchestra leader Cab Calloway, who like Ellington was a frequent headliner at the Cotton Club in Harlem* (Library of Congress)

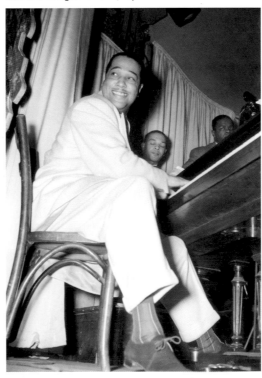

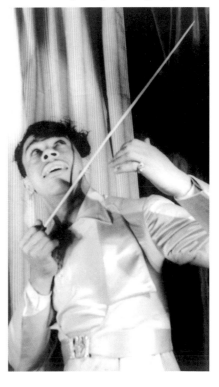

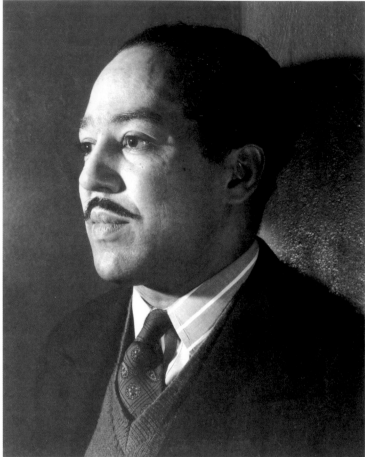

Langston Hughes (Library of Congress)

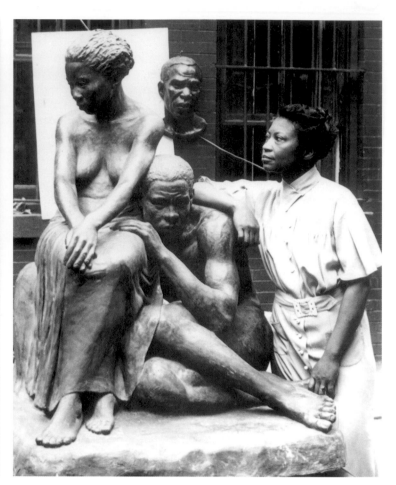

Augusta Savage with one of her sculptures (National Archives)

class, and the divisions between rural and urban black communities.

Toomer, a native of Washington, D.C., is best known for his novel *Cane* (1923), a tale of southern life that experimented with radical new forms of fictional narrative. *Cane* is considered one of the most important novels of 20th-century American literature, influencing the works of Alice Walker, Toni Morrison, and other black novelists to come.

A native of Kentucky, Cullen lived in New York City as a teenager, graduated from Harvard in 1927, and returned to Harlem to write poetry and help edit *Opportunity*. In such poetry volumes as *Copper Sun* and *The Ballad of the Brown Girl*, Cullen fused jazz and blues motifs with the written word.

Hurston, who was born in Alabama in 1891 and reared in rural Florida, attended Howard University, before moving to Harlem in 1925. An anthropologist and novelist, she is famous for her pioneering studies of black folklore. Her best-known work, however, is the novel *Their Eyes Were Watching God* (1938), the story of the life and loves of a rural African-American woman.

Still, amidst this plethora of talent, the dominant figure of the Harlem Renaissance remains Langston Hughes. Born in Joplin, Missouri, in 1902, Hughes was first raised by his grandmother in Kansas and, as a teenager, lived with his mother in Cleveland. A poet even in high school, Hughes had his first piece, "The Negro Speaks of Rivers," published in *Crisis* when he was just 19; it remains one of his most beloved poems to this day. Attending Columbia University, Hughes soon dropped out, drawn by the artistic excitement of nearby Harlem. (He would eventually receive his college degree from Lincoln University in Pennsylvania.) In 1930, he published his first novel, *Not Without Laughter*. Up to his death in 1967, Hughes remained prolific and versatile, putting out short story collections (*The Ways of White Folks*, 1934), plays (*Mulatto*, 1935, which is among the longest-running black plays in Broadway history), memoirs (*The Big Sea*, 1940), and weekly columns for the *Chicago Defender* for more than 20 years.

Some of more prominent visual artists of the Harlem Renaissance included Augusta Savage and Aaron Douglas. Born in rural Florida in 1892, Savage studi

A SELECTIVE INTRODUCTION TO JAZZ

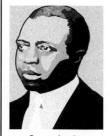 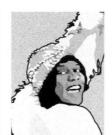 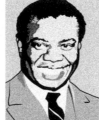 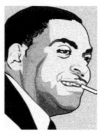 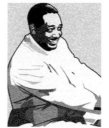 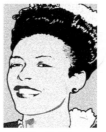 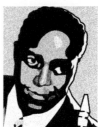

| Scott Joplin | Louis Armstrong | Bessie Smith | Fats Waller | Duke Ellington | Billie Holiday | Charlie Parker |

Louis Armstrong, who was widely regarded in his lifetime as not only the worldwide Ambassador of Jazz, but also one of its most revolutionary geniuses, once said, "If you have to ask what jazz is, you'll never understand." In its essence, however, jazz can be described as highly improvisational music that stresses syncopated rhythms and ensemble playing featuring weaving and contrasting elements. With roots in the West African rhythms and American slave field hollers and spirituals that formed the blues, jazz also has roots in European brass marching band music, ragtime, and other popular music of the late 19th and early 20th centuries. The chart below attempts to single out some of the major styles and figures that helped to shape the music during the first half of the 20th century.

Style	Description	Era	Selected Major Figures
Minstrelsy	Music and comedy, mainly featuring whites in blackface, performing African-American songs, jokes, and impersonations for segregated audiences. Minstrelsy also provided work for a few blacks, such as Bert Williams, the first black recording star.	1890s–1920s	Bert Williams (1874–1922) Al Jolson (1885–1950) Emmett Miller (1900–1962)
Ragtime	Classically based, rhythmically bouncy music.	1890s–1910s	Scott Joplin (1868–1917) James Reese Europe (1881–1919)
New Orleans Traditional	The first true jazz style, born in New Orleans, and featuring use of clarinet and tuba. Commonly heard in celebrations and funerals. Dixieland jazz, an upbeat offshoot, added banjo to the mix.	1900s–1920s	Jelly Roll Morton (1890–1941) Louis Armstrong (1900–1971)
Female Blues Vocals/ Vaudeville Blues	Blues and pop vocal music set to jazz instrumentation, featured in the black vaudeville circuit of the 1920s and early 1930s. Although shows incorporated comedy performed by group acts, headliners were usually solo female vocalists, such as Bessie Smith.	1920s–1930s	Ma Rainey (1886–1939) Bessie Smith (1894–1937) Mamie Smith (1883–1946)
Harlem Stride	Highly rhythmic piano music.	1920s–1930s	James P. Johnson (1894–1955) Willie "The Lion" Smith (1897–1973) Fats Waller (1904–1943)
Swing/Big Band	Lush instrumental adaptations of popular song, played for dancing. The first jazz style to reach national audiences through radio and film soundtracks.	1930s–1940s	Duke Ellington (1899–1974) Benny Goodman (1909–1986)
Jazz Vocals	Classic vocalists interpreting popular standards and originals in a jazz style.	1930s–1950s	Billie Holiday (1915–1959) Ella Fitzgerald (1918–1996)
Bebop	A complex, innovative style emphasizing fast, highly improvised solos, and a stripped-down rhythm section. Often seen as a reaction against conventional Big Band orchestration.	1940s–1950s	Charlie "Bird" Parker (1920–1955) Dizzy Gillespie (1917–1993)

The

SCOTTSBORO BOYS MUST NOT DIE!

MASS SCOTTSBORO DEFENSE MEETING

At St. Mark's M. E. Church
137th Street and St. Nicholas Avenue

Friday Eve., April 14th, 8 P. M.

Protest the infamous death verdict rendered by
an all-white jury at Decatur, Alabama against
HAYWOOD PATTERSON

The Meeting will be addressed by:
Mrs. JANIE PATTERSON, mother of Haywood Patterson,
victim of the lynch verdict; SAMUEL LEIBOWITZ, chief counsel for the defense; JOSEPH BRODSKY, defense counsel;
WILLIAM PATTERSON, National Secretary of the I. L. D.;
RICHARD B. MOORE; Dr. LORENZO KING; WM. KELLEY
of the Amsterdam News; and others.

THUNDER YOUR INDIGNATION AGAINST THE JUDICIAL MURDER
OF INNOCENT NEGRO CHILDREN!

COME TO THE MASS PROTEST MEETING

AT ST. MARK'S M. E. CHURCH
137th Street and St. Nicholas Avenue

FRIDAY EVENING, APRIL 14th, 8 P.M.

Emergency Scottsboro Defense Committee
119 West 135th Street, New York City

*Flyer in support of the Scottsboro Boys
(Library of Congress)*

sculpting at Cooper Union in New York City, where she caught the attention of DuBois and Garvey. She even carved busts of them. After a brief sojourn in Paris, Savage returned to New York and opened the Savage School of Arts and Crafts in Harlem in 1932, where she taught classes and influenced future generations of black artists. Douglas, a native of Kansas, moved to Harlem in 1925 where he produced paintings and illustrations in the popular art deco style of the day. Perhaps Douglas's best known works are the illustrations he did for *God's Trombones: Seven Negro Sermons in Verse*, a collection of poetry based on the rhetoric of black preachers.

Like many great artistic movements, the Harlem Renaissance was relatively short-lived, a creature of a particular time and place. For all the excitement they generated at the time—as well as all of the deserved scholarly attention they have drawn in recent decades—the writers and artists of the Harlem Renaissance were often culturally and socially divorced from the needs and aspirations of the larger black community, an ironic situation given their desire to find an artistic voice that spoke for black America. Unable to connect with a black population that remained largely rural even during the Great Migration, they were dependent on white patronage for much of their livelihood and audience. When the economic climate soured following the stock market crash of 1929, white patronage dried up, leaving Harlem's writers and artists bereft. It would take the civil rights movement of the post–World War II era—and its emphasis on black cultural and historical studies—to revive interest in this greatest flowering of African-American artistic and literary talent.

THE GREAT DEPRESSION

As historians and economists have frequently noted, the great economic boom of the 1920s did not affect all U.S. citizens equally. The rural United States, for example, where about half the population lived, remained mired in recession throughout the decade. Having expanded production to meet the demands of World War I—and to take advantage of inflation—farmers were caught with excess capacity when the war ended, resulting in a predictable collapse in commodity prices. With fully 80 percent of blacks living on farms as late as 1930, the ongoing agricultural slump hit them particularly hard. Fewer than 20 percent owned

land and the per capita income was roughly $200 a year among rural blacks less than a third that for urban whites. Nor were things much better in urban areas, where blacks were confined to the lowest-paying factory jobs, when they could find them. Unemployment rates among African Americans remained stubbornly high throughout the decade. The difference, then, between the Roaring Twenties and the depression of the 1930s was not nearly as sharp for the African-American community as the white. As one unemployed African-American worker noted in the 1930s, "it didn't mean too much to the [black man], the Great American Depression, as you call it. There was no such thing. The best he could be was a janitor or a shoeshine boy. It only became official when it hit the white man." Or as Langston Hughes put it, "the Depression brought everybody down a peg or two. And the Negroes had but few pegs to fall."

HARD TIMES

Still, the Great Depression hit the black community with a double force. Not only were black workers subject to the same economic forces as whites, but they were often singled out for the first firings. By 1932, at the depth of the depression, approximately one half the black work force in most of the major industrial cities of the Northeast and Midwest were without jobs. In Pittsburgh, for example, the black unemployment rate in 1933 was 48 percent for blacks and 31 percent for whites. It is estimated that nearly one out of three African-American families in 1932 was receiving some form of public assistance to get by.

Yet even as most African Americans—like much of working America—were victims of the rising unemployment and waves of bankruptcies and foreclosures that accompanied the worst economic downturn in the nation's history—overall, output fell by 50 percent and corporate profits by 90 percent between 1929 and 1933—they were also targeted for attack by angry and frustrated whites. Across the South, lynchings of blacks—which had steadily fallen through the 1920s to just seven in 1929—rose once again, to 20 in 1930 and 24 in 1933. Ironically, it was a case in which lynchings were avoided that focused the nation's attention—as it had not been since Reconstruction times—on the violence directed against southern blacks.

The incident began on March 25, 1931, when a freight train pulled into the small town of Scottsboro, Alabama. Like many

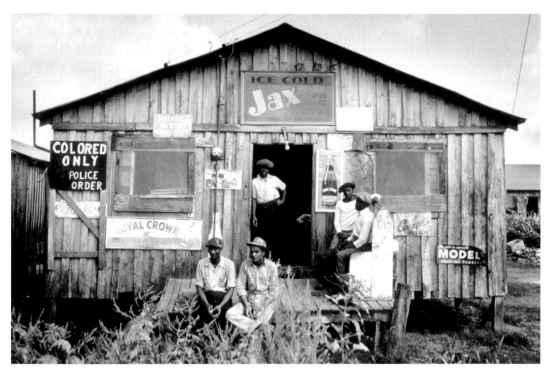

"Colored only" store, 1920s (National Archives)

such transports during the Great Depression, it was full of hoboes looking for work and fleeing hard times. A fight between white and black transients had been reported. As sheriff's deputies met the train and arrested nine black men, things turned decidedly ugly. Two white women suddenly came forward claiming they had been raped by the nine men. There was no worse accusation that could face a black man in the South in those days than being accused of sullying the purity and chastity of white southern womanhood. Racist myths about uncontrolled black male lust for white female flesh had always been one of the main justifications white southerners employed to defend their system of racial oppression. The scene in Scottsboro that day seemed ripe for multiple lynchings. Yet somehow the deputies held off the gathering mob and threw the men in jail.

The trial was a farce. An all-white jury and a white judge took almost no time—and heard virtually no corroborating evidence for the women's accusations—to find the men guilty and to sentence eight to death. (A ninth escaped the death penalty because he was a minor.) The Scottsboro case would probably have been just another case of racially prejudiced southern justice had it not been for the International Labor Defense (ILD), a labor group closely tied to the Communist Party of the U.S.A. (CPUSA) then experiencing an upsurge in membership and influence due to the collapse of the nation's capitalist economy.

Bringing expert lawyers to bear, the ILD helped convince the Supreme Court to overturn the convictions and require a new trial, on the grounds the men had been denied adequate legal counsel. Despite the fact that the women's stories were riddled with contradictions—one of them eventually recanted her story—five of the men were convicted again, this time to long prison sentences. However, the cases dragged on for years, drawing the attention of the black press and public and the NAACP, which had initially been slow to react. Eventually, four of the convicted men were paroled in 1944, while one escaped to Michigan where the governor refused to extradite him back to Alabama.

The Scottsboro case helped galvanize black political activism at a moment in time when the nation's politics as a whole were undergoing one of the most dramatic transformations in history. In 1932, Democrat Franklin Roosevelt—promising a "new deal" for the American people—was elected president. Upon his inauguration in March of the following year—perhaps, the lowest point of the Great Depression—the new president launched an unprecedented set of programs designed to save the nation's capitalist economy and put people back to work. A wide range of new programs—involving banking, manufacturing, and agriculture—were proposed and passed by a pro–New Deal Congress. The Federal Emergency Relief Administration doled out money to hungry families, while

WORLD WAR II

THE HOMEFRONT

Although triggered in the United States by the crash of the stock market in 1929, the Great Depression was a global economic catastrophe that seemed to have its greatest impact on the most industrialized countries: Great Britain, the United States, Japan, and Germany. Like any great economic upheaval, the worldwide depression of the 1930s created political turmoil in the countries most affected by it. But where the long democratic traditions of England and the United States allowed those nations to weather the slump with their governing institutions largely intact—if greatly expanded to meet the emergency—the same was not the case with Germany and Japan. Both had little in the way of a democratic history and thus were vulnerable to dictators and militarists who argued that authoritarianism and conquest was the only way out of the depression. Adding to Germany's burden were the damage to the nation's industrial infrastructure in World War I and the huge reparations that the Treaty of Versailles forced the German government to pay following the war. In 1933, the same year Roosevelt became president, Germany installed Adolf Hitler and his Nazi Party to power. Two years earlier, the militarist government of Japan had invaded the Chinese province of Manchuria. In 1935, Italy—under the control of fascist dictator Benito Mussolini since the 1920s—launched a brutal war of conquest against Ethiopia, Africa's last remaining independent country, except for Liberia.

Moreover, Hitler, Mussolini, and the Japanese justified their authoritarianism and aggression with racism. Each claimed that its own people were racially superior to others. In the case of the Japanese and especially the Germans, this ideology led to horrifying events. Japan perpetrated numerous massacres against the Chinese, while the Germans slaughtered millions of Slavic peoples, communists, and homosexuals and—most horrifying of all—attempted to wipe both the Jewish and Roma (Gypsy) peoples from the face of Europe. The struggle against these brutal regimes—which the United States belatedly joined in 1941 after the Japanese attack on Peal Harbor, and partly justified as a crusade against racial intolerance—would have a critical effect on the postwar civil rights movement in the United States. Meanwhile, as American industry began to gear up for the global conflict, a nascent civil rights struggle was brewing over issues of economic justice.

Most historians agree that for all the innovation of the New Deal, the Great Depression finally ended because of World War II. Indeed, the amount of money the federal government pumped into the economy for the war effort dwarfed all of the programs of the New Deal combined. Unemployment—which still stood at more than 17 percent in 1939—dropped into single digits in 1941, as industry began pumping out armaments for Great Britain and the Soviet Union, the two major powers fighting Nazi Germany prior to Pearl Harbor. But for African Americans, the economic situation hardly improved. In the early years of the depression, they had been the first fired; now, as the country pulled out of the slump, it seemed like they were the last hired. For example, just 240 of the nation's 100,000 aircraft workers were black in 1940, and most of those served in janitorial positions.

To address these economic inequalities, A. Philip Randolph—head of the Brotherhood of Sleeping Car Porters, the nation's largest black trade union—called for a march on Washington in the summer of 1941. Randolph, who questioned Roosevelt's commitment to civil rights, hoped that a mass demonstration might embarrass the president into action. He was right. Just days before the march's scheduled date of July 1, Roosevelt issued Executive Order 8002, banning "discrimination in the employment of workers in defense industries or government because of race, creed, color, or national origin." To implement the order, the president established the Fair Employment Practices Committee (FEPC) within the Office of Production Management, one of the key agencies involved in coordinating the wartime economy.

Still, neither Executive Order 8002 nor the FEPC was especially effective in battling discrimination. With little power to force compliance, the FEPC resolved only about one-third of the 8,000 complaints it received. Indeed, the fact that African Americans came to represent some 8 percent of all defense workers by 1944—the peak year for war-related production—had much more to do with industry's desperate need for manpower than FEPC enforcement. Moreover, the same forces that led to white backlash against blacks in World War I recurred. The Great Migration of blacks from the rural South to the urban North accelerated in the war years. This led to competition for scarce housing in industrial areas which set off riots in no less than 47 cities in 1943, including one in Detroit that left 25 blacks and nine whites dead.

And yet in many encouraging ways, World War II was different from the previous conflict. For one thing, black leaders were far more assertive in demanding equal rights and fighting discrimination, pointing out the obvious parallels between Nazi anti-Semitism and American racism in their "Double V" campaign (victory against fascism abroad and victory over racism at home). Membership in the NAACP grew from around 50,000 in 1940 to more than 450,000 by 1945. And in 1942, Randolph established the Congress of Racial Equality (CORE), a more militant organization that eschewed the lobbying and legal tactics of older black organizations for a more direct, confrontational approach that included street protests and sit-ins. Presaging later civil rights–era actions, CORE forced a number of Washington restaurants to integrate, after picketing them with the slogan: "Are You for Hitler's Way or the American Way? Make Up Your Mind!" The war years also saw the publication of the most important academic study ever conducted on American racial relations—Gunnar Myrdal's 1944 *An American Dilemma: The Negro Problem and Modern Democracy*, a pathbreaking book that got many white Americans thinking about the problems of racism for the first time.

AFRICAN AMERICANS IN UNIFORM

Despite the awareness by military planners that the manpower resources needed to defeat the Axis powers—Germany, Italy, and Japan—would be immense, discrimination nevertheless prevailed, at least at first. On the eve of America's entry into World War II, the army's mobilization plan allowed for just 6 percent of recruits to be black, about half their number in the total population. And, needless to say, there was no mention of integrating the armed forces. Most blacks were expected to fill menial support and supply positions. Yet, as the war progressed, things began to change and the history of African Americans in World War II offered a litany of firsts.

Messman Dorie Miller's story, though exceptional, captured the mixed record of blacks in the Second World War. Though ineligible for military training, Miller took over an anti-aircraft gun at Pearl Harbor, shooting down at least two and possibly more Japanese fighter planes. Ignored by the Navy, Miller was finally awarded the

Navy Cross after a campaign on his behalf was conducted by the nation's black press. Yet, when his ship—the aircraft carrier USS *Liscome Bay*—was sunk a year later, Miller was still a messman. Indeed, the Navy—which had a proud tradition of integrated crews through the Civil War—was the slowest to promote African Americans in its ranks and did not commission its first black officers until 1944.

The army was a bit quicker to act. In 1941, it moved to integrate its officers' candidate school and by July 1944 prohibited discrimination in transportation and recreational facilities at all its bases, although bases in the South were sometimes slow to implement the policy. At one in Texas, it took a courageous individual refusing to move to the back of the bus—and facing a court-martial for his action—to end segregation. His name was Jackie Robinson, the man who would go on to integrate major league baseball after the war. But it took the pressure of combat—specifically, the desperate Battle of the Bulge, Hitler's last-ditch effort in December 1944 to forestall Allied victory—to bring the first-ever integration of combat units. But perhaps the most illustrious achievement of African-American soldiers in World War II took place neither on sea or land but in the air.

Ever since the rise of military aviation in World War I, African Americans had demanded admission and training as airmen. These demands were dismissed out of hand. A 1925 Army War College study even offered "scientific proof" that blacks lacked the cranial capacity to operate sophisticated machinery like airplanes. It was not until 1939 that the government—in expanding the air corps generally—authorized expenditures for pilot training programs at several black colleges, including Tuskegee Institute, although only for support services

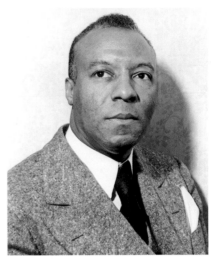

A. Philip Randolph (Library of Congress)

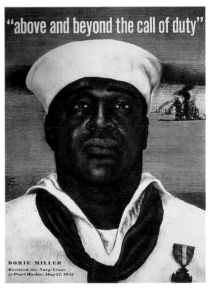

Dorie Miller, a messman in the U.S. Navy, was awarded the Navy Cross for his heroism at Pearl Harbor. This poster, issued by the federal government, commemorates his actions. (National Archives)

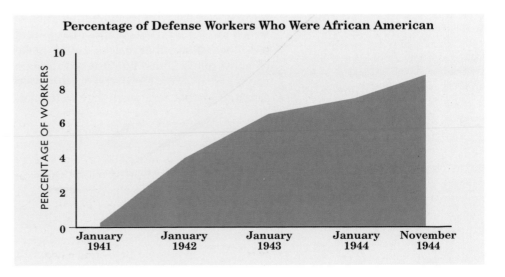

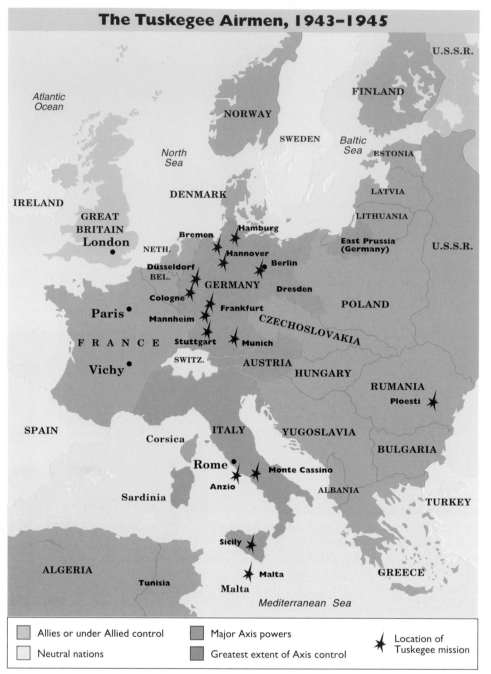

The Tuskegee Airmen, 1943–1945

ly permitted into combat, they remained in segregated units. Not surprisingly, the extra training made them especially effective pilots. By war's end, the all-black 332nd bomber escort group—of which the Tuskegee airmen were a part—could claim a perfect record. In 1,578 missions and 15,552 sorties, they never lost a single bomber. The commander of the 332nd—Benjamin O. Davis—would go on to become the nation's first black three-star general.

Yet despite the many firsts and break-throughs, the military remained a distinctly inhospitable place for African Americans during World War II. At no time did blacks constitute more than 8.7 percent of military personnel, and only 15 percent of all blacks in uniform ever served in combat. In the navy, just 5 percent of sailors were African-American. And as late as the start of the Korean War, there were less than 1,100 blacks in the Marine Corps, and nearly half of these were stewards. The situation in the officer corps was even more dismal. Of the approximately one million African Americans to enter the military services in World War II, just 7,000 became officers. While roughly one in six whites in the Army Air Corps were officers, the ratio among blacks was one in 90.

Still, World War II had a catalytic effect on racial relations both in the American military and in American society at large. The crusade against the racial superiority doctrines of Imperial Japan and Nazi Germany could not help but force some white Americans to question the racial practices in their own country. And, as in the Civil War, patriotism and military service contributed to a sense of pride in the black community and galvanized convictions that legal and political equality was their right as Americans. Moreover, the economic gains made by blacks during the war years—as well as in the prosperous decades to follow—created a confidence to take on the challenge of political activism. It is not too much to say that the great civil rights movement of the postwar era was born on the battlefields, army bases, defense plants, and home-front of World War II.

and not for combat. Still, resistance to the idea of black pilots persisted. Whites refused to serve with them and the army—which ran the air corps in those days—still did not believe that blacks could make effective pilots. Thus, the Tuskegee airmen continued to train long after whites were sent into combat and, when they were final-

THE CIVIL RIGHTS YEARS
African Americans in the Late 20th Century

One of the great ironies of African-American history concerns war, specifically the two costliest conflicts in this nation's history, the Civil War and World War II. Bloody as they were for soldiers of all races, in the end both conflicts helped to dramatically reshape African-American life for the better. The first ended slavery and set the stage for the civil rights program of the Reconstruction era; the second ushered in the modern civil rights era. In both wars, the need for black soldiers helped break down some of the institutional barriers to civil rights within the armed forces themselves. In addition, black valor on the battlefield won respect from all but the most prejudiced whites. Both wars were also fought—at least in part—in the name of freedom and human rights and against the forces of slavery and totalitarianism. A crusade abroad for basic human rights could not help but affect the cause of human rights at home.

THE BIRTH OF A MOVEMENT

There has also been an economic dividend for blacks in wartime. With its upward effect on cotton prices, the Civil War helped lift many African Americans from the abject poverty of slavery to a certain degree of prosperity as sharecroppers, if only temporarily. And World War II—with its enormous demand for manpower, as well as its upward effect on the value of agricultural commodities—offered unprecedented prosperity for civilian African Americans, both

An African-American moviegoer arriving at a segregated theater (National Archives)

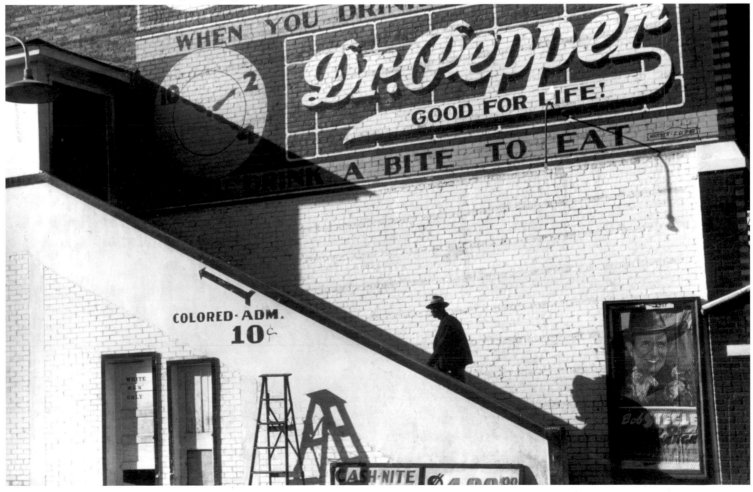

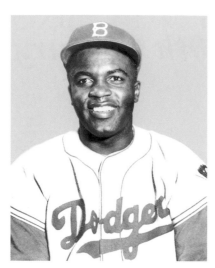

Jackie Robinson (Library of Congress)

for those who sought work in northern factories and those who remained on southern farms. The confidence engendered by this economic bounty—as well as the ideals for which the war was fought—combined to set in motion the most powerful social struggle in 20th-century American history: the civil rights movement.

JACKIE ROBINSON AND THE INTEGRATION OF BASEBALL

It is impossible to find a single date to mark the onset of something as profound and organic as the civil rights movement. The *Scottsboro* case of the early 1930s, the formation of the Southern Tenant Farmers Union in 1934, or the establishment of the Fair Employment Practices Committee in 1941 all come to mind as suggestions. But, perhaps, the best place to mark the starting point of the modern civil rights movement is with "America's favorite pastime"—baseball.

Baseball in the 1940s—as in most of the 20th century—was the all-American pastime, a game of New England origins that spread to the rest of the country through the army camps of the Civil War. In its early days as an organized sport just after the Civil War, baseball remained integrated, with black and white players competing together. But by the latter part of the 19th century, a rigid color line kept black players off white teams and black teams out of the white leagues. This exclusion, however, did not stop African-American athletes from playing professional baseball; they organized their own teams and leagues instead. Like many of the early white teams, the first black baseball squad was established by a business—New York's Argyle Hotel—for its employees and, no doubt, a few ringers from outside. A year later, in 1886, the Southern League of Colored Base Ballists was formed. It failed financially, as did several others, until the establishment of the Negro National League and the Eastern Colored League in 1920 and 1923 respectively.

While these black teams often had to accept inferior facilities—and had trouble finding accommodations on the road—there was nothing second-class about the ball they played. At least three teams—the Kansas City Monarchs, the Pittsburgh Crawfords, and the Homestead (Pennsylvania) Grays—were competitive with the best white teams, according to many sportswriters. And the stars of the African-American leagues—including outfielder James "Cool Papa" Bell; pitcher Leroy "Satchel" Paige; and Josh Gibson, arguably the greatest hitter, white or black, in baseball history, with a .362 lifetime batting average—could easily have played in the majors but for the prejudice of the day. Indeed, Jackie Robinson himself—the man to finally break major league baseball's color line—played briefly for the Monarchs at the end of World War II.

Robinson was born to sharecropping parents in rural Georgia but was raised in Pasadena, California. He attended UCLA,

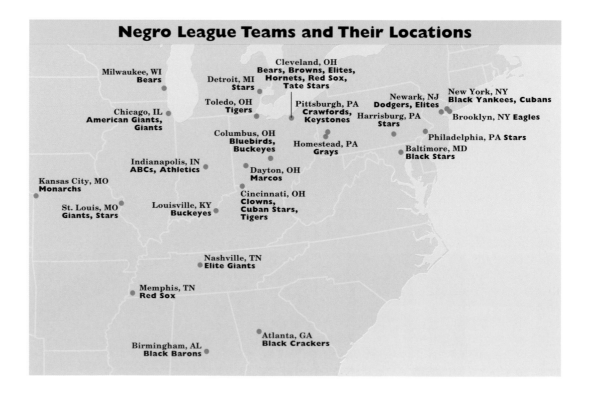

Negro League Teams and Their Locations

STARS OF THE NEGRO LEAGUES

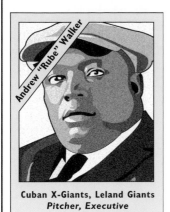

Cuban X-Giants, Leland Giants
Pitcher, Executive

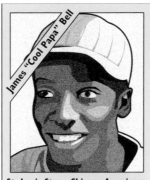

St. Louis Stars, Chicago Americans,
KC Monarchs, Pittsburgh Crawfords
Outfield

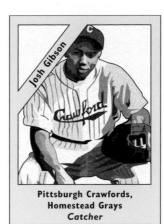

Pittsburgh Crawfords,
Homestead Grays
Catcher

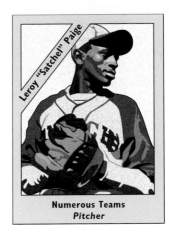

Numerous Teams
Pitcher

Andrew "Rube" Foster

Career: 1902–1926
Position: Pitcher, baseball
executive
Teams: Cuban X-Giants,
Leland Giants
Career Highlights: As a
player, he defeated the
Philadelphia A's star (and
future Hall of Famer) Rube
Waddell, thus earning his
nickname. As an executive he
is remembered as founder of
the Negro National League.

James "Cool Papa" Bell

Career: 1922–1946
Position: Outfielder
Teams: St. Louis Stars, Chicago Americans, Kansas City
Monarchs, Pittsburgh Crawfords
Career Highlights: A .330
lifetime hitter, Bell was so fast
that he onced scored from
first base on a single.

Josh Gibson

Career: 1929–1946
Position: Catcher
Teams: Pittsburgh Crawfords, Homestead Grays, Mexican and Puerto Rican teams
Career Highlights: With an
estimated 823 career home
runs, Gibson is thought top
have been an even more
prodigious home run hitter
than Hank Aaron or Babe
Ruth. He also hit for average—with a .440 average in
1938, and .521 in 1943.

Leroy "Satchel" Paige

Career: 1926–1950, 1965
Position: Pitcher
Teams: Numerous, including
major league baseball's Kansas
City Atheletics, at age 59
Career Highlights: Crowd-
pleasing theatrics. Perhaps the
most popular (white or black)
baseball player in America during the 1930s and 1940s. First
pitched in the major leagues in
1949.

where he lettered in four sports. Upon graduation, he accepted a position as an athletic
director with the National Youth Administration, a Great Depression–era agency that
offered employment and educational opportunities for young people. In 1942, Robinson
was drafted into the military andwas court-
martialed for refusing to sit in the back of an
army bus at Fort Hood, Texas. After the war,
as noted earlier, Robinson played a season in
the Negro Leagues before catching the eye of
Dodger general manager Branch Rickey. Not
only was Robinson a talented hitter and
infielder, he was also a man of upstanding
character and fortitude, two attributes that
would prove essential in challenging the
prejudice of white owners, white players,
and white fans.

Like many in major league baseball,
Rickey recognized the enormous well of talent in the Negro Leagues. But unlike most of
his colleagues, Rickey believed the time was
right to challenge the major league baseball
owners' unwritten "gentlemen's agreement"
to keep black players off their rosters. At a

secret 1945 meeting held to discuss the subject, Rickey's request to bring Robinson to
Brooklyn (where the Dodgers played until
their move to Los Angeles in 1958) was voted down unanimously by the owners. Rickey decided to challenge their decision, hiring
Robinson to play for the Montreal Royals, a
Dodger farm team, for 1946. His exceptional
stats there—.349 batting average and 112
runs scored—convinced Rickey that Robinson was professionally ready for the majors,
even if the majors were not ready for him.

In April 1947, "baseball's great experiment" began. Despite jeers from opposing
players and fans, Robinson proved an exceptional ballplayer, winning Rookie of the Year
honors that season and the National League
Most Valuable Player award in 1949. Other
Negro League stars soon joined Robinson,
including Willie Mays (often considered the
best all-around baseball player of all time),
Hank Aaron (lifetime homerun champion),
and Ernie Banks (winner of multiple baseball honors). Robinson's pioneering efforts
had an impact far beyond baseball. Today,

A CHRONOLOGY OF THE CIVIL RIGHTS ERA

June 1946	In the case *Morgan v. Commonwealth of Virginia*, the U.S. Supreme Court bans segregated seating on interstate buses.
July 1948	President Truman issues an executive order banning segregation in the armed forces.
May 1954	The U.S. Supreme Court issues its *Brown v. Board of Education* ruling, declaring segregation in public schools to be unconstitutional.
December 1955	The Montgomery Bus Boycott begins. It ends one year later with the desegration of the city's bus system.
March 1956	Ninety-six southern members of Congress sign a "Southern Manifesto," pledging their opposition to school desegregation.
January 1957	Martin Luther King Jr., Ralph Abernathy, Joseph Lowery, and Fred Shuttlesworth organize the Southern Christian Leadership Conference (SCLC).
September 1957	President Dwight D. Eisenhower sends troops to provide security for black students trying to integrate Little Rock, Arkansas, Central High School.
February 1960	Black college students stage sit-ins at segregated lunch counters in Greensboro, North Carolina. Sit-ins spread to eight other southern states.
April 1960	Student Non-Violent Coordinating Committee (SNCC) is organized in Raleigh, North Carolina.
May 1961	Black and white freedom riders test the compliance of integration on interstate buses by traveling together.
October 1962	James Meredith becomes the first black student to attend University of Mississippi; his enrollment leads to the most violent campus riot of the decade.
April 1963	Civil rights protests hit Birmingham, Alabama; from jail, King writes his famous "Letter from Birmingham Jail."
June 1963	Civil rights worker Medgar Evers is murdered in Mississippi.
August 1963	The March on Washington brings 250,000 to demonstrate for civil rights; King makes his famous "I Have a Dream" speech.
September 1963	Four children die in the firebombing of a black church in Birmingham.
June 1964	The Freedom Summer project to register voters begins in Mississippi; civil rights workers James Earl Chaney, Andrew Goodman, and Michael Schwerner are murdered.
July 1964	President Lyndon B. Johnson signs the Civil Rights Act of 1964; the Democratic Party refuses to seat the Mississippi Freedom Democratic Party delegation at the convention.
February 1965	SCLC organizes the Selma-Montgomery (Alabama) voting rights march; civil rights workers Jimmy Lee Jackson, Viola Liuzzo, and the Reverend James Reeb are murdered.
August 1965	President Johnson signs the Voting Rights Act; rioting breaks out in the Watts section of Los Angeles.

no less than 70 percent of National Football League players and fully 90 percent of the National Basketball Association players are African American. Still, segregation continues to mar professional sports, with team owners, management, and coaches still predominantly white.

INTEGRATION OF THE NATION'S MILITARY

With the possible exception of the integration of professional sports, the integration of the U.S. military represents the most successful—and one of the earliest—efforts to fully integrate a major institution in the nation's history, though the struggle was a long and difficult one. As noted in the previous chapter, a number of significant gains and firsts were achieved by African Americans in the armed forces during World War II. Yet, even at war's end, all branches of the military remained segregated and the generals and admirals seemed inclined to keep it that way. Military leaders in the mid-1940s feared that integration would stir up resentment among white soldiers and undermine combat readiness, a crucial consideration during a time of heightened cold war tensions. But the NAACP and other civil rights organizations maintained pressure on President and Commander-in-Chief Harry Truman who, in 1948, issued an executive order requiring integration of all branches of the military and the establish-

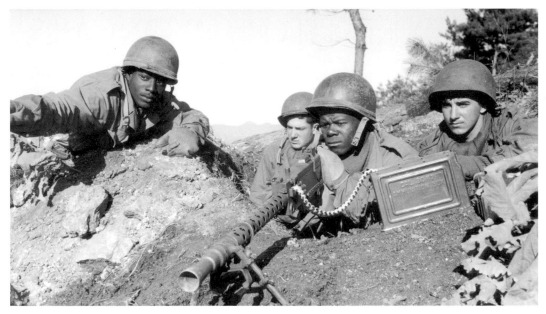

Integrated American troops in Korea (National Archives)

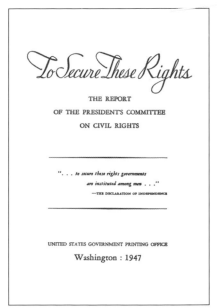

The commission report that recommended to President Harry S Truman that the U.S. military be desegregated (National Archives)

ment of the President's Committee on Equality of Treatment and Opportunity in the Armed Services to monitor civil rights progress.

Resistance was stiff at first, but the onset of the Korean War in 1950 accelerated the process. By war's end, more than 90 percent of all black troops were serving in integrated units. The most surprising progress came in the Marine Corps, often considered the most elite—and once the most racist—service within the armed forces of the United States. At war's outset, blacks represented just 1.4 percent of the 75,000-man corps; by the end of the Korean conflict in 1953, the Marine Corps was approaching full integration. Indeed, Marine Corps and other military leaders quickly learned what civil rights groups had been saying—and common sense indicated—all along. In the heat of battle, skin color faded to insignificance. By the Vietnam era of the 1960s, the ranks of enlisted men were fully integrated and, while the officer corps lagged behind, even there significant progress had been made.

Nonetheless, the Vietnam War offered up a different kind of civil rights problem. While African Americans represented roughly 11 percent of the total military force in the war zone, they accounted for fully 20 percent of all battlefield casualties. It was, one African-American soldier remarked, "the kind of integration that could kill you." Many civil rights leaders, including Martin Luther King Jr., employed such statistics to bolster their arguments in favor of ending American involvement in the war. King and other African-American critics of the war also criticized American policy in Vietnam

as an armed attack on a poor, nonwhite population—the Vietnamese—and as a drain on government financial resources that should have been spent on antipoverty programs.

Opposition to the Vietnam War was not limited to critics in the African-American community. The antiwar movement became a significant factor in not only shortening the war but also in the establishment of an all-volunteer military force. With higher unemployment levels, continued discrimination against them in private industry, and fewer economic opportunities in the rural South and inner-city North, blacks joined the military in far greater numbers than did whites. By 1981, fully one-third of the U.S. Army was African American, while the navy and air force lagged behind at just 12.6 and 16.5 percent respectively. In 1996, the figure for the armed forces as a whole totaled 21.9 percent, still significantly higher than the black proportion of the general population, which equaled roughly 12 percent the same year. Most notable was the progress made in the officer corps of the various branches of the service, an achievement symbolized by the accession to chairman of the Joint Chiefs of Staff—the military's highest uniformed position—of General Colin Powell, the son of West Indian immigrants of African heritage. As General Powell himself noted, "The Army was living the democratic idea ahead of the rest of America. Beginning in the fifties, less discrimination, a truer merit system, and leveler playing fields existed inside the gates of our military posts than in any southern city hall or northern corporation."

SELECTED SUPREME COURT DESEGREGATION CASES, 1938–1950

Year	Case	Background	Outcome
1938	*Missouri ex rel Gaines*	After Lloyd Gaines was denied admission to University of Missouri Law School because of his race, his lawyers took their case to the Supreme Court, arguing that, counter to the "separate but equal" doctrine, Gaines had been denied an equal opportunity to become a lawyer in Missouri.	Although the Court did not strike down *Plessy v. Ferguson*, it ruled that because Missouri had no all-black law school, either Gaines must be admitted or the state would have to build an "equal" all-black school.
1950	*Sweatt v. Painter*	Following the *Gaines* case, states were faced with the choice of admitting black students to graduate programs or building new all-black schools. In this case, H. Marion Sweatt, a University of Texas Law School applicant argued that although an all-black law school did exist, it was inferior to the white school.	Although the Court again refused to strike down *Plessy v. Ferguson*, it ruled that although the black school was separate, it was not equal. Sweatt, therefore, was allowed to enroll at the white school.
1950	*Henderson v. United States*	Elmer Henderson, a black man, had been separated from other diners on a train's dining car.	The Court ruled that dining cars on railroad cars had to end this Jim Crow practice.
1950	*McLaurin v. Oklahoma Board of Regents*	G.W. McLaurin was a black student who had been admitted to the all-white graduate school at University of Oklahoma. Once there, he was segregated from the rest of the student body by being forced to sit alone in classrooms, in the library, and in the cafeteria.	NAACP lawyers, led by Thurgood Marshall, brought his case to the Supreme Court, where the justices ruled that segregating black students was not allowed in classrooms or in any other graduate school facilities.

INTEGRATION OF THE NATION'S SCHOOLS

In marked contrast to the military—where, all things considered, civil rights progress came relatively smoothly and quickly—the integration of the nation's schools proved to be one of the slowest, most difficult, and most controversial civil rights efforts in U.S. history. There are several reasons for this. First, the military is a highly centralized institution built on obedience and loyalty; it is expected that all personnel will obey an order from a superior, especially the commander-in-chief. America's schools, on the other hand, are a local affair and federal interference—in the name of civil rights or almost anything else—is often resented. Second, most military personnel live on bases far from home where local prejudices are likely to have less of an effect than in schools, which are situated in people's own neighborhoods. And finally the military consists of adults while schools consist of children. Southern whites believed that they were defending their way of life when they stood against integration. And as raising children the way one chooses is one of the core values of the American way of life,

it is not surprising that southern whites—and white parents in general—were incensed by efforts to integrate local schools.

In fact, since Reconstruction times, southern schools had been kept strictly segregated, a fact of life legally enshrined by the 1896 *Plessy v. Ferguson* Supreme Court decision which allowed for "separate but equal" educational facilities. As noted earlier, the practice of segregation was more about the "separate" than the "equal." Alabama, for example, spent $36 per white pupil but just $10 per black in 1929. Beginning in the 1930s, however, the Court began to whittle away at *Plessy*, beginning at the highest reaches of the educational establishment. In the latter half of the decade, the states of Maryland and Missouri were forced to open up their law schools to black students, while Oklahoma was required to admit an African American to its graduate school of education.

Still, at the primary, secondary, and college levels, segregation remained strictly enforced. At a conference in 1948, the NAACP pledged itself to challenge this policy, putting its legal staff—headed by future Supreme Court justice Thurgood Marshall—on the case. There were many groups of plaintiffs to choose from in the early 1950s, but, confusing the issue, a number of southern state governments pledged themselves to improving black education. Moreover, the NAACP wanted a case where spending was roughly equal between black and white schools, in order to challenge directly the "separate" part of the *Plessy* decision. They chose the school district of Topeka, Kansas and, thus, in 1952 the most important case challenging school segregation in U.S. history was put in front of the Supreme Court as *Brown* (alphabetically, the first of the plaintiffs) *v. Board of Education* (of Topeka).

Marshall and his team of NAACP lawyers argued that segregation—or "separateness," as *Plessy v. Ferguson* called it—was inherently unequal even if the facilities for blacks and whites were identical down to the last nail. And because they were unequal, they were in violation of the equal protection clause of the 14th Amendment to the Constitution, an amendment ratified in the late 1860s to protect the newly won—and, then, quickly lost—civil rights of former slaves. Specifically, the lawyers argued, separate facilities for black schoolchildren ultimately created a second-class citizen.

To illustrate their point, they used the research of African-American sociologist Kenneth B. Clarke of Harvard University. Using two sets of dolls—one set with white features and one with black ones—Clarke asked black children to state their preferences. Virtually all chose the white dolls, which Clarke said indicated how segregated education lowers the self-esteem of black children, even when facilities at their schools matched those of whites'. That study—and the reasoned arguments of Marshall and the other NAACP lawyers—swayed the Court. Writing for the majority, Chief Justice Earl Warren argued that segregation "generates [in black children] a feeling of inferiority as to their status in the community that may affect their hearts and minds in a way unlikely to ever be undone." A year later, in a follow-up decision to the case commonly known as *Brown II*, the Court set out guidelines for dismantling segregated education in America.

But its choice of words—"with all deliberate speed"—was interpreted by many southern governments to mean "as slowly as possible." In 1956, more than 100 southern congressmen issued the "Southern Manifesto" denouncing *Brown* and urging their constituents to defy it. By early 1957, more than half a million southern whites had formed White Citizens' Councils, organizations bent on blocking the implementation of civil rights measures. Confederate symbols and flags were officially adopted by southern state governments as demonstrations of resistance. More extremist southerners flocked to the Ku Klux Klan, swelling its numbers to the highest level since the 1920s. As the 1957–1958 academic year loomed, both sides—the civil rights organizations on one side and white anti–civil rights groups on the other—appeared ready for a confrontation.

In September 1957, the Little Rock, Arkansas, school board attempted to integrate nine black students in Little Rock's Central High School, an all-white institution. The nine students were met by crowds of jeering white students and parents who shouted insults and threw stones. Film crews captured the events and broadcast them night after night to the nation's TV viewers. Meanwhile, Governor Orval Faubus called in the National Guard, not to protect the students but to bar them from the schoolhouse. The combination of public pressure resulting from the newscasts and Faubus's challenge to federal authority forced a very reluctant president Dwight Eisenhower to act, nationalizing the National Guard and sending in an additional 1,000 federal troops to integrate the school.

Central High School was integrated, but it remained a rarity. As late as 1960, less than 1 percent of southern blacks were attending integrated schools. Relatively consistent integration did not occur until the 1970s, and even then white resistance persisted. Across the South, white parents pulled their children out of integrated public schools and enrolled them in private segregated academies. And when the federal government order forced busing to achieve integration, whites—as well as some blacks—grew angry at having their children bused to schools miles away from their neighborhoods. Moreover, resistance to busing was not strictly a southern phenomenon, with the most widely publicized anti-busing protest movements of the 1970s occurring in Boston and Michigan.

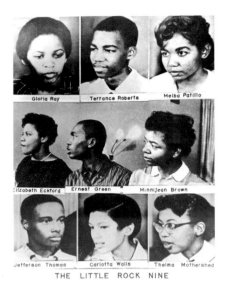

THE LITTLE ROCK NINE

Nine African-American teens desegregated Central High in Little Rock. The students are (top, left to right) Gloria Ray, Terrence Roberts, Melba Patillo, (center, left to right) Elizabeth Eckford, Ernest Green, Minnijean Brown, (bottom, left to right) Jefferson Thomas, Carlotta Walls, and Thelma Mothershed. (Library of Congress)

CIVIL RIGHTS PROTESTS

The integration of professional baseball, the *Brown* decision, and the events in Little Rock—important as they were—represented top-down gains for African Americans. That is to say, the efforts behind these

*"Little Nigger at Central High
Has got mighty free with his eye
Winks at white girls
Grabs their blond curls
Little nigger sure is anxious to die."*

—Printed on a card circulated among segregationist students in Little Rock, Arkansas

achievements were usually spearheaded by the NAACP and other national civil rights organizations, often based far from the South in Washington or northern urban centers. Yet, above all else, the civil rights movement of the 1950s and 1960s was a grassroots affair, originating among the regular black folk of the South, albeit aided by northern white and black supporters. If the civil rights movement is measured by the criteria of southern black initiative and leadership—a bottom-up movement, as it were—then its origins go back to a simple but remarkable event of December 2, 1955.

MONTGOMERY BUS BOYCOTT

Rosa Parks—a Montgomery, Alabama seamstress and a member of the local NAACP chapter—was coming home from work on the bus one evening when she was asked to give up her seat to a white man, as per bus company rules and southern custom and law. Segregation of public facilities had been widespread throughout the South since the late 19th century and represent-

ed—in its indignity and even cruelty—a daily reminder to African Americans of their second-class status in society. This time, however, Parks refused to surrender her seat. While it is true that Parks's act of resistance was spontaneous, it was equally the case that local black civil rights activists—of whom Parks was one—were looking for an occasion to challenge Montgomery's segregation statutes. As a respected community leader, Parks represented the perfect candidate to rally around. Thus, the day after Parks's arrest for "disorderly conduct," the Women's Political Council, a local black women's civic group led by Jo Ann Robinson, issued 52,000 fliers calling for a one-day bus boycott to coincide with Parks's trial on December 5.

Meanwhile, after bailing Parks out of jail, local labor leader E. D. Nixon called two Montgomery ministers, Ralph Abernathy of the First Baptist Church and Martin Luther King Jr. of the Dexter Avenue Baptist Church, and told them of her arrest. This turn to centers of faith was not unusual, as the black church represented one of the few independent African-American

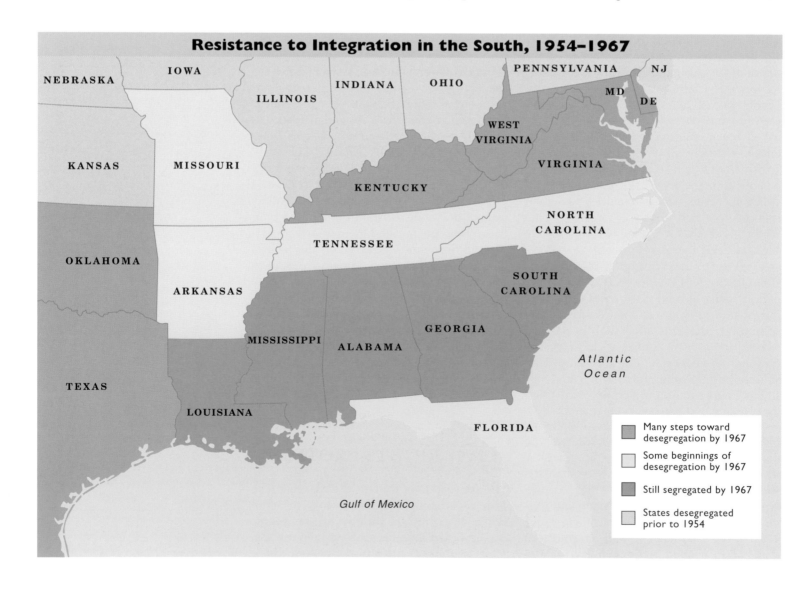

Resistance to Integration in the South, 1954–1967

Legend:
- Many steps toward desegregation by 1967
- Some beginnings of desegregation by 1967
- Still segregated by 1967
- States desegregated prior to 1954

institutions in most southern localities. Indeed, black churches were more than simply places of worship; they often engaged in civic and even political activities. And black churchmen—often more educated and worldly than most of their parishioners—traditionally served as community leaders in the black South. That was certainly the case with Abernathy and King. A graduate of Alabama State College, Abernathy became one of the founders of the Southern Christian Leadership Conference (SCLC) in 1957, among the leading civil rights organizations in the South. King had earned a Ph.D. in theology at Boston University before accepting his post at the Dexter Avenue Baptist Church. The central figure of the civil rights movement for more than a decade, King would go on to cofound the SCLC, fight segregation and discrimination across the South, lead the largest civil rights march in American history, and win the Nobel Peace Prize for his efforts, all before being assassinated in 1968.

But in December 1955, King's focus was local—the Montgomery boycott. On December 5, the city's buses—usually full of black workers on their way to jobs in factories and white homes—ran almost entirely empty. White officials—convinced "Negro goon squads" were intimidating black riders—dispatched police to restore order. But there were no goon squads; the boycott had the support of the vast majority of Montgomery's black community. When Parks was found guilty of violating the city's segregation ordinances, the boycott leaders organized the Montgomery Improvement Association (MIA), elected King as its president, and called for a continuing boycott to force an end to segregation on city buses. "There comes a time," King told an audience of 7,000 at the Holt Street Baptist Church, "when people get tired of being trampled over by the iron feet of oppression."

Reflecting King's philosophy of nonviolence—which he had adopted from the teachings of Mohandas K. Gandhi, leader of the anticolonial movement in India—the MIA peacefully resisted police intimidation and white violence. As teams of black cab drivers and carpoolers were organized to take people to work—and routinely harassed and arrested for driving too fast or too slow—King and other black leaders met with Montgomery bus officials. But their demands—for an end to segregation and more black drivers—fell on deaf ears. White supremacists in the area—believing, incorrectly, that the movement was being orchestrated by outsiders including communists—targeted local black leaders, setting off bombs at their homes and churches. The following spring, Montgomery officials issued arrest warrants for King and other

Rosa Parks being fingerprinted by a Montgomery, Alabama policeman following her arrest (Library of Congress)

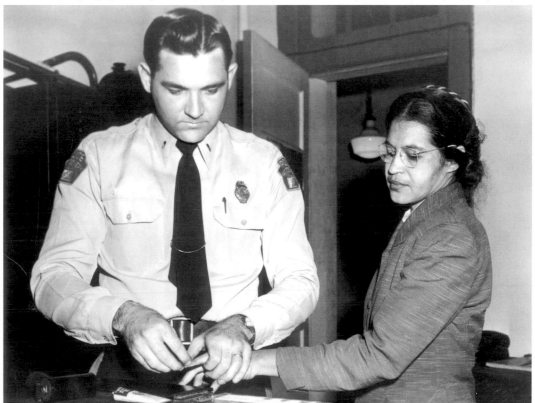

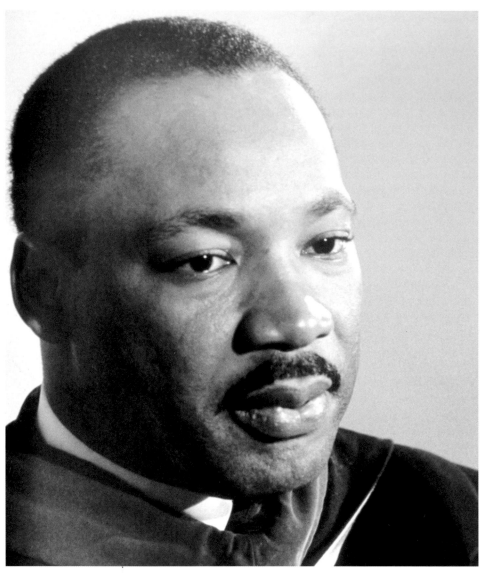

Martin Luther King Jr. (Library of Congress)

black leaders for organizing a boycott "without just cause or legal excuse." But when the arrestees turned themselves in, the national press came to cover the event.

By the summer, the civil rights movement had become a page one newspaper story, and King had appeared on the cover of *Time* and the *New York Times Magazine*. In June, a federal court ruled that segregated seating was unconstitutional, and although the case was appealed to the U.S. Supreme Court, the high court voted on December 20, 1956 to support the lower court's decision. Parks, Abernathy, King, the MIA, and the black community of Montgomery had won. As future events would bear out, the implications of the boycott were enormous—for the African-American community, the South, and the nation as a whole. "We have gained a new sense of dignity and destiny," King wrote. "We have discovered a new and powerful weapon—nonviolent resistance."

LUNCH COUNTER SIT-IN MOVEMENT

If the Montgomery bus boycott began as a spontaneous act of resistance, the lunch counter sit-ins—the next civil rights protest to gain national attention—were carefully planned and orchestrated. Like virtually all stores in the South, the Greensboro, North Carolina, Woolworth's maintained a strict segregationist policy. Blacks could shop there, but they were not permitted to eat at its lunch counter. It was a particularly insulting policy as it implied that blacks might somehow contaminate whites by their presence. And lunch counter segregation was only the tip of the iceberg; movie theaters, hotels, and restaurants of all kinds usually barred blacks or offered them distinctly inferior and separate sections. Nor was this policy always confined to the South. After black Hollywood movie star Dorothy Dandridge swam in a Las Vegas pool, the hotel drained and refilled it with water before allowing white patrons back in.

On February 5, 1960, four students from the all-black North Carolina Agricultural and Technical College—Ezell Blair Jr., Franklin McCain, Joseph McNeill, and David Richmond—sat down at the Woolworth's counter in Greensboro and ordered lunch. The staff refused to serve them and the four sat at the counter until the store closed, returning each morning for the next five days. As word of the protests spread, mobs of angry whites showed up, verbally and even physically abusing the students. Still, the four persisted, encouraged by hundreds of supporters on the streets outside. Over the course of 1960, the tactic of sit-ins would spread to no less than 126 towns and cities across the South, involving 50,000 participants. The most effective protests occurred in Nashville where the local student movement sat in at virtually all of the city's lunch counters, forcing storeowners to integrate their businesses.

While met by white violence and police intimidation—more than 36,000 protesters were jailed for disturbing the peace in 1960—the sit-ins proved very effective, as they cost the stores money. Not only did the protests disturb shoppers—and lead to a loss of black patronage—but TV and newspaper coverage spread the word across the country, sparking boycotts of Woolworth's and other chain stores in northern cities as well. Older leaders of the civil rights movement soon realized the effectiveness of student idealism and activism, as well as

A CHRONOLOGY OF THE CAREER OF MARTIN LUTHER KING JR.

1951–1955   Attends Boston University doctoral program; earns Ph.D. in theology

1953   Marries Coretta Scott, a student at the New England Conservatory of Music

1954   Is appointed minister of Dexter Avenue Baptist Church in Montgomery, Alabama

1955–1956   Leads a successful one-year boycott of Montgomery's bus system

1957   In early January, helps organize Southern Christian Leadership Conference (SCLC); a bomb is thrown at the King house, but it does not explode.

1958   Meets with President Dwight D. Eisenhower at the White House; he is arrested in Montgomery (first charged with loitering, a charge that is dropped and replaced with "failure to obey an officer"). King publishes *Strive Toward Freedom*, an account of the Montgomery bus boycott. While on tour to promote the book, he is stabbed in the chest. His condition is serious but not critical.

1960   Is arrested in February on charges that he failed to pay his Alabama state taxes in 1956 and 1958. He is later acquitted by an all-white jury. In June, he meets with President John F. Kennedy. In December he is arrested at an Atlanta sit-in.

1961   Arrives in Albany, Georgia, to participate in an unsuccessful desegregation campaign. In December, he is arrested in Albany for obstructing the sidewalk and leading a parade without a permit.

1962   Is arrested again, at a July prayer vigil in Albany, and charged with failure to obey a police officer, obstructing the sidewalk, and disorderly conduct. In October, he meets once more with President Kennedy.

1963   In March and April, leads sit-in demonstrations in Birmingham, Alabama. In jail, he writes his "Letter from Birmingham Jail." That summer he leads the historic March on Washington and delivers his famous "I Have a Dream" speech.

1964   Joins demonstrations in St. Augustine, Florida, in May and June and is arrested. His book *We Can't Wait* is released in June, and in July, he attends the ceremony at which President Lyndon Johnson signs the Civil Rights Act of 1964. In September, he meets with Pope Paul VI at the Vatican, and, in December, he receives the Nobel Peace Prize in Oslo, Norway.

1965   The Southern Christian Leadership Conference organizes a civil rights march from Selma to Montgomery, Alabama. On March 7, the marchers are beaten by Alabama state troopers when they attempt to cross Selma's Edmund Pettus Bridge. Two weeks later, joined by 3,000 supporters from around the nation, and protected by federal troops, they begin their march again. En route, they are joined by another 25,000 supporters. When he and the other marchers reach Selma, King addresses the marchers from the Montgomery capitol building.

1966   In Chicago, meets with Elijah Mohammed, leader of the Nation of Islam, and leads an unsuccessful protest against job discrimination, poor schools, and slum housing

1967   King's book *Where Do We Go From Here* is published. At a speech in Chicago, he denounces the war in Vietnam. In November, he announces that the SCLC will launch a Poor People's Campaign to address the problems of poor blacks and whites.

1968   Is assassinated after leading a sanitation workers strike in Memphis

THE FREEDOM RIDES, 1961

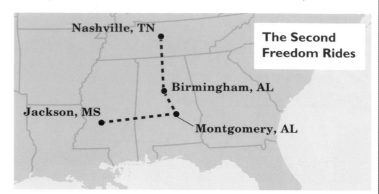

The First Freedom Rides

Washington, DC
Richmond, VA
Petersburg, VA
Lynchburg, VA

Charlotte, NC
Winnesboro, SC   Rock Hill, SC
Atlanta, GA   Camden, SC
Birmingham, AL   Sumter, SC
                        Anniston, AL
(by plane)   Montgomery, AL

New Orleans

The Second Freedom Rides

Nashville, TN

Birmingham, AL

Jackson, MS

Montgomery, AL

May 4 Seven blacks and six whites leave Washington, D.C., on one Greyhound bus and one Trailways bus.

May 4-7 The buses travel through Richmond, Petersburg, and Lynchburg, Virginia. At each stop both black and white riders use "whites only" lunch counters and bathrooms without incident.

May 7 Freedom rider Charles Perkins, an African American, attempts to get a shoe shine in a whites-only barbershop at a Charlotte, North Carolina, bus station. Although he is refused service, he remains in the shop until police place him under arrest.

May 9 In Rock Hill, South Carolina, a band of whites beat John Lewis after he attempts to enter the bus station waiting room. Albert Bigelow is also beaten. Although the police make no arrests, they allow riders to enter the waiting room.

May 11 In Winnesboro, South Carolina, freedom riders James Peck and Henry Thomas are arrested for attempting to integrate a bus station lunch counter.

May 11–13 The buses travel through Sumter and Camden, South Carolina, and Augusta and Athens, Georgia, without incident before arriving in Atlanta, where the riders regroup in preparation for the next leg of the journey—into Alabama and Mississippi.

May 14 Outside Anniston, Alabama, the Greyhound is surrounded by a mob, who break windows and slash the bus tires. One member of the mob tosses a torch through a window, filling the bus with smoke. As riders try to flee the bus, the crowd attempts to hold the doors shut, before beating passengers as they escape. The local hospital refuses to treat the injured riders. An hour later, the Trailways bus arrives in Anniston, where its passengers are also beaten before the bus leaves for Birmingham. There, whites board and attempt to force all blacks to the back of the bus. When two white riders attempt to intervene, they too are beaten. One, a 61-year old retired teacher named Walter Bergman, is left close to death, with permanent brain damage. The other needs 56 stitches in the head.

May 15–17 Despite the attack, the riders vow to continue on to Montgomery, Alabama. When no driver will take them, the group abandons its plans. The Justice Department arranges for the freedom riders to fly to New Orleans, Louisiana. Although a bomb threat delays takeoff, the group flies to New Orleans.

May 17 Convinced that ending the freedom rides would reward racists for their violence, Diane Nash, head of SNCC's Nashville, Tennessee chapter, organizes a new group of freedom riders. Their bus leaves Nashville, bound for Birmingham, Alabama.

May 18 The freedom riders arrive in Birmingham. They are arrested and begin a prison hunger strike. Police respond by driving the riders 150 miles north to the Tennessee border and dropping them off near the state line. Diane Nash sends a car to pick them up and bring them back to Birmingham. There, they eat for the first time in two days and head for the bus station.

May 19 The state of Alabama issues an injunction to prevent "entry into and travel within the State of Alabama, and engaging in the so-called 'freedom ride' and other acts of conduct calculated to provoke breaches of the peace."

May 20 The freedom riders wait in the Birmingham bus station until a driver agrees to take them to Montgomery. They are met there by an angry crowd of several hundred, who begin to assault them with clubs. One passenger has flammable liquid tossed on him and his clothes are set on fire. Assistant Attorney General John Siegenthaler, sent by the Kennedy administration to monitor the situation, is knocked unconscious after he attempts to assist one fleeing woman. Montgomery police allow the riot to continue for an hour before dispersing the crowd. In Washington, Attorney General Robert Kennedy orders 350 U.S. marshals into Alabama to quiet the situation.

May 21 U.S. marshals begin to arrive in Alabama. Martin Luther King Jr. flies into Mongomery. Governor John Patterson of Alabama threatens to arrest the marshals if they interfere, adding that the freedom rides were inspired by communists. That evening, a white mob forms outside of Reverend Ralph Abernathy's First Baptist Church, trapping inside 1,500 African Americans who are meeting there.

May 23 King, Abernathy, and Nash, as well as James Farmer and John Lewis of CORE, announce that the freedom rides will resume.

May 24 Escorted by Alabama National Guardsmen and the highway patrol, the riders leave Alabama for Jackson, Mississippi. When they arrive, Jackson police arrest take them. Two days later, they are convicted and given suspended sentences. The riders elect to remain in jail, at notorious Parchman Penitentiary, where they remain for almost a month before they are released.

international outrage at southern practices. As events in Birmingham would soon prove, white segregationists had failed to learn the same lesson.

BIRMINGHAM, 1963

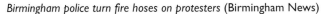

In 1963, King and the SCLC decided to turn their attention to Birmingham, Alabama's largest city and one of the industrial centers of the South. Local civil rights leader Fred Shuttlesworth, minister of the city's First Baptist Church, labeled it "the most segregated city in the United States." For six years, since civil rights organizers had begun to protest racial conditions in the city, there had been 18 unsolved bombings in the black community, earning the city the nickname "Bombingham." In early spring, the SCLC launched Project C (for "confrontation"), a series of demonstrations that brought thousands to downtown streets to protest the segregation and hiring practices of local department stores.

Civil rights activists were familiar with rough police tactics, but they had never seen anything like Birmingham. Under the leadership of Commissioner Eugene "Bull" Connor, the city's police used attack dogs, electric cattle prods, and high pressure fire hoses capable of stripping the bark off trees against the protesters, many of them children who had taken leave from school to participate. Once again, TV cameras were on hand to convey images of peaceful demonstrators being met with overwhelming violence for simply demanding their constitutional rights. As President John F. Kennedy noted, "the civil rights movement should thank God for Bull Connor. He's helped it as much as Abraham Lincoln." After securing a court order barring further demonstrations, Connor arrested King. While in jail, the SCLC leader penned a response to a group of white clergymen who criticized him for moving too fast on civil rights. "[I have] yet to engage in a direct-action campaign that was 'well-timed' in view of those who have not suffered unduly from the disease of segregation," King wrote in his famous essay "Letter from Birmingham City Jail." "For years now, I have heard the word 'Wait!' ring in the ear of every Negro with piercing familiarity. This 'Wait' has almost always meant 'Never.'" Meanwhile, protesters continued to pour into the streets and continued to be arrested, with more than 2,000 in jail by May.

With the city on the verge of a full-scale race riot, local business leaders asked the Kennedy administration to intervene. A federal mediator negotiated an agreement calling for an end to segregation in downtown stores. More bombings prompted the dispatch of federal troops. Birmingham proved a watershed for Kennedy on civil rights. Although widely supported by black voters, the young president had been reluctant to return the favor during his first few years in office. He and his attorney general,

Birmingham police turn fire hoses on protesters (Birmingham News)

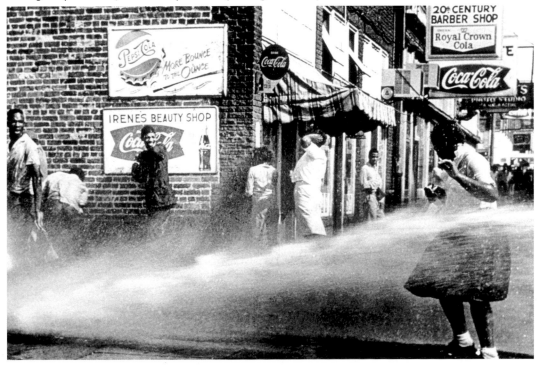

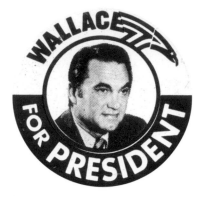

Segregationist Alabama governor George Wallace ran for president in both 1968 and 1972. (private collection)

MAJOR CIVIL RIGHTS ORGANIZATIONS

NAACP Legal Defense and Educational Fund
DATE FOUNDED: 1939
MAJOR LEADER: Thurgood Marshall
AIMS: To use the courts to fight discrimination and segregation
ACCOMPLISHMENTS: Helped win *Brown v. Board of Education* ruling outlawing segregation in public education

Congress of Racial Equality (CORE)
DATE FOUNDED: 1942
MAJOR LEADERS: James Farmer, Roy Innes
AIMS: To fight discrimination and racism through sit-ins and other nonviolent direct action
ACCOMPLISHMENTS: Sponsored freedom rides to end segregation in interstate transport

Southern Christian Leadership Conference (SCLC)
DATE FOUNDED: 1957
MAJOR LEADERS: Martin Luther King Jr., Ralph Abernathy
AIMS: To work for civil rights through direct nonviolent action
ACCOMPLISHMENTS: Helped get the 1965 Voting Rights Act passed

Student Non-Violent Coordinating Commitee (SNCC)
DATE FOUNDED: 1960
MAJOR LEADERS: John Lewis, Stokely Carmichael
AIMS: To fight segregation and discrimination through direct action, including jail-ins
ACCOMPLISHMENTS: Helped register voters during Freedom Summer in Mississippi; fought to integrate delegations at the Democratic National Convention

Black Panthers
DATE FOUNDED: 1966
MAJOR LEADERS: Bobby Seale, Huey Newton
AIMS: To fight racism in northern cities; defend the black community against racist police officers; provide social services for inner-city black communities
ACCOMPLISHMENTS: Established several day-care centers and clinics in black communities

brother Robert Kennedy, had even asked the Federal Bureau of Investigation to conduct surveillance on King's private life, leading to revelations of extramarital affairs by the civil rights leader. Most important, like Franklin Roosevelt before him, Kennedy had an ambitious legislative agenda and feared alienating conservative southern Democrats in Congress. But the gathering momentum of the civil rights movement—and fears that internationally broadcast images of American racism were hurting the country's image at a crucial moment in the cold war—prompted Kennedy to act. On June 12—the day Alabama governor George Wallace stood in the doorway of the University of Alabama to bar newly admitted black students—Kennedy went on national TV to announce a major federal initiative to enforce anti-segregation court rulings. Yet that very same evening came news of another act of white violence—the murder of Mississippi NAACP organizer Medgar Evers.

MARCH ON WASHINGTON

To rally support for Kennedy's proposal, as well as to demonstrate the broad coalition of forces that stood behind the civil rights movement, leaders of the "big six" organizations decided to sponsor a massive march on Washington for the summer of 1963. The six included Whitney Young of the National Urban League (NUL); Roy Wilkins, head of the NAACP; James Farmer, founder and president of the CORE; SNCC head John Lewis; and King of the SCLC. But while these leaders put the march together, the idea came from the old warhorse of the civil rights movement, A. Philip Randolph, president of the Brotherhood of Sleeping Car Porters and Negro American Labor

Council. As noted in the previous chapter, Randolph had planned a civil rights march on Washington in 1941 but was dissuaded when President Roosevelt signed legislation creating the Fair Employment Practices Committee to assure equal opportunities for African Americans in the burgeoning defense industry.

In December 1962, Randolph met with Rustin, a civil rights veteran famous for his early freedom ride in the 1940s, to discuss a new march to coincide with the 100th anniversary of the Emancipation Proclamation. As a labor leader, Randolph wanted to focus on jobs but Rustin suggested "freedom." In June, King—in the midst of his Birmingham struggle—signed on, urging that the march be used as an expression of the strength of the growing civil rights movement. Still, there remained deep divisions in the movement about the efficacy of such an action. More conservative civil rights organizations like the NAACP and the NUL insisted that the march be nonviolent and nonconfrontational. Younger and more militant members of CORE and SNCC

wanted to incorporate civil disobedience and more forceful language in the declarations surrounding the march. But King— increasingly the man other civil rights activists looked to for leadership—sided with the conservative groups. Soon, liberal white religious organizations—like the National Council of Churches, the National Conference of Catholic for Interracial Justice, and the American Jewish Congress— had come on board.

Working out of offices in Harlem, Rustin—now the chief organizer of the march—organized the complicated logistics of transportation, health and safety, and publicity—all on a limited budget made possible by thousands of small cash contributions and the sale of buttons. There were the normal organizational fears that few people would show up and the march would be a washout. But in the days leading up to August 28, tens of thousands of people poured into Washington by car, rail, and plane. One man even roller-skated there from Chicago. The sheer size of the crowd—some 250,000 persons attended—

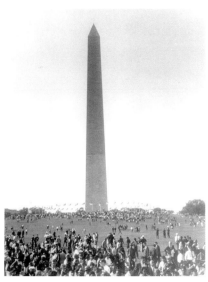

The March on Washington (Library of Congress)

Dr. King and fellow marchers in Washington. King can be seen second from the left, in the front row. (Library of Congress)

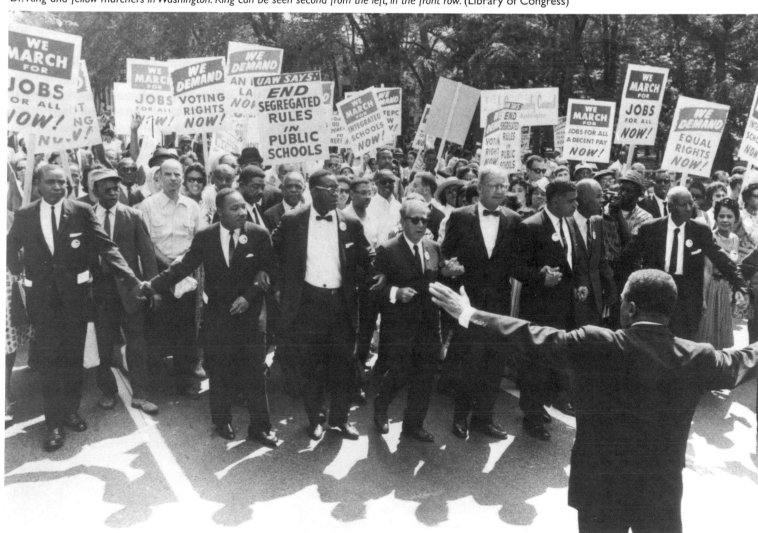

The Selma to Montgomery March, March 21-25, 1965

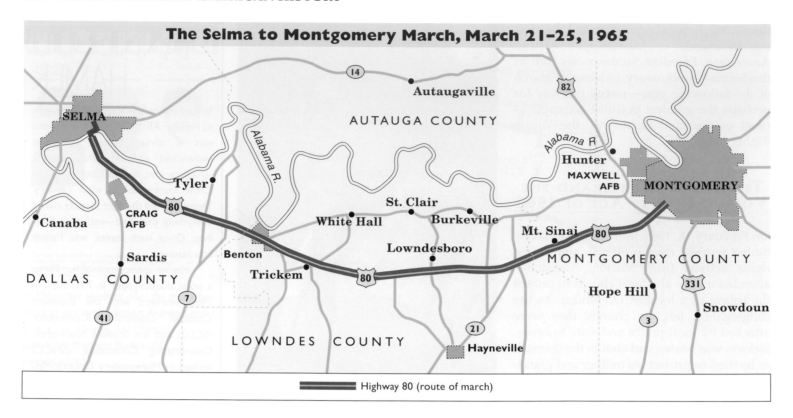

Highway 80 (route of march)

Eight days later, President Johnson himself went on national TV to announce that he was submitting a comprehensive voting rights bill to Congress. "Their cause," he said of the marchers, "must be our cause, too. Because it's not just Negroes, but it's really all of us who must overcome the crippling legacy of bigotry and injustice." Appearing to speak to Wallace and other white Alabamans, he insisted, "It is

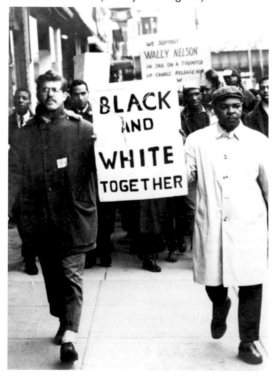

Marchers in Selma (Library of Congress)

wrong—deadly wrong, to deny any of your fellow Americans the right to vote in this country." Then, borrowing the rallying cry of the movement, he ended his speech, "And, we shall overcome." Never before had a president identified himself so closely and unapologetically with the cause of civil rights. King, it was said, cried as he listened to the speech. On March 21—accompanied by federal marshals and troops—King led 25,000 people across the Edmund Pettus Bridge and all the way to Montgomery without any violent incidents to speak of. They camped out along the way and reached Montgomery on March 25.

The Voting Rights Act signed into law by President Johnson on August 6, 1965 was the second and last major piece of legislation of the civil rights era. It was a sweeping and powerful bill that banned literacy tests and put Washington in the business of voter registration for the first time, by sending federal examiners to register voters in any county where more than 50 percent of the voting age population failed to show up on the registration lists. Together with the 24th Amendment of 1964, which banned poll taxes, the act ended all the legal ruses that southern states had employed to stop blacks from registering to vote.

Together, the Voting Rights Act of 1965 and the Civil Rights Act of 1964 fulfilled the promises of equal protection made by the 14th Amendment during Reconstruction. They reversed nearly a century of Jim Crow laws, though it would take another decade

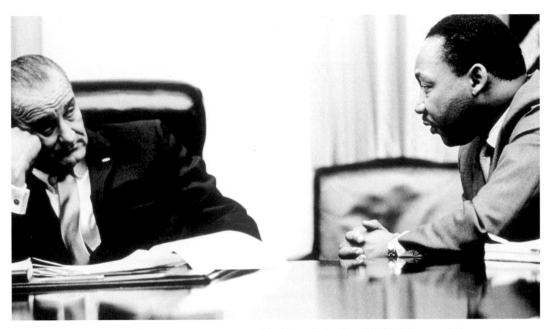

King confers with President Johnson prior to passage of the Voting Rights Act of 1965. (Library of Congress)

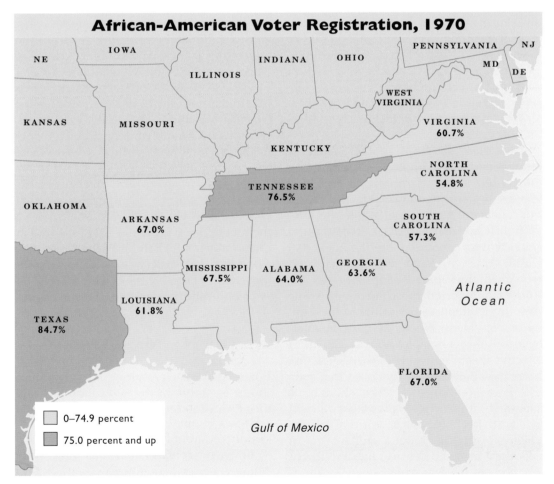

The map above reflects the percentages of African Americans registered to vote in the South in 1970.

or so to finally end the practice of southern segregation. But just as these bills represented the high water mark of civil rights legislation, so too the Selma-Montgomery [ ] marked the culmination of nonvio- [ ] as the centerpiece of the civil [ ] Less than six months later—

and just five days after Johnson signed the Voting Rights Act—a city as far from Alabama and Mississippi as it could be would explode in violence. The Watts Riots of Los Angeles—born of a more subtle de facto segregation—that is, segregation through practice rather than law—and triggered by routine police brutality—signaled a new and more violent phase of black unrest, and one that was not confined to the South.

MALCOLM X AND THE RISE OF BLACK NATIONALISM

Throughout the 20th century, two conflicting tendencies have permeated African-American political thought. One traces its lineage back to the writings of W. E. B. DuBois and the founding ideals of the NAACP: an integrated, multiracial United States, free of prejudice and discrimination, where African Americans enjoy equality of economic opportunity and full political participation. The means to reach these ends included political advocacy, nonviolent protest, Christian love, an appeal to constitutional protections, rigorous use of the legal system, and an acceptance of liberal, well-meaning whites within the ranks of the movement. The integrationist tendency, as it has been called, reached its highest peak in the civil rights movement of the 1950s and early 1960s and found its greatest leader—and martyr—in the Reverend Martin Luther King Jr.

But there has been another school of thought and action among black activists in this century, one that traces its lineage back to Marcus Garvey and his Universal Negro Improvement Association. While the integrationist approach to black freedom and equality was premised on the idea that white America could be changed and redeemed, the separatist approach—as it is sometimes referred to—condemned white America as unalterably hostile to the aspirations of blacks. Where the integrationists believed that nonviolence was the most effective means to deal with white violence, black nationalists—who believed that even the best-intentioned whites should be excluded on principle—advocated "a fight fire with fire" approach, not a Christian turning of the cheek but a militant and, if necessary, armed defense of life and liberty. The ends of the two schools were as different as their means. With white America irredeemably racist, nationalists argued, blacks must withdraw into their own social, economic, and political space. This separatist tendency achieved its own peak—in the Black Power movement of the late 1960s and early 1970s—and found its greatest leader—and martyr—in Malcolm X.

The two movements existed in an uneasy tension with each other, characterized by the mutual respect and mutual suspicion in which King and Malcolm held each other. Deep down both shared fundamental ideals: political equality for blacks, racial self-respect and dignity, and economic justice. Indeed, both shared a basic distrust of capitalism as the best means to achieve economic equality. And each admired the undeniable bravery of the other. But they disagreed about much, too. King felt that the nationalists—by engendering fear in whites—were in danger of provoking violent retribution against themselves and the black community generally. For his part, Malcolm ridiculed the nonviolent ideals of the integrationists as futile and even self-destructive. He likened the differences between the two tendencies to the old divisions of the plantation South. The integrationists, he said, were the "house niggers" who—feeling privileged by living in the master's house—identified with it and hoped to ameliorate its worst aspects. The nationalists, on the other hand, were the "fieldhands," living separate and apart from whites, with no illusion of ever being accepted in the white man's world.

However much one accepts or rejects the metaphor, there was an underlying truth to Malcolm's point—the two movements were fundamentally different, both in the physical and spiritual sense. Where the civil rights movement came out of the rural (and urban) South, the separatists were largely a northern and urban phenomenon. And where the integrationists placed their faith in a Christian god, separatists often looked to Allah and Islam, which—along with Marcus Garvey's Back-to-Africa movement of the 1920s—is where the history of 20th-century black nationalism begins.

THE NATION OF ISLAM

When Africans were brought to American shores as slaves in the 17th and 18th centuries, most practiced local ancestor-based indiginous faiths, while a minority followed Islam. Traumatized by the enslavement process, severed from their local cultural traditions, mixed together with Africans of varied backgrounds, thrust headlong into a dominant European-based society, and often worked to the point of exhaustion and death, the vast majority of enslaved Africans in North America lost touch with their African faiths or Islam, embracing Christianity in its stead. For hundreds of years, through slavery a nominal freedom they won in the African Americans utilized faith to sustain their spirit and hopes for a better life in the next world, even as they developed Christian institutions that served as centers of cultural, political, and social life in this one.

But to Wallace Fard, a door-to-door silk salesperson in early 1930s Detroit, Christianity represented the faith of the oppressor, and its worship by African Americans a symbol of their exile and servitude. While pitching his wares, Fard also preached a new Islamic-based faith. Islam held several attractions. Although tainted by its own connections to the slave trade, Islam was not associated in most African-American eyes with racism. Indeed, it was an alternative faith to Christianity, with the two in historically hostile competition with each other. At the same time, Islam was related to Christianity (it considered the Bible a holy book and Jesus a prophet, though not the son of God), so it was not entirely unfamiliar to African Americans. And finally, perhaps foremost among its many doctrines, it preached an equality of mankind, in submission to an almighty god, Allah. But Fard's Islam was hardly orthodox; it was heavily infused with biblical scripture (which was often employed to criticize Christianity), an Afrocentric view of humanity's creation, and denunciations of western civilization and white people, whom Fard called "blue-eyed devils."

Like many new religions, it began informally. But as it grew in numbers, it developed both written texts and an organizational infrastructure. Fard called the new faith the Nation of Islam (NOI) because he hoped to create an "independent" black Islamic nation—not necessarily geographically removed from America—but spiritually, culturally, and even economically separate. Fard wrote two manuals to guide the faithful and established two schools—for men and women—to teach the precepts of the faith. He also created a kind of religious police force—the Fruits of Islam—who acted as his bodyguards and enforced NOI laws.

With its militancy and strong antiwhite message, the NOI soon attracted the attention of white authorities, who tried to frame Fard in 1931 for a murder committed by one of his followers. Fearing prison, or worse, Fard prepared his right-hand man Elijah Muhammad (born Elijah Poole) for leadership. But the transfer of power did not go smoothly; the NOI split into two mutually suspicious groups and Muhammad led his followers to Chicago where they established the Temple of Islam Number 2 as the faith's national headquarters. Under

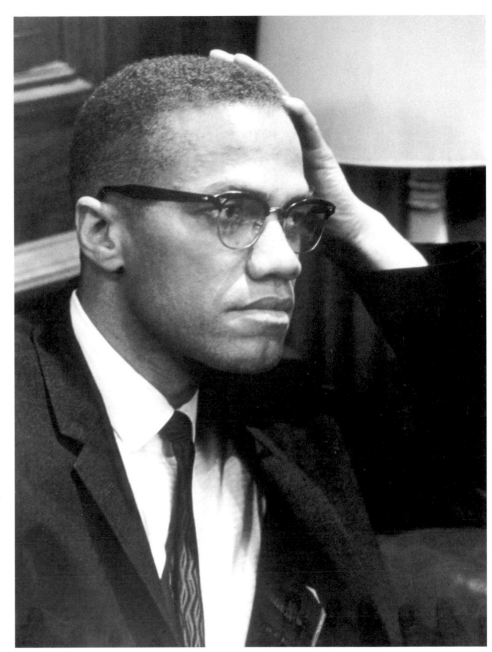

Malcolm X (Library of Congress)

Muhammad, the NOI grew rapidly, attracting legions of urban blacks, newly arrived from the rural South. Bewildered and frightened by their new environment, many found solace in NOI teaching and its emphasis on a highly structured way of life. The NOI preached the sanctity of marriage and family and, like its parent faith, Islam, advocated strict behavioral rules about diet, hygiene, and abstinence from alcohol and drugs. Muhammad emphasized both the importance of women—he maintained Fard's female schools—and their subservience to men, a principle that would come to be heavily criticized, not only during the women's liberation movement in the 1970s, but for decades to come.

At the same time, Muhammad put Fard's ideas about economic nationalism

THE BASIC TENETS OF THE NATION OF ISLAM

Although the Nation of Islam has roots in the Islamic faith, and shares some of its principles, it is an entirely separate religion. Below, some of the main tenets of each are discussed.

Basic Tenets of Islam

1. Islam's central feature is its devotion to the Koran, believed to be the revelation of God, or Allah, to the prophet Muhammad.
2. Allah is all powerful, just, loving, merciful, and good.
3. No creature is to be compared to Allah, for Allah is preeminent.
4. Allah has made revelations known through a series of chosen prophets, and when man has fallen away from these revelations, Allah has sent new prophets.
5. Early prophets included Adam, Noah, Abraham, Moses, and Jesus. Muhammad is the last prophet and when man falls from him, the end of the world will arrive.
6. Christians and Jews have corrupted the meaning of the Old Testament.
7. Muslims are forbidden to touch or eat pork, drink wine, gamble, or commit usury, fraud, or slander. They are also forbidden to make images.
8. The Muslim has five duties, which are as follows: First, once in his life, a follower must say with absolute acceptance, "There is no god but God and Muhammad is his prophet"; second, he must pray five times a day; third, he must give alms generously; fourth, he must keep the fast of Ramadan; and fifth, once in his life, if he is able, he must make a pilgrimage to Mecca.

Basic Tenets of the Nation of Islam

1. W. D. Fard was an incarnation of Allah who had come to free the "Lost-Found Nation of Islam in the West," or African Americans.
2. By listening to Fard, African Americans will learn the truth about themselves, defeat their white "slave masters," and be restored to a position of primacy among the world's peoples.
3. According to the teachings of Elijah Muhammad, and later Louis Farrakhan, black men are destined by Allah to assume their rightful cultural and political leadership of the earth.
4. Christianity is a white man's plot to enslave nonwhites.
5. The white race is a race of devils, whose reign is soon coming to an end.
6. In preparation for the final battle between good and evil, there is a need for blacks to work together to heal their fallen, such as drug addicts and criminals, and to strive for economic independence from white society.
7. Adherents of the Nation of Islam are prohibited from touching or eating pork, using intoxicants, and practicing sexual promiscuity.

into practice. With their adherence to principles of clean-living and hard work, black Muslims were often economically successful and most donated a large portion of their salary to the NOI. This allowed it to build more than 100 temples nationwide which, in turn, supported shops, restaurants and other small businesses in black neighborhoods. During the 1930s and the 1940s, the Nation of Islam became an institution within much of urban black America and began to adopt the trappings of the nationalism it preached. The Nation of Islam adopted a flag, an anthem, and salutes and it periodically conducted military parades. It was, in the description of one historian, a kind of "military theocracy." Unlike integrationist organizations, such as the NAACP, it offered more than politics; it offered an alternative way of life, free from whites. Its rituals, its emphasis on black pride, and its insistence on clean-living often appealed to those African Americans most victimized by white society—particularly the ghetto poor and prisoners. In the late 1940s, the Nation of Islam recruited its most famous convert—an imprisoned former drug dealer and petty thief named Malcolm Little. After joining the Nation of Islam, Little changed his name—to Malcolm X.

MALCOLM X AND BLACK NATIONALISM

In many ways, Malcolm X's story is the classic American tale of a person remaking their life after hitting rock bottom. And, in his redemption from a life of crime to a life dedicated to a fight for racial justice, he has inspired millions of black—and white—Americans. He grew up in a household shattered by the effects of white racism. Born in Omaha in 1925, Malcolm's father—Earl Little—was a local Baptist preacher and disciple of Marcus Garvey. While Earl's beliefs influenced his son, they also got the family in trouble with the Ku Klux Klan, which burned their new home in Lansing, Michigan to the ground. Later, Earl was killed under mysterious circumstances, allegedly being forced under a streetcar by white toughs. Louisa—Malcolm's mother—

was committed to a mental institution and the children were placed in foster homes, with Malcolm ending up the ward of a racist white couple. In his early teens, he fled Michigan for Boston, where he moved into the home of his half-sister Ella.

In the black Roxbury district of Boston, Malcolm discovered a world of people who lived by their wits and enjoyed all of the diversions of urban life. Malcolm danced the popular lindy hop, wore loud and colorful zoot suits and had his hair "conked" (or straightened), the latter decision one he would condemn later in life as a sad and self-degrading attempt to look more white. While not particularly political, he could not help hearing about the World War II–era, antiblack race riots in Detroit and elsewhere and did his best to avoid the draft into a "white man's war." To support himself, Malcolm soon turned to crime, including drug-dealing, pimping, and gambling, a way of life he continued after his move to Harlem. In 1946, however, Malcolm was arrested and convicted for burglary and other crimes and sent to prison.

It was in prison that Malcolm found the NOI and dedicated himself to the teachings of Wallace Fard and the leadership of Elijah Muhammad. In the NOI tradition, he immediately set out to improve himself, delving deeply into the Bible and the Koran, and reading widely in literature and history. To improve his vocabulary, he once read a dictionary from cover to cover. First an acolyte, Malcolm soon became an advocate, preaching the message of the NOI and honing his rhetorical skills. He even led the prison's debating team to victory over a squad from the Massachusetts Institute of Technology (MIT), arguing against capital punishment.

In 1952, Malcolm was released from prison and went to work for the NOI. He also changed his name. Calling his surname "Little" a "white man's name," he adopted "X" to symbolize his lost African heritage. (After his pilgrimage to Mecca in 1964, he adopted the Islamic name El-Hajj Malik El-Shabazz.) With his intense energy and charisma, his fiery rhetoric, and his devotion to Elijah Muhammad, Malcolm quickly rose within the NOI ranks, becoming minister of its Harlem temple and founder of its first national newspaper, *Muhammad Speaks*. Indeed, Malcolm's introduction into NOI leadership circles came at a fortuitous moment. For years on the cutting edge of black militancy, the NOI found itself in the mid-1950s competing with the civil rights movement for the hearts and minds of African Americans. Speaking around the country and through the media, Malcolm denounced the integrationist ideals of King and other civil rights leaders. "It is not integration that Negroes in America want," he insisted, "it is human dignity." Why, he asked, should blacks strive to fit into a society that detested them when they could use their talents building an independent black "nation"?

In 1958, Malcolm married Betty Sanders (later Betty Shabazz), a fellow NOI disciple, and would eventually father four daughters. Like his beloved Muhammad, Malcolm believed in traditional gender roles and insisted that his wife not overstep her bounds as mother and homemaker. Yet, in other ways, Malcolm was creating a certain intellectual distance between himself and Muhammad in the late 1950s. He questioned the latter's firm belief that all white people were "devils," and he quietly broke with the NOI's principle of not becoming involved in politics. Malcolm supported boycotts and marches called by civil rights organizations and increasingly became an advocate of the decolonization of nonwhite peoples around the world. He especially came to advocate pan-Africanism—a political belief that preached the unity of black people around the world—after a trip to the continent in 1959.

This independence of thought and action did not sit well with Muhammad, who feared that his famous follower's popularity was eclipsing his own and he began looking for ways to reassert his authority. The opportunity arose in November 1963, with President Kennedy's assassination. Asked by a reporter for his thoughts on the events in Dallas, Malcolm said it was a case of "the chickens coming home to roost," meaning Kennedy's unwillingness to stop racist violence in the South had created the conditions for his own murder in a southern state. The uproar that greeted these remarks led Muhammad to demand Malcolm make no more public statements. This move—combined with disturbing revelations that Muhammad had fathered several illegitimate children—led Malcolm to make a formal break with the NOI. On March 8, 1964, he announced both his resignation and his founding of a new Islamic movement—the Muslim Mosque, Inc.—which would commit itself to political activism and cooperation with civil rights leaders.

He also took time off to make the pilgrimage to Mecca, a requirement of all able-bodied Muslims, and to several newly independent African countries. Both had a profound impact on the last remaining year of his life. Claiming to have witnessed the

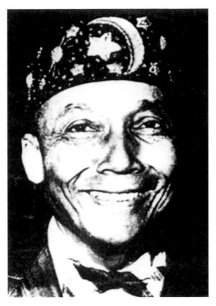

Elijah Muhammad (Library of Congress)

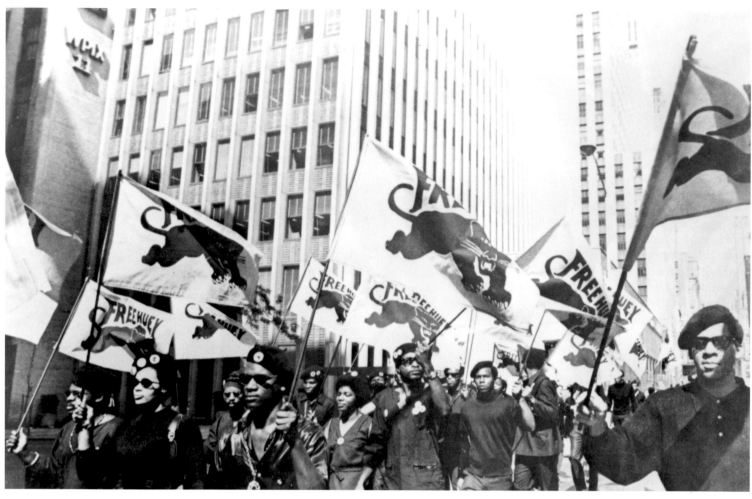

Black Panthers march in New York. (New York Public Library)

THE BLACK PANTHER PARTY PROGRAM

1. We want freedom. We want power to determine the destiny of our Black Community.
2. We want full employment for our people.
3. We want an end to the robbery by the white man of our Black Community.
4. We want decent housing, fit for shelter of human beings.
5. We want education for our people that exposes the true nature of this decadent American society. We want education that teaches us our true history and our role in the present-day society.
6. We want all Black men to be exempt from military service.
7. We want an immediate end to POLICE BRUTALITY and MURDER of Black people.
8. We want freedom for all Black men held in federal, state, county, and city prisons and jails.
9. We want all Black people when brought to trial to be tried in a court by a jury of their peer group or people from their Black communities, as defined by the Constitution of the United States.
10. We want land, bread, housing, education, clothing, justice, and peace. And as our major political objective, a United Nations–supervised plebiscite to be held throughout the Black colony in which only Black colonial subjects will be allowed to participate, for the purpose of determining the will of Black people as to their national destiny.

march to protest the shooting of James Meredith, the University of Mississippi's first African-American student. While marching, Carmichael and other SNCC members took up the call-and-response chant: "What do you want? . . . Black Power!" The media immediately focused on this

militancy as a new angle on the civil rights movement story.

In fact, the Black Power ideology had been coalescing for over a year and involved much more than a political strategy of economic self-reliance and independent black politics. In the tradition of many

1960s-era protest movements, it offered a cultural agenda as well. For many African Americans like poet Amiri Baraka (LeRoi Jones), it meant a pride in black America's African heritage. While black intellectuals called for a resurrection of afrocentric literature and arts—as well as demanding the establishment of black studies courses and departments at universities—ordinary African Americans expressed the Black Power message by sporting the Afro hairstyle, characterized by a round shape and tight curls, and wearing dashikis, a billowing and colorful West African upper garment. As the popular expression of the day had it, "black is beautiful."

Yet many veteran civil rights leaders had mixed feelings about Black Power. King, for one, appreciated its emphasis on African pride but feared it would commit the "error of building a distrust for all white people" and stray from the path of peaceful protest. Indeed, a leading proponent of Black Power and a future SNCC chairman—H. Rap Brown—was quoted as saying "violence is as American as apple pie." But perhaps the most serious challenge to King's integrationist, nonviolent philosophy came not from his SNCC allies in the South, but from a radical new organization arising on the West Coast—the Black Panther Party (BPP).

The Panthers were founded in Oakland, California, in October 1966 by activists Huey Newton and Bobby Seale who became, respectively, the new organization's defense minister and chairman. As with most urban African Americans in the North and West, the party itself had southern roots. For example, its logo, a crouched black panther, was adopted from the Lowndes County (Alabama) Freedom Organization, a black political party founded by Carmichael and SNCC in March 1966. The symbolic connection aside, the BPP had a very different agenda, advocating black self-defense—particularly against the police—and the restructuring of U.S. society along more economically, politically, and socially egalitarian lines.

In a ten-point program, Newton and Seale demanded—among other things—"full employment;" "decent housing, fit for shelter of human beings;" exemption for blacks from military service; an end to police brutality; and "the power to determine the destiny of our Black Community." More than just a political party and a self-defense organization, the Panthers also organized food, health, and education programs in the many black communities where they operated. While not admitting

A CHRONOLOGY OF THE BLACK PANTHER PARTY

1966

October 15	Huey Newton and Bobby Seale organize the Black Panther Party and draft a ten-point program for economic, social, and political development in black neighborhoods.

1967

January 1	The party opens its first official headquarters in Oakland, California.
February 21	Betty Shabazz, widow of Malcolm X, visits San Francisco; the Panthers provide armed security; they are stopped by police but cite their right to bear arms and are not arrested.
April 27	The first issue of the Panther paper, *Black Community News Service*, is published.
May 21	The Panthers show up in the state capital of Sacramento bearing arms; they read a statement, proclaiming their right to bear arms.
June 29	Stokely Carmichael, former chair of Student Non-Violent Coordinating Committee (SNCC), joins the Panthers.
October 28	Returning home from a party, Newton is stopped by police; a shootout erupts and an officer is killed; Newton is wounded and charged with murder, though no gun is found on his person.

1968

February 17–18	Two "Free Huey" rallies, featuring H. Rap Brown and Stokely Carmichael, lead to an alliance between SNCC and the Panthers.
March 4	FBI issues secret memos to fight Panthers.
April 4	Martin Luther King Jr. is assassinated; the Panthers plead for calm in Oakland.
April 6	Panther Bobby Hutton is killed by police; Eldridge Cleaver is wounded.
September 28	Newton is sentenced to 2–15 years; Oakland police officers, outraged by the light sentence, shoot out the windows of the Panther headquarters.

1969

January 17	Two leaders of the Southern California Panther Party are slain; police conduct raids on several Panther offices in Los Angeles.
April 2	Twenty-one Panthers in New York City are arrested for conspiring to bomb local department stores; all are acquitted in May 1971.
July 18–21	The Panthers sponsor an anti-fascist conference in Oakland, attended by SNCC, the Young Lords, and the Students for a Democratic Society.
December 4	Panther leaders Fred Hampton and Mark Clarke are slain by Chicago police.

1970

January 9	The Boston Panther Party starts free clothing program.
July 25	The Panther Party office in Omaha is bombed.
August 5	Newton is released from jail.
August 7	Hoping to liberate his brother George, Panther Jonathan Jackson assaults a courtroom in Marin County, California; Jackson, two other Panthers and the judge are killed in the shootout.
September 3	Panther leader Cleaver opens an international section in Algeria.
November 7	Southern California Panthers start a free breakfast program; they provide 1,700 meals a week to the poor.

1971

January 16	The Panthers establish a legal assistance program in Toledo, Ohio; the Chicago Panthers start a door-to-door health program.
August 21	Panther leader George Jackson is slain in San Quentin prison; guards say he was trying to escape.
February	Newton publishes *To Die For The People*.

1974

Summer	Newton goes into exile in Cuba to avoid trial for murder of a female barroom customer.
Fall	After converting to born-again Christianity, Cleaver returns to the United States from Algeria.

whites into their ranks, the Panthers nevertheless established alliances with the antiwar movement, including the Students for a Democratic Society, and the radical Weather Underground. Just eight months after its founding, the Panthers drew national media attention when they showed up in Sacramento, California's capital, to protest a law that banned the bearing of arms in public. Wearing their uniform black berets and black leather jackets, the Panthers also came armed with rifles. Seale and 30 others—including future Panther leader Eldridge Cleaver—were arrested.

From that moment, the BPP became the most controversial and widely feared organization in the country, at least as far as the white community and the government was concerned. This became especially the case after nationwide urban rioting in the summers of 1967 and 1968 which some police officials blamed on the Panthers. Calling the group the "greatest threat to internal security in the country," FBI director J. Edgar Hoover launched COINTELPRO (short for counterintelligence program). Using infiltrators, informers, and agents provocateurs (spies who would break the law on purpose to implicate the party), the FBI worked with local police to destroy the organization. By 1970, more than 25 Panthers had been killed by police, including activists Fred Hampton and Mark Clark, killed in a raid on the party's Chicago headquarters in December 1969. Hundreds of others were prosecuted for a range of crimes and either sent to prison or forced into exile, such as Cleaver who escaped to Cuba. No less than 21 BPP members in New York were charged with conspiring to kill police officers, blow up buildings, and even assassinate President Nixon. Many of the charges were based on the testimony of informants with criminal records, and a number of convictions—including Newton's for the shooting of an Oakland police officer—were overthrown on appeal.

Ironically, the BPP's commitment to a broad multiracial alliance of revolutionary groups served to isolate it. Its connections to SNCC—formed during the "Free Huey (Newton)" crusade of 1968—came apart over the former's decision to end all ties to white activists, as did the BPP's relationship with US, a Southern California-based black nationalist organization founded by Maulana Karenga, the creator of the Kwaanza holiday. Indeed, this latter break turned fatal when the two groups fought a gun battle on the UCLA campus that left two Panthers dead. With much of its leadership imprisoned, in exile, or dead, the BPP shifted to a less confrontational style and agenda in the early 1970s, epitomized by Seale's near-successful run for the mayoralty of Oakland. Despite such efforts, the Panthers continued to decline, a victim of isolation from other black political organizations and unprecedented government repression.

VIOLENCE IN THE STREETS

The growth of organizations like the Nation of Islam and the Black Panthers reflected, in part, a massive demographic shift within black America. Continuing a trend that began in the early part of the century, rural African Americans from the South had been making their way to urban centers in the North and West in ever greater numbers. By 1960, more than 40 percent of all U.S. blacks lived outside the South and nearly 75 percent resided in cities. There they faced very different challenges. While legal segregation was rare, de facto separation of the races was a way of life. Most urban blacks lived in ghettoes, poor inner-city neighborhoods that had once been inhabited by immigrants from southern and eastern Europe. But as these white ethnics prospered, they often moved to the suburbs, a trend accelerated by a phenomenon known as "white flight." As blacks moved in, whites—fearful of racial mixing and convinced that the presence of African Americans drove down housing values—left. Left in the wake of "white flight" were predominantly black and Hispanic communities, where jobs, social services, and local businesses grew increasingly scarce.

Adding to the plight were poorly thought through urban renewal programs. Interstate highways were extended through minority communities, dividing and destroying neighborhoods, while hundreds of thousands of poor blacks and Hispanics were crowded into soulless high-rise towers. The results were predictable: high unemployment, alcoholism, drug abuse, crime, and a growing sense of frustration. The response of local police forces did not help. Largely made up of white ethnics, police departments around the country—sometimes openly racist and nearly always insensitive to blacks whose personal history made them suspicious of authority—used increasingly intrusive and even brutal tactics to maintain order in the ghettoes. The frustration of inner-city black communities was boiling over by the mid-1960s.

The first great explosion of African-American anger erupted in Los Angeles. On

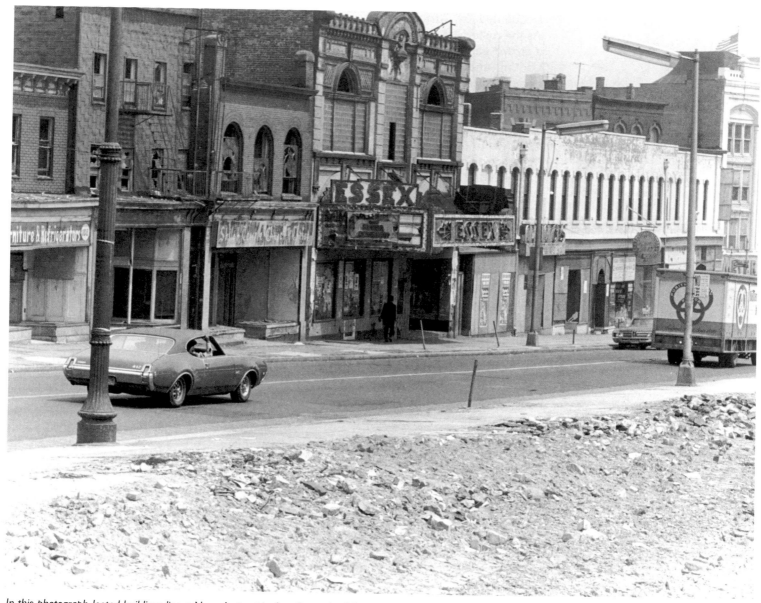

In this photograph, looted buildings line a Newark street in the aftermath of the July 1967 rioting. It took more than 4,000 police and National Guard troops to end the violence. (Library of Congress)

the evening of August 11, 1965—in the midst of a summer heat wave—police officers arrested an African-American man for drunk-driving in the predominantly black community of Watts. As crowds taunted the police, one of the officers—according to eyewitnesses—began hitting people with his baton. As word of the alleged police brutality spread through the community, rioting erupted. By the next day, hundreds of area stores and businesses had been looted and torched. With some 35,000 people taking part in the unrest, it took more than 16,000 police, sheriff's deputies, and National Guardsmen to return the area to calm. But the five days of violence had left 34 dead, 1,000 wounded, and some $200 million in property damage. The "long, hot summers" of the 1960s had begun. In 1966, rioting tore through Cleveland and Nashville. The following year, full-scale

rioting broke out in Washington, Atlanta, Chicago, Newark, and, most violent of all, Detroit.

Motown—as it was called—offered the quintessential urban black experience. Drawn to the high-wage automobile industry, rural southern blacks had been flocking to Detroit since the second decade of the 20th century. During World War II, major riots broke out between whites and blacks over scarce housing, leaving 34 dead. Despite the violence, and with the auto industry booming, blacks continued to move there through the 1950s and 1960s, as whites slowly made their way out. While employment remained low, a lack of black businesses, poor housing, dilapidated schools, and, most troubling, ongoing police abuses fueled a sense of frustration and anger. On the morning of July 23, police raided a bar in a black neighborhood

SELECTED AFRICAN-AMERICAN ATHLETES, 1968–PRESENT

Muhammad Ali (1942–) Born Cassius Clay, Ali changed his name in 1964 after joining the Nation of Islam. During his career, which ended in 1981, he won three heavyweight championships and one lightweight championship, winning approximately 100 fights and losing only five. In 1967, he was stripped of his first heavyweight title and banned from boxing for three years for his refusal to be drafted for military service in the Vietnam War. He regained the title in 1974, and then again in 1978.

Julius "Dr. J" Erving (1950–) Erving began his basketball career as an undergraduate free agent with the Virginia Squires if the ABA. When the ABA and the NBA merged in 1976, Erving joined the Philadelphia 76ers, with whom he remained for the next 11 years. Selected as an All-Star in every year of his NBA career, Erving also won the Most Valuable Player in 1981 and led the 76ers to the NBA championship in 1983.

Ken Griffey Jr. (1969–) The son of outfielder Ken Griffey Sr., "Junior" Griffey was born to play baseball. When Griffey began playing professionally at age 19, he and his father became the first father-son team to play in the majors at the same time. Since then, he has reached the 400 hundred home run mark faster than any other player in history, hitting 50 home runs in two different seasons and leading the American League in home runs for three consecutive seasons.

Michael "Air" Jordan (1963–) Drafted by the Chicago Bulls after his junior year of college, Jordan earned the nickname "Air" for his ability to leap great distances. In 1991, 1992, and 1993, he led the Bulls to championships. Prior to the 1993–1994 season, his father was mysteriously murdered, and Jordan retired. During his time away from basketball, Jordan joined a minor league baseball team, but he returned to basketball prior to the 1995 playoffs. He led his team to the world championship two more times before retiring for good in 1998.

Jackie Joyner-Kersee (1962–) On a basketball scholarship to the University of California, Los Angeles, Jackie Joyner met her future husband and track coach Bob Kersee. He convinced her to concentrate on track and field rather than basketball and helped her train for the heptathlon—an event that combines seven different running, jumping, and throwing events. Joyner-Kersee excelled in the event. At the 1988 Olympics, she won a gold in the heplathlon and a gold in the long jump. She won another for the heplathlon in 1992.

Walter "Sweetness" Payton (1954–1999) After having set a Jackson State University record for points scored, Payton joined the NFL's Chicago Bears. In his second season he made the Pro Bowl team for the first of nine times. In 1977, the running back ran a career-high 1,852 yards, helping the Bears reach the playoffs for the first time in 14 years. In 1993, Payton was inducted into the Football Hall of Fame.

Venus and Serena Williams (1980– and 1981–) The youngest two of five daughters, Venus and Serena Williams were raised by their father to excel at tennis. Venus, who turned pro in 1994 at age 14, won her first singles title in 1998 at the IGA Tennis Classic. She also won the women's singles championship at Wimbleton in 2000. In 1999, Serena won her first WTA career title in the Open Gaz de France. Her winning streak was stopped by her older sister at the Lipton Championships. Later that year, Serena became the first black woman to win the Grand Slam singles title at the U.S. Open since Althea Gibson in 1958.

Eldrick "Tiger" Woods (1975–) On June 15, 1997, 21-year-old Tiger Woods reached number one on the Official World Gold Ranking in his 42nd week as a professional golfer, becoming the youngest top-ranked golfer ever. Since his debut, Woods has won more than 20 championships, including the 1999 PGA Championship. Woods, whose father is of mixed African-American and white heritage and whose mother is Thai, is both the first African American and the first Asian American to win a major golf championship.

white allies—northern Republicans in the 19th century and white liberals in the 20th—either lose interest or grow hostile to new demands for racial justice and equality. This political falling-out was followed by judicial retreat. In both centuries, the courts whittled away at pro–civil rights decisions and laws rendered or passed during the high-water periods of Reconstruction and the civil rights movement. In the first period, the Supreme Court authored a series of rulings that undermined federal enforcement of civil rights legislation and legitimated segregation. In the second, the courts stepped in to invalidate affirmative action laws designed to assure minorities equal representation in many of the nation's institutions.

Still, too much can be made of these parallels. The white reaction of the late 19th century was far more virulent than that of the 20th century, with openly racist attitudes and thinking entering the mainstream. Similarly, the judicial backlash against civil rights legislation was far more extreme in the earlier period, placing southern blacks in a legal position just short of slavery. Yet, while the extent of the 19th century white backlash against African American civil rights gains was far greater than its 20th century counterpart, the pattern of black assertiveness and white reaction remains the same. And whereas this process was confined to the South in the 19th century, it became—because of the Great Migration of blacks northward throughout much of the century—a national phenomenon in the 20th century.

SCHOOL DESEGREGATION AND BUSING

The year 1968 was critical in the history of U.S. racial relations. In April, Martin Luther King Jr. was assassinated in Memphis, leading to rioting in inner cities across the country. Two months later, Senator Robert Kennedy—a Democratic aspirant for the presidency and one of the few national figures who appealed to both white and black voters—was gunned down in Los Angeles. Meanwhile, gaining ground in the Democratic presidential contest was Alabama governor George Wallace, whose calls for "law and order" were seen by many as a barely concealed appeal to white voters angry at black protesters and inner-city rioting. While Wallace would not win the nomination—he eventually ran as a third party candidate, winning 46 electoral votes in the South—his impact on U.S. politics and

Cities with Failed Desegregation Policies Since 1994

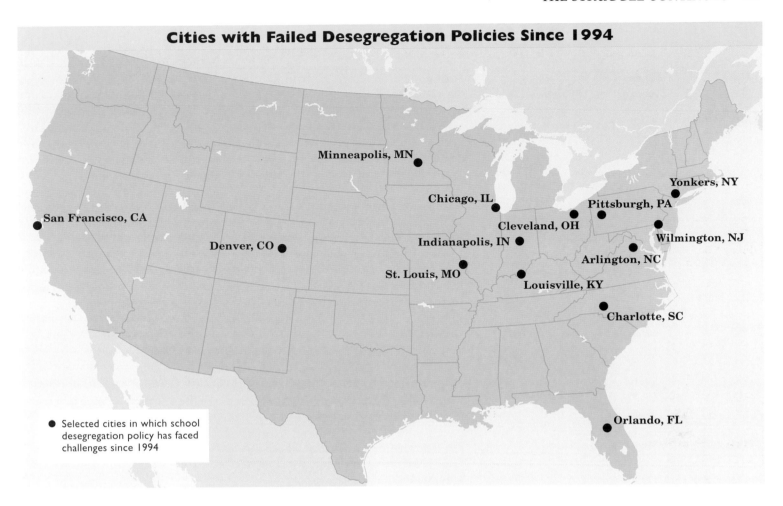

Minneapolis, MN

San Francisco, CA

Chicago, IL

Yonkers, NY

Pittsburgh, PA

Cleveland, OH

Denver, CO

Indianapolis, IN

Wilmington, NJ

Arlington, NC

St. Louis, MO

Louisville, KY

Charlotte, SC

Orlando, FL

● Selected cities in which school desegregation policy has faced challenges since 1994

racial relations would be felt for decades to come.

With the Democrats in disarray over the Vietnam War—and their national convention in Chicago marred by protests and police brutality—Republican candidate Richard Nixon won the presidency in a close contest against Vice President Hubert Humphrey. Adopting a page from Wallace's political playbook, Nixon made "law and order" the centerpiece of his campaign. That is to say, realizing that he had little chance of winning black and white liberal voters, Nixon openly appealed to those he called "the silent majority"—white suburban voters frustrated and angry with the perceived breakdown in social order caused, in their minds, by hippies, antiwar protesters, and, above all else, black radical activists.

Thus, upon coming to office, Nixon had no intention and no interest in furthering the civil rights agenda advanced by his Democratic predecessors Kennedy and Johnson. Indeed, internal memos within the Nixon White House that were leaked to the press in 1971 used the term "benign neglect" to describe the administration's approach to African Americans generally and to civil rights specifically. All manner of social programs launched by Johnson to fight poverty had their budgets cut, including the Office of Economic Opportunity, which included numerous programs designed to train and find employment for poor and minority citizens. Nixon also moved to put more conservative judges on the nation's courts, though his first attempt to do so on the Supreme Court backfired, after it was revealed that one of his appointees—G. Harrold Carswell—had worked to prevent the integration of a golf course in his native Florida. In the end, though, Nixon's strategy of moving the court to the right succeeded, as his appointees who won Senate confirmation— particularly Chief Justice William Rehnquist—were generally hostile to expanding the federal government's role in the enforcement of civil rights. This policy would continue and even accelerate during the Republican administrations of Ronald Reagan and George Bush during the 1980s and early 1990s.

Still, most of the federal courts remained in the hands of pro–civil rights liberals throughout the Nixon administration. And many of them, frustrated at the glacial pace in which local and state governments moved to implement the *Brown v. Board of Education* decision of 1954—which called for integration of the nation's schools

MAJOR DESEGREGATION COURT CASES

Year	Case	Ruling
1954	Brown v. Board of Education	Outlawed school segregation and declared racially separate schools inherently unequal.
1971	Swann v. Charlotte-Board of Education	Held that federal courts could order that students be bused from one neighborhood to another in order to desegregate Mecklenburg schools. At the same time, the court ruled that once legally enforced segregation was eliminated, single-race schools were permitted, as long as agencies of the government had not deliberately resegregated them.
1974	Millikin v. Bradley	After a federal court order that the city of Detroit would have to integrate its schools with 53 surrounding districts, the Supreme Court overturned the decision, stating that suburban districts could not be ordered to desegregate a city's schools unless those suburbs had been involved in illegally segregating them in the first place. In his dissenting opinion, Justice Thurgood Marshall, who had successfully argued the Brown v. Board of Education case 30 years earlier, argued that the ruling would permit "our great metropolitan areas to be divided up each into two cities—one black and one white."
1990	Board of Education of Oklahoma	Declared that a school district may be declared "unitary," or be freed from court supervision, once it eliminates the vestiges of segregation "to the extent practicable."
1992	Freeman v. Pitts	Stated that districts can be declared "unitary" "before full compliance has been achieved in every area of school operations." To do so, a district must demonstrate a "good faith commitment" to the desegregation program.
1995	Missouri v. Jenkins	The Supreme Court overturned the decision of a federal judge who ordered the Kansas City, Missouri School District to create a system of "magnet schools" to attract white suburban students to inner-city schools.

This cartoon pokes fun at President Richard Nixon, who occupied the White House when the implementation of federally mandated busing began. (Library of Congress)

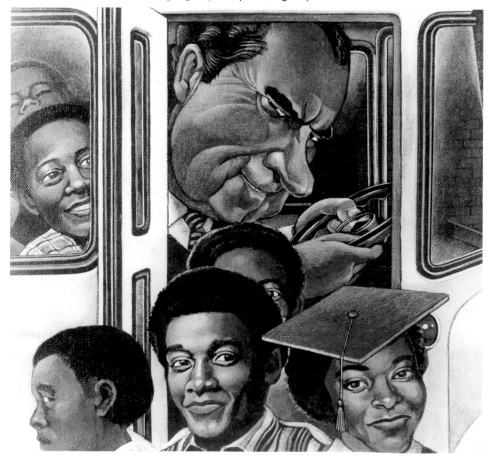

"with all deliberate speed"—began to force the issue. In 1971, a federal judge ordered the Charlotte-Mecklenburg school district in North Carolina to desegregate by means of busing children. Specifically, children in predominantly or all-black schools would be bused out of their neighborhood to predominantly or all-white schools in other parts of the district. A more radical plan to force the amalgamation of predominantly black inner-city and predominantly white suburban school districts into one unit, however, was rejected by the court in 1974. Yet, in the same decision, the court upheld the decision that largely racially segregated systems would have to use busing to integrate their schools.

Ironically, one such system was Boston. The center of antislave and abolitionist sentiment before the Civil War and one of the most liberal cities in America, Boston was also among the most segregated. Beginning in the 1960s, black civil rights activists and white liberal politicians had moved to integrate the city's schools and, in 1965, the state legislature passed the Massachusetts Racial Imbalance Act to do just that. Then, in the late 1960s and early 1970s, integrationist forces developed plans for "ma-

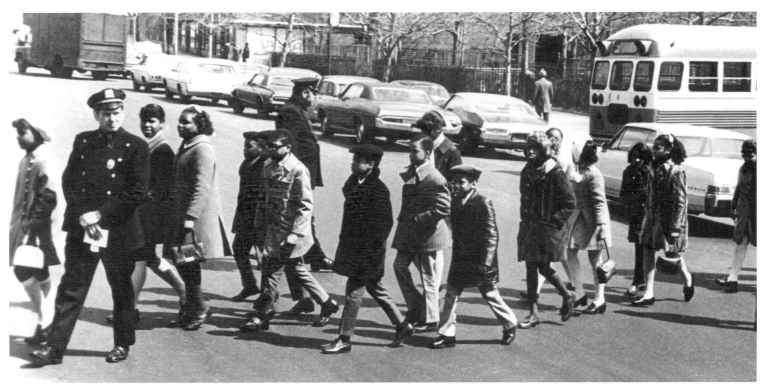

Policemen escort African-American children off a bus into school. (Library of Congress)

schools, or schools with extra funding and services designed to draw white and black students from around the city. There was even talk of forming a single district, uniting white suburban and black urban schools. But all of these plans met with resistance, particularly from the residents of the Irish-American working class enclave of South Boston. This led judge Arthur Garrity to issue a court order in 1974 calling for the busing of students from the predominantly black neighborhood of Roxbury to South Boston High School. Meant to be a stopgap measure only, the order was bitterly resented by South Boston residents.

In scenes reminiscent of the integration of Little Rock, Arkansas's Central High School in 1957, the first black students arriving at South Boston High in the fall of 1974 were greeted by white residents shouting racial obscenities and throwing rotten eggs and stones. Only the presence of hundreds of armed riot police prevented white mobs from attacking the students and destroying the buses. (In Michigan around the same time, school buses used for integration were indeed torched by whites.) And although integration occurred, tensions within the school remained high for years. As Phyllis Ellison, one of the first African-American students at South Boston High, recalled, "the black students sat on one side of the classes. The white students sat on the other side. . . . In the lunchrooms, the black students sat on one side. The

white students sat on the other. . . . If the blacks wanted to play basketball, the whites wanted to play volleyball. So we never played together."

Ellison's observations reflected the fundamental obstacle to integration in post–civil rights era America. Although it had taken a great struggle and cost the lives of dozens of courageous black (and white) citizens, ending legal segregation and discrimination had been relatively straightforward. The Constitution was clear on the matter and the power of the federal government eventually trumped the resistance of racist state governments in the South. Yet it was one thing to force the integration of schools where students were kept apart by law; it was quite another to integrate schools and neighborhoods where the segregation resulted from settlement patterns that had emerged over generations. In the end, court-ordered busing solved little in Boston as many white parents pulled their children out of the public schools and put them into largely segregated religious or private ones, thereby reinforcing segregation in the city's schools. By the late 1970s, an increasingly conservative federal court system backed away from busing as a means to integrate the nation's schools.

Ultimately, the failure of busing pointed out the profound difficulties of trying to undo centuries of racism and discrimination through laws and court orders. That is to say, once overtly racist legislation was eliminated from the nation's law books, the far more difficult—but just as morally and constitutionally necessary—task of redressing historically racist patterns in housing, college enrollment, business, and employment began. The method employed by the government to do this was called "affirmative action." And while it did not meet with the same violent resistance as busing did, it nevertheless was resented by many whites.

AFFIRMATIVE ACTION

Throughout the 1950s and early 1960s, civil rights leaders had emphasized that their goal for America was a "color-blind" society or, to put it in King's mellifluous phrasing, a nation where a person would "not be judged by the color of their skin but by the content of their character." Nonetheless, by the mid-1960s, King and other civil rights leaders had come to recognize that centuries of racist attitudes and discriminatory practices could not be undone as easily as all that. As President Johnson noted in 1965, "[y]ou do not take a person who for years has been hobbled by chains and . . . bring him up to the starting line of a race and then say, 'you are free to compete with all the others' and still justly believe that you have been completely fair." As early as 1969, the Nixon administration—as noted above, not normally associated with civil rights initiatives—instituted the first federal affirmative action program. Called the Philadelphia Plan, it required companies seeking federal contracts to develop goals for hiring minority employees.

In 1971, the Supreme Court—still largely controlled by liberal appointees—ruled that Title VII of the 1964 Civil Rights Act—

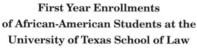

KEY MOMENTS IN THE AFFIRMATIVE ACTION DEBATE

First Year Enrollments of African-American Students at the University of Texas School of Law

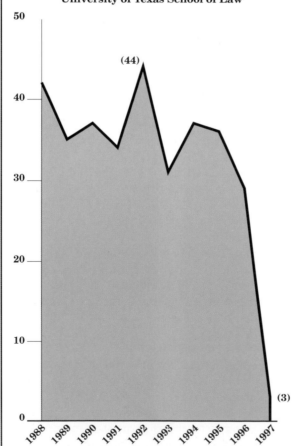

Source: University of Texas

The *Bakke* Decision (1978)
In 1978, Allan Bakke, a white applicant to the University of California at Davis School of Medicine, was denied admission due to the school's affirmative action policy. He sued on the grounds that his outstanding academic record was ignored through "reverse discrimination." In 1978, the U.S. Supreme Court ruled in his favor, and ordered the university to enroll him.

Proposition 209 (1996)
This California law prohibits the state, local governments, districts, public universities, colleges, and schools from giving preferential treatment to any individual or group in public employment, public education, or public contracting on the basis of race, sex, color, ethnicity, or national origin.

The *Hopwood* Ruling (1996)
In 1996, the *Hopwood* decision in Texas forbade the University of Texas from accounting for race in law school admissions. As more graduate programs enforced race-neutral admissions policies, the number of African-American enrollees declined. In top MBA programs, for example, the number of African Americans admitted decreased significantly.

which banned discrimination in employment and public accommodations—also outlawed "practices that are fair in [legal] form but discriminatory in operation." By that, the court meant to say that even if a predominantly white business had violated no laws in its hiring practices, it was still guilty of discrimination. Thus, to avoid discrimination lawsuits, it should move to redress past hiring practices by specifically seeking out minority applicants. (In 1972, Title VII was expanded to educational institutions as well.)

For all its noble intentions, however, affirmative action was problematic in practice. It raised legal and constitutional problems because programs or policies that favored African Americans at the expense of the civil rights of whites would obviously not pass constitutional muster. The courts, then, were forced to deal with a thicket of complicated legal cases arising from affirmative action. During the 1970s, the Supreme Court generally ruled in favor of affirmative action, but only on very narrow grounds. In the 1979 *United Steelworkers v. Weber* decision, the court permitted the continuation of a training program that gave preference to minorities so long as it remained short-term and voluntary. But when it came to quotas—that is, the establishment of numerical goals for minority hiring or enrollment—the Court was less agreeable. In the landmark 1978 *Regents of the University of California v. Bakke* ruling, the Court decided that a quota system that set aside a certain number of places for minority students at the University of California at Davis School of Medicine was unconstitutional in principle and discriminatory in practice against white applicants.

As conservative justices appointed by Republican presidents Ronald Reagan and George Bush began to take their place on the Court's bench during the 1980s and early 1990s, rulings further limited the use of affirmative action. In the 1986 *Wygant v. Jackson Board of Education* ruling, the court threw out a plan that protected minority teachers from layoffs at the expense of white teachers with more seniority. Then, in 1989, the Court ruled that local governments do not have the power to create "set-asides" or quotas for minority businesses competing for government contracts. Six years later, the justices ruled that even federally mandated "set-asides"—in this case, a law that required 10 percent of contracts on federal highway construction projects be reserved for businesses owned by "socially and economically disadvantaged individuals"—were unconstitutional unless they were "narrowly tailored" to serve a "compelling government interest."

At the same time, proponents of affirmative action faced more than just legal and constitutional hurdles, they faced major political opposition as well. While many white Americans could appreciate the principles upon which affirmative action was based—and even support such programs in the abstract—affirmative action in practice rubbed many people the wrong way. First, it seemed to be a case of "two wrongs not making a right." If redressing past discrimination against blacks meant present discrimination against whites then the vast majority of the latter were against it. This became obvious during the 1980s, when downsizing corporations and governments laid off millions of workers. As it became more difficult to find employment, many whites came to believe—despite the evidence of much higher unemployment rates among minority workers—that they faced discrimination because of affirmative action. Second, affirmative action seemed to violate the fundamental principle of equality before the law upon which the country had been founded. Although, as many African Americans pointed out, whites—who had not only tolerated racial inequality for centuries but positively benefited from it—only raised a ruckus about equal rights when they felt their own rights were being threatened.

Still, the bottom line remained; white people dominated the political process and no politician who wanted to remain in office could effectively ignore their rising sense of resentment. In 1995, the regents of the University of California voted to end all affirmative action programs in hiring and employment. A year later, a federal district court ordered the same thing in Texas. Defenders of affirmative action found little solace in the fact that their direst warnings—that black and Hispanic enrollment in the two state university systems would drop precipitously—proved correct. Meanwhile, California governor Pete Wilson—who had pressured the regents in their decision—worked to expand his crusade against affirmative action statewide. In 1996, he helped sponsor Proposition 209, a successful ballot referendum that put a stop to all state-sponsored affirmative action programs. While many supporters of affirmative action feared that 209 represented the start of a nationwide move to outlaw all affirmative action legislation, it turned out not to be the case. Legislatures in at least 13 states have voted down or refused to act on bills modeled after the California initiative,

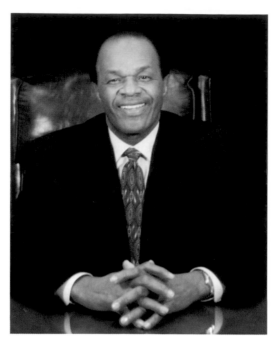

Marion Barry (Courtesy of Marion Barry)

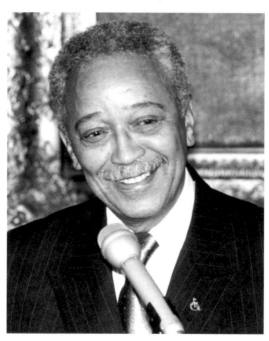

David Dinkins (Mayor's Office, New York City)

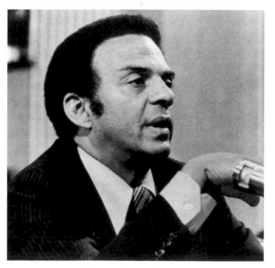

Andrew Young (Library of Congress)

try. Unlike Detroit, Bradley's Los Angeles was a predominantly white city at the time, and the largest minority was Mexican American. Although racial tensions were still sore eight years after the Watts riots, Los Angeles was nevertheless emerging as a global city, a trend Bradley encouraged through his conservative, pro-business policies. Ironically, though he saw himself as a builder and a racial healer, Bradley presided over the most violent and destructive episode in the city's history, the massive rioting that followed the acquittal of the four policemen accused of beating black motorist Rodney King. Within one year of the riots, Bradley decided not to run for a sixth term.

Another long-serving black mayor—Marion Barry of Washington, D.C.—had a far more checkered career than his counterparts in Detroit and Los Angeles. Born poor in the rural South, Barry was the first in his family to attend college. He went on to become an activist in various civil rights organizations, helping to stage nonviolent sit-ins at segregated Nashville restaurants. In 1965, Barry moved to the nation's capital where he organized youth groups and a political coalition trying to win more home rule for the district, which was largely run by Congress at the time. In 1974, he was elected to the city council and then ran successfully for mayor in 1978, winning with support from many of the city's liberal whites. Barry proved a poor administrator, however, and the city soon found itself in a fiscal crisis. Yet it was his personal shortcomings that led to his downfall. Caught in 1990 smoking crack cocaine by FBI cameras, Barry was removed from office and sent to jail. Upon his release from jail six months later, he began a remarkable political comeback, winning a seat on the city council and then the mayoralty once again in 1994, claiming he had experienced religious redemption. But a fiscal crisis led Congress to reassert its control over the city's budget and the voters to turn him out of office.

Although serving far shorter terms in office, mayors Harold Washington of Chicago and David Dinkins of New York City also had significant impacts on their cities. A longtime Democratic politician, Washington had served in the Illinois legislature and the U.S. Congress before winning the mayor's office in 1983. Left-leaning and blunt-spoken, Washington moved to diversify city government and city contracting, bringing many women and minorities into his governing coalition. A successful politician with a bright future ahead of him, Washington's life was cut short in 1987 by a fatal heart attack. Two years later, in 1989, David Dinkins, a longtime Democratic politician in city government, was elected mayor of the nation's largest city. A civil and dignified man, Dinkins was accused of indecision and mismanagement, especially when he failed to respond to racial flare-ups. He was defeated after just one term in 1993. Since the early 1990s, and the defeats or retirements of Young, Bradley, Barry, and Dinkins, most of the nation's cities are once again governed by white mayors.

AFRICAN AMERICANS IN CONGRESS

Throughout most of its history, the U.S. Congress has been largely a white man's institution. Of the 11,000 representatives who have served there since 1789, less than 100 have been African American. Their history has often been divided into two waves. The first occurred during and after Reconstruction, when some 22 African Americans —20 congressmen and two senators—represented southern states with large black constituencies. With the fall of Reconstruction in 1877, black membership in Congress dwindled to a handful, with the last representative—George White of North Carolina—leaving office in 1901.

From that year until 1929, when Republican Oscar DePriest of Chicago was elected, not a single African American served in the U.S. Congress, even though black Americans represented some 12 percent of the total U.S. population.

The second wave of African-American congressional representation was different from the first in a number of ways. First, unlike the sudden burst of black political power during Reconstruction, it took several decades for black representatives to establish themselves as a significant presence in Congress. Second, Oscar DePriest notwithstanding, most black congressional representatives in the 20th century have been members of the Democratic party. And third, African-American congressional representation began in northern urban rather southern rural districts.

Of the black representatives from the pre–civil rights era, the most important and best-known was Adam Clayton Powell Jr. of New York City's Harlem. The son of a well-known local minister, Powell served on the New York City Council before assuming his seat in Congress in 1945. An outspoken critic of racial segregation and discrimination, he became the first African American to chair a major congressional

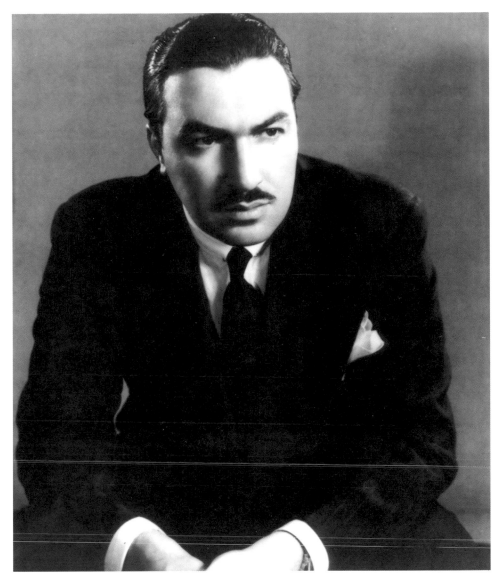

Adam Clayton Powell Jr. (Library of Congress)

committee—Education and Labor—and was instrumental in the passage of the Medicaid, Medicare, and Head Start programs of the 1960s. Plagued by scandal in the 1960s, however, Powell was denied his seat by an act of Congress. Although he won it back on an appeal to the Supreme Court, he was badly weakened politically and lost his seat to Charles Rangel in 1970, who remains Harlem's congressional representative to this day.

In the wake of the civil rights movement—and the Voting Rights Act of 1965—black representation in Congress increased significantly, and spread to southern states. (At the same time, the only two black senators of the modern era—Republican Edward Brooke of Massachusetts and Democrat Carol Mosely-Braun of Illinois—have come from urban-dominated northern states.) In addition, the early 1970s witnessed the arrival of the first black women representatives in Congress. First came

that figure had more than doubled to over 16 percent by 1999. For the population as a whole, the figures were 17 and 23 percent respectively. In other words, black college graduation rates were less than half that of the population as a whole in 1980, but more than 60 percent by 1999. While more than 15 percent of blacks in their 30s had college degrees in 1996, less than 10 percent of those over the age of 60 had them. Meanwhile, roughly 23 percent of blacks aged 18 to 21 were attending college in the late 1990s, while the figure for the population as a whole was 25 percent, a statistically negligible difference. Of course, income—as well as race—is an important factor in determining who goes to college. While 40 percent of black families with college-aged children

(i.e., 18 to 24) had one or more of them in college in 1995, that rate fell to about 20 percent for families with incomes under $20,000 annually, and rose to about 65 percent for families with incomes of $75,000 a year or higher.

HEALTH

While the gap between white and black educational levels has been and is likely to keep closing, the same cannot be said of the health gap, particularly for African-American males. For example, a black male child born in the year 2000 is likely to live just 64.6 years, while a white male can expect to make it to his 73rd birthday, nearly a decade

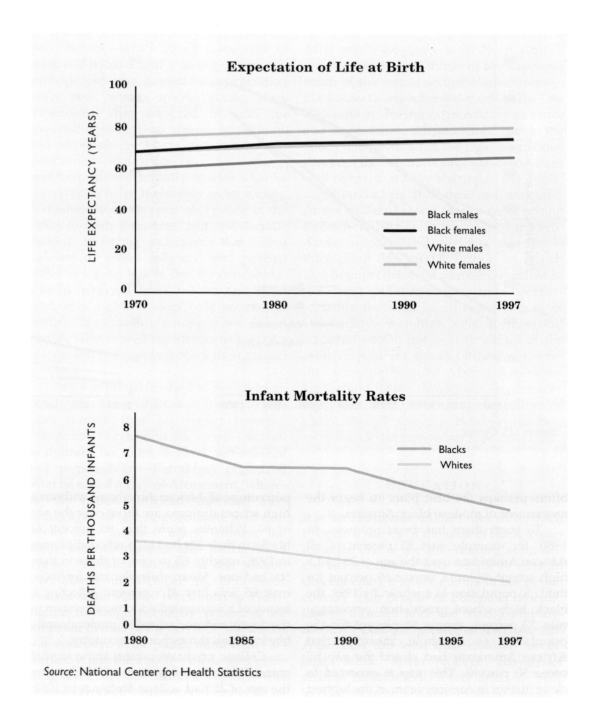

Source: National Center for Health Statistics

TOP TEN CAUSES OF DEATH:
African-American Versus General Population

African Americans	Death Rate	All Americans	Death Rate
1. Heart disease	227.4	1. Heart disease	268.2
2. Cancer	177.7	2. Cancer	200.3
3. Cerebrovascular diseases	53.0	3. Cerebrovascular diseases	58.6
4. Accidents	37.2	4. Pulmonary diseases	41.7
5. Diabetes	33.0	5. Accidents	36.2
6. Homicide	24.5	6. Pneumonia and influenza	34.0
7. Pneumonia and influenza	24.2	7. Diabetes	24.0
8. Pulmonary diseases	20.9	8. Suicide	11.3
9. HIV/AIDS	14.1	9. Kidney diseases	9.7
10. Conditions occurring at birth	14.1	10. Liver diseases	9.3

Note: Death rate equals number of deaths per 100,000
Source: U.S. Census

longer. Nor is there much of a gain in age projections for those who do make it to retirement age. White males aged 65 in the year 2000 can expect to live more than 15 percent longer than black males of the same age. For females, the racial health gap is not as large. Black females born in the year 2000 can expect to live to be nearly 75, while white females will live to be about 80, a gap of just half a decade. Similarly, black women aged 65 in the year 2000 can expect to live nearly another 18 years, while white women will live another 19.5 years on average, a gap of less than two years.

In other health-related areas, the racial gap is far wider. For example, infant mortality rates among blacks in the mid-1990s were 16.5 per 100,000 live births versus just 6.8 for whites, or about 140 percent higher. Similarly, low birthweight babies were more prevalent in the black population (13.2 percent) than among whites (6.1 percent). In virtually every other category, the picture remains the same. Blacks had a rate of death from cardiovascular disease 50 percent higher than whites and they were nearly twice as likely to die from stroke. The most glaring discrepancies, however, emerged in the areas of violence and sexually transmitted disease. At 40.9 per 100,000 persons, blacks were nearly seven times more likely to be murdered than whites.

And with a rate of 93.3 per 100,000, African Americans were more than six times more likely to be suffering from AIDS. The only health index where blacks outscored whites was suicide. While whites killed themselves at a rate of 12 personsper 100,000, blacks did so at a rate of just 7.2 per 100,000 in the mid-1990s.

Suicides aside, there are a number of factors that help explain why African-American health indices lag so badly behind those of whites. First, and perhaps, foremost is poverty. While less than 17 percent of white children under the age of 18 lived in poverty, the rate for black youths was nearly 44 percent in the mid-1990s. Poverty and lack of steady employment also means less health care coverage. White children were 50 percent less likely to be without health insurance than black children in 1996. While for all age groups the gap was smaller between white and black, it was still significant, with blacks nearly 40 percent more likely not to have health insurance coverage of some kind. Not surprisingly, this translates into lower physician contact rates. Blacks were 21.5 percent less likely to have visited a doctor's office over the course of a year than whites. At the same time, they were more than 60 percent more likely to have physician contact in a hospital, indicating that blacks tended to

SELECTED AFRICAN-AMERICAN ACTORS

Angela Bassett (1958–) Bassett decided that she wanted to be an actress after seeing a production of *Of Mice and Men* when she was a junior in high school. After receiving her master's degree in drama from Yale, Bassett moved to New York City where she was cast in Broadway plays *Ma Rainey's Black Bottom* and *Joe Turner's Come and Gone*. Eager to enter into film and television, Bassett weathered many rejections and poor roles until she was cast in John Singleton's film *Boyz N the Hood* (1991). Her success in film has continued with roles in *Malcolm X* opposite Denzel Washington and her Academy Award–nominated role as singer Tina Turner in *What's Love Got to Do With It* (1993).

Halle Berry (1968–) As a little girl, Berry was teased for having a white mother and a black father. The need to be accepted became very important to her. While in high school, she was class president, a cheerleader, and prom queen. Following high school, she joined the beauty pageant circle after winning the Miss Ohio title. Berry soon turned her attention from modeling to television. After a few fluffy situation comedy parts, Berry was cast as a crack addict in Spike Lee's *Jungle Fever* (1991). While not a huge role, it gave Berry her first opportunity to prove her acting talent. She has since starred in many television and film roles, including *Boomerang* (1993) with Eddie Murphy and *Bulworth* (1999) with Warren Beatty. In 1999, she fulfilled a personal dream by starring in and producing the HBO biopic, *Introducing Dorothy Dandridge*.

Bill Cosby (1937–) Raised in a poor Philadelphia neighborhood, Cosby loved to practice comedy routines on his mother. He especially liked to incorporate tales of his friends Fat Albert, Old Weird Harold, and Dumb Donald among others into his skits. Cosby pursued a career in comedy and in 1963 landed a guest spot on *The Tonight Show*. It was the peak of the civil rights era, but unlike other black comedians, Cosby chose not to base his jokes on race, but on experiences common to everyone. Since his television debut, Cosby has found no limit to his success with endeavors ranging from the 1960s espionage thriller *I Spy* to the 1970s children's cartoon *Fat Albert and the Cosby Kids*, to the 1980s hit sitcom *The Cosby Show*.

Morgan Freeman (1937–) Freeman's long and impressive career has included theater, television, and film. Beginning in the mid-1960s, Freeman performed in plays ranging from musicals to contemporary dramas to Shakespeare. He branched into television during the 1970s on the PBS show *The Electric Company*. In 1987, he received his first Academy Award nomination for his work in *Street Smart*. Two years later he received a second nomination for *Driving Miss Daisy*. Freeman has been one of the few African-American actors to be awarded roles that were not specifically written for a black actor.

Whoopi Goldberg (1949–) A native of New York City, Goldberg was born Caryn Johnson. In 1974, she moved to California and created the stage name Whoopi Goldberg. There she helped found the San Diego Repertory Theatre and in 1983 went on tour with her solo piece, *The Spook Show*. The show, in which she played four characters, later moved to Broadway and helped Goldberg advance into film. Her debut in *The Color Purple*, based on Alice Walker's novel, won her an Academy Award nomi-

nation. Since then she has not only won an Academy Award (for her role in the film *Ghost*), but has also hosted the Academy Awards three times and successfully relaunched the television game show *Hollywood Squares*.

Eddie Murphy (1961–) At the age of 15, Murphy began is stand-up comedy career. The New York native joined the cast of *Saturday Night Live* in 1980, at age 19 and made his parodies of Mr. Rogers, a grown-up Buckwheat, and Bill Cosby famous. The success of his feature film debut *48 Hrs* (1982) established him as one of the leading black actors in Hollywood. Murphy's success continued for the next decade, before beginning to stall in the early 1990s as his bad boy-image started to grow old. Murphy proved successfully revived his career in 1996, however, with the hit comedy *The Nutty Professor*.

Richard Pryor (1940–) Born in Peoria, Illinois, Pryor grew up in a brothel run by his grandparents and dropped out of school by the ninth grade. One of his teachers noticed Pryor's comedic talent and encouraged him to pursue a career in show business. Initially, Pryor, like Bill Cosby, told jokes that avoided politics and race, but as he began to develop his own style, his humor grew more political, sometimes raunchy or bitter, and ceaselessly honest. Pryor covered topics ranging from race to women and drugs to social commentary. He soon brought his comedic talents to film, starring in almost 40 movies throughout his career, including *Lady Sings the Blues* (1971) and *Bustin' Loose* (1981). Pryor's live routines, for which he is best known, are also captured in *Richard Pryor Live On Stage* (1979) and *Richard Pryor Live On Sunset Strip* (1982). In 1998, Pryor received the American Humor Mark Twain Prize, but was too weak to perform at the ceremony due to an ongoing battle with multiple sclerosis.

Will "Fresh Prince" Smith (1968–) As a grade schools student, Smith earned the nickname "Prince" from his teachers for his smooth-talking

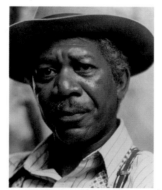

Morgan Freeman (Movie Star News)

charm. Smith used the name "Fresh Prince" when he started a career as a rapper. After achieving musical success, he turned his attention to acting in 1990 and landed the lead in the television sitcom *Fresh Prince of Bel Air*, which remained on the air for six seasons. Smith proved to be an actor with a wide range of ability, from his serious role on *Six Degrees of Separation* (1993) to a comedic one in *Men in Black* (1997) to action hero in *Enemy of the State* (1999) and *Wild Wild West* (1999). He has also returned to his music career, releasing award-winning albums *Big Willie Style* (1997) and *Willenium* (1999).

Denzel Washington (1954–) Although Washington earned his first break in show business on the television series *St. Elsewhere*, his diverse, but powerful film roles are what made him one of Hollywood's great leading men. He won an Academy Award for Best Supporting Actor for his portrayal of a runaway slave in *Glory* (1989). During the 1990s, Washington starred in three Spike Lee movies, most notably as the lead in *Malcolm X* (1992), for which he received a Best Actor nomination. Roles in films including *Crimson Tide* (1995) proved his success as an action star. At the 2000 Academy Awards, he earned his second Best Actor nomination for his work in *The Hurricane*, a film based on the life of boxer Rubin Carter.

become the world's largest African American–owned publishing company. Other divisions of the company include Fashion Fair Cosmetics, Supreme Beauty Products, Ebony Fashion Fair, and Johnson Publishing Company Books Division. John H. Johnson is publisher, chairperson, and CEO. His wife, Eunice W. Johnson, is secretary and treasurer of Johnson Publishing Company and producer-director of the Ebony Fashion Fair—one of the world's largest traveling fashion shows.

Another prominent black media executive is Robert L. Johnson. In 1979 Johnson and his wife Sheila Crump Johnson founded Black Entertainment Television (BET), the nation's first and only black-owned cable network.

In finance, Reginald Lewis established himself as a major player. In 1983 he set up the TLC Group as a vehicle to buy and sell companies. In one of his first major transactions, he bought a failing company for $22.5 million and after four years restored it to such financial success that it sold for $90 million. In 1987 Lewis pulled one of the greatest leveraged buyouts of an international company when he bought Beatrice, a French food company, for $985 million.

Among other leaders in the financial services industry are E. Stanley O'Neal, the executive vice president and cohead of Merrill Lynch's corporate and institutional client group, and Franklin D. Raines, who became the the first African American to head a major Fortune 500 corporation when selected chairman and CEO of Fannie Mae.

Not all senior African-American executives are men, of course. In the mid-1990s, Sylvia Rhone became chairperson and CEO of Elektra Entertainment Group, a major record label that represents a multiracial roster of musicians.

Probably the most famous example of a successful black business woman is Oprah Winfrey. Winfrey received her first media job while she was still in high school working at a local radio station. As she prepared to graduate from college, she accepted a position as a TV newscaster in Tennessee. Work as a cohost on the TV show *People Are Talking* soon followed and in 1985 a station in Chicago offered Winfrey her own talk show. Soon *The Oprah Winfrey Show* began national syndication and Winfrey soon became a household name. One of the highest paid television personalities in America, Winfrey has acted in films and also runs her own production company, Harpo (Oprah spelled backward), as well as Oprah's Book Club, through which she spotlights favorite books on a segment of her television show.

The club's influence has enormous influence on the American book publishing industry, with a spot on her program generally guaranteeing best-seller status for any book. In 1998 Winfrey became the first African-American woman to purchase a film or television studio, and in 2000, she launched a new women's magazine, known simply as *O*.

MULTICULTURAL BLACK AMERICA

While Americans of African descent have been making modest gains in education and income since the beginning of the 1980s, a far more profound cultural shift has been occurring in the African-American community over the past few decades. As with the country as a whole, black America is becoming more multicultural, with thousands of new immigrants of African descent arriving from the Caribbean and Africa itself. There are a number of factors that explain why more people of African descent are moving to America. Rising educational levels around the Caribbean, for example, have created a culture of rising expectations, a trend that the prevalence of U.S. culture in the region contributes to. In places like Jamaica, this has produced something of a brain drain, as professionals seek out better paying positions in the United States. But jobs alone are only part of the picture. Increasingly, many young people from the Caribbean—and particularly from the English-speaking islands—are flocking to U.S. institutions of higher learning. Other factors promoting immigration from the Caribbean and Africa include more convenient and faster transport than in the past, lower ticket prices, and the communications revolution. E-mail and falling long-distance phone rates make it easier and cheaper for people to keep in touch with families and friends back home.

There are also push factors behind the rising tide of immigration from the Caribbean and Africa. War and civil unrest, for example, have prompted thousands of Haitians to take their chances of making it to the United States in unseaworthy craft. Although probably fewer than 85,000 people immigrated to the United States from Haiti during the 1960s and 1970s—a time of relative stability in that impoverished land—roughly double that number came to this country between 1981 and 1997, a period of civil war, death squad killings, and a U.S. military intervention. Still, poverty and

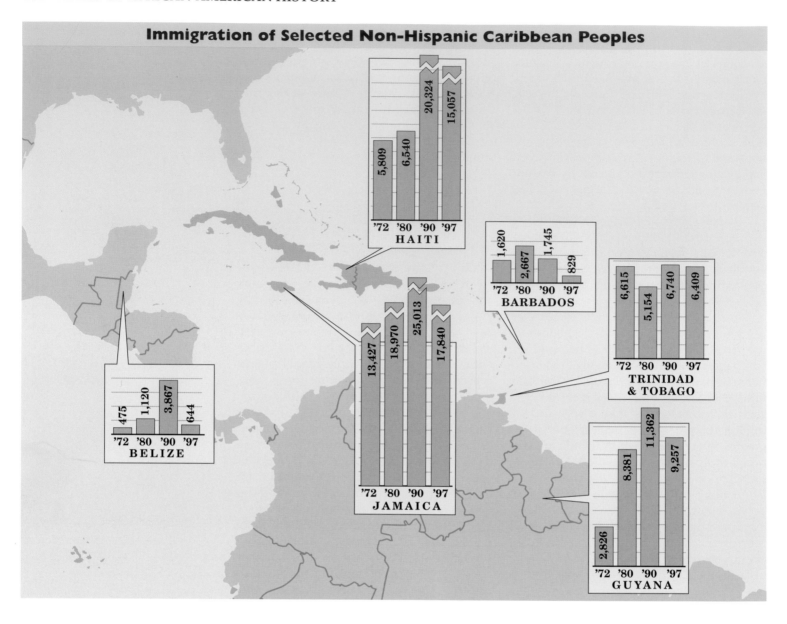

Immigration of Selected Non-Hispanic Caribbean Peoples

HAITI — '72: 5,809 | '80: 6,540 | '90: 20,324 | '97: 15,057

BARBADOS — '72: 1,620 | '80: 2,667 | '90: 1,745 | '97: 829

TRINIDAD & TOBAGO — '72: 6,615 | '80: 5,154 | '90: 6,740 | '97: 6,409

BELIZE — '72: 475 | '80: 1,120 | '90: 3,867 | '97: 644

JAMAICA — '72: 13,427 | '80: 18,970 | '90: 25,013 | '97: 17,840

GUYANA — '72: 2,826 | '80: 8,381 | '90: 11,362 | '97: 9,257

---

a lack of job opportunities continue to be the main causes of the immigration of African and Caribbean peoples. Africa, in particular, has suffered from economic stagnation since the late 1970s, when immigration from that continent began to increase.

Meanwhile, the impact of Caribbean and African immigrants on U.S. culture—and particularly on African-American culture—has been profound. The various kinds of music produced in these regions, for example, has influenced popular music in the United States. Moreover, immigrants of African descent have added yet another piece to the ethno-cultural mosaic of many U.S. cities. The annual West Indian Day parade in Brooklyn, for instance—held every Labor Day weekend—routinely draws more than half a million participants and viewers. Immigrants from the Caribbean and Africa have made their impact felt, economically, too. Like other newcomers, they have brought with them an ambition to succeed, a willingness to

take financial risks, a commitment to hard work, and an entrepreneurial drive that has helped revive many urban neighborhoods.

Of course, the arrival of so many newcomers of African descent has not been without its problems. Many face the same racism that African Americans have experienced for centuries. As mentioned earlier, two well-publicized police killings in New York in 1999 and 2000—of West African immigrant Amadou Diallo and Haitian-American Patrick Dorismond respectively—highlighted the difficulties facing these African and Caribbean newcomers. Moreover, the arrival of so many non-Americans of African descent has created tensions with the black American community itself. As was the case a century ago between white native-born Americans and new arrivals from Eastern and Southern Europe, blacks born in the United States often feel that immigrants of African descent are willing to work harder and for less, driving down wages and taking jobs. Meanwhile, many

Immigration from Africa by Country

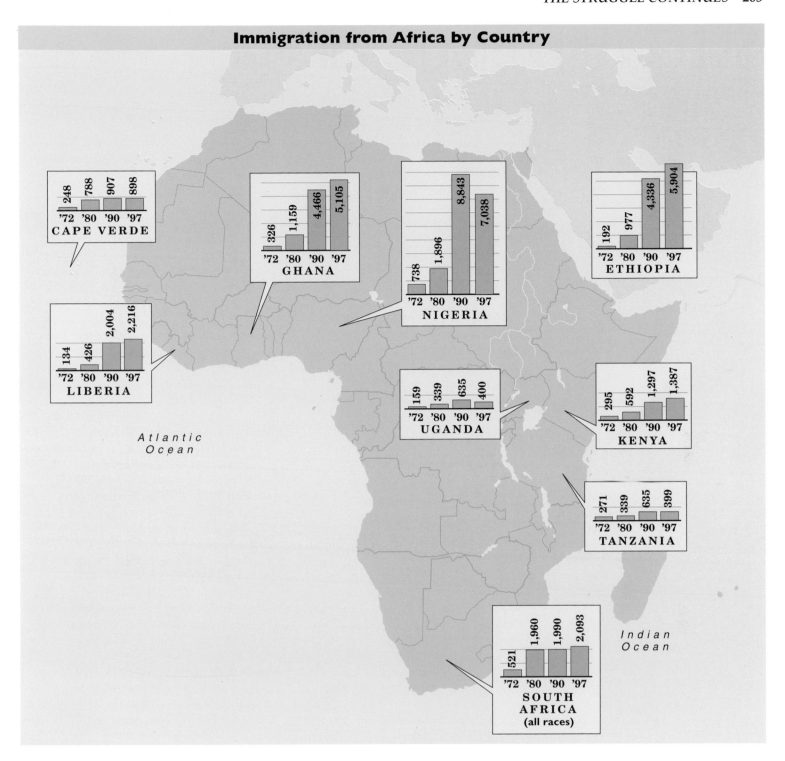

CAPE VERDE
'72	'80	'90	'97
248	788	907	898

GHANA
'72	'80	'90	'97
326	1,159	4,466	5,105

NIGERIA
'72	'80	'90	'97
738	1,896	8,843	7,038

ETHIOPIA
'72	'80	'90	'97
192	977	4,336	5,904

LIBERIA
'72	'80	'90	'97
134	426	2,004	2,216

UGANDA
'72	'80	'90	'97
159	339	635	400

KENYA
'72	'80	'90	'97
295	592	1,297	1,387

TANZANIA
'72	'80	'90	'97
271	339	635	399

SOUTH AFRICA (all races)
'72	'80	'90	'97
521	1,960	1,990	2,093

Atlantic Ocean

Indian Ocean

new arrivals feel unwelcomed and looked down upon by black Americans as ignorant and uncultured.

Still, for all the tensions between black Americans and black immigrants—and for all difficulties facing the latter as they adjust to life in their new home—one thing is clear. The arrival of immigrants of African descent—along with their more numerous Hispanic and Asian compatriots—is changing the nature of race relations in the United States. As the new categories listed in recent censuses indicate, the United States can no longer look at itself as a country neatly divided between white and black.

What is more, African Americans are feeling the impact of the new immigration more directly than whites. Concentrated in the same large metropolitan areas that attract the majority of immigrants, African Americans find themselves interacting with a diversity of new peoples. At the same time, immigrants—and particularly their more Americanized offspring—are being influenced by urban black culture. Whatever this cross-fertilization of world and African-American people produces, it will shape all of American culture—and through America's media empire, world culture—for much of the 21st century.

SELECTED BIBLIOGRAPHY

Andrews, William L., and Henry Lewis Gates Jr. *Slave Narratives*. New York: Library of America, 2000.

Appiah, Kwame Anthony, and Henry Lewis Gates Jr. *Africana: The Encyclopedia of the African and African American Experience*. New York: Basic Civitas Books, 1999.

Asante, Molefi K., and Mark T. Mattson. *Historical and Cultural Atlas of African Americans*. New York: Macmillan, 1991.

Bancroft, Frederic. *Slave-Trading in the Old South*, 2nd ed. Columbia: University of South Carolina Press, 1996.

Barbeau, Arthur, and Florette Henri. *The Unknown Soldiers: African American Troops in World War I*. New York: Da Capo, 1996.

Barraclough, Geoffrey, ed. *The Times Atlas of World History*, 4th ed. Maplewood, NJ: Hammond, 1993.

Beckles, Hilary, and Verene Shepherd, eds. *Caribbean Slave Society and Economy: A Student Reader*. New York: New Press, 1991.

Bennett, Lerone Jr. *Pioneers in Protest*. Chicago: Johnson Publishing, 1968.

Berlin, Ira. *Many Thousands Gone: The First Two Centuries of Slavery in North America*. Cambridge, MA: Harvard University Press, 2000.

Bernstein, Iver. *The New York City Draft Riots*. Oxford: Oxford University Press, 1990.

Black Church Burning Update. "List of Burned Black Churches." Available online. URL: http://stepshow.com/churches/list.html. Updated on June 26, 1996.

Blanchard, Peter. *Slavery and Abolition in Early Republican Peru*. Wilmington, DE: Scholarly Press, Inc., 1992.

Boley, George. *Liberia: The Rise and Fall of the First Republic*. New York: St. Martin's Press, 1983.

Bolster, Jeffrey W. *Black Jacks*. Cambridge, MA: Harvard University Press, 1997.

Boyd, Herb, and Lance Tooks. *Black Panthers for Beginners*. New York: Writers and Readings Publishing, 1995.

Branch, Taylor. *Parting the Waters*. New York: Simon & Schuster, 1989.

———. *Pillar of Fire*. New York: Simon & Schuster, 1998.

Braxton, Greg, and Jim Newton. "Looting and Fires Ravage L.A." *The Los Angeles Times*. Available online. URL: http://www.latimes.com/HOME/REPORTS/RIOTS/0501lede.htm. Posted on May 1, 1992.

Charters, Samuel. *The Roots of the Blues: An African Search*. New York: Da Capo, 1991.

Chase, Judith Wragg. *Afro-American Art & Craft*. New York: Van Nostrand Reinhold, 1971.

Clark, Dick, and Larry Lester. *The Negro Leagues Book*. Cooperstown, NY: Society for American Baseball Research, 1994.

Conrad, Earl. *Harriet Tubman*. Washington, DC: Associated Publishers, Inc., 1990.

Conrad, Robert Edgar. *World of Sorrow: The African Slave Trade to Brazil*. Baton Rouge: Louisiana State University Press, 1986.

Courlander, Harold. *A Treasury of Afro-American Folklore*, 2nd ed. New York: Marlowe & Company, 1996.

Covington, James. *The Seminoles of Florida*. Gainesville: University Press of Florida, 1993.

Cowan, Tom, and Jack Maguire. *Timelines of African-American History: Five Hundred Years of Black Achievement*. New York: Berkley Publishing Group, 1994.

Dance, Daryl Cumber. *Shuckin' and Jivin'*. Bloomington: Indiana University Press, 1987.

de Queiros Mattoso, Katia. *To Be a Slave in Brazil*. New Brunswick, NJ: Rutgers University Press, 1987.

DiBacco, Thomas V. *The History of the United States*. Boston: Houghton Mifflin, 1991.

DjeDje, Jacqueline Cogdell. *Turn Up the Volume!: A Celebration of African Music*. Berkeley: University of California Press, 1998.

Diop, Cheidh Anta. *Civilization or Barbarism: An Authentic Anthropology*. Brooklyn, NY: Lawrence Books, 1991.

Dodd, Donald. *Historical Statistics of the United States*. Westport, CT: Greenwood Publishing Group, Inc., 1993.

DuBois, W. E. B. *Souls of Black Folk*. New York: NAL/Dutton, 1995.

Duncan, Russell. *Entrepreneur for Equality: Governor Rufus Bollack, Commerce and Race in Post-Civil War Georgia*. Athens: University of Georgia Press, 1994.

Ellis, Joseph. *American Sphinx: The Character of Thomas Jefferson*. New York: Vintage Books, 1998.

Etis, David. *Economic Growth and the Ending of the Transatlantic Slave Trade*. Oxford: Oxford University Press, 1989.

Farmer, James. *Lay Bare the Heart*. Fort Worth: Texas Christian University Press, 1998.

Finkelman, Paul. *Slavery in the Courtroom: An Annotated Bibliography of American Cases*. Washington: Lawbook Exchange, 1996.

Fogel, Robert, and Stanley Engerman. *Time on the Cross: The Economics of American Negro Slavery*. New York: W.W. Norton & Co., 1994.

Foner, Eric. *Reconstruction*. New York: HarperCollins, 1989.

Foner, Eric, and John Garraty. *The Reader's Companion to American History*. Boston: Houghton Mifflin, 1991.

Freeman-Grenville, G. S. P. *The New Atlas of African History*. New York: Simon & Schuster, 1991.

Gale Research. *The African American Almanac*, 8th ed. Detroit: Gale Research, 1998.

Garrow, David. *Bearing the Cross: Martin Luther King, Jr. and the Southern Christian Leadership Conference, 1955–1968*. New York: William Morrow, 1999.

Gilje, Paul. *Rioting in America*. Bloomington: Indiana University Press, 1996.

Glatthaar, Joseph. *Forged in Battle*. New York: NAL/Dutton, 1990.

Grofman, Bernard, and Davidson, Chandler, eds. *Controversies in Minority Voting: The Voting Rights Act in Perspective*. Washington, DC: Brookings Institution, 1991.

Hamilton, Kenneth M. *Black Towns and Profit: Promotion and Development in the Trans-Appalachian West, 1877–1915*. Urbana: University of Illinois Press, 1991.

Handy, W. C., ed. *Blues: An Anthology*. New York: Da Capo, 1990.

Harlan, Louis, ed. *The Booker T. Washington Papers*. Vol. 14. Urbana: University of Illinois Press, 1989.

Harley, Sharon. *The Timetables of African-American History*. New York: Simon & Schuster, 1995.

Henretta, James, et al. *America's History*. New York: Worth Publishers, 1993.

Herold, Erich. *African Art*. London: Hamlyn, 1990.

Holloway, Joseph, and Winifred Vass. *The African Heritage of American English*. Bloomington: Indiana University Press, 1993.

Horton, Carrel, et al. *Statistical Record of Black America*. Detroit: Gale Research Inc., 1990.

Hughes, Langston, and Arna Bontemps. *The Book of Negro Folklore*. New York: Dodd, Mead and Company, 1958.

Hughes, Langston, et al. *A Pictorial History of African Americans*, 6th ed. New York: Crown Publishing, 1995.

Jackson, Kenneth, ed. *Encyclopedia of the City of New York*. New Haven, CT: Yale University Press, 1995.

Jacobs, Donald K., ed. *Courage and Conscience: Black and White Abolitionists in Boston*. Bloomington: Indiana University Press, 1993.

James, Cyril L. R. *The Black Jacobins*, 2nd ed. New York: Vintage Books, 1989.

Jones, Evan. *American Food: The Gastronomic Story*. New York: Vintage Books, 1981.

Jones, Howard. *Mutiny on the Amistad*. Oxford: Oxford University Press, 1997.

Karasch, Mary. *Slave Life in Rio de Janeiro, 1808–1850*. Princeton, NJ: Princeton University Press, 1987.

Katz, William Loren. *The Black West: A Documentary and Pictorial History of the African-American Role in the Westward Expansion of United States*. New York: Simon & Schuster, 1996.

Kelley, Robin D. G., and Earl Lewis. *To Make Ourselves Anew: A History of African Americans*. New York: Oxford University Press, 2000.

Kibbe, Jennifer, and David Hauck. *Leaving South Africa*. Washington, DC: South Africa Review Service, 1988.

Klein, Herbert. *African Slavery in Latin America and the Caribbean*. Oxford: Oxford University Press, 1988.

Kunen, James S. "The End of Integration." *Time Magazine*. Vol. 147, No. 18. Available online. URL: http://cgi.pathfinder.com/time/magazine/archive/1996/dom/960429/cover.html. Posted April 29, 1996.

Lane, Roger, and John J. Turner, eds. *Riot, Rout and Tumult: Readings in American Social and Political Violence*. Westport, CT: Greenwood Publishing Group, 1978.

Lewis, David Levering. *W. E. B. DuBois: Biography of a Race, 1868–1919*. New York: Henry Holt and Co., 1994.

———. *W. E. B. DuBois: The Fight for Equality and the American Century, 1919–1963*. New York: Henry Holt and Co., 2000.

Lieberman, Paul, and Dean E. Murphy. "Bush Ordering Troops to L.A." *The Los Angeles Times*. Available online. URL: http://www.latimes.com/HOME/REPORTS/RIOTS/0502lede.htm. Posted on May 2, 1992.

Lindsey, Howard O. *A History of Black America*. Greenwich, CT: Brompton Books, 1994.

Lloyd, Christopher. *The Navy and the Slave Trade: The Suppression of the African Slave Trade in the Nineteenth Century*. New York: Longman, 1968.

Lowe, Richard. *Republicans and Reconstruction in Virginia*. Charlottesville: University of Virginia Press, 1991.

Lowery, Charles. *Encyclopedia of African-American Civil Rights from Emancipation to the Present*. New York: Greenwood Press, 1992.

Luker, Ralph. *Historical Dictionary of the Civil Rights Movement*. Lanham, MD: Scarecrow Press, 1996.

Margo, Robert. *Race and Schooling in the South, 1880–1950: An Economic History*. Chicago: University of Chicago Press, 1991.

McKay, John, et al. *A History of World Societies*, 5th ed. Boston: Houghton Mifflin, 1999.

McLester, Cedric. *Kwanzaa: Everything You Always Wanted to Know but Didn't Know Where to Ask*. New York: Gumbs & Thomas, 1994.

McPherson, James. *Ordeal by Fire: The Civil War and Reconstruction*. New York: Knopf, 1992.

MelaNet. "What is Kwanzaa?" MelaNet's Kwanzaa Information Center. Available online. URL: http://www.melanet.com/kwanzaa.whatis.html#TOC. Downloaded October 28, 1998.

Mills, Thornton J., III. "Challenge and Response in the Montgomery Bus Boycott of 1955–1956." *Alabama Review* 33, no. 3 (July 1980): 153–235.

Moore, Jesse Thomas, Jr. *A Search for Equality: The National Urban League, 1910–1961*. University Park: Pennsylvania State University Press, 1989.

Morgan, Edmund. *American Slavery, American Freedom: The Ordeal of Colonia Virginia*. New York: W.W. Norton & Co., 1995.

Morgan, Philip D. *Slave Counterpoint: Black Culture in the Eighteenth Century Chesapeake*. Charlotte: University of North Carolina Press, 1998.

Morris, Robert. *Reading, 'Riting, and Reconstruction: The Education of Freedmen in the South, 1861–1870*. Chicago: University of Chicago Press, 1976.

Mosley, Walter. *Workin' on the Chain Gang: Shaking off the Dead Hand of History*. New York: Ballantine Books, 2000.

Moskos, Charles. "Success Story: Blacks in the Military." *The Atlantic Monthly* 257 (May 1986): 64–72.

Oates, Stephen B. *To Purge This Land with Blood: A Biography of John Brown*. Amherst: University of Massachusetts Press, 1990.

Packenham, Thomas. *The Scramble for Africa, 1876–1912*. New York: Random House, 1991.

Painter, Nell. *Exodusters: Black Migration to Kansas after Reconstruction*. New York: W.W. Norton & Co., 1992.

Payne, Charles M. *I've Got the Light of Freedom: The Organizing Tradition and the Mississippi Freedom Struggle*. Berkeley: University of California Press, 1999.

Perry, Regenia A. *Free Within Ourselves: African-American Artists in the Collection of the National Museum of Art*. Washington, DC; San Francisco, CA: National Museum of American Art in association with Pomegranate Art Books, Inc., 1992.

Pescatello, Ann, ed. *The African in Latin America*. New York: Knopf, 1975.

Peterson, Carrell, et al. *Statistical Record of Black America*. Detroit: Gale Research, 1990.

Peterson, Robert W. *Only the Ball Was White*. Oxford: Oxford University Press, 1992.

Peirce, Paul Skeels. *The Freedmen's Bureau: A Chapter in the History of Reconstruction*. Irvine, CA: Reprint Services Corporation, 1991.

Ploski, Harry, and James Williams, eds. *Encyclopedia of African-American History*. New York: Macmillan Library Reference USA, 1996.

Porter, Kenneth. *The Black Seminoles*. Gainesville: University Press of Florida, 1996.

Powledge, Fred. *Free at Last: The Civil Rights Movement and the People Who Made It*. Boston: Little, Brown, 1991.

Price, Richard, ed. *Maroon Societies,* 3rd ed. Baltimore: Johns Hopkins University Press, 1996.

Ransom, Roger, and Richard Sutch. *One Kind of Freedom: The Economic Consequences of Emancipation,* 2nd ed. New York: Cambridge University Press, 2000.

Ripley, C. Peter, ed. *Witness for Freedom*. Chapel Hill: University of North Carolina Press, 1993.

Roberts, Bari-Ellen, and Jack E. White. *Roberts vs. Texaco: A True Story of Race and Corporate America*. New York: Avon Books, 1996.

Roebuck, Julian, and Murty Komander. *Historically Black Colleges and Universities*. Westport, CT: Greenwood Publishing Group, 1993.

Rogosin, Donn. *Invisible Men*. New York: Kodansha America, Inc., 1995.

Rummel, Jack. *Malcom X: Militant Black Leader*. New York: Chelsea House Publishers, 1991.

Salzman, Jack, et al. *Encyclopedia of African-American History.* New York: Macmillan Library Reference USA, 1996.

Saxon, Lyle, et al., eds. *Gumbo Ya-Ya*. Gretna, LA: Pelican Publishing Company, 1988.

Savitt, Todd. *Medicine and Slavery: The Diseases and Health Care of Blacks in Antebellum Virginia*. Urbana: University of Illinois Press, 1978.

Schubert, Frank. *Black Valor: Buffalo Soldiers and the Medal of Honor, 1870–1898*. Wilmington, DE: Scholarly Resources, 1997.

Serrano, Richard A., and Tracy Wilkinson. "All 4 King Beating Acquitted." *The Los Angeles Times*. Available online. URL: http://www.latimes.com/ HOME/NEWS/REPORTS/RIOTS/0403lede.htm. Posted on April 30, 1992.

Shick, Tom. *Behold the Promised Land: A History of Afro-American Settler Society in Nineteenth Century Liberia*. Baltimore: Johns Hopkins University Press, 1980.

Shrader, Charles Reginald, ed. *Reference Guide to United States Military History, 1919–1945*. New York: Facts On File, Inc., 1994.

Slenes, R. *Demography and Economics of Brazilian Slavery, 1850–1888*. Ann Arbor, MI: University Microfilms, 1976.

Smith, Carter, ed. *The Black Experience*. New York: Facts On File, Inc., 1990.

Stanley, Jerry Hurry. *Freedom: African Americans in Gold Rush California*. New York: Crown Publishing, 2000.

Stewart, Jeffrey. *1001 Things Everyone Should Know About African American History*. New York: Doubleday and Co., 1998.

Tadman, Michael. *Speculators and Slaves: Masters, Traders, and Slaves in the Old South*. Madison: University of Wisconsin Press, 1996.

Thomas, Velma Maia. *Freedom's Children: The Passage from Emancipation to the Great Migration*. New York: Crown Publishing, 2000.

Thompson, Richard. *A History of South Africa*. New Haven, CT: Yale University Press, 1995.

Trelease, Allen. *White Terror: The Ku Klux Klan Conspiracy and Southern Reconstruction*. Baton Rouge: Louisiana State University Press, 1995.

U.S. Census Bureau. *Annual Yearbook*. Washington, DC: Government Printing Office, 1996.

———. *Historical Statistics of the United States*. Washington, DC: Government Printing Office, 1975.

———. *Reports*. Washington, DC: Government Printing Office, 1900, 1910, 1920, 1930, 1940, 1950.

———. *Statistical Abstracts*. Washington, DC: Government Printing Office, 1974, 1976.

U.S. Department of Agriculture. "1890 Land Grant Institutions and Tuskegee University." Available online. URL: http: www.reeusda.gov/1890/1890inst.htm. Downloaded October 29, 1998.

U.S. Department of Education. *Historically Black Colleges and Universities*. Washington, DC: Government Printing Office, 1996.

Washington Post. "Denny's Owners Settle with Minority Groups." Seattletimes.com. Available online. URL: http://archives.seattletimes.com/cgi-bin/texis/web/vortex/display?storyID=8077&query=Denny%27s. Posted on January 16, 1997.

Watson, Steven. *The Harlem Renaissance: Hub of African-American Culture, 1920–1930*. New York: Pantheon Books, 1996.

Werner, Craig Hansen. *Change is Gonna Come: Music, Race, and the Soul of America*. New York: Plume, 1999.

West, Cornel, and Henry Lewis Gates Jr. *The African-American Century: How Black Americans Have Shaped Our Country*. New York: Free Press, 2000.

Williams, Juan. *Eyes on the Prize: America's Civil Rights Years, 1954–1965.* New York: Viking Penguin, 1987.

Wilson, Christine. *All Shook Up.* Jackson: Mississippi Department of Archives and History, 1995.

Wise, Stephen R. *Gate of Hell: Campaign for Charleston Harbor 1863.* Columbia: University of South Carolina Press, 1994.

Wolters, Raymond. *Negroes and the Great Depression.* Westport, CT: Greenwood Publishing Group, 1970.

Woodward, C. Vann. *The Strange Career of Jim Crow.* Oxford: Oxford University Press, 1972.

Zips, Werner. *Schwartze Rebellion.* Vienna: Promedia, 1993.

INDEX